BATES' *Guide to*
Physical Examination
AND History Taking

BATES' *Guide to* Physical Examination

AND History Taking

TWELFTH EDITION

Lynn S. Bickley, MD, FACP
Clinical Professor of Internal Medicine
School of Medicine
University of New Mexico
Albuquerque, New Mexico

Peter G. Szilagyi, MD, MPH
Professor of Pediatrics and Executive Vice-Chair
Department of Pediatrics
University of California at Los Angeles (UCLA)
Los Angeles, California

Guest Editor

Richard M. Hoffman, MD, MPH, FACP
Professor of Internal Medicine and Epidemiology
Director, Division of General Internal Medicine
University of Iowa Carver College of Medicine
Iowa City, Iowa

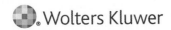

Philadelphia • Baltimore • New York • London
Buenos Aires • Hong Kong • Sydney • Tokyo

Acquisitions Editor: Crystal Taylor
Product Development Editor: Greg Nicholl
Marketing Manager: Michael McMahon
Production Project Manager: Cynthia Rudy
Design Coordinator: Holly McLaughlin
Art Director: Jennifer Clements
Illustrator: Body Scientific International
Manufacturing Coordinator: Margie Orzech
Prepress Vendor: Aptara, Inc.

Twelfth Edition

9 8 7 6 5 4 3 2

Printed in China

Library of Congress Cataloging-in-Publication Data
Names: Bickley, Lynn S., author. | Szilagyi, Peter G., author. | Hoffman,
    Richard M., editor.
Title: Bates' guide to physical examination and history taking / Lynn S.
    Bickley, Peter G. Szilagyi ; guest editor, Richard M. Hoffman.
Other titles: Guide to physical examination and history taking
Description: Twelfth edition. | Philadelphia : Wolters Kluwer, [2017] |
    Includes bibliographical references and index.
Identifiers: LCCN 2016018376 | ISBN 9781469893419 (alk. paper)
Subjects: | MESH: Physical Examination—methods | Medical History
    Taking–methods
Classification: LCC RC76 | NLM WB 205 | DDC 616.07/54—dc23
LC record available at https://lccn.loc.gov/2016018376

We would like to dedicate this book to all our

students, trainees, and mentees who have

taught us the true value of both

the science and the

art of medicine.

Faculty Reviewers

J.D. Bartleson Jr., MD
Associate Professor of Neurology
Mayo Clinic
Rochester, Minnesota

John D. Bartlett, MD
Assistant Clinical Professor of Ophthalmology
Jules Stein Eye Institute
David Geffen School of Medicine
Los Angeles, California

Amy E. Blatt, MD
Assistant Professor
Department of Medicine
School of Medicine and Dentistry
University of Rochester Medical Center
Rochester, New York

Adam Brodsky, MD
Associate Professor
Medical Director, Geriatric Psychiatry Services
Department of Psychiatry and Behavioral Sciences
School of Medicine
University of New Mexico Psychiatric Center &
    Sandoval Regional Medical Center
Albuquerque, New Mexico

Thomas M. Carroll, MD, PhD
Assistant Professor
Department of Medicine and Palliative Care
School of Medicine and Dentistry
University of Rochester Medical Center
Rochester, New York

Adam J. Doyle, MD
Assistant Professor
Department of Surgery
School of Medicine and Dentistry
University of Rochester Medical Center
Rochester, New York

Amit Garg, MD, FAAD
Associate Professor and Founding Chair
Department of Dermatology
Hofstra Northwell School of Medicine
Northwell Health
Manhasset, New York

Catherine F. Gracey, MD
Associate Professor
Department of Medicine
School of Medicine and Dentistry
University of Rochester Medical Center
Rochester, New York

Carla Herman, MD, MPH
Chief
Division of Geriatrics and Palliative Medicine
Professor
Department of Internal Medicine
School of Medicine
University of New Mexico
Albuquerque, New Mexico

Mark Landig, OD
Division of Cataract & Refractive Surgery
Jules Stein Eye Institute
David Geffen School of Medicine
Los Angeles, California

Helen R. Levey, DO, MPH
PGY5 Resident in Urology
School of Medicine and Dentistry
University of Rochester Medical Center
Rochester, New York

Patrick McCleskey, MD
Dermatologist
Kaiser Permanente Oakland Medical Center
Oakland, California

Jeanne H.S. O'Brien, MD
Associate Professor
Department of Urology
School of Medicine and Dentistry
University of Rochester Medical Center
Rochester, New York

Alec B. O'Connor, MD, MPH
Director, Internal Medicine Residency
Associate Professor
Department of Medicine
School of Medicine and Dentistry
University of Rochester Medical Center
Rochester, New York

A. Andrew Rudmann, MD
Associate Professor
Department of Medicine
School of Medicine and Dentistry
University of Rochester Medical Center
Rochester, New York

Moira A. Szilagyi, MD, PhD
Professor of Pediatrics
University of California at Los Angeles (UCLA)
Los Angeles, California

Loralei Lacina Thornburg, MD
Associate Professor
Department of Obstetrics and Gynecology
School of Medicine and Dentistry
University of Rochester Medical Center
Rochester, New York

Scott A. Vogelgesang, MD
Director, Division of Immunology
Clinical Professor
Department of Internal Medicine–Immunology
University of Iowa Carver College of Medicine
Iowa City, Iowa

Brian P. Watkins, MD, MS, FACS
Partner
Genesee Surgical Associates
Rochester, New York

Paula Zozzaro-Smith, DO
Fellow of Maternal-Fetal Medicine
Department of Obstetrics and Gynecology
University of Rochester Medical Center
Rochester, New York

STUDENT REVIEWERS

Ayala Danzig
University of Rochester School of Medicine and Dentistry

Benjamin Edmonds
University of Central Florida College of Medicine

Nicholas PN Goldstein
University of Rochester School of Medicine and Dentistry

Preface

Bates' Guide to Physical Examination and History Taking is designed for medical, physician assistant, nurse practitioner, and other students who are learning to interview patients, perform their physical examination, and apply clinical reasoning and shared decision making to their assessment and plan, based on a sound understanding of clinical evidence. The twelfth edition has many new features to facilitate student learning. As with previous editions, these changes spring from three sources: the feedback and reviews of students, teachers, and faculty; our commitment to making the book easier to read and more efficient to use; and the abundant new evidence that supports the techniques of examination, interviewing, and health promotion.

Throughout the twelfth edition, we emphasize common or important problems rather than the rare or esoteric, though at times we include unusual findings that are classic or life threatening. We encourage students to study the strong evidence base that informs each chapter and to carefully review the clinical guidelines and citations from the health care literature.

Special Features and Highlights

In this edition we have introduced *clinical pearls*, printed in blue, to highlight key points. We have also used color to highlight textboxes so students and teachers can quickly find important summaries of clinical conditions and tips for challenging examination techniques such as inspecting the fundus or measuring the jugular venous pressure. Many of the figures are new or have been updated and, for the first time, all figures are numbered with captions to make them easier to locate and reference in both the print and electronic editions.

Organization

The book comprises three units: *Foundations of Health Assessment, Regional Examinations*, and *Special Populations*.

Unit 1, *Foundations of Health Assessment*, includes chapters on clinical proficiency, assessing clinical evidence, and interviewing and health history. These chapters follow a logical sequence that begins with an overview of the components of patient evaluation, followed by important concepts in assessment of clinical evidence and clinical decision making, and the artful task of gathering the history.

■ Chapter 1, *Foundations for Clinical Proficiency*, features an overview of history taking, physical examination, and now includes the assessment and plan, and a sample patient record. This chapter describes the differences between subjective and objective data and symptoms and signs, and provides a model for sequencing the examination that optimizes patient comfort. It presents guidelines for creating a clear, succinct, and well-organized patient record.

■ Chapter 2, *Evaluating Clinical Evidence*, has been entirely rewritten in the twelfth edition by Dr. Richard Hoffman and clarifies key concepts to ensure student understanding of the history and physical examination as diagnostic tests; tools for evaluating diagnostic tests such as sensitivity, specificity, positive and negative predictive values, and likelihood ratios; types of studies that inform recommendations for health promotion; and an approach to critical appraisal of the clinical literatures and types of bias.

■ Chapter 3, *Interviewing and the Health History*, describes the differences between a comprehensive and focused health history, and between the fluid exchange of the interview and its transformation into the structured format of the written health history. It presents the techniques of skilled and advanced interviewing, the sequence and context of the interview, including its cultural dimensions, and foundational concepts of ethics and professionalism. It clarifies the transition from the open-ended interviewing of the Present Illness (and Personal and Social History) to the direct questions of the Past Medical History and Family History to the closed-ended "yes–no" questions of the Review of Systems. This chapter emphasizes the importance of *masterful listening*, so easily sacrificed to the time pressures of office and hospital care. It mirrors the precepts of Sir William Osler…for therapeutic relationships, always "Listen to your patient. He is telling you the diagnosis," and "The good physician treats the disease. The great physician treats the patient who has the disease."

Unit 2, *Regional Examinations* covers the regional examinations from "head to toe." The 14 chapters in this unit have been thoroughly updated and contain a review of anatomy and physiology, the common symptoms encountered in the health history, important topics for health promotion and counseling, detailed descriptions and images of techniques of examination, a sample written record, comparative tables of abnormalities, and conclude with extensive references from the recent clinical literature. Chapters with the most significant revisions are highlighted below.

■ Chapter 4, *Beginning the Physical Examination: General Survey, Vital Signs, and Pain*, contains updates on obesity and nutrition counseling, and new standards for measuring blood pressure from the *Joint National Committee on Prevention, Detection, Evaluation, and Treatment of High Blood Pressure VII Report (JNC 8)*.

■ Chapter 5, *Behavior and Mental Status*, has been substantially revised according to the *Diagnostic and Statistical Manual of Mental Disorders*, 5th Edition (*DSM-5*) of 2013.

■ Chapter 6, *The Skin, Hair, and Nails*, has been entirely rewritten for the twelfth edition by Dr. Patrick McCleskey and Dr. Amit Garg to improve the framework for assessing common lesions and abnormalities and the quality of its teaching photographs, and to align this chapter with recommendations of the American Academy of Dermatology for student learners.

■ Chapter 9, *The Cardiovascular System*, has detailed new evidence about risk factor screening, new clinical guidelines, and the complexities of assessing hypertension.

■ Chapter 16, *The Musculoskeletal System*, contains a more systematic approach to the musculoskeletal examination and an updated classification of maneuvers to assess the shoulder, with reference to likelihood ratios for abnormalities whenever permitted by the clinical literature.

Other notable features include discussion of new screening guidelines for breast cancer, prostate cancer, colon cancer, Papanicolaou smears, and stroke risk factors as well as updated information on sexually transmitted diseases.

Unit 3, *Special Populations* includes chapters covering special stages in the life cycle—infancy through adolescence, pregnancy, and aging.

■ Chapter 18, *Assessing Children: Infancy through Adolescence*, includes an increased emphasis on health promotion and child development, as well as the many tables and figures that highlight key concepts.

■ Chapter 19, *The Pregnant Woman*, updates health promotion and counseling topics such as nutrition, weight gain, immunizations, substance abuse, and intimate partner violence.

■ Chapter 20, *The Older Adult*, presents new information on frailty, when to screen, immunizations and cancer screening, the spectrum of cognitive decline and dementia screening tests, and the new algorithm for falls prevention from the Centers for Disease Control and Prevention. This chapter and Chapter 17, *The Nervous System*, also explore the challenging complexities of distinguishing delirium, dementia, and depression.

Additional Resources

Bates' Pocket Guide to Physical Examination and History Taking

As a companion to Bates' twelfth edition, we recommend *Bates' Pocket Guide to Physical Examination and History Taking, Eighth edition*. The *Pocket Guide* is an abbreviated version of the Bates' twelfth edition textbook, which is designed for portability and convenience at the bedside. Return to the textbook whenever more comprehensive study and understanding are needed.

Bates' Visual Guide to Physical Examination

The Bates' Visual Guide to Physical Examination (www.batesvisualguide.com), refilmed in 2013, is a key adjunct for mastering the many techniques of physical examination. This series of 18 videos displays seasoned clinicians conducting each of the regional examinations and demonstrates visually the varying techniques of inspection, palpation, percussion, and auscultation in the regional examinations and special populations. We encourage students to study the written chapters and videos in tandem, often numerous times.

For students preparing for clinical testing, the Visual Guide includes 10 Objective Structured Clinical Examinations (or OSCEs), which shows students evaluating patients with common clinical problems in standard OSCE formats, interspersed with questions to guide learning key points. These OSCEs cover:

1. Chest Pain
2. Abdominal Pain
3. Sore Throat
4. Knee Pain
5. Cough
6. Vomit
7. Amenorrhea
8. Falls
9. Back Pain
10. Shortness of Breath

Acknowledgments

Bates' Guide to Physical Examination and History Taking, now in its twelfth edition, spans an evolution of four decades. Drs. Barbara Bates and Robert Hoekelman, colleagues in internal medicine and pediatrics at the University of Rochester School of Medicine and Dentistry, launched the first edition in 1974 as a hands-on manual for medical and advanced practice nursing students learning to master the physical examination of adults and children. With clear prose and black and white drawings, they devoted 18 chapters to the techniques of regional examination for adults and children. They devised the classic format of the *Bates' Guide* still present today—black explanatory text in the major column, examples of abnormalities in red in the minor column, and comparative tables of abnormalities at the end of each chapter. Dr. Bickley became chief editor and author for the seventh edition, joined by Dr. Szilagyi for the eighth edition. By then the *Bates' Guide* contained additional sections on anatomy and physiology and new chapters on interviewing, the approach to symptoms, the mental status examination, and clinical thinking from data to plan.

Over the next four editions Drs. Bickley and Szilagyi added many features to make *Bates' Guide* useful to student learners. They introduced health history and health promotion and counseling sections in each chapter, and have increasingly accommodated the evidence-based medicine "revolution" with updated health promotion and counseling sections in each edition that cite major studies and clinical guidelines; examples of abnormalities, tables, and footnotes and references reflecting advances in the clinical literature; and now a new chapter on evaluating clinical evidence.

In this edition with pleasure and esteem the authors welcome Dr. Richard Hoffman, Professor of Internal Medicine and Epidemiology and Director of the Division of General Internal Medicine at the University of Iowa Carver College of Medicine/Iowa City VA Medical Center, as guest editor. Dr. Hoffman is Associate Editor for the American College of Physicians (ACP) Journal Club, and has been a peer reviewer for a number of prostate screening guidelines, authored two Cochrane reviews, and writes and reviews for UpToDate.

Each edition of the *Bates' Guide* builds on an extensive review process, with many thanks due. First, the publisher surveys students and faculty about the merits of each chapter. Summaries of their responses provide helpful recommendations for subsequent revisions. Then the authors elicit intensive chapter critiques and updates from faculty at health sciences schools across the country, listed in the Reviewers section to follow. For their valuable insights and intense focus on this edition, the authors especially commend Dr. Richard Hoffman for his lucid presentation of the complex concepts governing evaluation of clinical evidence in

Chapter 2, Dr. Patrick McCleskey for rewriting Chapter 6 and presenting a new paradigm for assessing skin lesions with many new teaching photographs, assisted by Dr. Amit Garg. Drs. John Bartlett and Mark Landig for their review of the head and neck examination in Chapter 7, Dr. J.D. Bartleson for refining the always challenging fundamentals of the examination of the nervous system in Chapter 17, and Drs. Carla Herman and John Robertson for their useful scrutiny of new developments in the evaluation of older adults in Chapter 20. We also appreciate the assistance of Dr. Alec O'Connor in locating skilled faculty reviewers for many of the adult examination chapters and making important contributions to revisions of Chapter 8. Several reviewers made valued additions to the assessment of children and adolescents in Chapter 18—Dr. Moira Szilagyi and medical students Nicholas Goldstein and Ayala Danzig.

To compose and produce the *Bates' Guide* requires the deft touch of a maestro. Newly revised chapters must be reviewed, author queries issued and answered, and photos and illustrations checked and rechecked for teaching style and accuracy. Text, textboxes, examples of abnormalities, and images all must be carefully aligned. Each page is designed to hold reader appeal, highlight key points, and facilitate student learning. For his untiring craft and dedication, we especially thank Greg Nicholl, Senior Product Development Editor at Wolters Kluwer, who has woven these many strands into a coherent and exemplary text. We commend Kelly Horvath who assisted Greg with line-by-line review and careful annotations to prepare the book for the compositor, and Chris Miller of Aptara who turned complex text documents into corrected print proofs ready for publication. Early in the editing process and preceding Greg Nicholl, Stephanie Roulias was a conscientious collaborator who set many of the editing processes for the twelfth edition in motion. Crystal Taylor has been an astute manager of acquisitions for the Bates' Suite of teaching materials, contracting, and marketing. The publishing team brings invaluable talent to the tradition of excellence that has made the *Bates' Guide* a premier text for students learning the time-honored skills of patient assessment and care.

How To Use
Bates' Guide To Physical Examination And History Taking

The twelfth edition of *Bates' Guide to Physical Examination and History Taking* is your comprehensive guide to learning to effectively conduct the health interview and physical examination. This section introduces you to the features and learning tools that will lead to successful health assessments, regional examinations, and working with special patient populations.

At the start of every chapter, you will see a list of additional learning resources that complement the book in order to build your knowledge and confidence in history taking and examination. The *Bates' Visual Guide to Physical Examination* offers over 8 hours of video content and delivers head-to-toe and systems-based physical examination techniques. When used alongside the book, you have a complete learning solution for preparedness for the boards and patient encounters.

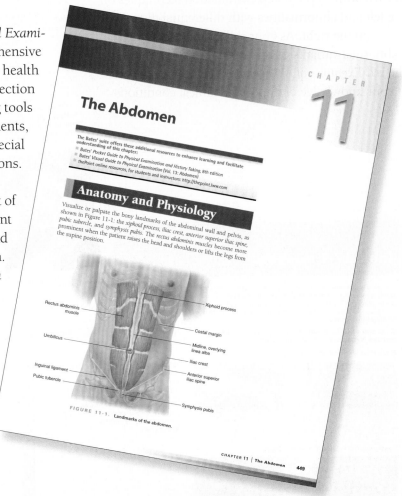

Clinical Pearls—NEW!

Be sure to pay special attention to the clinical pearls, printed in **blue**. These clinical comments provide practical "pearls" that enhance your understanding of the assessment techniques.

with a personal or family history of multiple or dysplastic nevi or previous melanoma. Patients who have a clinical skin examination within the 3 years prior to a melanoma diagnosis have thinner melanomas than those who did not have a clinical skin examination.[20] Both new and changing nevi should be closely examined, as at least half of melanomas arise *de novo* from isolated melanocytes rather than pre-existing nevi. Also consider "opportunistic screening" as part of the complete physical examination for patients with significant sun exposure and patients over age 50 years without prior skin examination or who live alone.

Since the USPSTF review, an important German study of over 350,000 patients reported that full-body primary care screening with dermatology referrals for concerning lesions reduced melanoma mortality by more than 47%.[21] Survival from melanoma strongly correlates with tumor thickness. Two further studies demonstrate that patients receiving skin examinations are more likely to have thinner melanomas.[20,22]

Detecting melanoma requires practice and knowledge of how benign nevi change over time, often going from flat to raised or acquiring additional brown pigment. Studies have shown that even limited clinician training makes a difference in detection: patients of primary care providers who spent 1.5 hours completing an online tutorial improved diagnostic accuracy. Similar studies show such training results in thinner melanomas than patients of providers without such training.[23–26]

Screening for Melanoma: The ABCDEs. Clinicians should apply the ABCE-EFG method when screening moles for melanoma (this does not apply for non-melanocytic lesions like seborrheic keratoses). The sensitivity of this tool for detecting melanoma ranges from 43% to 97%, and specificity ranges from 36% to 100%; diagnostic accuracy depends on how many criteria are used

Turn to Tables 6-4 through 6-6 on pp. 197–203 showing rough, pink, and brown nevi and their mimics.

Review the ABCDE-EFG rule and photographs in Table 6-6, pp. 200–203, which provide additional helpful identifiers and comparisons of benign brown lesions with melanoma.

Examples of Abnormalities

Once again, *Bates' Guide to Physical Examination and History Taking* offers an easy-to-follow two-column format with step-by-step examination techniques on the left and abnormalities with differential diagnoses on the right. As your skills progress, study the abnormal variants of common physical findings in the red *Examples of Abnormalities* column to deepen your knowledge of important clinical conditions.

Cranial Nerves III, IV, and VI—Oculomotor, Trochlear, and Abducens. Test the *extraocular movements* in the six cardinal directions of gaze, and look for loss of conjugate movements in any of the six directions, which causes *diplopia*. Ask the patient which direction makes the diplopia worse and inspect the eye closely for asymmetric deviation of movement. Determine if the diplopia is *monocular* or *binocular* by asking the patient to cover one eye, then the other.

Check convergence of the eyes.

See Chapter 7, Head and Neck (pp. 237–238) for a more detailed discussion of testing extraocular movements.

See Table 7-11, Dysconjugate Gaze, p. 278. Monocular diplopia is seen in local problems with glasses or contact lenses, cataracts, astigmatism, or ptosis. Binocular diplopia occurs in CN III, IV, and VI neuropathy (40% of patients), and eye muscle disorders from myasthenia gravis, trauma, thyroid ophthalmopathy, and internuclear ophthalmoplegia.[86]

Identify any *nystagmus*, an involuntary jerking movement of the eyes with quick and slow components. Note the direction of gaze in which it appears, the plane of the nystagmus (horizontal, vertical, rotary, or mixed), and the direction of the quick and slow components. Nystagmus is named for the direction of the quick component. Ask the patient to fix his or her vision on a distant object and observe if the nystagmus increases or decreases.

See Table 17-7, Nystagmus, pp. 785–786. Nystagmus is seen in *cerebellar disease*, especially with gait ataxia and dysarthria (increases with retinal fixation), and *vestibular disorders* (decreases with retinal fixation); and in *internuclear ophthalmoplegia*.

Look for *ptosis* (drooping of the upper eyelids). A slight difference in the width of the palpebral fissures is a normal variant in approximately one third of patients.

Ptosis is seen in *3rd nerve palsy* (CN III), *Horner syndrome* (ptosis, miosis, forehead anhidrosis), or *myasthenia gravis*.

Cranial Nerve V—Trigeminal

Motor. While palpating the temporal and masseter muscles in turn, ask the patient to firmly clench the teeth (Figs. 17-9 and 17-10). Note the strength of muscle contraction. Ask the patient to open and move the jaw from side to side.

Difficulty clenching the jaw or moving it to the opposite side suggests masseter and lateral pterygoid weakness, respectively. Jaw deviation during opening points to weakness on the deviating side.

Look for unilateral weakness in CN V pontine lesions; bilateral weakness in bilateral hemispheric disease.

CNS patterns from stroke include ipsilateral facial and body sensory loss from contralateral cortical or thalamic lesions; ipsilateral face, but contralateral body sensory loss in brainstem lesions.

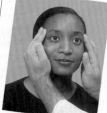

FIGURE 17-9. Palpate the temporal muscles.

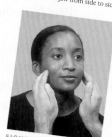

FIGURE 17-10. Palpate the masseter muscles.

Table 17-7 Nystagmus

Nystagmus is a rhythmic oscillation of the eyes, analogous to a tremor in other parts of the body. It has numerous causes, including impairment of vision in early life, disorders of the labyrinth and the cerebellar system, and drug toxicity. Nystagmus occurs normally when a person watches a rapidly moving object (e.g., a passing train). Study the three characteristics of nystagmus described in this table so that you can correctly identify the type of nystagmus. Then refer to the References for differential diagnoses.

Direction of Gaze in Which Nystagmus Appears
Example: Nystagmus on Right Lateral Gaze

Nystagmus Present (Right Lateral Gaze)

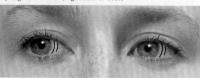

Although nystagmus may be present in all directions of gaze, it may appear or become accentuated only on deviation of the eyes (e.g., to the side or upward). On extreme lateral gaze, the normal person may show a few beats resembling nystagmus. Avoid making assessments in such extreme positions, and *observe for nystagmus only within the field of full binocular vision.*

Nystagmus Not Present (Left Lateral Gaze)

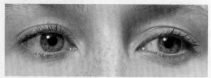

Direction of the Quick and Slow Phases
Example: Left-Beating Nystagmus—a Quick Jerk to the Left in Each Eye, then a Slow Drift to the Right

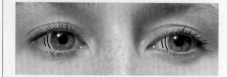

Nystagmus usually has both slow and fast movements, but is defined by its fast phase. For example, if the eyes jerk quickly to the patient's left and drift back slowly to the right, the patient is said to have *left-beating nystagmus*. Occasionally, nystagmus consists only of coarse oscillations without quick and slow components, described as *pendular.*

(continued)

To further sharpen your clinical acumen, turn to the end-of-chapter *Tables of Abnormalities*, which allow you to compare and contrast clinical conditions in a convenient single table format.

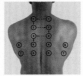

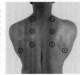
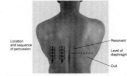

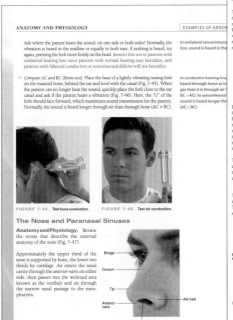
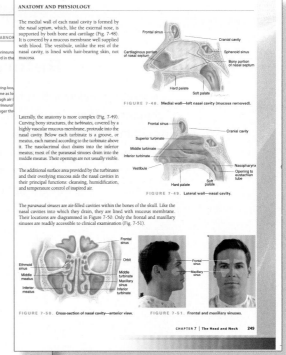

Examination Techniques

The *Techniques of Examination* sections are where you will learn the crucial and relevant examinations you will perform every day. Additional *Special Techniques* offer the examination approach for more uncommon conditions and special circumstances.

Photographs and Illustrations

The art program includes detailed, full-color photographs, drawings, and diagrams, some new or revised, to further illustrate key points in the text. They will enhance your learning potential by providing accurate and realistic representations.

And now, each figure has a figure number and caption to make the figures easier to find and understand.

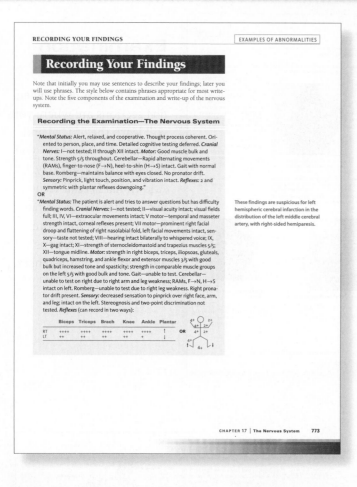

Recording Your Findings

Note that initially you may use sentences to describe your findings; later you will use phrases. The style below contains phrases appropriate for most write-ups. Note the five components of the examination and write-up of the nervous system.

Recording the Examination—The Nervous System

"*Mental Status:* Alert, relaxed, and cooperative. Thought process coherent. Oriented to person, place, and time. Detailed cognitive testing deferred. *Cranial Nerves:* I—not tested; II through XII intact. *Motor:* Good muscle bulk and tone. Strength 5/5 throughout. Cerebellar—Rapid alternating movements (RAMs), finger-to-nose (F→N), heel-to-shin (H→S) intact. Gait with normal base. Romberg—maintains balance with eyes closed. No pronator drift. *Sensory:* Pinprick, light touch, position, and vibration intact. *Reflexes:* 2 and symmetric with plantar reflexes downgoing."

OR

"*Mental Status:* The patient is alert and tries to answer questions but has difficulty finding words. *Cranial Nerves:* I—not tested; II—visual acuity intact; visual fields full; III, IV, VI—extraocular movements intact; V motor—temporal and masseter strength intact, corneal reflexes present; VII motor—prominent right facial droop and flattening of right nasolabial fold, left facial movements intact, sensory—taste not tested; VIII—hearing intact bilaterally to whispered voice; IX, X—gag intact; XI—strength of sternocleidomastoid and trapezius muscles 5/5; XII—tongue midline. *Motor:* strength in right biceps, triceps, iliopsoas, gluteals, quadriceps, hamstring, and ankle flexor and extensor muscles 3/5 with good bulk but increased tone and spasticity; strength in comparable muscle groups on the left 5/5 with good bulk and tone. Gait—unable to test. Cerebellar—unable to test on right due to right arm and leg weakness; RAMs, F→N, H→S intact on left. Romberg—unable to test due to right leg weakness. Right pronator drift present. *Sensory:* decreased sensation to pinprick over right face, arm, and leg; intact on the left. Stereognosis and two-point discrimination not tested. *Reflexes* (can record in two ways):

	Biceps	Triceps	Brach	Knee	Ankle	Plantar
RT	++++	++++	++++	++++	++++	↑
LT	++	++	++	++	+	↓

These findings are suspicious for left hemispheric cerebral infarction in the distribution of the left middle cerebral artery, with right-sided hemiparesis.

Recording Your Findings

Constructing a well-organized clinical record must clearly display important clinical information and your clinical reasoning and plan. You will gain this skill and learn the descriptive vocabulary of physical findings in the *Recording Your Findings* section of each of the regional examination and special populations' chapters.

References

Consult the *References* at the end of the chapters to deepen your knowledge of important clinical conditions. The habit of searching the clinical literature will serve you and your patients well throughout your career.

References

1. Clark D 3rd, Ahmed MI, Dell'italia LJ, et al. An argument for reviving the disappearing skill of cardiac auscultation. *Cleve Clin J Med.* 2012;79:536.
2. Delora A. The decline of cardiac auscultation: 'the ball of the match point is poised on the net'. *J Cardiovasc Med.* 2008;9:1173.
3. Markel H. The stethoscope and the art of listening. *N Engl J Med.* 2006;354:551.
4. Simel DL. Time, now, to recover the fun in the physical examination rather than abandon it. *Arch Intern Med.* 2006;166:603.
5. Vukanovic-Criley JM, Hovanesyan A, Criley SR, et al. Confidential testing of cardiac examination competency in cardiology and noncardiology faculty and trainees: a multicenter study. *Clin Cardiol.* 2010;33:738.
6. Wayne DB, Butter J, Cohen ER, et al. Setting defensible standards for cardiac auscultation skills in medical students. *Acad Med.* 2009;84(10 Suppl):S94.
7. Marcus G, Vessey J, Jordan MV, et al. Relationship between accurate auscultation of a clinically useful third heart sound and level of experience. *Arch Intern Med.* 2006;166:617.
8. Vukanovic-Criley JM, Criley S, Warde CM, et al. Competency in cardiac examination skills in medical students, trainees, physicians, and faculty. A multicenter study. *Arch Intern Med.* 2006;166:610.
9. March SK, Bedynek JL Jr, Chizner MA. Teaching cardiac auscultation: effectiveness of a patient-centered teaching conference on improving cardiac auscultatory skills. *Mayo Clin Proc.* 2005; 80;1443.
10. RuDusky BM. Auscultation and Don Quixote. *Chest.* 2005;127: 1869.
11. Mangione S. Cardiac auscultatory skills of physicians-in-training:

20. Saxena A, Barrett MJ, Patel AR, et al. Merging old school methods with new technology to improve skills in cardiac auscultation. *Semin Med Pract.* 2008;11:21.
21. Vukanovic-Criley JM, Boker JR, Criley SR, et al. Using virtual patients to improve cardiac examination competency in medical students. *Clin Cardiol.* 2008;31:334.
22. Barrett MJ, Lacey CS, Sekara AE, et al. Mastering cardiac murmurs. The power of repetition. *Chest.* 2004;126:470.
23. Lee E, Michaels AD, Selvester RH, et al. Frequency of diastolic third and fourth heart sounds with myocardial ischemia induced during percutaneous coronary intervention. *J Electrocardiol.* 2009;42:39.
24. Marcus GM, Gerber IL, McKeown BH, et al. Association between phonocardiographic third and four heart sound and objective measure of left ventricular function. *JAMA.* 2005;293:2238.
25. Shah SJ, Marcus GM, Gerber IL, et al. Physiology of the third heart sound: novel insights from tissue Doppler imaging. *J Am Soc Echocardiogr.* 2008;21:394.
26. Shah SJ, Nakamura K, Marcus GM, et al. Association of the fourth heart sound with increased left ventricular end-diastolic stiffness. *J Card Fail.* 2008;14:431.
27. Shah SJ, Michaels AD. Hemodynamic correlates of the third heart sound and systolic time intervals. *Congest Heart Fail.* 2006;12(4 suppl 1):8.
28. O'Rourke RA, Braunwald E. Ch 209, Physical examination of the cardiovascular system. In *Harrison's Principles of Internal Medicine.* 16th ed. New York: McGraw-Hill; 2005:1307.
29. Yancy CW, Jessup M, Bozkurt B, et al. 2013 AACF/AHA Guideline for the Management of Heart Failure. *J Am College Cardiol.* 2013; 62:e148.
30. Vinayak AG, Levitt J, Gehlbach B, et al. Usefulness of the external jugular vein examination in detecting abnormal central venous pressure in critically ill patients. *Arch Int Med.* 2006;166:2132.

Contents

UNIT 3

Special Populations 797

CHAPTER 18

Assessing Children: Infancy through Adolescence 799

List of Tables

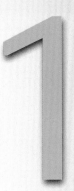

Foundations of Health Assessment

Foundations for Clinical Proficiency

The techniques of physical examination and history taking that you are about to learn embody the time-honored skills of healing and patient care. Gathering a sensitive and nuanced history and performing a thorough and accurate examination deepen your relationships with patients, focus your assessment, and set the guideposts that direct your clinical decision making (Fig. 1-1). The quality of your history and physical examination lays the foundation for patient assessment, your recommendations for care, and your choices for further evaluation and testing. As you become an accomplished clinician, you will continually polish these important relational and clinical skills.

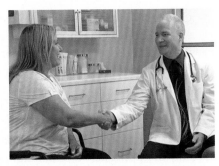

FIGURE 1-1. The importance of establishing rapport.

With practice, you will meet the challenge of integrating the essential elements of clinical care: empathic listening; the ability to interview patients of all ages, moods, and backgrounds; the techniques for examining the different body systems; levels of illness; and, finally, the process of clinical reasoning leading to your diagnosis and plan. Your experience with history taking and physical examination will grow, and will trigger the steps of clinical reasoning from the first moments of the patient encounter: identifying symptoms and abnormal findings; linking findings to underlying pathophysiology or psychopathology; and establishing and testing a set of explanatory hypotheses. Working through these steps will reveal the multifaceted profile of the patient before you. Paradoxically, the skills that allow you to assess all patients also shape the clinical portrait of the unique human being entrusted to your care. The physical examination is more than a means of gathering data and generating hypotheses for causality and testing. It is vital to the "formation of the [clinician]–patient bond, the beginning of a therapeutic partnership and the healing process (Fig. 1-2)."[1]

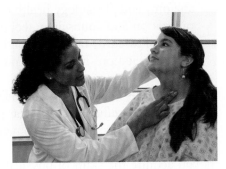

FIGURE 1-2. The skilled physical examination.

This chapter, revised in this edition, provides a guide to clinical proficiency in four critical areas: the *Health History*; the *Physical Examination*; *Clinical*

Reasoning, Assessment, and Plan; and *The Quality Clinical Record.* It describes the components of the health history and how to organize the patient's story; and it gives an overview of the physical examination with a sequence for ensuring patient comfort that briefly describes techniques of examination for each component of the physical examination, from the General Survey through the Nervous System. In this edition, the chapter also includes *Clinical Reasoning, Assessment, and Plan,* and *The Quality Clinical Record.* The new Chapter 2, Evaluating Clinical Evidence, provides the analytic tools for evaluating tests, guidelines, and the clinical literature that will ensure best practices and lifelong clinical learning. Chapter 3, Interviewing and the Health History, completes the foundational chapters that prepare you for performing the physical examination. You will learn the techniques of physical examination in Chapters 4 through 17. Each chapter is evidence based and includes citations from the clinical literature for easy reference so that you can continue to expand your knowledge. Beginning with Chapter 4, sections on *Health Promotion and Counseling: Evidence and Recommendations* review current clinical guidelines for preventive care.

The Bates' Guide to Physical Examination and History Taking follows the sequence described below:

- *Chapter 2, Evaluating Clinical Evidence,* discusses the history and physical examination as diagnostic tools, evaluation of the validity and reproducibility of diagnostic tests, health promotion, critical appraisal of the clinical research, and grading criteria for clinical guidelines.

- *Chapter 3, Interviewing and the Health History,* expands on the essential, varied, and often complex skills of building patient rapport and eliciting the patient's story. It addresses basic and advanced interviewing techniques and the approach to challenging patients as well as cultural competence and professionalism.

- *Chapters 4 to 17* are regional examination chapters, which detail the pertinent anatomy and physiology, health history, evidence-based guidelines for health promotion and counseling, techniques of examination, and the written record, followed by tables comparing common symptoms and physical findings and citations from the literature.

- *Chapters 18 to 20* extend and adapt the elements of the adult history and physical examination to special populations: newborns, infants, children, and adolescents; pregnant women; and older adults.

As you acquire the skills of physical examination and history taking, you will move to active patient assessment, gradually at first, but then with growing confidence and expertise, and ultimately clinical competence. From mastery of these skills and the mutual trust and respect of caring patient relationships emerge the timeless rewards of the clinical professions.

Patient Assessment: Comprehensive or Focused

Determining the Scope of Your Assessment

At the outset of each patient encounter, you will face the common questions, "How much should I do?" and "Should my assessment be comprehensive or focused?" For patients you are seeing for the first time in the office or hospital, you will usually choose to conduct a *comprehensive assessment,* which includes all the elements of the health history and the complete physical examination. In many situations, a more flexible *focused* or *problem-oriented assessment* is appropriate, particularly for patients you know well returning for routine care, or those with specific "urgent care" concerns like sore throat or knee pain. You will adjust the scope of your history and physical examination to the situation at hand, keeping several factors in mind: the magnitude and severity of the patient's problems; the need for thoroughness; the clinical setting—inpatient or outpatient, primary or subspecialty care; and the time available. Skill in all the components of a comprehensive assessment allows you to select the elements that are most pertinent to the patient's concerns, yet meet clinical standards for best practice and diagnostic accuracy.

The History and Physical Examination: Comprehensive or Focused?

Comprehensive Assessment	Focused Assessment
Is appropriate for new patients in the office or hospital	Is appropriate for established patients, especially during routine or urgent care visits
Provides fundamental and personalized knowledge about the patient	Addresses focused concerns or symptoms
Strengthens the clinician–patient relationship	Assesses symptoms restricted to a specific body system
Helps identify or rule out physical causes related to patient concerns	Applies examination methods relevant to assessing the concern or problem as thoroughly and carefully as possible
Provides a baseline for future assessments	
Creates a platform for health promotion through education and counseling	
Develops proficiency in the essential skills of physical examination	

As you can see, the *comprehensive examination* does more than assess body systems. It is a source of fundamental and personalized knowledge about the patient that strengthens the clinician–patient relationship. Most people seeking care have specific worries or symptoms. The comprehensive examination provides a more complete basis for assessing these concerns and answering patient questions.

For the *focused examination,* you will select the methods relevant to thorough assessment of the targeted problem. The patient's symptoms, age, and health history help determine the scope of the focused examination, as does your knowledge of disease patterns. Of all the patients with sore throat, for example, you will need to decide who may have infectious mononucleosis and warrants careful palpation of the liver and spleen and who, by contrast, has a common cold amenable to a more focused examination of the head, neck, and lungs. The clinical reasoning that underlies and guides such decisions is discussed later in this chapter.

What about the *routine clinical check-up,* or *periodic health examination*? Numerous studies have scrutinized the usefulness of the annual well-patient visit for screening and prevention of illness, in contrast to evaluation of symptoms, without coming to a clear consensus.[2–10] A growing body of evidence documents the utility of many components of the physical examination, its vital role in decision making, and its potential for savings through decreased testing.[11–15] Validated examination techniques include blood pressure measurement, assessment of central venous pressure from the jugular venous pulse, listening to the heart for evidence of valvular disease, detection of hepatic and splenic enlargement, and the pelvic examination with Papanicolaou (Pap) smears. Various consensus panels and expert advisory groups have further expanded recommendations for examination and screening, which will be addressed in the regional examination chapters.

What about the newer evidence about the physical examination itself and its relationship to advanced diagnostic testing? Recent studies view the *physical examination findings* themselves as *diagnostic tests* and have begun to validate their value by identifying their test characteristics using Bayes' theorem and the evidence-based tools described in Chapter 2, Evaluating Clinical Evidence.[16,17] Over time, "the rational clinical examination" is expected to improve diagnostic decision making, especially as national competencies and best teaching practices for physical examination skills become better understood.[11,18] Meanwhile, the physical examination yields "the intangible benefits of more time spent … communicating with patients,"[18] a unique therapeutic relationship, more accurate diagnoses, and more selective assessments and plans of care.[1,11]

Subjective Versus Objective Data

As you acquire the techniques of history taking and physical examination, remember the important differences between *subjective information* and *objective information,* summarized in the table below. *Symptoms* are subjective concerns, or what the patient tells you. *Signs* are considered one type of objective information, or what you observe. Knowing these differences helps you group together the different types of patient information. These distinctions are equally important for organizing written and oral presentations about patients into a logical and understandable format.

Differences Between Subjective and Objective Data

Subjective Data	Objective Data
What the patient tells you	What you detect during the examination, laboratory information, and test data
The *symptoms* and history, from Chief Complaint through Review of Systems	All physical examination findings, or *signs*
Example: Mrs. G. is a 54-year-old hairdresser who reports pressure over her left chest "like an elephant sitting there," which goes into her left neck and arm.	*Example:* Mrs. G. is an older, overweight white female, who is pleasant and cooperative. Height 5′4″, weight 150 lbs, BMI 26, BP 160/80, HR 96 and regular, respiratory rate 24, temperature 97.5 °F

The Comprehensive Adult Health History

Components of the Comprehensive Health History

- Identifying data and source of the history; reliability
- Chief complaint(s)
- Present illness
- Past history
- Family history
- Personal and social history
- Review of systems

See Chapter 18, Assessing Children: Infancy Through Adolescence, for the comprehensive history and examination of infants, children, and adolescents, pp. 799–925.

As you will learn in Chapter 3, Interviewing and the Health History, when you talk with patients, the health history rarely emerges in this order. The interview is more fluid; you will closely follow the patient's cues to elicit the patient's narrative of illness, provide empathy, and strengthen rapport. You will quickly learn where to fit different aspects of the patient's story into the more formal format of the oral presentation and written record. You will transform the patient's language and story into the components of the health history familiar to all members of the health care team. This restructuring organizes your clinical reasoning and provides a template for your expanding clinical expertise.

As you begin your clinical journey, review the components of the adult health history, then study the more detailed explanations that follow.

Overview: Components of the Adult Health History

Identifying Data	*Identifying data*—such as age, gender, occupation, marital status
	Source of the history—usually the patient, but can be a family member or friend, letter of referral, or the clinical record
	If appropriate, establish the *source of referral,* because a written report may be needed
Reliability	Varies according to the patient's memory, trust, and mood
Chief Complaint(s)	The one or more symptoms or concerns causing the patient to seek care
Present Illness	Amplifies the *Chief Complaint;* describes how each symptom developed
	Includes patient's thoughts and feelings about the illness
	Pulls in relevant portions of the *Review of Systems,* called "pertinent positives and negatives" (see p. 11)
	May include *medications, allergies,* and *tobacco use* and *alcohol,* which are frequently pertinent to the present illness
Past History	Lists childhood illnesses
	Lists adult illnesses with dates for events in at least four categories: medical, surgical, obstetric/gynecologic, and psychiatric
	Includes health maintenance practices such as immunizations, screening tests, lifestyle issues, and home safety
Family History	Outlines or diagrams age and health, or age and cause of death, of siblings, parents, and grandparents
	Documents presence or absence of specific illnesses in family, such as hypertension, diabetes, or type of cancer
Personal and Social History	Describes educational level, family of origin, current household, personal interests, and lifestyle
Review of Systems	Documents presence or absence of common symptoms related to each of the major body systems

The Comprehensive Adult Health History—Further Description

Initial Information

Date and Time of History. The date is always important. Be sure to document the time you evaluate the patient, especially in urgent, emergent, or hospital settings.

Identifying Data. These include age, gender, marital status, and occupation. The **source of history** or **referral** can be the patient, a family member or friend, an officer, a consultant, or the clinical record. Identifying the *source of referral* helps you assess the quality of the referral information, questions you may need to address in your assessment and written response.

Reliability. Document this information, if relevant. This judgment reflects the quality of the information provided by the patient and is usually made at the end of the interview. For example, "The patient is vague when describing symptoms, and the details are confusing," or, "The patient is a reliable historian."

Chief Complaint(s).
Make every attempt to quote the patient's own words. For example, "My stomach hurts and I feel awful." If patients have no specific complaints, report their reason for the visit, such as "I have come for my regular check-up" or "I've been admitted for a thorough evaluation of my heart."

Present Illness.
This *Present Illness* is a complete, clear, and chronologic description of the problems prompting the patient's visit, including the onset of the problem, the setting in which it developed, its manifestations, and any treatments to date.

- Each principal symptom should be well characterized, and should include the seven attributes of a symptom: (1) location; (2) quality; (3) quantity or severity; (4) timing, including onset, duration, and frequency; (5) the setting in which it occurs; (6) factors that have aggravated or relieved the symptom; and (7) associated manifestations. It is also important to query the "pertinent positives" and "pertinent negatives" drawn from sections of the Review of Systems that are relevant to the Chief Complaint(s). The presence or absence of these additional symptoms helps you generate the differential diagnosis, which includes the most likely and, at times, the most serious diagnoses, even if less likely, which could explain the patient's condition.

See discussion of the seven attributes of a symptom in Chapter 3, Interviewing and the Health History, pp. 65–108.

- Other information is frequently relevant, such as risk factors for coronary artery disease in patients with chest pain, or current medications in patients with syncope.

- The *Present Illness* should reveal the patient's responses to his or her symptoms and what effect the illness has had on the patient's life. Always remember, *the data flow spontaneously from the patient, but the task of oral and written organization is yours.*

- Patients often have more than one symptom or concern. Each *symptom* merits its own paragraph and a full description.

- Medications should be noted, including name, dose, route, and frequency of use. Also, list home remedies, nonprescription drugs, vitamins, mineral or herbal supplements, oral contraceptives, and medicines borrowed from family members or friends. Ask patients to bring in all their medications so that you can see exactly what they take.

■ **Allergies,** including *specific reactions* to each medication, such as rash or nausea, must be recorded, as well as allergies to foods, insects, or environmental factors.

■ Note **tobacco use,** including the type. Cigarettes are often reported in pack-years (a person who has smoked 1½ packs a day for 12 years has an 18-pack/year history). If someone has quit, note for how long.

■ **Alcohol** and **drug use** should always be investigated and is often pertinent to the *Presenting Illness.*

See Chapter 3, Interviewing and the Health History, for suggested questions about alcohol and drug use, pp. 65–108.

Past History

■ **Childhood Illnesses:** These include measles, rubella, mumps, whooping cough, chickenpox, rheumatic fever, scarlet fever, and polio. Also included are any chronic childhood illnesses.

■ **Adult Illnesses:** Provide information relative to **Adult Illnesses** in each of the four areas:

  ■ *Medical:* Illnesses such as diabetes, hypertension, hepatitis, asthma, and human immunodeficiency virus (HIV); hospitalizations; number and gender of sexual partners; and risk-taking sexual practices

  ■ *Surgical:* Dates, indications, and types of operations

  ■ *Obstetric/Gynecologic:* Obstetric history, menstrual history, methods of contraception, and sexual function

  ■ *Psychiatric:* Illness and time frame, diagnoses, hospitalizations, and treatments

■ **Health Maintenance:** Cover selected aspects of *Health Maintenance,* especially immunizations and screening tests. For *immunizations,* find out whether the patient has received vaccines for tetanus, pertussis, diphtheria, polio, measles, rubella, mumps, influenza, varicella, hepatitis B virus (HBV), human papilloma virus (HPV), meningococcal disease, *Haemophilus influenzae* type B, pneumococci, and herpes zoster. For *screening tests,* review tuberculin tests, Pap smears, mammograms, stool tests for occult blood, colonoscopy and cholesterol tests, together with results and when they were last performed. If the patient does not know this information, written permission may be needed to obtain prior clinical records.

Family History. Under *Family History,* outline or diagram the age and health, or age and cause of death, of each immediate relative including parents, grandparents, siblings, children, and grandchildren. *Review each of the following conditions and record whether they are present or absent in the family:* hypertension, coronary artery disease, elevated cholesterol levels, stroke, diabetes, thyroid or renal disease, arthritis, tuberculosis, asthma or lung disease, headache, seizure disorder, mental illness, suicide, substance abuse, and allergies, as well as symptoms reported by the patient. Ask about any history of breast, ovarian, colon, or prostate cancer. Ask about any genetically transmitted diseases.

Personal and Social History.   The *Personal and Social History* captures the patient's personality and interests, sources of support, coping style, strengths, and concerns. It should include occupation and the last year of schooling; home situation and significant others; sources of stress, both recent and long-term; important life experiences such as military service, job history, financial situation, and retirement; leisure activities; religious affiliation and spiritual beliefs; and activities of daily living (ADLs). Baseline level of function is particularly important in older or disabled patients. The *Personal and Social History* includes lifestyle habits that promote health or create risk, such as *exercise and diet,* including frequency of exercise, usual daily food intake, dietary supplements or restrictions, and use of coffee, tea, and other caffeinated beverages, and *safety measures,* including use of seat belts, bicycle helmets, sunblock, smoke detectors, and other devices related to specific hazards. Include *sexual orientation and practices* and any *alternative health care practices.* Avoid restricting the *Personal and Social History* to only tobacco, drug, and alcohol use. An expanded *Personal and Social History* personalizes your relationship with the patient and builds rapport.

See pp. 970–971 for the ADLs frequently assessed in older adults.

You will learn to intersperse personal and social questions throughout the interview to make the patient feel more at ease.

Review of Systems

Tips for Eliciting the Review of Systems

- Understanding and using *Review of Systems* questions may seem challenging at first. These "yes-no" questions should come at the end of the interview. Think about asking a series of questions going from "head to toe." It is helpful to prepare the patient by saying, "The next part of the history may feel like a hundred questions, but it is important to make sure we have not missed anything." Most *Review of Systems* questions pertain to symptoms, but on occasion, some clinicians include diseases like pneumonia or tuberculosis.
- Note that as you elicit the Present Illness, you may also draw on Review of Systems questions related to system(s) relevant to the Chief Complaint to establish "pertinent positives and negatives" that help clarify the diagnosis. For example, after a full description of chest pain, you may ask, "Do you have any history of high blood pressure ... palpitations ... shortness of breath ... swelling in your ankles or feet?" or even move to questions from the *Respiratory* or *Gastrointestinal Review of Systems.*

See Chapter 3, Interviewing and the Health History, for discussion of the role of pertinent positives and negatives in establishing the differential diagnosis, p. 80.

Start with a fairly general question as you address each of the different systems, then shift to more specific questions about systems that may be of concern. Examples of starting questions are, "How are your ears and hearing?" "How about your lungs and breathing?" "Any trouble with your heart?" "How is your digestion?" "How about your bowels?" The need for additional questions will vary depending on the patient's age, complaints, and general state of health and your clinical judgment.

■ The *Review of Systems* questions may uncover problems that the patient has overlooked, particularly in areas unrelated to the *Present Illness*. Significant health events, such as past surgery, hospitalization for a major prior illness, or a parent's death, require full exploration. Keep your technique flexible. Remember that major health events discovered during the Review of Systems should be moved to the Present Illness or Past History in your write-up.

■ Some experienced clinicians do the *Review of Systems* during the physical examination, asking about the ears, for example, as they examine them. If the patient has only a few symptoms, this combination can be efficient. If there are multiple symptoms, however, this can disrupt the flow of both the history and the examination, and necessary note taking becomes awkward.

Listed below is a standard series of *Review-of-System* questions. As you gain experience, these "yes or no" questions will take no more than several minutes. For each regional "system" ask: "Have you ever had any...?"

The Review of Systems

General: Usual weight, recent weight change, clothing that fits more tightly or loosely than before; weakness, fatigue, or fever.

Skin: Rashes, lumps, sores, itching, dryness, changes in color; changes in hair or nails; changes in size or color of moles.

Head, Eyes, Ears, Nose, Throat (HEENT):
   Head: Headache, head injury, dizziness, lightheadedness.
   Eyes: Vision, glasses or contact lenses, last examination, pain, redness, excessive tearing, double or blurred vision, spots, specks, flashing lights, glaucoma, cataracts.
   Ears: Hearing, tinnitus, vertigo, earaches, infection, discharge. If hearing is decreased, use or nonuse of hearing aids.
   Nose and sinuses: Frequent colds, nasal stuffiness, discharge, or itching, hay fever, nosebleeds, sinus trouble.
   Throat (or mouth and pharynx): Condition of teeth and gums, bleeding gums, dentures, if any, and how they fit, last dental examination, sore tongue, dry mouth, frequent sore throats, hoarseness.

Neck: "Swollen glands," goiter, lumps, pain, or stiffness in the neck.

Breasts: Lumps, pain, or discomfort, nipple discharge, self-examination practices.

Respiratory: Cough, sputum (color, quantity; presence of blood or hemoptysis), shortness of breath (dyspnea), wheezing, pain with a deep breath (pleuritic pain), last chest x-ray. You may wish to include asthma, bronchitis, emphysema, pneumonia, and tuberculosis.

Cardiovascular: "Heart trouble"; high blood pressure; rheumatic fever; heart murmurs; chest pain or discomfort; palpitations; shortness of breath; need to use pillows at night to ease breathing (orthopnea); need to sit up at night to ease

(continued)

The Review of Systems (*continued*)

breathing (paroxysmal nocturnal dyspnea); swelling in the hands, ankles, or feet (edema); results of past electrocardiograms or other cardiovascular tests.

Gastrointestinal: Trouble swallowing, heartburn, appetite, nausea. Bowel movements, stool color and size, change in bowel habits, pain with defecation, rectal bleeding or black or tarry stools, hemorrhoids, constipation, diarrhea. Abdominal pain, food intolerance, excessive belching or passing of gas. Jaundice, liver, or gallbladder trouble; hepatitis.

Peripheral vascular: Intermittent leg pain with exertion (claudication); leg cramps; varicose veins; past clots in the veins; swelling in calves, legs, or feet; color change in fingertips or toes during cold weather; swelling with redness or tenderness.

Urinary: Frequency of urination, polyuria, nocturia, urgency, burning or pain during urination, blood in the urine (hematuria), urinary infections, kidney or flank pain, kidney stones, ureteral colic, suprapubic pain, incontinence; in males, reduced caliber or force of the urinary stream, hesitancy, dribbling.

Genital: *Male:* Hernias, discharge from or sores on the penis, testicular pain or masses, scrotal pain or swelling, history of sexually transmitted infections and their treatments. Sexual habits, interest, function, satisfaction, birth control methods, condom use, and problems. Concerns about HIV infection. *Female:* Age at menarche, regularity, frequency, and duration of periods, amount of bleeding; bleeding between periods or after intercourse, last menstrual period, dysmenorrhea, premenstrual tension. Age at menopause, menopausal symptoms, postmenopausal bleeding. If the patient was born before 1971, exposure to diethylstilbestrol (DES) from maternal use during pregnancy (linked to cervical carcinoma). Vaginal discharge, itching, sores, lumps, sexually transmitted infections and treatments. Number of pregnancies, number and type of deliveries, number of abortions (spontaneous and induced), complications of pregnancy, birth-control methods. Sexual preference, interest, function, satisfaction, any problems, including dyspareunia. Concerns about HIV infection.

Musculoskeletal: Muscle or joint pain, stiffness, arthritis, gout, backache. If present, describe location of affected joints or muscles, any swelling, redness, pain, tenderness, stiffness, weakness, or limitation of motion or activity; include timing of symptoms (e.g., morning or evening), duration, and any history of trauma. Neck or low back pain. Joint pain with systemic symptoms such as fever, chills, rash, anorexia, weight loss, or weakness.

Psychiatric: Nervousness, tension, mood, including depression, memory change, suicidal ideation, suicide plans or attempts. Past counseling, psychotherapy, or psychiatric admissions.

Neurologic: Changes in mood, attention, or speech; changes in orientation, memory, insight, or judgment; headache, dizziness, vertigo, fainting, blackouts; weakness, paralysis, numbness or loss of sensation, tingling or "pins and needles," tremors or other involuntary movements, seizures.

Hematologic: Anemia, easy bruising or bleeding, past transfusions, transfusion reactions.

Endocrine: "Thyroid trouble," heat or cold intolerance, excessive sweating, excessive thirst or hunger, polyuria, change in glove or shoe size.

The Comprehensive Physical Examination

Beginning the Examination: Setting the Stage

Before you begin the adult physical examination, take time to prepare for the tasks ahead. Think through your approach to the patient, your professional demeanor, and how to make the patient feel comfortable and relaxed. Review the measures that promote the patient's physical comfort and make any adjustments needed in the environment.

See Chapter 18, Assessing Children: Infancy Through Adolescence, for comprehensive pediatric health histories, pp. 799–925.

Steps in Preparing for the Physical Examination

1. Reflect on your approach to the patient.
2. Adjust the lighting and the environment.
3. Check your equipment.
4. Make the patient comfortable.
5. Observe standard and universal precautions.
6. Choose the sequence, scope, and positioning of examination.

Reflect on Your Approach to the Patient. As you greet the patient, identify yourself as a student. Appear calm and organized even when you feel inexperienced. It is common to forget part of the examination, especially at first. Simply examine that area out of sequence. It is not unusual to go back to the patient later and ask to check one or two items that you might have overlooked.

Beginners need to spend more time than seasoned clinicians on selected portions of the examination, such as the funduscopic examination or cardiac auscultation. To avoid alarming the patient, warn the patient ahead of time by saying, for example, "I would like to spend extra time listening to your heart and the heart sounds, but this doesn't mean I hear anything wrong."

Many patients view the physical examination with some anxiety. They feel vulnerable, physically exposed, apprehensive about possible pain, and uneasy about what the clinician may find. At the same time, they appreciate your concern about their health and respond to your attention. With this in mind, the skillful clinician is thorough without wasting time, systematic but flexible and gentle, yet not afraid to cause discomfort should this be required. The skillful clinician examines each region of the body, and at the same time senses the whole patient, notes the wince or worried glance, and shares information that calms, explains, and reassures.

As a beginner, avoid interpreting your findings. You are not the patient's primary caregiver, and your views may be premature or wrong. As you grow in experience and responsibility, sharing findings will become more appropriate. If the patient has specific concerns, discuss them with your teachers. At times, you may discover abnormalities such as an ominous mass or a deep ulceration. Always avoid showing distaste, alarm, or other negative reactions.

Adjust the Lighting and the Environment. Several environmental factors affect the caliber of your examination. For the best results, it is important to "set the stage" so that both you and the patient are comfortable. Awkward positioning makes assessing physical findings more difficult for both you and the patient. Take the time to adjust the bed to a convenient height (but be sure to lower it when finished), and ask the patient to move toward you, turn over, or shift position whenever this makes the examination of selected areas of the body easier.

Good lighting and a quiet environment enhance what you see and hear but may be hard to arrange. Do the best you can. If a television interferes with auscultating heart sounds, politely ask the nearby patient to lower the volume, and remember to thank the patient as you leave.

Tangential lighting is optimal for inspecting structures such as the jugular venous pulse, the thyroid gland, and the apical impulse of the heart (Fig. 1-3). It casts light across body surfaces that throw contours, elevations, and depressions, whether moving or stationary, into sharper relief. When light is *perpendicular* to the surface or diffuse, shadows are reduced and subtle undulations across the surface are lost (Fig. 1-4). Experiment with focused tangential lighting across the tendons on the back of your hand; try to see the pulsations of the radial artery at your wrist.

Check Your Equipment. Equipment necessary for the physical examination includes the following:

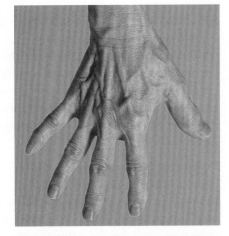

FIGURE 1-3. **Tangential lighting.**

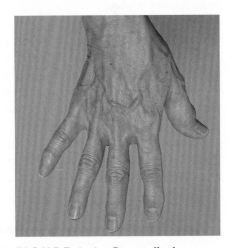

FIGURE 1-4. **Perpendicular lighting.**

Equipment for the Physical Examination

- An ophthalmoscope and an otoscope. If you are examining children, the otoscope could allow pneumatic otoscopy.
- A flashlight or penlight
- Tongue depressors
- A ruler and a flexible tape measure, preferably marked in centimeters
- Often a thermometer
- A watch with a second hand
- A sphygmomanometer
- A stethoscope with the following characteristics:
  - Ear tips that fit snugly and painlessly. To get this fit, choose ear tips of the proper size, align the ear pieces with the angle of your ear canals, and adjust the spring of the connecting metal band to a comfortable tightness.
  - Thick-walled tubing as short as feasible to maximize the transmission of sound: ~30 cm (12 inches), if possible, and no longer than 38 cm (15 inches)
  - A bell and a diaphragm with a good changeover mechanism
- A visual acuity card
- A reflex hammer
- Tuning forks, both 128 Hz and 512 Hz

(continued)

Equipment for the Physical Examination (continued)

- Cotton swabs, safety pins, or other disposable objects for testing sensation and two-point discrimination
- Cotton for testing the sense of light touch
- Two test tubes (optional) for testing temperature sensation
- Gloves and lubricant for oral, vaginal, and rectal examinations
- Vaginal specula and equipment for cytologic and bacteriologic studies
- Paper and pen or pencil, or desktop or laptop computer

Make the Patient Comfortable

Patient Privacy and Comfort. Your access to the patient's body is a unique and time-honored privilege of your role as a clinician. Showing sensitivity to privacy and patient modesty must be ingrained in your professional behavior and conveys respect for the patient's vulnerability. Close nearby doors, draw the curtains in the hospital or examining room, and wash your hands carefully before the examination begins.

During the examination, be aware of the patient's feelings and any discomfort. Respond to the patient's facial expressions and even ask, "Are you okay?" or "Is this painful?" to elicit unexpressed worries or sources of pain. Adjusting the angle of the bed or examining table, rearranging the pillows, or adding blankets for warmth demonstrates that you are attentive to the patient's well-being.

Draping the Patient. You will acquire the art of *draping the patient* with the gown or draw sheet as you learn each segment of the examination in the chapters ahead.

Tips for Draping the Patient

- Your goal is to visualize one area of the body at a time. This preserves the patient's modesty and helps you focus on the area being examined.
- With the patient sitting, for example, untie the gown in back to better listen to the lungs.
- For the breast examination, uncover the right breast but keep the left chest draped. Redrape the right chest, then uncover the left chest and proceed to examine the left breast and heart.
- For the abdominal examination, only the abdomen should be exposed. Adjust the gown to cover the chest and place the sheet or drape at the inguinal level. To help the patient prepare for potentially awkward segments of the examination, briefly describe your plans before starting, for example, "Now I am going to move your gown so I can check the pulse in your groin area," or "Because you mentioned irritation, I am going to inspect your perirectal area."

Courteous Clear Instructions. Make sure your instructions to the patient at each step in the examination are courteous and clear. For example, "I would like to examine your heart now, so please lie down," or "Now I am going to check your abdomen." Let the patient know if you anticipate embarrassment or discomfort.

Keeping the Patient Informed.   As you proceed with the examination, talk with the patient to see if he or she wants to know about your findings. Is the patient curious about the lung findings or your method for assessing the liver or spleen?

When you have completed the examination, tell the patient your general impressions and what to expect next. For hospitalized patients, make sure the patient is comfortable and rearrange the immediate environment to the patient's satisfaction. Be sure to lower the bed to avoid risk of falls and raise the bedrails. As you leave, wash your hands, clean your equipment, and dispose of any waste materials.

Observe Standard and Universal Precautions.   The Centers for Disease Control and Prevention (CDC) have issued several guidelines to protect patients and examiners from the spread of infectious disease. All clinicians examining patients are advised to study and observe these precautions at the CDC websites. Advisories for standard and methicillin-resistant *Staphylococcus aureus* (*MRSA*) precautions and for universal precautions are summarized below.[19–23]

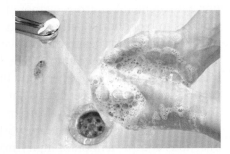

FIGURE 1-5.   Handwashing is a standard precaution.

Standard and MRSA precautions. Standard precautions are based on the principle that all blood, body fluids, secretions, excretions (except sweat), nonintact skin, and mucous membranes may contain transmissible infectious agents. Standard precautions apply to all patients in any setting. They include hand hygiene (Fig. 1-5); use of personal protective equipment (gloves; gowns; and mouth, nose, and eye protection) (Fig. 1-6); safe injection practices; safe handling of contaminated equipment or surfaces; respiratory hygiene and cough etiquette; patient isolation criteria; and precautions relating to equipment, toys, solid surfaces, and laundry handling. Because hand hygiene practices have been shown to reduce the transmission of multidrug-resistant organisms, especially MRSA and vancomycin-resistant enterococcus (VRE),[19] the CDC hygiene recommendations are reproduced below. White coats and stethoscopes also harbor bacteria and should be cleaned frequently.[24,25]

CDC Recommendations for Hand Hygiene

1. Key situations where hand hygiene should be performed include:
   a. before touching a patient, even if gloves are worn;
   b. before exiting the patient's care area after touching the patient or the patient's immediate environment;
   c. after contact with blood, body fluids, or excretions, or wound dressings;
   d. prior to performing an aseptic task (e.g., placing an intravenous drip, preparing an injection);
   e. if hands are moving from a contaminated-body site to a clean-body site during patient care; and
   f. after glove removal.

(continued)

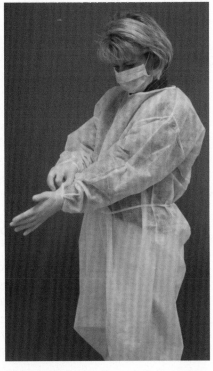

FIGURE 1-6.   Personal protective equipment.

CDC Recommendations for Hand Hygiene (continued)

2. Use soap and water when hands are visibly soiled (e.g., blood, body fluids), or after caring for patients with known or suspected infectious diarrhea (e.g., *Clostridium difficile,* norovirus). Otherwise, the preferred method of hand decontamination is with an alcohol-based hand rub.

Source: CDC. Guide to infection prevention in outpatient settings. Minimum expectations for safe care. May 2011. Available at http://www.cdc.gov/HAI/settings/outpatient/outpatient-care-guide-lines.html. Accessed March 1, 2015.

Universal precautions. Universal precautions are a set of guidelines designed to prevent parenteral, mucous membrane, and noncontact exposures of health care workers to bloodborne pathogens, including HIV and HBV. Immunization with the HBV vaccine for health care workers with exposure to blood is an important adjunct to universal precautions. The following fluids are considered potentially infectious: all blood and other body fluids containing visible blood, semen, and vaginal secretions and cerebrospinal, synovial, pleural, peritoneal, pericardial, and amniotic fluids. Protective barriers include gloves, gowns, aprons, masks, and protective eyewear. All health care workers should follow the precautions for safe injections and prevention of injury from needlesticks, scalpels, and other sharp instruments and devices. Report to your health service immediately if such injury occurs.

Choose the Sequence, Scope, and Positioning of the Examination

The Cardinal Techniques of Examination.

As you begin the examination, study the four cardinal techniques of examination. Plan your sequence and scope of examination and how you will position the patient.

The physical examination relies on four classic techniques: inspection, palpation, percussion, and auscultation. You will learn in later chapters about additional maneuvers that are important in amplifying physical diagnosis, such as having the patient lean forward to better detect the murmur of aortic regurgitation or balloting the patella to check for joint effusion.

Cardinal Techniques of Examination

Inspection	Close observation of the details of the patient's appearance, behavior, and movement such as facial expression, mood, body habitus and conditioning, skin conditions such as petechiae or ecchymoses, eye movements, pharyngeal color, symmetry of thorax, height of jugular venous pulsations, abdominal contour, lower extremity edema, and gait.

(continued)

Cardinal Techniques of Examination (*continued*)

Palpation	Tactile pressure from the palmar fingers or fingerpads to assess areas of skin elevation, depression, warmth, or tenderness, lymph nodes, pulses, contours and sizes of organs and masses, and crepitus in the joints.
Percussion	Use of the striking or *plexor finger,* usually the third, to deliver a rapid tap or blow against the distal *pleximeter finger,* usually the distal third finger of the left hand laid against the surface of the chest or abdomen, to evoke a sound wave such as resonance or dullness from the underlying tissue or organs. This sound wave also generates a tactile vibration against the pleximeter finger.
Auscultation	Use of the diaphragm and bell of the stethoscope to detect the characteristics of heart, lung, and bowel sounds, including location, timing, duration, pitch, and intensity. For the heart, this involves sounds from closure of the four valves, extra sounds from blood flow into the atria and ventricles, and murmurs. Auscultation also permits detection of bruits or turbulence over arterial vessels.

Sequence of Examination. The key to a thorough and accurate physical examination is developing a systematic sequence of examination. Organize your comprehensive or focused examination around three general goals:

- Maximize the patient's comfort.

- Avoid unnecessary changes in position.

- Enhance clinical efficiency.

In general, move from "head to toe." Avoid examining the patient's feet, for example, before checking the face or mouth. You will quickly see that some segments of the examination are best assessed when the patient is sitting, such as examination of the head and neck and the thorax and lungs, whereas others are best obtained with the patient supine, such as the cardiovascular and abdominal examinations.

As you review the Techniques of Examination on the following pages, note that clinicians vary in where they place different segments of the examination, especially examinations of the musculoskeletal system and the nervous system. Some of these options are indicated in red in the right-hand column. Suggestions for patient positioning during the different segments of the examination are also indicated in the right-hand column in red.

With practice, you will develop your own sequence of examination, keeping the need for thoroughness and patient comfort in mind. At first, you may need notes to remind you what to look for, but over time, this sequence will become habitual and remind you to return to segments of the examination you may have skipped, helping you to be complete.

Examining from the Patient's Right Side. This book recommends examining the patient from the patient's right side, moving to the opposite side or foot of the bed or examining table as necessary. This is the standard position for the physical examination and has several advantages compared with the left side: Estimates of jugular venous pressure are more reliable, the palpating hand rests more comfortably on the apical impulse, the right kidney is more frequently palpable than the left, and examining tables are frequently positioned to accommodate a right-handed approach.

Left-handed students are encouraged to adopt right-sided positioning, even it may seem awkward. The left hand can still be used for percussing or for holding instruments such as the otoscope or reflex hammer.

Review the proposed physical examination sequence in Figure 1-6, which meets the three goals of patient comfort, minimal changes in positioning, and efficiency.

The Physical Examination: Suggested Sequence and Positioning

- General survey
- Vital signs
- Skin: upper torso, anterior and posterior
- Head and neck, including thyroid and lymph nodes
- *Optional:* nervous system (mental status, cranial nerves, upper extremity motor strength, bulk, tone, cerebellar function)
- Thorax and lungs
- Breasts
- Musculoskeletal as indicated: upper extremities
- Cardiovascular, including jugular venous pressure (JVP), carotid upstrokes and bruits, point of maximal impulse (PMI), S$_1$, S$_2$; murmurs, extra sounds
- Cardiovascular, for S$_3$ and murmur of mitral stenosis
- Cardiovascular, for murmur of aortic insufficiency
- *Optional:* thorax and lungs—anterior
- Breasts and axillae
- Abdomen
- Peripheral vascular

- *Optional:* skin—lower torso and extremities
- Nervous system: lower extremity motor strength, bulk, tone, sensation; reflexes; Babinski reflex
- Musculoskeletal, as indicated
- *Optional:* skin, anterior and posterior
- *Optional:* nervous system, including gait
- *Optional:* musculoskeletal, comprehensive
- *Women:* pelvic and rectal examination
- *Men:* prostate and rectal examination

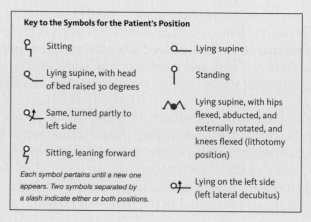

Key to the Symbols for the Patient's Position

Sitting	Lying supine
Lying supine, with head of bed raised 30 degrees	Standing
Same, turned partly to left side	Lying supine, with hips flexed, abducted, and externally rotated, and knees flexed (lithotomy position)
Sitting, leaning forward	

Each symbol pertains until a new one appears. Two symbols separated by a slash indicate either or both positions.

Lying on the left side (left lateral decubitus)

Examining the Patient at Bedrest. Often you will need to examine a patient *at bedrest,* especially in the hospital, where patients frequently cannot sit up in bed or stand. This often dictates changes in your sequence of examination. You can examine the head, neck, and anterior chest with the patient lying supine.

Then, roll the patient onto each side to listen to the lungs, examine the back, and inspect the skin. Roll the patient back and finish the rest of the examination with the patient again supine.

The Physical Examination—"Head to Toe"

General Survey.   Observe the patient's general state of health, height, build, and sexual development. Obtain the patient's height and weight. Note posture, motor activity, and gait; dress, grooming, and personal hygiene; and any odors of the body or breath. Watch the patient's facial expressions and note manner, affect, and reactions to people and the environment. Listen to the patient's speech, and note the state of awareness or level of consciousness.

Close observation begins at the outset of the patient encounter and continues throughout the history and physical examination.

Vital Signs.   Measure the blood pressure. Count the pulse and respiratory rate. If indicated, measure the body temperature.

The **patient is sitting** on the edge of the bed or examining table. Stand in front of the patient, moving to either side as needed.

Skin.   Observe the skin of the face and its characteristics. Assess skin moisture or dryness and temperature. Identify any lesions, noting their location, distribution, arrangement, type, and color. Inspect and palpate the hair and nails. Study both surfaces of the patient's hands. Continue your assessment of the skin as you examine the other body regions.

Head, Eyes, Ears, Nose, Throat (HEENT).   *Head:* Examine the hair, scalp, skull, and face. *Eyes:* Check visual acuity and screen the visual fields. Note the position and alignment of the eyes. Observe the eyelids and inspect the sclera and conjunctiva of each eye. With oblique lighting, inspect each cornea, iris, and lens. Compare the pupils, and test their reactions to light. Assess the extraocular movements. With an ophthalmoscope, inspect the ocular fundi. *Ears:* Inspect the auricles, canals, and drums. Check auditory acuity. If acuity is diminished, check lateralization (Weber test) and compare air and bone conduction (Rinne test). *Nose and sinuses:* Examine the external nose; using a light and a nasal speculum, inspect the nasal mucosa, septum, and turbinates. Palpate for tenderness of the frontal and maxillary sinuses. *Throat (or mouth and pharynx):* Inspect the lips, oral mucosa, gums, teeth, tongue, palate, tonsils, and pharynx. (*You may wish to assess the cranial nerves during this portion of the examination.*)

The room should be darkened for the ophthalmoscopic examination. This promotes pupillary dilation and visibility of the fundi.

Neck.   Inspect and palpate the cervical lymph nodes. Note any masses or unusual pulsations in the neck. Feel for any deviation of the trachea. Observe the sound and effort of the patient's breathing. Inspect and palpate the thyroid gland.

Move behind the sitting patient to feel the thyroid gland and to examine the back, posterior thorax, and lungs.

Back.   Inspect and palpate the spine and muscles of the back. Observe shoulder height for symmetry.

Posterior Thorax and Lungs.   Inspect and palpate the spine and muscles of the *upper* back. Inspect, palpate, and percuss the chest. Identify the level of diaphragmatic dullness on each side. Listen to the breath sounds; identify any adventitious (or added) sounds, and, if indicated, listen to the transmitted voice sounds (see pp. 326–327).

Breasts, Axillae, and Epitrochlear Nodes.   In a woman, inspect the breasts with her arms relaxed, then elevated, and then with her hands pressed on her hips. In either sex, inspect the axillae and feel for the axillary nodes. Feel for the epitrochlear nodes.

A Note on the Musculoskeletal System.   By this time, you have made preliminary observations of the musculoskeletal system. You have inspected the hands, surveyed the upper back, and, in women, made a fair estimate of the shoulders' range of motion. If indicated, *with the patient still sitting,* examine the hands, arms, shoulders, neck, and temporomandibular joints. Inspect and palpate the joints and check their range of motion. *(You may choose to examine upper extremity muscle bulk, tone, strength, and reflexes at this time, or wait until later.)*

Palpate the breasts, while at the same time continuing your inspection.

Anterior Thorax and Lungs.   Inspect, palpate, and percuss the chest. Listen to the breath sounds, any adventitious sounds, and, if indicated, transmitted voice sounds.

Cardiovascular System.   Observe the jugular venous pulsations and measure the jugular venous pressure in relation to the sternal angle. Inspect and palpate the carotid pulsations. Listen for carotid bruits.

Elevate the head of the bed to ~30° for the cardiovascular examination, adjusting as necessary to see the jugular venous pulsations.

Inspect and palpate the precordium. Note the location, diameter, amplitude, and duration of the apical impulse. Listen at each auscultatory area with the diaphragm of the stethoscope. Listen at the apex and the lower sternal border with the bell. Listen for the first and second heart sounds and for physiologic splitting of the second heart sound. Listen for any abnormal heart sounds or murmurs.

Abdomen.   Inspect, auscultate, and percuss the abdomen. Palpate lightly, then deeply. Assess the liver and spleen by percussion and then palpation. Try to palpate the kidneys. Palpate the aorta and its pulsations. If you suspect kidney infection, percuss posteriorly over the costovertebral angles.

Lower Extremities.   Examine the legs, assessing three systems while the patient is still supine. Each of these three systems can be further assessed when the patient stands.

With the patient supine:

- *Peripheral vascular system.* Palpate the femoral pulses and, if indicated, the popliteal pulses. Palpate the inguinal lymph nodes. Inspect for lower extremity edema, discoloration, or ulcers. Palpate for pitting edema.

The patient is **still sitting.** Move to the front again.

The patient position is supine. Ask the patient to lie down. You should stand at the *right side* of the patient's bed.

Ask the patient to roll partly onto the left side while you listen at the apex for an S_3 or *mitral stenosis.* The patient should sit, lean forward, and exhale while you listen for the murmur of *aortic regurgitation.*

Lower the head of the bed to the flat position. **The patient should be supine.**

The patient is **supine.**

■ *Musculoskeletal system.* Note any deformities or enlarged joints. If indicated, palpate the joints, check their range of motion, and perform any necessary maneuvers.

■ *Nervous system.* Assess lower extremity muscle bulk, tone, and strength; also assess sensation and reflexes. Observe any abnormal movements.

With the patient standing:

■ *Peripheral vascular system.* Inspect for varicose veins.

■ *Musculoskeletal system.* Examine the alignment of the spine and its range of motion, the alignment of the legs, and the feet.

■ *Genitalia and hernias in men.* Examine the penis and scrotal contents and check for hernias.

■ *Nervous system.* Observe the patient's gait and ability to walk heel-to-toe, walk on the toes, walk on the heels, hop in place, and do shallow knee bends. Do a Romberg test and check for pronator drift.

The patient is standing. You can sit on a chair or stool.

Nervous System. The complete examination of the nervous system can also be done at the end of the examination. It consists of the five segments: *mental status, cranial nerves* (including funduscopic examination), *motor system, sensory system,* and *reflexes.*

The patient is sitting or supine.

Mental Status. If indicated and not done during the interview, assess the patient's orientation, mood, thought process, thought content, abnormal perceptions, insight and judgment, memory and attention, information and vocabulary, calculating abilities, abstract thinking, and constructional ability.

Cranial Nerves. If not already examined, check sense of smell, strength of the temporal and masseter muscles, corneal reflexes, facial movements, gag reflex, and strength of the trapezia and sternocleidomastoid muscles.

Motor System. Assess muscle bulk, tone, and strength of major muscle groups. *Cerebellar function:* rapid alternating movements (RAMs), point-to-point movements, such as finger-to-nose (F → N) and heel-to-shin (H → S), gait.

Sensory System. Assess pain, temperature, light touch, vibration, and discrimination. Compare right with left sides and distal with proximal areas on the limbs.

Reflexes. Including biceps, triceps, brachioradialis, patellar, Achilles deep tendon reflexes; also plantar reflexes or Babinski response (see pp. 758–764).

Additional Examinations. The *rectal* and *genital* examinations are often performed at the end of the physical examination. Patient positioning is as indicated.

Genital and Rectal Examination in Men. Inspect the sacrococcygeal and perianal areas. Palpate the anal canal, rectum, and prostate. If the patient cannot stand, examine the genitalia before doing the rectal examination.

Genital and Rectal Examinations in Women. Examine the external genitalia, vagina, and cervix, with a chaperone when needed. Obtain a Pap smear. Palpate the uterus and adnexa bimanually. Perform the rectal examination if indicated.

The patient is **lying on his left side for the rectal examination (or standing and bending forward).**

The patient is **supine in the lithotomy position.** You should be seated during examination with the speculum, then standing during bimanual examination of the uterus, adnexa (and rectum as indicated).

Clinical Reasoning, Assessment, and Plan

After completing the history and physical examination, you reach the critical step of formulating your *Assessment* and *Plan* (Figs. 1-7 and 1-8). Using sound clinical reasoning, you must analyze your findings and identify the patient's problems. You must share your impressions with the patient, eliciting any concerns and making sure that he or she understands and agrees to the steps ahead. Finally, you must document your findings in the patient's record in a succinct legible format that communicates the patient's story and physical findings, and the rationale for your assessment and plan, to other members of the health care team. As you make clinical decisions, you will turn to clinical evidence, calling on your knowledge of sensitivity, specificity, predictive value, and the analytical tools detailed in Chapter 2, Evaluating Clinical Evidence.

The comprehensive health history and physical examination form the foundation of your clinical *Assessment.* The *subjective data* of the health history and the *objective data* from the physical examination and testing are primarily descriptive and factual. As you move to Assessment, you go beyond description and observation to analysis and interpretation. You select and cluster relevant pieces of information, analyze their significance, and try to explain them logically using principles of biopsychosocial and bioclinical science. Your clinical reasoning process is pivotal to how you interpret the patient's history and physical examination, single out problems identified in the *Assessment,* and move from each problem to its action plan (Fig. 1-9).

The *Plan* is often wide ranging and incorporates patient education, changes in medications, needed tests, referrals to other clinicians, and return visits for counseling and support. However, a successful *Plan* does more than just describe the approach to a problem. It includes the patient's responses to the problems identified and to the diagnostic and therapeutic interventions that you recommend. It requires good interpersonal skills and sensitivity to the patient's goals, economic means, competing responsibilities, and family structure and dynamics.

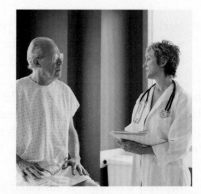

FIGURE 1-7. Discuss the assessment.

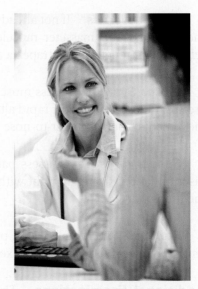

FIGURE 1-8. Share the plan.

Clinical Reasoning and Assessment

Because assessment takes place in the clinician's mind, the process of clinical reasoning may seem opaque and even mysterious to beginning students. Experienced clinicians often think quickly, with little overt or conscious effort. They differ widely in personal style, communication skills, clinical training, experience, and expertise. Some clinicians may find it difficult to explain the logic behind their clinical thinking. As an active learner, you will be expected to ask teachers and clinicians to elaborate on the fine points of their clinical reasoning and decision making.[26,27]

Cognitive psychologists have shown that clinicians use three types of reasoning for clinical problem solving: pattern recognition, development of schemas, and application of relevant basic and clinical science.[29-34] As you gain experience, your clinical reasoning will begin at the outset of the patient encounter, not at the end. Study the steps described here, then apply them to the *Case of Mrs. N.* that follows. Think about these steps as you see your first patients. As with all patients, focus on determining "What explains this patient's concerns?" and "What are the findings, problems, and diagnoses?"[17,35]

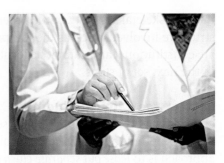

FIGURE 1-9. Apply clinical reasoning.

For clinical examples of excellent and faulty reasoning and strategies to avoid cognitive errors, turn to Kassirer et al., *Learning Clinical Reasoning.*[28]

Steps for Identifying Problems and Making Diagnoses

1. Identify abnormal findings.
2. Localize findings anatomically.
3. Cluster the clinical findings.
4. Search for the probable cause of the findings.
5. Cluster the clinical data.
6. Generate hypotheses about the causes of the patient's problems.
7. Test the hypotheses and establish a working diagnosis.

Identify Abnormal Findings. Make a list of the patient's *symptoms*, the *signs* you observed during the physical examination, and any laboratory reports available to you.

Localize These Findings Anatomically. Often, this step is straightforward. The symptom of scratchy throat and the sign of an erythematous inflamed posterior pharynx, for example, clearly localize the problem to the pharynx. A complaint of headache leads you quickly to the structures of the skull and brain. Other symptoms, however, may present greater difficulty. Chest pain, for example, can originate in the coronary arteries, the stomach and esophagus, or the muscles and bones of the thorax. If the pain is exertional and relieved by rest, either the heart or the musculoskeletal components of the chest wall may be involved. If the patient notes pain only when carrying groceries with the left arm, the musculoskeletal system becomes the likely culprit.

When localizing findings, be as specific as your data allow; however, you may have to settle for a body region, such as the chest, or a body system, such as the musculoskeletal system. On the other hand, you may be able to define the exact structure involved, such as the left pectoral muscle. Some symptoms and signs are constitutional and cannot be localized, such as fatigue or fever, but are useful in the next set of steps.

Cluster the Clinical Findings.   It is often challenging to decide whether clinical data fit into one problem or several problems. If there is a relatively long list of symptoms and signs, and an equally long list of potential explanations, one approach is to *tease out separate clusters of observations and analyze one cluster at a time.* Several clinical characteristics may help.

- *Patient age:* The patient's *age* may help; younger adults are more likely to have a single disease, whereas older adults tend to have multiple diseases.

- *Timing of symptoms:* The *timing* of symptoms is often useful. For example, an episode of pharyngitis 6 weeks ago is probably unrelated to the fever, chills, pleuritic chest pain, and cough that prompted an office visit today. To use timing effectively, you need to know the natural history of various diseases and conditions. A yellow penile discharge followed 3 weeks later by a painless penile ulcer suggests two problems: gonorrhea and primary syphilis. In contrast, a penile ulcer followed in 6 weeks by a maculopapular skin rash and generalized lymphadenopathy suggest two stages of the same problem: primary and secondary syphilis.

- *Involvement of different body systems:* Involvement of the *different body systems* may help group clinical data. If symptoms and signs occur in a single system, one disease may explain them. Problems in different, apparently unrelated, systems often require more than one explanation. Again, knowledge of disease patterns is necessary. For example, you might decide to group a patient's high blood pressure and sustained apical impulse together with flame-shaped retinal hemorrhages, place them in the cardiovascular system, and label the constellation "hypertensive cardiovascular disease with hypertensive retinopathy." You would develop another explanation for the patient's mild fever, left lower quadrant tenderness, and diarrhea.

- *Multisystem conditions:* With experience, you will become increasingly adept at recognizing *multisystem conditions* and building plausible explanations that link manifestations that are seemingly unrelated. To explain cough, hemoptysis, and weight loss in a 60-year-old plumber who has smoked cigarettes for 40 years, you would rank lung cancer high in your differential diagnosis. You might support your diagnosis with your observation of the patient's cyanotic nailbeds. With experience and continued reading, you will recognize that his other symptoms and signs fall under the same diagnosis. Dysphagia would reflect extension of the cancer to the esophagus, pupillary asymmetry would suggest pressure on the cervical sympathetic chain, and jaundice could result from metastases to the liver. In another example of multisystem disease, a young man who presents with odynophagia, fever, weight loss, purplish skin lesions, leukoplakia, generalized lymphadenopathy, and chronic diarrhea is likely to have acquired immune deficiency syndrome (AIDS). Related risk factors should be explored promptly.

■ *Key questions:* You can also *ask a series of key questions* that may steer your thinking in one direction and allow you to temporarily ignore the others. For example, you may ask what produces and relieves the patient's chest pain. If the answer is exercise and rest, you can focus on the cardiovascular and musculoskeletal systems and set the gastrointestinal (GI) system aside. If the pain is more epigastric, burning, and occurs only after meals, you can logically focus on the GI tract. A series of discriminating questions helps you analyze the clinical data and reach logical explanations.

Search for the Probable Cause of the Findings. Patient complaints often stem from a *pathologic process* involving diseases of a body system or structure. These processes are commonly classified as congenital, inflammatory or infectious, immunologic, neoplastic, metabolic, nutritional, degenerative, vascular, traumatic, and toxic. Possible pathologic causes of headache, for example, include sinus infection, concussion from trauma, subarachnoid hemorrhage, or even compression from a brain tumor. Fever and stiff neck, or nuchal rigidity, are two of the classic signs of headache from meningitis. Even without other signs, such as rash or papilledema, they strongly suggest an infectious process.

Other problems are *pathophysiologic,* reflecting derangements of biologic functions, such as heart failure or migraine headache. Still other problems are *psychopathologic,* such as disorders of mood like depression or headache as an expression of a somatic symptom disorder.

Generate Hypotheses About the Causes of the Patient's Problem. Draw on the full range of your knowledge and experience, and read widely. It is at this point that reading about diseases and abnormalities is most useful. By consulting the clinical literature, you embark on the lifelong goal of *evidence-based decision making and clinical practice.*[14,36–39] At first, your hypotheses may not be highly specific, but proceed as far as your knowledge and available data allow, observing the steps below.

Steps for Generating Clinical Hypotheses

1. *Select the most specific and critical findings to support your hypothesis.* If the patient reports "the worst headache of her life," nausea, and vomiting, for example, and you find altered mental status, papilledema, and meningismus, build your hypothesis around elevated intracranial pressure rather than GI disorders.
2. *Match your findings against all the conditions that can produce them.* Using your knowledge of the structures and processes involved, you can match your patient's papilledema with a list of conditions affecting intracranial pressure. Or you can compare the symptoms and signs associated with the patient's headache with the various infectious, vascular, metabolic, or neoplastic conditions that might produce this clinical picture.
3. *Eliminate the diagnostic possibilities that fail to explain the findings.* You might consider cluster headache as a cause of Mrs. N.'s headaches (see

(*continued*)

Steps for Generating Clinical Hypotheses (continued)

The Case of Mrs. N., pp. 30–36), but eliminate this hypothesis because it fails to explain the patient's throbbing bifrontal localization with associated nausea and vomiting. Also, the pain pattern is atypical for cluster headache—it is not unilateral, boring, or occurring repetitively at the same time over a period of days, nor is it associated with lacrimation or rhinorrhea.

4. *Weigh the competing possibilities and select the most likely diagnosis.* You are looking for a close match between the patient's clinical presentation and a typical case of a given condition. Other clues help in this selection. The *statistical probability* of a given disease in a patient of this age, sex, ethnic group, habits, lifestyle, and locality should greatly influence your selection. You should consider the possibilities of osteoarthritis and metastatic prostate cancer in a 70-year-old man with back pain, for example, but not in a 25-year-old woman with the same complaint. The *timing of the patient's illness* also makes a difference. Headache in the setting of fever, rash, and stiff neck that develops suddenly over 24 hours suggests quite a different problem than recurrent headache over a period of years associated with stress, visual scotoma, and nausea and vomiting relieved by rest.

5. *Give special attention to potentially life-threatening conditions.* Your goal is to minimize the risk of missing unusual or infrequent conditions such as meningococcal meningitis, bacterial endocarditis, pulmonary embolus, or subdural hematoma that are particularly ominous. One rule of thumb is always to include "the worst case scenario" in your differential diagnosis and make sure you have ruled out this possibility based on your findings and patient assessment.

See Chapter 2, Evaluating Clinical Evidence, pp. 45–64.

Test Your Hypotheses. Now that you have made a hypothesis about the patient's problem, you are ready to *test your hypothesis.* You are likely to need further history, additional maneuvers on physical examination, or laboratory studies or x-rays to confirm or rule out your tentative diagnosis or to clarify which of two or three possible diagnoses are most likely. When the diagnosis seems clear-cut—a simple upper respiratory infection or a case of hives, for example—these steps may not be necessary.

Establish a Working Diagnosis. Establish a working definition of the problem at the highest level of explicitness and certainty that the data allow. You may be limited to a symptom, such as "tension headache, cause unknown." At other times, you can define a problem more specifically based on its anatomy, disease process, or cause. Examples include "bacterial meningitis, pneumococcal," "subarachnoid hemorrhage, left temporoparietal lobe," or "hypertensive cardiovascular disease with left ventricular dilatation and heart failure."

Although most diagnoses are based on the identification of abnormal structures, disease processes, and clinical syndromes, patients frequently have clinically unexplained symptoms. You may not be able to move beyond simple descriptive categories such as "fatigue" or "anorexia." Other problems relate to stressful events in the patient's life such as losing a job or a family member that increase the risk for subsequent illness. Identifying these events and helping the patient develop coping strategies are just as important as managing a headache or a duodenal ulcer.

Another increasingly prominent item on problem lists is *Health Maintenance*. Routinely listing Health Maintenance helps you track several important health concerns more effectively: immunizations, screening tests such as mammograms or colonoscopies, instructions regarding nutrition and breast or testicular self-examinations, recommendations about exercise or use of seat belts, and responses to important life events.

Using Shared Decision-Making to Develop a Plan

Identify and record a *Plan* for each patient problem. Your *Plan* flows logically from the problems or diagnoses you have identified. Specify the next steps for each problem. These steps range from tests and procedures to subspecialty consultations to new or changed medications to arranging a family meeting. You will find that you follow many of the same diagnoses over time; however, your *Plan* is often more fluid, encompassing changes and modifications that emerge from each patient visit. The *Plan* should make reference to diagnosis, treatments, and patient education. It is important to discuss your assessment with the patient before finalizing the *Plan* and proceeding with further testing or evaluation, ensuring the patient's active participation in the plan of care (Fig. 1-10). It is critical to both obtain patient agreement and encourage patient participation in decision-making whenever possible. These practices promote optimal therapy, adherence to treatment, and patient satisfaction, especially since there is often no single "right" plan, but a range of variations and options. You may need to explain your recommendations several times to make sure the patient agrees to and understands what lies ahead.

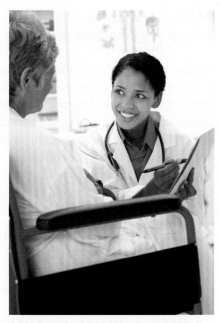

FIGURE 1-10. **Make sure the patient agrees with the plan.**

See Chapter 5, Behavior and Mental Status, section on "Medically Unexplained Symptoms," pp. 149–150.

The Quality Clinical Record: The Case of Mrs. N.

The *clinical record* serves a dual purpose—it reflects your analysis of the patient's health status, and it documents the unique features of the patient's history, examination, laboratory and test results, assessment, and plan in a formal written format (Fig. 1-11). In a well-constructed record, each problem in the *Assessment* is listed in order of priority with an explanation of supporting findings and a differential diagnosis, followed by a *Plan* for addressing that problem. The patient record facilitates clinical reasoning, promotes communication and coordination among the professionals who care for your patient, and documents the patient's problems and management for medicolegal purposes.

Compose the clinical record as soon after seeing the patient as possible, before your findings fade from memory. At first you may take notes, but work toward recording each segment of the health history during the interview, leaving spaces

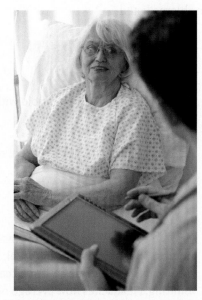

FIGURE 1-11. **Compose a well-constructed record.**

for filling in details later. Jot down blood pressure, heart rate, and key abnormal findings to prompt your recall when you complete the record later.

See Table 1-1, p. 41, for a Sample Progress Note for the follow-up visit of Mrs. N.

Almost all clinical information is subject to error. Patients forget to mention symptoms, confuse the events of their illness, avoid recounting embarrassing facts, and may slant their stories to what they believe the clinician wants to hear. Clinicians misinterpret patient statements, overlook information, fail to ask "the one key question," jump prematurely to conclusions and diagnoses, or forget an important part of the examination, such as the funduscopic examination in a woman with headache, leading to diagnostic errors.[40-48] You can avoid some of these errors by acquiring the habits summarized below.

Tips for Ensuring Quality Patient Data

- Ask open-ended questions and listen carefully to the patient's story.
- Craft a thorough and systematic sequence to history taking and physical examination.
- Keep an open mind toward both the patient and the clinical data.
- Always include "the worst-case scenario" in your list of possible explanations of the patient's problem, and make sure it can be safely eliminated.
- Analyze any mistakes in data collection or interpretation.
- Confer with colleagues and review the pertinent clinical literature to clarify uncertainties.
- Apply the principles of evaluating clinical evidence to patient information and testing.

Study the case of Mrs. N. and scrutinize the history, physical examination, assessment, and plan. Note the standard format of the clinical record. Apply your own clinical reasoning to the findings presented and begin to analyze the patient's concerns. See if you agree with the Assessment and Plan and the priority of the problems listed.

The Case of Mrs. N.

8/25/16 11:00 AM
Mrs. N. is a pleasant, 54-year-old widowed saleswoman residing in Espanola, New Mexico.
Referral. None
Source and Reliability. Self-referred; seems reliable.

Chief Complaint
"My head aches."

Present Illness
Mrs. N. reports increasing problems with frontal headaches over the past 3 months. These are usually bifrontal, throbbing, and mild to moderately severe. She has missed work on several occasions because of associated nausea and vomiting. Headaches now average once a week, usually related to stress, and

(continued)

The Case of Mrs. N. (*continued*)

last 4 to 6 hours. They are relieved by sleep and putting a damp towel over her forehead. There is little relief from aspirin. There are no associated visual changes, motor-sensory deficits, or paresthesias.

She had headaches with nausea and vomiting beginning at age 15 years. These recurred throughout her mid-20s, then decreased to one every 2 or 3 months, and almost disappeared.

The patient reports increased pressure at work from a demanding supervisor; she is also worried about her daughter (see *Personal and Social History*). She thinks her headaches may be like those in the past, but wants to be sure because her mother had a headache just before she died of a stroke. She is concerned because her headaches interfere with her work and make her irritable with her family. She eats three meals a day and drinks three cups of coffee a day and tea at night.

Medications. Acetaminophen, 1 to 2 tablets every 4 to 6 hours as needed. "Water pill" in the past for ankle swelling, none recently.

Allergies. Ampicillin causes rash.

Tobacco. About 1 pack of cigarettes per day since age 18 (36 pack-years).

Alcohol/drugs. Wine on rare occasions. No illicit drugs.

Past History

Childhood Illnesses: Measles, chickenpox. No scarlet fever or rheumatic fever.

Adult Illnesses: Medical: Pyelonephritis, 1998, with fever and right flank pain; treated with ampicillin; developed generalized rash with itching several days later. Reports x-rays were normal; no recurrence of infection.

Surgical: Tonsillectomy, age 6; appendectomy, age 13. Sutures for laceration, 2001, after stepping on glass. *Ob/Gyn:* 3–3–0–3, with normal vaginal deliveries. Three living children. Menarche age 12. Last menses 6 months ago. Little interest in sex, and not sexually active. No concerns about HIV infection. *Psychiatric:* None.

Gravida (G)-Parity (# of deliveries)
(P)-Miscarriages (M)-Living (L), or
G-P-M-L 3–3–0–3

Health Maintenance: Immunizations: Oral polio vaccine, year uncertain; tetanus shots × 2, 1982, followed with booster 1 year later; flu vaccine, 2000, no reaction. *Screening tests:* Last Pap smear, 2014, normal. No mammograms to date.

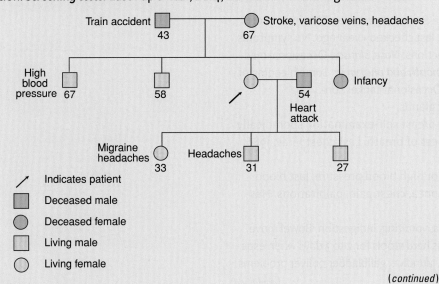

Train accident 43 — Stroke, varicose veins, headaches 67

High blood pressure 67 | 58 | / (patient) | 54 Heart attack | Infancy

Migraine headaches 33 | Headaches 31 | 27

/   Indicates patient
■   Deceased male
●   Deceased female
□   Living male
○   Living female

(*continued*)

The Case of Mrs. N. (*continued*)

Family History

The family history is depicted above.

Father died at age 43 years in a train accident. Mother died at age 67 years from stroke; had varicose veins, headaches.

One brother, age 61 years, with hypertension, otherwise well; one brother, age 58 years, well except for mild arthritis; one sister, died in infancy of unknown cause.

Husband died at age 54 of heart attack

Daughter, age 33 years, with migraine headaches, otherwise well; son, age 31 years, with headaches; son, age 27 years, well.

No family history of diabetes, tuberculosis, heart or kidney disease, cancer, anemia, epilepsy, or mental illness.

The Family History can be recorded as a diagram or a narrative. The diagram is more helpful for tracing genetic disorders. The negatives from the family history should follow either format.

Personal and Social History

Born and raised in Las Cruces, finished high school, married at age 19 years. Worked as sales clerk for 2 years, then moved with husband to Espanola, had three children. Returned to work 15 years ago to improve family finances. Children all married. Four years ago Mr. N. died suddenly of a heart attack, leaving little savings. Mrs. N. has moved to a small apartment to be near daughter, Isabel. Isabel's husband, John, has an alcohol problem. Mrs. N.'s apartment is now a haven for Isabel and her two children, Kevin, age 6 years, and Lucia, age 3 years. Mrs. N. feels responsible for helping them; she feels tense and nervous, but denies depression. She has friends, but rarely discusses family problems: "I'd rather keep them to myself. I don't like gossip." No church or other organizational support. She is typically up at 7:00 AM, works 9:00 AM to 5:30 PM, and eats dinner alone.

Exercise and diet. Gets little exercise. Diet high in carbohydrates.

Safety measures. Uses seat belt regularly. Uses sunblock. Medications kept in an unlocked medicine cabinet. Cleaning solutions in unlocked cabinet below sink. Mr. N.'s shotgun and box of shells in unlocked closet upstairs.

Review of Systems

General: Has gained 10 lbs in the past 4 years.

Skin: No rashes or other changes.

Head, Eyes, Ears, Nose, Throat (HEENT): See *Present Illness. Head:* No history of head injury. *Eyes:* Reading glasses for 5 years, last checked 1 year ago. No symptoms. *Ears:* Hearing good. No tinnitus, vertigo, infections. *Nose, sinuses:* Occasional mild cold. No hay fever, sinus trouble. *Throat (or mouth and pharynx):* Some bleeding of gums recently. Last dental visit 2 years ago. Occasional canker sore.

Neck: No lumps, goiter, pain. No swollen glands.

Breasts: No lumps, pain, discharge. Does breast self-examination sporadically.

Respiratory: No cough, wheezing, shortness of breath. Last chest x-ray, 1986, St. Mary's Hospital; unremarkable.

Cardiovascular: No known heart disease or high blood pressure; last blood pressure taken in 2007. No dyspnea, orthopnea, chest pain, palpitations. Has never had an electrocardiogram (ECG).

Gastrointestinal: Appetite good; no nausea, vomiting, indigestion. Bowel movement about once daily, though sometimes has hard stools for 2 to 3 days when especially tense; no diarrhea or bleeding. No pain, jaundice, gallbladder or liver problems.

(*continued*)

The Case of Mrs. N. (*continued*)

Urinary: No frequency, dysuria, hematuria, or recent flank pain; nocturia × 1, large volume. *Occasionally loses urine when coughing.

Genital: No vaginal or pelvic infections. No dyspareunia.

Peripheral vascular: Varicose veins appeared in both legs during first pregnancy. For 10 years, has had swollen ankles after prolonged standing; wears light elastic support hose; tried "water pill" 5 months ago, but it didn't help much; no history of phlebitis or leg pain.

Musculoskeletal: Mild low backaches, often at the end of the workday; no radiation into the legs; used to do back exercises, but not now. No other joint pain.

Psychiatric: No history of depression or treatment for psychiatric disorders. (See also *Present Illness* and *Personal and Social History.*)

Neurologic: No fainting, seizures, motor or sensory loss. Memory good.

Hematologic: Except for bleeding gums, no easy bleeding. No anemia.

Endocrine: No known thyroid disorders or heat or cold intolerance. No symptoms or history of diabetes.

PHYSICAL EXAMINATION

Mrs. N. is a short, overweight, middle-aged woman, who is animated and responds quickly to questions. She is somewhat tense, with moist, cold hands. Her hair is well groomed. Her color is good, and she lies flat without discomfort.

Vital signs: Ht (without shoes) 157 cm (5′2″). Wt (dressed) 65 kg (143 lb). BMI 26. BP 164/98 right arm, supine; 160/96 left arm, supine; 152/88 right arm, supine with wide cuff. Heart rate (HR) 88 and regular. Respiratory rate (RR) 18. Temperature (oral) 98.6 °F.

Skin: Palms cold and moist, but color good. Scattered cherry angiomas over upper trunk. Nails without clubbing, cyanosis.

Head, Eyes, Ears, Nose, Throat (HEENT):   *Head:* Hair of average texture. Scalp without lesions, normocephalic/atraumatic (NC/AT). *Eyes:* Vision 20/30 in each eye. Visual fields full by confrontation. Conjunctiva pink; sclera white. Pupils 4 mm constricting to 2 mm, round, regular, equally reactive to light. Extraocular movements intact. Disc margins sharp, without hemorrhages, exudates. No arteriolar narrowing or A-V nicking. *Ears:* Wax partially obscures right tympanic membrane (TM); left canal clear, TM with good cone of light. Acuity good to whispered voice. Weber midline. AC > BC. *Nose:* Mucosa pink, septum midline. No sinus tenderness. *Mouth:* Oral mucosa pink. Several interdental papillae red, slightly swollen. Dentition good. Tongue midline, with 3 × 4 mm shallow white ulcer on red base on undersurface near tip; tender but not indurated. Tonsils absent. Pharynx without exudates.

Neck: Neck supple. Trachea midline. Thyroid isthmus barely palpable, lobes not felt.

Lymph nodes: Small (<1 cm), soft, nontender, and mobile tonsillar and posterior cervical nodes bilaterally. No axillary or epitrochlear nodes. Several small inguinal nodes bilaterally, soft and nontender.

Thorax and lungs: Thorax symmetric with good excursion. Lungs resonant. Breath sounds vesicular with no added sounds. Diaphragms descend 4 cm bilaterally.

(continued)

The Case of Mrs. N. (continued)

Cardiovascular: Jugular venous pressure 1 cm above the sternal angle, with head of examining table raised to 30°. Carotid upstrokes brisk, without bruits. Apical impulse discrete and tapping, barely palpable in the 5th left interspace, 8 cm lateral to the midsternal line. Good S_1, S_2; no S_3 or S_4. A II/VI medium-pitched midsystolic murmur at the 2nd right interspace; does not radiate to the neck. No diastolic murmurs.

Breasts: Pendulous, symmetric. No masses; nipples without discharge.

Abdomen: Protuberant. Well-healed scar, right lower quadrant. Bowel sounds active. No tenderness or masses. Liver span 7 cm in right midclavicular line; edge smooth, palpable 1 cm below right costal margin (RCM). Spleen and kidneys not felt. No costovertebral angle tenderness (CVAT).

Genitalia: External genitalia without lesions. Mild cystocele at introitus on straining. Vaginal mucosa pink. Cervix pink, parous, and without discharge. Uterus anterior, midline, smooth, not enlarged. Adnexa not palpated due to obesity and poor relaxation. No cervical or adnexal tenderness. Pap smear taken. Rectovaginal wall intact.

Rectal: Rectal vault without masses. Stool brown, negative for fecal blood.

Extremities: Warm and without edema. Calves supple, nontender.

Peripheral vascular: Trace edema at both ankles. Moderate varicosities of saphenous veins both in lower extremities. No stasis pigmentation or ulcers. Pulses (2+ = brisk, or normal):

	Radial	Femoral	Popliteal	Dorsalis Pedis	Posterior Tibial
RT	2+	2+	2+	2+	2+
LT	2+	2+	2+	Absent	2+

Musculoskeletal: No joint deformities. Good range of motion in hands, wrists, elbows, shoulders, spine, hips, knees, ankles.

Neurologic: Mental Status: Tense, but alert and cooperative. Thought coherent. Oriented to person, place, and time. *Cranial nerves:* II to XII intact.

Motor: Good muscle bulk and tone. Strength 5/5 throughout. *Cerebellar:* RAMs, point-to-point movements intact. Gait stable, fluid. *Sensory:* Pinprick, light touch, position sense, vibration, and stereognosis intact. Romberg negative.

Reflexes:

	Biceps	Triceps	Brachio-radialis	Patellar	Achilles	Plantar
RT	2+	2+	2+	2+	1+	↓
LT	2+	2+	2+	2+/2+	1+	↓

OR

See Muscle Strength Grading, p. 743.

Two methods for recording reflexes may be used: a tabular form or a stick picture diagram; 2+ = brisk, or normal. See p. 758 for system for grading reflexes.

(continued)

The Case of Mrs. N. (*continued*)

ASSESSMENT AND PLAN

1. **Migraine headaches:** A 54-year-old woman with migraine headaches since childhood, with a throbbing vascular pattern and frequent nausea and vomiting. Headaches are associated with stress and relieved by sleep and cold compresses. There is no papilledema, and there are no motor or sensory deficits on the neurologic examination. The differential diagnosis includes tension headache, also associated with stress, but there is no relief with massage, and the pain is more throbbing than aching. There are no fever, stiff neck, or focal findings to suggest meningitis, and the lifelong recurrent pattern makes subarachnoid hemorrhage unlikely (usually described as "the worst headache of my life").

   Plan:
   - Discuss features of migraine versus tension headaches.
   - Discuss biofeedback and stress management.
   - Advise patient to avoid caffeine, including coffee, colas, and other carbonated beverages.
   - Start nonsteroidal anti-inflammatory drugs (NSAIDs) for headache, as needed.
   - If needed next visit, begin prophylactic medication if headaches are occurring more than 2 days a week or 8 days a month.

2. **Elevated blood pressure:** Systolic hypertension is present. May be related to anxiety from first visit. No evidence of end-organ damage to retina or heart.

   Plan:
   - Discuss standards for assessing blood pressure.
   - Recheck blood pressure in 1 month.
   - Check basic metabolic panel; review urinalysis.
   - Discuss weight reduction and exercise programs (see #4).
   - Reduce salt intake.

3. **Cystocele with occasional stress incontinence:** Cystocele on pelvic examination, probably related to bladder relaxation. Patient is perimenopausal. Incontinence reported with coughing, suggesting alteration in bladder neck anatomy. No dysuria, fever, flank pain. Not taking any contributing medications. Usually involves small amounts of urine, no dribbling, so doubt urge or overflow incontinence.

   Plan:
   - Explain cause of stress incontinence.
   - Review urinalysis.
   - Recommend Kegel exercises.
   - Consider topical estrogen cream to vagina during next visit if no improvement.

(*continued*)

The Case of Mrs. N. (continued)

4. **Overweight:** Patient 5'2", weighs 143 lbs. BMI is ~26.
   Plan:
   - Explore diet history, ask patient to keep food intake diary.
   - Explore motivation to lose weight, set target for weight loss by next visit.
   - Schedule visit with dietitian.
   - Discuss exercise program, specifically, walking 30 minutes most days a week.

5. **Family stress:** Son-in-law with alcohol problem; daughter and grandchildren seeking refuge in patient's apartment, leading to tensions in these relationships. Patient also has financial constraints. Stress currently situational. No current evidence of major depression.
   Plan:
   - Explore patient's views on strategies to cope with stress.
   - Explore sources of support, including Al-Anon for daughter and financial counseling for patient.
   - Continue to monitor for depression.

6. **Occasional musculoskeletal low back pain:** Usually with prolonged standing. No history of trauma or motor vehicle accident. Pain does not radiate; no tenderness or motor-sensory deficits on examination. Doubt disc or nerve root compression, trochanteric bursitis, sacroiliitis.
   Plan:
   - Review benefits of weight loss and exercises to strengthen low back muscles.

7. **Tobacco abuse:** 1 pack per day for 36 years.
   Plan:
   - Check peak flow or FEV_1/FVC on office spirometry.
   - Give strong warning to stop smoking.
   - Offer referral to tobacco cessation program.
   - Offer patch, current treatment to enhance abstinence.

8. **Varicose veins, lower extremities:** No complaints currently.

9. **History of right pyelonephritis:** 1998.

10. **Ampicillin allergy:** Developed rash, but no other allergic reaction.

11. **Health maintenance:** Last Pap smear 2014; has never had a mammogram.
    Plan:
    - Schedule mammogram.
    - Pap smear sent today.
    - Provide three cards to test for fecal blood; next visit, discuss screening colonoscopy.
    - Suggest dental care for mild gingivitis.
    - Advise patient to move medications and caustic cleaning agents to locked cabinet above shoulder height. Urge patient to move gun and cartridges to a locked gun cabinet.

See Chapter 3, Interviewing and the Health History, section on Motivational Interviewing, p. 81, and Table 3-1, Motivational Interviewing: A Clinical Example, p. 104.

The Importance of the Problem List

After you complete the clinical record, it is good clinical practice to generate a *Problem List* that summarizes the patient's problems that can be placed in the front of the office or hospital chart. *List the most active and serious problems first, and record their date of onset.* Some clinicians make separate lists for active or inactive problems; others make one list in order of priority. A good *Problem List* helps you to individualize the patient's care. On follow-up visits, the *Problem List* provides a quick summary of the patient's clinical history and a reminder to review the status of problems the patient may not mention. An accurate *Problem List* allows better population management of patients, by using EHRs to track patients with specific problems, recall patients who are behind on appointments, and follow up on specific issues. The *Problem List* also allows other members of the health care team to learn about the patient's health status at a glance.

A sample *Problem List* for Mrs. N. is provided below. You may wish to number each problem and use the number to refer to specific problems in subsequent notes.

Clinicians organize problem lists differently, even for the same patient. Problems can be symptoms, signs, past health events such as a hospital admission or surgery, or diagnoses. You might choose different entries from those above. Good lists vary in emphasis, length, and detail, depending on the clinician's philosophy, specialty, and role as a provider. Some clinicians would find this list too long. Others would be more explicit about "family stress" or "varicose veins."

Problem List: The Case of Mrs. N.

Date	Problem No.	Problem
8/25/16	1	Migraine headaches
	2	Elevated blood pressure
	3	Cystocele with occasional stress incontinence
	4	Overweight
	5	Family stress
	6	Low back pain
	7	Tobacco abuse since age 18 years
	8	Varicose veins
	9	History of right pyelonephritis: 1998
	10	Allergy to ampicillin
	11	Health maintenance

The list illustrated here includes problems that need attention now, like Mrs. N.'s headaches, as well as problems that need future observation and attention, such as her blood pressure and cystocele. Listing the allergy to ampicillin reminds you not to prescribe medications in the penicillin family. Some symptoms such as canker sores and hard stools do not appear on this list because they are minor concerns and do not require attention during this visit. Problem lists with too many relatively insignificant items are distracting. If these symptoms increase in importance, they can be added at a later visit.

Recording Your Findings

A clear, well-organized clinical record is one of the most important adjuncts to patient care. Your goal is a clear, concise, but comprehensive report that documents key findings and communicates your assessment in a succinct and *legible* format to clinicians, consultants, and other members of the health care team.

Regardless of your experience, adopting certain principles will help you organize a good record. Think especially about the *order and readability* of the record and the *amount of detail* needed. How much detail to include often varies at different points in training. As a student, you may wish (or be required) to be quite detailed. This builds your descriptive skills, vocabulary, and speed. Later, the pressures of workload and time management will lead to less but more focused detail. A good record always provides sufficient evidence from the history, physical examination, and laboratory findings to support all the problems or diagnoses identified.

Checklist to Ensure a Quality Clinical Record

Is the Order Clear?
Order is imperative. Make sure that readers can easily find specific points of information. Keep the *subjective* items of the history, for example, in the history; do not let them stray into the physical examination. Did you:

* Make the headings clear?
* Accent your organization with indentations and spacing?
* Arrange the *Present Illness* in chronologic order, starting with the current episode, then filling in relevant background information?

Do the Data Included Contribute Directly to the Assessment?
Spell out the supporting evidence, both positive and negative, for each problem or diagnosis. Make sure there is sufficient detail to support your differential diagnosis and plan.

Are Pertinent Negatives Specifically Described?
Often, portions of the history or examination suggest that an abnormality might exist or develop in that area. For example, for the patient with notable bruises, record the "pertinent negatives," such as the absence of injury or violence, familial bleeding disorders, or medications or nutritional deficits that might lead to bruising. For the patient who is depressed but not suicidal, recording both facts is important. In the patient with a transient mood swing, on the other hand, a comment on suicide is unnecessary.

Are There Overgeneralizations or Omissions of Important Data?
Remember that data not recorded are data lost. No matter how vividly you can recall clinical details today, you will probably not remember them in a few months. The phrase "neurologic exam negative," even in your own handwriting, may leave you wondering in a few months' time, "Did I really check the reflexes?"

(continued)

Checklist to Ensure a Quality Clinical Record *(continued)*

Is There Too Much Detail?

Is there excess information or redundancy? Is important information buried in a mass of detail, to be discovered by only the most persistent reader? Make your descriptions concise. "Cervix pink and smooth" indicates you saw no redness, ulcers, nodules, masses, cysts, or other suspicious lesions, but this description is shorter and more easily read. You can omit unimportant structures even though you examined them, such as normal eyebrows and eyelashes.

Omit most of your negative findings unless they relate directly to the patient's complaints or specific exclusions in your differential diagnosis. *Instead, concentrate on major negative findings* such as "no heart murmurs."

Is the Written Style Succinct? Are Phrases, Short Words, and Abbreviations Used Appropriately? Is Data Unnecessarily Repeated?

Omit repetitive introductory phrases such as "The patient reports no..." because readers assume the patient is the source of the history unless otherwise specified.

- Using words or brief phrases instead of whole sentences is common, but abbreviations and symbols should be used only if they are readily understood. Use shorter words when possible such as "felt" for "palpated" or "heard" for "auscultated." Omit unnecessary words, such as those in parentheses in the examples below. This saves valuable time and space. For example, "Cervix is pink (in color)." "Lungs are resonant (to percussion)." "Liver is tender (to palpation)." "Both (right and left) ears with cerumen." "II/IV systolic ejection murmur (audible)." "Thorax symmetric (bilaterally)."
- Describe what you observed, not what you did. "Optic discs seen" is less informative than "disc margins sharp."

Are Diagrams and Precise Measurements Included Where Appropriate?

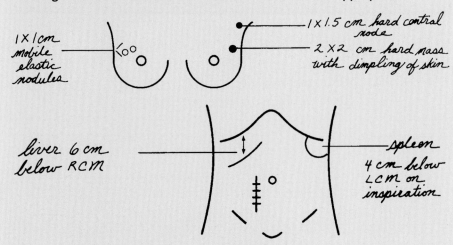

Diagrams add greatly to the clarity of the record.

(continued)

Checklist to Ensure a Quality
Clinical Record (*continued*)

To ensure accurate evaluations and future comparisons, make measurements in centimeters, not in fruits, nuts, or vegetables.

- "1 × 1 cm lymph node" versus a "pea-sized lymph node…"
- Or "2 × 2 cm mass on the left lobe of the prostate" versus a "walnut-sized prostate mass."

Is the Tone of the Write-up Neutral and Professional?
It is important to be objective. Hostile or disapproving comments have no place in the patient's record. Never use inflammatory or demeaning words or punctuation.

Comments such as "Patient DRUNK and LATE TO CLINIC AGAIN!!" are unprofessional and set a bad example for other clinicians reading the chart. They also might prove difficult to defend in a legal setting.

Table 1-1 Sample Progress Note

A month later, Mrs. N. returns for a follow-up visit. The format of the office or hospital progress note is quite variable, but it should meet the same standards as the initial assessment. The note should be clear, sufficiently detailed, and easy to follow. It should reflect your clinical reasoning and delineate your assessment and plan. Be sure to learn the documentation standards for billing in your institution, because this can affect the detail and type of information needed in your progress notes.

The note below follows the SOAP format: **S**ubjective, **O**bjective, **A**ssessment, and **P**lan. You will see many other styles, some focused on the "patient-centered" record.[49] The four categories of the SOAP note are often implied and not spelled out, as in the note below.

9/25/16

Mrs. N. returns for follow-up of her migraine headaches. She has had fewer headaches since reducing her intake of caffeine. She is now drinking decaffeinated coffee and has stopped drinking tea. She has joined a support group and started exercising to reduce stress. She is still having one to two headaches a month with some nausea, but they are less severe and generally relieved with NSAIDs. She denies any fever, stiff neck, associated visual changes, motor-sensory deficits, or paresthesias.

She has been checking her blood pressure at home. It is running about 150/90. She is walking 30 minutes three times a week in her neighborhood and has reduced her daily caloric intake. She has been unable to stop smoking. She has been doing the Kegel exercises, but still has some leakage with coughing or laughing.

Medications: Motrin 400 mg up to three times daily as needed for headache.
Allergies: Ampicillin causes rash.
Tobacco: 1 pack per day since age 18 years.

Physical Examination: Pleasant, overweight, middle-aged woman, who is animated and somewhat tense. Ht 157 cm (5' 2"). Wt 63 kg (140 lbs). BMI 26. BP 150/90. HR 86 and regular. RR 16. Afebrile.

Skin: No suspicious nevi. **HEENT:** Normocephalic, atraumatic. Pharynx without exudates. **Neck:** Supple, without thyromegaly. **Lymph nodes:** No lymphadenopathy. **Lungs:** Resonant and clear. **CV:** JVP 6 cm above the right atrium; carotid upstrokes brisk, no bruits. Good S_1, S_2. No murmurs heard today. No S_3, S_4. **Abdomen:** Active bowel sounds. Soft, nontender, no hepatosplenomegaly. **Extremities:** Without edema.

Labs: Basic metabolic panel and urinalysis from 8/25/16 unremarkable. Pap smear normal.

Impression and Plan

1. Migraine headaches—now down to one to two per month due to reductions in caffeinated beverages and stress. Headaches are responding to NSAIDs.
   - Will defer daily prophylactic medication for now because patient is having fewer than three headaches per month and feels better.
   - Affirm need to stop smoking and to continue exercise program.
   - Affirm patient's participation in support group to reduce stress.
2. Elevated blood pressure—BP remains elevated at 150/90.
   - Will initiate therapy with a diuretic.
   - Patient to take blood pressure three times a week at home and bring recordings to next office visit.
3. Cystocele with occasional stress incontinence—stress incontinence improved with Kegel exercises but still with some urine leakage. Urinalysis from last visit—no infection.
   - Initiate vaginal estrogen cream.
   - Continue Kegel exercises.
4. Overweight—has lost ~4 lbs.
   - Continue exercise.
   - Review diet history; affirm weight reduction.
5. Family stress—patient handling this better. See Plans above.
6. Occasional low back pain—no complaints today.
7. Tobacco abuse—see Plans above. Will start medication.
8. Health maintenance—Pap smear sent last visit. Mammogram scheduled. Colonoscopy recommended.

References

1. Verghese A, Horwitz RI. In praise of the physical examination. *BMJ.* 2009;339:b5448.

2. U.S. Preventive Services Task Force. Guide to Clinical Preventive Services 2014. Recommendations of the U.S. Preventive Services Task Force. June 2014. Available at http://www.ahrq.gov/professionals/clinicians-providers/guidelines-recommendations/guide/. See also U.S. Preventive Services Task Force: Recommendations for Primary Care Practice. December 2013. Available at http://www.uspreventiveservicestaskforce.org/Page/Name/recommendations Accessed February 27, 2015.

3. Sussman J, Beyth RJ. Society of General Internal Medicine, Choosing Wisely: Five Things Physicians and Patients Should Question, Don't Perform Routine General Health Checks for Asymptomatic Adults. ABIM Foundations Choosing Wisely Campaign Published online http://www.choosingwisely.org/doctor-patient-lists/society-of-general-internal-medicine/, 2013. Available at https://www.google.com/#q=Society+of+general+internal+medicine+-+choosing+wisely+Sussman+Beyth. Accessed March 18, 2015.

4. Krogsboll LT, Jorgensen KJ, Gronhoj Larsen C, et al. General health checks in adults for reducing morbidity and mortality from disease: Cochrane systematic review and meta-analysis. *BMJ.* 2012;345:e7191.

5. Chacko KM, Anderson RJ. The annual physical examination: important or time to abandon? *Am J Med.* 2007;120:581.

6. Boulware LE, Marinopoulos S, Phillips KA, et al. Systematic review: the value of the periodic health evaluation. *Ann Intern Med.* 2007;146:289.

7. Culica D, Rohrer J, Ward M, et al. Medical check-ups: who does not get them. *Am J Public Health.* 2002;92:88.

8. Laine C. The annual physical examination: needless ritual or necessary routine? *Ann Intern Med.* 2002;136:701.

9. Oboler SK, Prochazka AV, Gonzales R, et al. Public expectations and attitudes for annual physical examinations and testing. *Ann Intern Med.* 2002;136:652.

10. Hesrud DD. Clinical preventive medicine in primary care: background and practice. Rational and current preventive practice. *Mayo Clin Proc.* 2000;75:165.

11. Mookherjee S, Pheatt MA, Ranji SR, et al. Physical examination education in graduate medical education—a systematic review of the literature. *J Gen Int Med.* 2013;28:1090.

12. Reilly BM. Physical examination in the care of medical inpatients: an observational study. *Lancet.* 2003;362:1100.

13. Simel DL, Rennie D. The clinical examination. An agenda to make it more rational. *JAMA.* 1997;277:572.

14. Sackett DL. A primer on the precision and accuracy of the clinical examination. *JAMA.* 1992;267:2638.

15. Evidence-Based Working Group. Evidence-based medicine. A new approach to teaching the practice of medicine. *JAMA.* 1992;268:2420.

16. Herrie SR, Corbett EC, Fagan MJ, et al. Bayes' theorem and the physical examination: probability assessment and diagnostic decision-making. *Acad Med.* 2011;85:618.

17. McGee S. *Evidence-based Physical Diagnosis.* 3rd ed. Philadelphia, PA: Elsevier Saunders; 2012.

18. Smith MA, Burton WM, Mackay M. Development, impact, and measurement of enhanced physical diagnosis skills. *Adv Health Sci Educ Theory Pract.* 2009;14:547.

19. Centers for Disease Control and Prevention (CDC). Standard precautions. Guidelines for isolation precautions: preventing transmission of infectious agents in healthcare settings 2007. Updated October 2007. Available at http://www.cdc.gov/hicpac/2007IP/007isolationPrecautions.html. Accessed March 1, 2015.

20. Centers for Disease Control and Prevention. Guide to infection prevention in outpatient settings. Minimum expectations for safe care. May 2011. Available at http://www.cdc.gov/HAI/settings/outpatient/outpatient-care-guidelines.html. Accessed March 1, 2015.

21. Centers for Disease Control and Prevention. Hand Hygiene in Healthcare Settings. Updated January 2015. At http://www.cdc.gov/handhygiene/. Accessed March 1, 2015.

22. Centers for Disease Control and Prevention. Precautions to prevent the spread of MRSA in healthcare settings. Updated September 2014. Available at http://www.cdc.gov/mrsa/healthcare/clinicians/precautions.html. Accessed March 1, 2015.

23. Centers for Disease Control and Prevention. Bloodborne infectious diseases: HIV/AIDS, Hepatitis B, Hepatitis C. Universal precautions for the prevention for transmission of bloodborne infections, p. 66. Updated December 2011. Available at http://www.cdc.gov/niosh/topics/bbp/universal.html. Accessed March 1, 2105.

24. Bearman G, Bryant K, Leekha S, et al. Healthcare personnel attire in non-operating-room settings. *Infect Control Hosp Epidemiol.* 2014;35:107.

25. Treakle AM, Thom KA, Furuno JP, et al. Bacterial contamination of health care workers' white coats. *Am J Infect Control.* 2009;37:101.

26. Peterson MC, Holbrook JH, Von Hales DE, et al. Contributions of the history, physical examination, and laboratory investigation in making medical diagnoses. *West J Med.* 1992;156:163.

27. Hampton JR, Harrison MJ, Mitchell JR, et al. Relative contributions of history-taking, physical examination, and laboratory investigation to diagnosis and management of medical outpatients. *Br Med J.* 1975;2(5969):486.

28. Kassirer JP. Teaching clinical reasoning: case-based and coached. *Acad Med.* 2010;85:1118.

29. Kassirer J, Wong J, Kopelman R. *Learning Clinical Reasoning.* 2nd ed. Philadelphia, PA: Wolters Kluwer/Lippincott Williams & Wilkins; 2010.

30. Norman GR, Eva KW. Diagnostic error and clinical reasoning. *Med Educ.* 2010;44:94.

31. Bowen J. Educational strategies to promote clinical diagnostic reasoning. *New Engl J Med.* 2006;355:2217.

32. Coderre S, Mandin H, Harasym P, et al. Diagnostic reasoning strategies and diagnostic success. *Med Educ.* 2003;37:695.

33. Elstein A, Schwarz A. Clinical problem solving and diagnosis decision making: selective review of the cognitive literature. *Br Med J.* 2002;324(7339):729.

34. Norman G. Research in clinical reasoning: past history and current trends. *Med Educ.* 2005;39:418.

35. Schneiderman H, Peixoto AJ. *Bedside Diagnosis. An Annotated Bibliography of Literature on Physical Examination and Interviewing,* 3rd ed. Philadelphia, PA: American College of Physicians; 1997.

36. Simel DL, Rennie D. *The Rational Clinical Examination: Evidence-Based Clinical Diagnosis.* New York: McGraw Hill; 2009.

REFERENCES

37. Guyatt G, Rennie D, Meade M. *Users' Guide to the Medical Literature: A Manual for Evidence-Based Clinical Practice.* New York: McGraw-Hill Medical; 2008.

38. Fletcher RH, Fletcher SW, Fletcher G. *Clinical Epidemiology: The Essentials.* 5th ed. Philadelphia, PA: Lippincott Williams & Wilkins; 2014.

39. Sackett DL. *Evidence-based Medicine: How to Practice and Teach EBM.* 2nd ed. New York: Churchill Livingstone; 2000.

40. Montiero SM, Norman G. Diagnostic reasoning: where we've been, where we're going. *Teach Learn Med.* 2013;25(Suppl 1):S26.

41. Ely JW, Graber ML, Croskerry P. Checklists to reduce diagnostic errors. *Acad Med.* 2011;86:307.

42. Reilly JB, Odgie AR, Von Feldt JM, et al. Teaching about how doctors think: a longitudinal curriculum in cognitive bias and diagnostic error for residents. *BMJ Qual Saf.* 2013;22:1044.

43. Dubeau CE, Voytovich AE, Rippey RM. Premature conclusions in the diagnosis of iron-deficiency anemia: cause and effect. *Med Decis Making.* 1986;6:169.

44. Kuhn GJ. Diagnostic errors. *Acad Emerg Med.* 2002;9:740.

45. Graber ML, Franklin N, Gordon R. Diagnostic error in internal medicine. *Arch Intern Med.* 2005;165:1493.

46. Redelmeier DA. Improving patient care: the cognitive psychology of missed diagnoses. *Ann Intern Med.* 2005;142:115.

47. Berner ES, Graber ML. Overconfidence as a cause of diagnostic error in medicine. *Am J Med.* 2008;121:S2.

48. Newman-Toker DE, Pronovost PJ. Diagnostic errors—the next frontier for patient safety. *JAMA.* 2009;301:1060.

49. Donnelly WJ. Viewpoint: patient-centered medical care requires a patient-centered medical record. *Acad Med.* 2005;80:33.

Evaluating Clinical Evidence

The Bates' suite offers these additional resources to enhance learning and facilitate understanding of this chapter:

- Bates' *Pocket Guide to Physical Examination and History Taking,* 8th edition
- Bates' *Visual Guide to Physical Examination* (All Volumes)
- thePoint online resources, for students and instructors: http://thepoint.lww.com

Excellence in clinical care requires integrating clinical expertise, patient preferences, and the best available clinical evidence.[1]

Carefully study the clear descriptions of how the history and physical examination can be viewed as diagnostic tests; how to assess the accuracy of laboratory tests, radiographic imaging, and diagnostic procedures; and how to evaluate clinical research studies and disease prevention guidelines. Mastering these analytic skills will improve your clinical practice and ensure that your assessments and recommendations are based on the best clinical evidence (Fig. 2-1).

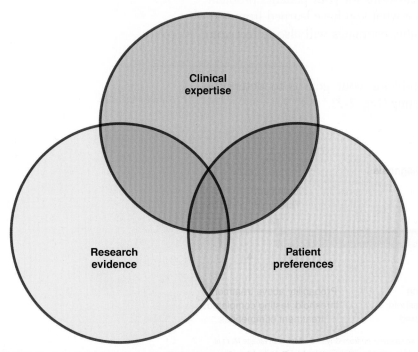

FIGURE 2-1. **Evidence-based clinical practice Venn diagram.** (Adapted with permission from Haynes RB, Sackett DL, Gray JM, et al. Transferring evidence from research into practice: 1. The role of clinical care research evidence in clinical decisions. *ACP J Club.* 1996;125:A14–A16.)

You will develop your clinical expertise as you learn about and practice your clinical discipline, enabling you to more efficiently make diagnoses and identify potential interventions. Chapter 3 addresses strategies for engaging patients in health care decisions, recognizing that patients bring individualized preferences, concerns, and expectations to the clinical encounter. Elements of the history and physical examination can be considered diagnostic tests, whose accuracy can be evaluated according to criteria presented later in this chapter. Throughout the regional examination chapters, you will find evidence-based recommendations for health promotion interventions, especially screening and prevention. These recommendations are also based on evidence from the clinical literature that can be evaluated according to criteria presented in this chapter.

The History and Physical Examination as Diagnostic Tests

The process of diagnostic reasoning begins with the history. As you learn about your patient, you will start to develop a *differential diagnosis*. This is a list of potential causes for the patient's problems and the length of the list will reflect your uncertainty about the possible explanation for a given problem. Your list will start with the most likely explanation, but will also include other plausible diagnoses, particularly those that have serious consequences if undiagnosed and untreated. You will assign probabilities to the various diagnoses that correspond to how likely you consider them to be explanations for your patient's problem. For now, these probabilities will be based on what you have learned from textbooks and lectures. In time, these probability estimates will also reflect your clinical experience.

When you begin approaching clinical problems your goal is to determine whether you need to perform additional testing (Fig. 2-2).[2]

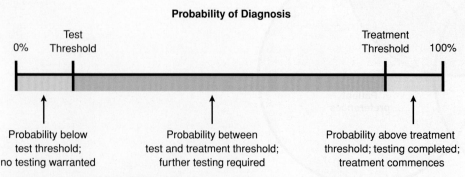

FIGURE 2-2. Probability revisions. (Adapted with permission from Guyatt G, Rennie D, Meade M, et al. *Users' Guides to the Medical Literature.* 2nd ed. New York, NY: McGraw-Hill Company; 2008; Chapter 14, Figure 14-2.)

If your probability for a disease based on your history and examination is very high (i.e., exceeds the treatment threshold), then you can move ahead and initiate treatment. Conversely, if your probability for a disease is very low (i.e., below the test threshold), then you do not need further testing. The area between the test and treatment thresholds represents *clinical uncertainty,* and you need further testing to revise probabilities and guide your clinical management. The expectation is that test results will enable you to cross a test-treatment threshold. You should understand that these test-treatment thresholds are not set in stone and will vary based on the potential adverse effects of the treatment and the seriousness of the condition. For example, you will require a much higher treatment threshold (confidence that the patient has a high probability of having the disease) for initiating cancer chemotherapy compared to prescribing an antibiotic for a urinary tract infection. You would require a much lower test threshold (confidence that the patient has a low probability of having the disease) when excluding ischemic heart disease than bacterial sinusitis. However, knowing whether a test result will achieve that effect can be challenging and requires you to understand how to evaluate the performance of a diagnostic test.

Evaluating Diagnostic Tests

You can turn to the clinical literature to determine how results from diagnostic tests—which include elements of the clinical history and physical examination, as well as laboratory tests, radiographic imaging, and procedures—can be used to revise probabilities. Two concepts in evaluating diagnostic tests will be explored: the *validity* of the findings and the *reproducibility* of the test results.

Validity

The initial step in evaluating a diagnostic test is to determine whether it provides valid results. *Does the test accurately identify whether a patient has a disease?* This involves comparing the test against a *gold standard*—the best measure of whether a patient has disease. This could be a biopsy to evaluate a lung nodule, a structured psychiatric examination to evaluate a patient for depression, or a colonoscopy to evaluate a patient with a positive stool blood test.

The *2 × 2 table* is the basic format for evaluating the performance characteristics of a diagnostic test, which means how much the test results revise probabilities for disease.

There are two columns—patients with disease present and patients with disease absent. These categorizations are based on the gold standard test. The two rows correspond to positive and negative test results. The four cells (a, b, c, d) correspond to true positives, false positives, false negatives, and true negatives, respectively.[3]

Setting up the 2 × 2 Table

	Gold Standard: Disease Present	Gold Standard: Disease Absent
Test positive	a True positive	b False positive
Test negative	c False negative	d True negative

Sensitivity and Specificity.   The first test statistics to estimate are *sensitivity* and *specificity*.

Sensitivity and Specificity

- **Sensitivity** is the probability that a person with disease has a positive test. This is represented as a/(a + c) in the disease present column of the 2 × 2 table. Sensitivity is also known as the true positive rate.
- **Specificity** is the probability that a non-diseased person has a negative test, represented as d/(b + d) in the disease absent column of the 2 × 2 table. Specificity is also known as the true negative rate.
- *Examples.* An example of these statistics would be the probability that spleno-megaly (see Chapter 11, p. 479) is associated with percussion dullness below the left costal margin (sensitivity). Conversely, the probability that a patient without splenomegaly will have percussion dullness is the false positive rate (1 – specificity) for this physical maneuver.

Knowing the sensitivity and specificity of a test does not necessarily help you make clinical decisions because they are statistics based on knowing whether the patient has disease. However, there are two exceptions. A negative result from a test with a high sensitivity (i.e., a very low false-negative rate) usually excludes disease. This is represented by the acronym SnNOUT—a Sensitive test with a Negative result rules OUT disease. Conversely, a positive result in a test with high specificity (e.g., a very low false-positive rate) usually indicates disease. This is represented by the acronym SpPIN—a Specific test with a Positive result rules IN disease.[4]

Positive and Negative Predictive Values.   The typical clinical scenario faced by clinicians involves determining whether a patient actually has disease based on a test result that is either positive or negative. The relevant test statis-tics here are the *positive* and *negative predictive values.*[3]

Positive and Negative Predictive Values

- The **positive predictive value (PPV)** is the probability that a person with a positive test has disease, represented as a/(a + b) from the test positive row in the 2 × 2 table.

    An example of this statistic is found in prostate cancer screening (see Chapter 15, p. 612), where a man with a PSA value greater than 4.0 ng/mL has only a 30% probability of having prostate cancer found on biopsy.[5]

- The **negative predictive value (NPV)** is the probability that a person with a negative test does not have disease, represented as d/(c + d) in the test negative row in the 2 × 2 table.

    Among men with a PSA level of 4.0 ng/mL or below, 85% are found to be cancer-free on biopsy.[6]

Prevalence of Disease.   Although the predictive value statistics seem intuitively useful, they will vary substantially according to the *prevalence of disease* (i.e., the proportion of patients in the disease present column). The prevalence is based on the characteristics of the patient population and the clinical setting. For example, the prevalence of many diseases will usually be higher among older patients and among patients being seen in specialist clinics or at referral hospitals.

The box below shows a 2 × 2 table where both the sensitivity and specificity of the diagnostic test are 90% and the prevalence (proportion of subjects that have the disease) is 10%. The positive predictive value calculated from the test positive row of the table would be 90/180 = 50%. This means that half of the people with a positive test have disease.

Predictive Values: Prevalence of 10% with Sensitivity and Specificity = 90%

	Disease Present	Disease Absent	Total
Test positive	a 90	b 90	180
Test negative	c 10	d 810	820
Total	100	900	1,000

Sensitivity = a/(a + c) = 90/100 or 90%; specificity = d/(b + d) = 810/900 = 90%

Positive predictive value = a/(a + b) = 90/180 = 50%

However, if the sensitivity and specificity remained the same, but prevalence was only 1%, then the cells would look very different.

Predictive Values: Prevalence of 1% with Sensitivity and Specificity = 90%

	Disease Present	Disease Absent	Total
Test positive	a 9	b 99	108
Test negative	c 1	d 891	892
Total	10	990	1,000

Sensitivity = a/(a + c) = 9/10 or 90%; specificity = d/(b + d) = 891/990 = 90%

Positive predictive value = a/(a + b) = 9/108 = 8.3%

Now the positive predictive value calculated from the test positive row of the table would be 9/108 = 8.3%. The consequence is that the great majority of positive tests are false positives—meaning that most of the subjects who undergo gold standard tests (which are usually invasive, expensive, and potentially harmful) will not have disease. This has implications for patient safety and resource allocation because clinicians want to limit the number of non-diseased patients who undergo gold standard tests. However, as shown by the example, predictive values will not necessarily provide us with sufficient guidance for using tests across populations with differing disease prevalence.

Likelihood Ratios. Fortunately, there are other ways to evaluate the performance of a diagnostic test that can account for the varying disease prevalence observed in different patient populations. One way uses *likelihood ratio* statistics, defined as the probability of obtaining a given test result in a diseased patient divided by the probability of obtaining a given test result in a non-diseased patient.[3,7] The likelihood ratio tells us how much a test result changes the pre-test disease probability (prevalence) to the post-test disease probability.

In the simplest case, we will assume that the test result is either positive or negative. Therefore, the *likelihood ratio for a positive test* is the ratio of getting a positive test result in a diseased person divided by the probability of getting a positive test result in a non-diseased person. From the 2 × 2 table, we see that this is the same as saying the ratio of the true positive rate (sensitivity) over the false positive rate (1 – specificity). A higher value (much >1) indicates that a positive test is much more likely to be coming from a diseased person than from a non-diseased person, increasing our confidence that a person with a positive result has disease.

The *likelihood ratio for a negative test* is the ratio of the probability of getting a negative test result in a diseased person divided by the probability of getting a negative test result in a non-diseased person.[7] From the 2 × 2 table, we see that this is the same as saying the ratio of the false negative rate (1 – sensitivity) divided by the true negative rate (specificity). A lower value (much <1) indicates that the negative test is much more likely to be coming from a non-diseased person than from a diseased person, increasing our confidence that a person with a negative result does not have disease.

The box below shows how to interpret likelihood ratios based on how much a test result changes the pre- to post-test probabilities for disease.[8]

Interpreting Likelihood Ratios

Likelihood Ratios[a]	Effect on Pre- to Post-Test Probability
LRs > 10 or < 0.1	Generate large changes
LRs 5–10 or 0.1–0.2	Generate moderate changes
LRs 2–5 and 0.5–0.2	Generate small (sometimes important) changes
LRs 1–2 and 0.5–1	Alter the probability to a small degree (rarely important)

[a]Likelihood ratios >1 are associated with positive results and an increased probability for disease. Likelihood ratios <1 are associated with negative results and a decreased probability of disease. A test with a likelihood ratio of 1 provides no additional information about the probability of disease.

We will show how likelihood ratios can be used to revise probabilities for disease with the example of breast cancer screening.

How Likely Is It That a Woman with Abnormal Mammogram Has Breast Cancer?

A 57-year-old woman at average risk for breast cancer has an abnormal mammogram. She wants to know the probability that she has breast cancer. The literature states that the baseline risk (prevalence) is 1%, the sensitivity of mammography is 90%, and the specificity is 91%.

Bayes Theorem. One way to use likelihood ratios to revise probabilities for disease is with the Bayes theorem.[4] This theorem requires converting the estimated prevalence (pre-test probability) to odds using the equation:

$$\text{Pre-test odds} = \text{pre-test probability}/(1 - \text{pre-test probability})$$

The pre-test odds are multiplied by the likelihood ratio to estimate the post-test odds using the following equation:

$$\text{Post-test odds} = \text{pre-test odds} \times \text{likelihood ratio}$$

The post-test odds are then converted to a probability using the equation:

$$\text{Post-test probability} = \text{post-test odds}/(1 + \text{post-test odds})$$

For the example, the 1% prevalence represents the pre-test probability; this means that the pre-test odds are 0.01/0.99 or 0.01. The likelihood ratio for a positive test is sensitivity/(1 − specificity), which is 90%/9% = 10. The pre-test odds are multiplied by this likelihood ratio (0.01 × 10) to give post-test odds of 0.10. The post-test odds are converted [0.1/(1 + 0.1)] to a post-test probability of about 9%.

Fagan Nomogram.   If you are more comfortable thinking in terms of probability of having disease, then the Fagan nomogram may be an easier way for you to use likelihood ratios (Fig. 2-3).[9] With this nomogram, you read the pre-test probabilities from the line on the left, then take a straight edge and draw a line from the pre-test probability through the likelihood ratio in the middle line, and then read the post-test probability on the line on the right.

You can also use the Fagan nomogram to answer the mammography question (Fig 2-3). The pre-test probability (prevalence) = 1% and the likelihood for a

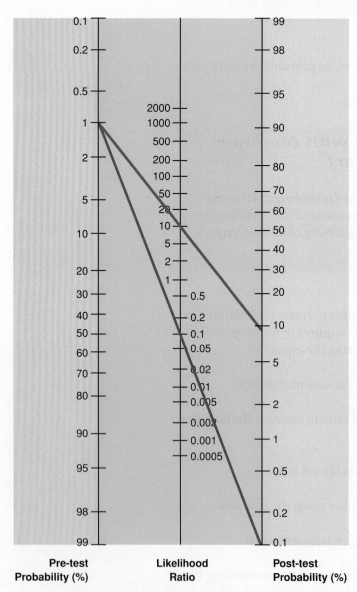

FIGURE 2-3. Fagan nomogram. (Adapted with permission from Fagan TJ. Letter: nomogram for Bayes theorem. *N Engl J Med.* 1975;293:257.)

positive test [sensitivity/(1 − specificity)] = 10. The blue line corresponds to the case of a positive test with a post-test probability of about 9%. If the mammogram result was negative (red line), then the likelihood ratio for a negative test [(1 − sensitivity)/specificity] would be 10%/91% = 0.11 and the post-test probability for breast cancer would be 0.1%.

Natural Frequencies.   Using frequency statements is another, perhaps more intuitive, alternative to likelihood ratios for determining how a test result will change the probability of disease.[9,10] *Natural frequencies* represent the joint frequency of two events, such as the number of patients with disease and the number who have a positive test result. Start by taking a large number of people (e.g., 100 or 1,000, depending upon the prevalence) and break the number down into natural frequencies (i.e., how many of the people have disease, how many with disease will test positive, how many without disease will test positive).

Natural Frequencies to Answer the Mammography Question

We can use natural frequencies to answer the mammography question by creating a 2 × 2 table based on a population of 1,000 women. The 1% prevalence means that 10 women will have breast cancer. The sensitivity of 90% means that 9 of the women with breast cancer will have an abnormal mammogram. The specificity of 91% means that 89 of the 990 women without breast cancer will still have an abnormal mammogram. The probability that a woman with an abnormal mammogram will have breast cancer is 9/(9 + 89) = about 9%.

Mammogram Result	Breast Cancer	No Breast Cancer	Total
Positive	9	89	98
Negative	1	901	902
	10	990	1,000

Data compiled from Gigerenzer G. What are natural frequencies? *BMJ*. 2011;343:d6386.

Reproducibility

Kappa Score.   Another characteristic of a diagnostic test is *reproducibility*.[3] An important aspect of evaluating diagnostic elements of the history or physical examination is determining the reproducibility of the findings for diagnosing a clinical disorder. When, for example, two clinicians examine a patient, they may not always agree upon the presence of a given finding. This raises the question of whether this finding is useful for diagnosing a clinical disorder. By chance, if many patients are being examined, there will be a certain amount of agreement between the two clinicians. Understanding whether there is agreement well beyond chance, though, is important in knowing whether the

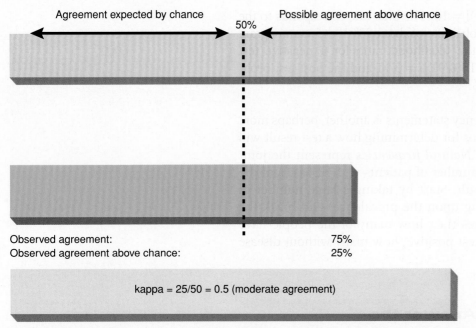

Agreement expected by chance | Possible agreement above chance

50%

Observed agreement: 75%
Observed agreement above chance: 25%

kappa = 25/50 = 0.5 (moderate agreement)

FIGURE 2-4. **Kappa scores.** (Adapted with permission from McGinn T, Wyer PC, Newman TB, et al. Tips for learners of evidence-based medicine: 3. Measures of observer variability [kappa statistic]. *CMAJ.* 2004;171:1369–1379.)

finding is useful enough to support clinical decision making. The *kappa score* measures the amount of agreement that occurs beyond chance (Fig. 2-4).[12] The box shows how to interpret Kappa values.

Interpreting Kappa Values

Value of Kappa	Strength of Agreement
<0.20	Poor
0.21–0.40	Fair
0.41–0.60	Moderate
0.61–0.80	Good
0.81–1.00	Excellent

Understanding Measure of Agreement between Different Observers. The clinicians agree 75% of the time that a patient has an abnormal physical finding. The expected agreement based on chance is 50%. This means that the potential agreement beyond chance is 50% and the actual observer agreement beyond chance is 25%. The kappa level is then 25%/50% = 0.5, which indicates moderate agreement.

Precision. In the context of reproducibility, *precision* refers to being able to apply the same test to the same unchanged person and obtain the same results.[4] Precision is often used when referring to laboratory tests. For example, when measuring a troponin level for cardiac ischemia, clinicians might use a particular cutoff level to decide whether to admit a patient to a coronary care unit. If the test results are imprecise, this could lead to admitting a patient without ischemic heart disease or sending a patient home with an ischemic event. A statistical test used to characterize precision is the *coefficient of variation*, defined as the standard deviation divided by the mean value. Lower values indicate greater precision.

Health Promotion

Throughout the book you will find health promotion sections that make recommendations for *primary prevention* (interventions designed to prevent disease) as well as *secondary prevention* (screening tests designed to find disease or disease processes at an early, asymptomatic stage). The rationale for secondary prevention is that treatment for early-stage disease is often more effective than treatment for later-stage disease. These health promotion recommendations are based on guidelines issued by professional organizations. We highlight guidelines that are evidence-based, such as those produced by the U.S. Preventive Services Task Force (USPSTF).[13] Such guidelines consider the quality of the evidence and the strength of the recommendation to either provide or withhold the intervention.[14] The strongest health promotion recommendations are based on results from randomized controlled trials (or syntheses of multiple such trials) of therapy or prevention.

The randomized controlled trial design reduces bias, thereby increasing the validity of the results. Observational studies are more likely to have biased results, and expert opinions may be offered in the absence of evidence. When searching for evidence-based information, you should select the highest level of available evidence (e.g., systematic reviews of high-quality randomized controlled studies) (Fig. 2-5).[15]

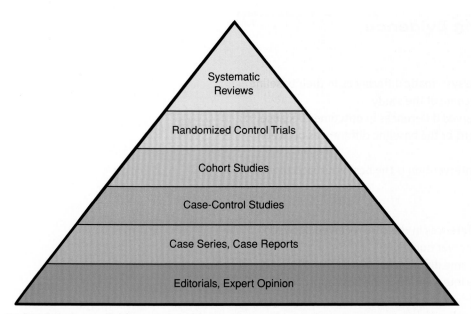

FIGURE 2-5. Evidence pyramid. (Adapted with permission from Sackett DL, Straus SE, Richardson WS, et al. *Evidence-Based Medicine: How to Practice and Teach EBM.* 2nd ed. Edinburgh: Churchill Livingstone; 2000.)

Critical Appraisal

During your health care training, it is essential that you learn the process of *critically appraising* the clinical literature in order to be able to interpret new studies and guidelines as they appear throughout your professional career.

A widely accepted process for critically appraising the clinical literature has been developed by The Evidence Based Working Group.[16] These experts in epidemiology, or the study of disease in populations, created a rigorous and standardized approach for evaluating studies. This approach has been applied to a wide range of clinical topics, including therapeutic and prevention trials, diagnostic tests, meta-analysis, cost-effectiveness analyses, and practice guidelines. This approach asks three basic questions:

1. Are the results valid (can you believe them)?

2. What are the results (magnitude and precision)?

3. How can you apply the results to patient care?

Understanding Bias

When evaluating study results, it is important to have a thorough understanding of bias, which is a systematic error in conducting a study that threatens the validity of the results. Studies with a low risk of bias provide the most valid evidence for clinical decision making and health promotion interventions. The key sources of bias in clinical research are selection bias, performance bias, detection bias, and attrition bias.[17]

Types of Biases Affecting Evidence

Selection Bias

- Occurs when comparison groups have systematic differences in their baseline characteristics that can affect the outcome of the study
- Creates problems in interpreting observed differences in outcomes because they could result from the interventions or the baseline differences between groups
- Randomly allocating subjects to the intervention is the best approach to minimizing this bias

Performance Bias

- Occurs when there are systematic differences in the care received between comparison groups (other than the intervention)
- Creates problems in interpreting outcome differences
- Blinding subjects and providers to the intervention is the best approach to minimizing this bias

(continued)

Types of Biases Affecting Evidence (*continued*)

Detection Bias

- Occurs when there are systematic differences in efforts to diagnose or ascertain an outcome
- Blinding outcomes assessors (ensuring that they are unaware of the intervention received by the subject) is the best approach to minimizing this bias

Attrition Bias

- Occurs when there are systematic differences in the comparison groups in the number of subjects who do not complete the study
- Failing to account for these differences can lead to incorrectly estimating the effectiveness of an intervention
- Using an intention-to-treat analysis, where all analyses consider all subjects who were assigned to a comparison group, regardless of whether they received or completed the intervention, can minimize this bias

Results

Assessing Performance of a Treatment or Prevention Intervention. Other issues to consider in evaluating the quality of the literature include *results* and *generalizability.* We have discussed the results found in studies of diagnostic tests. Guidelines for health promotion are usually based on clinical trials of therapy or prevention. Results from these studies are also calculated from a 2 × 2 table where the columns correspond to whether the subject developed the outcome and the rows correspond to whether the subject received (or was exposed to) the intervention. The statistics used to characterize the performance of a treatment or prevention intervention include relative risks, relative risk differences (can be a reduction or increase, reflecting benefit or harm), absolute risk differences (can be a reduction or increase, reflecting benefit or harm), numbers needed to treat, and numbers needed to harm.[18]

2 × 2 Tables for Evaluating Studies of Treatment or Prevention

	Event Occurred	No Event	Total
Experimental group	a	b	a + b
Control group	c	d	c + d

Calculating these statistics from the 2 × 2 table begins with determining probabilities for outcomes.

- The probability that an intervention subject had the outcome is described by a/(a + b) from row 1 (experimental group); this also called the *experimental event rate (EER)*.

- The probability that a control subject had the outcome is c/(c + d) from row 2 (control group), or the *control event rate (CER)*.

- The *relative risk,* the probability of an outcome in the intervention group compared to the probability of an outcome in the control group, is expressed as the EER/CER.

- The *relative risk difference* is defined as |CER − EER|/CER × 100% or 100% − the relative risk, which describes the proportion of baseline risk is reduced/increased by the therapy.

- The *absolute risk difference,* the difference in outcome rates between the comparisons groups, is expressed by the |CER − EER|.

- The reciprocal of the absolute risk difference (reported as a fraction) is the *number of subjects who need to be treated* over a specific period of time to prevent one outcome. If the intervention actually increases the risk for a bad outcome, then this statistic becomes the *number needed to harm.*

Measuring Treatment Effectiveness.   An example of these calculations is based on the hypothetical results of a study comparing the effects of a new drug, CardioProtect (CP) versus a widely used drug, CareStandard (CS) shown below. This 1-year randomized controlled trial compared patients who survived a recent myocardial infarction to see whether the new drug would reduce the outcome of a cardiovascular event, defined as fatal or non-fatal myocardial infarction or cerebrovascular event. The drugs were coated so that patients and providers could not tell them apart. Subjects receiving the CP are the experimental group, and the EER = 10 events among 100 subjects = 0.10. The control group received CS and the CER was 30 events among 100 subjects = 0.30. The relative risk of having a cardiovascular event among the CP group compared to the CS group is 0.10/0.30 = 0.33, or 33%. The relative risk reduction is 1 − 0.33 = 0.67, or 67%, meaning that the risk of a cardiovascular event among the CP group is 67% lower than in the CS group. CP led to a reduction in cardiovascular events, so we use the absolute risk reduction, which is reported as a decimal: 0.3 − 0.1 = 0.2. The reciprocal of this value (1/0.2) gives us a number needed to treat of 5—meaning that for every 5 patients who receive CP instead of CS there will be one fewer event. The number needed to treat is always based on a specific period of time, so that we should say that we need to treat 5 patients for 1 year with CP compared to CS to prevent one cardiovascular event.

Example of 2 × 2 Tables for Evaluating Studies of Treatment or Prevention

	Cardiovascular Event	No Event	Total
CardioProtect	10	90	100
CareStandard	30	70	100

Generalizability

The final point to consider when evaluating the quality of the literature is whether the results are generalizable (e.g., whether the study results can be applied to your patients). To make this determination, you need to first look at the *demographics of the study subjects* (e.g., age, gender, race/ethnicity, socioeconomic status, clinical conditions). Then, you need to determine whether the demographics are similar enough to your patient to make the results applicable. You also need to determine whether the *intervention is feasible* in your setting. *Do you have the clinical expertise, technology, and capacity to offer the intervention?* Most importantly, you need to consider the *range of potential benefits and harm* associated with the intervention and decide whether the intervention is acceptable for your patient.

Guideline Recommendations

There are many approaches for rating the strength of recommendations and we will discuss several grading systems.

United States Preventive Services Task Force (USPSTF) Approach. The USPSTF assigns 1 of 5 ratings to its recommendations (Table 2-1). It also assigns a level of certainty regarding net benefit (Table 2-2).

Grading of Recommendations, Assessment, Development, and Evaluation (GRADE). The GRADE process rates the quality of the evidence and grades the strength of recommendations in clinical guidelines.[19] Developed by an international group of guideline writers and evidence experts, the primary goals of GRADE are to (1) clearly separate the quality of the evidence and the strength of the recommendations and (2) provide clear, pragmatic interpretations of strong versus weak recommendations.

High-quality evidence that the benefit of an intervention outweighs the harm warrants a strong recommendation and suggests that further research is unlikely to change confidence in the estimated effect. Meanwhile, uncertainty about the trade-offs between benefits and harm (e.g., due to low-quality evidence or closely balanced risks and benefits) warrants a weak recommendation.

The American College of Chest Physicians (AACP) also developed a grading system used by many organizations.[20] The system classifies the quality of evidence as high (grade A), moderate (grade B), or low (grade C) based on study design, consistency of the results, and directness of the evidence. The system classifies the strength of the recommendation as strong (grade 1) or weak (grade 2) based on the estimated balance between benefits, risks, burdens, cost, and the degree of confidence in the estimates. Table 2-3 provides more detail on the criteria and definitions.

The health promotion sections will indicate the level of evidence behind the various recommendations.

Looking Ahead

This chapter introduces the concept of evidence-based clinical practice, showing how to bring clinical evidence to patient care. Physical examination maneuvers and elements of the clinical history can be seen as diagnostic tests and we have shown how to evaluate their diagnostic performance. Information on diagnostic performance will be further provided throughout the book. We also discussed the evidence behind clinical guidelines and how a good guideline should characterize that evidence and indicate the strength of recommendations to implement an intervention. We will provide this information when describing guidelines in the Health Promotion and Counseling sections of each of the regional examination chapters.

Table 2-1 U.S. Preventive Service Task Force Ratings: Grade Definitions and Implications for Practice

Grade	Definition	Suggestions for Practice
A	The USPSTF recommends the service. There is high certainty that the net benefit is substantial.	Offer or provide this service.
B	The USPSTF recommends the service. There is high certainty that the net benefit is moderate or there is moderate certainty that the net benefit is moderate to substantial.	Offer or provide this service.
C	The USPSTF recommends selectively offering or providing this service to individual patients based on professional judgment and patient preferences. There is at least moderate certainty that the net benefit is small.	Offer or provide this service for selected patients depending on individual circumstances.
D	The USPSTF recommends against the service. There is moderate or high certainty that the service has no net benefit or that the harms outweigh the benefits.	Discourage the use of this service.
I	The USPSTF concludes that the current evidence is insufficient to assess the balance of benefits and harms of the service. Evidence is lacking, of poor quality, or conflicting, and the balance of benefits and harms cannot be determined.	If the service is offered, patients should understand the uncertainty about the balance of benefits and harms.

The USPSTF defines *certainty* as the "likelihood that the USPSTF assessment of the net benefit of a preventive service is correct." The *net benefit* is defined as benefit minus harm of the preventive service as implemented in a general, primary care population.

Source: Grade Definitions. U.S. Preventive Services Task Force. October 2014. http://www.uspreventiveservicestaskforce.org/Page/Name/grade-definitions.

Table 2-2 U.S. Preventive Services Task Force Levels of Certainty Regarding Benefit

Level of Certainty	Description
High	The available evidence usually includes consistent results from well-designed, well-conducted studies in representative primary care populations. These studies assess the effects of the preventive service on health outcomes. This conclusion is therefore unlikely to be strongly affected by the results of future studies.
Moderate	The available evidence is sufficient to determine the effects of the preventive service on health outcomes, but confidence in the estimate is constrained by such factors as: ■ The number, size, or quality of individual studies. ■ Inconsistency of findings across individual studies. ■ Limited generalizability of findings to routine primary care practice. ■ Lack of coherence in the chain of evidence. As more information becomes available, the magnitude or direction of the observed effect could change, and this change may be large enough to alter the conclusion.
Low	The available evidence is insufficient to assess effects on health outcomes. Evidence is insufficient because of: ■ The limited number or size of studies. ■ Important flaws in study design or methods. ■ Inconsistency of findings across individual studies. ■ Gaps in the chain of evidence. ■ Findings not generalizable to routine primary care practice. ■ Lack of information on important health outcomes. More information may allow estimation of effects on health outcomes.

Source: Update on Methods: Estimating Certainty and Magnitude of Net Benefit. U.S. Preventive Services Task Force. February 2014. http://www.uspreventiveservicestaskforce.org/Page/Name/update-on-methods-estimating-certainty-and-magnitude-of-net-benefit.

Table 2-3 American College of Chest Physicians: Grading Recommendations

Grade of Recommendation/ Description	Benefit vs. Risk and Burdens	Methodological Quality of Supporting Evidence	Implications
1A/Strong recommendation; high-quality evidence	Benefits clearly outweigh risk and burdens, or vice versa	RCTs without important limitations or overwhelming evidence from observational studies	Strong recommendation; can apply to most patients in most circumstances without reservation
1B/Strong recommendation; moderate-quality evidence	Benefits clearly outweigh risk and burdens, or vice versa	RCTs with important limitations (inconsistent results, methodological flaws, indirect, or imprecise) or exceptionally strong evidence from observational studies	Strong recommendation; can apply to most patients in most circumstances without reservation
1C/Strong recommendation; low-quality or very low-quality evidence	Benefits clearly outweigh risk and burdens, or vice versa	Observational studies or case series	Strong recommendation but may change when higher-quality evidence becomes available
2A/Weak recommendation; high-quality evidence	Benefits closely balanced with risk and burdens	RCTs without important limitations or overwhelming evidence from observational studies	Weak recommendation; best action may differ depending on circumstances or patients' societal values
2B/Weak recommendation; moderate-quality evidence	Benefits closely balanced with risk and burdens	RCTs with important limitations (inconsistent results, methodological flaws, indirect, or imprecise) or exceptionally strong evidence from observational studies	Weak recommendation; best action may differ depending on circumstances or patients' societal values
2C/Weak recommendation; low-quality or very-low-quality evidence	Uncertainty in the estimates of benefits, risks, and burden; benefits, risks, and burdens may be closely balanced	Observational studies or case series	Very weak recommendation; other alternatives may be equally reasonable

Source: Guyatt G, Gutterman D, et al. Grading strength of recommendations and quality of evidence in clinical guidelines: report from an American college of chest physicians task force. *Chest.* 2006;129(1):174.

References

1. Haynes RB, Sackett DL, Gray JM, et al. Transferring evidence from research into practice: 1. The role of clinical care research evidence in clinical decisions. *ACP J Club.* 1996;125(3):A14.

2. Richardson WS, Wilson M, Guyatt G. The process of diagnosis. In: Guyatt G, Rennie D, eds. *Users' Guides to the Medical Literature.* 2nd ed. Chicago, IL: American Medical Association; 2008.

3. Jaeschke R, Guyatt G, Lijmer J. Diagnostic tests. In: Guyatt G, Rennie D, eds. *Users' Guides to the Medical Literature.* 2nd ed. Chicago, IL: American Medical Association; 2008.

4. Sackett DL, Haynes RB, Guyatt GH, et al. *Clinical Epidemiology. A Basic Science for Clinical Medicine.* 2nd ed. Boston, MA: Little, Brown and Company; 1991.

5. Wolf AM, Wender RC, Etzioni RB, et al; American Cancer Society Prostate Cancer Advisory Committee. American Cancer Society guideline for the early detection of prostate cancer: update 2010. *CA Cancer J Clin.* 2010;60(2):70.

6. Thompson IM, Pauler DK, Goodman PJ, et al. Prevalence of prostate cancer among men with a prostate-specific antigen level < or = 4.0 ng per milliliter. *N Engl J Med.* 2004;350(22):2239.

7. Richardson WS, Wilson MC, Keitz SA, et al. Tips for teachers of evidence-based medicine: making sense of diagnostic test results using likelihood ratios. *J Gen Intern Med.* 2008;23(1):87.

8. Jaeschke R, Guyatt GH, Sackett DL. Users' Guides to the Medical Literature. III. How to use an article about a diagnostic test. B. What are the results and will they help me in caring for my patients? The Evidence-Based Medicine Working Group. *JAMA.* 1994;271(9):703.

9. Fagan TJ. Nomogram for Bayes theorem. *N Engl J Med.* 1975; 293:257.

10. Gigerenzer G. What are natural frequencies? *BMJ.* 2011;343:d6386.

11. Gigerenzer G, Gaissmaier W, Kurz-Milcke E, et al. Helping doctors and patients make sense of health statistics. *Psychol Sci Public Interest.* 2008;8(2):53.

12. McGinn T, Guyatt G, Cook R, et al. Diagnosis. Measuring agreement beyond chance. In: Guyatt G, Rennie D, eds. *AMA's Users' Guides to the Medical Literature: A Manual for Evidence-Based Clinical Practice.* 2nd ed. Chicago, IL: American Medical Association; 2008.

13. *Home.* U.S. Preventive Services Task Force. January 2016. http://www.uspreventiveservicestaskforce.org/Page/Name/home.

14. *Grade Definitions.* U.S. Preventive Services Task Force. October 2014. http://www.uspreventiveservicestaskforce.org/Page/Name/grade-definitions.

15. Guyatt GH, Sackett DL, Sinclair JC, et al. Users' Guides to the Medical Literature. IX. A method for grading health care recommendations. Evidence-Based Medicine Working Group. *JAMA.* 1995;274(22):1800.

16. Guyatt G, Rennie D, Meade M, et al. *Users' Guides to the Medical Literature.* 2nd ed. New York, NY: McGraw-Hill Company; 2008.

17. Jüni P, Altman DG, Egger M. Systematic reviews in health care: Assessing the quality of controlled clinical trials. *BMJ* 2001;323:42.

18. Jaeschke R, Guyatt G, Barratt A, et al. *Therapy and Understanding the Results. Users' Guides to the Medical Literature.* 2nd ed. Chicago, IL: American Medical Association; 2008.

19. Guyatt G, Oxman AD, Akl EA, et al. GRADE guidelines: 1. Introduction-GRADE evidence profiles and summary of findings tables. *J Clin Epidemiol.* 2011;64(4):383.

20. Guyatt G, Gutterman D, Baumann MH, et al. Grading strength of recommendations and quality of evidence in clinical guidelines: report from an American college of chest physicians task force. *Chest.* 2006;129(1):174.

Interviewing and the Health History

The Bates' suite offers these additional resources to enhance learning and facilitate understanding of this chapter:

- Bates' *Pocket Guide to Physical Examination and History Taking*, 8th edition
- Bates' *Visual Guide to Physical Examination* (All Volumes)
- thePoint online resources, for students and instructors: http://thepoint.lww.com

The health history interview is a conversation with a purpose. As you learn to elicit the patient's story, you will draw on many of the interpersonal skills that you use every day, but with unique and important differences. In social conversation, you freely express your own views and are responsible only for yourself. In contrast, the primary goals of the patient interview are to *listen* and to improve the well-being of the patient through a trusting and supportive relationship (Fig. 3-1).

Relating effectively with patients is among the most valued skills of clinical care. For the patient, "a feeling of connectedness...of being deeply heard and understood...is the very heart of healing."[1] For the clinician, this deeper relationship enriches the rewards of patient care.[2–4] High-quality patient–clinician communication has also been shown to improve patient outcomes, decrease symptoms, improve functional status, reduce litigation, and decrease errors.[5–7] The interview is also the most commonly performed clinical intervention, occurring thousands of times in a clinician's career. These are all salient and compelling reasons to develop expertise in this skill (Fig. 3-2).

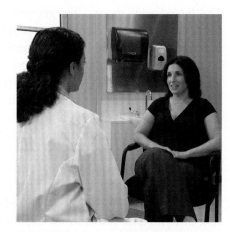

FIGURE 3-1. History-taking involves empathic listening.

This chapter introduces you to the essentials of interviewing and establishing trust, the foundations of your therapeutic alliance with patients. At first, you will focus on gathering information, but with experience and empathic listening, you will allow the patient's story to unfold in its most authentic and detailed form.

Interviewing is both a skill and an art. Skilled interviewing is both *patient-centered* and *clinician-centered*. The clinician must focus on the patient to elicit the full story of the patient's symptoms, but the clinician must also interpret key information to reach an assessment and plan. Patient-centered interviews "recognize the importance of patients' expressions of personal concerns, feelings, and emotions" and evoke "the personal context of the patient's symptoms and disease."[8] Experts have defined patient-centered interviewing as "following the patient's lead to understand their thoughts, ideas, concerns and requests, without adding

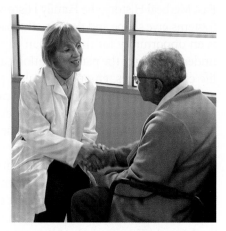

FIGURE 3-2. Establish connections with patients.

additional information from the clinician's perspective." In contrast, in the more symptom-focused, clinician-centered approach, the clinician "takes charge of the interaction to meet her or his own need to acquire the symptoms, their details, and other data that will help her or him identify a disease," which can bypass the personal dimensions of the illness.[8,9] Evidence suggests that the patient is best served by integrating these interviewing styles, leading to a more complete picture of the patient's illness and allowing clinicians to more fully convey the caring attributes of "respect, empathy, humility and sensitivity."[8,10] Current evidence shows that this approach is not only more satisfying for the patient and the clinician, but also more effective in achieving desired health outcomes (Fig. 3-3).[11,12]

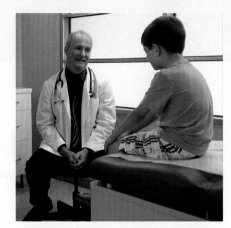

FIGURE 3-3. **Interviewing is symptom- and patient-focused.**

The *interviewing process* is quite different from the *format of the health history,* presented in Chapter 1. The *interview* is more than just a series of questions; it requires a highly refined sensitivity to the patient's feelings and behavioral cues. The *health history format* provides an important framework for organizing the patient's story into various categories pertinent to the patient's present, past, and family health. The interview and the health history format have distinct but complementary purposes. Keep these differences in mind as you learn the techniques of skilled interviewing.

The *interviewing process* that generates the patient's story is fluid and draws on numerous relational skills to respond effectively to patient cues, feelings, and concerns. The adaptability of the interviewer has been compared to the improvisation of jazz musicians who listen attentively to notes and themes and play to each other's cues. This "in-the-moment" flexibility lets the interviewer adapt to the patient's leads as the story unfolds.[13] The interview should be "open-ended," drawing on a range of techniques to cue patients to tell their stories—active listening, guided questioning, nonverbal affirmation, empathic responses, validation, reassurance, and partnering. These techniques are especially valuable when eliciting the patient's chief concerns and the History of the Present Illness.

The *health history format* is a structured framework for organizing patient information in written or verbal form. This format focuses your attention on the specific kinds of information you need to obtain, facilitates clinical reasoning, and standardizes communication to other health care providers involved in the patient's care. The Past Medical History, the Family History, Personal and Social History, and Review of Systems give shape and depth to the patient's story. The Personal and Social History is an opportunity for the clinician to see the patient as a person and gain deeper understanding of the patient's outlook and background. Learning about the patient's life circumstances, emotional health, perception of health care, health behaviors, and access to and utilization of health care strengthens your therapeutic alliance and improves health outcomes.[14] Make every effort to limit the "clinician-centered," closed-ended "yes-no" questions to the Review of Systems.

Above all, skilled interviewing requires your lifelong commitment to masterful *listening,* easily sacrificed to the time pressures of daily health care. In the words of Sir William Osler, one of our greatest clinicians and co-founder of Johns Hopkins School of Medicine in 1893: "Listen to your patient. He is telling you the diagnosis" and "The good physician treats the disease; the great physician treats the patient who has the disease."

Different Kinds of Health Histories

As you learned in Chapter 1, the scope and detail of the history depends on the patient's needs and concerns, your goals for the encounter, and the clinical setting (inpatient or outpatient, the amount of time available, primary care or subspecialty).

See Chapter 1, Overview: Physical Examination and History Taking, pp. 3–43.

- For new patients, in most settings, you will do a *comprehensive health history*.

- For patients seeking care for specific concerns, for example, cough or painful urination, a more limited interview tailored to that specific problem may be indicated; this is sometimes known as a *focused* or *problem-oriented history*.

- For patients seeking care for ongoing or chronic problems, focusing on the patient's self-management, response to treatment, functional capacity, and quality of life is most appropriate.[15]

- Patients frequently schedule health maintenance visits with the more focused goals of keeping up screening examinations or discussing concerns about smoking, weight loss, or sexual behavior.

- A specialist may need a more comprehensive history to evaluate a problem with numerous possible causes.

By knowing the content and relevance of the different components of the comprehensive health history, you are able to select the elements most pertinent to the visit and shared goals for the patient's health. This chapter sets guideposts for interviewing and the health history, outlined below.

Chapter Overview

The Fundamentals of Skilled Interviewing
- The Techniques of Skilled Interviewing: Active listening. Empathic responses. Guided questioning. Nonverbal communication. Validation. Reassurance. Partnering. Summarization. Transitions. Empowering the patient.

The Sequence and Context of the Interview
- Preparation: Reviewing the clinical record. Setting goals for the interview. Reviewing your clinical behavior and appearance. Adjusting the environment.
- The Sequence of the Interview: Greeting the patient and establishing rapport. Taking notes. Establishing the agenda for the interview. Inviting the patient's story. Identifying and responding to emotional cues. Expanding and clarifying the patient's story. Generating and testing diagnostic hypotheses. Sharing the treatment plan. Closing the interview and the visit. Taking time for self-reflection.
- The Cultural Context of the Interview: Demonstrating cultural humility—a changing paradigm.

(continued)

Chapter Overview (continued)

Advanced Interviewing

- Challenging Patients: The silent patient. The confusing patient. The patient with impaired capacity. The talkative patient. The angry or disruptive patient. The patient with a language barrier. The patient with low literacy or low health literacy. The hearing impaired patient. The blind patient. The patient with limited intelligence. The patient seeking personal advice. The seductive patient.
- Sensitive Topics: The sexual history. The mental health history. Alcohol and prescribed and illicit drug use. Intimate partner and family violence. Death and dying.

Ethics and Professionalism

The Fundamentals of Skilled Interviewing

You may have many reasons for choosing to enter the health care professions, but building effective and healing relationships is undoubtedly paramount. "Those who suffer empower healers to witness, explain, and relieve their suffering."[2] This section describes the fundamental techniques of therapeutic interviewing, the timeless skills you will continually polish as you care for patients. These skills require practice and feedback from your teachers so that you can monitor your progress. Over time, you will learn to select the techniques best suited to the ever-changing dynamics of human behavior in your patient relationships. Key among these techniques are active listening and empathy, the golden links to a therapeutic alliance.

Skilled Interviewing Techniques

- Active listening
- Empathic responses
- Guided questioning
- Nonverbal communication
- Validation
- Reassurance
- Partnering
- Summarization
- Transitions
- Empowering the patient

Active Listening. *Active listening* lies at the heart of the patient interview. Active listening means closely attending to what the patient is communicating, connecting to the patient's emotional state, and using verbal and nonverbal skills to encourage the patient to expand on his or her feelings and concerns. Active listening allows you to relate to those concerns at multiple levels of the patient's experience.[16] This takes practice. It is easy to drift into thinking about your next question or possible diagnoses and lose your concentration on the patient's story. Focus on what the patient is telling you, both verbally and nonverbally. Sometimes your body language tells a different story from your words.

Empathic Responses.   Empathic responses are vital to patient rapport and healing.[17,18] Empathy has been described as the capacity to identify with the patient and feel the patient's pain as your own, then respond in a supportive manner.[19] Empathy "requires a willingness to suffer some of the patient's pain in the sharing of suffering that is vital to healing."[20] As patients talk with you, they may convey, in their words or facial expressions, feelings they have not consciously acknowledged. These feelings are crucial to understanding their illnesses. To express empathy, you must first recognize the patient's feelings, then actively move toward and elicit emotional content.[21,22] At first, exploring these feelings may make you feel uncomfortable, but your empathic responses will deepen mutual trust.

When you sense unexpressed feelings from the patient's face, voice, behavior or words, gently ask: "How do you feel about that?" or "That seems to trouble you, can you say more?" Sometimes a patient's response may not correspond to your initial assumptions. Responding to a patient that the death of a parent must be upsetting, when in fact the death relieved the patient of a heavy emotional burden, reflects your interpretation, not what the patient feels. Instead, you can ask: "You have lost your father. What has that been like for you?" It is better to ask the patient to expand or clarify a point than assume you understand. Empathy may also be nonverbal—placing your hand on the patient's arm or offering tissues when the patient is crying. Unless you affirm your concern, important dimensions of the patient's experience may go untapped.

Once the patient has shared these feelings, reply with understanding and acceptance. Your responses may be as simple as: "I cannot imagine how hard this must be for you" or "That sounds upsetting" or "You must be feeling sad." For a response to be empathic, it must convey that you feel what the patient is feeling.

Guided Questioning: Options for Expanding and Clarifying the Patient's Story.
There are several ways to elicit more information without changing the flow of the patient's story. Your goal is to facilitate full communication, in the patient's own words, without interruption. Guided questions show your sustained interest in the patient's feelings and deepest disclosures (Fig. 3-4). They help you avoid questions that prestructure or even shut down the patient's responses. A series of "yes-no" questions makes the patient feel more restricted and passive, leading to significant loss of detail. Instead, use guided questioning to absorb the patient's full story.

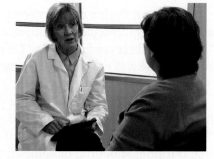

FIGURE 3-4.   **Employ guided questioning.**

For further practice see Smith, *Patient-Centered Interviewing.*[8]

Techniques of Guided Questioning

- Moving from open-ended to focused questions
- Using questioning that elicits a graded response
- Asking a series of questions, one at a time
- Offering multiple choices for answers
- Clarifying what the patient means
- Encouraging with continuers
- Using echoing

Moving from Open-Ended to Focused Questions. Your questions should flow from general to specific. Think about a cone, open at the top, then tapering to a focal point. Start with the most general questions like, "How can I help?" or "What brings you in today?" Then move to still open, but more focused, questions like, "Can you tell me more about what happened when you took the medicine?" Then pose closed questions like, "Did the new medicine cause any problems?"

Begin with a truly open-ended question that does not prefigure an answer. A possible sequence might be:

> "Tell me about your chest discomfort." (Pause)
> "What else?" (Pause)
> "Where did you feel it?" (Pause) "Show me."
> "Anywhere else?" (Pause) "Did it travel anywhere?" (Pause) "To which arm?"

Avoid *leading questions* that already contain an answer or suggested response like: "Has your pain been improving?" or "You don't have any blood in your stools, do you?" If you ask "Is your pain like a pressure?" and the patient answers yes, the patient's response is truncated instead of what he or she experienced. Adopt the more neutral "Please describe your pain."

Questioning That Elicits a Graded Response. Ask questions that require *a graded response* rather than a yes-no answer. "How many steps can you climb before you get short of breath?" is better than "Do you get short of breath climbing stairs?"

Asking a Series of Questions, One at a Time. Be sure to *ask one question at a time.* "Any tuberculosis, pleurisy, asthma, bronchitis, pneumonia?" may prompt "No" out of sheer confusion. Try "Do you have any of the following problems?" Be sure to pause and establish eye contact as you list each problem.

Offering Multiple Choices for Answers. Sometimes, patients need help describing their symptoms. To minimize bias, *offer multiple-choice answers:* "Which of the following words best describes your pain: aching, sharp, pressing, burning, shooting, or something else?" Almost any specific question can contrast two possible answers. "Do you bring up any phlegm with your cough, or is it dry?"

Clarifying What the Patient Means. Sometimes the patient's history is difficult to understand. It is better to acknowledge confusion than to act like the story makes sense. To understand what the patient means, you need to *request clarification,* as in "Tell me exactly what you mean by 'the flu'" or "You said you were behaving just like your mother. What did you mean?" Taking time for clarification reassures the patient that you want to understand his or her story and builds your therapeutic relationship.

Encouraging with Continuers. Without even speaking, you can use posture, gestures, or words to encourage the patient to say more. Pausing and nodding your head, or remaining silent, yet attentive and relaxed, is a *cue for the patient to continue*. Leaning forward, making eye contact, and using phrases like "Mm-hmm," or "Go on," or "I'm listening" all enhance the flow of the patient's story.

Echoing. Simply repeating the patient's last words, or *echoing,* encourages the patient to elaborate on details and feelings. Echoing also demonstrates careful listening and a subtle connection with the patient by using the same words. For example:

> Patient: "The pain got worse and began to spread." (Pause)
> Response: "Spread?" (Pause)
> Patient: "Yes, it went to my shoulder and down my left arm to the fingers. It was so bad that I thought I was going to die." (Pause)
> Response: "Going to die?"
> Patient: "Yes, it was just like the pain my father had when he had his heart attack, and I was afraid the same thing was happening to me."

This reflective technique helped to reveal not only the location and severity of the pain but also its meaning to the patient. It did not bias the story or interrupt the patient's train of thought.

Nonverbal Communication. Both clinicians and patients continuously display nonverbal communication that provides important clues to our underlying feelings. Being sensitive to nonverbal cues allows you to "read the patient" more effectively and send messages of your own. Pay close attention to eye contact, facial expression, posture, head position and movement such as shaking or nodding, interpersonal distance, and placement of the arms or legs—crossed, neutral, or open. Be aware that some forms of nonverbal communication are universal, but many are culturally bound.

Just as mirroring your posture shows the patient's sense of connection, matching your position to the patient's can transmit increased rapport. You can also mirror the patient's *paralanguage,* or qualities of speech, such as pacing, tone, and volume. Moving closer or making physical contact like placing your hand on the patient's shoulder conveys empathy and can help the patient gain control of upsetting feelings. The first step to using this important technique is to notice nonverbal behaviors and bring them to conscious level.

Validation. Another way to affirm the patient is to validate the legitimacy of his or her emotional experience. A patient caught in a car accident, even if uninjured, may still feel very distressed. Saying something like, "Your accident must have been very scary. Car accidents are always unsettling because they remind us how vulnerable we are. Perhaps that explains why you still feel upset," validates the patient's response as legitimate and understandable.

Reassurance. When patients are anxious or upset, it is tempting to provide reassurance like "Don't worry. Everything is going to be all right." Although this is common in social interactions, for clinicians, such comments may be premature and counterproductive. Depending on the actual situation, they may even be misleading and block further disclosure. The patient may sense that you are uncomfortable handling anxiety or fail to appreciate the depth of the distress.

The first step to effective reassurance is simply identifying and acknowledging the patient's feelings. For example, you might simply say, "You seem upset today." This promotes a feeling of connection. Meaningful reassurance comes later, after you have completed the interview, the physical examination, and perhaps some laboratory tests. At that point, you can explain what you think is happening and deal openly with any concerns. Reassurance is more appropriate when the patient feels that problems have been fully understood and are being addressed.

Partnering.   When building rapport with patients, express your commitment to an ongoing relationship. Make patients feel that no matter what happens, you will continue to provide their care. Even as a student, especially in a hospital setting, this support can make a big difference.

Summarization.   Giving a capsule summary of the patient's story during the course of the interview serves several purposes. It communicates that you have been listening carefully. It identifies what you know and what you don't know. "Now, let me make sure that I have the full story. You said you've had a cough for 3 days, that it's especially bad at night, and that you have started to bring up yellow phlegm. You have not had a fever or felt short of breath, but you do feel congested, with difficulty breathing through your nose." Following with an attentive pause, or asking "Anything else?" lets the patient add other information and corrects any misunderstandings.

You can use summarization at different points in the interview to structure the visit, especially at times of transition (see below). This technique also allows you to organize your clinical reasoning and convey your thinking to the patient, making the relationship more collaborative. It also helps learners when they draw a blank on what to ask next.

Transitions.   Patients may be apprehensive during a health care visit. To put them more at ease, tell them when you are changing directions during the interview. Just like signs along the highway, "signposting" transitions help prepare patients for what comes next. As you move through the history and on to the physical examination, orient the patient with brief transitional phrases like "Now I'd like to ask some questions about your past health." Make clear what the patient should expect or do next. "Before we move on to reviewing all your medications, was there anything else about past health problems?" "Now I would like to examine you. I will step out for a few minutes. Please undress and put on this gown."

Empowering the Patient.   The clinician–patient relationship is inherently unequal. Your feelings of inexperience as a student predictably change over time as you grow in clinical experience. Patients, however, have many reasons to feel vulnerable. They may be in pain or worried about a symptom. They may feel overwhelmed by even scheduling a visit, a task you might take for granted.

Differences of gender, ethnicity, race, or socioeconomic status contribute to the power asymmetry of the relationship. Ultimately, however, patients are responsible for their own care.[23] When you empower patients to ask questions, express their concerns, and probe your recommendations, they are most likely to adopt your advice, make lifestyle changes, or take medications as prescribed (Fig. 3-5).[21]

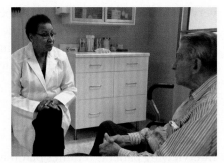

FIGURE 3-5. **Share power with patients.**

Listed below are techniques for sharing power with your patients. Although many have already been discussed, reinforcing patients' responsibility for their health is fundamental and worth summarizing here.

Empowering the Patient: Techniques for Sharing Power

- Evoke the patient's perspective.
- Convey interest in the person, not just the problem.
- Follow the patient's leads.
- Elicit and validate emotional content.
- Share information with the patient, especially at transition points during the visit.
- Make your clinical reasoning transparent to the patient.
- Reveal the limits of your knowledge.

The Sequence and Context of the Interview

Preparation, Sequence, and Cultural Context

Preparation: Reviewing the clinical record. Setting goals for the interview. Reviewing your clinical behavior and appearance. Adjusting the environment.

The Sequence of the Interview: Greeting the patient and establishing rapport. Establishing the agenda for the interview. Inviting the patient's story. Exploring the patient's perspective. Identifying and responding to emotional cues. Expanding and clarifying the patient's story. Generating and testing diagnostic hypotheses. Sharing the treatment plan. Closing the interview and the visit. Taking time for self-reflection.

The Cultural Context of the Interview: Demonstrating cultural humility—a changing paradigm.

Now that you have learned the fundamentals of skilled interviewing, you are ready to start the interview. First, prepare for the interview by reviewing the record and setting goals for the interview ahead. Check your appearance. Make sure the patient is comfortable and the environment is conducive to the very personal information soon to be shared. You will find that each interview has its own rhythm and sequence. Master the steps described. Finally, the interview has important societal dimensions. Reflect on any biases you have that color your reactions to the patient and the therapeutic alliance you need to create.

Preparation

Interviewing patients requires planning. As you begin, consider several steps that are crucial to success.

Reviewing the Clinical Record.   Before seeing the patient, review the clinical record (Fig. 3-6). This provides important background information and suggests areas you need to explore. Review identifying data such as age, gender, address, and insurance. Look at the problem list and the patient's medications and allergies. Even though the clinical record usually contains past diagnoses and treatments, you need to make your own assessment based on what you learn from the visit ahead. The clinical record is compiled from many observers. Data may be incomplete or even disagree with what the patient tells you. Correcting discrepancies in the record is important for the patient's care.

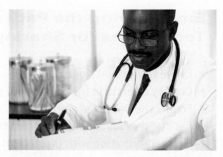

FIGURE 3-6. **Review records and set goals.**

Setting Goals for the Interview.   Before you talk with the patient, clarify your goals for the interview. As a student, your primary purpose may be to complete a comprehensive history required for your rotation. As a practicing clinician, your goals can range from assessing a new concern, to treatment follow-up, to completing forms. *The clinician must balance these provider-centered goals with patient-centered goals,* weighing multiple agendas arising from the needs of the patient, the patient's family, and health care agencies and facilities. Taking a few minutes to think about your goals makes it easier to align your priorities with the patient's agenda.[24]

Reviewing Your Clinical Behavior and Appearance.   Just as you carefully observe the patient, the patient will be watching you. Consciously or not, you send messages through both your words and your behavior. Posture, gestures, eye contact, and tone of voice all convey the extent of your interest, attention, acceptance, and understanding. The skilled interviewer seems calm and unhurried, even when time is limited. Patients sense when you are preoccupied. It is important to learn to focus and give the patient your full attention. Patients are also sensitive to any implied disapproval, embarrassment, impatience, or boredom and to behaviors that condescend, stereotype, criticize, or belittle. Professionalism requires equanimity and "unconditional positive regard" to nurture healing relationships.[25] Your appearance is also important. Patients find cleanliness, neatness, conservative dress, and a name tag reassuring. Remember to keep *the patient's perspective* in mind if you want to build the patient's trust.

Adjusting the Environment.   Make the interview setting as private and comfortable as possible. You may have to talk with the patient in surroundings like a two-bed room or the corridor of a busy emergency department. Making the environment as confidential as possible improves communication. If there are privacy curtains, try to pull them shut. Suggest moving to an empty room instead of talking in a waiting area. Adjust the room temperature for the patient's comfort. *As the clinician, it is part of your role to make the patient more comfortable.* These efforts are always worth the time.

The Sequence of the Interview

In general, an interview moves through several stages. Throughout this sequence, as the clinician you must remain attuned to the patient's feelings, help the patient express them, respond to their content, and validate their significance. As a student, you will concentrate primarily on eliciting the patient's story and creating a shared understanding of the patient's concerns. Later on, as a practicing clinician, reaching agreement on a plan for further evaluation and treatment becomes more important. Whether the interview is comprehensive or focused, pay close attention to the patient's feelings and affect, always working on strengthening the relationship as you move through the typical sequence that follows. Including the patient's feelings, ideas, and expectations leads to therapeutic interventions best suited to the patient's needs, coping skills, and life circumstances.

Greeting the Patient and Establishing Rapport. The initial moments of your encounter lay the foundation for your ongoing relationship. How you greet the patient and other visitors in the room, provide for the patient's comfort, and arrange the physical setting all shape the patient's first impressions.

As you begin, *greet the patient by name and introduce yourself,* giving your own name. If possible, shake hands with the patient. If this is the first contact, explain your role, your status as a student, and how you will be involved in the patient's care. Introduce yourself during future meetings until you are sure the patient knows who you are: "Good morning, Mr. Peters. I am Susannah Velasquez, a third-year clinical student. You may remember me. I was here yesterday talking with you about your heart problems. I am part of the clinical team taking care of you."

In general, use a formal title to address the patient, Mr. O'Neil or Ms. Washington for example.[25] Except with children or adolescents, avoid first names until you have specific permission. Calling a patient "dear" or overly familiar names can depersonalize and demean. If you are unsure how to pronounce the patient's name, don't be afraid to ask. You can say, "I am afraid of mispronouncing your name. Could you say it for me?" Then repeat it to make sure that you heard it correctly.

When visitors are in the room, acknowledge and greet each one in turn, inquiring about each person's name and relationship to the patient. Whenever visitors are present, *you are obligated to maintain the patient's confidentiality.* Let the patient decide if visitors or family members should stay in the room, and ask for the patient's permission before conducting the interview in front of them. For example, "I am comfortable with having your sister stay for the interview, Mrs. Jones, but I want to make sure that this is what you want" or "Is it better if I speak to you alone or with your sister present?" For sensitive questions, you may need to arrange another time to be with the patient alone.

See Chapter 18, Assessing Children, Infancy Through Adolescence, for discussion of visitors present during pediatric visits, pp. 765–891.

Always be attuned to the patient's comfort. In the office or clinic, help the patient find a place for coats and belongings. In the hospital, after greeting the patient, ask how the patient is feeling and if you are coming at a convenient time. Arranging the bed to make the patient more comfortable or waiting a few minutes while the patient says goodbye to visitors or finishes in the bathroom shows that you are attentive to the patient's needs. In any setting, look for signs of discomfort, such as shifting position or facial expressions of pain or anxiety. Attend to these signs first to promote trust and provide enough comfort for the interview to proceed.

Consider the best way to *arrange the room* and how close you should be to the patient. Remember that cultural background and individual taste influence preferences about interpersonal space. Choose a distance that facilitates conversation and allows good eye contact (Fig. 3-7). You should probably be within several feet, close enough to hear and be heard clearly. Pull up a chair and, if possible, sit at eye level with the patient. Move physical barriers like bed railings or bedside tables out of the way. In an outpatient setting, sitting on a rolling stool, for example, allows you to change distances in response to patient cues. Avoid arrangements that convey disrespect, like interviewing a woman already positioned for a pelvic examination or talking through a bathroom door. Lighting also makes a difference. If you sit between a patient and a bright light or window the patient may have to squint to see you, lending the interaction an air of interrogation.

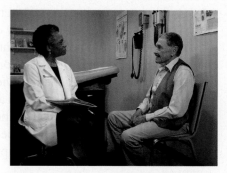

FIGURE 3-7. Choose a distance that facilitates conversation and eye contact.

As you begin the interview, give the patient your undivided attention. Spend enough time on small talk to put the patient at ease, and avoid looking down to take notes, read the chart, or scan a computer screen. Show interest in the patient as a unique individual. You can begin by asking, "So that I can get to know you, tell me about yourself."[26]

Taking Notes. As a novice, you may need to write down much of what you learn during the interview. Experienced clinicians usually recall much of the interview without any notes, but few remember all the details of a comprehensive history. Jot down short phrases, specific dates, or words; but do not let note taking or the laptop screen distract you from the patient. Maintain good eye contact. If the patient is talking about sensitive or disturbing material, put down your pen or move away from the keyboard. For patients who find note taking uncomfortable, explore their concerns and explain your need to make an accurate record. When using an electronic health record, face the patient directly as you elicit the patient's story, maintaining good eye contact and observing nonverbal behaviors; turn to the screen only after engaging the patient in the goals for the visit. Look up at the patient as often as possible, readjusting your screen and position if needed.[27]

Establishing the Agenda. Once you have established rapport, you are ready to pursue the patient's reason for seeking care, traditionally called the *chief complaint.* In the ambulatory setting, where there are often three or four reasons for the visit, the phrase *presenting problem(s)* may be preferable. One benefit to this phrase is that it does not characterize the patient as a complainer. Begin with open-ended questions that allow full freedom of response: "What are your special concerns today?", "How can I help you?", or "Are there specific concerns that prompted your appointment today?" These questions encourage the patient to talk about any kinds of concerns, not just clinical ones. Note that the first problem the patient mentions may not be the one that is most important.[28] Often, patients give one reason for the visit to the nurse and another to you. For some visits, patients do not have a specific concern and only "want a check-up."

Identifying all the concerns at the outset allows you and the patient to decide which ones are most pressing and which ones can be postponed to a later visit. Questions such as "Is there anything else?", "Have we got everything?", or "Is there anything we missed?" help you uncover the patient's full agenda and "the real reason" for the visit. You may want to address different goals, like discussing an elevated blood pressure or an abnormal test result. Identifying the full agenda protects time for the most important issues. However, even negotiating the agenda at the outset does not avert "oh by the way" concerns that suddenly emerge at the end of the visit.

Inviting the Patient's Story. Once you have prioritized the agenda, invite the patient's story by asking about the foremost concern, "Tell me more about…" Encourage patients to tell their stories in their own words, using an open-ended approach. Avoid biasing the patient's story—do not inject new information or interrupt. Instead, use active listening skills: lean forward as you listen; add continuers such as nodding your head and phrases like "uh huh," "go on," or "I see." Train yourself to follow the patient's leads. If you ask specific questions prematurely, you risk suppressing details in the patient's own words. Studies show that clinicians wait only 18 seconds before they interrupt.[28] Once interrupted, patients usually do not resume their stories. After the patient's initial description, explore the patient's story in more depth. Ask, *"How would you describe the pain?", "What happened next?",* or *"What else did you notice?"* so that the patient enriches important details.

See pp. 70–71 for discussions of *continuers.*

Exploring the Patient's Perspective. The *disease/illness distinction model* helps elucidate the different yet complementary perspectives of the clinician and the patient.[29] *Disease* is the explanation that the *clinician* uses to organize symptoms that leads to a clinical diagnosis. *Illness* is a construct that explains how the *patient* experiences the disease, including its effects on relationships, function, and sense of well-being. Many factors may shape this experience, including prior personal or family health, its impact on everyday life, the patient's outlook, style of coping, and expectations about care. *The clinical interview needs to incorporate both these views of reality.* The melding of these two perspectives forms the basis for planning evaluation and treatment.

See pp. 69–71 for discussions of *guided questioning.*

Even a straightforward concern like sore throat can illustrate these divergent views. The patient may be worried about pain and difficulty swallowing, missing time from work, or a cousin who was hospitalized with tonsillitis. The clinician may focus on specific points in the history that differentiate streptococcal pharyngitis from other etiologies, or on a questionable history of allergy to penicillin. To understand the patient's perspective, the clinician needs to explore the four domains below. This information is crucial to patient satisfaction and patient compliance.[8,30]

Exploring the Patient's Perspective (F-I-F-E)

- The patient's **F**eelings, including fears or concerns, about the problem
- The patient's **I**deas about the nature and the cause of the problem
- The effect of the problem on the patient's life and **F**unction
- The patient's **E**xpectations of the disease, of the clinician, or of health care, often based on prior personal or family experiences

To explore the patient's perspective, use different types of questions. To uncover the patient's feelings, ask, "What concerns you most about the pain?" or "How has this been for you?" For views about the cause of the problem, ask, "Why do you think you have this [stomachache]?" You might ask, "What have you tried to help?" since these choices suggest how the patient perceives the cause. Some patients worry that their pain is a symptom of serious disease. Others just want relief. To determine how the illness affects the patient's lifestyle, particularly if the illness is chronic, ask, "What did you do before that you can't do now? How has your [backache, shortness of breath, etc.] affected you? Your life at home? Your social activities? Your role as a parent? Your function in intimate relationships? The way you feel about yourself as a person?" To find out what the patient expects from you or from the encounter in general, consider asking, "I am glad the pain is almost gone, how specifically can I help you now?" Even if the pain is gone, the patient may still need a work excuse to take to an employer. A mnemonic for the patient's perspective on the illness is FIFE—*Feelings, Ideas*, effect on *Function*, and *Expectations*.

Identifying and Responding to the Patient's Emotional Cues.

Illness is often accompanied by emotional distress; 30% to 40% of patients have anxiety and depression in primary care practices.[31] Visits tend to be longer when clinicians miss emotional clues. Patients may withhold their true concerns in up to 75% of acute care visits even though they give clues to these concerns that are direct, indirect, verbal, nonverbal, or disguised as related ideas or emotions.[32] Check on these clues and feelings by asking, "How did you feel about that?" or "Many people would be frustrated by something like this." See the box below for a taxonomy of the clues about the patient's perspective on illness.

Clues to the Patient's Perspective on Illness

- Direct statement(s) by the patient of explanations, emotions, expectations, and effects of the illness
- Expression of feelings about the illness without naming the illness
- Attempts to explain or understand symptoms
- Speech clues (e.g., repetition, prolonged reflective pauses)
- Sharing a personal story
- Behavioral clues indicative of unidentified concerns, dissatisfaction, or unmet needs such as reluctance to accept recommendations, seeking a second opinion, or early return appointment

Source: Lang F, Floyd MR, Beine KL. Clues to patients' explanations and concerns about their illnesses: a call for active listening. *Arch Fam Med.* 2000;9:222.

Learn to respond attentively to emotional cues using techniques like reflection, feedback, and "continuers" that convey support. A mnemonic for responding to emotional cues is **NURSE**: **N**ame—"That sounds like a scary experience"; **U**nderstand or legitimize—"It's understandable that you feel that way"; **R**espect—"You've done better than most people would with this"; **S**upport—"I will continue to work with you on this"; and **E**xplore—"How else were you feeling about it?"[33,34]

Expanding and Clarifying the Patient's Story.   As you elicit the patient's story, you must diligently clarify the attributes of each symptom, including context, associations, and chronology. For pain and many other symptoms, understanding these essential characteristics, summarized as the *seven attributes of a symptom,* is critical.

To pursue the seven attributes, two mnemonics may help:

- **OLD CARTS,** or **O**nset, **L**ocation, **D**uration, **C**haracter, **A**ggravating/**A**lleviating Factors, **R**adiation, and **T**iming, *or*

- **OPQRST,** or **O**nset, **P**alliating/**P**rovoking Factors, **Q**uality, **R**adiation, **S**ite, and **T**iming

The Seven Attributes of a Symptom

1. *Location.* Where is it? Does it radiate?
2. *Quality.* What is it like?
3. *Quantity or severity.* How bad is it? (For pain, ask for a rating on a scale of 1 to 10.)
4. *Timing.* When did (does) it start? How long does it last? How often does it come?
5. *Onset (setting in which symptom occurs).* Include environmental factors, personal activities, emotional reactions, or other circumstances that may have contributed to the illness.
6. *Remitting or exacerbating factors.* Is there anything that makes it better or worse?
7. *Associated manifestations.* Have you noticed anything else that accompanies it?

Whenever possible, *repeat back the patient's words and expressions* as the history unfolds, to affirm the patient's experience as you clarify what he or she means. Although using clinical terminology is tempting, these terms can leave patients confused and frustrated. Be aware of how easily jargon like "take a history" and "work you up" can creep into your discussions. Choose plain language for reflecting back the patient's story, for example, "You said there was 'a heavy weight' on your chest. Can you tell me more about that?" Or, to help clarify the meaning of a patient symptom by offering a choice of responses, ask, "You mentioned you were light-headed. Did you feel like fainting or that your legs were just weak?" It is highly important to establish *the sequence and time course* of each of the patient's symptoms to ensure that your assessments are based on a fully accurate history. To establish the correct chronological order, ask questions like "What then?" or "What happened next?" or "Please start at the beginning, or the last time you felt well, and go step by step." To fill in specific details, vary the types of questions and interviewing techniques that you use, including focused questions for information that is still missing. *In general, an interview moves back and forth from open-ended questions to increasingly focused questions and then on to another open-ended question, returning the lead in the interview to the patient.*

See Skilled Interviewing Techniques and discussion of focused questions, pp. 68–73.

Generating and Testing Diagnostic Hypotheses. As you gain experience listening to patient concerns, you will deepen your skills of clinical reasoning. You will *generate and test diagnostic hypotheses* about which disease process might be present. Identifying all the features of each symptom is fundamental to recognizing patterns of disease and to generating the *differential diagnosis.* It is important to fully flesh out the patient's story. This avoids the common trap of *premature closure,* or shutting down the patient's story too quickly, which can lead to errors in diagnosis.[35]

It is helpful to visualize the process of evoking a full description of each symptom as "the cone" (Fig. 3-8).

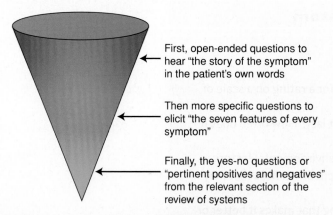

First, open-ended questions to hear "the story of the symptom" in the patient's own words

Then more specific questions to elicit "the seven features of every symptom"

Finally, the yes-no questions or "pertinent positives and negatives" from the relevant section of the review of systems

FIGURE 3-8. **Gather a full description of each symptom.**

For example, in a patient with a cough, the yes-no questions would come from the Respiratory section of the Review of Systems, on p. 12.

Each symptom has its own "cone," which becomes a paragraph in the History of Present Illness in the written record.

Questions about clusters of symptoms in common clinical entities are also found in "The Health History" section of each of the regional physical examination chapters. The interview is your primary source of evidence for and against various diagnostic possibilities. The challenge is to avoid a clinician-centered agenda, letting focused questions take over that obscure the patient's perspective and limit your opportunity to create an empathic therapeutic connection.

Sharing the Treatment Plan. Learning about the disease and conceptualizing the illness allow you and the patient to create a shared picture of the patient's problems. This multifaceted picture then forms the basis for planning further evaluation (e.g., physical examination, laboratory tests, consultations) and negotiating a treatment plan. *Shared decision-making* has been called the pinnacle of patient-centered care.[36] Experts recommend a three-step process: introducing choices and describing options using patient decision support tools when available; exploring patient preferences; and moving to a decision, checking that the patient is ready to make a decision and offering more time, if needed.[37]

Behavior Change and Motivational Interviewing. Many of your patient visits will close with a discussion of behavior changes needed to optimize health or treat illness. These could include a change in diet, exercise habits, cessation of smoking or drinking, adherence to medication regimens, or self-management strategies, among others.[38] Advanced techniques such as motivational interviewing and the therapeutic use of the clinician–patient relationship are beyond the scope of this book. Nonetheless, it is worthwhile to introduce the principles of motivational interviewing, a set of well-documented techniques that improve health outcomes, especially for patients with substance abuse.[39] Motivational interviewing helps patients "to say why and how they might change, and is based on the use of a guiding style" of interviewing, rather than direct advice. It engages patients to express the pros and cons of a given behavior.[40] Motivational interviewing makes the assumption that many patients already know what is best for them and helps them confront their ambivalence to change.[41] Using three core skills empowers *the patient* to provide ideas, solutions, and a timetable for change, as shown in the following table.

See Table 3-1, Motivational Interviewing: A Clinical Example, p. 104.

The Guiding Style of Motivational Interviewing

1. "Ask" open-ended questions—invite the patient to consider how and why they might change.
2. "Listen" to understand your patient's experience—"capture" their account with brief summaries or reflective listening statements such as "quitting smoking feels beyond you at the moment"; these express empathy, encourage the patient to elaborate, and are often the best way to respond to resistance.
3. "Inform"—by asking permission to provide information, and then asking what the implications might be for the patient.

Source: Quoted directly from Rollnick S, Butler CC, Kinnersly P, et al. Motivational Interviewing. *BMJ.* 2010;340:1242.

See Table 3-2, Brief Action Planning (BAP)—A Self-Management Support Tool, p. 105.

Closing the Interview and the Visit. You may find that ending the health history interview, and later concluding the visit, are difficult. Patients often have many questions, and if you have done your job well, they feel engaged and affirmed as they talk with you. Let the patient know that the end of the interview or the visit is approaching to allow time for any final questions. Make sure the patient understands the mutual plans you have developed. For example, before gathering your papers or standing to leave the room, you can say, "We need to stop now. Do you have any questions about what we've covered?" As you close, summarizing plans for future evaluation, treatments, and follow-up is helpful. A useful technique to assess the patient's understanding is to "teach back," whereby you invite the patient to tell you, in his or her own words, the plan of care. An example would be: "Could you please tell me what you understand is our plan of care?"[42,43]

The patient should have a chance to ask any final questions, but the last few minutes are not a good time to bring up new topics. If this happens and the concern is not life threatening, simply assure the patient of your interest and make plans to address the problem at a future time. "That knee pain sounds concerning. Why don't you make an appointment for next week so we can discuss it?" Reaffirming your ongoing commitment to the patient's health shows your involvement and esteem.

Taking Time for Self-Reflection. The role of self-reflection, or mindfulness, in developing clinical empathy cannot be overemphasized. Mindfulness refers to the state of being "purposefully and nonjudgmentally attentive to [one's] own experience, thoughts, and feelings."[44] As you encounter people of diverse ages, gender identities, social class, race, and ethnicity, being consistently respectful and open to individual differences is an ongoing challenge of clinical care. Because we bring our own values, assumptions, and biases to every encounter, we must look inward to see how our own expectations and reactions affect what we hear and how we behave. *Self-reflection is a continual part of professional development in clinical work. It brings a deepening personal awareness to our work with patients. This personal awareness is one of the most rewarding aspects of patient care.*[45]

The Cultural Context of the Interview

Demonstrating Cultural Humility—A Changing Paradigm.
Communicating effectively with patients from every background has always been an important professional skill. Nonetheless, the disparities in risks of disease, morbidity, and mortality are marked and broadly documented across different population groups, reflecting inequities in health care access, income level, type of insurance, educational level, language proficiency, and provider decision making.[46,47] To moderate these disparities, clinicians are increasingly urged to engage in self-reflection, critical thinking, and cultural humility as they experience diversity in their clinical practices.[48–50]

See Chapters 4 to 20, sections on Health Promotion and Counseling: Evidence and Recommendations and selected notations in the Examples of Abnormalities columns.

Cultural competence is commonly viewed as "a set of attitudes, skills, behaviors, and policies that enable organizations and staff to work effectively in cross-cultural situations. It reflects the ability to acquire and use knowledge of the health-related beliefs, attitudes, practices, and communication patterns of clients and their families to improve services, strengthen programs, increase community participation, and close the gaps in health status among diverse population groups."[51] Culturally competent care requires "understanding of and respect for the cultures, traditions, and practices of a community."[52] For example, Asians and Pacific Islanders for Reproductive Health have cited environmental toxins as threats to food safety, and the

Native American Women's Health Education Resource Center has included sovereignty and the right to parent as Native Americans in their agendas for health.

Experts caution that too often, cultural competence is reduced to a static decontextualized set of traits and beliefs for particular ethnic groups that objectifies patients as "other," implicitly reinforcing the perspectives of the dominant, often Western, culture.[53] Instead, "culture is ever-changing and always being revised within the dynamic context of its enactment." However, "this dynamic is often compromised by various sociocultural mismatches between patients and providers."[54] Such mismatches arise from clinicians' lack of knowledge about patient beliefs and lived experiences as well as unintentional or intentional enactment of stereotypes and bias during patient encounters.

Instead, move toward the precepts of *cultural humility*. Cultural humility is defined as a "process that requires humility as individuals continually engage in self-reflection and self-critique as lifelong learners and reflective practitioners."[54] It is a process that includes "the difficult work of examining cultural beliefs and cultural systems of both patients and providers to locate the points of cultural dissonance or synergy that contribute to patients' health outcomes."[55] It calls for clinicians to "bring into check the power imbalances that exist in the dynamics of (clinician)–patient communication" and maintain mutually respectful and dynamic partnerships with patients and communities. To attain these attributes, seek out the more effective training models that continue to emerge.[56–60]

Begin your commitment to self-reflective practice by studying the vignettes that follow. These examples illustrate how cultural differences and unconscious bias can unwittingly lead to poor communication and poor patient outcomes.

Cultural Humility: Scenario 1

A 28-year-old taxi driver from Ghana who had recently moved to the United States complained to a friend about U.S. clinical care. He had gone to the clinic because of fever and fatigue. He described being weighed, having his temperature taken, and having a cloth wrapped tightly, to the point of pain, around his arm. The clinician, a 36-year-old woman from Washington, D.C., asked the patient many questions, examined him, and wanted to take blood, which the patient had refused. The patient's final comment was "…and she didn't even give me chloroquine!"—his primary reason for seeking care. The man from Ghana was expecting few questions, no examination, and treatment for malaria, which is what fever usually means in Ghana.

In this example, cross-cultural miscommunication is understandable and thus less threatening to explore. Unconscious bias leading to miscommunication, however, occurs in many clinical interactions. Consider the scenario below that is closer to daily practice.

Cultural Humility: Scenario 2

A 16-year-old high school student came to the local teen health center because of painful menstrual cramps that interfered with her concentration at school. She was dressed in a tight top and short skirt and had multiple piercings. The 30-year-old male clinician asked the following questions: "Are you passing all of your classes? What kind of job do you want after high school? What kind of birth control do you want?" The teen felt pressured into accepting birth control pills, even though she had clearly stated that she had never had intercourse and planned to postpone it until she got married. She was an honor student planning to go to college, but the clinician did not elicit these goals. The clinician glossed over her cramps by saying, "Oh, you can just take some ibuprofen. Cramps usually get better as you get older." The patient will not take the birth control pills that were prescribed, nor will she seek health care soon again. She experienced the encounter as an interrogation, so failed to gain trust in her clinician. In addition, the clinician's questions made assumptions about her life and did not show respect for her health concerns. Even though the provider pursued important psychosocial domains, she received ineffective health care because of conflicting cultural values and clinician bias.

In both of these cases, the failure stems from mistaken assumptions or biases. In the first case, the clinician did not consider the many variables affecting patient beliefs about health and expectations for care. In the second case, the clinician allowed stereotypes to dictate the agenda instead of listening to the patient and respecting her as an individual. Each of us has our own cultural background and our own biases. These do not simply fade away as we become clinicians.

As you provide care for an ever-expanding and diverse group of patients, you must recognize how culture shapes not only the patient's beliefs, but also your own. *Culture* is the system of shared ideas, rules, and meanings that influences how we view the world, experience it emotionally, and behave in relation to other people. It can be understood as the "lens" through which we perceive and make sense out of the world we inhabit. The meaning of culture is much broader than the term "ethnicity." Cultural systems are not limited to minority groups; they emerge in many social groupings, including clinical professionals.

Avoid letting personal impressions about cultural groups turn into professional stereotyping. For example, you may have heard that Hispanic patients are more dramatic when they express pain. Recognize that this is a stereotype. Evaluate each patient as an individual, not decreasing the dose of analgesics, but staying attuned to your reactions to the patient's style. Work on an informed clinical approach to each patient by consciously acknowledging your own values and biases, developing communication skills that transcend cultural differences, and building therapeutic partnerships based on respect for each patient's life experience. This type of framework, described in the next section, will allow you to approach each patient as a unique individual.

The Three Dimensions of Cultural Humility

1. *Self-awareness.* Learn about your own biases; we all have them.
2. *Respectful communication.* Work to eliminate assumptions about what is "normal." Learn directly from your patients; they are the experts on their culture and illness.
3. *Collaborative partnerships.* Build your patient relationships on respect and mutually acceptable plans.

Self-Awareness. Start by exploring your own cultural identity. How do you describe yourself in terms of ethnicity, class, region or country of origin, religion, and political affiliation? Don't forget the characteristics we often take for granted—gender, life roles, sexual orientation, physical ability, and race—especially if we belong to majority groups. What aspects of your family of origin do you identify with, and how are you different from your family of origin? How do these identities influence your beliefs and behaviors?

A more challenging task is to bring our own values and biases to a conscious level. *Values* are the standards we use to measure our own and others' beliefs and behaviors. *Biases* are the attitudes or feelings that we attach to perceived differences. Being attuned to difference is normal; in fact, in the distant past, reacting to differences may have ensured survival. Instinctively knowing members of one's own group is a survival skill that we may have outgrown as a society, but that is still actively at work.

Feeling guilty about our biases makes them hard to recognize and acknowledge. Start with less threatening constructs, like the way an individual relates to time, a culturally determined phenomenon. Are you always on time—a positive value in the dominant Western culture? Or do you tend to run a little late? How do you feel about people whose habits are opposite to yours? Next time you attend a meeting or class, notice who is early, on time, or late. Is it predictable? Think about the role of physical appearance. Do you consider yourself thin, mid-size, or heavy? How do you feel about your weight? What does prevailing U.S. culture teach us to value in physique? How do you feel about people who have different weights?

Respectful Communication. Given the complexities of global society, no one can possibly know the health beliefs and practices of every culture and subculture. Let your patients be the experts on their own unique cultural perspectives. Even if patients have trouble describing their values or beliefs, they can often respond to specific questions. Find out about the patient's cultural background. Maintain an open, respectful, and inquiring attitude. "What did you hope to get from this visit?" If you have established rapport and trust, patients will be willing to teach you. Be aware of questions that contain assumptions. And always be ready to acknowledge your areas of ignorance or bias. "I know very little about Ghana. What would have happened at a clinic there if you had these concerns?" Or, with the second patient and with much more difficulty, "I mistakenly made assumptions about you that are not right.

Use some of the same questions discussed earlier in Sharing the Treatment Plan, pp. 80–81.

I apologize. Would you be willing to tell me more about yourself and your future goals?"

Learning about the patient's specific culture broadens the areas you, as a clinician, need to explore. Do some reading about the life experiences of individuals in ethnic or racial groups who live in your area. There may be historic reasons for loss of trust in clinicians or health care.[60] Go to movies filmed in foreign countries, which can help you better understand different cultures. Learn about the explicit health agendas of different consumer groups. Talk with different kinds of healers and learn about their practices. Most importantly, be open to learning from each patient. Do not assume that your impressions about a given cultural group apply to the individual before you.

Collaborative Partnerships. Through continual work on self-awareness and seeing through the "lens" of others, the clinician lays the foundation for the collaborative relationship that best supports the patient's health. Communication based on trust, respect, and your own willingness to re-examine assumptions allows patients to be more open to expressing views that diverge from the dominant culture. They may have strong feelings such as anger or shame. You, the clinician, must be willing to listen to and validate these emotions, and not let your own feelings of discomfort or time pressure prevent you from exploring painful areas. Be willing to re-examine your beliefs about the "right approach" to clinical care in a given situation. Make every effort to be flexible as you develop shared plans that reflect patients' knowledge about their best interests that are congruent with both their beliefs and effective clinical care. Remember that if the patient stops listening, fails to follow your advice, or does not return, your care has not been successful.

Advanced Interviewing

Interviewing the Challenging Patient

As you spend time inviting patient stories, you will find that some patients are more difficult to interview than others. For some clinicians, a quiet patient might seem difficult, for others, a patient who is more assertive. Being aware of your reactions helps develop your clinical skills. Your success in eliciting the history from different types of patients grows with experience, but take into account your own stressors, such as fatigue, mood, and overwork. Self-care is also important in caring for others. Even if a patient is challenging, *always remember the importance of listening to the patient and clarifying his or her concerns.*

The Silent Patient. Novice interviewers often feel uncomfortable with periods of silence and try to keep the conversation going. Silence has many meanings. Patients fall silent to collect their thoughts, remember details, or decide if they can trust you with certain information. Periods of silence usually seem longer to the clinician than the patient. Be attentive and respectful, and encourage the patient to continue when ready. Watch the patient closely for nonverbal cues, such as difficulty controlling emotions. Being comfortable with periods of silence may be therapeutic, prompting the patient to reveal deeper feelings.

Patients with depression or dementia may seem subdued and lose their usual affect, giving only short answers to questions, then falling silent. If you have already tried guided questioning, try shifting to more direct inquiry about symptoms of depression, or begin an exploratory mental status examination.

See Chapter 5, Behavior and Mental Status, pp. 147–171.

At times, silence may be the patient's response to how you are asking questions. Are you asking too many short-answer questions in rapid succession? Have you offended the patient by showing disapproval or criticism? Have you failed to recognize an overwhelming symptom such as pain, nausea, or shortness of breath? If so, you may need to ask the patient directly, "You seem very quiet. Have I done something to upset you?"

The Confusing Patient. Some patient stories are confusing and do not seem to make sense. Just as you develop a differential diagnosis from the symptoms of the Present Illness, keep several possibilities in mind as you assess why the story is confusing. It may be the patient's style, and by using your skills of guiding questions, clarification, and summarizing, you can put together a coherent story. Watch for an underlying issue, however, that is interfering with communication.

Some patients present a confusing array of *multiple symptoms*. They seem to have every symptom that you ask about, or "a positive review of systems." With these patients, focus on the context of the symptom, emphasizing the patient's perspective (see pp. 77–78), and guide the interview into a psychosocial assessment.

See Chapter 5, Behavior and Mental Status, Medically Unexplained Symptoms, pp. 149–150, and Table 5-1, Somatic Symptom and Related Disorders, p. 169.

At other times, you may feel baffled and frustrated because the history is vague, and ideas are poorly connected and hard to follow. Even with careful wording, you cannot prompt clear answers to your questions. The patient may seem peculiar, distant, aloof, or inappropriate. Symptoms may seem bizarre: "My fingernails feel too heavy" or "My stomach knots up like a snake." Perhaps there is a mental status change like psychosis or delirium, a mental illness such as schizophrenia, or a neurologic disorder. Consider delirium in acutely ill or intoxicated patients and dementia in the elderly. Their histories are inconsistent and dates are hard to follow. Some may even confabulate to fill in the gaps in their memories.

See Table 20-2, Delirium and Dementia, p. 1001.

If you suspect a psychiatric or neurologic disorder, gathering a detailed history can tire and frustrate both you and the patient. Shift to the mental status examination, focusing on level of consciousness, orientation, memory, and capacity to understand. You can ease this transition by asking questions like "When was your last appointment at the clinic? Let's see…that was about how long ago?" "Your address now is…?…and your phone number?" You can confirm these responses in the chart or ask permission to speak with family members or friends to obtain their perspectives.

See Chapter 5, Behavior and Mental Status, The Mental Status Examination, pp. 147–171.

The Patient with Altered Cognition. Some patients cannot provide their own histories because of delirium, dementia, or mental health conditions.

Others are unable to remember certain parts of the history, such as events related to a febrile illness or a seizure. Under these circumstances, you will need to obtain historical information from other sources such as family members or caregivers. Always seek the best-informed source. Apply the basic principles of interviewing to your conversations with relatives or friends. Find a private place to talk. Introduce yourself, state your purpose, inquire how they are feeling under the circumstances, and recognize and acknowledge their concerns. As you listen to their accounts, assess their credibility in light of the quality of their relationship with the patient. Establish how they know the patient. For example, when a child is brought in for health care, the accompanying adult may not be the parent or caregiver, but just the most available driver. Remember that while you are gathering information about the history, you should not disclose information about the patient unless the informant is the health care proxy or has a durable power of attorney for health care, or you have permission from the patient. Learn the tenets of the Health Insurance Portability and Accountability Act (HIPAA) passed by Congress in 1996, which sets strict standards for disclosure for both institutions and providers when sharing patient information.[61]

Some patients can provide a history, but lack the ability to make informed health care decisions. You then need to determine whether a patient has "decision-making capacity," which is the ability to understand information related to health, weigh choices and their consequences, reason through the options, and communicate a choice. *Capacity* is a clinical designation and can be assessed by clinicians, whereas *competence* is a legal designation and can only be decided by a court. If a patient lacks capacity to make a health care decision, then identify the health care proxy or the agent with power of attorney for health care. If the patient had not identified a surrogate decision-maker, then that role may shift to a spouse or family member. It is critical to remember that decision-making capacity is both "temporal and situational":[62] It can fluctuate depending on the condition of the patient and the complexity of the decision involved. A patient who is quite ill may be unable to make decisions about care, but can regain capacity with clinical improvement. A patient may be unable to make a complex decision, but still able to make simple decisions. Even if patients lack capacity for certain decisions, it is still important to seek their input, as they may have definite opinions about their care.

Elements of Decision-Making Capacity

Patients must have the ability to:

- Understand the relevant information about proposed diagnostic tests or treatment,
- Appreciate their situation (including their underlying values and current clinical situation),
- Use reason to make a decision, and
- Communicate their choice.

Source: Sessums LL, Zembrzuska H, Jackson JL. Does This Patient Have Medical Decision-Making Capacity? *JAMA*. 2011;306:420.

The Aid to Capacity Evaluation (ACE)[63] is an instrument that has been validated against a gold standard, is free and available online, can be performed in less than 30 minutes, and uses the patient's actual clinical scenario in the evaluation.

The Talkative Patient.   The garrulous rambling patient is also challenging. Faced with limited time to "get the whole story," you may grow impatient, even exasperated. Although this problem has no perfect solution, several techniques are helpful. Give the patient free rein for the first 5 or 10 minutes, while listening closely. Perhaps the patient simply needs a good listener and is expressing pent-up concerns, or just enjoys telling stories. Does the patient seem obsessively detailed? Is the patient unduly anxious or apprehensive? Is there flight of ideas or a disorganized thought process that suggests a thought disorder?

Focus on what seems most important to the patient. Show your interest by asking questions in those areas. Interrupt only if necessary, but be courteous. Learn to set limits when needed, since part of your task is structuring the interview to gain important information about the patient's health. A brief summary may help you change the subject, yet validate any concerns. "Let me make sure that I understand. You have described many concerns. In particular, I heard about two different kinds of pain, one on your left side that goes into your groin and is fairly new, and one in your upper abdomen after you eat that you have had for months. Let's focus just on the side pain first. Can you tell me what it feels like?" Or you can ask the patient, "What is your #1 concern today?"

See Summarization, p. 72.

Finally, avoid showing impatience. If time runs out, explain the need for a second visit and prepare the patient by setting a time limit. "I know we have much more to talk about. Can you come again next week? We will have a 30-minute visit then."

The Crying Patient.   Crying signals strong emotions, ranging from sadness to anger or frustration. Pausing, gentle probing, or responding with empathy gives the patient permission to cry. Usually crying is therapeutic, as is your quiet acceptance of the patient's distress. Offer a tissue and wait for the patient to recover. Make a supportive remark like "I am glad you were able to express your feelings." Most patients will soon compose themselves and resume their story. Crying makes many clinicians uncomfortable. If this is true for you, learn how to accept displays of emotion so you can support patients at these moving and significant times.

The Angry or Disruptive Patient.   Many patients have reasons to be angry: They are ill, they have suffered a loss, they have lost control of their health, or they feel overwhelmed by the health care system.[26] They may direct this anger toward you. It is possible that their anger at you is justified...were you late for your appointment, inconsiderate, insensitive, or angry yourself? If so, acknowledge the situation and try to make amends. More often, however, patients displace their anger onto the clinician as a reflection of their frustration or pain.

Learn to accept angry feelings from patients without getting angry in return or retreating from the patient's affect.[64] Avoid reinforcing criticism of other clinicians, the clinical setting, or the hospital, even if you feel sympathetic. You can validate patients' feelings without agreeing with their reasons. "I understand that you felt frustrated by answering the same questions over and over. Repeating the same information to everyone on the team can seem unnecessary when you are sick." After the patient has calmed down, help the patient to work through his or her angry feelings and move on to other concerns.

Some angry patients become overtly disruptive, belligerent, or out of control. Before approaching such patients, alert the security staff; ensuring a safe environment is one of your responsibilities. Stay calm and avoid being confrontational. Keep your posture relaxed and nonthreatening. At first, do not try to make disruptive patients lower their voices or stop threatening you or the staff. Listen carefully. Try to understand what they are saying. Once you have established rapport, gently suggest moving to a more private location.

The Patient with a Language Barrier. Nothing makes the importance of the history more evident than being unable to communicate with the patient, an increasingly common experience. In 2011, the Census Bureau reported that more than 60 million Americans speak a language other than English at home. Of these, more than 20% have limited English proficiency. Spanish is the primary non-English language, spoken by 37 million Americans.[65] These individuals are less likely to have regular primary or preventive care and more likely to experience dissatisfaction and adverse outcomes from clinical errors. Learning to work with qualified interpreters is essential for optimal outcomes and cost-effective care.[66–70] Experts take this one step further, "If it isn't culturally and linguistically appropriate, it isn't health care."[71]

If your patient speaks a different language, make every effort to find a trained interpreter. A few words of clinical Spanish may enhance rapport, but they are no substitute for the full story. Even if you are fluent, you may miss important nuances in the meanings of certain words.[72] Recruiting family members as translators is equally hazardous—it may violate confidentiality, and information may be incomplete, misleading, or harmful. Lengthy patient explanations may be telescoped into a few words, omitting significant details. The ideal interpreter is a "cultural navigator" who is neutral and trained in both languages and cultures.[73,74] However, even trained interpreters may be unfamiliar with the multiple subcultures in many societies.

When you work with an interpreter, begin by establishing rapport and reviewing the information that will be most useful. Ask the interpreter to translate everything, not to condense or summarize. Make your questions clear, short, and simple. Help the interpreter by outlining your goals for each segment of the history. After going over your plans, arrange the seating so that you have easy eye contact with the patient. Then speak directly to the patient... "How long have you been sick?" rather than "How long has the patient been sick?" Having the interpreter sit close to the patient, or even behind you, keeps you from turning your head back and forth.

When available, bilingual written questionnaires are invaluable, especially for the review of systems. First, however, be sure that patients can read in their language; otherwise, ask the interpreter for help. In some clinical settings, use speakerphone translators, if available.

Guidelines for Working with an Interpreter: "INTERPRET"

I   Introductions: Make sure to introduce all the individuals in the room. During the introduction, include information as to the roles individuals will play.

N   Note Goals: Note the goals of the interview. What is the diagnosis? What will the treatment entail? Will there be any follow-up?

T   Transparency: Let the patient know that everything said will be interpreted throughout the session.

E   Ethics: Use qualified interpreters (not family members or children) when conducting an interview. Qualified interpreters allow the patient to maintain autonomy and make informed decisions about his or her care.

R   Respect Beliefs: Limited English Proficient (LEP) patients may have cultural beliefs that need to be taken into account as well. The interpreter may be able to serve as a cultural broker and help explain any cultural beliefs that may exist.

P   Patient Focus: The patient should remain the focus of the encounter. Providers should interact with the patient and not the interpreter. Make sure to ask and address any questions the patient may have before ending the encounter. If you don't have trained interpreters on staff, the patient may not be able to call in with questions.

R   Retain Control: It is important as the provider that you remain in control of the interaction and not let the patient or the interpreter take over the conversation.

E   Explain: Use simple language and short sentences when working with an interpreter. This will ensure that comparable words can be found in the second language and that all the information can be conveyed clearly.

T   Thanks: Thank the interpreter and the patient for their time. On the chart, note that the patient needs an interpreter and who served as an interpreter this time.

Source: U.S. Department of Health and Human Services. INTERPRET tool: working with interpreters in cultural settings. Available at https://www.google.com/#q = USDHHS+Interpret+Tool. Accessed January 11, 2015.

The Patient with Low Literacy or Low Health Literacy.   Before giving written instructions, assess the patient's *ability to read.* More than 14% of Americans, or 30 million people, are unable to read basic documents.[75] Low literacy may explain why the patient has not taken medications or followed your recommendations.

To detect low literacy, you can ask about years completed in school, or "How is your reading?" You can ask "How comfortable are you with filling out health forms?" or check how well the patient reads written instructions. One rapid screen is to hand the patient a written text upside down—most patients will turn the page around immediately. Many patients are embarrassed about reading poorly. Be sensitive to their quandary, and do not confuse their degree of literacy with level of intelligence. Explore the reasons for impaired literacy—language barriers, learning disorders, poor vision, or level of education.

Research shows that low *health literacy*, affecting 80 million Americans, leads to poor health outcomes and impaired use of health services.[76] Health literacy goes beyond just reading. It includes the practical skills the patient needs to navigate the health care environment: print literacy, or the ability to interpret information in documents; numeracy, or the ability to use quantitative information for tasks like interpreting food labels or adhering to medication regimens; and oral literacy, or the ability to speak and listen effectively.

The Patient with Hearing Loss. Approximately 9% of the U.S. population is deaf or hard of hearing. This population "is a heterogeneous group that includes persons who have varying degrees of hearing loss, use multiple languages, and belong to different cultures. Solutions to providing health care to one group from (this) population do not necessarily apply to the other groups. Factors that must be considered with this population include degree of hearing loss, age of onset of loss, preferred language, and psychological issues."[77] Communication and trust are special challenges, and the risk of miscommunication is high.[78] Even hearing-impaired patients who use English may not follow standard English usage.

Find out the patient's preferred method of communication. Learn whether the patient belongs to the deaf culture or the hearing culture, when the hearing loss occurred relative to the development of speech and language, and the kinds of schools the patient attended. Review responses to written question-naires. Patients may use American Sign Language (ASL), a unique language with its own syntax. These patients typically have a low English reading level and prefer having certified ASL interpreters present during their visits.[77] Other patients may use varying combinations of signs and speech. If working with an interpreter, adopt the principles identified earlier. Alternatively, time-consuming handwritten questions and answers may be the only solution.

Partial hearing deficits vary. If the patient has a hearing aid, find out if the patient is using it. Make sure it is working. For patients with unilateral hearing loss, sit on the hearing side. A person who is *hard of hearing* may not be aware of the problem, a situation you will have to address tactfully. Eliminate back-ground noise from the television or hallway. Face patients who can read lips directly, in good light. Patients should put on their glasses to see cues that help them understand you. Speak at a normal volume and rate. Avoid letting your voice trail off at the ends of sentences, covering your mouth, or looking down at papers while speaking. Emphasize key points first. Even the best lip readers comprehend only a part of what you say, so asking them to "teach back" is important. When closing, write out your instructions for them to take home.

The Patient with Impaired Vision. With blind patients, shake hands to establish contact and explain who you are and why you are there. If the room is unfamiliar, orient the patient to the surroundings and report if anyone else is present. If helpful, adjust the light. Encourage visually impaired patients to wear glasses whenever possible. Spend more time on verbal explanations because postures and gestures are unseen.

The Patient with Limited Intelligence. Patients of moderately limited intelligence can usually give adequate histories. If you suspect a disability, pay special attention to the patient's school record and ability to function independently. How far have such patients gone in school? If they didn't finish, why not? What kinds of courses have they taken? How did they do? Has any testing been done? Are they living alone? Do they need assistance with activities like transportation or shopping? The sexual history is equally important and often overlooked. Find out if the patient is sexually active and provide information about pregnancy or sexually transmitted infections (STIs), if needed.

If you are unsure about the patient's level of intelligence, transition to the mental status examination and assess simple calculations, vocabulary, memory, and abstract thinking.

See Chapter 5, Behavior and Mental Status, pp. 147–171.

For patients with severe mental retardation, turn to family or caregivers for the history, but always show interest in the patient first. Establish rapport, make eye contact, and engage in simple conversation. As with children, avoid "talking down" or condescending behavior. The patient, family members, caregivers, or friends will appreciate your respect.

The Patient with Personal Problems.   Patients may ask you for advice about personal problems that fall outside the range of your clinical expertise. Should the patient quit a stressful job, for example, or move out of state? Instead of responding, ask about what alternatives that the patient has considered, related pros and cons, and others who have provided advice. Letting the patient talk through the problem with you is more therapeutic than giving your own opinions.

The Seductive Patient.   Clinicians occasionally find themselves physically attracted to their patients. Similarly, patients may make sexual overtures or exhibit flirtatious behavior. The emotional and physical intimacy of the clinician–patient relationship can lend itself to these sexual feelings.

If you become aware of such feelings, bring them to conscious level to keep them from affecting your professional behavior. Denial can heighten the risk of responding inappropriately. *Any sexual contact or romantic relationship with patients is unethical;* keep your relationship with the patient within professional bounds, and seek help if you need it.[79–82]

When patients are seductive, you may be tempted to ignore their behavior because you are not sure it really happened, or you are just hoping it will go away. Calmly but firmly set clear limits that your relationship is professional, not personal. If necessary, leave the room and find a chaperone before you continue the visit. Think carefully about your own behavior. Has your clothing or demeanor been inappropriate? Have you been overly warm with the patient? It is your responsibility to evaluate and avoid sending any misleading signals to the patient.

Sensitive Topics

Clinicians talk with patients about many sensitive topics. These discussions can be awkward when you are inexperienced or assessing patients you do not know well. Even seasoned clinicians are inhibited by societal constraints when discussing certain subjects: abuse of alcohol or drugs, sexual practices, death and dying, financial concerns, racial and ethnic bias, domestic violence, psychiatric illness, physical deformity, bowel function, and others. Many of these topics trigger strong personal responses related to family, cultural, and societal values. Mental illness, drug use during pregnancy, and same-sex practices are examples of issues that may evoke biases that affect your interaction with the patient (Fig. 3-9).

Several basic principles can help guide your response to sensitive topics:

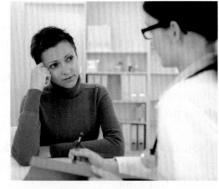

FIGURE 3-9. **Maintain a nonjudgmental manner.**

Guidelines for Broaching Sensitive Topics

- *The single most important rule is to be nonjudgmental.* Your role is to learn from the patient and help the patient achieve better health. Acceptance is the best way to reach this goal.
- *Explain why you need to know certain information.* This makes patients less apprehensive. For example, say to patients, "Because sexual practices put people at risk for certain diseases, I ask all of my patients the following questions."
- Find opening questions for sensitive topics and learn the specific kinds of information needed for your shared assessment and plan.
- Consciously acknowledge whatever discomfort you are feeling. Denying your discomfort may lead you to avoid the topic altogether.

Look into strategies that help make you more comfortable when discussing sensitive areas. These include reading about these topics in clinical and lay literature; talking with colleagues and teachers about your concerns; taking courses that help you explore your feelings and reactions; and ultimately, reflecting on your own life experience. Take advantage of all these resources. If possible, listen to experienced clinicians as they approach these issues with patients, then practice similar techniques in your own discussions. Over time, your level of comfort will grow and expand.

The Sexual History. Exploring the sexual history can be life-saving. Sexual behaviors determine risks for pregnancy, STIs, and human immunodeficiency virus (HIV); good interviewing helps prevent or reduce these risks.[83,84] Sexual practices may be directly related to the patient's symptoms and integral to both diagnosis and treatment. Many patients express their concerns more freely when you ask about sexual health. In addition, sexual dysfunction may result from medications or clinical issues that can be readily corrected.

You can elicit the sexual history at multiple points in the interview. If the chief complaint involves genitourinary symptoms, include questions about sexual health as part of "expanding and clarifying" the patient's story. For women, you can ask these questions during the Obstetric/Gynecologic section of the Past Medical History. You can include the sexual history in discussions about Health Maintenance, or in the Personal and Social History as you explore lifestyle issues and important relationships. In a comprehensive history, you can also ask about sexual practices during the Review of Systems. Do not forget to cover the sexual history in older patients and patients with disability or chronic illness.

An orienting sentence or two is often helpful. "To assess your risk for various diseases, I need to ask you some questions about your sexual health and practices" or "I routinely ask all patients about their sexual function." For more specific complaints you might state, "To figure out why you have this discharge and what we should do, I need to ask some questions about your sexual activity." If you are matter-of-fact, the patient is more likely to follow your lead. *Use specific language.* Refer to genitalia with explicit words such as penis or vagina and avoid phrases like "private parts." Choose words that are understandable and explain what you mean. "By intercourse, I mean when a man inserts his penis into a woman's vagina."

Also ask about satisfaction with sexual activity. Review the examples of questions that follow. These questions are designed to help patients reveal their concerns.

See specific questions in Chapter 13, Male Genitalia and Hernias, pp. 541–563, and Chapter 14, Female Genitalia, pp. 565–606.

The Sexual History: Sample Questions

- "When was the last time you had intimate physical contact with someone?" "Did that contact include sexual intercourse?" The term "sexually active" can be ambiguous. Patients have been known to reply, "No, I just lie there."
- "Do you have sex with men, women, or both?" Patients may have same-sex partners, yet not consider themselves gay, lesbian, or bisexual. Some gay and lesbian patients have had opposite-sex partners.
- "How many sexual partners have you had in the last 6 months? In the last 5 years? In your lifetime?" These questions make it easy for the patient to acknowledge multiple partners. Ask, "Have you had any new partners in the past 6 months?" If patients question why this information is important, explain that new partners or multiple partners over a lifetime can raise the risk for STIs. Ask about routine use of condoms. "How often do you use condoms?" is an open-ended question that does not presume an answer.
- It is important to ask all patients, "Do you have any concerns about HIV infection or AIDS?" since infection can occur in the absence of risk factors.

Note that these questions make no assumptions about marital status, sexual preference, or attitudes about pregnancy or contraception. Listen to each of the patient's responses, and invite additional history as indicated. To elicit information about sexual behaviors, you will need to ask more specific and focused questions than in other parts of the interview.

The Mental Health History. Cultural constructs of mental and physical illness vary widely, leading to differences in social acceptance and attitudes. Think how easy it is for patients to talk about diabetes and taking insulin compared with discussing schizophrenia and using psychotropic medications. Ask open-ended questions initially. "Have you ever had any problem with emotional or mental illnesses?" Then move to more specific questions such as "Have you ever seen a counselor or psychotherapist?" "Have you ever taken medication for a mental health condition?" "Have you ever been hospitalized for an emotional or mental health problem?" "What about members of your family?"

For patients with depression or thought disorders such as schizophrenia, take a careful history of their symptoms and course of illness. Watch for mood changes or symptoms such as fatigue, unusual tearfulness, appetite or weight changes, insomnia, and vague somatic complaints. Two validated screening questions for depression are: "Over the past 2 weeks, have you felt down, depressed, or hopeless?" and "Over the past 2 weeks, have you felt little interest or pleasure in doing things?"[85] If the patient seems depressed, always ask about suicide: "Have you ever thought about hurting yourself or ending your life?" As with chest pain, you must evaluate severity—both depression and angina are potentially lethal.

Turn to Chapter 5, Behavior and Mental Status, for discussions of depression, suicidality, and psychotic disorders, pp. 147–171.

Many patients with psychotic disorders like schizophrenia are living in the community and can tell you about their diagnoses, symptoms, hospitalizations, and current medications. Investigate whether their symptoms and level of function are stable and review their support systems and plan of care.

Alcohol and Prescription and Illicit Drugs. Many clinicians hesitate to ask patients about excess use of alcohol and prescribed or illicit drugs. The prevalence of substance abuse and dependence remains high. In 2013, 21.6 million Americans, or 8.2% of persons aged 12 years and older, were classified with a substance abuse or dependence disorder, including 14.7 million people with alcohol abuse or dependence, 2.6 million with alcohol *and* illicit drug abuse or dependence, and 4.3 million with illicit drug abuse or dependence. Abuse of prescribed pain medications is also increasing, now numbering about 1.9 million people.[86] Roughly 28% of Americans aged 12 years or older report binge or heavy drinking, and almost 3%, or 7 million, have used prescription drugs for nonclinical reasons, especially pain relievers, stimulants, and antidepressants.[39,87,88] The high prevalence of substance abuse makes it is essential to routinely assess current and past use of alcohol and drugs, patterns of use, and family history. Be familiar with current definitions of addiction, dependence, and tolerance.

Addiction, Physical Dependence, and Tolerance

Tolerance: A state of adaptation in which exposure to a drug induces changes that result in a diminution of one or more of the drug's effects over time.

Physical Dependence: A state of adaptation that is manifested by a drug class-specific withdrawal syndrome that can be produced by abrupt cessation, rapid dose reduction, decreasing blood level of the drug, and/or administration of an antagonist.

Addiction: A primary, chronic, neurobiologic disease, with genetic, psychosocial, and environmental factors influencing its development and manifestations. It is characterized by behaviors that include one or more of the following: impaired control over drug use, compulsive use, continued use despite harm, and craving.

Source: American Pain Society. Definitions Related to the Use of Opioids for the Treatment of Pain. A consensus statement from the American Academy of Pain Medicine, the American Pain Society, and the American Society of Addiction Medicine, 2001. Available at http://www.asam.org/docs/public-policy-statements/1opioid-definitions-consensus-2-011.pdf?sfvrsn=0. Accessed January 13, 2015.

Alcohol. Questions about alcohol and other drugs follow naturally after questions about caffeine and cigarettes. "Tell me about your use of alcohol" is an opening query that avoids the easy yes-no response. Remember that some patients do not consider wine or beer as "alcohol." Positive answers to two additional questions are highly suspicious for problem-drinking: "Have you ever had a drinking problem?" and "When was your last drink?", especially if the night before.[89] The most widely used screening questions are the *CAGE* questions about *C*utting down, *A*nnoyance when criticized, *G*uilty feelings, and *E*ye-openers. The CAGE Questionnaire is readily available online.

Two or more affirmative answers to the CAGE Questionnaire suggest alcohol misuse and have a sensitivity that ranges from 43% to 94% and specificity ranging from 70% to 96%.[90,91] Several well-validated short screening tests, such as the MAST (Michigan Alcohol Screening Test) and the AUDIT (Alcohol Use Disorders Identification Test), are also helpful.[92] If you detect misuse, ask about blackouts (loss of memory about events during drinking), seizures, accidents or injuries while drinking, job problems, and conflict in personal relationships.

Illicit Drugs. The National Institute on Drug Abuse recommends first asking a highly sensitive and specific single question: "How many times in the past year have you used an illegal drug or used a prescription medication for non-clinical reasons?"[93,94] If there is a positive response, ask specifically about non-clinical use of illicit and prescription drugs: "In your lifetime have you ever used: marijuana; cocaine; prescription stimulants; methamphetamines; sedatives or sleeping pills; hallucinogens like lysergic acid diethylamide (LSD), ecstasy, mushrooms…; street opioids like heroin or opium; prescription opioids like fentanyl, oxycodone, hydrocodone…; or other substances." For those answering yes, a series of further questions is recommended.[93]

Another approach is to modify the CAGE questions by adding "or drugs" to each question. Once you identify substance abuse, probe further with questions like "Are you always able to control your use of drugs?" "Have you had any bad reactions?" "What happened…Any drug-related accidents, injuries, or arrests? Job or family problems?"…"Have you ever tried to quit? Tell me about it."

Intimate Partner Violence and Domestic Violence. Intimate partner violence is the leading cause of serious injury and the second leading cause of death among U.S. women of reproductive age.[95] Each year, more than 12 million U.S. women and men experience rape, physical violence, or stalking by an intimate partner; these are groups that experience high rates of mental health disorders and substance abuse.[96,97] Prevalence varies from 20% in general practice settings to over 30% in emergency rooms and orthopedic clinics.[98–100] The U.S. Preventive Services Task Force and the American College of Obstetricians and Gynecologist recommend routine screening of all women of childbearing age for intimate partner violence and providing or referring those who screen positive for intervention services.[101,102] Elders are also highly vulnerable to neglect and abuse.[103–105]

Sensitive interviewing is essential, since even with skilled inquiry, only 25% of patients disclose their abuse experience.[106,107] The type of questioning is important. Experts recommend beginning with normalizing statements such as

National Institute of Alcohol Abuse and Alcoholism Definitions of Drinking at Low Risk for Developing and Alcohol Use Disorder

- Men: no more than 4 drinks on a single day or 14 drinks a week
- Women: no more than 3 drinks on a single day or 7 drinks a week
- Healthy adults over age 65 years and not taking medications: no more than 3 drinks on a single day or 7 drinks a week
- 1 drink is defined as 12 ounces of beer, 5 ounces of wine, or 1.5 ounces of spirits

Source: National Institute of Alcohol Abuse and Alcoholism, Drinking levels defined. Available at http://www.niaaa.nih.gov/alcohol-health/overview-alcohol-consumption/moderate-binge-drinking. Accessed January 14, 2015.

"Because abuse is common in many women's lives, I've begun to ask about it routinely." Disclosure is more likely when probing questions lead and then in-depth direct questions follow. "Are you in a relationship where you have been hit or threatened?" with a pause to encourage the patient to respond. If the patient says no, continue with "Has anyone ever treated you badly or made you do things you don't want to?" or "Is there anyone you are afraid of?" or "Have you ever been hit, kicked, punched, or hurt by someone you know?" Following disclosure, empathic validating and nonjudgmental responses are critical, but currently occur less than half the time.

Clues to Physical and Sexual Abuse. Be alert to the unspoken clues to abuse, often present in the growing numbers of victims of human sex trafficking in the United States and internationally, estimated at 50,000 women and children annually in the United States alone.[108,109]

See also Chapter 18, Assessing Children, Infancy Through Adolescence, Table 18-11, Physical Signs of Sexual Abuse, p. 921.

Clues to Physical and Sexual Abuse

- Injuries that are unexplained, seem inconsistent with the patient's story, are concealed by the patient, or cause embarrassment
- Delay in getting treatment for trauma
- History of repeated injuries or "accidents"
- Presence of alcohol or drug abuse in patient or partner
- Partner tries to dominate the visit, will not leave the room, or seems unusually anxious or solicitous
- Pregnancy at a young age; multiple partners
- Repeated vaginal infections and STIs
- Difficulty walking or sitting due to genital/anal pain
- Vaginal lacerations or bruises
- Fear of the pelvic examination or physical contact
- Fear of leaving the examination room

When you suspect abuse, it is important to spend part of the visit alone with the patient. You can use the transition to the physical examination as a reason to ask others to leave the room. If the patient is also resistant, do not force the situation, potentially placing the victim in jeopardy. Be attuned to diagnoses that have a higher association with abuse, such as pregnancy and somatic symptom disorder.

To begin screening for child abuse, ask parents about their approach to discipline. Ask how they cope with a baby who will not stop crying or a child who misbehaves: "Most parents get very upset when their baby cries (or their child has been naughty). How do you feel when your baby cries?" "What do you do when your baby won't stop crying?" "Do you have any fears that you might hurt your child?"

See Chapter 18, Assessing Children: Infancy Through Adolescence, pp. 799–925.

Death and the Dying Patient. There is a growing and important emphasis in health care education on improving care for dying patients and their families. Many studies have advanced our understanding of palliative care and set standards for quality care.[110,111] Even as beginning students, working through your own feelings about death and dying and acquiring basic skills to ensure good

For discussion of end-of-life decision-making, grief and bereavement, and advance directives, turn to Chapter 20, The Older Adult, pp. 975–976.

communication are important, as you will come into contact with patients of all ages near the end of their lives. Studies show that clinicians are still not communicating effectively with patients and families about how to manage symptoms and their preferences for care. Clinician interventions that improve symptoms and avoid hospitalization reduce grief and bereavement, improve outcomes and quality of care, reduce costs, and sometimes even prolong survival.[111–113]

For those facing death and their survivors, there are overlapping and sometimes prolonged phases of anticipatory grief and bereavement.[114] Kübler-Ross provided the classical description of the stages in our response to loss or the anticipatory grief of impending death: denial and isolation, anger, bargaining, depression or sadness, and acceptance.[115] These stages may occur sequentially or in any order or combination. Offer openings for patients and family members to talk about their feelings and ask questions. As defined by the World Health Organization, your goal is "the prevention and relief of suffering by means of early identification and impeccable assessment and treatment of pain and other problems, physical, psychosocial, and spiritual."[116] Ask, "I wonder if you have concerns about your illness? ... your pain? ... your preferences for treatment?" Provide the information requested and demonstrate your commitment to support and coordinate the patient's care throughout the illness. Dying patients rarely want to talk about their illnesses at each encounter, nor do they wish to confide in everyone they meet. If they wish to stay at a social level, respect their preferences. A smile, a touch, an inquiry about a family member, a comment on the day's events, or even gentle humor conveys your concern and responsiveness.

Clarifying the patient's wishes about treatment at the end of life is an important responsibility. Failing to facilitate end-of-life decision-making is widely viewed as a flaw in clinical care. The health status of the patient and the health care setting often determine what needs to be discussed. For patients who are acutely ill and in the hospital, discussions about how to respond to a cardiac or respiratory arrest are usually mandatory. Asking about *Do Not Resuscitate (DNR) status* is often difficult if you have not had a previous relationship with the patient or are unsure of the patient's understanding of the illness. The media give many patients an unrealistic view of the effectiveness of resuscitation. Explore, "What experiences have you had with the death of a close friend or relative?" "What do you know about cardiopulmonary resuscitation (CPR)?" Educate patients about the likely success of CPR, especially if they are chronically ill or advanced in age. Assure them that relieving pain and taking care of their spiritual and physical needs will be a priority.

In general, it is important to encourage any adult, but especially the elderly or chronically ill, to establish a *health proxy* who can act as the patient's health decision maker. This part of the interview can be a "values history" that identifies what is important to the patient and makes life worth living, and when living would no longer be worthwhile. Ask how patients spend their time every day, what they enjoy, and what they look forward to. Make sure to clarify the meaning of statements like, "You said that you don't want to be a burden to your family. What exactly do you mean by that?" Explore the patient's religious or spiritual beliefs so that you and the patient can make the most appropriate decisions about health care.

See discussion of the Patient with Altered Cognition, pp. 87–89.

Ethics and Professionalism

Clinical ethics come into play scores of times each day in almost every patient interaction.[117–119] The power of clinician–patient communication calls for guidance beyond our innate sense of morality.[120] *Ethics* are a set of principles crafted through reflection and discussion to define right and wrong. *Clinical ethics,* which guide our professional behavior, are neither static nor simple, but several principles have guided clinicians throughout the ages. Although often your sense of right and wrong may be all that you need, even as students, you will face decisions that call for the application of ethical principles.

Some of the traditional and still fundamental maxims embedded in the healing professions are listed below. This body of ethics has been termed *"principalism."* As the field of clinical ethics expands, other ethical systems come in use: *utilitarianism,* or providing the greatest good for the greatest number, building on the work of John Stuart Mill; *feminist ethics,* which invoke problems of marginalization of social groups; *casuistry,* or the analysis of paradigmatic prior cases as relevant; and *communitarianism,* which emphasizes the interests of communities and societies over individuals and social responsibilities bearing on the need to maintain the institutions of civil society.[121]

Building Blocks of Professional Ethics in Patient Care

- *Nonmaleficence or primum non nocere* is commonly stated as, "First, do no harm." In the context of the interview, giving information that is incorrect or not really related to the patient's problem can do harm. Avoiding relevant topics or creating barriers to open communication can also do harm.
- *Beneficence* is the dictum that the clinician acts in the best interest of the patient.
- *Autonomy* reminds us that informed patients have the right to make their own clinical decisions. This principle has become increasingly important over time and is consistent with collaborative rather than paternalistic clinician–patient relationships.
- *Confidentiality* can be one of the most challenging principles. As a clinician, you are obligated not to repeat what you learn from or know about a patient. This privacy is fundamental to our professional relationships with patients. In the flurry of daily patient care, it is all too easy to let something slip. You must be on your guard. Note that some frameworks posit *Justice* as the fourth critical principle, namely that all patients be treated fairly with equitable distribution of health care resources.[122]

As students, you are exposed to some of the ethical challenges that you will encounter later as practicing clinicians. However, there are dilemmas unique to students that you will face from the time that you begin taking care of patients. The following vignettes capture some common experiences. They raise a variety of interconnected ethical and practical issues.

Ethics and Professionalism: Scenario 1

You are a third-year clinical student on your first clinical rotation in the hospital. It is late in the evening when you are finally assigned to the patient you are to "work up" and present the next day at preceptor rounds. You go to the patient's room and find the patient exhausted from the day's events and ready to settle down for the night. You know that your intern and attending physician have already done their evaluations. Do you proceed with a history and physical that is likely to take 1 to 2 hours? Is this process only for your education? Do you ask permission before you start? What do you include?

Here you are confronted with the tension between *the need to learn by doing* and *doing no harm to patients*. There is a utilitarian ethical principle that reminds us that if clinicians-in-training do not learn, there will be no future caregivers. Yet, the dictums to do no harm and prioritize what is in the patient's best interests are clearly in conflict with that future need. This dilemma will arise often while you are a student.

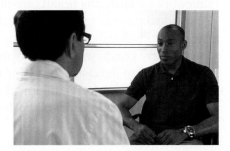

The means to address this ethical dilemma is to obtain *informed consent*. Always make sure the patient realizes that you are in training and new at patient evaluation (Fig. 3-10). It is impressive how often patients willingly let students be involved in their care; it is an opportunity for patients to give back to their caregivers. Even when clinical activities appear purely for educational purposes, there may be a benefit to the patient. Multiple caregivers provide multiple perspectives, and the experience of being heard and having a special advocate can be therapeutic.

FIGURE 3-10. Obtain informed consent from patients when needed.

Ethics and Professionalism: Scenario 2

It is after 10 PM, and you and your resident are on the way to complete the required advance directives form with a frail, elderly patient who was admitted earlier that day with bilateral pneumonia. The form, which includes a discussion of DNR orders, must be completed before the team can sign out and leave for the day. Just then, your resident is paged to an emergency and asks you to go ahead and meet with the patient to complete the form; the resident will cosign it later. You had a lecture on advance directives and end-of-life discussions in your first year of training, but have never seen a clinician discuss these issues with a patient. You have not yet met the patient, nor have you had a chance to really look at the form. What should you do? Do you inform the resident that you have never done this before or even seen it done? Do you inform the patient that this is totally new for you? Who should decide whether you are competent to do this independently?

In this situation, you are being asked to take responsibility for clinical care that exceeds your level of comfort and perhaps your competence. This can happen in a number of situations, such as being asked to evaluate a clinical situation without proper back-up or to draw blood or start an IV before practicing under supervision. You may have many of the following thoughts about this patient: "the patient needs to have this completed before going to sleep and so will benefit"; "the risk to the patient from discussing advance directives is minimal"; "you are pretty good with elderly patients and think that you might be able to do this"; "what if the patient actually arrests that night and you are responsible for what happens?"; and finally, "if you bother the resident now, he or she will be angry and that may affect your evaluation." There is educational value in being pushed to the limits of your knowledge to solve problems and to gain confidence in functioning independently. But what is the right thing to do in this situation?

The principles listed on page 100 only partially help you sort this out, because only part of your quandary relates to your relationship with the patient. Much of the tension in this scenario involves the dynamics of a health care team and your role as a team member. You are there to help with the work, but you are primarily there to learn. Current formulations of clinical ethics address those issues and others. One such formulation is the *Tavistock Principles*.[123] These principles construct a framework for analyzing health care situations that extend beyond our direct care of individual patients to complicated choices about the interactions of health care teams and the distribution of resources for the well-being of society. A broadly representative group, which initially met in Tavistock Square in London in 1998, has continued to develop an evolving document of ethical principles for guiding health care behavior for both individuals and institutions across the health care spectrum. A current iteration of the Tavistock Principles follows.

The Tavistock Principles

Rights: People have a right to health and health care.
Balance: Care of the individual patient is central, but the health of populations is also our concern.
Comprehensiveness: In addition to treating illness, we have an obligation to ease suffering, minimize disability, prevent disease, and promote health.
Cooperation: Health care succeeds only if we cooperate with those we serve, each other, and those in other sectors.
Improvement: Improving health care is a serious and continuing responsibility.
Safety: Do no harm.
Openness: Being open, honest, and trustworthy is vital in health care.

In the second scenario, think about the Tavistock Principles of *openness and cooperation,* in addition to the balance between *do no harm* and *beneficence.* You need to work with your team in a way that is honest and reliable to do the best for the patient (Fig. 3-11). You can also see that there are no clear or easy answers in such situations. What responses are available to you to address these and other quandaries?

You need to reflect on your beliefs and assess your level of comfort with a given situation. Sometimes there may be alternative solutions. For example, in Scenario 1,

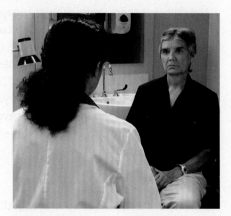

FIGURE 3-11. Apply ethical principles to difficult decisions.

the patient may really be willing to have the history and physical examination at that late hour, or perhaps you can negotiate a time for the next morning. In Scenario 2, you might find another person who is more qualified to complete the form or supervise you. Alternatively, you may choose to go ahead and complete the form, focusing on open communication, and alerting the patient to your inexperience while obtaining the patient's consent. You will need to choose when situations warrant voicing your concerns, even at the risk of a bad evaluation.

Seek coaching on how to express your reservations in a way that ensures that they will be heard. As a clinical student, you will need settings for discussing these immediately relevant ethical dilemmas with other students and with more senior trainees and faculty. Small groups that are structured to address these kinds of issues are particularly useful in providing validation and support. Take advantage of such opportunities whenever possible.

Ethics and Professionalism: Scenario 3

You are the student on the clinical team that has been taking care of Ms. Robbins, a 64-year-old woman admitted for an evaluation of weight loss and weakness. During the hospitalization, she had a biopsy of a mass in her chest in addition to many other tests. You have gotten to know her well, spending a lot of time with her to answer questions, explain procedures, and learn about her and her family. You have discussed her fears about what "they" will find and know that she likes to know everything possible about her health and clinical care. You have even heard her express frustration with her attending physician at not always getting the "straight story." It is late Friday afternoon, but you promised Ms. Robbins that you would come by one more time before the weekend and let her know if her biopsy results were back yet. Just before you go to her room, the resident tells you that the pathology is back from her biopsy and shows metastatic cancer, but the attending physician does not want the team to say anything until he comes in on Monday.

What are you going to do? You feel that it is wrong to avoid the situation by not going to her room. You also believe that the patient's preference and anxiety are best served by not waiting for 3 days. You do not want to go against the attending physician's clear instructions, however, because you respect the fact that it is his patient.

In this situation, telling the patient about her biopsy results is dictated by several ethical principles: the patient's best interests, autonomy, and your integrity. The other part of the ethical dilemma concerns communicating your plan to the attending. Sometimes, the most challenging part of such dilemmas tests your will to follow through with the right course of action. Although it may appear to be a lose–lose situation, a respectful and honest discussion with the attending, articulating what is in the patient's best interest, will usually be heard. Enlist the support of your resident or other helpful attendings if that is possible. Learning how to navigate difficult discussions will be a useful professional skill.

Table 3-1 Motivational Interviewing: A Clinical Example

The police brought a 40-year-old woman to the psychiatric emergency room because while intoxicated she threatened to kill her partner and herself. She had no history of violence or of legal or psychiatric problems. When she became sober the next day, she reported calmly that she was an alcoholic and was not violent and had no intention of hurting herself. She wanted to be discharged. The typical psychiatric approach to this problem would be a combination of education and confrontation; the psychiatrist would explain the dangers of alcoholism to the patient and encourage her to seek treatment, handing her a list of alcohol treatment centers.

In contrast, the actual motivational interviewing (MI) conversation proceeded like this:

Patient: I am an alcoholic and don't want to change. I am not dangerous; just let me go home now.

Psychiatrist: OK, that's what we'll do. We can't force you to change. Can I just ask you a few questions and then we'll let you out of here?

(MI: Respect for autonomy—the psychiatrist respects the individual's right to change or not make a change; collaboration—the psychiatrist is equal to the patient in power and asks permission for further inquiry.)

Patient: OK.

Psychiatrist: I am interested in learning a little about your drinking. I understand you don't want to change. So I am assuming that the alcohol is mostly a good thing in your life. I am wondering if there is anything not so good about the alcohol in your life?

(MI: Elicit ambivalence)

Patient: Well, they said my liver is not so good anymore. It's going to fail if I don't stop drinking.

Psychiatrist: OK, so that sounds like one part of the drinking that is not so good.

(MI: Explore ambivalence)

Patient: Right.

Psychiatrist: But it doesn't sound important enough to make you want to change. I'm guessing that you don't care so much whether your liver fails or not.

(MI: Not at all sarcastic here; really respecting her autonomy)

Patient: Well, I can't live without a liver.

Psychiatrist: OK. Then it sounds like you don't care much whether you live or die.

(MI: Again, not at all sarcastic; simply reflecting content and respecting autonomy)

Patient: No way! I love life!

Psychiatrist: Well, I'm not sure I understand then. On the one hand, you are very sure that you are not going to stop drinking, yet you also say you love life and don't want your liver to fail.

(MI: Develop discrepancy. Elicit change talk.)

Patient: Well, I know I'm going to have to cut down or stop sometime. This is just not the time.

Psychiatrist: OK. I hear what you are saying. You want to stop drinking at some point, to save your liver and save your life—it's just not the right time now.

(MI: Listen, understand, express empathy, and reflect feelings; respect autonomy.)

Patient: Right.

Psychiatrist: OK. Can I ask another question or two?…If you do think you're going to stop at some point, I wonder what thoughts you've had about when and how you would like to stop drinking? Would you want or need any help if and when you decided to cut down or stop drinking?

(MI: Open questions for understanding; encourage change talk.)

Source: Cole S, Bogenschutz M, Hungerford M. Motivational interviewing and psychiatry: use in addiction treatment, risky drinking and routine practice. *Focus* IX:42–52, 2011.

Table 3-2 Brief Action Planning (BAP)—A Self-Management Support Tool

Brief Action Planning is structured around three core questions

1. _____ Elicit person's preferences/desires for behavior change.

   "Is there anything you would like to do for your health in the next week or two?"

   _____ What?

   _____ Where?

   _____ When?

   _____ How often?

   _____ Elicit commitment statement

   "Just to make sure we understand each other, would you please tell me back what you've decided to do?"

2. _____ Evaluate confidence

   "I wonder how confident you feel about carrying out your plan. Considering a scale of 0 to 10, where '0' means you are not at all confident and '10' means you are very confident, about how confident do you feel?"

   (If the confidence level is less than 7, problem-solve how to overcome barriers or adjust the plan. *"5 is great. A lot higher than zero. I wonder if there is any way we might modify the plan to get you to a level of '7' or more? Maybe we could make the goal a little easier, or you could ask for help from a friend or family member, or even think of something else that might help you feel more confident?"*

3. _____ Arrange a follow-up (or accountability).

   "Sounds like a plan that's going to work for you. When would you like to check in with me to review how you're doing with your plan?"

Source: Steven Cole, Damara Gutnick, Connie Davis, Kathy Reims, Mary Cole BAP is a registered trademark of Steven Cole. ©2004–2012. Stevecolemd@gmail. com. All rights reserved. BAP may be used in clinical practice, research, and education without permission. For further information, go to www.ComprehensiveMI. com and www.centreCMI.ca. See also Gutnick D, Reims K, et al. Brief Action Planning to facilitate behavior change and support for self-management. *JCOM* 2014;1:17. Available at http://www.centrecmi.ca/about-us/publications/. Accessed January 19, 2015. Originally developed circa 2004 by Steven Cole, with contributions by Mary Cole. Current version was developed with contributions from Damara Gutnick, Connie Davis, and Kathy Reims.

References

1. Suchman AL, Matthews DA. What makes the patient doctor relationship therapeutic? Exploring the connectional dimension of medical care. *Ann Intern Med.* 1988;108:125.

2. Matthews DA, Suchman AL, Branch WT. Making "connexions": enhancing the therapeutic potential of patient-clinician relationships. *Ann Intern Med.* 1993;118:973.

3. Larson EB, Yao X. Clinical empathy as emotional labor in the patient-physician relationship. *JAMA.* 2005;293:1100.

4. Krasner MS, Epstein RM, Beckman H, et al. Association of an educational program in mindful communication with burnout, empathy, and attitudes among primary care physicians. *JAMA.* 2009;302:1284.

5. Stewart MA. Effective physician-patient communication and health outcomes: a review. *CMAJ.* 1995;152:1423.

6. Dambha H, Griffin S, Kinmonth AL. Patient-centered care in general practice. InnovAIT, 0(0),1. doi:10.1177/1755738014544482.

7. Reiss H, Kraft-Todd G. E.M.P.A.T.H.Y.: A tool to enhance nonverbal communication between clinicians and their patients. *Acad Med.* 2014;89:1108.

8. Fortin AH VI, Dwamena FC, Frankel RM, et al. *Smith's Patient-Centered Interviewing. An Evidence-Based Method.* 3rd ed. Philadelphia, PA: McGraw Hill; 2012.

9. Smith RC. An evidence-based infrastructure for patient-centered interviewing. In: Frankel FM, Quill TE, McDaniel SH eds. *The Biopsychosocial Approach: Past, Present, and Future.* Rochester, NY: University of Rochester Press; 2003:149.

10. Haidet P, Paterniti DA. "Building" a History Rather Than "Taking" One: A Perspective on Information Sharing During the Medical Interview. *Arch Intern Med.* 2003;163:1134.

11. Stewart M. Questions about patient-centered care: answers from quantitative research. In: Stewart M, et al. eds. *Patient-centered Medicine: Transforming the Clinical Method.* Abington, UK: Radcliffe Medical Press; 2003:263.

12. Atlas SJ, Grant RW, Ferris TG, et al. Patient-physician connectedness and the quality of primary care. *Ann Intern Med.* 2009;150:325.

13. Haidet P. Jazz and the "Art" of Medicine: Improvisation in the Medical Encounter. *Ann Fam Med.* 2007;5:164.

14. Behfourouz HL, Drain PK, Rhatigan JJ. Rethinking the social history. *N Engl J Med.* 2014;371:1277.

15. Wagner EH, Austin BT, Korff MV. Organizing care for patients with chronic illness. *Milbank Q.* 1996;74:511.

16. Coulehan JL, Block MR. *The Medical Interview: Mastering Skills for Clinical Practice.* 5th ed. Philadelphia, PA: F.A. Davis Company; 2006.

17. Halpern J. What is clinical empathy? *J Gen Intern Med.* 2003;18:670.

18. Halpern J. Empathy and patient-physician conflicts. *J Gen Intern Med.* 2007;22:696.

19. Buckman R, Tulsky JA, Rodin G. Empathic responses in clinical practice: intuition or tuition? *CMAJ.* 2011;183:569.

20. Egnew TR. Suffering, meaning, and healing: challenges of contemporary medicine. *Ann Fam Med.* 2009;2:170.

21. Batt-Rawden SA, Chisholm MS, Anton B, et al. Teaching empathy to medical students: an updated, systematic review. *Acad Med.* 2013;88:1171.

22. Epner DE, Baile W. Difficult conversations: teaching medical oncology trainees communication skills one hour at a time. *Acad Med.* 2014;89:578.

23. Lipkin M Jr, Putnam SM, Lazare A, et al. eds. *The Medical Interview: Clinical Care, Education, and Research.* New York: Springer-Verlag; 1995.

24. Tomsik PE, Witt AM, Raddock ML, et al. How well do physician and patient visit priorities align? *J Fam Prac.* 2014;63:E8.

25. Makoul G, Zick A, Green M. An evidence-based perspective on greetings in medical encounters. *Arch Int Med.* 2007;167:1172.

26. Platt FW, Gaspar DL, Coulehan JL, et al. "Tell me about yourself": the patient-centered interview. *Ann Intern Med.* 2001;134:1079.

27. Ventres W, Kooienga S, Vuvkovic N, et al. Physicians, patients and the electronic health record: an ethnographic analysis. *Ann Fam Med.* 2006;4:124.

28. Beckman HB, Frankel RM. The effect of physician behavior on the collection of data. *Ann Intern Med.* 1984;101:692.

29. Kleinman A, Eisenberg L, Good B. Culture, illness, and care: clinical lessons from anthropological and cross-cultural research. *Ann Intern Med.* 1978;88:251.

30. Mausch L, Farber S, Greer HT. Design, dissemination, and evaluation of an advanced communication elective at seven U.S. medical schools. *Acad Med.* 2013;88:843.

31. Jackson JL, Passamonti M, Kroenke K. Outcome and impact of mental disorders in primary care at 5 years. *Psychosom Med.* 2007;69:270.

32. Lang F, Floyd MR, Beine KL. Clues to patients' explanations and concerns about their illnesses: a call for active listening. *Arch Fam Med.* 2000;9:222.

33. Communication: What do patients want and need? *J Oncol Pract.* 2008;4(5):249. doi:10.1200/JOP.0856501 PMCID: PMC2794010

34. Pollak KI, Arnold RM, Jeffreys AS, et al. Oncologist communication about emotion during visits with patients with advanced cancer. *J Clin Oncol.* 2007;25(36):5748.

35. Croskerry P. The importance of cognitive errors in diagnosis and strategies to minimize them. *Acad Med.* 2003;78:775.

36. Barry MJ, Edgman-Levitan S. Shared decision making–pinnacle of patient-centered care. *New Engl J Med.* 2012;366:780.

37. Elwyn G, Frosch D, Thomson R, et al. Shared decision-making: a model for clinical practice. *J Gen Int Med.* 2012;27:1361.

38. Rollnick S, Butler CC, Kinnersly P, et al. Motivational interviewing. *BMJ.* 2010;340:c1900.

39. Cole S, Bogenschutz M, Hungerford M. Motivational interviewing and psychiatry: use in addiction treatment, risky drinking and routine practice. *Focus.* 2011;IX:42.

40. Hettema J, Steele J, Miller WR. Motivational interviewing. *Ann Rev Clin Psychol.* 2005;1:91.

41. Lundahl B, Moleni T, Burke BL, et al. Motivational interviewing in medical care settings: a systematic review and meta-analysis of randomized controlled trial. *Patient Educ Couns.* 2013;93:157.

42. Kripalani S, Jackson AT, Schnipper JL, et al. Promoting effective transitions of care at hospital discharge: A review of key issues for hospitalists. *J Hosp Med.* 2007;2:314.

43. Kemp EC, Floyd MR, McCord-Duncan E, et al. Patients prefer the method of "Tell back-collaborative inquiry" to assess understanding of medical information. *J Am Board Fam Med.* 2008;21:24.

44. Epstein RM. Mindful practice. *JAMA.* 1999;282:833.

45. Beach MC, Roter D, Korthuis PT, et al. A multicenter study of physician mindfulness and health care quality. *Ann Fam Med.* 2013;11:421.

46. Smedley BA, Stith AY, Nelson AR, eds. *Committee on Understanding and Eliminating Racial and Ethnic Disparities in Health Care. Unequal Treatment: Confronting Racial and Ethnic Disparities in Health Care.* Washington, DC: Institute of Medicine; 2003.

47. Agency for Healthcare Research and Quality. U.S. Department of Health and Human Services. 2013 National Healthcare Disparities

REFERENCES

Report. Available at http://www.ahrq.gov/research/findings/nhqrdr/nhdr13/index.html. Accessed January 17, 2015.

48. Like RC. Educating clinicians about cultural competence and disparities in health and health care. *J Contin Educ Health Prof.* 2011;31:196.

49. Boutin-Foster C, Foster JC, Konopasek L. Viewpoint: physician, know thyself: the professional culture of medicine as a framework for teaching cultural competence. *Acad Med.* 2008;83:106.

50. Teal CR, Street RL. Critical elements of culturally competent communication in the medical encounter: a review and model. *Soc Sci Med.* 2009;68:533.

51. Management Sciences for Health. The Providers' Guide to Quality and Culture. What is cultural competence. Available at http://erc.msh.org/mainpage.cfm?file=1.0.htm&module=provider&language=English. Accessed January 17, 2015.

52. Silliman J, Fried MG, Ross L, et al. *Ch. 1, Women of Color and Their Struggles for Reproductive Justice, in Undivided Rights–Women of Color Organize for Reproductive Justice.* Cambridge, MA: South End Press; 2004:6.

53. Kumas-Tan Z, Beagan B, Loppie C, et al. Measures of cultural competence: examining hidden assumptions. *Acad Med.* 2007;82:548.

54. Tervalon M, Murray-Garcia J. Cultural humility versus cultural competence: a critical distinction in defining physician training outcomes in multicultural education. *J Health Care Poor Underserved.* 1998;9:117.

55. Tervalon M. Components of culture in health for medical students' education. *Acad Med.* 2003;78:570.

56. Smith WR, Betancourt JR, Wynia MK, et al. Recommendations for teaching about racial and ethnic disparities in health and health care. *Ann Intern Med.* 2007;147:654.

57. Center for Cultural Competence. Georgetown University Center for Child and Human Development. Available at http://nccc.georgetown.edu/index.html. See also Self Assessments at http://nccc.georgetown.edu/resources/assessments.html, Accessed January 18, 2015.

58. Juarez JA, Marvel K, Brezinski KL, et al. Bridging the gap: a curriculum to teach residents cultural humility. *Fam Med.* 2006;38:97.

59. National Consortium for Multicultural Education for Health Professionals. Available at http://culturalmeded.stanford.edu./ Accessed January 18, 2015.

60. Jacobs EA, Rolle I, Ferrans CE, et al. Understanding African Americans' views of the trustworthiness of physicians. *J Gen Intern Med.* 2006;21:642.

61. Office for Civil Rights–Health Insurance Portability and Accountability Act of 1996 (HIPAA), U.S. Department of Health and Human Services. Available at http://www.hhs.gov/ocr/privacy/index.html. Accessed January 18, 2015.

62. Sessums LL, Zembrzuska H, Jackson JL. Does this patient have medical decision-making capacity? *JAMA.* 2011;306:420.

63. Joint Centre for Bioethics, University of Toronto. The Aid to Capacity Evaluation (ACE). At http://www.jcb.utoronto.ca/tools/ace_download.shtml. Accessed January 15, 2015.

64. Markowitz JC, Milrod BL. The importance of responding to negative affect in psychotherapies. *Am J Psychiatry.* 2011;168:124.

65. Ryan C. American Community Survey Reports, United States Census Bureau. Language use in the United States, 2011. Issued August 2013. Available at www.census.gov/prod/2013oubs/acc-22.pdg. Accessed January 18, 2015.

66. Karliner LS, Jacobs EA, Chen AH, et al. Do professional interpreters improve clinical care for patients with limited English proficiency? A systematic review of the literature. *Health Serv Res.* 2007;42:727.

67. Thompson DA, Hernandez RG, Cowden JD, et al. Caring for patients with limited English proficiency: are residents prepared to use medical interpreters? *Acad Med.* 2013;88:1485.

68. Schyve PM. Language differences as a barrier to quantity and safety in health care: the Joint Commission perspective. *J Gen Int Med.* 2007;22(Suppl 2):360.

69. Jacobs EA, Sadowski LS, Rathous PJ. The impact of enhanced interpreter service intervention on hospital costs and patient satisfaction. *J Gen Intern Med.* 2007;22 (Suppl 2):306.

70. Hardt E, Jacobs EA, Chen A. Insights into the problems that language barriers may pose for the medical interview. *J Gen Intern Med.* 2006;21:1357.

71. Office of Minority Health, Department of Health and Human Services. Think Cultural Health. CLAS Standards; Communication Tools. Available at https://www.thinkculturalhealth.hhs.gov/content/clas.asp. Accessed January 18, 2015.

72. Brady AK. Medical Spanish. *Ann Intern Med.* 2010;152:127.

73. Gregg J, Saha S. Communicative competence: a framework for understanding language barriers in health care. *J Gen Int Med.* 2007;22(Suppl 2):368.

74. Saha S, Fernandez A. Language barriers in health care. *J Gen Int Med.* 2007;22(Suppl 2):281.

75. National Center for Education Statistics. National Assessment of Health Literacy, 2003 Survey. Available at http://nces.ed.gov/naal/kf_demographics.asp. Accessed January 19, 2015.

76. Berkman ND, Sheridan SL, Donahue KE, et al. Low health literacy and health outcomes: an updated systematic review. *Ann Intern Med.* 2011;155:97.

77. Meador HE, Zazove P. Health care interactions with deaf culture. *J Am Board Fam Pract.* 2005;18:218.

78. Barnett S, Klein JD, Pollard RQ Jr, et al. Community participatory research with deaf sign language users to identify health inequities. *Am J Public Health.* 2011;101:2235.

79. Committee on Ethics, American College of Obstetricians and Gynecologists. ACOG Committee Opinion No. 373: Sexual misconduct. *Obstet Gynecol.* 2007;110(2 Pt 1):441.

80. Nadelson C, Notman MT. Boundaries in the doctor-patient relationship. *Theor Med Bioeth.* 2002;23:191.

81. Gabbard GO, Nadelson C. Professional boundaries in the physician-patient relationship. *JAMA.* 1995;273(18):1445.

82. Council on Ethical and Judicial Affairs. American Medical Association: sexual misconduct in the practice of medicine. *JAMA.* 1991;266:2741.

83. Coverdale JH, Franz CP, Balon R, et al. Teaching sexual history-taking: a systematic review of educational programs. *Acad Med.* 2011;86:1590.

84. Shindel AW, Ando KA, Nelson CJ, et al. Medical student sexuality: How sexual experience and sexuality training impact U.S. and Canadian medical students' comfort in dealing with patients' sexuality in clinical practice. *Acad Med.* 2010;85:1321.

85. U.S. Preventive Services Task Force. Screening for depression: recommendations and rationale. 2002 (update pending). Available at http://www.uspreventiveservicestaskforce.org/Page/Document/RecommendationStatementFinal/depression-in-adults-screening. Accessed January 19, 2015.

86. Substance Abuse and Mental Health Services Administration, Department of Health and Human Services. Results from the 2013 National Survey on Drug Use and Health: Summary of National Findings. Available at http://www.samhsa.gov/data/sites/default/files/NSDUHresultsPDFWHTML2013/Web/NSDUHresults2013.pdf. Accessed January 15, 2015.

87. Medline Plus, National Institutes of Health. Prescription drug abuse: a fast-growing problem. Available at http://www.nlm.nih.gov/medlineplus/magazine/issues/fall11/articles/fall11pg21.html. Accessed January 19, 2015.

88. American Pain Society. Definitions Related to the Use of Opioids for the Treatment of Pain. A consensus statement from the American Academy of Pain Medicine, the American Pain Society, and the American Society of Addiction Medicine, 2001. Available at http://www.asam.org/docs/publicy-policy-statements/1opioid-definitions-consensus-2–011.pdf?sfvrsn=0. Accessed January 15, 2015.

89. Cyr MG, Wartman SA. The effectiveness of routine screening questions in the detection of alcoholism. *JAMA.* 1988;259:51.

90. U.S. Preventive Services Task Force. Screening and behavioral counseling interventions in primary care to reduce alcohol misuse: recommendation statement. May 2013. Available at http://www.uspreventiveservicestaskforce.org/Page/Document/RecommendationStatementFinal/alcohol-misuse-screening-and-behavioral-counseling-interventions-in-primary-care. Accessed January 19, 2015.

91. Ewing JA. Detecting alcoholism: the CAGE questionnaire. *JAMA.* 1984;252:1905.

92. Friedman PD. Clinical practice. Alcohol use in adults. *New Engl J Med.* 2013;368:325.

93. National Institute on Drug Abuse. Screening for drug use in general medical settings. Updated March 2102. Available at http://www.drugabuse.gov/publications/resource-guide-screening-drug-use-in-general-medical-settings/nida-quick-screen. Accessed January 19, 2015.

94. Smith PC, Schmidt SM, Allensworth-Davies D, et al. A single-question screening test for drug use in primary care. *Arch Intern Med.* 2010;170:1155.

95. Hewitt LN, Bhavsar P, Phelan HA. The secrets women keep: intimate partner violence screening in the female trauma patient. *J Trauma.* 2011;70:320.

96. Centers for Disease Control and Prevention. Understanding intimate partner violence. Fact sheet 2014. Available at http://www.cdc.gov/violenceprevention/pub/ipv_factsheet.html. Accessed January 19, 2015.

97. Ahmad F, Hogg-Johnson S, Stewart DR, at al. Computer-assisted screening for intimate partner violence and control: a randomized trial. *Ann Intern Med.* 2009;151:93.

98. Rees S, Silove D, Chey T, et al. Lifetime prevalence of gender-based violence in women and the relationship with mental disorders and psychosocial function. *JAMA.* 2011;306:513.

99. Daugherty JD, Houry DE. Intimate partner violence screening in the emergency department. *J Postgrad Med.* 2008;54(4):301.

100. Praise Investigators, Sprague S, Bhandari M, et al. Prevalence of abuse and intimate partner violence surgical evaluation (PRAISE) in orthopaedic fracture clinics: a multinational prevalence study. *Lancet.* 2013;382:866.

101. U.S. Preventive Services Task Force. Intimate partner violence and abuse of elderly and vulnerable adults: screening. January 2013. Available at http://www.uspreventiveservicestaskforce.org/Page/Document/RecommendationStatementFinal/intimate-partner-violence-and-abuse-of-elderly-and-vulnerable-adults-screening. Accessed January 19, 2015.

102. Moracco KE, Cole TB. Preventing intimate partner violence. Screening is not enough. *JAMA.* 2009;302:568.

103. Acierno R, Hernandez MA, Amstadter AB, et al. Prevalence and correlates of emotional, physical, sexual, and financial abuse and potential neglect in the United States: the National Elder Mistreatment Study. *Am J Public Health.* 2010;100(2):292.

104. Samaras N, Chevalley T, Samaras D, et al. Older patients in the emergency department: a review. *Ann Emerg Med.* 2010;56:261.

105. Mosqueda L, Dong X. Elder abuse and self-neglect: "I don't care anything about going to the doctor, to be honest…". *JAMA.* 2011;306:532.

106. Alpert EJ. Addressing domestic violence: the (long) road ahead. *Ann Intern Med.* 2007;147:666.

107. World Health Organization. Responding to intimate partner violence and sexual violence against women. WHO clinical and policy guidelines, 2013. Available at http://www.who.int/reproductivehealth/publications/violence/9789241548595/en/. Accessed January 19, 2015.

108. Hossain M, Zimmerman C, Abas M, et al. The relationship of trauma to mental disorders among trafficked and sexually exploited girls and women. *Am J Public Health.* 2010;100:2442.

109. Logan TK, Walker R, Hunt G. Understanding human trafficking in the United States. *Trauma Violence Abuse.* 2009;10:3.

110. National Consensus Project for Quality Palliative Care. Clinical practice guidelines for quality palliative care. 3rd ed. 2013. Available at http://www.nationalconsensusproject.org/guidelines_download2.aspx. Accessed January 14, 2015.

111. Agency for Healthcare Research and Quality. Improving health care and palliative care for advanced and serious illness. Closing the quality gap. October 2012. Available at http://www.ahrq.gov/research/findings/evidence-based-reports/gappallcaretp.html. Accessed January 14, 2015.

112. Bakitas M, Lyons KD, Hegel MT, et al. Effects of a palliative care intervention on clinical outcomes in patients with advanced cancer: the Project ENABLE II randomized controlled trial. *JAMA.* 2009;302:741.

113. Casarett D, Pickard A, Bailey FA, et al. Do palliative consultations improve patient outcomes? *J Am Geriatr Soc.* 2008;56:593.

114. Maciejewski PK, Zhang B, Block SD, et al. An empirical examination of the stage theory of grief. *JAMA.* 2007;297:16.

115. Kübler-Ross E. *On Death and Dying.* New York: Macmillan; 1997.

116. World Health Organization. WHO Definition of Palliative Care. Available at http://www.who.int/cancer/palliative/definition/en/. Accessed January 14, 2015.

117. Manthous CA. Introducing the primer of medical ethics. *Chest.* 2006;130:1640.

118. Carrese JA, Sugarman J. The inescapable relevance of bioethics for the practicing clinician. *Chest.* 2006;1230:1864.

119. Swetz KM, Crowley ME, Hook C, et al. Report of 255 clinical ethics consultations and review of the literature. *Mayo Clin Proc.* 2007;82:686.

120. ABIM Foundation, American Board of Internal Medicine, ACP-ASIM Foundation, American College of Physicians-American Society of Internal Medicine, European Federation of Internal Medicine. Medical professionalism in the new millennium: a physician charter. *Ann Intern Med.* 2002;136:243.

121. Giordano J. *The Ethics Of Interventional Pain Management: Basic Concepts And Theories: Problems And Practice.* Lubbock, TX: Presentation, Texas Tech University Health Sciences Center; 2008.

122. *President's Commission for the Study of Ethical Problems in Medicine and Biomedical and Behavioral Research. Making health care decisions: The legal and ethical implications of informed consent in the patient-practitioner relationship.* Washington, DC: United States Government Printing Office; 1982.

123. Berwick D, Davidoff F, Hiatt H, et al. Refining and implementing the Tavistock principles for everybody in health care. *BMJ.* 2001;323(7313):616.

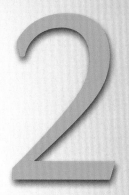

Regional Examinations

Beginning the Physical Examination: General Survey, Vital Signs, and Pain

The Bates' suite offers these additional resources to enhance learning and facilitate understanding of this chapter:

■ Bates' *Pocket Guide to Physical Examination and History Taking*, 8th edition
■ Bates' *Visual Guide to Physical Examination* (Vol. 5: General Survey and Vital Signs)
■ thePoint online resources, for students and instructors: http://thepoint.lww.com

Now that you have elicited the patient's concerns and formed a trusting relationship, you are ready to begin the physical examination. At first you may feel unsure of your skills, but through study and repetition, the physical examination will soon flow more smoothly, and you will shift your attention from technique and how to handle instruments to what you hear, see, and feel (Fig. 4-1). Touching the patient's body will seem more natural, and you will learn to minimize any discomfort to the patient (Fig. 4-2). As you gain proficiency, what once took between 1 and 2 hours will take considerably less time.

This chapter introduces the sections of the regional examination chapters you will find throughout the book: *The Health History* of Common and Concerning Symptoms (in this chapter, these are common constitutional symptoms); *Health Promotion and Counseling,* which focuses in this chapter on lifestyle components such as weight, nutrition, and exercise; then, *Techniques of Examination,* which include the initial elements of the physical examination, the General Survey, Vital Signs, and assessment of pain; followed by *Tables* and the *References.* The regional examination chapters, Chapters 6 through 20, begin with an additional section, *Anatomy and Physiology.*

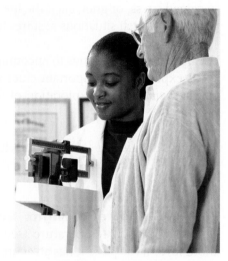

FIGURE 4-1. **The physical examination flows more efficiently with practice.**

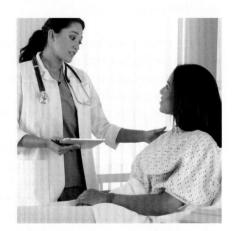

FIGURE 4-2. **The clinician's touch can reassure as well as assess.**

The Health History

Common or Concerning Symptoms

- Fatigue and weakness
- Fever, chills, night sweats
- Weight change
- Pain

Fatigue and Weakness. *Fatigue* is a nonspecific symptom with many causes. It refers to a sense of weariness or loss of energy that patients describe in various ways. "I don't feel like getting up in the morning"..."I don't have any energy"..."I can hardly get through the day"..."By the time I get to work, I feel as if I've done a day's work." Because fatigue is a normal response to hard work, sustained stress, or grief, elicit the life circumstances in which it occurs. Fatigue unrelated to such situations requires further investigation.

Use open-ended questions to encourage the patient to fully describe what he or she is experiencing. Important clues about etiology often emerge from a good psychosocial history, exploration of sleep patterns, and a thorough review of systems.

Weakness is different from fatigue. It denotes a demonstrable loss of muscle power and will be discussed later with other neurologic symptoms (see p. 723).

Fever, Chills, and Night Sweats. *Fever* refers to an abnormal elevation in body temperature (see p. 133 for definitions of normal). Ask about fever if the patient has an acute or chronic illness. Find out if the patient has measured his or her temperature. Has the patient felt feverish or unusually hot, noted excessive sweating, or felt chilly and cold? Try to distinguish between *feeling cold,* and a *shaking chill* with shivering throughout the body and chattering of teeth.

Feeling cold, goosebumps, and shivering accompany a rising temperature, whereas feeling hot and sweating accompanies a falling temperature. Normally, the body temperature rises during the day and falls during the night. When fever exaggerates this swing, *night sweats* occur. Malaise, headache, and pain in the muscles and joints often accompany fever.

Fever has many causes. Focus on the timing of the illness and its associated symptoms. Become familiar with patterns of infectious diseases that may affect your patient. Inquire about travel, contact with sick people, or other unusual exposures. Even medications may cause fever. By contrast, recent ingestion of aspirin, acetaminophen, corticosteroids, and nonsteroidal anti-inflammatory drugs may mask fever and affect the temperature recorded at the office visit.

Fatigue is a common symptom of depression and anxiety, but also consider *infections* (such as hepatitis, infectious mononucleosis, and tuberculosis); *endocrine disorders* (hypothyroidism, adrenal insufficiency, diabetes mellitus); heart failure; chronic disease of the lungs, kidneys, or liver; electrolyte imbalance; moderate to severe anemia; malignancies; nutritional deficits; and medications.

Weakness, especially if localized in a neuroanatomical pattern, suggests possible *neuropathy* or *myopathy.*

Recurrent shaking chills suggest more extreme swings in temperature and systemic *bacteremia.*

Feeling hot and sweating also accompany menopause. Night sweats occur in *tuberculosis* and *malignancy.*

In immunocompromised patients with sepsis, fever may be absent, low-grade, or drop below normal (*hypothermia*).

Weight Change.   Weight change results from changes in body tissues or body fluid. Good opening questions include "How often do you check your weight?" "How is it compared to a year ago?" If there are changes, ask, "Why do you think it has changed?" "What would you like to weigh?" If weight gain or loss appears to be a problem, ask about the amount of change, its timing, the setting in which it occurred, and any associated symptoms.

Weight gain occurs when caloric intake exceeds caloric expenditure over time, and typically results in increased body fat. Weight gain can also reflect abnormal accumulation of body fluids, particularly when the gain is very rapid.

Patients with a body mass index (BMI) of ≥25 to 29 are defined as *overweight;* those with a BMI ≥30 are considered *obese.* For these patients, plan a thorough assessment to avert the many associated risks of morbidity and mortality. Clarify the timing and evolution of the weight gain. Was the patient overweight as a child? Are the parents overweight? Ask about weight at life milestones like birth, kindergarten, high school or college graduation, military discharge, pregnancy, menopause, and retirement. Has a recent disability or surgery affected weight? What about depression or anxiety? Is there a change in sleep pattern or daytime drowsiness suspicious for sleep apnea?[1] Establish the level of physical activity and results of prior attempts at weight loss. Assess eating patterns and dietary preferences.

Review the patient's medications.

Explore any clinically significant *weight loss,* defined as loss of 5% or more of usual body weight over a 6-month period. Mechanisms include decreased food intake due to anorexia, depression, dysphagia, vomiting, abdominal pain, or financial difficulties; defective gastrointestinal absorption or inflammation; and increased metabolic requirements. Ask about abuse of alcohol, cocaine, amphetamines, or opiates, or withdrawal from marijuana, all associated with weight loss. Heavy smoking also suppresses appetite.

Assess food intake. Has it been normal, dropped, or even increased?

Rapid changes in weight, over a few days, suggest changes in body fluid, not tissue.

Edema from extravascular fluid retention is visible in *heart failure, nephrotic syndrome, liver failure,* and *venous stasis.*

See Classification of Overweight and Obesity by BMI on p. 116.

See Table 4-1, Obesity-Related Health Conditions, p. 139, and discussion on pp. 114–118.

Many drugs are associated with weight gain, such as: tricyclic antidepressants; insulin and sulfonylurea; contraceptives, glucocorticoids, and progestational steroids; mirtazapine and paroxetine; gabapentin and valproate; and propranolol.

Causes of weight loss include gastrointestinal diseases; endocrine disorders (*diabetes mellitus, hyperthyroidism, adrenal insufficiency*); chronic infections, HIV/AIDS; malignancy; chronic cardiac, pulmonary, or renal failure; depression; and *anorexia nervosa* or *bulimia.*

See Table 4-2, Eating Disorders and Excessively Low BMI, p. 140.

Weight loss with relatively high food intake suggests *diabetes mellitus, hyperthyroidism,* or *malabsorption.* Consider also binge eating (*bulimia*) with clandestine vomiting.

Pursue a thorough psychosocial history. Who cooks and shops for the patient? Where does the patient eat? With whom? Are there any problems with obtaining, storing, preparing, or chewing food? Does the patient avoid or restrict certain foods for medical, religious, or other reasons?

Poverty, old age, social isolation, physical disability, emotional or mental impairment, lack of teeth, ill-fitting dentures, alcoholism, and drug abuse increase risk of malnutrition.

Check the medication history.

Drugs associated with weight loss include anticonvulsants, antidepressants, levodopa, digoxin, metformin, and thyroid medication.[2]

Be alert for symptoms and signs of *malnutrition*. These may be subtle and non-specific, such as weakness, easy fatigability, cold intolerance, flaky dermatitis, and ankle swelling. Securing a good diet history of eating patterns and quantities is essential. Ask general questions about intake at different times throughout the day, such as "Tell me what you typically eat for lunch." "What do you eat for a snack?" "When?"

See Table 4-3, Nutrition Screening, p. 141.

Pain. Pain is one of the most common presenting symptoms in office practice. Each year, an estimated 100 million Americans experience chronic pain at a cost in medical care, disability, and work days lost of $560 to $635 million.[3,4] Acute pain affects another 12% of Americans annually.[5] The most frequent causes are low back pain, headache or migraine, and knee and neck pain; prevalence varies by race, ethnicity, and socioeconomic status. Localizing symptoms, "the seven attributes of every symptom," and the psychosocial history are essential to your physical examination, assessment, and a comprehensive management plan.

Turn to the section on Acute and Chronic Pain, pp. 134–137, at the end of this chapter for an approach to assessment and management.

Health Promotion and Counseling: Evidence and Recommendations

Important Topics for Health Promotion and Counseling

- Optimal weight, nutrition, and diet
- Blood pressure and dietary sodium
- Exercise

Optimal Weight, Nutrition, and Diet. Fewer than half of U.S. adults maintain a healthy weight, defined as a BMI between 18.5 and 24.9 kg/m². Obesity has increased in every segment of the U.S. population, regardless of age, gender, ethnicity, geographic area, or socioeconomic status. Review the alarming statistics about the epidemic of obesity nationally and worldwide in the table on the next page.[6–8]

See Calculating the BMI and Measuring the Waist Circumference, pp. 122–123.

Obesity at a Glance

- Nearly 69% of U.S. adults are overweight or obese (BMI ≥25 kg/m²), including 71% of men, 66% of women; overall, about 35% of U.S. adults are obese.
- About 15% of U.S. children and adolescents are overweight and 17% are obese.
- Health disparities: the prevalence of overweight or obesity varies by racial/ ethnic and socioeconomic groups:
  - Women: black women, 82%; Hispanic women, 77%; non-Hispanic white women, 63%.
  - Higher-income women are less likely to be obese than low-income women.
  - Men: Hispanic men, 79%; non-Hispanic white men, 71%; black men, 69%.
  - Youth ages 2 to 19 years: highest prevalence in Hispanic boys and girls (41%; 37%), black boys and girls (34%; 36%), children living in low-income, low-education, and higher-unemployment households.
- Overweight and obesity increase risk of heart disease, numerous types of cancers, type 2 diabetes, stroke, arthritis, sleep apnea, infertility, and depression. Obesity may increase risk of death.[9,10]
- More than 80% of people with type 2 diabetes and over 20% of people with hypertension are overweight or obese.
- Obesity is increasing worldwide, affecting an estimated 2.1 billion overweight and obese individuals.[11] The prevalence of overweight and obesity is higher in developed countries at all ages. In the world's poorest countries, poverty is associated with underweight and malnutrition; but poverty in a middle-income country adopting a Western lifestyle increases the risk of obesity.
- Only 65% of obese U.S. adults report that health care professionals have told them that they were overweight. Less than half report being advised by a health care professional to lose weight, though obese adults with diabetes are more likely to receive such advice.[12]

Sources: Go AS, Mozaffarian D, Roger VL, et al. Heart disease and stroke statistics–2014 update: a report from the American Heart Association. *Circulation.* 2014;129(3):e28; Ogden CL, Carroll MD, Kit BK, et al. Prevalence of childhood and adult obesity in the United States, 2011–2012. *JAMA.* 2014;311(8):806; Ogden CL, Carroll MD, Kit BK, et al. Prevalence of obesity among adults: United States, 2011–2012. *NCHS Data Brief.* 2013;(131):1; Centers for Disease Control and Prevention. Obesity and overweight. Data and statistics. Available at http://www.cdc.gov/obesity/data/index.html. Accessed December 1, 2014.

See Table 4-1, Obesity-Related Health Conditions, p. 139.

To promote optimal patient weight and nutrition, adopt the four-pronged approach outlined here. Reducing weight by even 5% to 10% can improve blood pressure, lipid levels, and glucose tolerance, and reduce the risk of diabetes or hypertension.

Four Steps to Promote Optimal Weight and Nutrition

1. Measure BMI and waist circumference; adults with a BMI ≥25 kg/m², men with waist circumferences >40 inches, and women with waist circumferences >35 inches are at increased risk for heart disease and obesity-related diseases. Measuring the waist-to-hip ratio (waist circumference divided by

(continued)

Four Steps to Promote Optimal Weight and Nutrition (continued)

hip circumference) may be a better risk predictor for individuals older than 75 years. Ratios >0.95 in men and >0.85 in women are considered elevated. Determine additional risk factors for cardiovascular diseases, including smoking, high blood pressure, high cholesterol, physical inactivity, and family history.

2. Assess dietary intake.
3. Assess the patient's motivation to change.
4. Provide counseling about nutrition and exercise.

Take advantage of the excellent resources available for patient assessment and counseling summarized in the following sections.[13] Review the role of weight in the growing prevalence of *metabolic syndrome,* present in about 34% of the U.S. population.[6]

See definition and discussion of *metabolic syndrome* in Chapter 9, Cardiovascular System, p. 370.

Step 1: Measure the BMI and Assess Risk Factors. Classify the BMI according to the national guidelines in the following table. If the BMI is *above 25 kg/m²,* assess the patient for *additional risk factors* for heart disease and other obesity-related diseases: hypertension, high low-density lipoprotein (LDL) cholesterol, low high-density lipoprotein (HDL) cholesterol, high triglycerides, high blood glucose, family history of premature heart disease, physical inactivity, and cigarette smoking. Patients with a BMI over 25 kg/m² and two or more risk factors should pursue weight loss—especially if the waist circumference is elevated.

Classification of Overweight and Obesity by BMI

	Obesity Class	BMI (kg/m²)
Underweight		<18.5
Normal		18.5–24.9
Overweight		25.0–29.9
Obesity	I	30.0–34.9
	II	35.0–39.9
Extreme obesity	III	≥40

Source: National Institutes of Health and National Heart, Lung, and Blood Institute: Clinical Guidelines on the Identification, Evaluation, and Treatment of Overweight and Obesity in Adults: The Evidence Report. NIH Publication 98–4083. June 1998. Available at http://www.nhlbi.nih.gov/guidelines/obesity/ob_gdlns.pdf. Accessed January 21, 2015.

Step 2: Assess Dietary Intake. Take a diet history and assess the patient's eating patterns. Select a brief screening tool and be sensitive to the impact of income and cultural preferences on what the patient chooses to eat.

See Table 4-3, Nutrition Screening, p. 141.

Step 3: Assess Motivation to Change. Once you have assessed BMI, risk factors, and dietary intake, address the patient's motivation to make lifestyle changes that promote weight loss. The Prochaska model helps tailor interventions to the patient's level of motivation to adopt new eating behaviors.

See Table 4-4, Obesity: Stages of Change Model and Assessing Readiness, p. 142.

Step 4: Provide Counseling About Nutrition and Exercise. You should be well informed about diet and nutrition as you counsel overweight patients, especially in light of the many and often contradictory diet options in the popular press. The U.S. Department of Agriculture released new dietary guidelines in 2010 to help clinicians and patients address the obesity epidemic more effectively.[14] The Department's new nutrition icon, MyPlate, is appealing and easy to understand (Fig. 4-3). Review the MyPlate website and the dietary guidelines report, as well as recent guides for identifying and managing overweight and obesity from the National Heart, Lung, and Blood Institute and the Agency for Healthcare Research and Quality.[10,15]

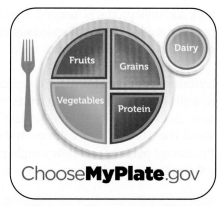

FIGURE 4-3. **The MyPlate icon helps patients understand nutrition.**
(U.S. Department of Agriculture.)

A key element of effective counseling is working with the patient to set reasonable goals. Experts note that patients often have a "dream weight" as much as 30% below initial body weight.[2] However, a 5% to 10% weight loss is more realistic and still proven to reduce risk of diabetes and other obesity-associated health problems. Educate your patients about common roadblocks to sustained weight loss: hitting a plateau due to feedback physiologic systems that maintain body homeostasis; poor adherence to diet due to increasing hunger over time as weight declines; and inhibition of leptin, a protein cytokine secreted and stored in fat cells that modulates hunger.[16] Use a full array of strategies to promote weight loss. A safe goal for weight loss is 0.5 to 2 lbs per week.

Strategies That Promote Weight Loss

- The most effective diets combine realistic weight loss goals with exercise and behavioral reinforcements.
- Encourage patients to walk 30 to 60 minutes 5 or more days a week, or a total of at least 150 minutes a week. Pedometers help patients match distance in steps with calories burned.
- The total calorie deficit goal, usually 500 to 1,000 kilocalories a day, is more important than the type of diet. Since many types of diets have been studied and appear to confer similar results, support the patient's preferences as long as they are reasonable.[17,18] Consider low-fat diets for those with dyslipidemias.
- Encourage proven behavioral habits such as portion-controlled meals, meal planning, food diaries, and activity records.
- Follow professional guidelines for pharmacologic therapies in patients having high weights and morbidities who do not respond to conventional treatment.[19]

If the BMI falls *below 18.5 kg/m²*, investigate possible anorexia, bulimia, or other serious medical conditions.

See Table 4-2, Eating Disorders and Excessively Low BMI, p. 140.

The *USDA Dietary Guidelines 2010* point out that to maintain caloric balance and achieve and sustain a healthy weight, most Americans need to lower their caloric intake and increase physical activity. The Guidelines emphasize consuming *nutrient-dense foods and beverages* such as vegetables, fruits, whole grains, fat-free or low-fat milk and milk products, seafood, lean meats and poultry, eggs, beans and peas, and nuts and seeds.[14] Intake of added sugars (primarily sweeteners), solid saturated and/ or trans fats, and refined grains make it difficult to achieve optimal nutrition.

Introduce your patients to the colorful "chooseMyPlate.gov" website and its easy-to-follow guides for selecting fruits, vegetables, grains, protein, and dairy products. Sodium intake should be less than 2,300 mg/day, saturated fatty acids should be ≤10% of total calories, and dietary cholesterol should be ≤300 mg/day. Encourage patients to follow simple practical tips for daily meals, the "10 Tips to a Great Plate" listed below.

10 Tips to a Great Plate

1. Balance calories.
2. Eat less.
3. Avoid oversized portions.
4. Eat nutrient-dense foods more often.
5. Make half the plate fruits and vegetables.
6. Switch to fat-free or low-fat milk.
7. Make half of grain intake whole grains.
8. Eat foods high in solid fats, salt, and added sugars less often.
9. Use the Nutrition Facts label to choose lower sodium versions of foods like soup, bread, and frozen meals.
10. Drink water or unsweetened beverages instead of sweetened soda, energy drinks, or sports drinks.

Source: Choose My Plate–10 Tips to a Great Plate. Available at www.choosemyplate.gov/food-groups/downloads/TenTips/DGTipsheet1ChooseMyPlate.pdf. Accessed January 21, 2015. U.S. Department of Agriculture.

Help adolescent females and women of childbearing age increase intake of iron, vitamin C, and folic acid. Assist adults older than 50 years to identify foods rich in vitamin B_{12}. Advise older adults and those with dark skin or low exposure to sunlight to increase intake of vitamin D.

See Table 4-5, Nutrition Counseling: Sources of Nutrients, p. 143.

Blood Pressure and Dietary Sodium.
Excess sodium intake can lead to hypertension, a major risk factor for cardiovascular disease. A meta-analysis concludes that a difference of 5 g of salt intake a day is linked to a 23% difference in the rate of stroke and a 17% difference in the rate of total cardiovascular disease.[20] The Institute of Medicine (IOM) has determined that a daily dietary intake of 2,300 mg of sodium is the tolerable upper intake level for adults.[21] However, the average sodium intake among Americans is 3,400 mg/day and over 90% of adults exceed the recommended upper intake level.[22] While reducing sodium intake to 1,500 mg provides better blood pressure control, the IOM found no evidence of benefit for overall health outcomes below the 2,300 mg level.[21] Even without achieving this level, reducing sodium intake by at least 1,000 mg/day lowers blood pressure.[23]

See Table 4-6, Patients with Hypertension: Recommended Changes in Diet, p. 143.

Because over 75% of consumed sodium comes from processed foods and *less than 10% of Americans consume 2,300 mg/day or less of recommended dietary sodium*, the

American Heart Association and the IOM have jointly recommended population-wide salt reduction measures including government standards for manufacturers, restaurants, and foodservice operators.[24,25] Advise patients to read the Nutrition Facts panel on food labels closely to help them adhere to the 2,300-mg/day guideline. Urge them to consider the well-investigated Dietary Approaches to Stop Hypertension, or DASH Eating Plan, for a model diet.[26]

Exercise.   Physical fitness is a key component of both weight control and weight loss. To achieve health benefits, adults should do at least 150 minutes (2 hours and 30 minutes) of moderate-intensity cardiorespiratory activity, for example, walking briskly at a pace of 3 to 4.5 miles (4.8 to 7.2 km) per hour, each week.[27,28] Patients can increase exercise by such simple measures as parking farther away from their place of work or using stairs instead of elevators. Alternatively, adults can engage in vigorous-intensity aerobic activity, such as jogging or running, for 75 minutes (1 hour and 15 minutes) each week. An equivalent combination of moderate- and vigorous-intensity aerobic activity is also beneficial. Greater health benefits can be achieved by increasing the frequency, duration, and/or intensity of physical activity.

Moderate and Vigorous Exercise

A 154-lb (69 kg) man who is 5'10" uses up approximately the number of calories listed doing each activity below. *Those who weigh more will use more calories, and those who weigh less will use fewer.* The calorie values listed include both calories used by the activity and calories used for normal body functioning.

	Approximate Calories Used by a 154-lb Man	
	In 1 hour	In 30 minutes
Moderate Physical Activities:		
Hiking	370	185
Light gardening/yard work	330	165
Dancing	330	165
Golf (walking and carrying clubs)	330	165
Bicycling (less than 10 miles per hour)	290	145
Walking (3.5 miles per hour)	280	140
Weight training (general light workout)	220	110
Stretching	180	90
Vigorous Physical Activities:		
Running/jogging (5 miles per hour)	590	295
Bicycling (more than 10 miles per hour)	590	295
Swimming (slow freestyle laps)	510	255
Aerobics	480	240
Walking (4.5 miles per hour)	460	230
Heavy yard work (chopping wood)	440	220
Weight lifting (vigorous effort)	440	220
Basketball (vigorous)	440	220

Source: U.S. Department of Agriculture: Choose MyPlate.gov. Physical Activity. How many calories does physical activity use? Modified June 2011. Available at http://www.choosemyplate.gov/food-groups/physicalactivity_calories_used_table.html. Accessed January 21, 2015.

The General Survey

The *General Survey* of the patient's appearance, height, and weight begins with the opening moments of the patient encounter, but your observations of the patient's appearance often crystallize as you start the physical examination. The best clinicians continually sharpen their powers of observation and description. As you talk with and examine the patient, heighten your focus on the patient's mood, build, and behavior. These details enrich and deepen your emerging clinical impression. Your goal is to describe the distinguishing features of the patient so clearly that colleagues can spot the patient in a crowd of strangers, avoiding clichés like "middle-aged gentleman" and the uninformative "in no acute distress."

Many factors contribute to the patient's body habitus: socioeconomic status, nutrition, genetic makeup, physical fitness, mood state, early illnesses, gender, geographic location, and age cohort. Nutritional status affects many of the characteristics you scrutinize during the *General Survey:* height and weight, blood pressure, posture, mood and alertness, facial coloration, dentition and condition of the tongue and gingiva, color of the nail beds, and muscle bulk, to name a few. Your assessment of height, weight, BMI, and risk for obesity should be routine for each patient in your clinical practice.

Recall your observations from the first moments of the encounter that you have been refining throughout your assessment. Does the patient hear you when greeted in the waiting room or examination room? Rise with ease? Walk easily or stiffly? If hospitalized when you first meet, what is the patient doing—sitting up and enjoying television?...or lying in bed?...What do you see on the bedside table—a magazine?...candy bars or chips?...a Bible or a rosary?...multiple beverage containers?...or nothing at all? Each observation raises questions or hypotheses to consider as your assessment unfolds.

General Appearance

Apparent State of Health.   Try to make a general judgment based on observations throughout the encounter. Support it with the significant details.

Is the patient acutely or chronically ill, frail, or fit and robust?

Level of Consciousness.   Is the patient awake, alert, and responsive to you and others in the environment? If not, promptly assess the level of consciousness.

See Chapter 17, The Nervous System, Level of Consciousness, pp. 768–769.

Signs of Distress.   Does the patient show evidence of the problems listed below?

- Cardiac or respiratory distress

Is there clutching of the chest, pallor, diaphoresis, labored breathing, wheezing, or coughing?

- Pain

Is there wincing, diaphoresis, protectiveness of a painful area, grimacing, or an unusual posture favoring one limb or region of the body?

■ Anxiety or depression

Are there anxious facial expressions, fidgety movements, cold moist palms, inexpressive or flat affect, poor eye contact, or psychomotor slowing? See Chapter 5, Behavior and Mental Status, pp. 147–171.

Skin Color and Obvious Lesions.   Inspect for any changes in skin color, scars, plaques, or nevi.

Pallor, cyanosis, jaundice, rashes, bruises, or mottling of the extremities should be pursued. See Chapter 6, The Skin, Hair, and Nails, pp. 173–214.

Dress, Grooming, and Personal Hygiene.   How is the patient dressed? Is the clothing suitable for the temperature and weather? Is it clean and appropriate to the setting?

Excess clothing may reflect the cold intolerance of *hypothyroidism,* hide skin rash or needle marks, mask anorexia, or signal personal lifestyle preferences.

Notice the patient's shoes. Are there cut-outs or holes? Are the shoes run-down?

Holes or slippers suggest gout, bunions, edema, or other painful foot conditions. Run-down shoes can contribute to foot and back pain, calluses, falls, and infection.

Is the patient wearing unusual jewelry? Are there body piercings?

Copper bracelets suggest joint pain. Tattoos and piercings can be associated with alcohol and drug use.[29]

Note the patient's hair, fingernails, and use of make-up. They may be clues to the patient's personality, mood, lifestyle, and self-regard.

"Grown-out" hair and nail polish suggest the length of a possible illness. Bitten fingernails may reflect stress.

Do personal hygiene and grooming seem appropriate for the patient's age, lifestyle, and occupation?

Neglected appearance may appear in *depression* and *dementia,* but should be compared with the patient's norm.

Facial Expression.   Observe the facial expression at rest, during conversation and social interactions, and during the physical examination. Watch closely for eye contact. Is it natural? . . . sustained and unblinking? . . . averted quickly? . . . absent?

Watch for the stare of *hyperthyroidism,* the immobile facies of *parkinsonism,* and the flat or sad affect of *depression.* Decreased eye contact may be cultural or suggest anxiety, fear, or sadness.

Odors of the Body and Breath.   Odors can be important diagnostic clues, like the fruity odor of diabetes or the scent of alcohol.

Breath odors can reveal the presence of alcohol or acetone (diabetes), pulmonary infections, uremia, or liver failure.

Never assume that alcohol on a patient's breath explains changes in mental status or neurologic findings.

These changes can have serious but treatable causes such as hypoglycemia, subdural hematoma, or postictal state.

Posture, Gait, and Motor Activity. What is the patient's preferred posture?

Patients often prefer sitting upright in *left-sided heart failure* and leaning forward with arms braced in *chronic obstructive pulmonary disease.*

Is the patient restless or quiet? How often does the patient change position?

Anxious patients appear agitated and restless. Patients in pain often avoid movement.

Is there any involuntary motor activity? Are some body parts immobile? Which ones?

Look for tremors, other involuntary movements, or paralysis. See Table 17-5, Tremors and Involuntary Movements, pp. 782–783.

Does the patient walk smoothly, with comfort, self-confidence, and balance, or is there a limp, fear of falling, loss of balance, or any movement disorder?

See Table 17-10, Abnormalities of Gait and Posture, p. 789. An impaired gait increases risk of falls.

Height and Weight. Measure the patient's height and weight with shoes removed to determine the BMI. Note any changes in height or weight over time.

Is the patient unusually short or tall? Is the build slender, muscular, or stocky? Is the body symmetric? Note the general body proportions.

Watch for very short stature in *Turner syndrome,* childhood renal failure, and *achondroplastic* and *hypopituitary dwarfism;* long limbs in proportion to the trunk in hypogonadism and *Marfan syndrome;* and height loss in *osteoporosis* and vertebral compression fractures.

Is the patient emaciated, slender, overweight, or obese? If the patient is obese, is the fat distributed evenly, concentrated over the upper torso, or settled around the hips?

There is generalized fat distribution in simple obesity and truncal fat with relatively thin limbs in *Cushing syndrome* and *metabolic syndrome.*

Make note of any weight changes.

Causes of weight loss include malignancy, *diabetes mellitus, hyperthyroidism,* chronic infection, depression, diuresis, and successful dieting.

Calculating the BMI. Use your measurements of height and weight to determine BMI. Body fat consists primarily of adipose in the form of triglycerides and is stored in subcutaneous, intra-abdominal, and intramuscular fat deposits that are difficult to measure directly. The BMI incorporates estimated but more accurate measures of body fat than weight alone. The National Institutes of

See discussion of Optimal Weight, Nutrition, and Diet, pp. 114–118.

Health caution that people who are very muscular can have a high BMI, but still be healthy. Likewise, the BMI for older adults and those with low muscle mass may appear inappropriately "normal."

To determine the BMI, choose the method best suited to your practice. Use a standard BMI table or the electronic medical record software, which frequently shows the BMI automatically.[30] You can also calculate the BMI using one of the methods shown below.

Methods to Calculate Body Mass Index (BMI)

Unit of Measure	Method of Calculation
Weight in pounds, height in inches	(1) Standard BMI Chart
	(2) $\left(\dfrac{\text{Weight (lbs)} \times 700^*}{\text{Height (inches)}} \right)$
Weight in kilograms, height in meters squared	(3) $\dfrac{\text{Weight (kg)}}{\text{Height (m}^2)}$
Either unit of measure	(4) "BMI Calculator" at http://www. nhlbi.nih.gov/health/educational/ lose_wt/BMI/bmicalc.htm

*Several organizations use 704.5, but the variation in BMI is negligible. Conversion formulas: 2.2 lb = 1 kg; 1 inch = 2.54 cm; 100 cm = 1 m.

Source: National Institutes of Health–National Heart, Lung, and Blood Institute: Calculate Your Body Mass Index. Available at: http://www.nhlbi.nih.gov/health/educational/lose_wt/BMI/bmicalc. htm. Accessed January 21, 2015.

Waist Circumference.   If the BMI is ≥ 35 kg/m^2, measure the patient's waist circumference just above the hips. Risk for diabetes, hypertension, and cardiovascular disease increases significantly if the waist circumference is *35 inches or more in women and 40 inches or more in men.*

The Vital Signs

The *Vital Signs*—blood pressure, heart rate, respiratory rate, and temperature— provide critical initial information that often influences the tempo and direction of your evaluation. If already recorded by office staff, review the Vital Signs promptly at the outset of the encounter. If the Vital Signs are abnormal, you will often retake them yourself during the visit.

Begin by measuring the blood pressure and the heart rate. Count the heart rate for one minute by palpating the *radial pulse* with your fingers, or by listening for the *apical pulse* with your stethoscope at the cardiac apex. Continue either of these techniques as you quietly count the *respiratory rate*, since once patients are

See Table 9-3, Abnormalities of the Arterial Pulse and Pressure Waves, p. 402.

alerted, their breathing patterns may change. The *temperature* may be taken in various sites, depending on the patient and the equipment available. Learn the techniques that ensure accuracy when you measure the vital signs, described in the pages to follow.

Blood Pressure

The Complexities of Measuring Blood Pressure.   The accuracy of blood pressure measurements varies according to *how* these measurements are taken. Office screening with manual and automated cuffs remains common, but elevated readings increasingly require confirmation with home and ambulatory monitoring. In its 2014 draft recommendations, the U.S. Preventive Services Task Force reported that 5% to 65% of elevated office blood pressures failed to be confirmed by ambulatory monitoring and recommended ambulatory blood pressure monitoring to confirm the diagnosis of hypertension.[31] Numerous studies show that ambulatory and home blood pressure monitoring are more predictive of cardiovascular disease and end organ damage than manual and automated measurements in the office.[32] Automated *ambulatory blood pressure monitoring* measures blood pressure at preset intervals over 24 to 48 hours, usually every 15 to 20 minutes during the day and 30 to 60 minutes during the night. It is now considered the reference standard for confirming elevated office blood pressures.[33]

Be familiar with the important features of the different methods for measuring blood pressure, summarized in the table below, since errors in office readings raise substantial risks of misdiagnosis and unnecessary treatment.

Methods for Measuring Blood Pressure

Method	Features
Auscultatory office blood pressure with aneroid or mercury blood pressure cuff (Fig. 4-4)	Common, inexpensive Subject to patient anxiety ("white coat hypertension"), observer technique, cuff recalibration every 6 months Requires measurements over several visits Ambulatory or home monitoring needed to detect masked hypertension Single measurements with sensitivity and specificity of 75% compared to ambulatory monitoring[34]
Automated oscillometric office blood pressure	Requires optimal patient positioning, cuff size and placement, and device calibration Takes multiple measurements over short period Requires confirmatory measurements to reduce misdiagnosis Comparable sensitivity and specificity to manual measurements[34]

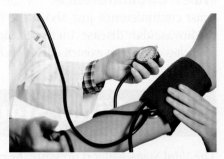

FIGURE 4-4. **Auscultatory blood pressure measurement with arm at heart level.**

(*continued*)

Methods for Measuring Blood Pressure (*continued*)

Method	Features
Home blood pressure monitoring	Accurate automated device applied by patient, easy to use, less expensive than ambulatory monitoring
	Acceptable alternative if ambulatory monitoring not feasible; more predictive of cardiovascular risk than office measurements[32]
	Requires patient education for accurate technique, repeated measurements (two morning, two evening readings daily for 1 week); nighttime readings not recorded[32]
	Detects *white coat hypertension*—present in 20%[32]
	Detects *masked hypertension*—present in 10% (blood pressure is higher than office readings)[32]
	Sensitivity 85%, specificity 62% compared to ambulatory monitoring[34]
Ambulatory blood pressure monitoring	Automated; clinical and research "gold standard"
	Provides 24-hour average blood pressures and averages of daytime (awake), nighttime (asleep), systolic, and diastolic blood pressures
	Shows whether nocturnal blood pressure "dips" (normal) or stays elevated (= cardiovascular disease risk factor)
	More expensive; may not be covered by insurance

If you recommend home blood pressure monitoring, advise patients about how to choose the best upper arm cuff for home use and have it recalibrated. Let them know that wrist and fingers monitors are popular but less accurate. Systolic pressure increases in more distal arteries, whereas diastolic pressure falls; and hydrostatic effects introduce errors due to differences in position relative to the heart.

Patient education about the correct use of home monitors is essential. Make sure patients understand all the steps needed to ensure accurate readings at home, as detailed in this section.

Definitions for Diagnosing Hypertension. Note the differences in the definitions of hypertension depending on the measurement method used.

Definitions of Hypertension

- Office manual or automated blood pressure based on the average of two readings on two separate occasions: ≥140/90[35,36]
- Home automated blood pressure: <135/85[32]
- Ambulatory automated blood pressure:[37]
  - 24-hour average: ≥ of 130/80
  - Daytime (awake) average: ≥135/85
  - Nighttime (asleep) average: >120/70

Types of Hypertension. Three types of hypertension are especially important to recognize: *white coat hypertension, masked hypertension,* and *nocturnal hypertension.* Suspicion of these entities and assessing the effects of treatment are indications for ambulatory blood pressure monitoring.

- *White coat hypertension (isolated clinic hypertension):* White coat hypertension is defined as blood pressure ≥140/90 in medical settings and mean awake ambulatory readings <135/85. This phenomenon, reported in up to 20% of patients with elevated office blood pressure, is important to identify since it carries normal to slightly increased cardiovascular risk and does not require treatment.[32,37] It is attributed to a conditioned anxiety response. Poor measurement technique, including rounding of measurements to zero, the presence of a physician or nurse, and even the prior diagnosis of hypertension can also substantially alter office readings. Replacing manual office measurements with an automated device that makes several readings with the patient seated alone in a quiet room has been shown to reduce the "white coat effect."[38]

- *Masked hypertension:* Masked hypertension, defined as office blood pressure <140/90, but an elevated daytime blood pressure of >135/85 on home or ambulatory testing, is more serious. Untreated adults with masked hypertension, an estimated 10% to 30% of the general population, have increased risk of cardiovascular disease and end-organ damage.[32,37]

- *Nocturnal hypertension:* Physiologic blood pressure "dipping" occurs in most patients at night as they shift from wakefulness to sleep. A nocturnal fall of <10% of daytime values is associated with poor cardiovascular outcomes and can only be identified on 24-hour ambulatory blood pressure monitoring. Two other patterns have poor cardiovascular outcomes, a nocturnal rising pattern and a marked nocturnal fall of >20% of daytime values.[37]

Choosing the Correct Blood Pressure Cuff (Sphygmomanometer). More than 76 million Americans have elevated blood pressure.[39] To detect blood pressure elevations, an accurate instrument is essential. Four types of office blood pressure devices are currently used: mercury, aneroid, electronic, and "hybrid," which combines features of both electronic and ambulatory devices. In hybrid devices, the mercury column is replaced by an electronic pressure gauge; blood pressure can be displayed as a simulated mercury column, an aneroid reading, or a digital readout. All measuring instruments should be routinely tested for accuracy using international protocols.[40,41]

Some offices continue to use mercury cuffs, although these are no longer commercially available. Experts recommend that mercury cuffs, now modified to minimize risk of environmental spill, can still be used for routine office measurements and evaluating the accuracy of nonmercury devices.[42]

Selecting the Correct Size Blood Pressure Cuff

It is important for clinicians and patients to use a cuff that fits the patient's arm. Follow the guidelines outlined here for selecting the correct size:

- Width of the inflatable bladder of the cuff should be about 40% of upper arm circumference (about 12 to 14 cm in the average adult).
- Length of the inflatable bladder should be about 80% of upper arm circumference (almost long enough to encircle the arm).
- The standard cuff is 12 × 23 cm, appropriate for arm circumferences up to 28 cm.

If the cuff is too *small* (narrow), the blood pressure will read *high;* if the cuff is too *large* (wide), the blood pressure will read *low* on a small arm and *high* on a large arm.

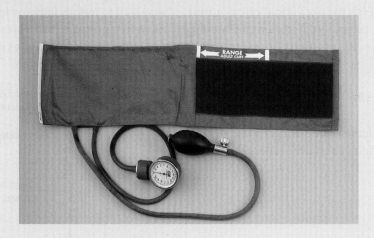

Making Accurate Blood Pressure Measurements. Take the time to make sure your BP measurement will be accurate. Proper technique is important and reduces the inherent variability arising from the patient or examiner, the equipment, and the procedure itself.[36]

Steps to Ensure Accurate Blood Pressure Measurement

1. The patient should avoid smoking, caffeine, or exercise for 30 minutes prior to measurement.
2. The examining room should be quiet and comfortably warm.
3. The patient should sit quietly for 5 minutes in a chair with feet on the floor, rather than on the examining table.
4. The arm selected should be *free of clothing,* fistulas for dialysis, scars from brachial artery cutdowns, or lymphedema from axillary node dissection or radiation therapy.
5. Palpate the brachial artery to confirm a viable pulse and position the arm so that the brachial artery, at the antecubital crease, is *at heart level*—roughly level with the fourth interspace at its junction with the sternum.
6. If the patient is seated, rest the arm on a table a little above the patient's waist; if standing, try to support the patient's arm at the midchest level.

If the brachial artery is *below* heart level, the blood pressure reading will be higher; if the brachial artery is above heart level, the reading will be lower.

Position the Cuff and Arm. With the arm at heart level, center the inflatable bladder over the brachial artery. The lower border of the cuff should be about 2.5 cm above the antecubital crease. Secure the cuff snugly. Slightly flex the patient's arm at the elbow.

A loose cuff or a bladder that balloons outside the cuff leads to falsely high readings.

Estimate the Systolic Pressure and Add 30 mm Hg. To decide how high to raise the cuff pressure, first estimate the systolic pressure by palpation. As you palpate the radial artery with the fingers of one hand, rapidly inflate the cuff until the radial pulse disappears. Read this pressure on the manometer and *add 30 mm Hg.* Using this sum for subsequent inflations prevents discomfort from unnecessarily high cuff pressures. It also avoids the occasional error caused by an *auscultatory gap*—a silent interval that may be present between the systolic and the diastolic pressures (Fig. 4-5). Deflate the cuff promptly and completely and wait for 15 to 30 seconds.

An unrecognized auscultatory gap may lead to serious underestimation of systolic pressure (150 instead of 200 in the example below) or overestimation of diastolic pressure.

Position the Stethoscope Bell Over the Brachial Artery. Now place the bell of a stethoscope lightly over the brachial artery, taking care to make an air seal with the full rim (Fig. 4-6). Because the sounds to be heard, the *Korotkoff sounds,* are relatively low in pitch, they are generally better heard with the bell.

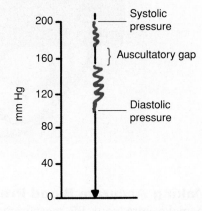

FIGURE 4-5. **Auscultatory gap.**

If you find an auscultatory gap, record your findings completely (e.g., 200/98 with an auscultatory gap from 170 to 150).

An auscultatory gap (Fig. 4-6) is associated with arterial stiffness and atherosclerotic disease.[43]

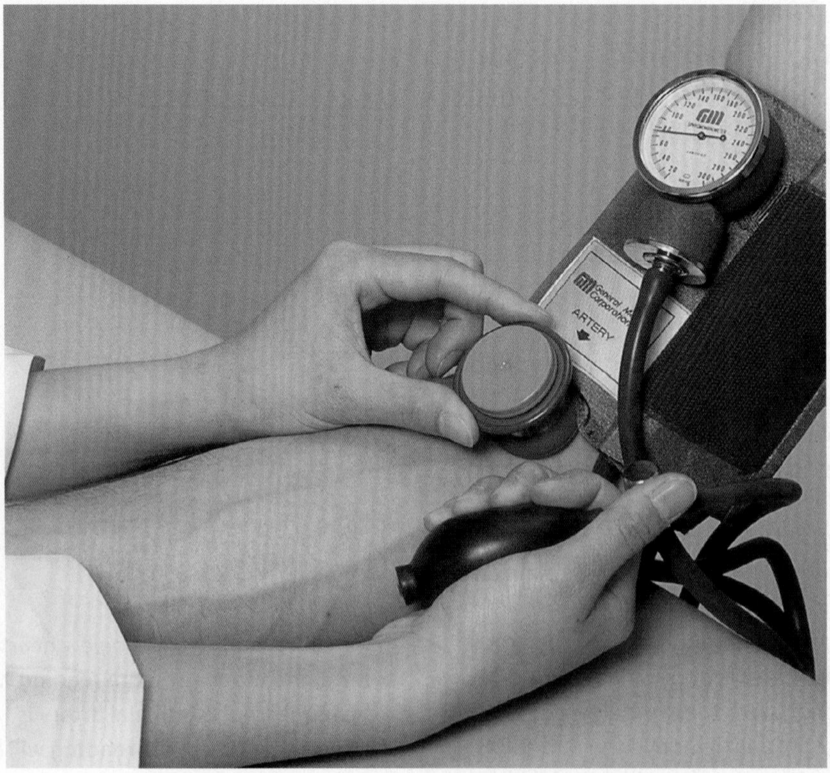

FIGURE 4-6. **Place the bell over the brachial artery.**

Identify the Systolic Blood Pressure. Inflate the cuff again rapidly to the target level, and then deflate the cuff slowly at a rate of about 2 to 3 mm Hg per second. Note the level when you hear the sounds of at least two consecutive beats. This is the *systolic pressure* (Fig. 4-7).

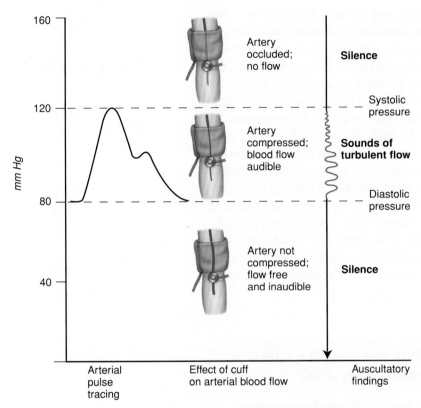

FIGURE 4-7. **Auscultating systolic and diastolic Koratkoff sounds.**

Identify the Diastolic Blood Pressure. Continue to deflate the cuff slowly until the sounds become muffled and disappear. To confirm the disappearance point, listen as the pressure falls another 10 to 20 mm Hg. Then deflate the cuff rapidly to zero. The disappearance point, which is usually only a few mm Hg below the muffling point, provides the best estimate of *diastolic pressure* (Fig. 4-7).

In some people, the muffling point and the disappearance point are farther apart. Occasionally, as in aortic regurgitation, the sounds never disappear. If the difference is 10 mm Hg or greater, record both figures (e.g., 154/80/68).

Average Two or More Readings. Read both the systolic and the diastolic levels to the nearest 2 mm Hg. *Wait 2 or more minutes and repeat.* Average your readings. If the first two readings differ by more than 5 mm Hg, take additional readings.

When using an aneroid instrument, hold the dial so that it faces you directly. Avoid slow or repetitive inflations of the cuff because the resulting venous congestion can cause false readings.

By making the sounds less audible, venous congestion may produce artificially low systolic and high diastolic pressures.

Measure Blood Pressure in Both Arms At Least Once. Normally, there may be a difference in pressure of 5 mm Hg and sometimes up to 10 mm Hg. Subsequent readings should be made on the arm with the higher pressure.

A pressure difference of more than 10 to 15 mm Hg occurs in *subclavian steal syndrome, supravalvular aortic stenosis,* and *aortic dissection,* and should be investigated.

Classification of Normal and Abnormal Blood Pressure. *The Seventh Joint National Committee on Prevention, Detection, Evaluation, and Treatment of High Blood Pressure Report* recommends using the mean of two or more properly measured seated blood pressure readings, taken on two or more office visits, for establishing of the blood pressure. The blood pressure measurement should be verified in the contralateral arm.[36] This report identifies four levels of systolic and diastolic hypertension, affirmed by the American Society of Hypertension in 2013.[44] Note that either component may be high. In 2013, the *Eighth Joint National Committee (JNC 8)* issued the JNC 8 report based on rigorous scientific review of clinical trial data.[35] This report focuses more narrowly on thresholds and goals for pharmacologic treatment. For patients ages ≥18 years to <60 years in the general population, JNC 8 recommends treatment to lower blood pressure for a diastolic blood pressure of ≥90 (strong evidence) and systolic blood pressure of ≥140 (expert opinion). For patients ages ≥60 years, JNC 8 recommends treatment for blood pressures ≥150/90. The JNC 8 report also recommends a higher treatment threshold than JNC 7 for patients with diabetes and chronic kidney disease (CKD), ≥140/90.

Blood Pressure Classification for Adults (JNC 8, American Society of Hypertension, JNC 7)[35,36,44]

Category	Systolic (mm Hg)	Diastolic (mm Hg)
Normal[36]	<120	<80
Prehypertension[36,44]	120–139	80–89
Stage 1 hypertension[35]		
Ages ≥18 to <60 years; diabetes or renal disease	140–159	90–99
Age ≥60 years[a]	150–159	90–99
Stage 2 hypertension[36,44]	≥160	≥100

[a]The American Society of Hypertension raises this cutoff to age ≥80 years.

Assessment of hypertension also includes its effects on target "end organs"—the eyes, heart, brain, and kidneys. Look for hypertensive retinopathy, left ventricular hypertrophy, and neurologic deficits suggesting stroke. Renal assessment requires urinalysis and blood tests of renal function.

When the systolic and diastolic levels fall in different categories, use the higher category. For example, 170/92 mm Hg is stage 2 hypertension; 135/98 mm Hg is stage 1 hypertension. In *isolated systolic hypertension,* systolic blood pressure is ≥140 mm Hg, and diastolic blood pressure is <90 mm Hg.

Treatment of *isolated systolic hypertension* in patients ages ≥60 years reduces mortality and complications from cardiovascular disease. The prevalence of isolated systolic hypertension in Americans ages 18 to 49 years is increasing, also placing them at higher cardiovascular risk.[45,46]

Low Blood Pressure. Interpret relatively low levels of blood pressure in the light of past readings and the patient's clinical state.

A pressure of 110/70 mm Hg would usually be normal, but could also indicate significant hypotension if past pressures have been high.

Orthostatic Hypotension. If indicated, assess *orthostatic hypotension*, common in older adults. Measure blood pressure and heart rate in two positions—*supine* after the patient is resting from 3 to 10 minutes, then within 3 minutes once the patient *stands up*. Normally, as the patient rises from the horizontal to the standing position, systolic pressure drops slightly or remains unchanged, whereas diastolic pressure rises slightly. Orthostatic hypotension is a drop in systolic blood pressure of at least 20 mm Hg or in diastolic blood pressure of at least 10 mm Hg within 3 minutes of standing.[47,48]

Causes of *orthostatic hypotension* include drugs, moderate or severe blood loss, prolonged bed rest, and diseases of the autonomic nervous system.

See Chapter 20, Physical Examination of the Older Adult, pp. 989–997.

Special Situations

Weak or Inaudible Korotkoff Sounds. Consider technical problems such as erroneous placement of your stethoscope, failure to make full skin contact with the bell, and venous engorgement of the patient's arm from repeated inflations of the cuff. Also consider the possibilities of vascular disease or shock. When you cannot hear Korotkoff sounds at all, alternative methods using a Doppler probe or direct arterial pressure tracings may be necessary.

In rare cases, patients are pulseless due to occlusive disease in the arteries of all the limbs from *Takayasu arteritis, giant cell arteritis,* or *atherosclerosis.*

White Coat Hypertension. Encourage the patient to relax and remeasure the blood pressure later in the encounter. Consider automated office readings or ambulatory recordings.

See definition of white coat hypertension on p. 126.

The Obese or Very Thin Patient. For the *obese arm,* use a cuff 16 cm in width. If the upper arm is short despite a large circumference, use a thigh cuff or a very long cuff. If the arm circumference is >50 cm and not amenable to use of a thigh cuff, wrap an appropriately sized cuff around the forearm, hold the forearm at heart level, and feel for the radial pulse.[42] Other options include using a Doppler probe at the radial artery or an oscillometric device. For the *very thin arm,* consider using a pediatric cuff.

Using a small cuff overestimates systolic blood pressure in obese patients.[49]

Arrhythmias. Irregular rhythms produce variations in pressure and therefore unreliable measurements. Ignore the effects of an occasional premature contraction. With frequent premature contractions or atrial fibrillation, determine the average of several observations and note that your measurements are approximate. Ambulatory monitoring for 2 to 24 hours is recommended.[42]

Detection of an irregularly irregular rhythm suggests *atrial fibrillation.* For all irregular patterns, obtain an ECG to identify the type of rhythm.

The Hypertensive Patient with Systolic Blood Pressure Higher in the Arms than in the Legs. Compare blood pressure in the arms and the legs and assess "femoral delay" at least once in every hypertensive patient.

- *Coarctation of the aorta* arises from narrowing of the thoracic aorta, usually distal to origin of the left subclavian artery, and classically presents with systolic hypertension greater in the arms than the legs. In normal patients, the systolic blood pressure should be 5 to 10 mm Hg higher in the lower extremities than in the arms.

In coarctation of the aorta and *occlusive aortic disease* there is systolic hypertension in the upper extremities and lower blood pressure in the legs, and diminished or delayed femoral pulses, sometimes termed *femoral delay.*[50]

- To determine blood pressure in the leg, use a wide, long thigh cuff that has a bladder size of 18 × 42 cm, and apply it to the midthigh. Center the bladder over the posterior surface, wrap it securely, and listen over the popliteal artery. If possible, the patient should be prone. Alternatively, ask the supine patient to flex one leg slightly, with the heel resting on the bed.

- Palpate the radial or brachial and the femoral pulses at the same time, and compare their volume and timing. Normally, volume is equal and the pulses occur simultaneously.

Heart Rate and Rhythm

Examine the arterial pulses, the heart rate and rhythm, and the amplitude and contour of the pulse wave.

Heart Rate. The radial pulse is commonly used to assess the heart rate (Fig. 4-8). With the pads of your index and middle fingers, compress the radial artery until a maximal pulsation is detected. If the rhythm is regular and the rate seems normal, count the rate for 30 seconds and multiply by 2. If the rate is unusually fast or slow, count for 60 seconds. The usual range of normal is 60 to 90 to 100 beats per minute.[51]

An elevated resting heart rate is associated with increased risk of cardiovascular disease and mortality.[52]

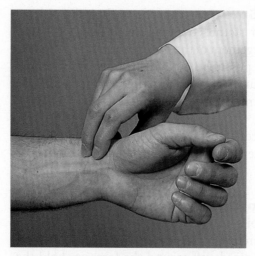

FIGURE 4-8. **Palpate the radial pulse.**

Rhythm. Begin by palpating the radial pulse. If there are any irregularities, assess the rhythm at the apex by listening with your stethoscope. Premature beats of low amplitude may not be transmitted to the peripheral pulses, leading to underestimates of the heart rate. Is the rhythm regular or irregular? If irregular, try to identify a pattern: (1) Do early beats appear in a basically regular rhythm? (2) Does the irregularity vary consistently with respiration? (3) Is the rhythm totally irregular?

See Table 9-1, Selected Heart Rates and Rhythms, p. 400, and Table 9-2, Selected Irregular Rhythms, p. 401.

Always check an ECG to identify the type of rhythm.

Respiratory Rate and Rhythm

Observe the *rate, rhythm, depth,* and *effort of breathing.* Count the number of respirations in 1 minute either by visual inspection or by subtly listening over the patient's trachea with your stethoscope during your examination of the head and neck or chest. Normally, adults take approximately 20 breaths per minute in a quiet, regular pattern. An occasional sigh is normal. Check to see if expiration is prolonged.

See Table 8-4, Abnormalities in Rate and Rhythm of Breathing, p. 335.

Prolonged expiration is common in COPD.

Temperature

The core body temperature, measured internally, is approximately 37°C (98.6°F) and fluctuates approximately 1°C over the course of the day. It is lowest in the early morning and highest in the afternoon and evening. Women have a wider range of normal temperature than men.[53]

Although the research gold standard for core body temperature is the blood temperature in the pulmonary artery, clinical practice relies on noninvasive oral, rectal, axillary, tympanic membrane, and temporal artery measurements.[44] Tympanic membrane and temporal artery temperatures use infrared thermometry.

■ *Oral and rectal temperature* measurements remain common. Oral temperatures are generally *lower* than the core body temperature. They are also *lower* than rectal temperatures by an average of 0.4 to 0.5°C (0.7 to 0.9°F), and *higher* than axillary temperatures by approximately 1°. *Axillary temperatures* take 5 to 10 minutes to register and are considered less accurate than other measurements.

■ *Tympanic membrane temperatures* can be more variable than oral or rectal temperatures. Studies vary in methodology, but suggest that in adults, *oral and temporal artery temperatures* correlate more closely with the pulmonary artery temperature, but are about 0.5°C lower.[54-56]

Oral Temperatures. For *oral temperatures,* options include electronic or glass thermometers. Due to breakage and mercury exposure, glass thermometers are being replaced by electronic thermometers. If using an *electronic thermometer,* carefully place the disposable cover over the probe and insert the thermometer under the tongue. Ask the patient to close both lips, and then watch closely for the digital readout. An accurate temperature recording usually takes about 10 seconds.

For *glass thermometers,* shake the thermometer down to 35°C (96°F) or below, insert it under the tongue, instruct the patient to close both lips, and wait for 3 to 5 minutes. Then read the thermometer, reinsert it for a minute, and read it again. If the temperature is still rising, repeat this procedure until the reading remains stable. Note that hot or cold liquids, and even smoking, can alter the temperature reading. In these situations, delay taking the temperature for 10 to 15 minutes.

Rectal Temperatures. For a *rectal temperature,* ask the patient to lie on one side with the hip flexed. Select a rectal thermometer with a stubby tip, lubricate it, and insert it about 3 cm to 4 cm (1.5 inches) into the anal canal, in a direction pointing to the umbilicus. Remove it after 3 minutes, then read. Alternatively, use an electronic thermometer after lubricating the probe cover. Wait about 10 seconds for the digital temperature recording to appear.

Fever, or *pyrexia,* refers to an elevated body temperature. *Hyperpyrexia* refers to extreme elevation in temperature, above 41.1°C (106°F), whereas *hypothermia* refers to an abnormally low temperature, below 35°C (95°F) rectally.

Causes of *fever* include infection, trauma such as surgery or crush injuries, malignancy, drug reactions, and immune disorders such as collagen vascular disease.

The chief cause of *hypothermia* is exposure to cold. Other causes include reduced movement as in paralysis, interference with vasoconstriction from sepsis or excess alcohol, starvation, hypothyroidism, and hypoglycemia. Older adults are especially susceptible to hypothermia and also less likely to develop fever.

Rapid respiratory rates tend to increase the discrepancy between oral and rectal temperatures. In these situations, rectal temperatures are more reliable.

Tympanic Membrane Temperatures.   The tympanic membrane shares the same blood supply as the hypothalamus, where temperature regulation occurs in the brain. Accurate temperature readings require access to the tympanic membrane. Make sure the external auditory canal is free of cerumen, which can lower temperature readings. Position the probe in the canal so that the infrared beam is aimed at the tympanic membrane, or otherwise the measurement will be invalid. Wait for 2 to 3 seconds until the digital temperature reading appears.

Temporal Artery Temperatures.   This method takes advantage of the location of the temporal artery, which branches off the external carotid artery and lies within a millimeter of the skin surface of the forehead, cheek, and behind the ear lobes. Place the probe against the center of the forehead, depress the infrared scanning button, and brush the device across the forehead, down the cheek, and behind an earlobe. Read the display, which records the highest measure temperature. Industry information suggests that combined forehead and behind-the-ear contact is more accurate than scanning only the forehead.

Acute and Chronic Pain

Assessing Acute and Chronic Pain

The International Association for the Study of Pain defines *pain* as "an unpleasant sensory and emotional experience" associated with tissue damage. The experience of pain is complex and multifactorial. Pain involves sensory, emotional, and cognitive processing, but may lack a specific physical etiology.[57]

Chronic pain is defined in several ways: pain not associated with cancer or other medical conditions that persists for more than 3 to 6 months; pain lasting more than 1 month beyond the course of an acute illness or injury; or pain recurring at intervals of months or years. Chronic noncancer pain affects an estimated 100 million Americans and 5% to 33% of patients in primary care settings.[58,59] More than 40% of patients report that their pain is poorly controlled. Treatment and management represent a growing concern to leading educators and professional societies, warranting a special report by the IOM in 2011 on *Relieving Pain in America, A Blueprint for Transforming Prevention, Care, Education, and Research*[58] and targeted interdisciplinary curricula.[60]

Adopt a multidisciplinary, measurement-based approach to assessing pain, carefully listening to the patient's story, the many features of pain, and contributing factors.[58,61]

The Patient's History.   Elicit the full history of the patient's pain, tailoring your approach to each patient's unique experience. Ask the patient to describe the pain and how it started. Is it related to a site of injury, movement, or time of day? What is the quality of the pain—sharp, dull, burning? Ask if the pain radiates or follows a particular pattern. What makes the pain better or worse? Pursue the seven features of pain, as you would with any symptom. Ask the patient to point to the pain because verbal descriptions can be imprecise.

Chronic pain may be a spectrum disorder related to mental health and somatic conditions. See Chapter 5, Behavior and Mental Status, Symptoms and Behavior, pp. 148–153.

Numerous validated brief screening tools are available for office use.[58,61]

See Chapter 3, The Seven Attributes of a Symptom, p. 79.

Ask about treatments that the patient has tried, including medications, physical therapy, and alternative medicines. A comprehensive medication history identifies drugs that interact with analgesics and reduce their efficacy.

Explore any comorbid conditions such as arthritis, diabetes, HIV/AIDS, substance abuse, sickle cell disease, or psychiatric disorders. These can have significant effects on the patient's experience of pain.

Chronic pain is the leading cause of disability and impaired performance at work. Inquire about the effects of pain on the patient's daily activities, mood, sleep, work, and sexual activity.

Assessing Severity of the Pain.   Use a consistent method to assess pain severity. Three scales are common: the Visual Analog Scale and two scales using ratings from 1 to 10—the Numeric Rating Scale and the Wong-Baker FACES Pain Rating Scale. Numerous more detailed multidimensional tools like the Brief Pain Inventory and the McGill Pain Questionnaire are also available, but take longer to administer.[62] The Wong-Baker FACES® Pain Raiting Scale can be used by children as well as patients with language barriers or cognitive impairment.[63] The Faces Pain Scale by the International Association for the Study of Pain[64] is reproduced in Figure 4-9.

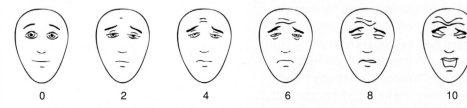

FIGURE 4-9.   **Pain rating scale. Explain to the person that each face is for a person who feels happy because he has no pain (hurt) or sad because he has some or a lot of pain. Face 0 is very happy because he doesn't hurt at all. Face 2 hurts just a little bit. Face 4 hurts a little more. Face 6 hurts even more. Face 8 hurts a whole lot. Face 10 hurts as much as you can imagine, although you don't have to be crying to feel this bad. Ask the person to choose the face that best describes how he is feeling.** (Faces Pain Scale—Revised (FPS-R). www.iasp-pain.org/fpsr. Copyright © 2001, International Association for the Study of Pain®. Reproduced with permission.)

Health Disparities.   Health disparities in pain treatment and delivery of care are well documented, ranging from lower use of analgesics in emergency rooms for African-American and Hispanic patients to disparities in use of analgesics for cancer, postoperative, and low back pain.[58] Studies show that clinician stereotypes, language barriers, and unconscious clinician biases in decision making all contribute to these disparities. Critique your own communication style, seek information and best practice standards, and improve your techniques of patient education and empowerment as first steps to ensure uniform and effective pain management.

See IOM report, *Unequal Treatment: Confronting Racial and Ethnic Disparities in Health Care*, 2002.[65]

Types of Pain.   Review the summary of types of pain on the next page to aid in your diagnosis and management.[66]

Types of Pain

Nociceptive (somatic)	Nociceptive (somatic) pain is linked to tissue damage to the skin, musculoskeletal system, or viscera (visceral pain), but the sensory nervous system is intact, as in arthritis or spinal stenosis. It can be acute or chronic. It is mediated by the afferent A-delta and C-fibers of the sensory system. The involved afferent nociceptors can be sensitized by inflammatory mediators and modulated by both psychological processes and neurotransmitters like endorphins, histamines, acetylcholine, serotonin, norepinephrine, and dopamine.
Neuropathic pain	*Neuropathic pain* is a direct consequence of a lesion or disease affecting the somatosensory system. Over time, neuropathic pain may become independent of the inciting injury, becoming burning, lancinating, or shock-like in quality, It may persist even after healing from the initial injury has occurred. Mechanisms postulated to evoke neuropathic pain include central nervous system brain or spinal cord injury from stroke or trauma; peripheral nervous system disorders causing entrapment or pressure on spinal nerves, plexuses, or peripheral nerves; and referred pain syndromes with increased or prolonged pain responses to inciting stimuli. These triggers appear to induce changes in pain signal processing through "neuronal plasticity," leading to pain that persists beyond healing from the initial injury.
Central sensitization	In *central sensitization pain,* there is alteration of central nervous system processing of sensation, leading to amplification of pain signals. There is a lower pain threshold to nonpainful stimuli, and the response to pain may be more severe than expected. Mechanisms are the subject of ongoing research. An example is fibromyalgia, which has a strong overlap with depression, anxiety, and somatization disorders and responds best to medications that modify neurotransmitters like serotonin and dopamine.
Psychogenic pain	*Psychogenic pain* involves the many factors that influence the patient's report of pain—psychiatric conditions like anxiety or depression, personality and coping style, cultural norms, and social support systems.
Idiopathic pain	*Idiopathic pain* is pain without an identifiable etiology.

Managing Chronic Pain. Managing pain is a complex clinical challenge. Experts recommend a stepped-care approach, with an emphasis on measurement and tracking tools to follow responses to treatment and referrals to specialists, summarized below.[67]

Managing Chronic Pain: Steps for Measurement-Based Care

Step 1: *Measure pain intensity and pain interference.* A validated two-item questionnaire is available for primary care asking patients to rate pain in the past month and interference with daily activities on a scale of 1 to 10.[61]

Step 2: *Measure mood.* Treatable depression, anxiety, and posttraumatic stress disorder (PTSD) frequently accompany chronic pain. The PHQ-4 is a 4-item questionnaire for detecting anxiety and depression.[68] The Primary Care-PTSD is a 4-question screen for PTSD.[69]

Step 3: *Measure the effect of pain on sleep.* Opioid doses correlate with sleep-disordered breathing and sleep apnea.

Step 4: Measure risk of co-occurring substance abuse, estimated at 18% to 30%.

Step 5: *Measure the opioid dose* and calculate the opioid dose equivalency using available web-based calculators.

Source: Tauben D. Chronic pain management: measurement-based stepped care solutions. Pain: Clinical Updates. International Association for the Study of Pain. December 2012. Available at http://www.iasp-pain.org/PublicationsNews/NewsletterIssue.aspx?ItemNumber=2064. Accessed January 28, 2015.

Treating pain requires sophisticated knowledge of nonopioid, opioid, and adjuvant analgesics and behavioral and physical therapy, areas that are beyond the scope of this book. Over recent decades, clinicians have become increasingly attentive to chronic pain in response to numerous guidelines for treatment and care. In parallel, prescriptions for some opioids have increased more than 800% in the past 10 years.[70] Roughly a third of all patients with chronic noncancer pain, or more than 3% of U.S. adults, take opioids, primarily for arthritis and low back pain.[71] At the same time, rates of death from opioid overdose among medically prescribed opioid users have climbed to 148 per 100,000.[72] Recent studies show that the death rate is directly related to the maximum prescribed dose of daily opioids. Risk of overdose increases more than four- to eightfold for patients taking the highest doses, namely 100 mg/day or more.[72,73] Risk factors for fatal overdose include age 65 years or older, depression, substance abuse, and concurrent benzodiazepine treatment. To avoid such hazards, make a commitment to acquiring skills in pain assessment and therapeutics, and take advantage of the validated substance abuse screening and brief intervention protocols that have been shown to reduce substance-use–related problems.[74–77]

Focus on the *Four A's* to monitor patient outcomes:
- **Analgesia**
- **Activities of daily living**
- **Adverse effects**
- **Aberrant drug-related behaviors**

See Chapter 3, Interviewing and the Health History, for definitions of tolerance, physical dependence, and addiction, p. 96.

Recording Your Findings

Your write-up of the physical examination begins with a general description of the patient's appearance, based on the General Survey. Note that initially you may use sentences to describe your findings; later you will use phrases. The style below contains phrases appropriate for most write-ups.

Recording the Physical Examination—The General Survey and Vital Signs

Choose vivid and graphic adjectives, as if you are painting a picture in words. Avoid clichés such as "well-developed," "well-nourished," or "in no acute distress," because they are too general to convey the special features of the patient before you.

Record the vital signs taken at the time of your examination rather than earlier in the day. (Common abbreviations for blood pressure, heart rate, and respiratory rate are self-explanatory.)

"Mrs. Scott is a young, healthy-appearing woman, well-groomed, fit, and cheerful. Height is 5'4", weight 135 lbs, BMI 24, BP 120/80, right and left arms, HR 72 and regular, RR 16, temperature 37.5°C."

OR

"Mr. Jones is an elderly man who looks pale and chronically ill. He is alert, with good eye contact but unable to speak more than two or three words at a time due to shortness of breath. He has intercostal muscle retraction when breathing and sits upright in bed. He is thin, with diffuse muscle wasting. Height is 6'2", weight 175 lbs, BP 160/95, right arm, HR 108 and irregular, RR 32 and labored, temperature 101.2°F."

These findings suggest exacerbation of *COPD*.

Table 4-1 Obesity-Related Health Conditions

Cardiovascular
- Hypertension
- Coronary artery disease
- Atrial fibrillation
- Heart failure
- Cor pulmonale
- Varicose veins

Endocrine
- Metabolic syndrome
- Type 2 diabetes
- Dyslipidemia
- Polycystic ovarian syndrome/androgenicity
- Amenorrhea/infertility/menstrual disorders

Gastrointestinal
- Gastroesophageal reflux disease (GERD)
- Nonalcoholic fatty liver disease (NAFLD)
- Cholelithiasis
- Hernias
- Cancer: colon, pancreas, esophagus, liver

Genitourinary
- Urinary stress incontinence
- Obesity-related glomerulopathy
- Hypogonadism (male)
- Cancer: breast, cervical, ovarian, uterine
- Pregnancy complications
- Nephrolithiasis, chronic renal disease

Integument
- Striae distensae (stretch marks)
- Status pigmentation of legs
- Lymphedema
- Cellulitis
- Intertrigo, carbuncles
- Acanthosis nigricans/skin tags

Musculoskeletal
- Hyperuricemia and gout
- Immobility
- Osteoarthritis (knees, hips)
- Low back pain

Neurologic
- Stroke
- Idiopathic intracranial hypertension
- Meralgia paresthetica

Psychological
- Depression/low self-esteem
- Body image disturbance
- Social stigmatization

Respiratory
- Dyspnea
- Obstructive sleep apnea
- Hypoventilation syndrome/Pickwickian syndrome
- Pulmonary embolism
- Asthma

Used with permission from Kushner RF. *Roadmaps for Clinical Practice: Case Studies in Disease Prevention and Health Promotion—Assessment and Management of Adult Obesity: A Primer for Physicians.* Chicago, IL: American Medical Association; 2003. © American Medical Association 2003. All Rights Reserved.

Table 4-2 Eating Disorders and Excessively Low BMI

In the United States, an estimated 5 to 10 million women and 1 million men suffer from eating disorders. The lifetime prevalence estimates for anorexia nervosa, bulimia nervosa, and binge eating disorders are 0.9%, 1.5%, and 3.5%, respectively, among women; and 0.3%, 0.5%, and 2.0%, respectively, among men. These severe disturbances of eating behavior are often difficult to detect, especially in teens wearing baggy clothes or in individuals who binge and then induce vomiting or evacuation. Be familiar with the two principal eating disorders, *anorexia nervosa* and *bulimia nervosa*. Both conditions are characterized by distorted perceptions of body image and weight. Early detection is important because prognosis improves when treatment occurs in the early stages of these disorders.

Clinical Features

Anorexia Nervosa	Bulimia Nervosa
<ul><li>Refusal to maintain minimally normal body weight (or BMI above 17.5 kg/m^2)</li><li>Afraid of gaining weight or becoming fat</li><li>Frequently starving but in denial; lacking insight</li><li>Often brought in by family members</li><li>May present as failure to make expected weight gains in childhood or adolescence, amenorrhea in women, loss of libido or potency in men</li><li>Associated with depressive symptoms such as depressed mood, irritability, social withdrawal, insomnia, decreased libido</li><li>Additional features supporting diagnosis: self-induced vomiting or purging, excessive exercise, use of appetite suppressants and/or diuretics</li><li>Biologic complications<ul><li>*Gynecological:* amenorrhea</li><li>*Endocrine:* hypercortisolemia, hypoglycemia, osteoporosis, euthyroid hypothyroxinemia</li><li>*Cardiovascular disorders:* bradycardia, hypotension, arrhythmias, cardiomyopathy</li><li>*Metabolic disorders:* hypokalemia, hypochloremic metabolic alkalosis, increased blood urea nitrogen (BUN), edema</li><li>*Other:* dry skin, dental caries, delayed gastric emptying, constipation, anemia, fatigue, weakness</li></ul></li></ul>	<ul><li>Repeated binge eating followed by self-induced vomiting, misuse of laxatives, diuretics or other medications, fasting, or excessive exercise</li><li>Often with normal weight</li><li>Overeating at least once a week during 3-month period; large amounts of food consumed in short period (~2 hrs)</li><li>Preoccupation with eating; craving and compulsion to eat; lack of control over eating; alternating with periods of starvation</li><li>Dread of fatness (usually leading to underweight)</li><li>Subtypes of<ul><li>*Purging:* bulimic episodes accompanied by self-induced vomiting or use of laxatives, diuretics, or enemas</li><li>*Nonpurging:* bulimic episodes accompanied by compensatory behavior such as fasting, or excessive exercising</li></ul></li><li>Biologic complications. See changes listed for anorexia nervosa, especially weakness, fatigue, mild cognitive disorder; also erosion of dental enamel, parotid gland swelling, pancreatitis, mild neuropathies, seizures, hypokalemia, hypochloremic metabolic acidosis, hypomagnesemia</li></ul>

Sources: Hudson JI, Hiripi E, Pope HG Jr, et al. The prevalence and correlates of eating disorders in the National Comorbidity Survey Replication. *Biol Psychiatry.* 2007;61:348; World Health Organization. *The ICD-10 Classification of Mental and Behavioral Disorders: Diagnostic Criteria for Research.* Geneva: World Health Organization, 1993; American Psychiatric Association. *DSM-5: Diagnostic and Statistical Manual of Mental Disorders.* 5th ed. Washington, DC: American Psychiatric Association, 2013; Andersen AE. Eating Disorders: In: Sadock BJ, Sadock VA, Ruiz P, eds. *Kaplan and Sadock's Comprehensive Textbook of Psychiatry.* 9th ed. New York, NY: Wolters Kluwer; Lippincott Williams & Wilkins, 2009.

Table 4-3 Nutrition Screening

Mini Nutritional Assessment
MNA®

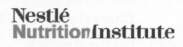

Last name: _____   First name: _____

Sex: _____   Age: _____   Weight, kg: _____   Height, cm: _____   Date: _____

Complete the screen by filling in the boxes with the appropriate numbers. Total the numbers for the final screening score.

Screening

A Has food intake declined over the past 3 months due to loss of appetite, digestive problems, chewing or swallowing difficulties?

0 = severe decrease in food intake
1 = moderate decrease in food intake
2 = no decrease in food intake ☐

B Weight loss during the last 3 months

0 = weight loss greater than 3 kg (6.6 lbs)
1 = does not know
2 = weight loss between 1 and 3 kg (2.2 and 6.6 lbs)
3 = no weight loss ☐

C Mobility

0 = bed or chair bound
1 = able to get out of bed / chair but does not go out
2 = goes out ☐

D Has suffered psychological stress or acute disease in the past 3 months?

0 = yes   2 = no ☐

E Neuropsychological problems

0 = severe dementia or depression
1 = mild dementia
2 = no psychological problems ☐

F1 Body Mass Index (BMI) (weight in kg) / (height in m)^2

0 = BMI less than 19
1 = BMI 19 to less than 21
2 = BMI 21 to less than 23
3 = BMI 23 or greater ☐

IF BMI IS NOT AVAILABLE, REPLACE QUESTION F1 WITH QUESTION F2.
DO NOT ANSWER QUESTION F2 IF QUESTION F1 IS ALREADY COMPLETED.

F2 Calf circumference (CC) in cm

0 = CC less than 31
3 = CC 31 or greater ☐

Screening score (max. 14 points)

12 - 14 points: Normal nutritional status
8 - 11 points: At risk of malnutrition
0 - 7 points: Malnourished ☐☐

References
1. Vellas B, Villars H, Abellan G, et al. Overview of the MNA® - Its History and Challenges. J Nutr Health Aging. 2006;10:456-465.
2. Rubenstein LZ, Harker JO, Salva A, Guigoz Y, Vellas B. Screening for Undernutrition in Geriatric Practice: Developing the Short-Form Mini Nutritional Assessment (MNA-SF). J. Geront. 2001; 56A: M366-377
3. Guigoz Y. The Mini-Nutritional Assessment (MNA®) Review of the Literature - What does it tell us? J Nutr Health Aging. 2006; 10:466-487.
4. Kaiser MJ, Bauer JM, Ramsch C, et al. Validation of the Mini Nutritional Assessment Short-Form (MNA®-SF): A practical tool for identification of nutritional status. J Nutr Health Aging. 2009; 13:782-788.
® Société des Produits Nestlé, S.A., Vevey, Switzerland, Trademark Owners © Nestlé, 1994, Revision 2009. N67200 12/99 10M
For more information: www.mna-elderly.com

Table 4-4 Obesity: Stages of Change Model and Assessing Readiness

Stage	Characteristic	Patient Verbal Cue	Appropriate Intervention	Sample Dialogue
Precontemplation	Unaware of problem, no interest in change	"I'm not really interested in weight loss. It's not a problem."	Provide information about health risks and benefits of weight loss	"Would you like to read some information about the health aspects of obesity?"
Contemplation	Aware of problem, beginning to think of changing	"I know I need to lose weight, but with all that's going on in my life right now, I'm not sure I can."	Help resolve ambivalence; discuss barriers	"Let's look at the benefits of weight loss, as well as what you may need to change."
Preparation	Realizes benefits of making changes and thinking about how to change	"I have to lose weight, and I'm planning to do that."	Teach behavior modification; provide education	"Let's take a closer look at how you can reduce some of the calories you eat and how to increase your activity during the day."
Action	Actively taking steps toward change	"I'm doing my best. This is harder than I thought."	Provide support and guidance, with a focus on the long term	"It's terrific that you're working so hard. What problems have you had so far? How have you solved them?"
Maintenance	Initial treatment goals reached	"I've learned a lot through this process."	Relapse control	"What situations continue to tempt you to overeat? What can be helpful for the next time you face such a situation?"

Sources: American Medical Association. Roadmaps for Clinical Practice—Case Studies in Disease Prevention and Health Promotion—Assessment and Management of Adult Obesity: A Primer for Physicians. Communication and Counseling Strategies. Booklet 8. Chicago, November 2003. Adapted from Prochaska JO, DiClemente CC. Toward a comprehensive model of change. In: Miller WR, ed. *Treating Addictive Behaviors*. New York, NY: Plenum, 1986:3.

Table 4-5 Nutrition Counseling: Sources of Nutrients

Nutrient	Food Source
Calcium	Dairy foods such as milk, natural cheeses, and yogurt Calcium-fortified cereals, fruit juice, soy milk, and tofu Dark green leafy vegetables like collard, turnip, and mustard greens; kale; bok choy Sardines
Iron	Lean meat, dark turkey meat, liver Clams, mussels, oysters, sardines, anchovies Iron-fortified cereals Enriched and whole grain bread Spinach, peas, lentil, turnip greens, and artichokes Dried prunes and raisins
Folate	Cooked dried beans and peas Oranges, orange juice Liver Spinach, mustard greens Black-eyed peas, lentils, okra, chick peas, peanuts Folate-fortified cereals
Vitamin D	Vitamin D–fortified milk, orange juice, and cereals Cod liver oil; swordfish, salmon, herring, mackerel, tuna, trout Egg yolk Mushrooms

Source: Adapted from U.S. Department of Agriculture and U.S. Department of Health and Human Services. Dietary Guidelines for Americans, 2010. Washington, DC: U.S. Government Printing Office; 2010; Choose MyPlate.gov. Available at http://www.choosemyplate.gov/index.html. Accessed December 15, 2014; Office of Dietary Supplements, National Institutes of Health. Dietary Supplement Fact Sheets: Calcium; Vitamin D. Available at http://ods.od.nih.gov/factsheets/list-all/. Accessed December 15, 2014.

Table 4-6 Patients with Hypertension: Recommended Changes in Diet

Dietary Change	Food Source
Increase foods high in potassium	Baked white or sweet potatoes, white beans, beet greens, soybeans, spinach, lentils, kidney beans Yogurt Tomato paste, juice, puree, and sauce Bananas, plantains, many dried fruits, orange juice
Decrease foods high in sodium	Canned foods (soups, tuna fish) Pretzels, potato chips, pizza, pickles, olives Many processed foods (frozen dinners, ketchup, mustard) Batter-fried foods Table salt, including for cooking

Source: Adapted from: U.S. Department of Agriculture and U.S. Department of Health and Human Services. Dietary Guidelines for Americans, 2010. Washington, D.C.: U.S. Government Printing Office; 2010; Choose MyPlate.gov. Available at http://www.choosemyplate.gov/index.html. Accessed December 15, 2014; Office of Dietary Supplements, National Institutes of Health. Dietary Supplement Fact Sheets: Calcium; Vitamin D. Available at http://ods.od.nih.gov/factsheets/list-all/. Accessed December 15, 2014.

References

1. Balachandran JS, Patel SR. In the clinic: obstructive sleep apnea. *Ann Intern Med.* 2014;161:ITC-1.

2. Bray GA, Wilson JF. In the clinic. Obesity. *Ann Intern Med.* 2008; 154:ITC4–1.

3. American Academy of Pain Medicine. AAPM Facts and Figures on Pain. Available at http://www.painmed.org/patientcenter/facts_on_pain.aspx. Accessed January 21, 2015.

4. Institute of Medicine of the National Academies Report. *Relieving Pain in America: A Blueprint for Transforming Prevention, Care, Education, and Research.* Washington, DC: The National Academies Press; 2011.

5. Riskowski JL. Associations of socioeconomic position and pain prevalence in the United States: findings from the National Health and Nutrition Examination Survey. *Pain Med.* 2014;15:1508.

6. Go AS, Mozaffarian D, Roger VL, et al. Heart disease and stroke statistics–2014 update: a report from the American Heart Association. *Circulation.* 2014;129(3):e28.

7. Ogden CL, Carroll MD, Kit BK, et al. Prevalence of childhood and adult obesity in the United States, 2011–2012. *JAMA.* 2014;311(8): 806.

8. May AL, Freedman D, Sherry B, et al. Obesity–United States, 1999–2010. *MMWR Surveill Summ.* 2013;62(Suppl 3):120.

9. Bogers RP, Bemelmans WJ, Hoogenveen RT, et al. Association of overweight with increased risk of coronary heart disease partly independent of blood pressure and cholesterol levels: a meta-analysis of 21 cohort studies including more than 300,000 persons. *Arch Intern Med.* 2007;167(16):1720.

10. National Heart, Lung, and Blood Institute (NHLBI), North American Association for the Study of Obesity (NAASO). *Practical Guide on the Identification, Evaluation, and Treatment of Overweight and Obesity in Adults.* Bethesda, MD: National Institutes of Health; 2000. Available at http://www.nhlbi.nih.gov/files/docs/guidelines/prctgd_c.pdf. Accessed January 21, 2015.

11. Ng M, Fleming T, Robinson M, et al. Global, regional, and national prevalence of overweight and obesity in children and adults during 1980–2013: a systematic analysis for the Global Burden of Disease Study 2013. *Lancet.* 2014;384(9945):766.

12. Schauer GL, Halperin AC, Mancl LA, et al. Health professional advice for smoking and weight in adults with and without diabetes: findings from BRFSS. *J Behav Med.* 2013;36:10.

13. Kushner RF, Ryan DH. Assessment and lifestyle management of patients with obesity: clinical recommendations from systematic reviews. *JAMA.* 2014;312:943.

14. U.S. Department of Agriculture, U.S. Department of Health and Human Services. *Dietary Guidelines for Americans, 2010.* Washington, DC: U.S. Government Printing Office; 2010. Available at http://www.cnpp.usda.gov/DietaryGuidelines. Accessed January 21, 2015.

15. Le Blanc E, O'Connor E, Whitlock EP, et al. Screening for and Management of Obesity and Overweight in Adults. Evidence Report No. 89. AHRQ Publication No. 11–05159-EF-1. Rockville, MD. Agency for Healthcare Research and Quality, October 2011. Available at http://www.ncbi.nlm.nih.gov/pubmedhealth/PMH0016399/. Accessed January 21, 2015.

16. Kelesidis T, Kelesidis I, Chou S, et al. Narrative review: the role of leptin in human physiology: emerging clinical applications. *Ann Intern Med.* 2010;152(2):93.

17. Foster GD, Wyatt HR, Hill JO, et al. Weight and metabolic outcomes after 2 years on a low-carbohydrate versus low-fat diet: a randomized trial. *Ann Intern Med.* 2010;153(3):147.

18. Sacks FM, Bray GA, Carey VJ, et al. Comparison of weight-loss diets with different compositions of fat, protein, and carbohydrates. *N Engl J Med.* 2009;360(9):859.

19. Lau DC, Douketis JD, Morrison KM, et al. 2006 Canadian clinical practice guidelines on the management and prevention of obesity in adults and children [summary]. *CMAJ.* 2007;176(8):S1.

20. Strazzullo P, D'Elia L, Kandala NB, et al. Salt intake, stroke, and cardiovascular disease: meta-analysis of prospective studies. *BMJ.* 2009;339:b4567.

21. Institute of Medicine. *Sodium Intake in Populations: Assessment of Evidence. Report Brief.* Washington, DC: The Institute of Medicine; 2013.

22. Centers for Disease Control and Prevention (CDC). Trends in the prevalence of excess dietary sodium intake—United States, 2003–2010. *MMWR Morb Mortal Wkly Rep.* 2013;62(50):1021.

23. Eckel RH, Jakicic JM, Ard JD, et al. 2013 AHA/ACC guideline on lifestyle management to reduce cardiovascular risk: a report of the American College of Cardiology/American Heart Association Task Force on Practice Guidelines. *Circulation.* 2014;129(25 Suppl 2):S76.

24. Appel LJ, Frohlich ED, Hall JE, et al. The importance of population-wide sodium reduction as a means to prevent cardiovascular disease and stroke: a call to action from the American Heart Association. *Circulation.* 2011;123(10):1138.

25. Institute of Medicine. *Strategies to Reduce Sodium Intake in the United States.* Washington, DC; 2010.

26. National Heart L, and Blood Institute. *Your Guide to Lowering Your Blood Pressure with DASH.* U.S. Department of Health and Human Services; 2006.

27. *2008 Physical Activity Guidelines for Americans.* Washington, DC: U.S. Department of Health and Human Services; 2008.

28. Garber CE, Blissmer B, Deschenes MR, et al. American College of Sports Medicine position stand. Quantity and quality of exercise for developing and maintaining cardiorespiratory, musculoskeletal, and neuromotor fitness in apparently healthy adults: guidance for prescribing exercise. *Med Sci Sports Exerc.* 2011;43(7):1334.

29. Laumann A, Derick A. Tattoos and body piercings in the United States: a national data set. *J Am Acad Dermatol.* 2006;55:413.

30. National Heart Lung Blood Institute, National Institutes of Health. Body Mass Index Tables 1 and 2. Available at: http://www.nhlbi.nih.gov/health/educational/lose_wt/BMI/bmi_tbl.htm. Accessed January 21, 2015.

31. U.S. Preventive Services Task Force. Draft Recommendation Statement: High Blood Pressure in Adults: Screening. December 2014. Available at http://www.uspreventiveservicestaskforce.org/Page/Document/RecommendationStatementDraft/hypertension-in-adults-screening-and-home-monitoring. Accessed January 28, 2015.

32. Pickering TG, Miller NH, Ogebegbe G, et al. Call to action on use and reimbursement for home blood pressure monitoring: executive Summary. A joint scientific statement from the American Heart Association, American Society of Hypertension, and Preventive Cardiovascular Nurses Association. *Hypertension.* 2008;52:1.

33. Piper MA, Evans CV, Burda BU, et al. Diagnostic and predictive accuracy of blood pressure screening methods with consideration of rescreening intervals: an updated systematic review for the U.S. Preventive Services Task force. *Ann Intern Med.* 2014;162(3):192.

34. Hodgkinson J, Mant J, Guo B, et al. Relative effectiveness of clinic and home blood pressure monitoring compared with ambulatory

REFERENCES

blood pressure monitoring in diagnosis of hypertension: systematic review. *BMJ.* 2011;342:d3621.

35. James PA, Oparil S, Carter BL, et al. 2014 Evidence-based guideline for the management of high blood pressure in adults–report from the panel members appointed to the Eighth Joint National Committee (JNC 8). *JAMA.* 2014;311:507.

36. Chobanian AV, Bakris GL, Black HR, et al. The Seventh Report of the Joint National Committee on Prevention, Detection, Evaluation, and Treatment of High Blood Pressure—The JNC 7 Report. *JAMA.* 2003;289:2560. Available at http://www.nhlbi.nih.gov/health-pro/guidelines/current/hypertension-jnc-7/complete-report. Accessed January 22, 2015.

37. O'Brien E, Parati G, Stergiou G, et al. European Society of Hypertension position paper on ambulatory blood pressure monitoring. *J Hypertens.* 2013;31:1731.

38. Myers MG, Godwin M, Dawes M, et al. Conventional versus automated measurement of blood pressure in primary care patients with systolic hypertension: randomised parallel design controlled trial. *BMJ.* 2011;342;d286. doi: 10.1136/bmj.d286.

39. Roger VL, Go AS, Lloyed-Jone DM, et al. Executive summary: heart disease and stroke statistics–2012 update: a report from the American Heart Association. *Circulation.* 2012;125:188.

40. O'Brien E, Asmar R, Beilin L, et al. European Society of Hypertension recommendations for conventional, ambulatory, and more blood pressure measurement. *J Hypertens.* 2005;21:821.

41. O'Brien E, Pickering T, Asmar R, et al. International protocol for validation of blood pressure measuring devices in adults. *Blood Press Monit.* 2002;7:3.

42. Pickering TG, Hall JE, Appel LJ, et al. Recommendations for blood pressure measurement in humans and experimental animals. Part 1: blood pressure measurement in humans: a statement for professionals from the Subcommittee of Professional and Public Education of the American Heart Association Council on High Blood Pressure Research. *Circulation.* 2005;111:697.

43. Cavallini MC, Roman MJ, Blank SG, et al. Association of the auscultatory gap with vascular disease in hypertensive patients. *Ann Intern Med.* 1996;124:877.

44. Weber MA, Schiffrin EL, White WB, et al. Clinical practice guidelines for the management of hypertension in the community: A statement by the American Society of Hypertension and the International Society of Hypertension. *J Clin Hypertens.* 2014;16:14.

45. Chobanian A. Isolated systolic hypertension in the elderly. *N Engl J Med.* 2007;357:789.

46. Yano Y, Stamler J, Garside DB, et al. Isolated systolic hypertension in young and middle-aged adults and 31-year risk for cardiovascular mortality. The Chicago Heart Association Detection Project in Industry Study. *J Am Coll Cardiol.* 2015;65:327.

47. Freeman R. Neurogenic orthostatic hypotension. *N Engl J Med.* 2008; 358:615.

48. Carslon JE. Assessment of orthostatic blood pressure: measurement technique and clinical applications. *South Med J.* 1999;92:167.

49. Fonseca-Reyes S, de Alba-García JG, Parra-Carrillo JZ, et al. Effect of standard cuff on blood pressure readings in patients with obese arms. How frequent are arms of a 'large circumference'? *Blood Press Monit.* 2003;8:101.

50. Warnes CA, Williams RG, Bashore TM, et al. ACC/AHA 2008 Guidelines for the Management of Adults with Congenital Heart Disease: a report of the American College of Cardiology/American Heart Association Task Force on Practice Guidelines. *Circulation.* 2008;52:1558.

51. Mason JW, Ramseth DJ, Chanter DO, et al. Electrocardiographic reference ranges derived from 79,743 ambulatory subjects. *J Electrocardiol.* 2007;40:228.

52. Aladin AI, Whelton SP, Al-Mallah MH, et al. Relation of resting heart rate to risk for all-cause mortality by gender after considering exercise capacity (the Henry Ford Exercise Testing Project). *Am J Cardiology.* 2014:114:1701.

53. Sund-Levander M, Forsberg C, Wahren LK. Normal oral, rectal, tympanic and axillary body temperature in adult men and women: a systematic literature review. *Scand J Caring Sci.* 2002;16:122.

54. Jeffries S, Wetherall M, Young P, et al. A systematic review of the accuracy of peripheral thermometry in estimated core temperatures among febrile critically ill patients. *Crit Care Resusc.* 2011;13:194.

55. Lawson L, Bridges EJ, Ballou I, et al. Accuracy and precision of noninvasive temperature measurement in adult intensive care patients. *Am J Crit Care.* 2007;16:485.

56. McCallum L, Higgins D. Measuring body temperature. *Nurs Times.* 2012;108:20.

57. International Association for the Study of Pain. IASP Taxonomy. Updated May 2012. Available at http://www.iasp-pain.org/Taxonomy?navItemNumber=576. Accessed January 28, 2015.

58. Institute of Medicine. Relieving Pain in America: A Blueprint for Transforming Prevention, Care, Education, and Research (2011). Available at http://www.nap.edu/download.php?record_id=13172. Accessed January 28, 2015.

59. Breuer B, Cruciani R, Portenoy RK. Pain management by primary care physicians, pain physicians, chiropractors, and acupuncturists: a national survey. *South Med J.* 2010;103:738.

60. International Association for the Study of Pain. IASP Interprofessional Pain Curriculum Online. Updated January 2014. Available at http://www.iasp-pain.org/Education/CurriculumDetail.aspx?ItemNumber = 2057. Accessed January 29, 2015.

61. Washington State Agency Medical Directors' Group. *Interagency Guideline On Opioid Dosing For Chronic Non-Cancer Pain: An Education Aid To Improve Care And Safety With Opioid Treatment.* Olympia, Washington: Washington State Department of labor and Industries, 2010. Available at http://www.agencymeddirectors.wa.gov/opioiddosing.asp. Accessed January 28, 2015.

62. Keller S, Bann CM, Dodd SL, et al. Validity of the brief pain inventory for use in documenting the outcomes of patients with noncancer pain. *Clin J Pain.* 2004;20:309.

63. Bieri D, Reeve R, Champion GD, et al. The Faces Pain Scale for the self-assessment of the severity of pain experienced by children: development, initial validation and preliminary investigation for ratio scale properties. *Pain.* 1990;41:139.

64. International Society for the Study of Pain. Faces Pain Scale–Revised Home. Updated September 2014. Available at http://www.iasp-pain.org/Education/Content.aspx?ItemNumber=1519&navItemNumber=577. Accessed January 28, 2015.

65. Smedley BR, Stith AY, Nelson AR, eds. *Committee on Understanding and Eliminating Racial and Ethnic Disparities in Health Care. Unequal Treatment: Confronting Racial and Ethnic Disparities in Health Care.* Washington, DC: National Academies Press; 2002.

66. Haanpaa M, Attal N, Backonja M, et al. NeuPSIG guidelines on neuropathic pain assessment. *Pain.* 2011;152:14.

67. Tauben D. Chronic pain management: measurement-based stepped care solutions. Pain: Clinical Updates. International Association for the Study of Pain. December 2012. Available at http://www.iasp-pain.org/PublicationsNews/NewsletterIssue.aspx?ItemNumber=2064. Accessed January 28, 2015.

REFERENCES

68. Kroenke K, Spitzer RL, Williams JB, et al. An ultra-brief screening scale for anxiety and depression: the PHQ-4. *Psychosomatics.* 2009;50:613.

69. Ouimette P, Wade M, Prins A, et al. Identifying PTSD in primary care: comparison of the Primary Care-PTSD screen (PC-PTSD) and the General Health Questionnaire-12 (GHQ). *J Anxiety Disord.* 2008;22:337.

70. McClellan TA, Turner BJ. Chronic non-cancer pain management and opioid overdose: time to change prescribing practices. *Ann Intern Med.* 2010;152:123.

71. Altman RD, Smith HS. Opioid therapy for osteoarthritis and chronic low back pain. *Postgrad Med.* 2010;122:87.

72. Dunn KM, Saunders KW, Rutter CM, et al. Opioid prescriptions for chronic pain and overdose. A cohort study. *Ann Intern Med.* 2010;152:85.

73. Bohnert AS, Valenstein M, Bair MJ, et al. Association between opioid prescribing patterns and opioid overdose-related deaths. *JAMA.* 2011;305:1315.

74. Madras BK, Compton WM, Avula D, et al. Screening, brief interventions, referral to treatment (SBIRT) for illicit drug and alcohol use at multiple healthcare sites: comparison at intake and 6 months later. *Drug Alcohol Depend.* 2009;99:280.

75. Gilron I, Watson PN, Cahill CM, et al. Neuropathic pain: a practical guide for the clinician. *CMAJ.* 2006;175:256.

76. Butler SF, Budman SH, Fernandez K, et al. Validations of a screener and opioid assessment measure for patients with chronic pain. *Pain.* 2004;112(1–2):65.

77. Webster LR, Webster RM. Predicting aberrant behaviors in opioid-treated patients: preliminary validation of the Opioid Risk Tool. *Pain Med.* 2005;6:432.

5

Behavior and Mental Status

The Bates' suite offers these additional resources to enhance learning and facilitate understanding of this chapter:

- Bates' *Pocket Guide to Physical Examination and History Taking*, 8th edition
- Bates' *Visual Guide to Physical Examination*
- thePoint online resources, for students and instructors: http://thepoint.lww.com

As clinicians, we are uniquely poised to detect clues to mental illness and harmful behavior through empathic listening and close observation. Nonetheless, these clues are often missed. Recognizing mental illness is especially important given its significant prevalence and morbidity, the high likelihood that it is treatable, the shortage of psychiatrists, and the increasing importance of primary care clinicians as the first to encounter the patient's distress.[1,2] The prevalence of mental health disorders in U.S. adults in 2012 was 18%, affecting 43.7 million people; yet, only 41% received treatment.[3] Even for those receiving care, adherence to treatment guidelines in primary care offices is <50% and disproportionately lower for ethnic minorities.[4–6]

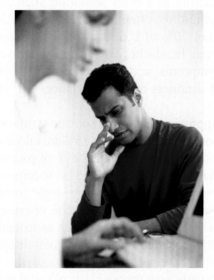

FIGURE 5-1. **Assessment of mental status can be challenging.**

Recognizing Mental Disorders

This chapter presents:

- Common symptoms and behaviors suggestive of mental health disorders
- Concepts that guide history taking and the general assessment of mental health
- Priorities for mental health promotion and counseling, and
- Components of the *mental status examination*, a structured framework for formal assessment of behavioral and mental health disorders, and a major component of the examination of the nervous system (Fig. 5-1).

See Chapter 17, The Nervous System, pp. 711–796.

Mental health disorders are commonly masked by other clinical conditions, calling for sensitive and careful inquiry. Learn to look for the interaction of anxiety and depression in patients with substance abuse, termed "dual diagnosis," because both must be treated for the patient to achieve optimal function. Watch for underlying psychiatric conditions in "difficult encounters" and patients with unexplained symptoms.[7] Explore the outlook of patients with chronic illness, a group that is especially vulnerable to depression and anxiety.[8] Finally, bear in mind that nearly half of those with any single mental disorder meet the criteria for one or more additional disorders, with severity strongly related to comorbidity.[9]

Symptoms and Behavior

Understanding Symptoms: What Do They Mean?

Changing Paradigms for Understanding Symptoms. Sorting the array of symptoms encountered in an office visit is an ongoing challenge. Unlike physical signs, symptoms are not observable. Traditionally, dualistic or binary explanatory models of symptoms have prevailed. Symptoms have been viewed as *psychological,* reflecting a mental or emotional state, or *physical,* relating to a body sensation such as pain, fatigue, or palpitations. Physical symptoms, often termed *somatic* in the mental health literature, prompt more than 50% of U.S. office visits.[10] Common somatic complaints include: pain from headache, backache, or musculoskeletal conditions; gastrointestinal symptoms; sexual or reproductive symptoms; and neurologic symptoms such as dizziness or loss of balance.

Approximately 5% of somatic symptoms are acute, triggering immediate evaluation.[11] Another 70% to 75% are minor or self-limited and resolve in 6 weeks. Nevertheless, approximately 25% of patients have persisting and recurrent symptoms that elude assessment and fail to improve. Overall, 30% of symptoms are *medically unexplained.* Some involve single complaints that persist longer than others, for example, back pain, headache, or musculoskeletal pain. Others present as clusters in *functional syndromes,* such as irritable bowel syndrome, fibromyalgia, chronic fatigue, temporomandibular joint disorder, and multiple chemical sensitivity.

Experts now propose that physical and psychological symptoms are interactive and represent "a varying mix of disease and nondisease input" that lies along a spectrum from medical to mental disorders.[11] Evidence shows that symptom etiology is often multifactorial, lacking a single cause; and that often, there are several related symptoms or symptom clusters rather than single complaints. The integrative continuum model leads to explanations that are less likely to be "simplified, reductionistic, or mechanistic." Watch for emerging schemas that place symptoms along a causative spectrum with five nodal points: symptoms like wheezing, with a clear medical cause; functional somatic syndromes like irritable bowel syndrome; "symptom-only diagnoses" such as low back pain; symptoms associated with psychological conditions, like fatigue in depression; and finally, medically unexplained symptoms.

Changes have also occurred in the classification of somatic syndromes in the *Diagnostic and Statistical Manual of Mental Disorders,* 5th Edition (*DSM-5*) of 2013. When patients have "distressing somatic symptoms plus abnormal thoughts, feelings, and behaviors in response to these symptoms," clinicians can

See Table 5-1, Somatic Symptom and Related Disorders, p. 169, for types of somatic symptom disorders and guidelines for management.

consider the diagnosis of *somatic symptom and related disorders*.[12] These patients have prominent somatic symptoms associated with significant distress and impairment and are seen more often in primary care and medical settings than in psychiatric and mental health settings. They may have accompanying medical disorders. The *DSM-5* notes that "a distinctive characteristic of the many individuals with somatic symptom disorder is not the somatic symptoms per se, but instead the way they present and interpret them." This change in diagnostic criteria emphasizes the presence of positive symptoms, and moves away from relying on medically unexplained symptoms and the absence of a medical cause, which can be difficult to determine. The prevalence of somatic symptom disorders is estimated at 5% to 7%.

Medically Unexplained Symptoms.   Patients with medically unexplained symptoms fall into heterogeneous groupings ranging from selected impairment to behaviors meeting *DSM-5* criteria for mood and somatic symptom disorders.[13,14] Many patients do not report symptoms of anxiety and depression, the most common mental health disorders in the general population, but focus on physical concerns instead (Fig. 5-2). Two-thirds of patients with depression, for example, present with physical complaints, and half report multiple unexplained or somatic symptoms.[14] Furthermore, functional syndromes have been shown to "frequently co-occur and share key symptoms and selected objective abnormalities."[15] Overlap rates for fibromyalgia and chronic fatigue syndrome in an analysis of 53 studies ranged from 34% to 70%. Failure to recognize the admixture of physical symptoms, functional syndromes, and common mental disorders—anxiety, depression, unexplained and somatoform symptoms, and substance abuse—add to the burden of patient undertreatment and poor quality of life. Authors of the first randomized controlled intervention trial for patients with medically unexplained symptoms advise viewing such symptoms as "a generalized warning sign of underlying psychological distress, of which depression is an advanced manifestation."[16]

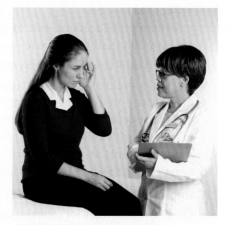

FIGURE 5-2. Clinicians often encounter symptoms not easily diagnosed.

The "Difficult Encounter."   Patients with unexplained and somatic symptoms are often frequent users of the health care system and labeled as "difficult patients." Patient depression and anxiety "make physician ratings of difficult encounters three times more likely, and somatization increases this likelihood nine-fold."[17] A growing literature reveals that 15% to 20% of primary care visits, or up to three to four visits a day, are considered difficult.[7] In the difficult encounter dyad, clinician factors have emerged that include job stress and burnout, anxiety and depression in the clinician, less clinical experience, and aversion to the psychosocial aspects of care.[18,19] Clinicians are urged to identify the many variables associated with these encounters, identify their own underlying negative emotions, adapt their approach and redirect the encounter, and explore what makes the encounter difficult with the patient.[20,21] In the words of an expert:

"Celebrate the well-navigated difficult encounter. Dealing with difficulty signifies mastery rather than weakness. Olympic dives are rated in terms of difficulty, as are mountain climbs, hiking trails, musical works, crossword puzzles, and highly technical procedures. Partnering with patients in the challenging aspects of their health, lives, or medical care is a stepping stone to surmounting together the difficult encounter."[7]

Mental Disorders and Unexplained Symptoms in Primary Care Settings

Mental Disorders in Primary Care

- Approximately 20% of primary care outpatients have mental disorders, but 50% to 75% of these disorders are undetected and untreated.[22,23]
- Prevalence of mental disorders in primary care settings is roughly as follows[22,24-26]:
  - Anxiety—20%
  - Mood disorders including dysthymia, depressive, and bipolar disorders—25%
  - Depression—10%
  - Somatoform disorders—10% to 15%
  - Alcohol and substance abuse—15% to 20%

Explained and Unexplained Symptoms

- Physical symptoms account for approximately 50% of office visits.
- Roughly one-third of physical symptoms are unexplained; in 20% to 25% of patients, physical symptoms become chronic or recurring.[10,14]
- In patients with *unexplained symptoms,* the prevalence of depression and anxiety exceeds 50% and increases with the total number of reported physical symptoms,[10,14] making detection and "dual diagnosis" important clinical goals.

Common Functional Syndromes

- Co-occurrence rates for *common functional syndromes* such as irritable bowel syndrome, fibromyalgia, chronic fatigue, temporomandibular joint disorder, and multiple chemical sensitivity reach 30% to 90%, depending on the disorders compared.[15]
- The prevalence of *symptom overlap* is high in the common functional syndromes namely, complaints of fatigue, sleep disturbance, musculoskeletal pain, headache, and gastrointestinal problems.
- The common functional syndromes also overlap in rates of functional impairment, psychiatric comorbidity, and response to cognitive and antidepressant therapy.

Mental Health Screening

Unexplained conditions lasting more than 6 weeks are increasingly recognized as chronic disorders that should prompt screening for depression, anxiety, or both. Because screening all patients is time consuming and expensive, experts recommend a two-tier approach: brief screening questions with high sensitivity and specificity for patients at risk, followed by more detailed investigation when indicated.

Several groups of patients warrant brief screening because of high risk of coexisting depression and anxiety. Recent studies have helped clarify *overlap symptoms* and *functional syndromes* and provide streamlined practical screening tools suitable for office care.[27] A well-established instrument to aid in office diagnosis is the PRIME-MD (Primary Care Evaluation of Mental Disorders); however, it contains 26 questions and takes up to 10 minutes to complete.[25] The *DSM-5* acknowledges the diagnostic challenges facing primary care providers and has reduced the total number of disorders as well as their subcategories in the reclassification of Somatic Symptoms and Related Disorders. Improved screening tools for office use and management will continue to emerge.

Patient Indications for Mental Health Screening

- Medically unexplained physical symptoms—more than half have depression or anxiety disorder
- Multiple physical or somatic symptoms or "high symptom count"
- High severity of the presenting somatic symptom
- Chronic pain
- Symptoms for more than 6 weeks
- Physician rating as a "difficult encounter"
- Recent stress
- Low self-rating of overall health
- Frequent use of health care services
- Substance abuse

Chronic pain may be a spectrum disorder in patients with anxiety, depression, or somatic symptoms. See Chapter 4, Beginning the Physical Examination: General Survey, Vital Signs, and Pain, pp. 111–146.

High-Yield Screening Questions for Office Practice

Depression
- Over the past 2 weeks, have you felt down, depressed, or hopeless?[22,28,29]
- Over the past 2 weeks, have you felt little interest or pleasure in doing things (anhedonia)?

Anxiety
Anxiety disorders include generalized anxiety disorder, social phobia, panic disorder, posttraumatic stress disorder, and acute stress disorder.[30–33]
- Over the past 2 weeks, have you been feeling nervous, anxious, or on edge?
- Over the past 2 weeks, have you been unable to stop or control worrying?
- Over the past 4 weeks, have you had an anxiety attack—suddenly feeling fear or panic?

Illness Anxiety Disorder (Replaces Hypochondriasis in *DSM-5*)
- Whiteley Index: 14-item self-rating scale[34,35]

Substance-Related and Addictive Disorders
- CAGE questions adapted for alcohol and drug abuse—see Chapter 3, Interviewing and the Health History, p. 97.

Multidimensional
- PRIME-MD (Primary Care Evaluation of Mental Disorders) for the five most common disorders in primary care: depression, anxiety, alcohol, somatoform, and eating disorders; 26-item patient questionnaire followed by clinician evaluation; takes approximately 10 minutes.[36]
- PRIME-MD Patient Health Questionnaire, available as patient health questionnaire for self-rating; takes approximately 3 minutes.[36]

Personality Disorders. Patients with personality disorders can also display problematic office behaviors that escape diagnosis. The *DSM-5* characterizes these disorders as "an enduring pattern of inner experience and behavior that deviates markedly from the expectations of the individual's culture, is pervasive and inflexible, has an onset in adolescence or early adulthood, is stable over time, and leads to distress or impairment." These patients have dysfunctional interpersonal coping styles that disrupt and destabilize their relationships, including those with health care providers. A recent study reports an overall prevalence of 9%, with prevalence of the three subcomponent clusters of 5.7% for odd and eccentric disorders; 1.5% for dramatic, emotional, or erratic disorders; and 6% for anxious or fearful disorders.[12] Personality disorders co-occur at high frequencies with alcohol and substance abuse and with the axis I disorders of depression, anxiety disorders, bipolar disorder, attention deficit hyperactivity disorder, autism spectrum disorders, anorexia nervosa, bulimia nervosa, and schizophrenia.[37] Note that *DSM-5* section II continues "the categorical perspective that personality disorders are qualitatively distinct clinical syndromes." Section III presents an alternative approach to guide further research, namely a dimensional perspective that characterizes personality disorders as "impairments in personality functioning and pathological personality traits" that "merge imperceptibly into normality and into one another." For more detailed diagnostic criteria, beyond the scope of this book, consult the *DSM-5*.

Personality Disorders: *DSM-5* Section II

Cluster/Personality Type	Characteristic Behavior Patterns
A: Odd or Eccentric Disorders	
• Paranoid	Distrust and suspiciousness
• Schizoid	Detachment from social relations with a restricted emotional range
• Schizotypal	Eccentricities in behavior and cognitive distortions; acute discomfort in close relationships
B: Dramatic, Emotional or Erratic Disorders	
• Antisocial	Disregard for, and violation of, the rights of others
• Borderline	Instability in interpersonal relationships, self-image and affective regulation; impulsivity
• Histrionic	Excessive emotionality and attention seeking
• Narcissistic	Persisting grandiosity, need for admiration and lack of empathy

(continued)

Personality Disorders: *DSM-5* Section II (*continued*)

Cluster/Personality Type	Characteristic Behavior Patterns
C: Anxious or Fearful Disorders	
• Avoidant	Social inhibition, feelings of inadequacy and hypersensitivity to negative evaluation
• Dependent	Submissive and clinging behavior related to an excessive need to be taken care of
• Obsessive–compulsive	Preoccupation with orderliness, perfectionism, and control

Note that in *DSM-5*, the dimensional model reduces these disorders to six categories: antisocial, avoidant, borderline, narcissistic, obsessive–compulsive, and schizotypal, and emphasizes self and interpersonal functioning.

Sources: Adapted from Schiffer RB. *Ch 420, Psychiatric disorders in medical practice, in Cecil Textbook of Medicine*, 22nd ed. Philadelphia: Saunders, 2004, p. 2628; American Psychiatric Association. *Diagnostic and Statistical Manual of Mental Disorders*, 5th Ed. Washington, DC: American Psychiatric Press, 2013.

Borderline Personality Disorder. Patients with borderline personality disorders are especially challenging. These patients show "a pervasive pattern of instability of interpersonal relationships, self-image, and affects, and marked impulsivity."[12] They make "frantic efforts to avoid real or imagined abandonment" and show recurrent suicidal behavior, gestures, or threats, or self-mutilating behavior. Prevalence in primary care practices is 6%, though the diagnosis is often missed.[38,39] More than 90% of patients with this disorder meet criteria for other personality disorders. Many have coexisting mood, anxiety, and substance abuse disorders. Presenting symptoms overlap with depression, anxiety, substance abuse, and eating disorders, which complicate diagnosis. In clinical settings, over 75% of those affected are women, and the disorder shows a strong genetic and familial pattern.[40] More than half lose their jobs because of interpersonal problems, and roughly one-third experience sexual abuse. Patients often report feeling depressed and empty, with mood swings that spiral out of control leading to feelings of rage, sadness, and anxiety. To clinicians, these patients may appear demanding, disruptive, or manipulative. Recognition of borderline features is essential for patient understanding, reduction of patient self-harm, and referral for expert evaluation.

The Health History

Common or Concerning Symptoms

- Changes in attention, mood, or speech
- Changes in insight, orientation, or memory
- Anxiety, panic, ritualistic behavior, and phobias
- Delirium or dementia

Overview.   As you interact with the patient, you will quickly observe the patient's level of *alertness* and *orientation*, and *mood, attention,* and *memory.* While the history unfolds, you will learn about the patient's *insight* and *judgment,* as well as any *recurring or unusual thoughts or perceptions.* These and other components of mood and cognition will alert you to conditions that require more detailed follow-up, including a formal mental status examination and possible referral.

Many of the terms pertinent to the mental health history and the mental status examination are familiar from social conversation. It is important to learn their precise meanings in the context of the formal evaluation of mental status, detailed in the box below.

See Techniques of Examination for the formal mental status examination on pp. 158–168.

Terminology: The Mental Status Examination

Level of Consciousness	Alertness or State of Awareness of the Environment
Attention	The ability to focus or concentrate over time on a particular stimulus or activity—an inattentive person is easily distractible and may have difficulty giving a history or responding to questions.
Memory	The process of registering or recording information, tested by asking for immediate repetition of material, followed by storage or retention of information. *Recent* or *short-term memory* covers minutes, hours, or days; *remote* or *long-term memory* refers to intervals of years.
Orientation	Awareness of personal identity, place, and time; requires both memory and attention
Perceptions	Sensory awareness of objects in the environment and their interrelationships (external stimuli); also refers to internal stimuli such as dreams or hallucinations.
Thought processes	The logic, coherence, and relevance of the patient's thought as it leads to selected goals; *how* people think
Thought content	*What* the patient thinks about, including level of insight and judgment
Insight	Awareness that symptoms or disturbed behaviors are normal or abnormal; for example, distinguishing between daydreams and hallucinations that seem real.
Judgment	Process of comparing and evaluating alternatives when deciding on a course of action; reflects values that may or may not be based on reality and social conventions or norms

(continued)

Terminology: The Mental Status Examination (continued)

Level of Consciousness	Alertness or State of Awareness of the Environment
Affect	A fluctuating pattern of observable behaviors that expresses subjective feelings or emotions through tone of voice, facial expression, and demeanor. Disturbed affect may be flat, blunted, labile, or inappropriate.
Mood	A more pervasive and sustained emotion that colors the person's perception of the world. (Affect is to mood as weather is to climate.) Mood may be euthymic (in the normal range), elevated, or dysphoric (unpleasant, possibly as sad, anxious, or irritable), for example.
Language	A complex symbolic system for expressing, receiving, and comprehending words; as with consciousness, attention, and memory, language is essential for assessing other mental functions
Higher cognitive functions	Assessed by vocabulary, fund of information, abstract thinking, calculations, construction of objects that have two or three dimensions

Attention, Mood, Speech, Insight, Orientation, Memory. Assess the patient's *level of consciousness; general appearance; mood,* including depression or mania; and *ability to pay attention, remember, understand,* and *speak.* Place the patient's vocabulary and general fund of information in the context of his or her cultural and educational background. The patient's account of illness and life circumstances often tells you about *insight and judgment.* If you suspect a problem in orientation and memory, you can ask, "Let's see, your last clinic appointment was when...?" "And the date today?" Try to integrate your evaluation of mental status into the history so it will seem less like an interrogation.

See Table 17-6, Disorders of Speech, p. 784.

Anxiety, Panic, Ritualistic Behavior, Phobias. Explore any unusual thoughts, preoccupations, beliefs, or perceptions as they come up during the interview. For example, excessive worry persisting over a 6-month period suggests a possible *anxiety disorder,* one of the most prevalent psychiatric conditions in the United States, with a lifetime prevalence of approximately 3%.[12] Over time, you will recognize some of its mimics: *panic disorder,* with recurrent panic attacks followed by a period of anxiety about further attacks; *obsessive–compulsive disorder,* with intrusive thoughts and ritualistic behaviors; *posttraumatic stress disorder,* characterized by re-experiencing, avoidance, persistent negative alterations in cognition and mood, and alterations in arousal and reactivity; and *social anxiety disorder,* with its marked anticipatory anxiety in social situations. Supplement your interview with questions in specific areas and pursue a formal mental status examination when indicated.

Compulsions, obsessions, phobias, and *anxieties* are seen in mood disorders. For official diagnostic criteria of anxiety disorders, see *Diagnostic and Statistical Manual of Mental Disorders (DSM-5).*

Neurocognitive Disorders: Delirium and Dementia. In the *DSM-5, delirium* and *dementia* fall under the new category of *neurocognitive disorders,* based on consultation with expert groups. Dementia is classified as a *major cognitive disorder;* a less severe level of cognitive impairment is now *mild neurocognitive disorder,* which applies to younger individuals with impairment from traumatic brain injury or HIV infection. The *DSM-5* retains the term *dementia,* however, due to widespread clinical usage. Helpful tables provide working definitions of each cognitive domain, with examples of symptoms related to everyday activities and related assessments.

A wide range of patients in clinical practice warrant assessment of mental status: patients with brain injury, psychiatric symptoms, or reports from family members of vague or changed behavior; patients with subtle behavioral changes, difficulty taking medications as prescribed, problems attending to household chores or paying bills, or loss of interest in their usual activities; and patients with change in orientation after surgery or during an acute illness. Identify these problems promptly because they impact family relationships, work status, and possible disability.

See Table 20-2, Neurocognitive Disorders: Delirium and Dementia, p. 1001.

See also discussions in Chapter 17, The Nervous System, pp. 711–796 and in Chapter 20, The Older Adult, pp. 955–1008.

Health Promotion and Counseling: Evidence and Recommendations

Important Topics for Health Promotion and Counseling

- Screening for depression and suicidality
- Screening for substance use disorders, including alcohol and prescription drugs

Mental health disorders impose a substantial burden of suffering.[41] About 1 in 5 U.S. adults (43.7 million) experience mental illness in a given year, with about 1 in 25 (9.6 million) experiencing serious mental illness (schizophrenia, major depression, or bipolar disorder). Depression and anxiety disorders are a common cause of hospitalization in the United States, and mental illness is associated with increased risks for chronic medical conditions, decreased life expectancy, disability, substance abuse, and suicide.

See Chapter 3, Interviewing and the Health History, pp. 65–108.

Mood Disorders and Depression. Depressive and bipolar disorders affect over 9% of the U.S. population.[42,43] About 16 million adult Americans, or almost 7%, have major depression, often with coexisting anxiety disorders and substance abuse. Depression is nearly twice as common in women as men; the prevalence of postpartum depression is 7% to 13%.[44] Depression frequently accompanies chronic medical illness. High-risk patients may have subtle early signs of depression, including low self-esteem, loss of pleasure in daily activities (*anhedonia*), sleep disorders, and difficulty concentrating or making decisions.

Look carefully for symptoms of depression in vulnerable patients, especially those who are young, female, single, divorced or separated, seriously or chronically ill, bereaved, or have other psychiatric disorders, including substance abuse. A personal or family history of depression also places patients at risk.

The U.S. Preventive Services Task Force (USPSTF) made a grade B recommendation in 2009 for depression screening in clinical settings that can provide care supports and accurate diagnosis, treatment, and follow-up.[28] Performing screening in less supportive settings received only a grade C recommendation. Asking two simple questions about mood and anhedonia appears to be as effective as using more detailed instruments. A positive test response has a sensitivity of 83% and a specificity of 92% for detecting major depression.[45] All positive screening tests warrant full diagnostic interviews. Failure to diagnose depression can have fatal consequences—the presence of an affective disorder is associated with an 11-fold increased risk for suicide.[46]

See screening questions on p. 151 and review screening tools readily available for office practice.

Suicide.   Suicide ranks as the 10th leading cause of death in the United States, accounting for nearly 40,000 deaths. Annually, there are almost 13 completed suicides per 100,000 population.[47–49] Suicide is the second leading cause of death among 15- to 24-year olds. Suicide rates are highest among those ages 45 to 54 years, followed by elderly adults ≥age 85 years. Men have suicide rates nearly four times higher than women, though women are three times more likely to attempt suicide. Men are most likely to use firearms to commit suicide, while women are most likely to use poison. Overall, suicides in non-Hispanic whites account for about 90% of all suicides, though American Indian/Alaska Native women ages 15 to 24 years have the highest suicide rates of any racial/ethnic group. An estimated 25 attempts are made for each death by suicide, with ratios of 100 to 200 to 1 among young adults. In 2011, nearly 16% of U.S. high school students reported that they had seriously considered attempting suicide in the previous year. Despite the public health burden of suicide, the USPSTF has concluded that the current evidence is insufficient to assess the balance of benefits and harms of screening for suicide risk in a primary care setting—a grade I recommendation,[50] but statistics underscore the importance of investigating patient clues and risk factors.

Substance Use Disorders, Including Alcohol and Prescription Drugs.   The harmful interactions between mental disorders and substance use disorders also present a major public health problem. The 2013 National Survey on Drug Use and Health showed that 23% of the U.S. population ages 12 years or older (60.1 million people) reported binge drinking, and over 6% reported heavy drinking.[41] Over 24 million Americans (9.4% of the population) reported use of an illicit drug during the month before the survey, including nearly 20 million marijuana users, 1.6 million cocaine users, and 6.5 million users of prescription drugs for nonmedical indications. Nearly 22 million persons aged 12 years or older were classified as having a substance use disorder based on *Diagnostic and Statistical Manual of Mental Disorders* (*DSM-IV*) criteria.[51] Only about 2.5 million of these individuals received treatment at a specialty facility for an illicit drug or alcohol problem. Rates of drug-induced deaths continue to increase and are highest among whites and American Indian/Alaska Natives. The Centers for Disease Control and Prevention reports that *prescription drugs* have replaced illicit drugs as a leading cause of drug-induced deaths.[52]

Every patient should be asked about alcohol use, substance abuse, and misuse of prescription drugs. The USPSTF has given a grade B recommendation to screening adults ages 18 years and older for alcohol misuse, and providing brief behavioral counseling for those engaging in risky or hazardous drinking.[53] However, the USPSTF has issued only a grade I (insufficient evidence) recommendation for screening for illicit drug use.[54]

See discussion of screening tools in Chapter 3, Interviewing and the Health History, Alcohol and Prescription and Illicit Drugs, pp. 96–97, and Chapter 11, Abdomen, Screening for Alcohol Abuse, pp. 464–466.

Techniques of Examination

The Mental Status Examination

- Appearance and behavior
- Speech and language
- Mood
- Thoughts and perceptions
- Cognition, including memory, attention, information and vocabulary, calculations, abstract thinking, and constructional ability

The assessment of mental status is challenging and complex. Changes in mental status warrant careful evaluation for underlying pathologic and pharmacologic causes. The patient's personality, psychodynamics, family and life experiences, and cultural background all come into play. Amplify your findings from the history and physical examination as you select all or part of the formal mental status examination for further testing. The Mental Status Examination is central to assessment in psychiatric practice. It is also a critical element in the assessment of the nervous system and the first segment of the nervous system write-up. Learn to describe the patient's mood, speech, behavior, and cognition and to relate these findings to your examination of the cranial nerves, motor and sensory systems, and reflexes.

The Mental Status Examination consists of five components: *appearance and behavior*; *speech and language*; *mood*; *thoughts and perceptions*; and *cognitive function*. Cognitive function includes orientation, attention, memory, attention, and higher cognitive functions such as information and vocabulary, calculations, abstract thinking, and constructional ability. Prepare the patient for formal testing and explain your rationale.

See Chapter 17, Nervous System, pp. 711–796, especially pp. 733–735 and Recording Your Findings, p. 773.

The format that follows should help structure your observations, but is not intended as a step-by-step guide. Be flexible, but thorough. In some situations, however, sequence is important. If the patient's consciousness, attention, comprehension of words, and ability to speak are impaired, assess these deficits promptly. If the patient cannot give a reliable history, testing most of the other mental functions will be difficult and merits an evaluation for acute causes.

Appearance and Behavior

Integrate the observations you have made throughout the history and physical examination, including the following.

Level of Consciousness.   Is the patient awake and alert? Does the patient understand your questions and respond appropriately and reasonably quickly, or tend to lose track of the topic, grow silent, or even fall asleep?

If the patient does not respond to your questions, escalate the stimulus in steps:

- Speak to the patient by name and in a loud voice.

- Shake the patient gently, like wakening a sleeper.

If there is no response to these stimuli, promptly assess the patient for stupor or coma—severe reductions in level of consciousness.

See the table on Level of Consciousness (Arousal), Chapter 17, The Nervous System, p. 769.

Lethargic patients are drowsy, but open their eyes and look at you, respond to questions, and then fall asleep.

Obtunded patients open their eyes and look at you, but respond slowly and are somewhat confused.

Posture and Motor Behavior.   Does the patient sit or lie quietly or prefer to walk around? Observe the patient's posture and ability to relax. Note the pace, range, and type of movement. Are movements voluntary and spontaneous? Are any limbs immobile? Are posture and motor activity affected by topics under discussion, type of activity, or who is in the room?

Look for tense posture, restlessness, and anxious fidgeting; the crying, pacing, and hand-wringing of *agitated depression;* the hopeless slumped posture and slowed movements of *depression;* the agitated and expansive movements of a *manic episode.*

Dress, Grooming, and Personal Hygiene.   How is the patient dressed? Is the clothing clean and presentable? Is it appropriate for the patient's age and social group? Note the grooming of the patient's hair, nails, teeth, skin, and, if present, beard. How do the grooming and hygiene compare with peers of comparable age, lifestyle, and socioeconomic group? Compare one side of the body with the other.

Grooming and personal hygiene may deteriorate in *depression, schizophrenia,* and *dementia.* Excessive fastidiousness may be seen in *obsessive–compulsive disorder.* One-sided neglect may result from a lesion in the opposite parietal cortex, usually the nondominant side.

Facial Expression.   Observe the face both at rest and during conversation. Watch for changes in expression. Are they appropriate for the topics being discussed? Or is the face relatively immobile throughout?

Note expressions of anxiety, depression, apathy, anger, elation, or facial immobility in parkinsonism.

Manner, Affect, and Relationship to People and Things.   Assess the patient's *affect,* or external expression of the inner emotional state. Is it appropriate to the topics being discussed? Or is the affect labile, blunted, or flat? Does it seem exaggerated at certain points? If so, how? Observe the patient's openness, approachability, and reactions to others and the surroundings. Does the patient hear or see things not present, or converse with someone who is not there?

Watch for the anger, hostility, suspiciousness, or evasiveness of patients with *paranoia;* the elation and euphoria of *mania;* the flat affect and remoteness of *schizophrenia;* the apathy (dulled affect with detachment and indifference) of *dementia;* and anxiety or depression. Hallucinations occur in schizophrenia, alcohol withdrawal, and systemic toxicity.

Speech and Language

Throughout the interview, note the following characteristics of the patient's speech.

Quantity.   Is the patient talkative or unusually silent? Are comments spontaneous, or limited to direct questions?

Rate.   Is speech fast or slow?

Note the slow speech of *depression;* the accelerated louder speech of *mania.*

Volume.   Is speech loud or soft?

Articulation of Words.   Are the words clear and distinct? Does the speech have a nasal quality?

Dysarthria refers to defective articulation. *Aphasia* is a disorder of language. *Dysphonia* results from impaired volume, quality, or pitch of the voice. See Table 17-6, Disorders of Speech, p. 784.

Fluency.   Fluency reflects the rate, flow, and melody of speech and the content and use of words. Watch for abnormalities of spontaneous speech such as:

- Hesitancies and gaps in the flow and rhythm of words

- Disturbed inflections, such as a monotone

- Circumlocutions, in which phrases or sentences are substituted for a word the person cannot think of, such as "what you write with" for "pen"

- Paraphasias, in which words are malformed ("I write with a den"), wrong ("I write with a bar"), or invented ("I write with a dar").

These abnormalities suggest *aphasia* from cerebrovascular infarction. Aphasia may be *receptive* (impaired comprehension with fluent speech) or *expressive* (with preserved comprehension and slow nonfluent speech).

If the patient's speech lacks meaning or fluency, proceed with further testing as outlined in the following box. A person who can write a correct sentence does not have aphasia.

Testing for Aphasia

Word Comprehension	Ask the patient to follow a one-stage command, such as "Point to your nose." Try a two-stage command: "Point to your mouth, then your knee."
Repetition	Ask the patient to repeat a phrase of one-syllable words (the most difficult repetition task): "No ifs, ands, or buts."
Naming	Ask the patient to name the parts of a watch.
Reading Comprehension	Ask the patient to read a paragraph aloud.
Writing	Ask the patient to write a sentence.

These questions help identify the type of aphasia. Check for deficits in vision, hearing, intelligence, and education which may affect responses. Two common kinds of aphasia—*expressive* (Broca aphasia) and *receptive* (Wernicke aphasia)—are compared in Table 17-6, Disorders of Speech, p. 784.

Mood

Ask the patient to describe his or her mood, including usual mood level and fluctuations related to life events. "How did you feel about that?" for example, or, more generally, "How is your overall mood?" The reports from family and friends may be of value.

Has the mood been intense and unchanging, or labile? How long has it lasted? Is it appropriate to the patient's situation? If depression, have there been episodes of an elevated mood, suggesting a bipolar disorder?

If you suspect depression, assess its severity and any risk of suicide. Ask...

- Do you feel discouraged or depressed?

- How low do you feel?

- What do you see for yourself in the future?

- Do you ever feel that life isn't worth living? Or that you want to be dead?

- Have you ever thought of killing yourself?

- How did (do) you think you would do it? Do you have a plan?

- What do you think would happen after you were dead?

It is your responsibility to ask directly about suicidal thoughts. This may be the only way to uncover suicidal ideation and plans that launch immediate intervention and treatment.

Moods range from sadness and melancholy; contentment, joy, euphoria, and elation; anger and rage; anxiety and worry; to detachment and indifference.

For official diagnostic criteria of depressive and bipolar disorders, see *Diagnostic and Statistical Manual of Mental Disorders* (*DSM-5*).

Thought and Perceptions

Thought Processes.   Assess the logic, relevance, organization, and coherence of the patient's thought processes throughout the interview. Does speech progress logically toward a goal? Listen for patterns of speech that suggest disorders of thought processes, as outlined in the box below.

Variations and Abnormalities in Thought Processes

Circumstantiality	The mildest thought disorder, consisting of speech with unnecessary detail, indirection, and delay in reaching the point. Some topics may have a meaningful connection. Many people without mental disorders have circumstantial speech.	Circumstantiality occurs in people with obsessions.
Derailment (loosening of associations)	"Tangential" speech with shifting topics that are loosely connected or unrelated. The patient is unaware of the lack of association.	Derailment is seen in schizophrenia, manic episodes, and other psychotic disorders.

(*continued*)

Variations and Abnormalities in Thought Processes (*continued*)

Flight of Ideas	An almost continuous flow of accelerated speech with abrupt changes from one topic to the next. Changes are based on understandable associations, plays on words, or distracting stimuli, but ideas are not well connected.	Flight of ideas is most frequently noted in *manic episodes*.
Neologisms	Invented or distorted words, or words with new and highly idiosyncratic meanings.	Neologisms are observed in schizophrenia, psychotic disorders, and aphasia.
Incoherence	Speech that is incomprehensible and illogical, with lack of meaningful connections, abrupt changes in topic, or disordered grammar or word use. Flight of ideas, when severe, may produce incoherence.	Incoherence is seen in severe psychotic disturbances (usually *schizophrenia*).
Blocking	Sudden interruption of speech in midsentence or before the idea is completed, attributed to "losing the thought." Blocking occurs in normal people.	Blocking may be striking in *schizophrenia*.
Confabulation	Fabrication of facts or events in response to questions, to fill in the gaps from impaired memory.	Confabulation is seen in Korsakoff syndrome from alcoholism.
Perseveration	Persistent repetition of words or ideas.	Perseveration occurs in *schizophrenia* and other *psychotic disorders*.
Echolalia	Repetition of the words and phrases of others.	Echolalia occurs in manic episodes and *schizophrenia*.
Clanging	Speech with choice of words based on sound, rather than meaning, as in rhyming and punning. For example, "Look at my eyes and nose, wise eyes and rosy nose. Two to one, the ayes have it!"	Clanging occurs in schizophrenia and manic episodes.

Thought Content.   To assess thought content, follow the patient's leads and cues rather than asking direct questions. For example, "You mentioned that a neighbor caused your entire illness. Can you tell me more about that?" Or, in another situation, "What do you think about at times like these?" For more focused inquiries, be tactful and accepting. "When people are upset like this, sometimes they can't keep certain thoughts out of their minds," or "...things seem unreal. Have you experienced anything like this?" In these ways, explore any of the patterns in the following box.

Abnormalities of Thought Content

Compulsions	Repetitive behaviors that the person feels driven to perform in response to an obsession, aimed at preventing or reducing anxiety or a dreaded event or situation; these behaviors are excessive and unrealistically connected to the provoking stimulus[12]	Compulsions, obsessions, phobias, and anxieties often occur in anxiety disorders. See *Diagnostic and Statistical Manual of Mental Disorders* (*DSM-5*).

(continued)

Abnormalities of Thought Content (*continued*)

Obsessions	Recurrent persistent thoughts, images, or urges experienced as intrusive and unwanted that the person tries to ignore, suppress, or neutralize with other thoughts or actions (for example, performing a compulsive behavior)
Phobias	Persistent irrational fears, accompanied by a compelling desire to avoid the provoking stimulus
Anxieties	Apprehensive anticipation of future danger or misfortune accompanied by feelings of worry, distress, and/or somatic symptoms of tension
Feelings of Unreality	A sense that the environment is strange, unreal, or remote
Feelings of Depersonalization	A sense that one's self or identity is different, changed, unreal; lost; or detached from one's mind or body
Delusions	False fixed personal beliefs that are not amenable to change in light of conflicting evidence; types of delusions include:

- *Persecutory*
- *Grandiose*
- *Jealous*
- *Erotomanic*—the belief than another person is in love with the individual
- *Somatic*—involves bodily functions or sensations
- *Unspecified*—includes delusions of reference without a prominent persecutory or grandiose component, or the belief that external events, objects, or people have a particular and unusual personal significance (for example, commands from the radio or television)

Delusions and feelings of unreality or depersonalization are often associated with *psychotic disorders*. For official diagnostic criteria of psychotic disorders, see *Diagnostic and Statistical Manual of Mental Disorders (DSM-5)*.

Delusions may also occur in delirium, severe mood disorders, and dementia.

Perceptions.   Pursue false perceptions. For example, "When you heard the voice speaking to you, what did it say? How did it make you feel?" Or, "After you've been drinking a lot, do you ever see things that aren't really there?" Or, "Sometimes after major surgery like yours, people hear peculiar or frightening things. Has anything like this happened to you?" In these ways, find out about the following abnormal perceptions.

Abnormalities of Perception

Illusions	Misinterpretations of real external stimuli, such as mistaking rustling leaves for the sound of voices.[12]
Hallucinations	Perception-like experiences that seem real but, unlike illusions, lack actual external stimulation. The person may or may not recognize the experiences as false. Hallucinations may be auditory, visual, olfactory, gustatory, tactile, or somatic. False perceptions associated with dreaming, falling asleep, and awakening are not classified as hallucinations.

Illusions may occur in grief reactions, *delirium*, acute and *posttraumatic stress disorders*, and *schizophrenia*.

Hallucinations may occur in *delirium*, *dementia* (less commonly), *posttraumatic stress disorder, schizophrenia,* and alcoholism.

Insight.   Some of your first questions to the patient often yield important information about insight: "What brings you to the hospital?" "What seems to be the trouble?" "What do you think is wrong?" Note whether the patient is aware that a particular mood, thought, or perception is abnormal or part of an illness.

Patients with psychotic disorders often lack insight into their illness. Denial of impairment may accompany some neurologic disorders.

Judgment.   Assess judgment by noting the patient's responses to family situations, jobs, use of money, and interpersonal conflicts. "How do you plan to get help after leaving the hospital?" "How are you going to manage if you lose your job?" "If your husband starts to abuse you again, what will you do?" "Who will take care of your financial affairs while you are in the nursing home?"

Judgment may be poor in delirium, dementia, intellectual disability, and psychotic states. Anxiety, mood disorders, intelligence, education, income, and cultural values also influence judgment.

Note whether decisions and actions are based on reality or impulse, wish fulfillment, or disordered thought content. What insights and values seem to underlie the patient's decisions and behavior? Allowing for cultural variations, how do these compare with a comparable mature adult? Because judgment reflects maturity, it may be variable and unpredictable during adolescence.

Cognitive Functions

Orientation.   You can usually assess orientation during the interview. For example, you can ask quite naturally for clarification about specific dates and times, the patient's address and telephone number, the names of family members, or the route to the hospital. At times, direct questions will be needed: "Can you tell me the time now…and what day it is?" Assess orientation to:

Disorientation is common when memory or attention is impaired, as in delirium.

- *Person*—the patient's name, and names of relatives and professional personnel

- *Time*—the time of day, day of the week, month, season, date and year, duration of hospitalization

- *Place*—the patient's residence, the names of the hospital, city, and state

Attention.   The following tests of attention are commonly used.

Digit Span.   Explain that you would like to test the patient's ability to concentrate, perhaps adding that this can be difficult if the patient is in pain or ill. Recite a series of digits, starting with two at a time and speaking each number clearly at a rate of about one per second. Ask the patient to repeat the numbers back to you. If this repetition is accurate, try a series of three numbers, then four, and so on as long as the patient responds correctly. Jot down the numbers as you say them to ensure your own accuracy. If the patient makes a mistake, try once more with another series of the same length. Stop after a second failure in a single series.

Causes of poor performance include *delirium, dementia, intellectual disability,* and performance anxiety.

When choosing digits, use street numbers, zip codes, telephone numbers, and other numerical sequences that are familiar to you, but avoid consecutive numbers, easily recognized dates, and sequences that are familiar to the patient.

Now, starting again with a series of two, ask the patient to repeat the numbers to you backward.

Normally, a person should be able to repeat correctly at least five digits forward and four backward.

Serial 7s.   Instruct the patient, "Starting from a hundred, subtract 7, and keep subtracting 7 . . . ." Note the effort required and the speed and accuracy of the responses. Writing down the answers helps you keep up with the arithmetic. Normally, a person can complete serial 7s in 1½ minutes, with fewer than four errors. If the patient cannot do serial 7s, try 3s or counting backward.

> Poor performance may result from delirium, the late stage of dementia, intellectual disability, anxiety, or depression. Also consider educational level.

Spelling Backward.   This can substitute for serial 7s. Say a five-letter word, spell it, for example, W-O-R-L-D, and ask the patient to spell it backward.

Remote Memory.   Inquire about birthdays, anniversaries, social security number, names of schools attended, jobs held, or past historical events such as wars relevant to the patient's past.

> Remote memory may be impaired in the late stage of *dementia.*

Recent Memory.   This can involve the events of the day. Ask questions with answers you can check against other sources to see if the patient is confabulating, or making up facts to compensate for a defective memory. These might include the day's weather or appointment time, current medications, or laboratory tests taken during the day.

> Recent memory is impaired in *dementia* and *delirium. Amnestic disorders* impair memory or new learning ability and reduce social or occupational functioning, but lack the global features of delirium or dementia. Anxiety, depression, and intellectual disability may also impair recent memory.

New Learning Ability.   Give the patient three or four words such as "83, Water Street, and blue," or "table, flower, green, and hamburger." Ask the patient to repeat them so that you know that the information has been heard and registered. This step, like digit span, tests registration and immediate recall. Then proceed to other parts of the examination. After 3 to 5 minutes, ask the patient to repeat the words. Note the accuracy of the response, awareness of whether it is correct, and any tendency to confabulate. Normally, a person should be able to remember the words.

Higher Cognitive Functions

Information and Vocabulary.   If observed clinically in the context of cultural and educational background, information and vocabulary provide a rough estimate of the patient's baseline abilities. Begin assessing fund of knowledge and vocabulary during the interview. Ask about work, hobbies, reading, favorite television programs, or current events. Start with simple questions, then move to more difficult questions. Note the person's grasp of information, complexity of the ideas, and choice of vocabulary.

> Information and vocabulary are relatively unaffected by psychiatric disorders except in severe cases. Testing helps distinguish adults with life-long intellectual impairment (whose information and vocabulary are limited) from those with mild or moderate *dementia* (whose information and vocabulary are fairly well preserved).

More directly, you can ask about specific facts such as:

- The name of the president, vice president, or governor

- The names of the last four or five presidents

- The names of five large cities in the country

Calculating Ability. Test the patient's ability to do arithmetical calculations, starting with simple addition ("What is 4 + 3?...8 + 7?") and multiplication ("What is 5 × 6?...9 × 7?"). Proceed to more difficult tasks using two-digit numbers ("15 + 12" or "25 × 6") or longer, written examples.

Poor performance suggests dementia or *aphasia*, but should be measured against the patient's fund of knowledge and education.

Alternatively, pose practical functionally important questions, like: "If something costs 78 cents and you give the clerk one dollar, how much should you get back?"

Abstract Thinking. Test the capacity to think abstractly in two ways.

Proverbs. Ask the patient what the following proverbs mean:

A stitch in time saves nine.

Don't count your chickens before they're hatched.

The proof of the pudding is in the eating.

A rolling stone gathers no moss.

The squeaky wheel gets the grease.

Concrete responses are common in people with intellectual disability, *delirium*, or *dementia*, but may also reflect limited education. Patients with *schizophrenia* may respond concretely or with personal and bizarre interpretations.

Note the relevance of the answers and their degree of concreteness or abstractness. For example, "You should sew a rip before it gets bigger" is concrete, whereas "Prompt attention to a problem prevents trouble" is abstract. Average patients should give abstract or semiabstract responses.

Similarities. Ask the patient to tell you how the following are alike:

An orange and an apple	A church and a theater
A cat and a mouse	A piano and a violin
A child and a dwarf	Wood and coal

Note the accuracy and relevance of the answers and their degree of concreteness or abstractness. For example, "A cat and a mouse are both animals" is abstract, "They both have tails" is concrete, and "A cat chases a mouse" is not relevant.

Constructional Ability. The task here is to copy figures of increasing complexity onto a piece of blank unlined paper. Show each figure one at a time and ask the patient to copy it as well as possible (Fig. 5-3).

With intact vision and motor ability, poor constructional ability suggests dementia or parietal lobe damage. Intellectual disability can also impair performance.

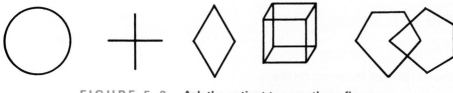

FIGURE 5-3. Ask the patient to copy these figures.

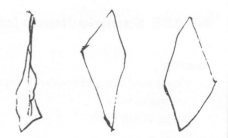

FIGURE 5-4. Poor, fair, and good shapes.

These three diamonds are rated poor, fair, and good (but not excellent).[55]

In another approach, ask the patient to draw a clock face complete with numbers and hands (Fig. 5-5).

FIGURE 5-5. Patient-drawn clock rated as excellent.

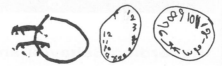

FIGURE 5-6. Poor, fair, and good clocks.

These three clocks are poor, fair, and good.[55]

Special Techniques

Mini-Mental State Examination (MMSE). This brief test has been widely used to screen for cognitive dysfunction or dementia, and follow their course over time. Although several versions are available on the internet, copyright permission for use and reproduction is required. For more detailed information regarding the MMSE, contact the publisher, Psychological Assessment Resources, Inc., 16204 North Florida Avenue, Lutz, Florida 33549, or online: http://www4.parinc.com/. Below are some sample questions.

MMSE Sample Items

Orientation to Time
   "What is the date?"

Registration
   "Listen carefully. I am going to say three words. You say them back after I stop. Ready? Here they are . . .
   APPLE (pause), PENNY (pause), TABLE (pause). Now repeat those words back to me." (Repeat up to five times, but score only the first trial.)

Naming
   "What is this?" (Point to a pencil or pen.)

(continued)

MMSE Sample Items (*continued*)

Reading

"Please read this and do what it says." (Show examinee the words on the stimulus form.)

CLOSE YOUR EYES

Recording Your Findings

Recording Behavior and Mental Status

"*Mental Status:* The patient is alert, well-groomed, and cheerful. Speech is fluent and words are clear. Thought processes are coherent, insight is good. The patient is oriented to person, place, and time. Serial 7s accurate; recent and remote memory intact. Calculations intact."

OR

"*Mental Status:* The patient appears sad and fatigued; clothes are wrinkled. Speech is slow and words are mumbled. Thought processes are coherent, but insight into current life reverses is limited. The patient is oriented to person, place, and time. Digit span, serial 7s, and calculations accurate, but responses delayed. Clock drawing is good."

These findings suggest depression.

Table 5-1 Somatic Symptom and Related Disorders

TYPES OF SOMATIC SYMPTOM AND RELATED DISORDERS

Type of Disorder	Diagnostic Features
Somatic symptom disorder	Somatic symptoms are either very distressing or result in significant disruption of functioning, as well as excessive and disproportionate thoughts, feelings, and behaviors related to those symptoms. Symptoms should be specific if with predominant pain.
Illness anxiety disorder	Preoccupation with having or acquiring a serious illness where somatic symptoms, if present, are only mild in intensity.
Conversion disorder	Syndrome of symptoms of deficits mimicking neurologic or medical illness in which psychological factors are judged to be of etiologic importance.
Psychological factors affecting other medical conditions	Presence of one or more clinically significant psychological or behavioral factors that adversely affect a medical condition by increasing the risk for suffering, death, or disability
Factitious disorder	Falsification of physical or psychological signs or symptoms, or induction of injury or disease, associated with identified deception. The individual presents himself or herself as ill, impaired, or injured even in the absence of external rewards.

Other Related Disorders or Behaviors

Body dysmorphic disorder	Preoccupation with one or more perceived defects or flaws in physical appearance that are not observable or appear only slight to others.
Dissociative disorder	Disruption of and/or discontinuity in the normal integration of consciousness, memory, identity, emotion, perception, body representation, motor control, and behavior.

Note to readers: Regarding tables in past editions on mood, anxiety, and psychotic disorders, per current *DSM-5* copyright, readers are referred to the *DSM-5* for further diagnostic information.

References

1. Olfson M, Kroenke K, Wang S, et al. Trends in office-based mental health care provided by psychiatrists and primary care physicians. *J Clin Psychiatry.* 2014;75:247.

2. Rief W, Hessel A, Braehler E. Somatization symptoms and hypochondriacal features in the general population. *Psychosomatic Medicine.* 2001;63:595.

3. Substance Abuse and Mental Health Services Administration. *Results from the 2012 National Survey on Drug Use and Health: Mental Health Findings.* Rockville, MD: NSDUH Series H-47, HHS Publication No. (SMA) 13–4805; 2013. Available at http://store.samhsa.gov/product/Results-from-the-2012-National-Survey-on-Drug-Use-and-Health-NSDUH-H-47-Mental-Health-Findings/SMA13–4805. Accessed Jan 30, 2015.

4. Hepner KA, Rowe M, Rost K, et al. The effect of adherence to practice guidelines on depression outcomes. *Ann Int Med.* 2007;147:320.

5. Gonzalez HM, Vega WA, Williams DR, et al. Depression care in the United States: too little for too few. *Arch Gen Psychiatry.* 2010;67:37.

6. Williams DR, González HM, Neighbors H. Prevalence and distribution of major depressive disorder in African Americans, Caribbean blacks, and non-Hispanic whites: results from the National Survey of American Life. *Arch Gen Psychiatry.* 2007;64:305.

7. Kroenke K. Unburdening the difficult clinical encounter. *Arch Intern Med.* 2009;169:333.

8. Strine TW, Mokdad AH, Balluz LS, et al. Depression and anxiety in the United States: findings from the 2006 Behavioral Risk Factor Surveillance System. *Psychiatr Serv.* 2008;59:1283.

9. Kessler RC, Chiu WT, Demler O, et al. Prevalence, severity, and comorbidity of twelve-month DSM-IV disorders in the National Comorbidity Survey Replication (NCS-R). *Arch Gen Psych.* 2005; 62:617.

10. Kroenke K. Patients presenting with somatic complaints: epidemiology, psychiatric comorbidity, and management. *Int J Methods Psychiatr Res.* 2003;12:34.

11. Kroenke K. A practical and evidence-based approach to common symptoms: a narrative review. *Ann Intern Med.* 2014;161:579.

12. American Psychiatric Association. *Diagnostic and Statistical Manual of Mental Disorders.* 5th ed. Washington, DC: American Psychiatric Press, 2013.

13. Dwamena FC, Lyles JS, Frankel RM, et al. In their own words: qualitative study of high-utilising primary care patients with medically unexplained symptoms. *BMC Fam Pract.* 2009;10:67.

14. Kroenke K. The interface between physical and psychological symptoms. Primary Care Companion. *J Clin Psychiatry.* 2003; 5(Suppl 7):11.

15. Aaron LA, Buchwald D. A review of the evidence for overlap among unexplained clinical conditions. *Ann Intern Med.* 2001; 134:868.

16. Smith RC, Lyles JS, Gardiner JC, et al. Primary care clinicians treat patients with medically unexplained symptoms: a randomized controlled trial. *J Gen Int Med.* 2006;21:671.

17. Jackson JL, Kroenke K. Managing somatization—medically unexplained should not mean medically ignored. *J Gen Int Med.* 2006; 21:797.

18. Hinchey SA, Jackson JL. A cohort study assessing difficult patient encounters in a walk-in primary care clinic, predictors and outcomes. *J Gen Intern Med.* 2011;26:588.

19. An PG, Rabatin JS, Manwell LB, et al. Burden of difficult encounters in primary care: data from the Minimizing Error, Maximizing Outcomes study. *Arch Intern Med.* 2009;169:410.

20. Lorenzetti CR, Jacques CH, Donovan C, et al. Managing difficult encounters: understanding physician, patient, and situational factors. *Am Fam Physician.* 2013;87:419.

21. Arciniegas DB, Beresford TP. Managing difficult interactions with patients in neurology practices: a practical approach. *Neurology.* 2010;75(18 Suppl 1):S39.

22. Staab JP, Datto CJ, Weinreig RM, et al. Detection and diagnosis of psychiatric disorders in primary medical care settings. *Med Clin N Am.* 2001;85:579.

23. Ansseau M, Dierick M, Buntinkxz F, et al. High prevalence of mental disorders in primary care. *J Affect Disord.* 2004;78:49.

24. Kroenke K, Spitzer RL, deGruy FV, et al. A symptom checklist for screen for somatoform disorders in primary care. *Psychosomatics.* 1998;39:263.

25. Spitzer RL, Kroenke K, Williams JB, et al. Validation and utility of a self-report version of PRIME-MD—the PHQ Primary Care Study. *JAMA.* 1999;282:1737.

26. Kroenke K, Sharpe M, Sykes R. Revising the classification of somatoform disorders: key questions and preliminary recommendations. *Psychosomatics.* 2007;48:277.

27. Primary Health Care Screeners. Updated December 2013. Free. Available at http://www.phqscreeners.com/overview.aspx. Accessed February 1, 2015.

28. U.S. Preventive Services Task Force. Screening for depression: recommendations and rationale. December 2009. Available at http://www.uspreventiveservicestaskforce.org/Page/Document/RecommendationStatementFinal/depression-in-adults-screening. Accessed February 1, 2015.

29. Whooley MA, Avins AL, Miranda J, et al. Case-finding instruments for depression. Two questions are as good as many. *J Gen Intern Med.* 1997;12:439.

30. Kroenke K, Spitzer RL, Williams JB, et al. An ultra-brief screening scale for anxiety and depression: the PHQ-4. *Psychosomatics.* 2009;50:613.

31. Spitzer RL, Kroenke K, Williams JB, et al. A brief measure for assessing generalized anxiety disorder: the GAD 7. *Arch Int Med.* 2006;166:1092.

32. Kroenke K, Spitzer RL, Williams JB, et al. Anxiety disorders in primary care: prevalence, impairment, comorbidity, and detection. *Ann Int Med.* 2007;146:317.

33. Lowe B, Grafe K, Zipfel S, et al. Detecting panic disorder in medical and psychosomatic outpatients—comparative validation of the Hospital Anxiety and Depression Scale, the Patient Health Questionnaire, a screening question, and physicians diagnosis. *J Psychosom Res.* 2003;55:515.

34. Conradt M, Cavanagh M, Franklin J, et al. Dimensionality of the Whiteley Index: assessment of hypochondriasis in an Australian sample of primary care patients. *J Psychosom Res.* 2006;60:137.

35. Pilowsky U. Dimensions of hypochondriasis. *Br J Psychiatry.* 1967;113:89.

36. Spitzer RL, Williams JB, Kroenke K, et al. Utility of a new procedure for diagnosing mental disorders in primary care. The PRIME-MD 1000 study. *JAMA.* 1994;272:1749.

37. Compton WM, Thomas YF, Stinson FS, et al. Prevalence, correlates, disability, and comorbidity of DSM-IV drug abuse and dependence in the United States—results from the national epidemiologic

REFERENCES

survey on alcohol and related conditions. *Arch Gen Psychiatry.* 2007;64:566–576.

38. Gross R, Olfson M, Gameroff M, et al. Borderline personality disorder in primary care. *Arch Int Med.* 2002;162:50.

39. Grant BF, Chou SP, Goldstein RB, et al. Prevalence, correlates, disability, and comorbidity of DSM-IV borderline personality disorder: results from the Wave 2 National Epidemiologic Survey on Alcohol and Related Conditions. *J Clin Psychiatry.* 2008;69:533.

40. Gunderson JG. Borderline personality disorder. *N Engl J Med.* 2011;364:2037.

41. Substance Abuse and Mental Health Services Administration, Center for Behavioral Health Statistics and Quality. *The NSDUH Report: Substance Use and Mental Health Estimates from the 2013 National Survey on Drug Use and Health: Overview of Findings.* Rockville, MD: Substance Abuse and Mental Health Services Administration; 2014. Available at http://store.samhsa.gov/shin/content//NSDUH14–0904/NSDUH14–0904.pdf.

42. National Institutes of Mental Health. Any Mental Illness (AMI) Among Adults. 2014. Available at http://www.nimh.nih.gov/health/statistics/prevalence/any-mental-illness-ami-among-adults.shtml. Accessed February 1, 2015.

43. National Institutes of Mental Health. Any Mood Disorder Among Adults. 2014. Available at http://www.nimh.nih.gov/health/statistics/prevalence/any-mood-disorder-among-adults.shtml

44. Gavin NI, Gaynes BN, Lohr KN, et al. Perinatal depression: a systematic review of prevalence and incidence. *Obstet Gynecol.* 2005; 106(5 Pt 1):1071.

45. Kroenke K, Spitzer RL, Williams JB. The Patient Health Questionnaire-2: validity of a two-item depression screener. *Med Care.* 2003;41:1284.

46. Li Z, Page A, Martin G, et al. Attributable risk of psychiatric and socio-economic factors for suicide from individual-level, population-based studies: a systematic review. *Soc Sci Med.* 2011;72:608.

47. U.S. Preventive Services Task Force. Screening for depression in adults: U.S. preventive services task force recommendation statement. *Ann Intern Med.* 2009;151(11):784–792.

48. American Institute of Suicidology. *Suicide in the USA—Based on 2011 Data.* Washington, DC, 2014. Available at http://www.suicidology.org/Portals/14/docs/Resources/FactSheets/2011/Suicide-USA2014.pdf. Accessed February 1, 2015.

49. Centers for Disease Control and Prevention. *Suicide Facts at a Glance.* Atlanta, GA, 2014. Available at http://www.cdc.gov/ViolencePrevention/pdf/Suicide-DataSheet-a.pdf. Accessed February 1, 2015.

50. LeFevre ML. Screening for suicide risk in adolescents, adults, and older adults in primary care: U.S. Preventive Services Task Force recommendation statement. *Ann Intern Med.* 2014;160:719.

51. American Psychiatric Association. *Diagnostic and statistical manual of mental disorders.* 4th ed. Text Revision. Washington, DC, 2000.

52. Mack KA. Drug-induced deaths—United States, 1999–2010. *MMWR Surveill Summ.* 2013;62(Suppl 3):161.

53. Moyer VA. Screening and behavioral counseling interventions in primary care to reduce alcohol misuse: U.S. preventive services task force recommendation statement. *Ann Intern Med.* 2013; 159:210.

54. U.S. Preventive Services Task Force. *Drug Use, Illicit: Screening.* Rockville, MD: 2008. Available at http://www.uspreventiveservicestaskforce.org/uspstf/uspsdrug.htm. Accessed February 1, 2015.

55. Strub RL, Black FW. *The Mental Status Examination in Neurology.* 2nd ed. Philadelphia, PA: FA Davis, 1985.

6

The Skin, Hair, and Nails

The Bates' suite offers these additional resources to enhance learning and facilitate understanding of this chapter:

- Bates' *Pocket Guide to Physical Examination and History Taking*, 8th edition
- Bates' *Visual Guide to Physical Examination* (Vol. 6: Skin)
- thePoint online resources, for students and instructors: http://thepoint.lww.com

In this edition, you will find a helpful new approach to examining the skin, hair, and nails and many new tables and photographs. This approach features careful history taking; thorough inspection and palpation of benign and suspicious lesions to better detect the three major skin cancers—*basal cell carcinoma* (*BCC*), *squamous cell carcinoma* (*SCC*), and *melanoma*; focused techniques for assessing changes in the hair and nails; accurate use of terminology to describe your findings; and visual familiarity with important common benign and malignant skin conditions. Updated information on skin cancer prevention and screening is found in the section on *Health Promotion and Counseling*.

Anatomy and Physiology

The skin keeps the body in homeostasis despite daily assaults from the environment. It retains body fluids while protecting underlying tissues from microorganisms, harmful substances, and radiation. It modulates body temperature and synthesizes vitamin D. Hair, nails, and sebaceous and sweat glands are considered appendages of the skin. The skin and its appendages undergo many changes during aging.

Turn to Chapter 20, The Older Adult, pp. 955–1008, to review skin changes with aging.

Skin

The skin is the heaviest single organ of the body, accounting for approximately 16% of body weight and covering an area of roughly 1.2 to 2.3/m². It contains three layers: the epidermis, the dermis, and the subcutaneous tissues.

The most superficial layer, the *epidermis,* is thin avascular keratinized epithelium consisting of two layers: an outer horny *stratum corneum* of dead keratinized cells; and an inner cellular layer, the *stratum basale* and the *stratum spinosum,* also known as the malpighian layer, where both melanin and keratin are formed. Migration from the inner to the outer layer takes approximately 1 month.

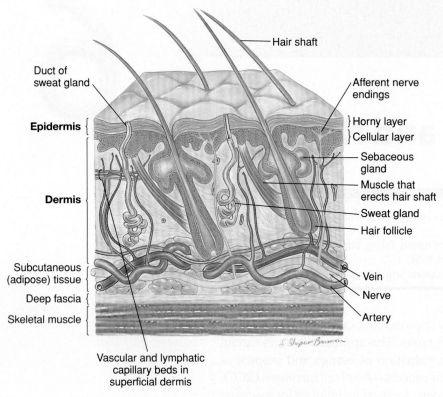

FIGURE 6-1. **Anatomy of the skin.**

The epidermis depends on the underlying vascularized *dermis* for nutrition. The dermis is a dense layer of interconnecting collagen and elastic fibers containing sebaceous glands, sweat glands, hair follicles, and most of the terminals of the cutaneous nerves (Fig. 6-1). Inferiorly, the dermis merges with *subcutaneous* fatty tissue, or *adipose tissue.*

Normal skin color depends on the amount and type of melanin, but is also influenced by underlying vascular structures, changing hemodynamics, and changes in carotene and bilirubin. The amount of *melanin,* a brownish pigment, is genetically determined and increased by exposure to sunlight. *Hemoglobin* in the red blood cells transports oxygen in the form of *oxyhemoglobin,* a bright red pigment in the arteries and capillaries that causes reddening of the skin. After passing through the capillary bed and releasing oxygen to the tissues, the darker bluer pigment of *deoxyhemoglobin* circulates in the veins. The scattering of light through the turbid superficial layers of the skin or blood vessels also makes the veins look bluer and less red than circulating venous blood.

Pallor indicates anemia.

Cyanosis, a blue color, can indicate decreased oxygen in the blood or decreased blood flow in response to a cold environment.

Carotene, a yellow pigment, is found in the subcutaneous fat and heavily keratinized areas such as the palms and soles. *Bilirubin,* a yellow-brown pigment, arises from the breakdown of heme in the red blood cells.

Jaundice, or yellowing of the skin, results from increased bilirubin.

Hair

Adults have two types of hair: *vellus hair,* which is short, fine, inconspicuous, and relatively unpigmented; and *terminal hair,* which is coarser, thicker, more conspicuous, and usually pigmented. Scalp hair and eyebrows are examples of terminal hair.

Nails

Nails protect the distal ends of the fingers and toes. The firm rectangular and usually curving *nail plate* gets its pink color from the vascular *nail bed* to which the plate is firmly attached (Figs. 6-2 and 6-3). Note the whitish moon, or *lunula,* and the free edge of the nail plate. Roughly one-fourth of the nail plate, the *nail root,* is covered by the proximal nail fold. The *cuticle* extends from the fold and, functioning as a seal, protects the space between the fold and the plate from external moisture. *Lateral nail folds* cover the sides of the nail plate. Note that the angle between the proximal nail fold and nail plate is normally less than 180°.

Fingernails grow approximately 0.1 mm daily; toenails grow more slowly.

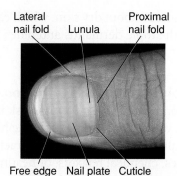

FIGURE 6-2. **Anatomy of the fingernail.**

Sebaceous Glands and Sweat Glands

Sebaceous glands produce a fatty substance secreted onto the skin surface through the hair follicles. These glands are present on all skin surfaces except the palms and soles.

Sweat glands are of two types: eccrine and apocrine. The *eccrine glands* are widely distributed, open directly onto the skin surface, and by their sweat production help to control body temperature. In contrast, the *apocrine glands* are found chiefly in the axillary and genital regions and usually open into hair follicles. Bacterial decomposition of apocrine sweat is responsible for adult body odor.

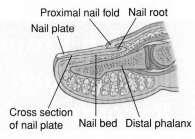

FIGURE 6-3. **Cross-section of fingernail.**

The Health History

Common or Concerning Symptoms

- Growths
- Rashes
- Hair loss or nail changes

Growths.   Start by asking if the patient is concerned about any new growths or rashes: "Have you noticed any changes in your skin? … your hair? … your nails?" "Have you had any rashes? … sores? … lumps? … itching?" If the patient reports a new growth, it is important to pursue the patient's personal and family history of skin cancer. Note the type, location, and date of any past skin cancer and ask about regular self-skin examination and use of sunscreen. Also ask "Has anyone in your family had a skin cancer removed? If so, who? Do you know what type of skin cancer—basal cell carcinoma, squamous cell carcinoma, or melanoma?" Document the response even if the patient does not know which type and counsel the patient about skin cancer prevention.

See discussion of prevention in Health Promotion and Counseling section, pp. 176–180.

Rashes.   For complaints of rash, ask about itching, the most important symptom when assessing rashes. Does itching precede the rash or follow the rash? For itchy rashes, ask about seasonal allergies with itching and watery eyes, asthma, and *atopic dermatitis,* often accompanied by rash on the inside of the elbows and knees in childhood. Can the patient sleep all night or does itching wake up the patient? For rashes, it is important to find out what type of moisturizer or over-the-counter products have been applied.

Causes of generalized itching, without apparent rash, include dry skin; pregnancy; uremia; jaundice; lymphomas and leukemia; drug reactions; and, less commonly, *polycythemia vera* and thyroid disease.

Also, ask about dry skin, which can cause itching and rash, especially in children with atopic dermatitis and older adults, due to loss of the natural moisture barrier in the epidermis.

Hair Loss or Nail Changes.   Patients often report hair loss or nail changes spontaneously. For *hair loss,* ask if there is hair thinning or hair shedding and, if so, where. If shedding, does the hair come out at the roots or break along the hair shafts? Ask about hair care practices like frequency of shampooing and use of dyes, chemical relaxers, or heating appliances. See Table 6-11, pp. 209–210, for normal patterns of hair loss in men and women and counsel affected patients appropriately. Be familiar with common *nail changes* such as onychomycosis, habit tic deformity, and melanonychia, shown in Table 6-12, pp. 211–212.

Encourage use of moisturizers to replace the lost moisture barrier. Some recommended brands even include sunscreen.[1,2]

The most common causes of diffuse hair thinning are male and female pattern baldness.

Hair shedding at the roots is common in telogen affluvium and alopecia areata. Hair breaks along the shaft suggest damage from hair care or *tinea capitis.*

Health Promotion and Counseling: Evidence and Recommendations

Important Topics for Health Promotion and Counseling

- Skin cancer prevention
- Skin cancer screening

Skin Cancer Prevention.   Clinicians play a vital role in educating patients about skin cancer prevention. Skin cancers are the most common cancers in the United States, affecting an estimated one in five Americans during their lifetime.[3] They are caused by a combination of genetic predisposition and ultraviolet radiation exposure. Fair-skinned individuals are at highest risk. The most common skin cancer is *basal cell carcinoma (BCC),* followed by *squamous cell carcinoma (SCC),* and *melanoma.*

Melanoma.   Although it is the least common skin cancer, *melanoma* is the most lethal due to its high rate of metastasis and high mortality at advanced stages, causing over 70% of skin cancer deaths.[4] The incidence of melanoma has more than doubled in the past three decades, the most rapid increase of any cancer.[5] Melanoma is now the fifth most frequently diagnosed cancer in men and the seventh most frequently diagnosed in women. In the United States in 2014, the estimated lifetime risk was 1 in 48 for whites (2%), 1 in 200 for Hispanics, and 1 in 1,000 for African Americans.[6]

Ask patients about the melanoma risk factors listed below, and use of the *Melanoma Risk Assessment Tool* developed by the National Cancer Institute, available at http://www.cancer.gov/melanomarisktool/. This tool assesses an individual's 5-year risk of developing melanoma based on geographic location, gender, race, age, history of blistering sunburns, complexion, number and size of moles, freckling, and sun damage. It is applicable up to age 70 years, but is not intended for patients with a family history of melanoma.

For discussion and examples of types of skin cancers, turn to the tables on pp. 197–203.

Risk Factors for Melanoma

- Personal or family history of previous melanoma[4,7–9]
- ≥50 common moles
- Atypical or large moles, especially if dysplastic
- Red or light hair
- *Solar lentigines* (acquired brown macules on sun-exposed areas)
- Freckles (inherited brown macules)
- Ultraviolet radiation from heavy sun exposure, sunlamps, or tanning booths
- Light eye or skin color, especially skin that freckles or burns easily
- Severe blistering sunburns in childhood
- Immunosuppression from human immunodeficiency virus (HIV) or from chemotherapy
- Personal history of nonmelanoma skin cancer

Avoiding Ultraviolet Radiation and Tanning Beds. Increasing life-time sun exposure correlates directly with increasing risk of skin cancer. Intermittent sun exposure appears to be more harmful than chronic exposure.[9] The best defense against skin cancers is to avoid ultraviolet radiation exposure by limiting time in the sun, avoiding midday sun, using sunscreen, and wearing sun-protective clothing with long sleeves and hats with wide brims. Advise patients to avoid indoor tanning, especially children, teens, and young adults. Use of indoor tanning beds, especially before age 35 years, increases risk of melanoma by as much as 75%.

In 2009, the International Agency for Research on Cancer classified ultraviolet-emitting tanning devices as "carcinogenic to humans."[10] Options for tanning include self-tanning products or sprays in conjunction with sunscreen. Targeted patient messages in primary care practices have been shown to amplify these sun-protective behaviors.[11,12] The U.S. Preventive Services Task Force (USPSTF) has made a grade B recommendation supporting behavioral counseling through minimizing ultraviolet radiation exposure in fair-skinned children, adolescents, and young adults aged 10 to 24 years and cites insufficient evidence, grade I, for counseling adults older than 24 years, but noted no harms associated with counseling.[13]

Regular Use of Sunscreen Prevents Skin Cancer. There are many myths about sunscreen. A landmark study in 2011 demonstrated that the regular use of sunscreen decreases the incidence of melanoma.[14] This well-designed study showed that when clinicians strongly encouraged use of sunscreen, patients were more likely to use it regularly and melanoma incidence declined.

Advise patients to use at least sun protective factor (SPF) 30 and broad-spectrum protection (Fig. 6-4). For water exposure, patients should use water-resistant sunscreens. New U.S. Food and Drug Administration labeling guidelines in 2011 make it easy to see these features on all bottles of sunscreen. Free information about protection and proper use of sunscreen are available from the AAD and the Skin Cancer Foundation.[15,16]

Signs of chronic sun damage include numerous *solar lentigines* on the shoulders and upper back, many melanocytic nevi, *solar elastosis* (yellow, thickened skin with bumps, wrinkles, or furrowing), *cutis rhomboidalis nuchae* (leathery thickened skin on the posterior neck), and *actinic purpura*. See Table 6-9, Signs of Sun Damage, on p. 206.

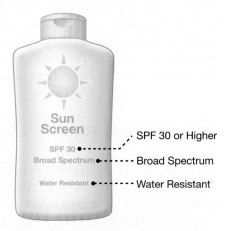

FIGURE 6-4. Advise use of broad spectrum sunscreen with SPF 30.

Skin Cancer Screening. Although the USPSTF found insufficient evidence (grade I) to recommend routine skin cancer screening by primary care physicians, it does advise clinicians to "remain alert for skin lesions with malignant features" during routine physical examinations and reference the ABCDE criteria.[17,18] The American Cancer Society (ACS) and the AAD recommend *full-body examinations* for patients over age 50 years or at high risk, because melanoma can appear in any location.[15,19] High-risk patients are those with a personal or family history of multiple or dysplastic nevi or previous melanoma. Patients who have a clinical skin examination within the 3 years prior to a melanoma diagnosis have thinner melanomas than those who did not have a clinical skin examination.[20] Both new and changing nevi should be closely examined, as at least half of melanomas arise *de novo* from isolated melanocytes rather than pre-existing nevi. Also consider "opportunistic screening" as part of the complete physical examination for patients with significant sun exposure and patients over age 50 years without prior skin examination or who live alone.

Since the USPSTF review, an important German study of over 350,000 patients reported that full-body primary care screening with dermatology referrals for concerning lesions reduced melanoma mortality by more than 47%.[21] Survival from melanoma strongly correlates with tumor thickness. Two further studies demonstrate that patients receiving skin examinations are more likely to have thinner melanomas.[20,22]

Detecting melanoma requires practice and knowledge of how benign nevi change over time, often going from flat to raised or acquiring additional brown pigment. Studies have shown that even limited clinician training makes a difference in detection: patients of primary care providers who spent 1.5 hours completing an online tutorial improved diagnostic accuracy. Similar studies show such training results in thinner melanomas than patients of providers without such training.[23–26]

Turn to Tables 6-4 through 6-6 on pp. 197–203 showing rough, pink, and brown nevi and their mimics.

Screening for Melanoma: The ABCDEs. Clinicians should apply the ABCE-EFG method when screening moles for melanoma (this does not apply for non-melanocytic lesions like seborrheic keratoses). The sensitivity of this tool for detecting melanoma ranges from 43% to 97%, and specificity ranges from 36% to 100%; diagnostic accuracy depends on how many criteria are used to define abnormality.[27] If two or more of these features are present, biopsy should be considered. The most sensitive is E, for evolution or change. Pay close attention to nevi that have changed rapidly based on objective evidence.

Review the ABCDE-EFG rule and photographs in Table 6-6, pp. 200–203, which provide additional helpful identifiers and comparisons of benign brown lesions with melanoma.

The ABCDE Rule

The ABCDE method has been used for many years to teach clinicians and patients about features suspicious for melanoma. If two or more of these are present, risk of melanoma increases and biopsy should be considered. Some have suggested adding EFG to help detect aggressive nodular melanomas.

(continued)

The ABCDE Rule (continued)

	Melanoma	Benign Nevus

Asymmetry
Of one side of mole compared to the other

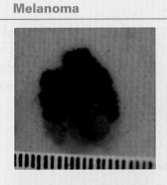
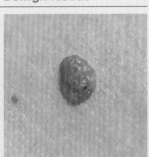

Border irregularity
Especially if ragged, notched, or blurred

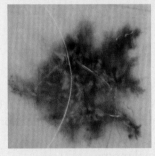
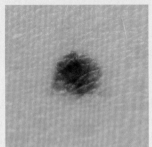

Color variations
More than two colors, especially blue-black, white (loss of pigment due to regression), or red (inflammatory reaction to abnormal cells)

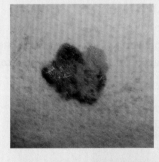
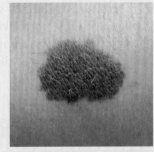

With the exception of a homogenous blue color in a blue nevus, blue or black color within a larger pigmented lesion is especially concerning for melanoma.

Diameter >6 mm
Approximately the size of a pencil eraser

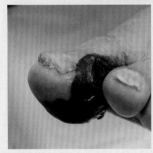
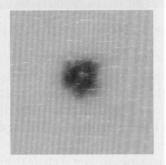

Early melanomas may be <6 mm, and many benign lesions are >6 mm.

(continued)

The ABCDE Rule (continued)

	Melanoma	Benign Nevus
Evolving Or changing rapidly in size, symptoms, or morphology	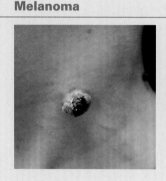	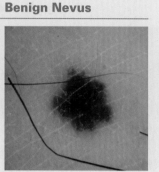

- **E**levated
- **F**irm to palpation
- **G**rowing progressively over several weeks

Evolution, or change, is the most sensitive of these criteria. A reliable history of change may prompt biopsy of a benign-appearing lesion.

Patient Screening: The Self Skin Examination. The AAD and the ACS recommend regular self-skin examination based on expert opinion.[15,28] Instruct patients with risk factors for skin cancer and melanoma, especially those with a history of high sun exposure, prior or family history of melanoma, and ≥50 moles or >5 to 10 atypical moles, to perform regular self-skin examinations. Patients who examine their skin regularly are more likely to have thinner melanomas, if detected.[24,29] Teach patients about the appearance of different skin cancers, making use of the excellent resources available on the internet.[15]

See Patient Instructions for Self Skin Examination, pp. 187–188.

Approximately half of melanomas are initially detected by patients or their partners.

Techniques of Examination

Full-Body and Integrated Skin Examinations

Perform a *full-body skin examination* in the context of the overall physical examination. Some patients at risk for melanoma, especially men over age 50 years, may not request this examination, so the general physical examination is an important opportunity to look for melanomas and other skin cancers, especially in areas patients find hard to see such as the back and posterior legs.

Inspect and palpate all skin lesions, focusing on key features that help distinguish if lesions are benign or suspicious for malignancy. Are they *raised, flat,* or *fluid-filled*? Are they *rough* or *smooth*? What about *color*? Is the lesion *pink* or *brown*? Measure the *size*. Is the size changing? Learn to describe each lesion accurately, using the terminology specified below. Changing moles, a history of skin cancer, and other risk factors all warrant a full-body skin examination.

See Tables 6-1 and 6-2 for examples and descriptions of primary skin lesions including flat, raised, fluid-filled, pustules, furuncles, nodules, cysts, wheals, and burrows (pp. 191–195); Table 6-3 for a safari of benign lesions (p. 196); and Tables 6-4 to 6-6 for rough, pink, and brown lesions and their mimics (pp. 197–203).

Even during routine examinations, you can pursue an *integrated skin examination* as you examine sun-exposed areas that are already easily accessible.

- When examining the head and neck, remember to inspect closely for skin cancers as well as common benign lesions such as *acne,* which can become scarring.

See Tables 6-7, Acne Vulgaris: Primary and Secondary Lesions, p. 204.

- Look at the arms and hands for *sun damage,* actinic keratoses, and SCCs, as well as normal findings. Educate the patient about such findings as *solar lentigines* and *seborrheic keratoses.*

See Table 6-9, Signs of Sun Damage, p. 206.

- When listening to the lungs, remove the shirt or open the gown and fully inspect the back for normal moles versus possible melanomas. Think about this approach throughout the physical examination. Note any vascular or purpuric lesions, petechiae, or eccymoses.

See Risk Factors for Melanoma on p. 177.

See Table 6-8, Vascular and Purpuric Lesions of the Skin, p. 205.

Integrating the skin examination into the physical examination and routinely recording your findings as part of the general write-up saves time and contributes to earlier detection of skin cancers, when they are easier to treat. Begin implementing this approach early in your training on each patient you examine, whether outpatient or inpatient. Instead of documenting what is not present on the skin, document what *is* present. This is the best way to learn to distinguish normal skin lesions from abnormal lesions and potential skin cancers. Systemic illnesses also have many associated skin findings.

See Table 6-10, Systemic Illnesses and Associated Skin Findings, pp. 207–208.

Preparing for the Examination

Lighting, Equipment, and Dermoscopy. Make sure there is adequate lighting. Good overhead ambient lighting or natural light from windows is usually adequate. You may wish to add a strong light source if the room is dark.

You will also need a small ruler or tape measure; these can often be obtained from packets containing disposable marking pens. In addition, a small magnifying glass allows you to examine lesions more closely. These tools help you document important features of skin lesions, such as size, shape, color, and texture.

Dermoscopy is an increasingly useful office practice for deciding whether a melanocytic lesion is benign or malignant. This handheld device provides cross-polarized or unpolarized light to visualize patterns of pigmentation or vascular structures. With adequate clinician training, use of dermoscopy improves the sensitivity and specificity of differentiating melanomas from benign lesions.[24,30]

The Patient Gown. Ask the patient to change into a gown with the opening in the back and clothes removed except for underwear (Fig. 6-5). This is the first requirement for the skin examination. Ask if the patient would like to have a chaperone present, especially when examination of the genital areas is anticipated.

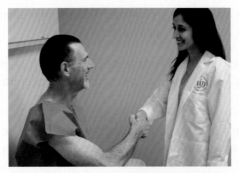

FIGURE 6-5. **The patient gown should open in the back.**

Handwashing. Before beginning the examination, cleanse your hands thoroughly. It is important for you to palpate lesions for texture, firmness, and scaliness. Because frequent handwashing increases the risk of irritant contact dermatitis, dermatologists recommend using hand sanitizers, which are less drying than soap and water. Explain that cleansing your hands ensures hygiene and an optimal examination. It is best to restrict use of gloves to touching wounds rather than throughout the examination so that the patient feels accepted. The power of professional and caring human touch can be therapeutic, especially for patients with stigmatizing diseases like psoriasis and HIV.

The Skin Examination

Important Terms for Describing Skin Lesions. It is important to use specific terminology to describe skin lesions and rashes. Good descriptions include each of the following elements: number, size, color, shape, texture, primary lesion, location, and configuration.

For example, for seborrheic keratosis, examine and record: "Multiple 5 mm to 2 cm tan to brown oval stuck-on flat-topped verrucous plaques on the back and abdomen, following skin tension lines." Note the description of each element: *number*, multiple; *size*, 5 mm–2 cm; *color*, tan to brown; *shape*, oval; *texture*, flat-topped verrucous; *location*, on the back and abdomen; and *configuration*, following skin tension lines.

Describing Skin Findings

- Primary lesion: Primary lesions are *flat* or *raised*.
  - *Flat:* You cannot palpate the lesion with your eyes closed.
    - *Macule:* Lesion is flat and <1 cm.
    - *Patch:* Lesion is flat and >1 cm.
  - *Raised:* You can palpate the lesion with eyes closed.
    - *Papule:* Lesion is raised, <1 cm, and not fluid filled.
    - *Plaque:* Lesion is raised, >1 cm, but not fluid filled.

(*continued*)

See Table 6-1, Describing Primary Skin Lesions: Flat, Raised, and Fluid-filled, pp. 191–193; Table 6-2, Additional Primary Lesions: Pustules, Furuncles, Nodules, Cysts, Wheals, Burrows, pp. 194–195; and Table 6-3, Dermatology Safari: Benign Skin Lesions, p. 196.

Describing Skin Findings (continued)

- *Vesicle:* Lesion is raised, <1 cm, and filled with fluid.
- *Bulla:* Lesion is raised, >1 cm, and fluid filled.
- Other primary lesions include erosions, ulcers, nodules, ecchymoses, petechiae, and palpable purpura.

- **Number:** Lesions can be solitary or multiple. If multiple, record how many. Also consider estimating the total number of the type of lesion you are describing.
- **Size:** Measure with a ruler in millimeters or centimeters. For oval lesions, measure in the long axis, then perpendicular to the axis.
- **Shape:** Some good words to learn are "circular," "oval," "annular" (ring-like, with central clearing), "nummular" (coin-like, no central clearing), and "polygonal."
- **Color:** Use your imagination and be creative. Refer to a color wheel, if needed. There are many shades of tan and brown, but start with tan, light brown, and dark brown if you are having trouble.
  - Use "skin-colored" to describe a lesion that is the same shade as the patient's skin.
  - For red lesions or rashes, blanch the lesion by pressing it firmly with your finger or a glass slide to see if the redness temporarily lightens then refills.

Blanching lesions are *erythematous* and suggest inflammation. Non-blanching lesions such as petechiae, purpura, and vascular structures (cherry angiomas, vascular malformations) are not erythematous, but rather bright red, purple, or violaceous. See Table 6-8, Vascular and Purpuric Lesions of the Skin, p. 205.

- **Texture:** Palpate the lesion to see if it is smooth, fleshy, verrucous or warty, or scaly (fine, keratotic, or greasy scale).

Scaling can be greasy, like *seborrheic dermatitis* or *seborrheic keratoses,* dry and fine like *tinea pedis,* or hard and keratotic like *actinic keratoses* or *SCC.*

- **Location:** Be as specific as possible. For single lesions, measure their distance from other landmarks (e.g., 1 cm lateral to left oral commissure).
- **Configuration:** Although not always necessary, describing patterns is often very helpful.

For more information and additional illustrations of each of these elements, LearnDerm is a free and very helpful website.[31]

Examples are *herpes zoster* with unilateral and dermatomal vesicles; *herpes simplex,* with grouped vesicles or pustules on an erythematous base; *tinea pedis* with annular lesions; and *poison ivy allergic contact dermatitis* with linear lesions.

Techniques of Examination—Patient Seated.   Choose one of two patient positions for performing the full-body skin examination. The patient can be seated or can lie supine, then prone. Plan to *examine the skin in the same order every time,* so you are less likely to skip part of the examination.

With the *patient seated* on the examining table, stand in front of the patient and adjust the table to a comfortable height. Start by examining the *hair and scalp* (Fig. 6-6). Separate the hair to examine the scalp from one side to the other. You may need to use your fingers or a cotton-tipped applicator ("Q-tip") to separate the hair to see the scalp (Fig. 6-7). Note the distribution, texture, and quantity of hair. Remember to inspect the ears.

Alopecia, or hair loss, can be diffuse, patchy, or total. Male and female pattern hair loss are normal with aging. Focal patches may be lost suddenly in *alopecia areata*. Refer scarring alopecia to a dermatologist.

Sparse hair is seen in hypothyroidism; fine, silky hair in hyperthyroidism. See Table 6-11, Hair Loss, pp. 209–210.

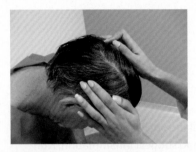

FIGURE 6-6. **Part the hair on the scalp.**

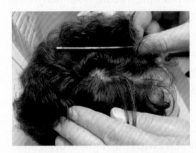

FIGURE 6-7. **Use fingers or an applicator to better visualize the scalp.**

Now inspect the *head and neck,* including the forehead; eyes including eyelids, conjunctivae, sclerae, eyelashes, and eyebrows; nose, cheeks, lips, oral cavity, and chin; and anterior neck (Figs. 6-8 to 6-10).

Look for signs of BCC on the face. See Table 6-5, Pink Lesions: Basal Cell Carcinoma and Its Mimics, pp. 198–199.

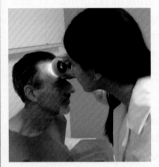

FIGURE 6-8. **Inspect the forehead.**

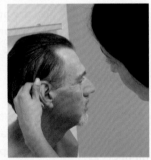

FIGURE 6-9. **Inspect the face, eyes, and ears.**

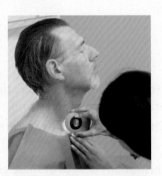

FIGURE 6-10. **Inspect the anterior neck.**

Move the gown to see each area. Ask permission first by saying, "I'd like to separate the gown to look at your back now. Is that okay?" (Fig. 6-11). Do this for every part of the body.

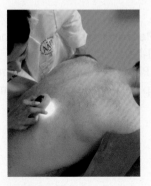

FIGURE 6-11. **Inspect the back.**

Now inspect the *shoulders, arms,* and *hands* (Fig. 6-12). Inspect and palpate the *fingernails* (Fig. 6-13). Note their color, shape, and any lesions. Longitudinal bands of pigment are normal in people with darker skin.

See Table 6-12, Findings In or Near the Nails, pp. 211–212.

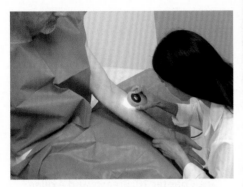

FIGURE 6-12. **Inspect the arms.**

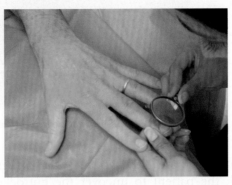

FIGURE 6-13. **Inspect and palpate the fingernails.**

Now inspect the *chest and abdomen* (Fig. 6-14), preparing the patient by saying, "Let's look at your upper chest and then your stomach area." The patient will generally help by lowering or raising the gown to expose these areas and covering up when you are finished (Fig. 6-15).

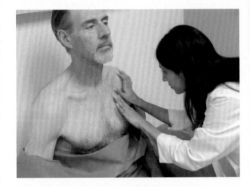

FIGURE 6-14. **Inspect the chest.**

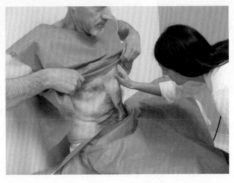

FIGURE 6-15. **Inspect the abdomen.**

Now let the patient know that you will be inspecting the *thighs* and *lower legs* (Fig. 6-16). You and the patient can work together to expose the skin in these areas, moving down to the *feet* and *toes* (Fig. 6-17). Inspect and palpate the *toenails,* and inspect the soles and between the toes (Figs. 6-18 and 6-19).

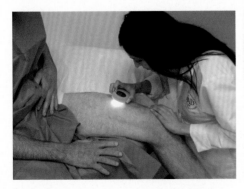

FIGURE 6-16. **Inspect the thighs.**

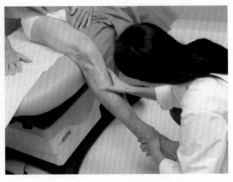

FIGURE 6-17. **Inspect the lower legs.**

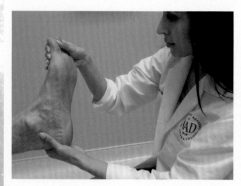

FIGURE 6-18. **Inspect the soles of the feet.**

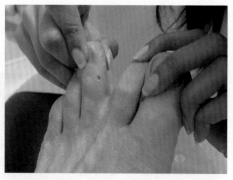

FIGURE 6-19. **Inspect between the toes.**

Now ask the patient to stand so that you inspect the *lower back* and *posterior legs* (Figs. 6-20 and 6-21). If needed, ask the patient to uncover the buttocks (Fig. 6-22). Examination of the *breasts* and *genitalia* may be saved for last. These examinations are described in other chapters. Remember to consider patient comfort, modesty, and use of a chaperone during these examinations.

See Chapter 10, Breasts and Axillae, pp. 419–447; Chapter 13, Male Genitalia, pp. 541–563; and Chapter 14, Female Genitalia, pp. 565–606.

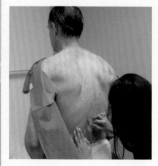

FIGURE 6-20. **Inspect the back.**

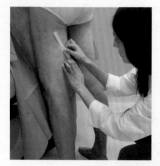

FIGURE 6-21. **Inspect the posterior legs.**

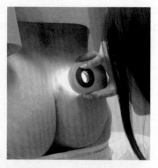

FIGURE 6-22. **Inspect the buttocks.**

Techniques of Examination—Patient Supine and Prone. Some clinicians prefer this positioning for more thorough examinations, although patients may feel it is more "clinical." Practice and feedback from patients will give you a sense of patient preferences.

Start with the patient *supine,* lying flat on the examination table. As with the seated position, start by inspecting the *scalp, face,* and *anterior neck* (Fig. 6-23). Next, move to the *shoulders, arms,* and *hands* (Fig. 6-24); then to the *chest* and

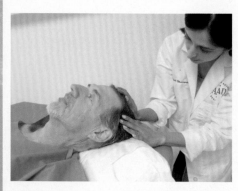

FIGURE 6-23. **Inspect the scalp.**

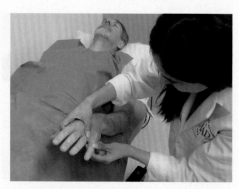

FIGURE 6-24. **Inspect the hands.**

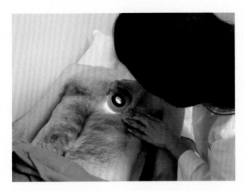

FIGURE 6-25. **Inspect the chest.**

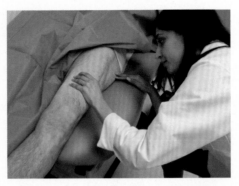

FIGURE 6-26. **Inspect the anterior thighs.**

abdomen (Fig. 6-25); *anterior thighs* (Fig. 6-26); and *lower legs, feet,* and, if appropriate, the *genitalia.* As noted previously, ask permission when moving the gown to expose different areas, and let the patient know which areas you will be examining next so the patient feels more involved in the examination.

Now ask the patient to turn over to the *prone* position, lying face down. Look at the *posterior scalp, posterior neck, back, posterior thighs, legs, soles of the feet,* and *buttocks* (if appropriate).

Special Techniques

Patient Instructions for the Self Skin-Examination. The AAD recommends regular self-examination of the skin using the techniques illustrated. The patient will need a full-length mirror, a hand-held mirror, and a well-lit room that provides privacy. Teach the patient the *ABCDE-EFG method* for assessing moles. Help them to identify melanomas by looking at photographs of benign and malignant nevi on easy-to-access websites, handouts, or tables in this chapter.

Review the ABCDE-EFG criteria on pp. 178–180.

Patient Instructions for Skin Self-Examination

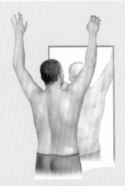

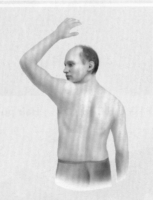

Examine your body front and back in the mirror, then look at your right and left sides with arms raised.

Bend elbows and look carefully at forearms, upper underarms, and palms.

(continued)

Patient Instructions for Skin Self-Examination (continued)

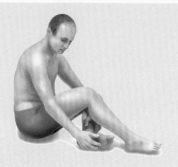

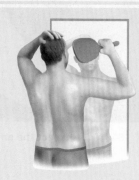

Look at the backs of your legs and feet, the spaces between your toes, and the soles.

Examine the back of your neck and scalp with a hand mirror. Part hair for a closer look.

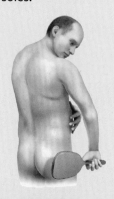

Finally, check your back and buttocks with a hand mirror.

Source: Adapted from American Academy of Dermatology. How to perform a self-exam. Available at https://www.aad.org/spot-skin-cancer/understanding-skin-cancer/how-do-i-check-my-skin/how-to-perform-a-self-exam. Accessed February 12, 2015.

Examining the Patient with Hair Loss. Based on the patient's history, start by examining the hair to determine the overall pattern of hair loss or hair thinning.[32] Inspect the scalp for erythema, scaling, pustules, tenderness, bogginess, and scarring. Look at the width of the hair part in various sections of the scalp. To examine the hair for shedding from the roots, perform a *hair pull test* by gently grasping 50 to 60 hairs with your thumb and index and middle fingers, pulling firmly away from the scalp (Fig. 6-27). If all the hairs have telogen bulbs, the most likely diagnosis is *telogen effluvium*. To examine the hair for fragility, perform the *tug test* by holding a group of hairs in one hand, pulling along the hair shafts with the other (Fig. 6-28); if any hairs break, it is abnormal.

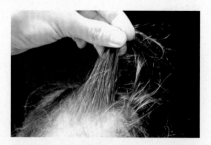

FIGURE 6-27. **Hair pull test.**

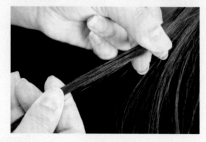

FIGURE 6-28. **Tug test.**

Most (97%) hair loss is nonscarring, but any scarring, namely shiny spots without any hair follicles on close examination with a magnifying glass, should prompt referral to dermatology for scalp biopsy.

Possible internal causes of diffuse nonscarring hair shedding in young women are *iron-deficiency anemia* and *hyper-* or *hypothyroidism*.

Evaluating the Bedbound Patient.   People confined to bed, especially when they are emaciated, elderly, or neurologically impaired, are particularly susceptible to skin damage and ulceration. *Pressure sores* result from sustained compression that obliterates arteriolar and capillary blood flow to the skin, and from shear forces created by body movements. When a person slides down in bed from a partially sitting position, for example, or is dragged rather than lifted up after being supine, rough movement can distort the soft tissues of the buttocks and close off the arteries and arterioles. Friction and moisture further increase the risk of abrasions and sores.

See Table 6-13, Pressure Ulcers, p. 213.

Assess every susceptible patient by carefully inspecting the skin that overlies the sacrum, buttocks, greater trochanters, knees, and heels. Roll the patient onto one side to see the low back and gluteal area best.

Local redness of the skin warns of impending necrosis, although some deep pressure sores develop without antecedent redness. Inspect closely for skin breaks and ulcers.

Recording Your Findings

Note that initially you may use sentences to describe your findings; later you will use phrases. The examples below contain phrases appropriate for most write-ups.

For more details about this terminology, turn to Techniques of Examination, pp. 182–183.

As stated on p. 182, use specific terms to describe skin lesions and rashes, including:

- *Number*—solitary or multiple; estimate of total number

- *Size*—measured in millimeters or centimeters

- *Color*—including erythematous if blanching; if nonblanching, vascular-like cherry angiomas and vascular malformations, petechiae, or purpura

- *Shape*—circular, oval, annular, nummular, or polygonal

- *Texture*—smooth, fleshy, verrucous or warty, keratotic; greasy if scaling

- *Primary lesion*—flat, a macule or patch; raised, a papule or plaque; or fluid filled, a vesicle or bulla (may also be erosions, ulcers, nodules, ecchymoses, petechiae, and palpable purpura)

- *Location*—including measured distance from other landmarks

- *Configuration*—grouped, annular, linear

Recording the Skin, Hair, and Nails Physical Examination

"Skin warm and dry. Nails without clubbing or cyanosis. Approximately 20 brown, round macules on upper back, chest, and arms, are all symmetric in pigmentation, none suspicious. No rash, petechiae, or ecchymoses."

OR

"Marked facial pallor, and circumoral cyanosis. Palms cold and moist. Cyanosis in nail beds of fingers and toes. Numerous palpable purpura on lower legs bilaterally."

OR

"Scattered stuck-on verrucous plaques on back and abdomen. Over 30 small round brown macules with symmetric pigmentation on back, chest, and arms. Single 1.2 × 1.6 cm asymmetric dark brown and black plaque with erythematous, uneven border, on left upper arm."

OR

"Facial plethora. Skin icteric. Many telangiectatic mats on chest and abdomen. Single 5 mm pearly papule with rolled border on left zygomatic cheek. Nails with clubbing but no cyanosis."

There are normal nevi and perfusion without any rashes or suspicious lesions.

These findings suggest central cyanosis and vasculitis.

These findings suggest normal seborrheic keratoses and benign nevi, but also a possible malignant melanoma.

These findings suggest probable end-stage liver disease and incidental BCC.

Table 6-1 Describing Primary Skin Lesions: Flat, Raised, and Fluid-Filled

Describe skin lesions accurately, including number, size, color, texture, shape, primary lesion, location, and configuration. This table identifies common primary skin lesions and includes classic descriptions of each lesion with the diagnosis in italics.

Flat Spots

If you run your finger over the lesion but do not feel the lesion, the lesion is *flat*. If a flat spot is small (<1 cm), it is a **macule**. If a flat spot is larger (>1 cm), it is a **patch**.

Macules (flat, small)

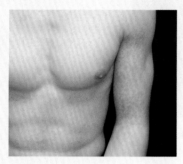

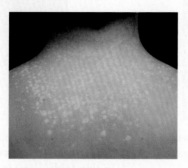

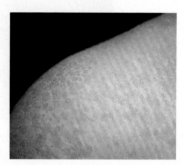

Multiple 3–8-mm erythematous confluent round **macules** on chest, back, and arms; *morbilliform drug eruption*

Multiple 2–5-mm hypopigmented, hyperpigmented, or tan round to oval **macules** on upper neck and back, upper chest, and arms with slight inducible scale on scraping (*tinea versicolor*)

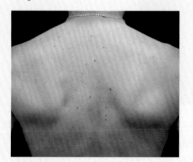

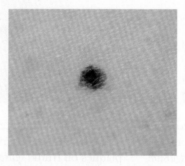

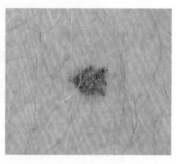

Multiple scattered 2–4-mm round and oval brown **macules**, symmetrically pigmented, on back and chest with reticular pattern on dermoscopy; *benign melanocytic nevi*

Solitary 6-mm dark brown round symmetric macule on upper back; *benign melanocytic nevus*

Solitary dark brown, blue-gray, and red 7-mm **macule** with irregular borders and fingerlike projections of pigment, on right forearm; *malignant melanoma*

Patches (flat, large)

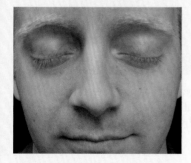

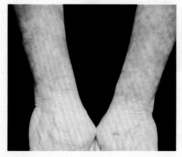

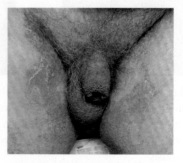

Bilaterally symmetric erythematous **patches** on central cheeks and eyebrows, some with overlying greasy scale; *seborrheic dermatitis*

Large confluent completely depigmented patches on dorsal hands and distal forearms; *vitiligo*

Bilateral erythematous, geographic patches with peripheral scaling, on inner thighs bilaterally, sparing the scrotum; *tinea cruris*

(continued)

Raised Spots

If you run your finger over the lesion and it is palpable above the skin, it is *raised*. If a raised spot is small (<1 cm), it is a **papule**. If a raised spot is larger (>1 cm), it is a **plaque**.

Papules (raised, small)

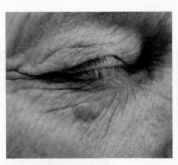

Solitary 7-mm oval pink pearly **papule** with overlying telangiectasias on right nasojugal fold; *basal cell carcinoma*

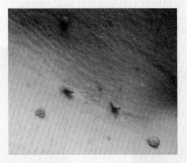

Multiple 2–4-mm soft, fleshy skin-colored to light brown **papules** on lateral neck and axillae in skin folds; *skin tags*

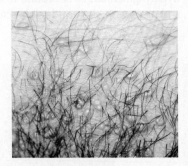

Multiple 3–5-mm pink firm smooth domed **papules** with central umbillications, in mons pubis, and on penile shaft; *molluscum contagiosum*

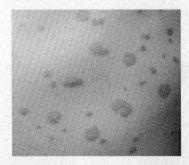

Scattered erythematous round drop-like, flat-topped well-circumscribed scaling **papules** and plaques on trunk; *guttate psoriasis*

Plaques (raised, large)

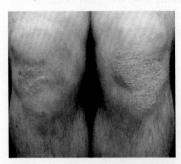

Scattered erythematous to bright pink well-circumscribed flat-topped **plaques** on extensor knees and elbows, with overlying silvery scale; *plaque psoriasis*

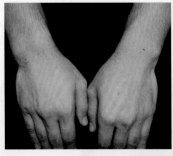

Bilateral erythematous, lichenified (thickened from rubbing) poorly circumscribed **plaques** on flexor wrists, antecubital fossae, and popliteal fossae; *atopic dermatitis*

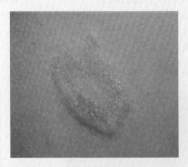

Single, oval, flat-topped superficial erythematous to skin-colored **plaque** on right abdomen; *herald patch of pityriasis rosea*

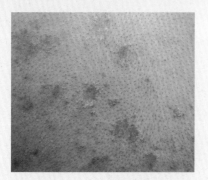

Multiple round to oval scaling violaceous **plaques** on abdomen and back; *pityriasis rosea*

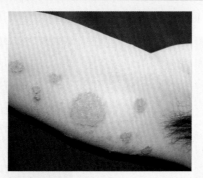

Multiple round coin-like eczematous **plaques** on arms, legs, and abdomen, with overlying dried transudate crust; *nummular dermatitis*

Fluid-filled Lesions

If the lesion is raised, filled with fluid, and small (<1 cm), it is a **vesicle**. If a fluid-filled spot is larger (>1 cm), it is a **bulla**.

Vesicles (fluid-filled, small)

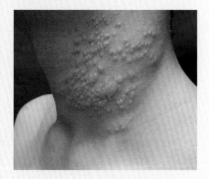

Multiple 2–4-mm **vesicles** and pustules on erythematous base, grouped together on left neck; *herpes simplex virus*

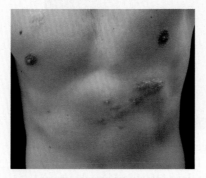

Grouped 2–5-mm **vesicles** on erythematous base on left upper abdomen and trunk in a dermatomal distribution that does not cross the midline; *herpes zoster or "shingles"*

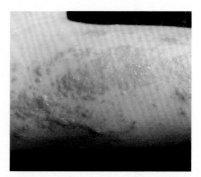

Scattered 2–5-mm erythematous papules and **vesicles** with transudate crust, some with linear arrays, on forearms, neck, and abdomen; *rhus dermatitis* or *allergic contact dermatitis* from poison ivy

Bullae (fluid-filled, large)

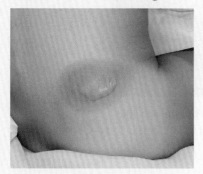

Solitary 8-cm dusky oval patch with smaller inner violaceous patch and central 3.5-cm tense **bulla,** on right posterior lower back; *bullous fixed drug eruption*

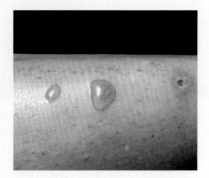

Several tense bullae on lower legs; *insect bites*

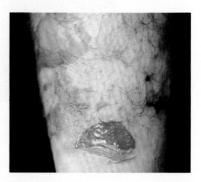

Many vesicles and tense **bullae** up to 4 cm, some having unroofed and left large (4-cm) erosions, on lower legs bilaterally up to the line of the top of combat boots; *an inherited skin fragility disorder*

Pustule: Small palpable collection of neutrophils or keratin that appears white

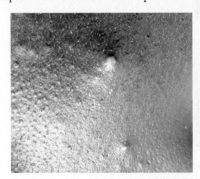

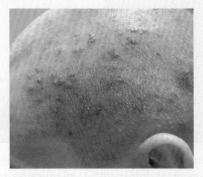

~15–20 **pustules** and acneiform papules on buccal and parotid cheeks bilaterally; *acne vulgaris*

~30 2–5-mm erythematous papules and **pustules** on frontal, temporal, and parietal scalp; *bacterial folliculitis*

Furuncle: Inflamed hair follicle; multiple furuncles together form a carbuncle

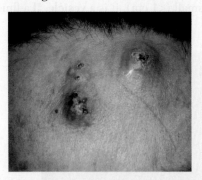

Two large (2-cm) **furuncles** on forehead, without fluctuance; *furunculosis* (Note: fluctuant deep infections are *abscesses*)

Nodule: Larger and deeper than a papule

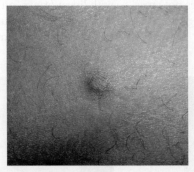

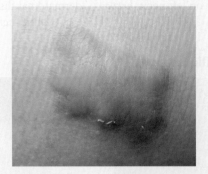

Solitary blue-brown 1.2-cm firm **nodule** with positive dimple sign and hyperpigmented rim on left lateral thigh; *dermatofibroma*

Solitary 4-cm pink and brown scar-like **nodule** on central chest at site of previous trauma; *keloid*

Subcutaneous mass/cyst: Whether mobile or fixed, cysts are encapsulated collections of fluid or semisolid

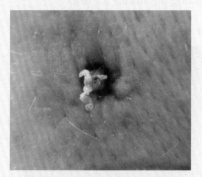

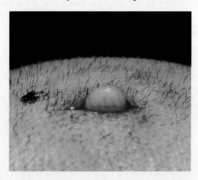

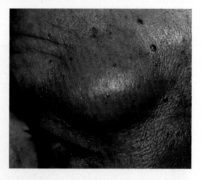

Solitary 2-cm tethered subcutaneous **cyst** with overlying punctum releasing caseous whitish yellow substance with foul odor; *epidermal inclusion cyst*

Three 6–8-mm mobile subcutaneous **cysts** on vertex scalp, that on excision reveal pearly white balls; *pilar cysts*

Solitary 9-cm mobile rubbery subcutaneous **mass** on left temple; *lipoma*

Wheal: Area of localized dermal edema that evanesces (comes and goes) within a period of 1–2 days; this is the essential primary lesion of *urticaria*

Burrow: Small linear or serpiginous pathways in the epidermis created by the scabies mite

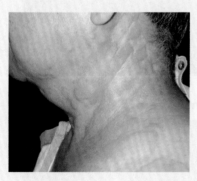

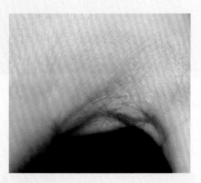

Many variably sized (1–10-cm) **wheals** on lateral neck, shoulders, abdomen, arms, and legs; *urticaria*

Multiple small (3–6-mm) erythematous papules on abdomen, buttocks, scrotum, and shaft and head of penis, with four **burrows** noted on interdigital web spaces; *scabies*

Table 6-3 Dermatology Safari: Benign Lesions

Practice makes perfect . . . Look for these common lesions during your clinical rotations. Perform a skin examination on as many patients as you can. If you are unsure about identifying the lesion, ask your instructors or attending physicians for help.

Cherry angiomas

Seborrheic keratosis

Solar lentigines

Benign melanocytic nevi

Dermatofibroma

Keloids

Epidermal inclusion cyst

Pilar cyst

Lipoma

Table 6-4 Rough Lesions: Actinic Keratoses, Squamous Cell Carcinoma, and Their Mimics

Patients commonly report feeling rough lesions. Many are benign, like *seborrheic keratoses* or *warts,* but *squamous cell carcinoma* (*SCC*) and its precursor *actinic keratosis* can also feel rough or keratotic. *SCC* most commonly arises on sun-damaged skin of the head, neck, and dorsal arms and hands and can metastasize if left untreated. It consists of more mature cells usually resembling the spinous layer of the epidermis and accounts for ~16% of skin cancers. If left untreated, *actinic keratoses* progress to SCC at a rate of about 1 in 1,000 per year. Counsel affected patients about sun avoidance and use of sunscreen and offer treatment to prevent progression to SCC.

Actinic Keratosis and Squamous Cell Carcinoma

Actinic keratosis

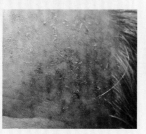 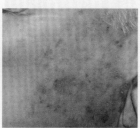

- Actinic keratosis after field therapy with 5-fluorouracil (left photo)
- Often easier to feel than to see
- Superficial keratotic papules "come and go" on sun-damaged skin

Cutaneous horn/keratotic scale

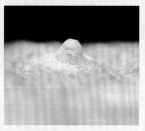 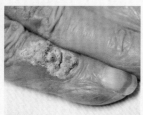

- The *protypic keratotic scale* of actinic keratoses and SCC is formed by keratin and can result in a cutaneous horn
- Cutaneous horns should generally be biopsied to rule out SCC

Squamous cell carcinoma

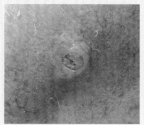 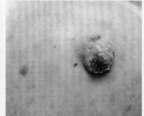

- Keratoacanthomas are SCCs that arise rapidly and have a crateriform center
- Often have a *smooth but firm border*
- SCCs can become quite large if left untreated (Note: *highest sites of metastasis are the scalp, lips, and ears*)

Mimics

Superficial xerosis or seborrheic dermatitis

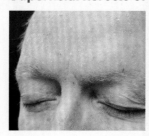

- May occur in same distribution on forehead, central face
- Scale is less keratotic and will improve with moisturizers, mild topical steroids

Warts

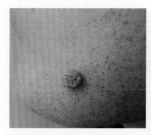 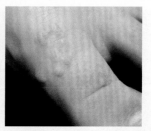

- Usually skin-colored to pink, texture more verrucous than keratotic
- May be filiform
- Often have hemorrhagic punctae that can be seen with a magnifying glass or dermatoscope

Seborrheic keratosis

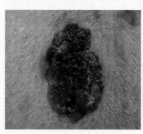 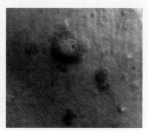

- Often have a verrucous texture
- Appear like a "stuck-on" or flattened ball of wax
- May crumble or bleed if picked
- Specific features on dermoscopy such as milia-like cysts or comedone-like openings are reassuring, if present
- May be erythematous if inflamed

Table 6-5 Pink Lesions: Basal Cell Carcinoma and Its Mimics

Basal cell carcinoma (BCC) is the most common cancer in the world. Fortunately, it rarely spreads to other parts of the body. Nonetheless, it can invade and destroy local tissues, causing significant morbidity to the eye, nose, or brain. BCC consists of immature cells similar to those in the basal layer of the epidermis, and account for roughly 80% of all skin cancers. BCCs should be biopsied for confirmation before treatment. Review the BCC features below and how they contrast with mimics that are benign.

Basal Cell Carcinomas

Mimics

Superficial basal cell carcinoma

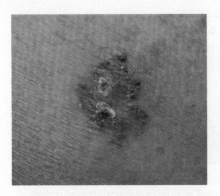

- Pink patch that does not heal
- May have focal scaling

Actinic keratosis and squamous cell carcinoma in situ

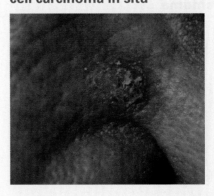

- Actinic keratosis or squamous cell carcinoma *in situ* usually has keratotic scaling

Nodular basal cell carcinoma

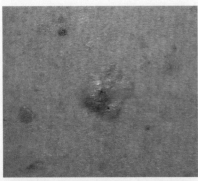

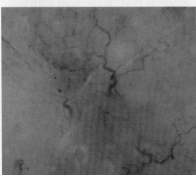

- Pink papule, often with translucent or pearly appearance and overlying telangiectasias
- May have focal pigmentation
- Dermoscopy shows arborizing vessels, focal pigment globules, and other specific patterns

Sebaceous hyperplasia

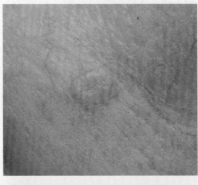

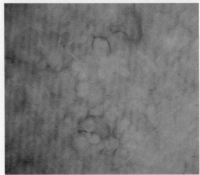

- Yellowish globular papules, often with central dell, on forehead and cheeks
- Dermoscopy shows telangiectasias that go around sebaceous glands rather than over them as in BCC

Basal Cell Carcinomas

Nodular basal cell carcinoma (*continued*)

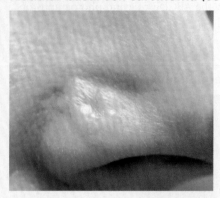

- 1 cm pearly pink plaque with central depression and overlying arborizing telangiectasias on nasal ala

Ulcerated basal cell carcinoma

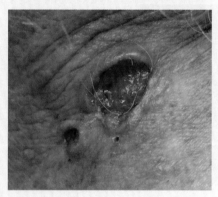

- Non-healing ulcer, resulting in *"rolled border"*

Mimics

Fibrous papule

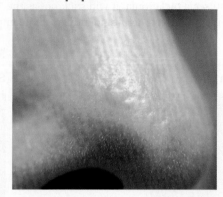

- Skin-colored to pink papule on the nose, without telangiectasias
- May become excoriated

Squamous cell carcinoma

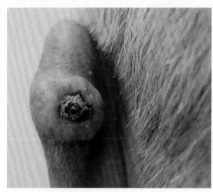

- May also be ulcerated
- Firmer at edges than BCC

Table 6-6 Brown Lesions: Melanoma and Its Mimics

Most patients have brown spots on their body surface if you look thoroughly. Although these are usually freckles, benign nevi, solar lentigines, or seborrheic keratoses, you and the patient must look closely for any that stand out as a possible *melanoma*. The best way to detect a melanoma is to do numerous skin examinations so that you recognize brown lesions that are benign. With enough practice, when you see a melanoma, it will stick out as the "ugly duckling." Review the ABCDE rule and photographs on pp. 178–180, which provide additional helpful identifiers and comparisons.

Melanomas	Mimics

Amelanotic melanoma

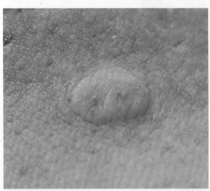

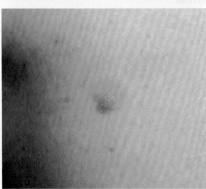

- Usually in very fair-skinned people
- *Evolution or rapid change* is the most important feature, because variegation or dark pigment is missing in this type

Skin tags or intradermal nevi

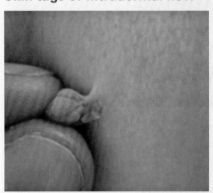

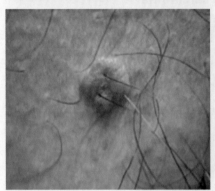

- Soft and fleshy
- Often around neck, axillae, or back
- Sessile nevi may have a hint of brown pigmentation

Melanoma *in situ*

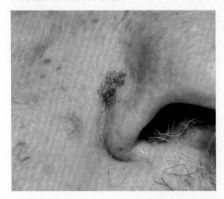

- On sun-exposed or sun-protected skin
- Look for ABCDE features

Solar lentigo

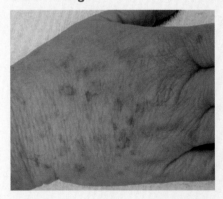

- On sun-exposed skin
- Light brown and uniform in color but may be asymmetric

Melanomas

Melanoma

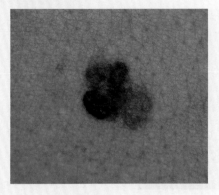

- May arise de novo or in existing nevi and exhibits ABCDEs
- Patients with many dysplastic nevi have increased risk of melanoma

Melanoma

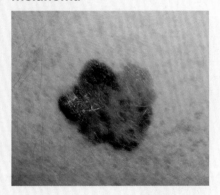

- May have *variegated color* (browns, red)
- Has melanocytic features on dermoscopy

Melanoma

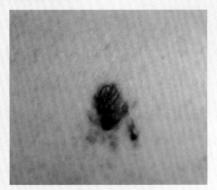

- May be uniform in color but *asymmetric*; key feature is *rapid change or Evolution*

Mimics

Dysplastic nevus

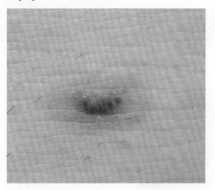

- May have macular base and papular central "fried egg" component
- Compare to the patient's other nevi and monitor changes

Inflamed seborrheic keratosis

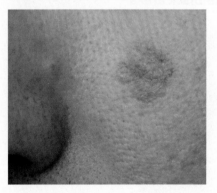

- Can sometimes mimic a melanoma if it has an erythematous base
- Dermoscopy helps the trained eye distinguish these

Seborrheic keratosis

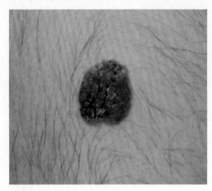

- Stuck-on and verrucous, may be darkly pigmented

(continued)

Table 6-6 Brown Lesions: Melanoma and Its Mimics (*Continued*)

Melanomas

Acral melanoma

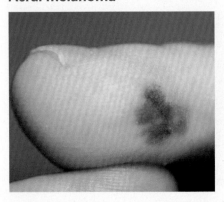

- Rapid change or evolution helps detect acral melanoma
- Consider biopsies if >7 mm, rapidly growing, or concerning features on dermoscopy

Melanoma with blue-black areas

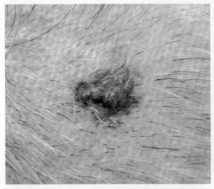

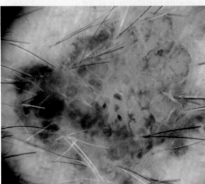

- *Blue-black areas* are concerning for melanoma, especially if they are asymmetric

Mimics

Acral nevus

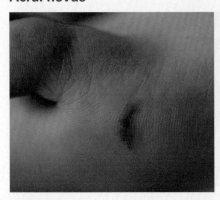

- Likely benign if <7 mm and has a reassurance pattern on dermoscopy, such as the parallel furrow or lattice patterns

Blue nevus

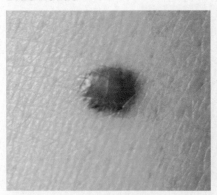

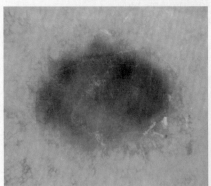

- Blue nevi have a homogenous blue-gray appearance, clinically and on dermoscopy

Finding the Ugly Duckling: As you evaluate changing brown lesions in the context of the patient's other nevi and lentigines, the "ugly duckling" is the nevus that looks different from the patient's other nevi. A patient may make many atypical nevi with surrounding macular components and central papular components, but they all look the same. Find the patient's *signature nevus,* then search for the ugly duckling that looks different from the patient's typical "signature" nevi.

Most dermatologists now rely on a dermatoscope to evaluate pigmented lesions, which allows them to detect melanomas when they are thinner. With training, dermoscopy can help distinguish nevi with reassuring patterns from possible early melanomas. Even without dermoscopy, however, a keen eye actively inspecting the skin for "ugly ducklings" is likely to detect melanomas when they arise.

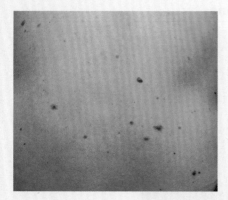 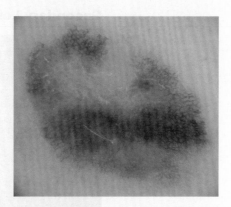

This patient has multiple atypical nevi, but the one on his right back just lateral to midline stands out as the "ugly duckling" because it has three colors; the white area showed melanoma in situ on biopsy.

Table 6-7 Acne Vulgaris—Primary and Secondary Lesions

Acne vulgaris is the most common cutaneous disorder in the United States, affecting more than 85% of adolescents.[33] Acne is a disorder of the pilosebaceous unit that involves proliferation of the keratinocytes at the opening of the follicle; increased production of sebum, stimulated by androgens, which combines with keratinocytes to plug the follicular opening; growth of *Propionibacterium acnes,* an anaerobic diphtheroid normally found on the skin; and inflammation from bacterial activity and release of free fatty acids and enzymes from activated neutrophils. Cosmetics, humidity, heavy sweating, and stress are contributing factors. Most recommendations for treatment of acne are divided along its morphologic subdivisions: comedonal (mild), inflammatory (moderate), and nodulocystic (severe).

Lesions appear in areas with the greatest number of sebaceous glands, namely the face, neck, chest, upper back, and upper arms. They may be primary, secondary, or mixed.

Primary Lesions	**Secondary Lesions**

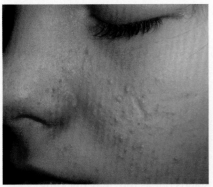

Mild Acne: Open and closed comedones, occasional papules

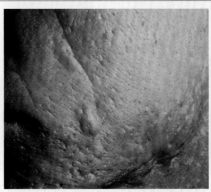

Acne with Pitting and Scars

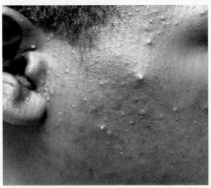

Moderate Acne: Comedones, papules, pustules

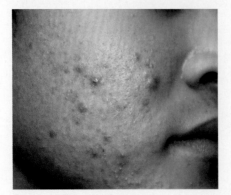

Severe Cystic Acne

Table 6-8 Vascular and Purpuric Lesions of the Skin

Vascular Lesions

	Spider Angioma[a]	Spider Vein[a]	Cherry Angioma
	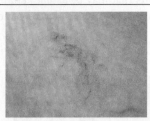		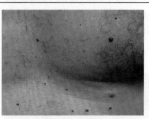
Color and Size	Fiery red; from very small to 2 cm	Bluish; size variable, from very small to several inches	Bright or ruby red; may become purplish with age; 1–3 mm
Shape	Central body, sometimes raised, surrounded by erythema and radiating legs	Variable; may resemble a spider or be linear, irregular, cascading	Round, flat, or sometimes raised; may be surrounded by a pale halo
Pulsatility and Effect of Pressure	Often seen in center of the spider when pressure with a glass slide is applied; pressure on the body causes blanching of the spider	Absent; pressure over the center does not cause blanching, but diffuse pressure blanches the veins	Absent; may show partial blanching, especially if pressure applied with edge of a pinpoint
Distribution	Face, neck, arms, and upper trunk; almost never below the waist	Most often on the legs, near veins; also on the anterior chest	Trunk; also extremities
Significance	Single spider angiomas are normal and are common on the face and chest; also seen in pregnancy and liver disease	Often accompanies increased pressure in the superficial veins, as in varicose veins	None; increases in size and numbers with aging

Purpuric Lesions

	Petechia/Purpura	Ecchymosis
	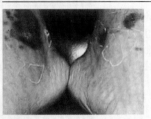	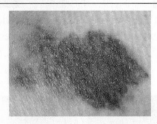
Color and Size	Deep red or reddish purple, fading away over time; petechia, 1–3 mm; purpura are larger	Purple or purplish blue, fading to green, yellow, and brown with time; ariable size, larger than petechiae, >3 mm
Shape	Rounded, sometimes irregular; flat	Rounded, oval, or irregular; may have a central subcutaneous flat nodule (a hematoma)
Pulsatility and Effect of Pressure	Absent; no effect from pressure	Absent; no effect from pressure
Distribution	Variable	Variable
Significance	Blood outside the vessels; may suggest a bleeding disorder or, if petechiae, emboli to skin; palpable purpura in *vasculitis*	Blood outside the vessels; often secondary to bruising or trauma; also seen in bleeding disorders

[a]These are telangiectasias, or dilated small vessels that look red or bluish.

Sources of photos: *Spider Angioma*—Marks R. Skin Disease in Old Age. Philadelphia: JB Lippincott, 1987; *Petechia/Purpura*—Kelley WN. Textbook of Internal Medicine. Philadelphia: JB Lippincott, 1989.

Table 6-9 Signs of Sun Damage

Sun damage is one of the most important clues that a patient is at risk of skin cancer. Study carefully the following indicators of sun damage accrued throughout life. These indicators should prompt close inspection for **pink lesions** that are possible *basal cell carcinomas*; **rough** or **keratotic lesions** that may be *actinic keratoses* or *squamous cell carcinomas*; or **asymmetric, multicolored,** or **changing lesions** that could be *melanoma*. Counsel affected patients about proper sun protection, not only for themselves but for their families.

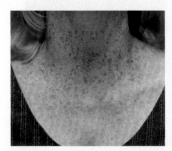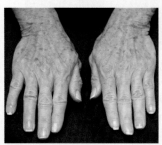

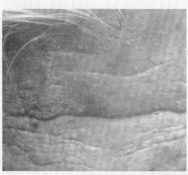

Solar lentigo: Bilaterally symmetric brown macules located on sun-exposed skin, including the face, shoulders, and arms and hands

Solar elastosis: Yellowish white macules or papules in sun-exposed skin, especially on the forehead

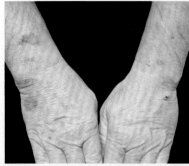

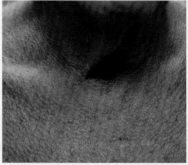

Actinic purpura: Ecchymoses limited to the dorsal forearms and hands but not extending above the "shirt sleeve" line on the upper arm

Poikiloderma: Red patches in sun-damaged areas, especially the V of the neck, and lateral neck (usually sparing the shadow inferior to the chin) with fine telangiectasias, and both hyper- and hypopigmentation

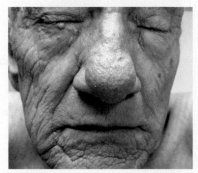

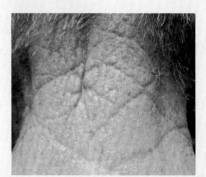

Wrinkles: Increased sun damage and tanning leads to deeper wrinkles at an earlier age

Cutis rhomboidalis nuchae: Deep wrinkles on the posterior neck that "criss-cross"

Table 6-10 Systemic Diseases and Associated Skin Findings

Systemic Disease	Associated Findings or Diagnoses
Addison disease	Hyperpigmentation of oral mucosa as well as sun-exposed skin, sites of trauma, and creases of palms and soles
Acquired immune deficiency syndrome	Human papillomavirus, herpes simplex virus, varicella zoster virus, cytomegalovirus, molluscum contagiosum, bacterial abscesses, mycobacterium (tuberculosis, leprae, avium) infections, candidiasis, deep fungal infections (cryptococcus, histoplasmosis), oral hairy leukoplakia, Kaposi sarcoma, oral and anal squamous cell carcinoma, acquired ichthyosis, severe psoriasis, severe seborrheic dermatitis, eosinophilic folliculitis
Chagas disease (American trypanosomiasis)	Unilateral conjunctivitis and lid edema associated with preauricular lymphadenopathy
Chronic renal disease	Pallor, xerosis, uremic frost, pruritus, "half and half" nails, calciphylaxis.
CREST syndrome	Calcinosis, Raynaud phenomenon, sclerodactyly, matted telangiectasias of face and hands (palms)
Crohn disease	Erythema nodosum, pyoderma gangrenosum, enterocutaneous fistulas, aphthous ulcers
Cushing disease	Striae, atrophy, purpura, ecchymoses, telangiectasias, acne, moon facies, buffalo hump, hypertrichosis
Dermatomyositis	Violaceous erythema as macules, patches or papules in periocular region (heliotrope), on interphalangeal joints (Gottron sign), and on upper back and shoulders (shawl sign); poikiloderma in sun-exposed areas; periungual telangiectasia, ragged cuticles (Samitz sign)
Diabetes	Pruritus, diabetic dermopathy, acanthosis nigricans, candidiasis, neuropathic ulcers, necrobiosis lipoidica, eruptive xanthomas
Disseminated intravascular coagulation	Purpura, petechiae, hemorrhagic bullae, induration, necrosis
Dyslipidemias	Xanthomas (tendon, eruptive, and tuberous), xanthelasma (may also occur in healthy people)
Gonococcemia	Purple to grey macules, papules or hemorrhagic pustules distributed over acral and periarticular surfaces
Hemochromatosis	Skin bronzing and hyperpigmentation
Hypothyroidism	Dry, rough, and pale skin; coarse and brittle hair; myxedema; alopecia (lateral third of the eyebrows to diffuse); skin cool to touch; thin and brittle nails
Hyperthyroidism	Warm, moist, soft, and velvety skin; thin and fine hair; alopecia; vitiligo; pretibial myxedema (in Graves disease); hyperpigmentation (local or generalized)
Infective endocarditis	Janeway lesions, Osler nodes, splinter hemorrhages, petechiae

(continued)

Table 6-10 Systemic Diseases and Associated Skin Findings (*Continued*)

Systemic Disease	Associated Findings or Diagnoses
Kawasaki disease	Mucosal erythema (lips, tongue, and pharynx), strawberry tongue, cherry red lips, polymorphous rash (primarily on trunk), erythema of palms and soles with later desquamation of fingertips
Liver disease	Jaundice, spider angiomas and other telangiectasias, palmar erythema, Terry nails, pruritus, purpura, caput medusae
Leukemia/lymphoma	Pallor, exfoliative erythroderma, nodules, petechiae, ecchymoses, pruritus, vasculitis, pyoderma gangrenosum, bullous diseases
Leukocytoclastic vasculitis (post-capillary venules)	Palpable purpura, purpuric wheals, hemorrhagic bullae in dependent areas
Lymphogranuloma venereum	Lymphadenopathy above and below Poupart ligament (groove sign)
Medium vessels vasculitides (e.g., polyarteritis nodosa, granulomatosis with polyangiitis, eosinophilic granulomatosis with polyangiitis, microscopic polyangiitis)	Livedo racemosa, purpuric nodules, ulcers
Meningococcemia	Angular or stellate purpuric patches and plaques with gunmetal gray center. Progresses to ecchymoses, bullae, necrosis
Neurofibromatoses 1 (von Recklinghausen syndrome)	Neurofibromas, café-au-lait spots, freckling in the axillae (Crowe sign), plexiform neurofibroma
Pancreatitis (hemorrhagic)	Bruising and induration over the costovertebral angle (Grey Turner sign), Cullen sign, panniculitis
Pancreatic carcinoma	Panniculitis, migratory thrombophlebitis (Trousseau sign)
Porphyria cutanea tarda	Photosensitivity with bullae and skin fragility on dorsal hands and forearms; bullae rupture and heal with scarring and milia; hypertrichosis of the face; bronzing of skin when associated with hemochromatosis
Pyoderma gangrenosum	Painful pustule quickly progressing to ragged ulcer with sharply marginated violaceous border and undermined edges
Rocky Mountain spotted fever	Pink or reddish papules progressing to purpuric papules; starts on wrists and ankles and spreads to palms and soles and then to trunk and face
Sarcoidosis	Red-brown plaques, often annular, typically involving the head and neck and especially the nose and ears; may show apple jelly color with dermoscopy
Systemic lupus erythematosus	Malar erythema (mid cheeks, spans bridge of nose), relative sparing of nasolabial folds, periungual erythema, interphalangeal erythema

Table 6-11 Hair Loss

When taking a complete history of hair loss, include the duration, acuity of onset, cause from decreased hair density or increased shedding, the pattern (diffuse or localized), medication history, hair care practices, and associated medical conditions or stressors. *Decrease in hair density* is usually caused by male or female pattern hair loss, but less commonly by scarring alopecias. *Hair shedding from the roots* is often caused by *telogen effluvium, alopecia areata, anagen effluvium* (insults to the hair shaft from exposure to agents like chemotherapy) or less commonly, scarring alopecias. Perform a hair pull test to look for the percentage of telogen hairs. *Hair shedding from breakage at the hair shaft* is often caused by *tinea capitis,* improper hair care, and less commonly hair shaft disorders or *anagen effluvium.* Perform a tug test to look for hair fragility. See Figures 6-27 and 6-28 on p. 188 for examples of the hair pull test and tug test.

Generalized or Diffuse Hair Loss

Male and female pattern hair loss affects over half of men by their 50 years of age, and over half of women by their 80 years of age. In men, look for frontal hairline regression and thinning on the posterior vertex; in women, look for thinning that spreads from the crown down without hairline regression. Severity is described by standardized classifications: Norwood-Hamilton (men) and Ludwig (women). The *hair pull test* is normal or only pulls a few hairs.

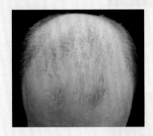

Male pattern hair loss (MPHL)

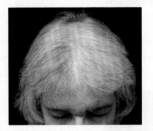

Female pattern hair loss (FPHL)

Telogen Effluvium and Anagen Effluvium

In *telogen effluvium,* overall, the patient's scalp and hair distribution appear normal, but a positive *hair pull test* reveals most hairs have telogen bulbs. In *anagen effluvium,* there is diffuse hair loss from the roots. The *hair pull test* shows few if any hairs with telogen bulbs.

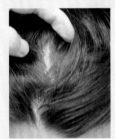

Normal hair part width in telogen effluvium

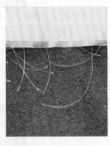

Positive hair pull test in telogen effluvium showing all hairs have telogen bulbs

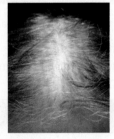

Anagen effluvium

Focal Hair Loss

Alopecia Areata

There is sudden onset of clearly demarcated, usually localized, round or oval patches of hair loss leaving smooth skin without hairs, in children and young adults. There is no visible scaling or erythema.

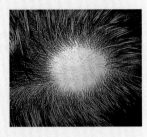

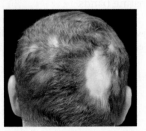

(continued)

Table 6-11 Hair Loss (*Continued*)

Tinea Capitis ("Ringworm")

There are round scaling patches of alopecia, mostly seen in children. There may be "black dots" of broken hairs and comma or corkscrew hairs on dermoscopy. Usually caused by *Trichophyton tonsurans* from humans, and less commonly, *Microsporum canis* from dogs or cats. Boggy plaques are called kerions.

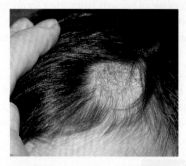
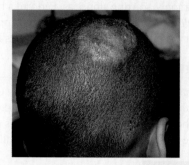

Scarring Alopecia

Scarring on the scalp is characterized by shiny skin, complete loss of hair follicles, and often, discoloration. Presence of any scarring should prompt referral to a dermatologist for possible scalp biopsy if the patient desires treatment. Examples of scarring alopecia include central centrifugal scarring alopecia and discoid lupus erythematosus, among others.

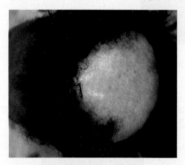
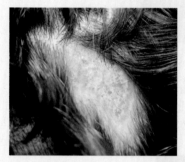

Central centrifugal scarring alopecia

Discoid lupus scarring alopecia

Hair Shaft Disorders

Patients with abnormal hair from birth, as in this patient with a genetic condition called monilethrix, should be referred to dermatology.

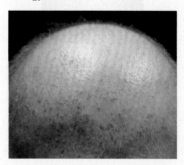
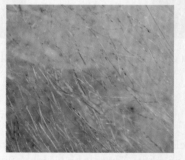

Hair shaft disorder with alternating bands

References: For a complete guide to evaluation of hair loss, review Mubki T, Rucnicka L, Olszewska M, et al. Evaluation and diagnosis of the hair loss patient. *J Am Acad Dermatol* 2014;71:415. *See also Hair Loss Help. Hair loss classifications. Available at http://www.hairlosshelp.com/hair_loss_research/hair_loss_charts. cfm. Accessed February 13, 2015.

Sources of photo: *Alopecia Areata [left]*—Hall JC. Sauer's Manual of Skin Diseases, 9th ed. Philadelphia: Lippincott Williams & Wilkins, 2006.

Table 6-12 Findings in or Near the Nails

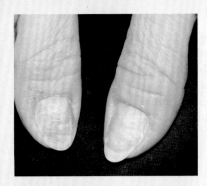

Paronychia

A superficial infection of the proximal and lateral nail folds adjacent to the nail plate. The nail folds are often red, swollen, and tender. Represents the most common infection of the hand, usually from *Staphylococcus aureus* or *Streptococcus* species, and may spread until it completely surrounds the nail plate. Creates a felon if it extends into the pulp space of the finger. Arises from local trauma due to nail biting, manicuring, or frequent hand immersion in water. Chronic infections may be related to *Candida*.

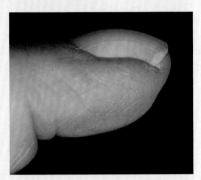

Clubbing of the Fingers

Clinically, a bulbous swelling of the soft tissue at the nail base, with loss of the normal angle between the nail and the proximal nail fold. The angle increases to 180° or more, and the nail bed feels spongy or floating. The mechanism is still unknown but involves vasodilatation with increased blood flow to the distal portion of the digits and changes in connective tissue, possibly from hypoxia, changes in innervation, genetics, or a platelet-derived growth factor from fragments of platelet clumps. Seen in congenital heart disease, interstitial lung disease and lung cancer, inflammatory bowel diseases, and malignancies.

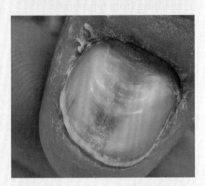

Habit Tic Deformity

There is depression of the central nail with a "Christmas tree" appearance from small horizontal depressions, resulting from repetitive trauma from rubbing the index finger over the thumb or vice versa. Pressure on the nail matrix causes the nail to grow out abnormally. Avoidance of the behavior leads to normal nail growth.

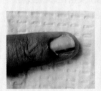

Melanonychia

Melanonychia is caused by increased pigmentation in the nail matrix, leading to a streak as the nail grows out. This may be a normal ethnic variation if found in multiple nails. A thin uniform streak may be caused by a nevus, but a wide streak, especially if growing or irregular, could represent a *subungual melanoma*.

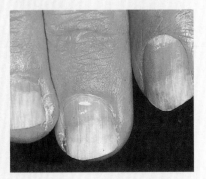

Onycholysis

A painless separation of the whitened opaque nail plate from the pinker translucent nail bed. Fingernails that extend past the fingertip are more likely to result in the traumatic shearing forces that produce onycholysis. Starts distally and progresses proximally, enlarging the free edge of the nail. Local causes include trauma from excess manicuring, psoriasis, fungal infection, and allergic reactions to nail cosmetics. Systemic causes include diabetes, anemia, photosensitive drug reactions, hyperthyroidism, peripheral ischemia, bronchiectasis, and syphilis.

(continued)

Table 6-12 Findings in or Near the Nails (*Continued*)

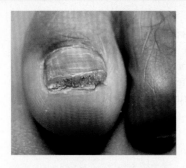

Onychomycosis

The most common cause of nail thickening and subungual debris is *onychomycosis,* most often from the dermatophyte *Trichophyton rubrum,* but also from other dermatophytes and some molds such as *Alternaria* and *Fusarium* species. Onychomycosis affects 1 in 5 over age 60. The best prevention is to treat and prevent *tinea pedis.* Only half of all nail dystrophies are caused by onychomycosis, so a positive fungal culture, potassium hydroxide exam, or pathologic evaluation of nail clippings is recommended before treating with oral antifungals.

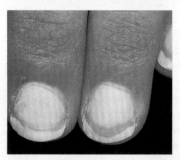

Terry Nails

Nail plate turns white with a ground-glass appearance, a distal band of reddish brown, and obliteration of the lunula. Commonly affects all fingers, although may appear in only one finger. Seen in liver disease, usually cirrhosis, heart failure, and diabetes. May arise from decreased vascularity and increased connective tissue in nail bed.

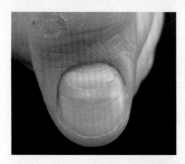

Transverse Linear Depressions (*Beau Lines*)

Transverse depressions of the nail plates, usually bilateral, resulting from temporary disruption of proximal nail growth from systemic illness. Timing of the illness may be estimated by measuring the distance from the line to the nail bed (nails grow approximately 1 mm every 6 to 10 days). Seen in severe illness, trauma, and cold exposure if Raynaud disease is present.

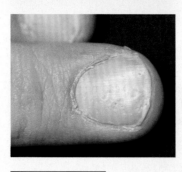

Pitting

Punctate depressions of the nail plate caused by defective layering of the superficial nail plate by the proximal nail matrix. Usually associated with psoriasis but also seen in Reiter syndrome, sarcoidosis, alopecia areata, and localized atopic or chemical dermatitis.

Sources of photos: *Onycholysis, Terry Nails*—Habif TP. Clinical Dermatology: A Color Guide to Diagnosis and Therapy, 2nd ed. St. Louis: CV Mosby, 1990.

Table 6-13 Pressure Ulcers

Pressure (*decubitus*) ulcers usually develop over bony prominences subject to unrelieved pressure, resulting in ischemic damage to underlying tissue. Prevention is important: inspect the skin thoroughly for *early warning signs of erythema that still blanches with pressure,* especially in patients with risk factors. Pressure ulcers form most commonly over the sacrum, ischial tuberosities, greater trochanters, and heels. A commonly applied staging system, based on depth of destroyed tissue, is illustrated below. Note that necrosis or eschar must be debrided before ulcers can be staged. Ulcers may not progress sequentially through the four stages.

Inspect ulcers for signs of infection (drainage, odor, cellulitis, or necrosis). Fever, chills, and pain suggest underlying *osteomyelitis.* Address the patient's overall health, including *comorbid conditions* such as vascular disease, diabetes, immune deficiencies, collagen vascular disease, malignancy, psychosis, or depression; nutritional status; pain and level of analgesia; risk for recurrence; psychosocial factors such as learning ability, social supports, and lifestyle; and evidence of polypharmacy, overmedication, or abuse of alcohol, tobacco, or illicit drugs.[34,35]

Risk Factors for Pressure Ulcers

- Decreased mobility, especially if accompanied by increased pressure or movement causing friction or shear stress
- Decreased sensation, from brain or spinal cord lesions or peripheral nerve disease
- Decreased blood flow from hypotension or microvascular disease such as diabetes or atherosclerosis
- Fecal or urinary incontinence
- Presence of fracture
- Poor nutritional status or low albumin

Stage I

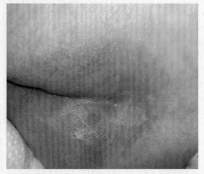

Stage II

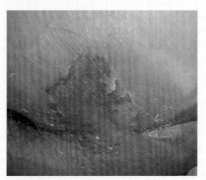

Presence of a reddened area that fails to blanch with pressure, and changes in temperature (warmth or coolness), consistency (firm or boggy), sensation (pain or itching), or color (red, blue, or purple on darker skin; red on lighter skin)

The skin forms a blister or sore. Partial-thickness skin loss or ulceration involving the epidermis, dermis, or both

Stage III

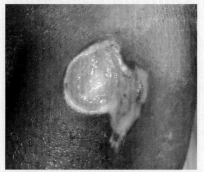

Stage IV

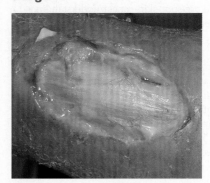

A crater appears in the skin, with full-thickness skin loss and damage to or necrosis of subcutaneous tissue that may extend to, but not through, underlying muscle

The pressure ulcer deepens. There is full-thickness skin loss, with destruction, tissue necrosis, or damage to underlying muscle, bone, and sometimes tendons and joints

Source: Used with permission of National Pressure Ulcer Advisory Panel, Washington, DC.

References

1. Eichenfeld LF, Tom WL, Berger TG, et al. Guidelines of care for the management of atopic dermatitis. *J Am Acad Dermatol.* 2014;71:116.
2. National Eczema Association. Available at http://nationaleczema.org/eczema-products/moisturizers/. Accessed October 27, 2014.
3. Stern RS. Prevalence of a history of skin cancer in 2007: results of an incidence-based model. *Arch Dermatol.* 2010;146:279.
4. Siegel R, Desantis C, Jemal A. Cancer statistics, 2015. *CA Cancer J Clin.* 2015;65:5.
5. Howlader N, Noone AM, Krapcho M, et al. *SEER Cancer Statistics Review, 1975–2011.* Bethesda, MD: National Cancer Institute; 2014.
6. American Cancer Society. Key statistics about Melanoma Skin Cancer. Available at http://www.cancer.org/cancer/skincancer-melanoma/detailedguide/melanoma-skin-cancer-key-statistics. Accessed February 2, 2015.
7. Naeyaert JM, Brochez L. Clinical practice. Dysplastic nevi. *N Engl J Med.* 2003;349:2233.
8. American Academy of Dermatology. Skin cancer. Available at https://www.aad.org/dermatology-a-to-z/diseases-and-treatments/q—t/skin-cancer. Accessed February 11, 2015.
9. National Cancer Institute. Genetics of Skin Cancer (PDQ®). Melanoma. Available at http://www.cancer.gov/cancertopics/pdq/genetics/skin/HealthProfessional/page4. Accessed February 14, 2015.
10. El Ghissassi F, Baan R, Straif K, et al. A review of human carcinogens—part D: radiation. *Lancet Oncol.* 2009;10:751.
11. Glanz K, Schoenfeld ER, Steffen A. A randomized trial of tailored skin cancer prevention messages for adults: Project SCAPE. *Am J Public Health.* 2010;100:735.
12. Lin JS, Eder M, Weinmann S. Behavioral counseling to prevent skin cancer: a systematic review for the U.S. Preventive Services Task Force. *Ann Intern Med.* 2011;154:190. See also http://www.ncbi.nlm.nih.gov/books/NBK53508/. Accessed February 15, 2015.
13. Moyer VA. Behavioral counseling to prevent skin cancer: U.S. Preventive Services Task Force recommendation statement. *Ann Intern Med.* 2012;157:59. See also http://www.uspreventiveservicestaskforce.org/Page/Topic/recommendation-summary/skin-cancer-counseling?ds=1&s=. Accessed February 15, 2015.
14. Green AC, Williams GM, Logan V, et al. Reduced melanoma after regular sunscreen use: randomized trial follow-up. *J Clin Oncol,* 2011;29:257.
15. American Academy of Dermatology. How do I prevent skin cancer. Available at https://www.aad.org/spot-skin-cancer/understanding-skin-cancer/how-do-i-prevent-skin-cancer. Accessed February 11, 2015.
16. Skin Cancer Foundation. Sun protection. Available at http://www.skincancer.org/prevention/sun-protection. Accessed February 15, 2015.
17. U.S. Preventive Services Task Force. Screening for skin cancer. Recommendation statement. *Ann Intern Med.* 2009;150:188. See also http://www.uspreventiveservicestaskforce.org/Page/Topic/recommendation-summary/skin-cancer-screening?ds=1&s=. Accessed February 15, 2015.
18. Wolff T, Tai E, Miller T. Screening for skin cancer: an update of the evidence for the U.S. Preventive Services Task Force. *Ann Intern Med.* 2009;150:194. See also http://www.ncbi.nlm.nih.gov/books/NBK34051/. Accessed February 15, 2015.
19. Siegel R, Desantis C, Jemal A. Colorectal cancer statistics, 2014. *CA Cancer J Clin.* 2014;64:104.
20. Aitken JF, Elwood M, Baade PD, et al. Clinical whole-body skin examination reduces the incidence of thick melanomas. *Int J Cancer.* 2010;126:450.
21. Katalinic A, Waldmann A, Weinstock MA, et al. Does skin cancer screening save lives? An observational study comparing trends in melanoma mortality in regions with and without screening. *Cancer.* 2012;118:5395.
22. Swetter SM, Pollitt RA, Johnson TM, et al. Behavioral determinants of successful early melanoma detection. *Cancer.* 2012;118:3725.
23. Grange F, Barbe L, Mas F, et al. The role of general practitioners in diagnosis of cutaneous melanoma: a population-based study in France. *Br J Dermatol.* 2012;167:1351.
24. Mayer JE, Swetter SM, Fu T, et al. Screening, early detection, education, and trends for melanoma: current status (2007–2013) and future directions, Parts I and II. *J Am Acad Dermatol.* 2014;71:599; 611.
25. Eide MJ, Asgari NM, Fletcher SW, et al. Effects on skills and practice from a web-based skin cancer course for primary care providers. *J Am Board Fam Med.* 2013;26:648.
26. Skinsight INFORMED Skin Cancer Education Series. Melanoma and Skin Cancer Early Detection. http://www.skinsight.com/info/for_professionals/skin-cancer-detection-informed/skin-cancer-education. Accessed February 15, 2015.
27. Abbasi NR, Shaw HM, Rigel DS, et al. Early diagnosis of cutaneous melanoma revisiting the ABCD criteria. *JAMA.* 2004;292:2771.
28. American Cancer Society. Skin exams. Available at http://www.cancer.org/cancer/skincancer-melanoma/moreinformation/skincancerpreventionandearlydetection/skin-cancer-prevention-and-early-detection-skin-exams. Accessed February 11, 2015.
29. McPherson M, Elwood M, English DR, et al. Presentation and detection of invasive melanoma in a high-risk population. *J Am Acad Dermatol.* 2006;54:783.
30. Zalaudek I, Kittler H, Marghoob AA, et al. Time required for a complete skin examination with and without dermoscopy: a prospective, randomized multicenter study. *Arch Dermatol.* 2008;144:509.
31. Learn Derm. http://www.visualdx.com/learnderm/. Accessed February 15, 2015.
32. Mubki T, Rucnicka L, Olszewska M, et al. Evaluate and diagnosis of the hair loss patient. *J Am Acad Dermatol.* 2014;71:415.
33. Thiboutot D, Gollnick H, Bettoli V, et al. New insights into the management of acne: an update from the Global Alliance to Improve Outcomes in Acne group. *J Am Acad Dermatol.* 2009;60(5 Suppl):S1.
34. Smith TE, Totten A, Hickam DH, et al. Pressure ulcer treatment strategies: a systemic comparative effectiveness review. *Ann Intern Med.* 2013;159:39.
35. VanGilder C, MacFarlane G, Meyer S, et al. Body mass index, weight, and pressure ulcer prevalence: an analysis of the 2006–2007 International Pressure Ulcer Prevalence Surveys. *J Nurs Care Qual.* 2009;24:127.

The Head and Neck

The Bates' suite offers these additional resources to enhance learning and facilitate understanding of this chapter:

- Bates' *Pocket Guide to Physical Examination and History Taking*, 8th edition
- Bates' *Visual Guide to Physical Examination* (Vol. 7: Head, Eyes, and Ears; Vol. 8: Nose, Mouth, and Neck)
- thePoint online resources, for students and instructors: http://thepoint.lww.com

Many critical structures like the sensory organs, cranial nerves (CNs), and major blood vessels originate in the head and neck. To help students integrate this complex anatomy and physiology with the skills of physical examination, this chapter follows a special format. The Health History and the Health Promotion and Counseling sections cover the "HEENT" components—Head, Eyes, Ear, Nose, and Throat—as a unit since head and neck symptoms, as well as prevention strategies, are often interconnected. However, Anatomy and Physiology and Techniques of Examination are grouped together in five combined sections due to the close linkage between anatomic structures and function and techniques of examination, especially for the examination of the eyes (Fig. 7-1).

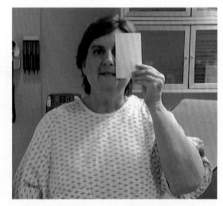

FIGURE 7-1. Test the complex anatomy and physiology of vision.

The Health History

Common or Concerning Symptoms

- Headache
- Change in vision: blurred vision, loss of vision, floaters, flashing lights
- Eye pain, redness, or tearing
- Double vision (diplopia)
- Hearing loss, earache, ringing in the ears (tinnitus)
- Dizziness and vertigo
- Nosebleed (epistaxis)
- Sore throat, hoarseness
- Swollen glands
- Goiter

Many symptoms of the head and neck represent common benign processes, but sometimes these symptoms reflect a serious underlying condition. Careful attention to the interview and physical examination, with a focus on features and findings that do not fit a typical benign pattern, can often distinguish a common condition of the head and neck from a serious underlying disease.

The Head

Headache is one of the most common symptoms in clinical practice, with a lifetime prevalence of 30% in the general population.[1,2] Among types of headaches, *tension headache* predominates, affecting half of all individuals during their lifetime.[3] Headaches are generally classified as *primary* (without an identified underlying disease) or *secondary* (with an identified underlying disease). However, every headache warrants careful evaluation for life-threatening secondary causes such as meningitis, subarachnoid hemorrhage, or mass lesion. Elicit a full description of every headache and its seven attributes (see p. 79). Is it unilateral or bilateral? Severe with sudden onset, like a thunderclap? Steady or throbbing? Continuous or intermittent? Is there an aura? Is the headache "typical" or is there something different?

Look for important signs ("red flags") that warn of headaches needing prompt investigation.

> See Tables 7-1 and 7-2 on Primary Headaches and Secondary Headaches and Cranial Neuralgias on pp. 267–269.
>
> *Primary headaches* include migraine, tension, cluster, and chronic daily headaches; *secondary headaches* arise from underlying structural, systemic, or infectious causes such as meningitis or subarachnoid hemorrhage and may be life-threatening.[4–6]
>
> The *International Classification of Headache Disorders,* now in its second iteration, continues to evolve.[5,7–9]

Headache Warning Signs

- Progressively frequent or severe over a 3-month period
- Sudden onset like a "thunderclap" or "the worst headache of my life"
- New onset after age 50 years
- Aggravated or relieved by change in position
- Precipitated by Valsalva maneuver or exertion
- Associated symptoms of fever, night sweats, or weight loss
- Presence of cancer, HIV infection, or pregnancy
- Recent head trauma
- Change in pattern from past headaches
- Lack of a similar headache in the past
- Associated papilledema, neck stiffness, or focal neurologic deficits

> Thunderclap headaches reaching maximal intensity over several minutes occur in 70% of patients with *subarachnoid hemorrhage,* and are often preceded by a *sentinel leak headache* from a vascular leak into the subarachnoid space.[10]

The three most important attributes of headache are its *severity,* its *chronologic pattern,* and its *associated symptoms.* Is the headache severe and of sudden onset? Does it intensify over several hours? Is it episodic? Or is it chronic or recurring? Is there a recent change in its pattern? Does the headache recur at the same time every day? What other symptoms, especially weakness or numbness in an arm or leg?

After your usual open-ended assessment, ask the patient to *point to the area of pain or discomfort.*

> If headache is severe and of sudden onset, consider *subarachnoid hemorrhage* or *meningitis.*[10]
>
> *Migraine* and *tension headaches* are episodic and tend to peak over several hours. New and persisting, progressively severe headaches raise concerns of *tumor, abscess,* or *mass lesion.*
>
> Unilateral headache occurs in *migraine and cluster headaches.*[4,11] Tension headaches often arise in the temporal areas; cluster headaches may be retro-orbital.

Ask about associated symptoms such as nausea and vomiting.

Nausea and vomiting are common with *migraine,* but also occur with *brain tumors* and *subarachnoid hemorrhage.*

Is there a prodrome of unusual feelings such as euphoria, craving for food, fatigue, or dizziness? Does the patient report an aura with neurologic symptoms, such as change in vision, numbness, or weakness?

Approximately 60% to 70% of patients with *migraine* have a symptom prodrome prior to onset. About a third experience a visual aura, such as spark photopsias (flashes of light), fortifications (zig-zag arcs of light), and scotomas (areas of visual loss with surrounding normal vision).

Note that, due to *increased risk of ischemic stroke and cardiovascular disease,* the World Health Association advises women with migraines over age 35 years and women with migraines with aura avoid use of estrogen–progestin contraceptives.[12–15]

Ask if coughing, sneezing, or changing the position of the head affects the headache. If head position affects the headache, ask if leaning forward or lying down increases the headache, or if lying down increases the headache.

Valsalva maneuvers and leaning forward may increase pain from *acute sinusitis.* Valsalva and lying down may increase pain from mass lesions due to changing intracranial pressure.

Is there any overuse of analgesics, ergotamines, or triptans?

Medication for overuse headache may cause headache if present ≥15 days a month for three months and reverts to <15 days a month when the medication is discontinued.[16]

Ask about family history.

Genetic inheritance is present in 30% to 50% of patients with migraine.[11,17]

The Eyes

Begin with open-ended questions such as "How is your vision?" and "Have you had any trouble with your eyes?" If the patient reports a change in vision, pursue the related details.

- Is vision worse during close work or at distances?

Difficulty with close work suggests *hyperopia* (farsightedness) or *presbyopia* (aging vision), or, if with distances, *myopia* (nearsightedness).

- Is there blurred vision? If yes, is the onset sudden or gradual? If sudden and unilateral, is the visual loss painless or painful?

If sudden visual loss is *unilateral and painless,* consider *vitreous hemorrhage* from diabetes or trauma, *macular degeneration, retinal detachment, retinal vein occlusion,* or *central retinal artery occlusion.*

If *painful,* causes are usually in the cornea and anterior chamber such as *corneal ulcer, uveitis, traumatic hyphema,* and *acute angle closure glaucoma.*[18–20] *Optic neuriti*s from multiple sclerosis may also be painful.[21] Immediate referral is warranted.[22,23]

■ Is the visual loss bilateral (sudden bilateral visual loss is rare)? If so, is it painful?

If *bilateral and painless,* consider vascular etiologies such as *giant-cell arteritis* or nonphysiologic causes. If *bilateral and painful,* consider chemical or radiation exposures.

■ Is the onset of bilateral visual loss gradual?

Gradual vision loss usually arises from *cataracts* or *macular degeneration.*

■ Location of visual loss may also be helpful. Is there blurring of the entire field of vision or only parts of it?

Slow central loss occurs in *nuclear cataract* (p. 276) and *macular degeneration*[24] (p. 242), peripheral loss in advanced *open-angle glaucoma* (p. 270), and one-sided loss with *hemianopsia* and *quadrantic defects* (p. 273).

■ If the visual field defect is partial, is it central, peripheral, or on only one side?

■ Are there specks in the vision or areas where the patient cannot see (*scotomas*)? If so, do they move around in the visual field with shifts in gaze or are they fixed?

Moving specks or strands suggest vitreous floaters; fixed defects, or *scotomas,* suggest lesions in the retina or visual pathways.

■ Are there lights flashing across the field of vision? Vitreous floaters may accompany this symptom.

Flashing lights with new vitreous floaters suggest detachment of the vitreous body from the retina. Prompt consultation is indicated.[25]

■ Does the patient wear glasses?

Ask about pain in or around the eyes, redness, and excessive tearing or watering.

A red painless eye is seen in *subconjunctival hemorrhage,* a red eye with a gritty sensation in *viral conjunctivitis.* A red painful eye is seen in *hyphema, episcleritis, acute angle closure glaucoma, herpes keratitis,* foreign body, *fungal keratitis,* and *sarcoid uveitis.*[26,27] See Table 7-3, Red Eyes, p. 270.

Check for double vision, or *diplopia.* If present, find out if the images are side by side (horizontal diplopia) or on top of each other (vertical diplopia). Does diplopia persist with one eye closed? Which eye is affected?

One kind of horizontal diplopia is physiologic. Hold one finger upright approximately 6 inches in front of your face, a second at arm's length. When you focus on either finger, the image of the other is double. A patient who notices this phenomenon can be reassured.

Diplopia is seen in lesions in the brainstem or cerebellum, and with weakness or paralysis of one or more extraocular muscles, as in *horizontal diplopia* from palsy of CN III or VI, or *vertical diplopia* from palsy of CN III or IV. Diplopia in one eye, with the other closed, suggests a problem in the cornea or lens.

The Ears

Opening questions are "How is your hearing?" and "Have you had any trouble with your ears?" If the patient has noticed a *hearing loss,* does it involve one or both ears? Did it start suddenly or gradually? What are the associated symptoms, if any?

Distinguish *conductive loss,* which results from problems in the external or middle ear, from *sensorineural loss,* resulting from problems in the inner ear, the cochlear nerve, or its central connections in the brain. Two questions may be helpful: Does the patient have special difficulty understanding people as they talk? What happens in a noisy environment?

Pursue symptoms associated with hearing loss, such as earache or vertigo to help sort out likely causes. Ask about medications that might affect hearing and about sustained exposure to loud noise.

Complaints of *earache,* or *pain in the ear,* are especially common. Ask about associated fever, sore throat, cough, and concurrent upper respiratory infection; if present, these heighten the likelihood of ear infection.

Ask about *discharge from the ear,* especially if associated with earache or trauma. Wax or debris in the ear is usually normal.

Tinnitus is a perceived sound that has no external stimulus—commonly, a musical ringing or a rushing or roaring noise in one or both ears. Tinnitus may accompany hearing loss and often remains unexplained. Occasionally, popping sounds originate in the temporomandibular joint, or sounds from the vessels in the neck may be audible.

Vertigo is the sensation of true rotational movement of the patient or the surroundings.[32] These sensations point primarily to a problem in the labyrinths of the inner ear, peripheral lesions of CN VIII, or lesions in its central pathways or nuclei in the brain.

Complaints of *dizziness* and *light-headedness* are challenging because they are often nonspecific and suggest a diverse set of conditions ranging from vertigo to presyncope, weakness, unsteadiness, and disequilibrium. Clarify by asking what the patient means by dizziness. Then ask, "Do you feel as if the room is spinning or tilting (vertigo)? Do your symptoms get worse when you move your head?" Then, "Do you feel as if you are going to fall or pass out (presyncope)?...Or do you feel you are unsteady or losing your balance (disequilibrium)?"

Hearing loss may also be congenital, from single gene mutations.[28,29]

People with *sensorineural loss* have trouble understanding speech, often complaining that others mumble; noisy environments make hearing worse. In *conductive loss,* noisy environments may help.

Medications that affect hearing include aminoglycosides, aspirin, NSAIDs, quinine, and furosemide.

Pain occurs in the external canal in *otitis externa* (inflammation of the external ear canal) and, deeper within the ear in *otitis media* (infection of the middle ear).[30] Pain in the ear may also be referred from other structures in the mouth, throat, or neck.

***Acute otitis externa* and *acute or chronic otitis media* with perforation usually present with yellow-green discharge.**

***Tinnitus* is a common symptom, increasing in frequency with age. When associated with hearing loss and vertigo, suspect *Ménière disease.*[31]**

See Table 7-4, Dizziness and Vertigo, p. 271.

See Table 7-4, Dizziness and Vertigo, p. 271, for distinguishing symptoms and time course.

If there is true vertigo, distinguish peripheral from central neurologic causes (see Chapter 17, see p. 722). Establish the time course of symptoms. Check for nausea, vomiting, double vision, and gait disturbance. Review the patient's medications. Proceed with a careful neurologic examination focusing on presence of nystagmus and focal neurologic signs.

Vertigo represents vestibular disease, usually from peripheral causes in the inner ear such as *benign positional vertigo, labyrinthitis, vestibular neuritis,* and *Ménière disease.* Ataxia, diplopia, and dysarthria signal central neurologic causes in the cerebellum or brainstem such as cerebral vascular disease or posterior fossa tumor; also consider *migraine.*[32] Feeling lightheaded, weak in the legs, or about to faint points to *presyncope* from arrhythmia, orthostatic hypotension, or vasovagal stimulation.

The Nose and Sinuses

Rhinorrhea refers to drainage from the nose and is often associated with *nasal congestion,* a sense of stuffiness or obstruction. These symptoms are frequently accompanied by sneezing, watery eyes, and throat discomfort, and itching in the eyes, nose, and throat.[33]

Causes include *viral infections, allergic rhinitis* ("hay fever"), and *vasomotor rhinitis.* Itching favors an allergic cause.

Do symptoms occur when colds are prevalent and last less than seven days? Do they occur during the same season each year when pollens are in the air? Are symptoms triggered by specific animal or environmental exposures? Are there indoor environmental triggers such as dust or animals?

Seasonal onset or environmental triggers suggest *allergic rhinitis.*

What remedies has the patient used? For how long? And how well do they work?

Drug-induced rhinitis occurs in excessive use of topical decongestants, or use of cocaine.

Is nasal or sinus congestion preceded by a viral upper respiratory tract infection (URI)? Is there purulent nasal discharge, loss of smell, tooth pain, or facial pain made worse by bending forward, ear pressure, cough, or fever?

Acute bacterial sinusitis, now termed *rhinosinusitis,* is unlikely until viral URI symptoms persist more than 7 days; both purulent drainage and facial pain should be present for diagnosis (sensitivity and specificity are above 50%).[34–36]

Ask about drugs that may induce nasal stuffiness.

Inquire about all medications or drugs, particularly oral contraceptives, reserpine, alcohol, and cocaine.

Is the nasal congestion only on one side?

Consider a deviated nasal septum, nasal polyp, foreign body, *Wegener granuloma,* or carcinoma.

Epistaxis is bleeding from the nasal passages. Bleeding can also originate in the paranasal sinuses or nasopharynx. Note that bleeding from posterior nasal structures may pass into the throat instead of out through the nostrils. Ask the patient to pinpoint the source of the bleeding. Is it from the nose, or has the patient actually coughed up blood (*hemoptysis*) or vomited blood (*hematemesis*)? These conditions have very different causes.

Local causes of epistaxis include trauma (especially nose-picking), inflammation, drying and crusting of the nasal mucosa, tumors, and foreign bodies.

Is epistaxis a recurrent problem? Has there been easy bruising or bleeding elsewhere in the body?

Anticoagulants, NSAIDs, vascular malformations, and coagulopathies can contribute to epistaxis.

The Mouth, Throat, and Neck

Sore throat or *pharyngitis* is a frequent complaint, usually associated with an acute URI. However, sometimes a sore throat is the only symptom.

Centor's clinical prediction rules for *streptococcal* and *Fusobacterium necrophorum pharyngitis* have been used in the past to help guide diagnosis and treatment of bacterial infection: fever history, tonsillar exudates, swollen tender anterior cervical adenopathy, and absence of cough. However, the sensitivity and specificity of these rules are less than 90%, calling their validity into question due to a high rate of unnecessary antibiotic use. Guidelines now recommend rapid antigen testing or throat culture for diagnosis and treatment.[37–39]

A *sore tongue* may result from local lesions as well as from systemic illness.

Abnormalities include *aphthous ulcers* (p. 298) and the sore smooth tongue of nutritional deficiency (p. 297).

Bleeding from the gums, especially when brushing teeth, is a common symptom. Ask about local lesions and any tendency to bleed or bruise elsewhere.

Bleeding gums are usually caused by *gingivitis* (p. 295).

Hoarseness refers to a change in voice quality, often described as husky, rough, harsh, or lower pitched than usual. Causes range from diseases of the larynx to extralaryngeal lesions that press on the laryngeal nerves.[40] Ask the patient about environmental allergies, acid reflux, smoking, alcohol use, and inhalation of fumes or other irritants. Also ask if the patient talks a great deal at work.

If hoarseness is acute, consider voice overuse, *acute viral laryngitis,* and possible neck trauma.

Is the problem chronic, lasting more than 2 weeks? Is there prolonged tobacco or alcohol use, cough or hemoptysis, weight loss, or unilateral throat pain?

If hoarseness lasts over 2 weeks, refer for laryngoscopy and consider causes such as *hypothyroidism,* reflux, vocal cord nodules, head and neck cancers including thyroid masses, and neurologic disorders like *Parkinson disease, amyotrophic lateral sclerosis,* or *myasthenia gravis.*

Ask "Have you noticed any swollen glands or lumps in your neck?" because patients are often more familiar with lay terms than with "*lymph nodes.*"

Enlarged tender lymph nodes commonly accompany *pharyngitis.*

Assess thyroid function and ask about any enlargement of the thyroid gland, or *goiter.* To evaluate thyroid function, ask about *temperature intolerance* and *sweating.* Opening questions include, "Do you prefer hot or cold weather?" "Do you dress more warmly or less warmly than other people?" "What about blankets … do you use more or fewer than others at home?" "Have you noticed any changes in the texture of your skin?" "Do you perspire more or less than others?" "Any new palpitations or change in weight?" Recall that as people grow older, they sweat less, have less tolerance for cold, and tend to prefer warmer environments.

With *goiter,* thyroid function may be increased, decreased, or normal; see Table 7-27, p. 299.

Intolerance to cold, weight gain, dry skin, and slowed heart rate point to *hypothyroidism;* intolerance to heat, weight loss, moist velvety skin, and palpitations point to *hyperthyroidism.* See Table 7-27, p. 299.

Health Promotion and Counseling: Evidence and Recommendations

Important Topics for Health Promotion and Counseling

- Loss of vision: cataracts, macular degeneration, glaucoma
- Hearing loss
- Oral health

Vision and hearing, critical senses for experiencing the world around us, are two areas of special importance for health promotion and counseling. Oral health, often overlooked, also merits clinical attention.

Loss of Vision.   An estimated 14 million Americans aged 12 years or older are considered visually impaired, defined as having a visual acuity of ≥20/50 in the better-seeing eye.[41] Vision disorders in healthy young adults are usually refractive errors. Older adults have more serious disorders, including cataracts, glaucoma, and age-related macular degeneration. The prevalence of visual impairment increases dramatically with age, rising from 5% in adults aged 40 to 49 to 26% of adults 80 years and older.[42] In older adults, visual impairment is associated with decreased functional capacity, poor quality of life, increased risk of fall and injuries, and loss of independent living. However, vision in ~80% of visually impaired Americans can be corrected.[41] Because onset can be gradual, those affected may not recognize their visual decline. Although acknowledging that numerous treatments can improve visual acuity, in 2009, the U.S. Preventive Services Task Force (USPSTF) found insufficient evidence to recommend screening by primary care physicians, assigning screening only a grade I recommendation.[43] In contrast, the American Academy of Ophthalmology strongly recommends a comprehensive medical eye examination for all adults every 1 to 2 years, depending on age and risk factors, including formal screening for visual acuity and glaucoma.[44] Assessing vision is a standard component of thorough physical examination. Ask patients about any problems with face recognition, reading, or performing regular tasks, and test acuity with the Snellen chart or a hand-held card. *Refer patients with an impairment of ≥20/50 or a one-line difference between the eyes.* Examine the lens and fundi to detect additional disorders.

Primary open-angle glaucoma (POAG) is a leading cause of visual impairment and blindness in the United States, affecting over 2.5 million adults, including roughly 2% of adults older than age 40 years.[45,46] Over half are unaware of having the disease. In POAG, there is gradual loss of vision in the peripheral visual fields, resulting from loss of retinal ganglion cell axons. Retinal examination reveals pallor and increasing size of the optic cup, which can enlarge to more than half the diameter of the optic disc. Risk factors include age ≥65 years, African American

See Chapter 20, Older Adult, pp. 955–1008.

See pp. 232–233 for testing acuity, using the Snellen eye chart, and examination techniques.

Look for clouding of the lens (*cataracts*), mottling of the macula, variations in retinal pigmentation, subretinal hemorrhage or exudates (*macular degeneration*), and change in color and size of the optic disc (*glaucoma*). See techniques for testing acuity and using the Snellen eye chart on p. 232.

ethnicity, diabetes, myopia, and ocular hypertension (intraocular pressure [IOP] is ≥21 mm Hg). Not all people with POAG have elevated IOP, and those with elevated IOP may not develop visual impairment. Further, diagnosis of optic disc enlargement is variable, even among experts. Nonetheless, glaucoma can be successfully treated with medical and surgical interventions, despite possible adverse events like eye irritation and cataracts. In 2013, the USPSTF found insufficient evidence for general glaucoma screening by primary care physicians due to the complexities of diagnosis and treatment, giving only a grade I recommendation.[46] However, the American Academy of Ophthalmology strongly recommends periodic glaucoma testing, especially for older and at-risk patients.[47]

Ultraviolet (UV) light can damage the eyes and cause skin cancers on the eyelids, including basal cell carcinoma, squamous cell carcinoma, and melanoma. In addition, there is some evidence that UV light is associated with the development of cataracts (the relation between UV light and glaucoma is less clear). Recommended preventive actions include use of sunscreen on the face and eyelids and wearing sunglasses during exposure to direct sunlight.[48]

Hearing Loss.   More than a third of adults older than 50 years—and 80% of those 80 years and older—have hearing loss.[42] However, this impairment, which often contributes to emotional isolation and social withdrawal, is frequently undetected. Unlike vision prerequisites for driving, there is no mandate for widespread hearing testing, and many older adults avoid using hearing aids. The USPSTF recommends screening adults 50 years of age and older.[42] Hearing loss can be accurately detected by a number of measures: a single-item screening test, namely asking patients if they have difficulty hearing; multi-item questionnaires such as the Hearing Handicap Inventory for the Elderly—Screening Version;[49] handheld audiometers; the clinical "whisper test"; or the finger rub test.[42] Aging is the most important risk factor for hearing loss and *presbycusis* is the most common age-related cause. In presbycusis, degenerating hair cells in the ear lead to gradually progressive hearing loss, particularly for high-frequency sounds. Other risk factors include congenital or familial hearing loss, syphilis, rubella, meningitis, diabetes, recurring inner ear infections, exposure to ototoxic agents, frequent use of headphones, and exposure to hazardous noise levels at work, leisure, or on the battlefield. Hearing aids can improve hearing and quality of life, but are more likely to be adopted by those who report hearing loss than those diagnosed clinically. Consequently, in 2012, the USPSTF concluded that the evidence for screening adults ≥age 50 years is insufficient, giving only a grade I recommendation.[50]

Oral Health.   Clinicians should play an active role in promoting oral health: up to 19% of children aged 2 to 19 years have untreated cavities, and about 5% of adults aged 40 to 59 years and 25% of those older than age 60 years have no teeth at all.[51,52] Nearly 50% of adults aged 30 years and above have some form or periodontal disease, including 8.5% with severe disease.[53] Risk factors for periodontal disease include low income, male gender, smoking, diabetes, and poor oral hygiene. Begin by carefully examining the mouth. Inspect the oral cavity for decayed or loose teeth, inflammation of the gingiva (*gingivitis*), and signs of periodontal disease such as bleeding, pus, recession of the gums, and bad breath. Inspect the mucous membranes, the palate, the oral floor, and the surfaces of the tongue for ulcers and *leukoplakia,* warning signs for oral cancer and HIV disease.

To improve oral health *counsel patients to adopt daily hygiene measures.* Use of fluoride-containing toothpastes reduces tooth decay, and brushing and flossing retard periodontal disease by removing bacterial plaques. Urge patients to *seek dental care at least annually* to receive the benefits of more specialized preventive care such as scaling, planing of roots, and topical fluorides.

Address diet and tobacco use. As with children, adults should avoid excessive intake of foods high in starches and refined sugars such as sucrose, which enhance attachment and colonization of cariogenic bacteria. Urge patients to avoid use of all tobacco products and to limit alcohol consumption to reduce risk of oral cancer.

Saliva cleanses and lubricates the mouth. Many medications reduce salivary flow, increasing risk for tooth decay, mucositis, and gum disease from xerostomia, especially for the elderly. If medications cannot be changed, recommend drinking higher amounts of water and chewing sugarless gum. For those wearing dentures, recommend removal and cleaning each night to reduce bacterial plaque and risk of malodor. Regular massage of the gums relieves soreness and pressure from dentures on the underlying soft tissue.

Oral Cancer. Over 40,000 cases of cancer of the oral cavity and oropharynx were diagnosed in 2014, and more than 8,000 deaths were caused by these cancers.[54] Tobacco and alcohol account for about 75% of oral cavity cancers.[55] Sexually transmitted infection with the human papillomavirus (HPV) affecting the tonsils, oropharynx, and base of the tongue is an increasingly important cause of oropharyngeal cancers, accounting for 80% to 95% of cases.[56] Risk for HPV infection is associated with age (highest prevalence among those aged 30 to 34 years and 60 to 64 years), male gender, a higher number of sexual partners, sexual behaviors (oral sex), and cigarette smoking.[57] The primary screening test for these cancers is examination of the oral cavity; a critical preventive strategy is HPV vaccination among age-eligible patients. However, in 2014, the USPSTF concluded that there was insufficient evidence to routinely screen asymptomatic adults (grade I recommendation).[50] The American Dental Association recommends that providers be aware of potentially malignant lesions during routine oral examinations, particularly among patients who use tobacco or consume excessive amounts of alcohol.[58]

Anatomy and Physiology and Techniques of Examination

The Head

Anatomy and Physiology. Regions of the head take their names from the underlying bones of the skull, for example, the frontal area. Knowing this anatomy helps to locate and describe physical findings (see Fig. 7-2).

Two paired salivary glands lie near the mandible: the *parotid gland,* superficial to and behind the mandible (both visible and palpable when enlarged), and the *submandibular gland,* located deep to the mandible. Feel for the latter as you press

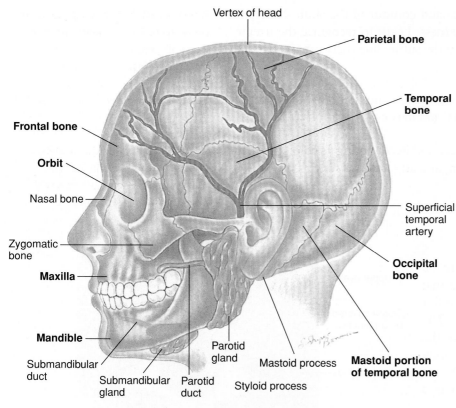

Vertex of head

Parietal bone

Temporal bone

Frontal bone

Orbit

Nasal bone

Superficial temporal artery

Zygomatic bone

Occipital bone

Maxilla

Mandible

Parotid gland

Submandibular duct

Mastoid portion of temporal bone

Submandibular gland

Parotid duct

Mastoid process

Styloid process

FIGURE 7-2. **Anatomy of the head.**

your tongue against your lower incisors. Its lobular surface can often be felt against the tightened muscle. The openings of the parotid and submandibular ducts are visible within the oral cavity (see p. 254).

The *superficial temporal artery* passes upward just in front of the ear, where it is readily palpable. In many normal people, especially thin and elderly ones, the tortuous course of one of its branches can be traced across the forehead.

Techniques of Examination. Because abnormalities under the hair are easily missed, ask if the patient has noticed anything wrong with the scalp or hair. Hairpieces and wigs should be removed. Examine the following.

The Hair. Note its quantity, distribution, texture, and any pattern of loss. You may see loose flakes of dandruff.

Fine hair is seen in *hyperthyroidism,* coarse hair in *hypothyroidism.* Tiny white ovoid granules that adhere to hairs may be nits (lice eggs).

The Scalp. Part the hair in several places and look for scaliness, lumps, nevi, or other lesions.

Look for redness and scaling that may indicate *seborrheic dermatitis or psoriasis;* soft lumps that may be *pilar cysts* (wens); and pigmented nevi that raise concern of *melanoma.* See Table 6-6, Brown Lesions—Melanoma and Its Mimics, pp. 200–203.

The Skull. Observe the general size and contour of the skull. Note any deformities, depressions, lumps, or tenderness. Learn to recognize the irregularities in a normal skull, such as those near the suture lines between the parietal and occipital bones.

The Face. Note the patient's facial expression and contours. Observe for asymmetry, involuntary movements, edema, and masses.

The Skin. Observe the skin on the face and head, noting its color, pigmentation, texture, thickness, hair distribution, and any lesions.

An enlarged skull may signify *hydrocephalus* or *Paget disease* of bone. Palpable tenderness or bony step-offs may be present after head trauma.

See Table 7-5, Selected Facies, p. 272.

Acne is common in adolescents. *Hirsutism* (excessive facial hair) may appear in some women with *polycystic ovary syndrome.*

The Eyes

Anatomy and Physiology. Identify the structures illustrated in Figure 7-3. Note that the upper eyelid covers a portion of the iris but does not normally overlay the pupil. The opening between the eyelids is called the *palpebral fissure.* The white sclera may look somewhat buff-colored at its periphery. Do not mistake this color for jaundice, which is a deeper yellow.

The *conjunctiva* is a clear mucous membrane with two easily visible components. The *bulbar conjunctiva* covers most of the anterior eyeball, adhering loosely to the underlying tissue. It meets the cornea at the *limbus.* The *palpebral conjunctiva* lines the eyelids. The two parts of the conjunctiva merge in a folded recess that permits movement of the eyeball.

Within the eyelids lie firm strips of connective tissue called *tarsal plates* (Fig. 7-4). Each plate contains a parallel row of *meibomian glands,* which open on the lid margin. The *levator palpebrae,* the muscle that raises the upper eyelid, is innervated by the oculomotor nerve, CN III. Smooth muscle, innervated by the sympathetic nervous system, also contributes to lid elevation.

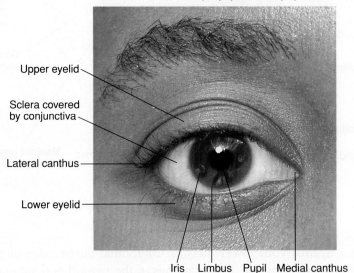

Upper eyelid

Sclera covered by conjunctiva

Lateral canthus

Lower eyelid

Iris Limbus Pupil Medial canthus

FIGURE 7-3. **Anatomy of the eye.**

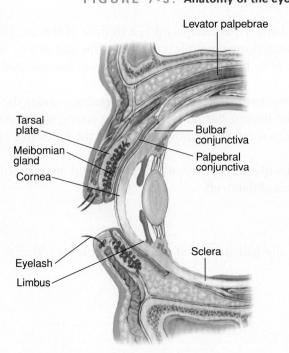

Levator palpebrae

Tarsal plate

Meibomian gland

Cornea

Bulbar conjunctiva

Palpebral conjunctiva

Eyelash

Limbus

Sclera

FIGURE 7-4. **Sagittal section of the anterior eye.**

A film of tear fluid protects the conjunctiva and cornea from drying, inhibits microbial growth, and gives a smooth optical surface to the cornea. This fluid comes from the meibomian glands, conjunctival glands, and lacrimal gland. The *lacrimal gland* lies mostly within the bony orbit, superior and lateral to the eyeball (Fig. 7-5). The tear fluid spreads across the eye and drains medially through two tiny holes called *lacrimal puncta*. The tears then pass into the *lacrimal sac* and on into the nose through the *nasolacrimal duct*. You can easily find a *punctum* atop the small elevation of the medial lower lid medially. The lacrimal sac rests in a small depression inside the bony orbit and is not visible.

The eyeball is a spherical structure that focuses light on the neurosensory elements within the retina. The muscles of the iris control pupillary size. Muscles of the *ciliary body* control the thickness of the lens, allowing the eye to focus on near or distant objects.

A clear liquid called *aqueous humor* fills the anterior and posterior chambers of the eye. Aqueous humor is produced by the *ciliary body*, circulates from the posterior chamber through the pupil into the anterior chamber, and drains out through the *canal of Schlemm*. This circulatory system helps to control the pressure inside the eye (Fig. 7-6).

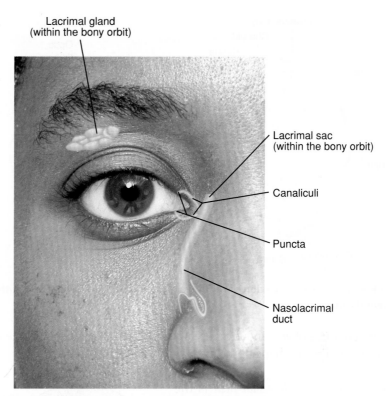

FIGURE 7-5. **Lacrimal gland, sac, and duct.**

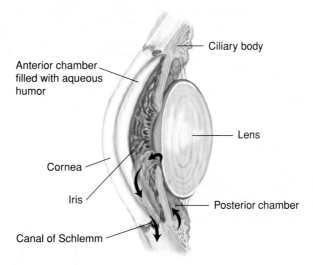

FIGURE 7-6. **Circulation of aqueous humor.**

The posterior portion of the eye that is seen through the ophthalmoscope is often called the *optic fundus* (Fig. 7-7). Structures here include the retina, choroid, fovea, macula, optic disc, and retinal vessels. The optic nerve with its retinal vessels enters the eyeball posteriorly, visible with an ophthalmoscope at the *optic disc*. Lateral and slightly inferior to the disc, there is a small depression in the retinal surface that marks the point of central vision. Around it is a darkened circular area called the *fovea*. The roughly circular *macula* surrounds the fovea, but has no discernible margins. You do not usually see the normal *vitreous body*,

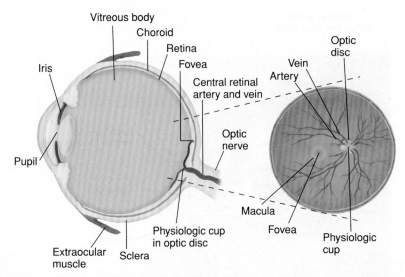

FIGURE 7-7. **Cross-section of right eye showing the fundus as seen with an ophthalmoscope.**

a transparent mass of gelatinous material that fills the eyeball behind the lens and helps to maintain the shape of the eye.

Visual Fields. A *visual field* is the entire area seen by an eye when it looks at a central point. Fields are conventionally diagrammed on circles from the patient's point of view. The center of the circle represents the focus of gaze. The circumference is 90° from the line of gaze. Each visual field, shown by the white areas in Figure 7-8, is divided into quadrants. Note that the fields extend farthest on the temporal sides. Visual fields are normally limited by the brows above, the cheeks below, and the nose medially. A lack of retinal receptors at the optic disc produces an oval blind spot in the normal field of each eye, 15° temporal to the line of gaze.

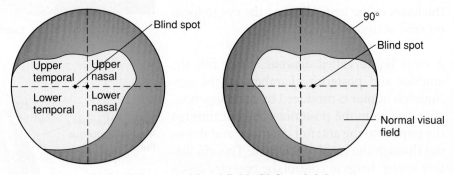

FIGURE 7-8. **Visual field of left and right eyes.**

When a person is using both eyes, the two visual fields overlap in an area of binocular vision. Laterally, vision is monocular (Fig. 7-9).

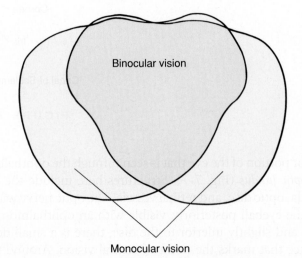

FIGURE 7-9. **Binocular field created by overlapping monocular fields.**

Visual Pathways. To see an image, light reflected from the target must pass through the pupil and be focused on photoreceptors in the retina. The image projected there is upside down and reversed right to left (Fig. 7-10). An image from the upper nasal visual field thus strikes the lower temporal quadrant of the retina.

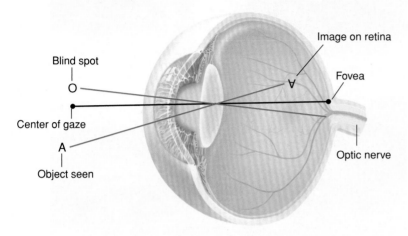

FIGURE 7-10. **Light pathway into the eye.**

Nerve impulses, stimulated by light, are conducted through the retina, optic nerve (CN II), and optic tract on each side, then on through a curving tract called the *optic radiation.* This ends in the visual cortex, a part of the occipital lobe.

Pupillary Reactions. Pupillary size changes in response to light and to the effort of focusing on a near object.

The Light Reaction. A light beam shining onto one retina causes pupillary constriction in both that eye, termed the *direct reaction* to light, and in the contralateral eye, the *consensual reaction to light.* The initial sensory pathways are similar to those described for vision: retina, optic nerve (CN II), and optic tract, which diverges in the midbrain. Impulses back to the constrictor muscles of the iris of each eye are transmitted through the oculomotor nerve, CN III (Fig. 7-11).

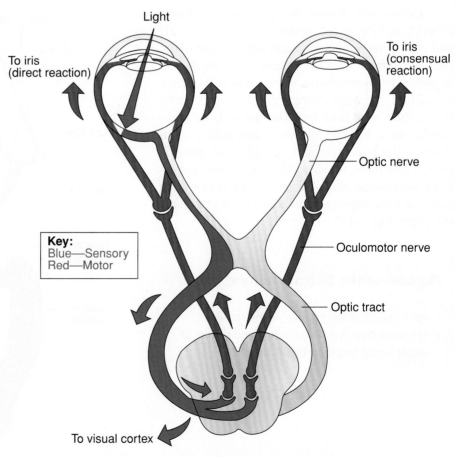

FIGURE 7-11. **Pathways of the light reaction.**

The Near Reaction. In the *near reaction,* when a person shifts gaze from a far object to a near object, the pupils constrict (Fig. 7-12). This response, like the light reaction, is mediated by the oculomotor nerve (CN III). Coincident with this *pupillary constriction,* but not part of it, are (1) *convergence* of the eyes, a medial rectus movement; and (2) *accommodation,* an increased convexity of the lenses caused by contraction of the ciliary muscles. In accommodation the change in shape of the lenses brings near objects into focus, but is not visible to the examiner.

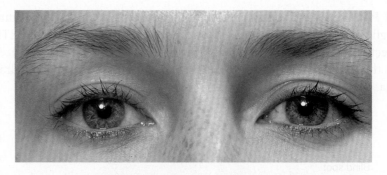

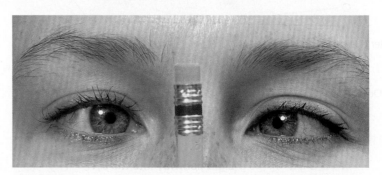

FIGURE 7-12. **The pupils constrict when the focus shifts to a close object.**

Autonomic Nerve Supply to the Eyes. Fibers travelling in the oculomotor nerve (CN III) and producing pupillary constriction are part of the parasympathetic nervous system. The iris is also supplied by sympathetic fibers. When these are stimulated, the pupil dilates, and the upper eyelid rises a little, as if from fear. The sympathetic pathway starts in the hypothalamus and passes down through the brainstem and cervical cord into the neck. From there, it follows the carotid artery or its branches into the orbit. A lesion anywhere along this pathway may impair sympathetic effects that dilate the pupil (Fig. 7-13).

Autonomic Stimulation

- Parasympathetics: Pupillary constriction
- Sympathetics: Pupillary dilation and raising of upper eyelid (superior tarsal muscle)

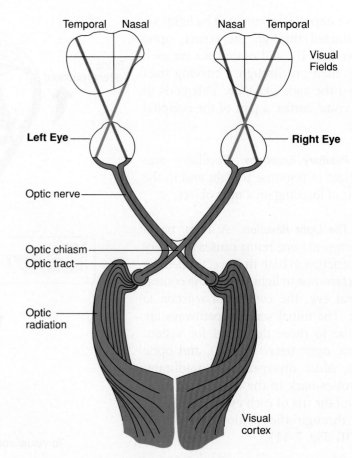

FIGURE 7-13. **Visual pathways from retina to visual cortex.**

Extraocular Movements. The coordinated action of six muscles, the four rectus and two oblique, control the eye. You can test the function of each muscle and its CN innervation by asking the patient to move the eye in the direction controlled by that muscle. There are six such *cardinal directions,* indicated by the lines in Figure 7-14. When a person looks down and to the right, for example, the right inferior rectus (CN III) is principally responsible for moving the right eye, whereas the left superior oblique (CN IV) is principally responsible for moving the left eye. If one of these muscles is paralyzed, the eye will deviate from its normal position in that direction of gaze and the eyes will no longer appear conjugate, or parallel.

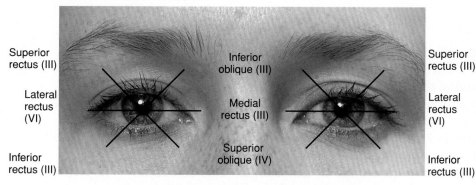

Superior rectus (III)

Inferior oblique (III)

Superior rectus (III)

Lateral rectus (VI)

Medial rectus (III)

Lateral rectus (VI)

Inferior rectus (III)

Superior oblique (IV)

Inferior rectus (III)

FIGURE 7-14. **Cardinal directions of gaze.**

CN IV (trochlear nerve) damage, due to head trauma, congenital causes, or central lesions, causes dysfunction of the superior oblique muscle, leading to *diplopia* (double vision).

Techniques of Examination

Important Areas of Examination

- Visual acuity
- Visual fields
- Conjunctiva and sclera
- Cornea, lens, and pupils
- Extraocular movements
- Fundi, including: Optic disc and cup, retina, and retinal vessels

Visual Acuity. To test the acuity of central vision, use a well-lit Snellen eye chart, if possible. Position the patient 20 feet from the chart. Patients who wear glasses other than for reading should put them on. Ask the patient to cover one eye with a card (to prevent looking through the fingers) and to read the smallest line of print possible. Coaxing to attempt the next line may improve performance. A patient who cannot read the largest letter should be positioned closer to the chart; note the intervening distance. Identify the smallest line of print where the patient can identify more than half the letters. Record the visual acuity designated at the side of this line, along with use of glasses, if any. Visual acuity is expressed as two numbers (e.g., 20/30): the first indicates the distance of the patient from the chart, and the second, the distance at which a normal eye can read the line of letters.[59]

Vision of 20/200 means that at 20 feet the patient can read print that a person with normal vision could read at 200 feet. The larger the second number, the worse the vision. "20/40 corrected" means the patient could read the 20/40 line with glasses (a correction).

Myopia (nearsightedness) causes focusing problems for distance vision.

Testing near vision with a hand-held card can help identify the need for reading glasses or bifocals in patients older than 45 years. You can also use this card to test visual acuity at the bedside. Held 14 inches from the patient's eyes, the card simulates a Snellen chart.

If you have no charts, screen visual acuity with any available print. If patients cannot read even the largest letters, test their ability to count your upraised fingers and distinguish light (such as your flashlight) from dark.

Presbyopia causes focusing problems for near vision, found in middle-aged and older adults. A presbyopic person often sees better when the card is farther away.

In the United States, a person is usually considered *legally blind* when vision in the better eye, corrected by glasses, is *20/200 or less*. Legal blindness also results from a constricted field of vision: 20° or less in the better eye.

Visual Fields by Confrontation. Confrontation testing of the visual fields is a valuable screening technique for detection of lesions in the anterior and posterior visual pathway. Recent studies recommend combining two tests to achieve the best results: the *static finger wiggle test* and the *kinetic red target test*.[60,61] Sensitivity and specificity of the two tests, when performed rigorously, compared to automated perimetry, is 78% and 90%; diagnostic accuracy improves with higher density and severity of field defects, irrespective of diagnosis.[60] Nevertheless, even relatively dense quadrantic or hemianopic visual field defects can be missed by confrontation screening tests. A formalized automated perimetry test such as the Humphrey visual field performed by an ophthalmologist is needed to make a definitive diagnosis of a visual field defect.

Refer patients with suspected visual field defects for ophthalmology evaluation. Causes of anterior pathway defects include *glaucoma, optic neuropathy, optic neuritis,* and *glioma.* Posterior pathway defects include stroke and chiasmal tumors.[62]

Static Finger Wiggle Test. Position yourself about an arm's length away from the patient. Close one eye and have the patient cover the opposite eye while staring at your open eye. So, for example, when the patient covers the left eye, to test the visual field of the patient's right eye you should cover your right eye to mimic the patent's field of view. Place your hands about 2 feet apart out of the patient's view, roughly lateral to the patient's ears (Fig. 7-15).

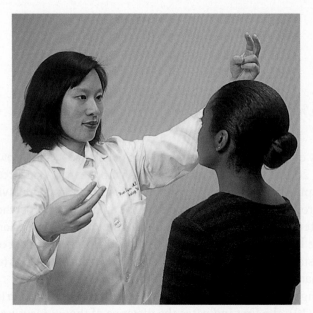

FIGURE 7-15. Static finger wiggle test.

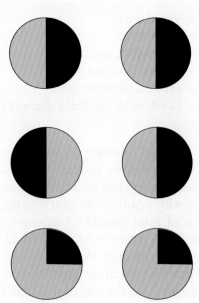

FIGURE 7-16. Visual field defects.

While in this position, wiggle your fingers and slowly bring your moving fingers forward into the patient's center of view. Ask the patient to tell you as soon as he or she sees your finger movement. Test each clock hour, or at least each quadrant. Test each eye individually and record the extent of visits in each area. Note any abnormal "field cuts" (Figs. 7-16 and 7-17).

Review these patterns in Table 7-6, Visual Field Defects, p. 273.

As an example, when the patient's left eye repeatedly does not see your fingers until they have crossed the line of gaze, a left *homonymous hemianopsia* is present. It is diagrammed from the patient's viewpoint.

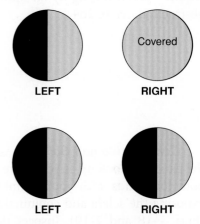

FIGURE 7-17. **A left homonymous hemianopsia may be established.**

Kinetic Red Target Test. Facing the patient, move a 5-mm red-topped pin inward from beyond the boundary of each quadrant along a line bisecting the horizontal and vertical meridians. Ask the patient when the pin first appears to be red.

An enlarged blind spot occurs in conditions affecting the optic nerve such as *glaucoma, optic neuritis,* and *papilledema.*[23]

Position and Alignment of the Eyes. Stand in front of the patient and survey the eyes for position and alignment. If one or both eyes seem to protrude, assess them from above (see p. 264).

Abnormalities include *esotropia* (inward deviation) or *exotropia* (outward deviation) of the eyes and also abnormal protrusion in *Graves disease* or ocular tumors.

Eyebrows. Inspect the eyebrows, noting their fullness, hair distribution, and any scaliness of the underlying skin.

Scaliness occurs in *seborrheic dermatitis,* lateral sparseness in *hypothyroidism.*

Eyelids. Note the position of the lids in relation to the eyeballs. Inspect for the following:

See Table 7-7, Variations and Abnormalities of the Eyelids, p. 274.

■ Width of the palpebral fissures

Upslanting palpebral fissures are noted in *Down syndrome.*

■ Edema of the lids

■ Color of the lids

Red inflamed lid margins occur in *blepharitis,* often with crusting.

■ Lesions

■ Condition and direction of the eyelashes

■ Adequacy of eyelid closure. Look for this especially when the eyes are unusually prominent, when there is facial paralysis, or when the patient is unconscious.

Failure of the eyelids to close exposes the corneas to serious damage.

Lacrimal Apparatus. Briefly inspect the regions of the lacrimal gland and lacrimal sac for swelling.

See Table 7-8, Lumps and Swellings in and Around the Eyes, p. 275.

Look for excessive tearing or dryness of the eyes. Assessment of dryness may require special testing by an ophthalmologist. To test for nasolacrimal duct obstruction, see p. 264.

Excessive tearing may be from increased production, caused by *conjunctival inflammation* or *corneal irritation,* or impaired drainage, caused by *ectropion* (p. 274) and *nasolacrimal duct obstruction.* Dryness from impaired secretion is seen in *Sjögren syndrome.*

Conjunctiva and Sclera. Ask the patient to look up as you depress both lower lids with your thumbs, exposing the sclera and conjunctiva (Figs. 7-18 and 7-19). Inspect the sclera and palpebral conjunctiva for color. Note the vascular pattern against the white scleral background. The slight vascularity of the sclera in Figures 7-18 and 7-20 is normal and present in most people.

Look for any nodules or swelling (Fig. 7-21).

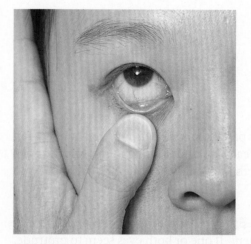

FIGURE 7-18. **Inspect the sclera and conjunctiva.**

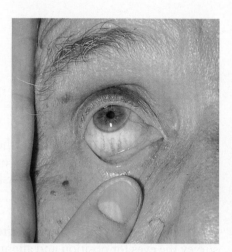

FIGURE 7-19. **A yellow sclera indicates jaundice.**

If you need a fuller view of the eye, rest your thumb and finger on the bones of the cheek and brow, respectively, and spread the lids (Fig. 7-20).

Ask the patient to look to each side and down. This technique gives you a good view of the sclera and bulbar conjunctiva, but not of the palpebral conjunctiva of the upper lid. For this, you need to evert the lid (see pp. 264–265).

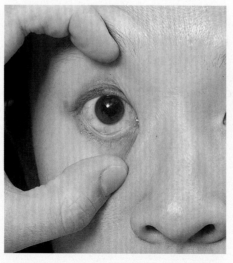

FIGURE 7-20. **Obtain a fuller view of the eye.**

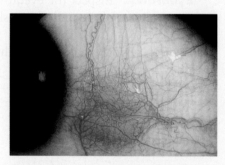

FIGURE 7-21. **Local redness is from nodular episcleritis.**

For comparisons, see Table 7-3, Red Eyes, p. 270.

Cornea and Lens. With oblique lighting, inspect the cornea of each eye for opacities. Note any opacities in the lens that may be visible through the pupil.

See Table 7-9, Opacities of the Cornea and Lens, p. 276.

Iris. At the same time, inspect each iris. The markings should be clearly defined. With your light shining directly from the temporal side, look for a crescentic shadow on the medial side of the iris (Fig. 7-22). Because the iris is normally fairly flat and forms a relatively open angle with the cornea, this lighting casts no shadow.

Occasionally, the iris bows abnormally far forward, forming a very narrow angle with the cornea. The light then casts a crescentic shadow as shown here.

This narrow angle increases the risk for acute *narrow-angle glaucoma* a sudden increase in IOP when drainage of the aqueous humor is blocked (see left upper diagram).

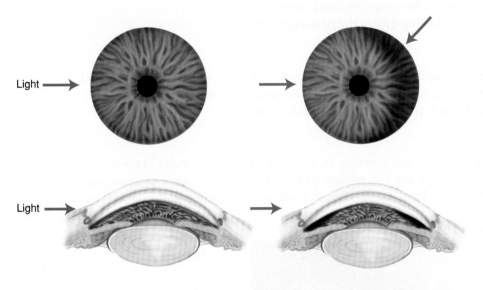

In *open-angle glaucoma,* the common form of glaucoma, the normal spatial relation between iris and cornea is preserved and the iris is fully lit.

FIGURE 7-22. **Light each eye from the side for inspection.**

Pupils. In a dim light, inspect the *size, shape,* and *symmetry* of both pupils. Measure the pupils with a card showing black circles of varying sizes, shown below, and test the light reaction. Note if the pupils are large (>5 mm), small (<3 mm), or unequal (Fig. 7-23).

Miosis refers to constriction of the pupils, *mydriasis* to dilation.

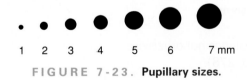

FIGURE 7-23. **Pupillary sizes.**

Simple *anisocoria,* or a difference in pupillary diameter of 0.4 mm or greater without a known pathologic cause, is visible in approximately 35% of healthy people, and rarely exceeds 1 mm.[63] Simple anisocoria is considered benign if it is equal in dim and bright light, and there is brisk pupillary constriction to light (the light reaction).

Compare benign anisocoria with *Horner syndrome, oculomotor nerve paralysis,* and *tonic pupil.* See Table 7-10, Pupillary Abnormalities, p. 277.

The Light Reaction. In dim light, test the *pupillary reaction to light.* Ask the patient to look into the distance, and shine a bright light obliquely into each pupil in turn. Both the distant gaze and the oblique lighting help to prevent a near reaction. Look for:

■ The *direct reaction* (pupillary constriction in the same eye)

■ The *consensual reaction* (pupillary constriction in the opposite eye)

Always darken the room and use a bright light before deciding that a light reaction is abnormal or absent.

The Near Reaction. If the reaction to light is impaired or questionable, test the *near reaction* in both dim and normal light. Testing one eye at a time makes it easier to concentrate on pupillary responses, without the distraction of EOM. Hold your finger or pencil about 10 cm from the patient's eye. Ask the patient to look alternately at it and into the distance directly behind it. Watch for pupillary constriction with near effort and convergence of the eyes. The third component of the near reaction, accommodation of the lens that brings the near object into focus, is not visible.

Compare the normal light reaction and near reaction of benign anisocoria with the constriction abnormalities of *tonic pupil* and *oculomotor nerve (CN III) paralysis* and the dilatation abnormalities of *Horner syndrome* and *Argyll Robertson pupils*.

Extraocular Muscles. Standing about 2 feet directly in front of the patient, shine a light into the patient's eyes and ask the patient to look at it. *Inspect the light reflection in the corneas.* They should be visible slightly nasal to the center of the pupils (Fig. 7-24).

> Testing the near reaction is helpful in diagnosing *Argyll Robertson* and *tonic (Adie) pupils* (see p. 277).

> See Table 7-10, Pupillary Abnormalities, p. 277.

> Asymmetry of the corneal reflections indicates a deviation from normal ocular alignment. A temporal light reflection on one cornea, for example, indicates a nasal deviation of that eye.

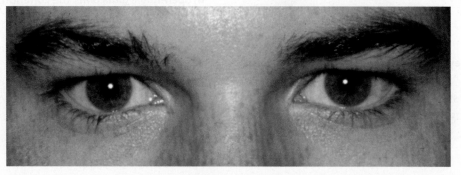

FIGURE 7-24. Inspect light reflection in the corneas.

A *cover–uncover test* may reveal a slight or latent muscle imbalance not otherwise seen; this is particularly useful in examining children (see p. 278).

Now assess the EOMs, looking for:

- The normal *conjugate movements* of the eyes in each direction. Note any deviation from normal, or *dysconjugate gaze.*

- *Nystagmus,* a fine rhythmic oscillation of the eyes. A few beats of nystagmus on extreme lateral gaze are normal. If you see this, bring your finger in to within the field of binocular vision and look again.

- *Lid lag* as the eyes move from up to down.

> See Table 7-11, Dysconjugate Gaze, p. 278.

> Sustained nystagmus within the binocular field of gaze is seen in congenital disorders, labyrinthitis, cerebellar disorders, and drug toxicity. See Table 17-7, Nystagmus, pp. 785–786.

> In the lid lag of *hyperthyroidism,* a rim of sclera is visible above the iris with downward gaze.

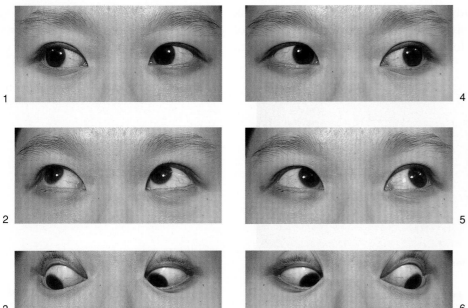

FIGURE 7-25. **Test extraocular movements.**

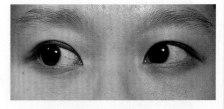

LOOKING RIGHT

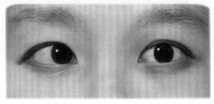

LOOKING LEFT

FIGURE 7-26. **CN VI paralysis.**

Test the Six EOMs. *Ask the patient to follow your finger or pencil* as you sweep through the six cardinal directions of gaze. Making a wide H in the air, lead the patient's gaze (Fig. 7-25):

1. to the patient's extreme right,

2. to the right and upward, and

3. down on the right; then

4. without pausing in the middle, to the extreme left,

5. to the left and upward, and

6. down on the left.

Pause during upward and lateral gaze to detect nystagmus. Move your finger or pencil at a comfortable distance from the patient. Because middle-aged or older adults may have difficulty focusing on near objects, increase this distance. Some patients move their heads to follow your finger. If necessary, hold the head in the proper midline position.

If you suspect lid lag or hyperthyroidism, ask the patient to follow your finger again as you move it slowly from up to down in the midline. The upper eyelid should overlap the iris slightly throughout this movement as shown in Figure 7-27. Figure 7-28 shows proptosis.

In paralysis of the left CN VI, illustrated above, the eyes are conjugate in right lateral gaze but not in left lateral gaze.

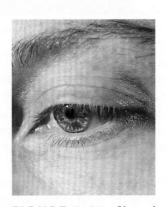

FIGURE 7-27. **Normal upper lid overlap.**

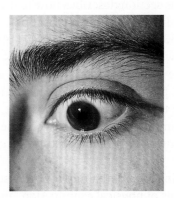

FIGURE 7-28. **Visible rim of sclera caused by proptosis.**

Note the rim of sclera from *proptosis*, an abnormal protrusion of the eyeballs in *hyperthyroidism*, leading to a characteristic "stare" on frontal gaze. If unilateral, consider an *orbital tumor* or *retrobulbar hemorrhage from trauma*.

Finally, if the near reaction has not already been tested, test for *convergence*. Ask the patient to follow your finger or pencil as you move it in toward the bridge of the nose. The converging eyes normally follow the object to within 5 cm to 8 cm of the nose (Fig. 7-29).

Convergence is poor in *hyperthyroidism*.

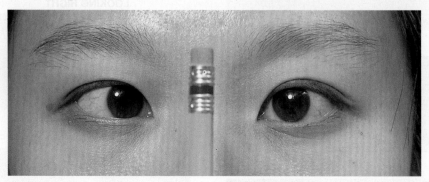

FIGURE 7-29. **Test for convergence.**

Ophthalmoscopic Examination. In general health care, examine your patients' eyes *without dilating their pupils*, which can obscure important neurologic findings. Therefore, your view is limited to the posterior structures of the retina. To see more peripheral structures, to evaluate the macula well, or to investigate unexplained visual loss, consider referral to ophthalmologists for pupillary dilatation with mydriatic drops.

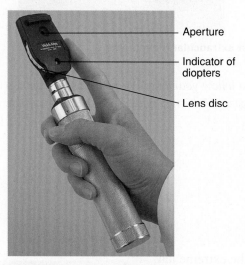

Aperture

Indicator of diopters

Lens disc

FIGURE 7-30. **Parts of the ophthalmoscope.**

Contraindications for mydriatic drops include (1) head injury and coma, since continuing observations of pupillary reactions are essential, and (2) any suspicion of narrow-angle glaucoma.

This section describes how to use the traditional ophthalmoscope (Fig. 7-30). Of note, some medical offices now use a *PanOptic ophthalmoscope*. The PanOptic ophthalmoscope allows clinicians to view the retina, even when the pupils are undilated. It provides a five-fold greater view of the fundus than the traditional ophthalmoscope, enables a 25° field of view, and increases the examining distance between the patient and the clinician. Since most clinical settings still use the traditional ophthalmoscope, emphasized here.

Using the ophthalmoscope to visualize the fundus is one of the most challenging skills of physical examination, and one of the most critical when assessing headache and changes in mental status. With feedback and dedicated practice of proper technique, the fundus, optic disc, and retinal vessels will come into focus. *Remove your glasses* unless you have marked nearsightedness or severe astigmatism, or your refractive error makes it difficult to see the fundi.

Review the components of the ophthalmoscope pictured above and follow the steps for using the ophthalmoscope. With commitment and repetition, your examination skills will improve over time.

Steps for Using the Ophthalmoscope

- Darken the room. Switch on the ophthalmoscope light and turn the lens disc until you see the large round beam of white light.* Shine the light on the back of your hand to check the type of light, its desired brightness, and the electrical charge of the ophthalmoscope.

- Turn the lens disc to the 0 diopter. (A diopter is a unit that measures the power of a lens to converge or diverge light.) At this diopter, the lens neither converges nor diverges light. Keep your finger on the edge of the lens disc so that you can turn the disc to focus the lens when you examine the fundus.

- Hold the ophthalmoscope in your right hand and use your right eye to examine the patient's right eye; hold it in your left hand and use your left eye to examine the patient's left eye. This keeps you from bumping the patient's nose and gives you more mobility and closer range for visualizing the fundus. With practice, you will become accustomed to using your nondominant eye.

- Hold the ophthalmoscope firmly braced against the medial aspect of your bony orbit, with the handle tilted laterally at about 20° slant from the vertical. Check to make sure you can see clearly through the aperture. *Instruct the patient to look* slightly up and *over your shoulder at a point directly ahead on the wall.*

- Place yourself about 15 inches away from the patient and at an angle *15° lateral to the patient's line of vision.* Shine the light beam on the pupil and look for the orange glow in the pupil—the *red reflex.* Note any opacities interrupting the red reflex.

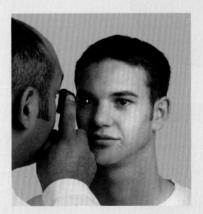

Examiner at 15-degree angle from patient's line of vision, eliciting red reflex.

- Now *place the thumb of your other hand across the patient's eyebrow,* which steadies your examining hand. Keeping the light beam focused on the red reflex, move in with the ophthalmoscope on the 15° angle toward the pupil until you are very close to it, almost touching the patient's eyelashes and the thumb of your other hand.
  - Try to keep both eyes open and relaxed, as if gazing into the distance, to help minimize any fluctuating blurriness as your eyes attempt to accommodate.
  - *You may need to lower the brightness of the light beam* to make the examination more comfortable for the patient, avoid *hippus* (spasm of the pupil), and improve your observations.

*Some clinicians like to use the large round beam for large pupils, and the small round beam for small pupils. The other beams are rarely helpful. The slitlike beam is sometimes used to assess elevations or concavities in the retina, the green (or red-free) beam to detect small red lesions, and the grid to make measurements. Ignore the last three lights and practice with the large or small round white beam.

Absence of a *red reflex* suggests an opacity of the lens (cataract) or, possibly, the vitreous (or even an artificial eye). Less commonly, a *detached retina* or, in children, a *retinoblastoma* may obscure this reflex.

Now you are ready to inspect the *optic disc* and the *retina*. The optic disc is a round, yellow-orange to creamy pink structure with a pink neuroretinal rim and central depression that often takes practice to locate. The ophthalmoscope magnifies the normal disc and retina about 15 times and the normal iris about 4 times. The optic disc actually measures about 1.5 mm. Follow the next steps for this important segment of the physical examination.

When the lens has been removed surgically, its magnifying effect is lost. Retinal structures then look much smaller than usual, and you can see a much larger expanse of the fundus.

Steps for Examining the Optic Disc and the Retina

The Optic Disc

- First, *locate the optic disc.* Look for the round yellowish-orange structure described above, or follow a blood vessel centrally until it enters the disc. The vessel size will help you. The vessel size becomes progressively larger at each branch point as you approach the disc.

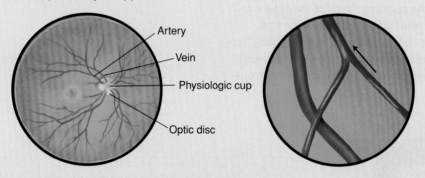

Artery
Vein
Physiologic cup
Optic disc

The optic disc and fundus.

- Now, *bring the optic disc into sharp focus* by adjusting the lens of your ophthalmoscope. If both you and the patient have no refractive errors, the retina should be in focus at 0 diopters.
- If structures are blurred, rotate the lens disc until you find the sharpest focus.

  For example, if the patient is myopic (nearsighted), rotate the lens disc counterclockwise to the minus diopters; in a hyperopic (farsighted) patient, move the disc clockwise to the plus diopters. You can correct your own refractive error in the same way.

- *Inspect the optic disc.* Note the following features:
  - *The sharpness or clarity of the disc outline.* The nasal portion of the disc margin may be somewhat blurred, a normal finding.
  - *The color of the disc,* normally yellowish orange to creamy pink. White or pigmented crescents may ring the disc, a normal finding.
  - *The size of the central physiologic cup,* if present. It is usually yellowish white. The horizontal diameter is usually less than half the horizontal diameter of the disc.
  - *The comparative symmetry* of the eyes and findings in the fundi.

In a *refractive error,* light rays from a distance do not focus on the retina. In *myopia,* they focus anterior to the retina, in *hyperopia,* posterior to it. Retinal structures in a myopic eye look larger than normal.

See Table 7-12, Normal Variations of the Optic Disc, p. 279, and Table 7-13, Abnormalities of the Optic Disc, p. 280.

An enlarged cup suggests *chronic open-angle glaucoma.*

(continued)

Steps for Examining the Optic Disc and the Retina (*continued*)

The Importance of Detecting Papilledema

Swelling of the optic disc and anterior bulging of the physiologic cup suggest *papilledema* (Fig. 7-31), which is associated with increased intracranial pressure. This pressure is transmitted to the optic nerve, causing stasis of axoplasmic flow, intra-axonal edema, and swelling of the optic nerve head. Papilledema signals serious disorders of the brain, such as meningitis, subarachnoid hemorrhage, trauma, and mass lesions, so searching for this important disorder is a priority during all your funduscopic examinations (see technique as described on prior page).

Inspect the fundus for *spontaneous venous pulsations* (SVPs), rhythmic variations in the caliber of the retinal veins as they cross the fundus (narrower in systole; wider in diastole), present in 90% of normal patients.

The Retina—Arteries, Veins, Fovea, and Macula

- *Inspect the retina,* including arteries and veins as they extend to the periphery, arteriovenous crossings, the fovea, and the macula. Distinguish arteries from veins based on the features listed below.

	Arteries	Veins
Color	Light red	Dark red
Size	Smaller (2/3 to 3/4 the diameter of veins)	Larger
Light reflex (*reflection*)	Bright	Inconspicuous or absent

- *Follow the vessels peripherally in each direction,* noting their relative sizes and the character of the arteriovenous crossings.

Identify any lesions of the surrounding *retina* and note their size, shape, color, and distribution. As you search the retina, move your head and instrument as a unit, using the patient's pupil as an imaginary fulcrum. At first, you may lose your view of the retina because your light falls out of the pupil, but you will improve with practice.

Lesions of the retina can be measured in terms of "disc diameters" from the optic disc.

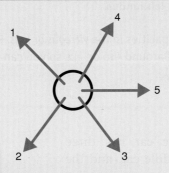

Sequence of inspection from disc to macula (left eye).

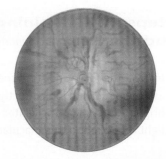

FIGURE 7-31. **Papilledema.**

Loss of SVPs occurs with high intracranial pressures (above 190 mm H_2O) that change the pressure gradient between cerebral spinal fluid pressure and intraocular pulse pressure in the optic disc. Other causes include *glaucoma* and *retinal vein occlusion*.[64,65]

See Tables 7-14 to 7-18 for information on retinal arteries and AV crossings, spots and streaks in the fundi, normal and hypertensive retinopathy, diabetic retinopathy, and light-colored spots in the fundi.

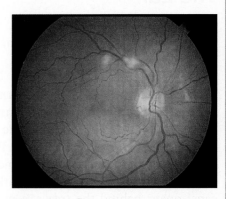

FIGURE 7-32. **Cotton-wool patches.**

Note the irregular patches, seen in diabetic and hypertensive retinopathy, between 11 and 12 o'clock, 1 to 2 disc diameters from the disc. Each measures about ½ by ½ disc diameters.

(*continued*)

Steps for Examining the Optic Disc and the Retina (*continued*)

- Inspect the *fovea* and surrounding *macula*. Direct your light beam laterally or ask the patient to look directly into the light. In younger people, the tiny bright reflection at the center of the fovea helps to orient you; shimmering light reflections in the macular area are common.

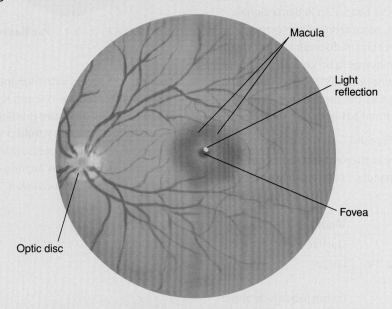

Structures of the left fundus.

- *Inspect the anterior structures*. Look for opacities in the *vitreous or lens*. Rotate the lens disc progressively to diopters of around +10 or +12, so you can focus on the more anterior structures in the eye.

Macular degeneration is an important cause of poor central vision in older adults. Types include *dry atrophic* (more common but less severe) and *wet exudative,* or neovascular. Cellular debris, called *drusen,* may be hard and sharply defined, as seen in Figure 7-33, or soft and confluent with altered pigmentation (see p. 285).

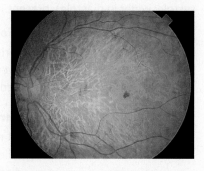

FIGURE 7-33. Hard drusen.

(Photo from Tasman W, Jaeger E (eds). *The Wills Eye Hospital Atlas of Clinical Ophthalmology,* 2nd ed. Philadelphia, Lippincott Williams & Wilkins, 2001.)

Vitreous floaters are dark specks or strands seen between the fundus and the lens. Cataracts are densities in the lens (see p. 276).

The Ear

Anatomy and Physiology. The ear has three compartments: the external ear, the middle ear, and the inner ear.

The External Ear. The *external ear* comprises the auricle and ear canal. The *auricle* consists chiefly of cartilage covered by skin and has a firm elastic consistency. Its prominent curved outer ridge is the *helix.* Parallel and anterior to the helix is another curved prominence, the *antihelix.* Inferiorly is the fleshy projection of the earlobe, or *lobule.* The ear canal opens behind the *tragus,* a nodular protrusion that points backward over the entrance to the canal (Fig. 7-34).

The *ear canal* curves inward and is approximately 24 mm long. Cartilage encases its outer two thirds. In this segment, the skin is hairy and contains glands that produce cerumen (wax). The inner third of the canal is surrounded by bone

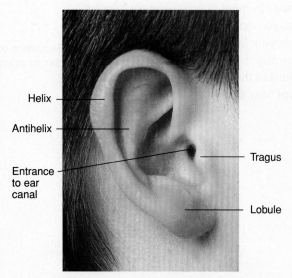

FIGURE 7-34. Anatomy of the external ear.

and lined by thin, hairless skin. Pressure on this latter area causes pain—a point to remember when you when you examine the ear. At the end of the ear canal lies the lateral *tympanic membrane,* or eardrum, marking the medial limit of the external ear. The external ear captures sound waves for transmission into the middle and inner ear (Fig. 7-35).

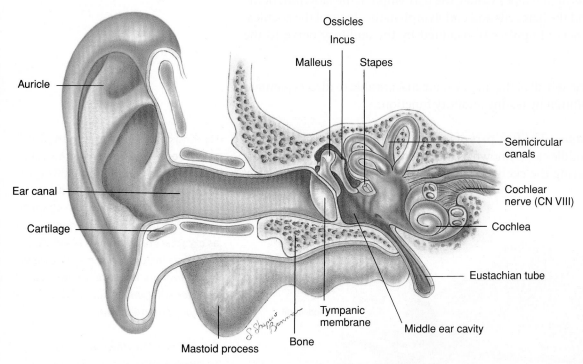

FIGURE 7-35. **Anatomy of middle and inner ear.**

Behind and below the ear canal is the mastoid portion of the temporal bone. The lowest portion of this bone, the *mastoid process,* is palpable behind the lobule.

The Middle Ear. In the air-filled middle ear, the *ossicles—the malleus, the incus, and the stapes—*transform sound vibrations into mechanical waves for the inner ear. The proximal end of the *eustachian tube* connects the middle ear to the nasopharynx.

Two of the ossicles are visible through the tympanic membrane, and are angled obliquely and held inward at its center by the *malleus* (Fig. 7-36). Find the *handle* and the *short process* of the malleus, the two chief landmarks. From the *umbo,* where the eardrum meets the tip of the malleus, a light reflection called the *cone of light* fans downward and anteriorly. Above the short process lies a small portion of the eardrum called the *pars flaccida.* The remainder of the drum is the *pars tensa.* Anterior and posterior malleolar folds, which extend obliquely upward from the short process, separate the pars flaccida from the pars tensa, but

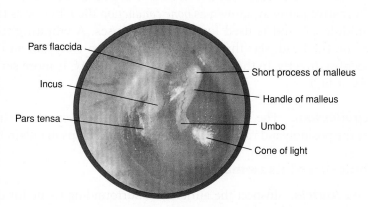

FIGURE 7-36. **Right eardrum.**

are usually invisible unless the eardrum is retracted. A second ossicle, the *incus,* can sometimes be seen through the drum.

The Inner Ear. The inner ear includes the *cochlea,* the *semicircular canals,* and the distal end of the *auditory nerve,* also known as the *vestibulocochlear nerve,* or *CN VIII.* Movements of the stapes vibrate the perilymph in the labyrinth of the semicircular canals and the hair cells and endolymph in the ducts of the cochlea, producing electrical nerve impulses transmitted by the auditory nerve to the brain.

Much of the middle ear and all of the inner ear are inaccessible to direct examination. Assess their condition by testing auditory function.

Hearing Pathways. The first part of the hearing pathway, from the external ear through the middle ear, is known as the *conductive phase.* The second part of the pathway, involving the cochlea and cochlear nerve, is the *sensorineural phase* (Fig. 7-37).

Hearing disorders of the external and middle ear cause *conductive hearing loss.* External ear causes include cerumen impaction, infection *(otitis externa),* trauma, *squamous cell carcinoma,* and benign bony growths such as *exostoses or osteomas.* Middle ear disorders include *otitis media, congenital conditions, cholesteatomas and otosclerosis, tumors, and perforation of the tympanic membrane.*

Disorders of the inner ear cause *sensorineural hearing loss* from congenital and hereditary conditions, *presbycusis,* viral infections such as *rubella* and *cytomegalovirus, Ménière disease,* noise exposure, ototoxic drug exposure, and *acoustic neuroma.*[44]

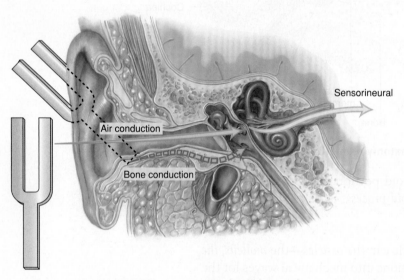

FIGURE 7-37. **Hearing pathways.**

Air conduction (AC) describes the normal first phase in the hearing pathway. An alternative pathway, known as *bone conduction (BC),* bypasses the external and middle ear and is used for testing purposes. A vibrating tuning fork, placed on the head, sets the bone of the skull into vibration and stimulates the cochlea directly. In those with normal hearing, AC is more sensitive than BC (AC > BC).

Equilibrium. The labyrinth of three semicircular canals in the inner ear senses the position and movements of the head and helps maintain balance.

Techniques of Examination

The Auricle. Inspect the auricle and surrounding tissue for deformities, lumps, or skin lesions.

See Table 7-19, Lumps on or Near the Ear, p. 286.

If ear pain, discharge, or inflammation is present, move the auricle up and down, press the tragus, and press firmly just behind the ear.

Ear Canal and Drum. To see the ear canal and drum, use an otoscope with the largest ear speculum that inserts easily into the canal. Position the patient's head so that you can see comfortably through the otoscope. To straighten the ear canal, grasp the auricle firmly but gently and pull it upward, backward, and slightly away from the head (Fig. 7-38).

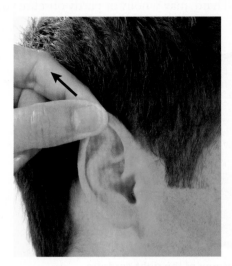

FIGURE 7-38. Straighten the ear canal to insert the otoscope.

Movement of the auricle and tragus (the "tug test") is painful in acute *otitis externa* (inflammation of the ear canal), but not in *otitis media* (inflammation of the middle ear). Tenderness behind the ear occurs in *otitis media*.

Holding the otoscope handle between your thumb and fingers, brace your hand against the patient's face (Fig. 7-39). Your hand and instrument can then follow unexpected movements by the patient. (If you are uncomfortable switching hands for the left ear, as shown in Figure 7-40, you may reach over that ear to pull it up and back with your left hand and hold the otoscope steady with your right hand as you gently insert the speculum.)

Insert the speculum gently into the ear canal, directing it somewhat down and forward and through the hairs, if any.

Nontender nodular swellings covered by normal skin deep in the ear canals suggest *exostoses* (Fig. 7-41). These are nonmalignant overgrowths which may obscure the drum.

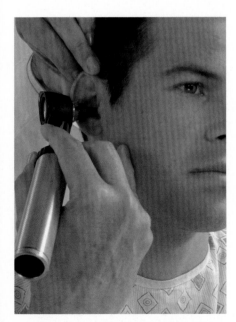

FIGURE 7-39. Brace your hand and gently insert the speculum.

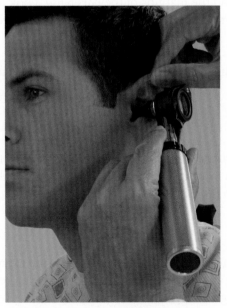

FIGURE 7-40. Insert the speculum at a slight downward angle.

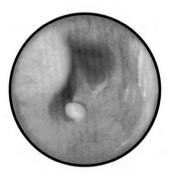

FIGURE 7-41. Exostosis.

Inspect the ear canal, noting any discharge, foreign bodies, redness of the skin, or swelling. Cerumen, which varies in color and consistency from yellow and flaky to brown and sticky or even to dark and hard, may wholly or partly obscure your view.

In acute *otitis externa* (Fig. 7-43), the canal is often swollen, narrowed, moist, pale, and tender. It may be reddened.

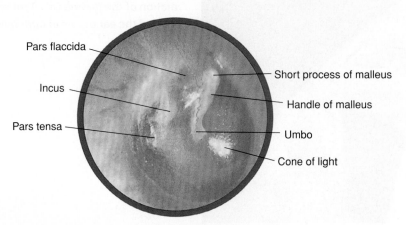

FIGURE 7-42. **Anatomy of the right eardrum.**

Labels: Pars flaccida, Incus, Pars tensa, Short process of malleus, Handle of malleus, Umbo, Cone of light

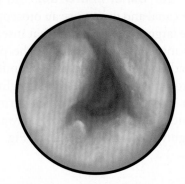

FIGURE 7-43. **Acute otitis externa.**

Inspect the eardrum, noting its color and contour (Fig. 7-42). The cone of light—usually easy to see—helps to orient you.

In *chronic otitis externa,* the skin of the canal is often thickened, red, and itchy.

Look for the red bulging drum of acute purulent *otitis media*[30] and for the amber drum of a serous effusion. See Table 7-20, Abnormalities of the Eardrum, pp. 287–288 and Table 18-7, Abnormalities of the Eyes, Ears, and Mouth, p. 916.

Identify the *handle of the malleus,* noting its position, and inspect the *short process of the malleus.*

An unusually prominent short process and a prominent handle that looks more horizontal suggest a retracted drum.

Gently move the speculum so that you can see as much of the drum as possible, including the *pars flaccida* superiorly and the margins of the *pars tensa.* Look for any perforations. The anterior and inferior margins of the drum may be obscured by the curving wall of the ear canal.

Mobility of the eardrum can be evaluated with a pneumatic otoscope (see p. 870).

A serous effusion, a thickened drum, or purulent *otitis media* may decrease mobility. If there is a perforation, there will be no mobility.

Testing Auditory Acuity—Whispered Voice Test. To begin screening, ask the patient "Do you feel you have a hearing loss or difficulty hearing?" If the patient reports hearing loss, proceed to the whispered voice test.

Patients who answer "yes" are twice as likely to have a hearing deficit; for patients who report normal hearing the likelihood of moderate to severe hearing impairment is only 0.13.[66]

The *whispered voice test* is a reliable screening test for hearing loss if the examiner uses a standard method of testing and exhales before whispering. For best results, follow the steps on the next page.

Sensitivity is 90% to 100% and specificity 70% to 87%.[66–69] This test detects significant hearing loss of greater than 30 decibels. A formal hearing test is still the gold standard.

Whispered Voice Test for Auditory Acuity

- Stand 2 feet behind the seated patient so that the patient cannot read your lips.[68]
- Occlude the nontest ear with a finger and gently rub the tragus in a circular motion to prevent transfer of sound to the nontest ear.
- Exhale a full breath before whispering to ensure a quiet voice.
- Whisper a combination of three numbers and letters, such as 3-U-1. Use a different number/letter combination for the other ear.
- Interpretation:
  - *Normal:* Patient repeats initial sequence correctly.
  - *Normal:* Patient responds incorrectly, so test a second time with a different number/letter combination; patient repeats at least three out of the possible six numbers and letters correctly.
  - *Abnormal:* Four of the six possible numbers and letters are incorrect. Conduct further testing by audiometry. (The Weber and Rinne tests are less accurate and precise.)[66]

Note that older adults with *presbycusis* have higher frequency hearing loss, making them more likely to miss consonants, which have higher frequency sounds than vowels.

Testing for Conductive Versus Neurosensory Hearing Loss: Tuning Fork Tests. For patients failing the whispered voice test, the Weber and Rinne fork tests may help determine if the hearing loss is conductive or sensorineural in origin. However, their precision, or test–retest reproducibility, and their accuracy compared to air–bone gap reference standards have been questioned.[66]

Note also that tuning fork tests do not distinguish normal hearing from bilateral sensorineural loss or from mixed conductive–sensorineural loss. Sensitivity of the Weber test is about 55%; specificity for sensorineural loss is about 79%, and for conductive loss, 92%. Sensitivity and specificity of the Rinne test are 60% to 90% and 95% to 98%.[70]

To conduct these tests, make sure the room is quiet, and *use a tuning fork of 512 Hz.* These frequencies fall within the range of conversational speech, namely 500 to 3,000 Hz and between 45 and 60 decibels.

Set the fork into light vibration by briskly stroking it between the thumb and index finger (—⤳) or by tapping it on your forearm just in front of your elbow.

- *Test for lateralization (Weber test).* Place the base of the lightly vibrating tuning fork firmly on top of the patient's head or on the midforehead (Fig. 7-44).

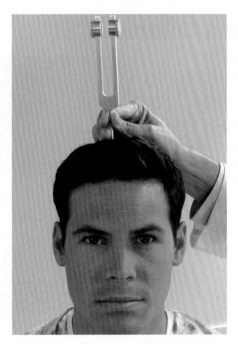

FIGURE 7-44. **Weber test.**

In unilateral *conductive hearing loss,* sound is heard in (lateralized to) the impaired ear. Explanations include *otosclerosis, otitis media,* perforation of the eardrum, and cerumen. See Table 7-21, Patterns of Hearing Loss, p. 289.

Ask where the patient hears the sound: on one side or both sides? Normally, the vibration is heard in the midline or equally in both ears. If nothing is heard, try again, pressing the fork more firmly on the head. Restrict this test to patients with unilateral hearing loss since patients with normal hearing may lateralize, and patients with bilateral conductive or sensorineural deficits will not lateralize.

In unilateral *sensorineural hearing loss*, sound is heard in the good ear.

■ *Compare AC and BC (Rinne test).* Place the base of a lightly vibrating tuning fork on the mastoid bone, behind the ear and level with the canal (Fig. 7-45). When the patient can no longer hear the sound, quickly place the fork close to the ear canal and ask if the patient hears a vibration (Fig. 7-46). Here, the "U" of the fork should face forward, which maximizes sound transmission for the patient. Normally, the sound is heard longer through air than through bone (AC > BC).

In *conductive hearing loss*, sound is heard through bone as long as or longer than it is through air (BC = AC or BC > AC). In *sensorineural hearing loss*, sound is heard longer through air (AC > BC).

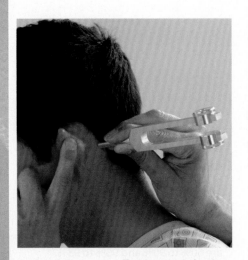

FIGURE 7-45. Test bone conduction.

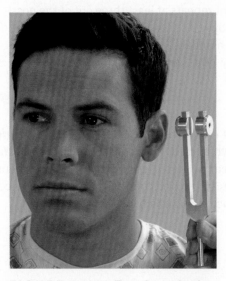

FIGURE 7-46. Test air conduction.

The Nose and Paranasal Sinuses

Anatomy and Physiology. Review the terms that describe the external anatomy of the nose (Fig. 7-47).

Approximately the upper third of the nose is supported by bone, the lower two thirds by cartilage. Air enters the nasal cavity through the *anterior naris* on either side, then passes into the widened area known as the *vestibule* and on through the narrow nasal passage to the naso-pharynx.

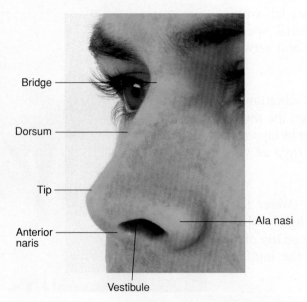

Bridge

Dorsum

Tip

Anterior naris

Ala nasi

Vestibule

FIGURE 7-47. External anatomy of the nose.

The medial wall of each nasal cavity is formed by the *nasal septum,* which, like the external nose, is supported by both bone and cartilage (Fig. 7-48). It is covered by a mucous membrane well supplied with blood. The vestibule, unlike the rest of the nasal cavity, is lined with hair-bearing skin, not mucosa.

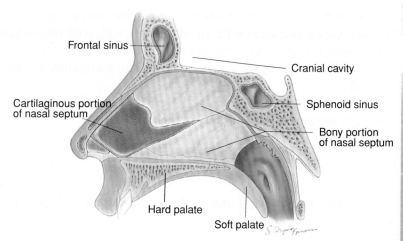

FIGURE 7-48. **Medial wall—left nasal cavity (mucosa removed).**

Laterally, the anatomy is more complex (Fig. 7-49). Curving bony structures, the *turbinates,* covered by a highly vascular mucous membrane, protrude into the nasal cavity. Below each turbinate is a groove, or meatus, each named according to the turbinate above it. The nasolacrimal duct drains into the inferior meatus; most of the paranasal sinuses drain into the middle meatus. Their openings are not usually visible.

The additional surface area provided by the turbinates and their overlying mucosa aids the nasal cavities in their principal functions: cleansing, humidification, and temperature control of inspired air.

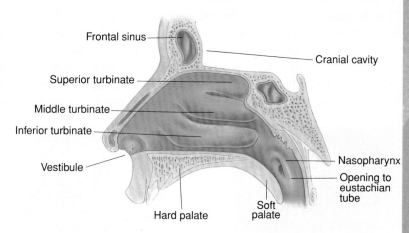

FIGURE 7-49. **Lateral wall—nasal cavity.**

The *paranasal sinuses* are air-filled cavities within the bones of the skull. Like the nasal cavities into which they drain, they are lined with mucous membrane. Their locations are diagrammed in Figure 7-50. Only the frontal and maxillary sinuses are readily accessible to clinical examination (Fig. 7-51).

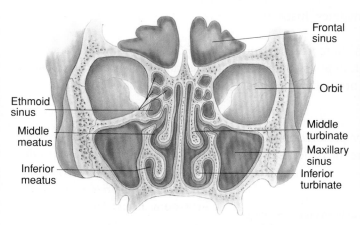

FIGURE 7-50. **Cross-section of nasal cavity—anterior view.**

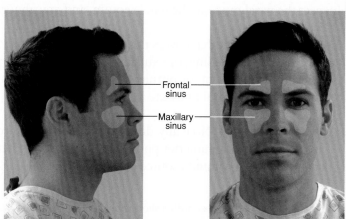

FIGURE 7-51. **Frontal and maxillary sinuses.**

Techniques of Examination. *Inspect the anterior and inferior surfaces of the nose.* Gentle pressure on the tip of the nose with your thumb usually widens the nostrils. Use a penlight or otoscope light to obtain a partial view of each nasal *vestibule.* If the nasal tip is tender, be gentle and manipulate the nose as little as possible.

Note any asymmetry or deformity of the nose.

Test for nasal obstruction, if indicated, by pressing on each ala nasi in turn and asking the patient to breathe in.

Inspect the inside of the nares with an otoscope and the largest available ear speculum.* Tilt the patient's head back a bit and insert the speculum gently into the vestibule of each nostril, avoiding contact with the sensitive nasal septum (Fig. 7-53). Hold the otoscope handle to one side to avoid the patient's chin and improve your mobility. By directing the speculum posteriorly, then upward in small steps, try to see the inferior and middle turbinates, the nasal septum, and the narrow nasal passage between them, as shown in Figure 7-54. Some asymmetry of the two sides is normal.

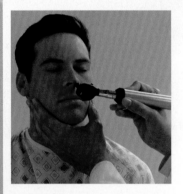

FIGURE 7-53. **Inspect inside the nares.**

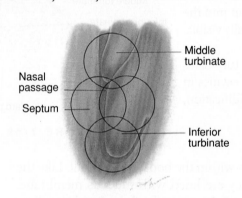

Nasal passage
Septum
Middle turbinate
Inferior turbinate

FIGURE 7-54. **Inferior and middle turbinates.**

Inspect the nasal mucosa, the nasal septum, and any abnormalities. Inspect:

- The *nasal mucosa* that covers the septum and turbinates. Note its color and any swelling, bleeding, or exudate. If exudate is present, note its character: clear, mucopurulent, or purulent. The nasal mucosa is normally somewhat redder than the oral mucosa.

- The *nasal septum.* Note any deviation, inflammation, or perforation of the septum. The lower anterior portion of the septum (where the patient's finger can reach) is a common source of *epistaxis* (nosebleed).

*A nasal illuminator, equipped with a short wide nasal speculum but lacking an otoscope's magnification, may also be used, but structures look much smaller. Otolaryngologists use special equipment not widely available in general practice.

Tenderness of the nasal tip or alae suggests local infection such as a furuncle, particularly if there is a small erythematous and swollen area.

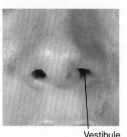

Vestibule

FIGURE 7-52. **Deviation of the lower septum.**

Deviation of the lower septum is common and may be easily visible, as in Figure 7-52. Deviation seldom obstructs air flow.

In *viral rhinitis,* the mucosa is reddened and swollen; in *allergic rhinitis,* it may be pale, bluish, or red.

Fresh blood or crusting may be seen. Causes of septal perforation include trauma, surgery, and intranasal use of cocaine or amphetamines, which also cause septal ulceration.

■ Any *abnormalities* such as ulcers or polyps.

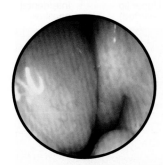

FIGURE 7-55. **Nasal polyps.**

Inspection of the nasal cavity through the anterior naris is usually limited to the vestibule, the anterior portion of the septum, and the lower and middle turbinates. Examination of posterior abnormalities requires a nasopharyngeal mirror and technique is beyond the scope of this book.

Place all nasal and ear specula outside your instrument case after use; then discard or clean and disinfect them appropriately. Check the policies of your institution.

Palpate for sinus tenderness. Press up on the *frontal sinuses* from under the bony brows, avoiding pressure on the eyes (Fig. 7-56). Then press up on the *maxillary sinuses* (Fig. 7-57).

Nasal polyps (Fig. 7-55) are pale saclike growths of inflamed tissue that can obstruct the air passage or sinuses, seen in *allergic rhinitis,* aspirin sensitivity, asthma, chronic sinus infections, and *cystic fibrosis.*[36]

Malignant tumors of the nasal cavity occur rarely, associated with exposure to tobacco or chronically inhaled toxins.

Local tenderness, together with symptoms such as facial pain, pressure or fullness, purulent nasal discharge, nasal obstructions, and smell disorder, especially when present for >7 days, suggest *acute bacterial rhonosinusitis* involving the frontal or maxillary sinuses.[34–36,71]

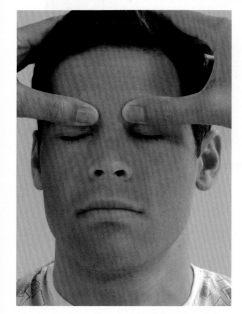

FIGURE 7-56. **Palpate the frontal sinuses.**

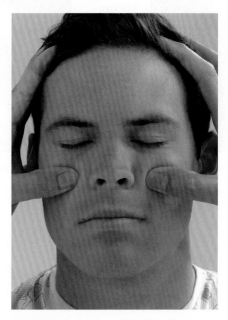

FIGURE 7-57. **Palpate the maxillary sinuses.**

Mouth and Pharynx

Anatomy and Physiology. The *lips* are muscular folds that surround the entrance to the mouth. When opened, the gums (gingiva) and teeth are visible (Fig. 7-58). Note the scalloped shape of the *gingival margins* and the pointed *interdental papillae.*

The *gingiva* is firmly attached to the teeth and to the maxilla and mandible in which they are seated. In lighter-skinned people, the gingiva is pale or coral pink and lightly stippled. In darker-skinned people, it may be diffusely or partly brown, as shown below. A midline mucosal fold, called a *labial frenulum,* connects each lip with the gingiva. A shallow *gingival sulcus* between the gum's thin margin and each tooth is not readily visible (but is probed and measured by dentists). Adjacent to the gingiva is the *alveolar mucosa,* which merges with the *labial mucosa* of the lip (Fig. 7-59).

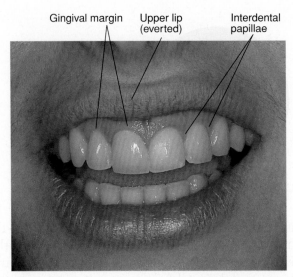

FIGURE 7-58. **Gingiva and interdental papillae.**

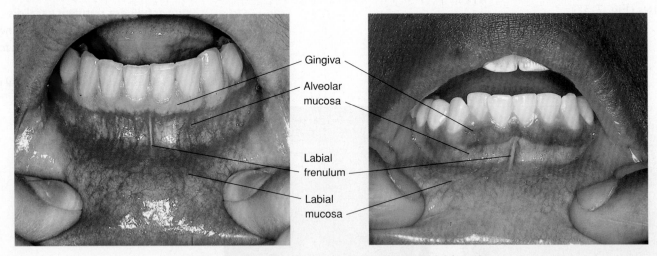

FIGURE 7-59. **Alveolar and labial mucosa, labial frenulum.**

Each tooth, composed chiefly of dentin, lies rooted in a bony socket with only its enamel-covered crown exposed. Small blood vessels and nerves enter the tooth through its apex and pass into the pulp canal and pulp chamber (Fig. 7-60).

Note that there are 32 adult teeth, conventionally numbered 1 to 16 right to left on the upper jaw and 17 to 32 left to right on the lower jaw (Fig. 7-61).

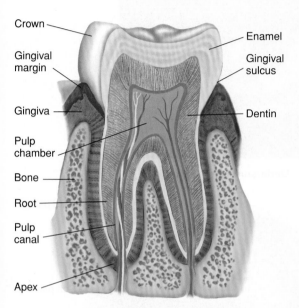

FIGURE 7-60. **Anatomy of a tooth.**

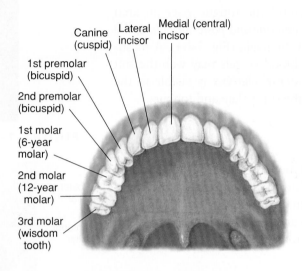

FIGURE 7-61. **Adult teeth.**

The dorsum of the *tongue* is covered with papillae, giving it a rough surface. Some of these papillae look like red dots, which contrast with the thin white coat that often covers the tongue. This patient has an erythematous posterior pharynx (Fig. 7-62).

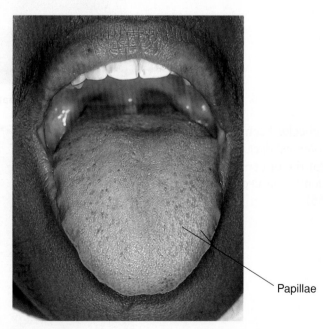

FIGURE 7-62. **Dorsal papillae of the tongue.**

The undersurface of the tongue has no papillae. Note the midline *lingual frenulum* that connects the tongue to the floor of the mouth and the *ducts of the submandibular gland* (Wharton ducts) which pass forward and medially (Fig. 7-63). They open on papillae that lie on each side of the lingual frenulum. The paired sublingual salivary glands lie just under the floor of the mouth mucosa.

Above and behind the tongue rises an arch formed by the *anterior* and *posterior pillars,* the *soft palate,* and the *uvula* (Fig. 7-64). A meshwork of small blood vessels may web the soft palate. The *posterior pharynx* is visible in the recess behind the soft palate and tongue.

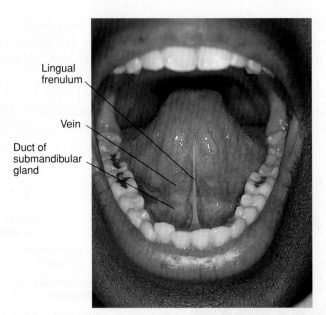

FIGURE 7-63. **Undersurface of the tongue.**

In Figure 7-64, note the right tonsil protruding from the hollowed *tonsillar fossa,* or cavity, between the anterior and posterior pillars. In adults, tonsils are often small or absent, as in the empty left tonsillar fossa.

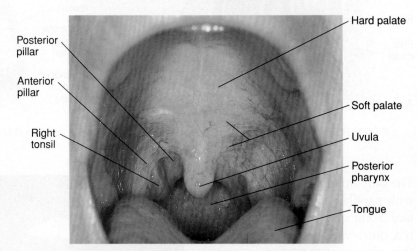

FIGURE 7-64. **Anatomy of the posterior pharynx.**

The *buccal mucosa* lines the cheeks. Each *parotid duct,* sometimes termed *Stensen duct,* opens onto the buccal mucosa near the upper second molar. Its location is frequently marked by its own small papilla (Fig. 7-65).

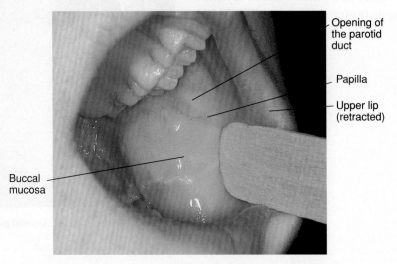

FIGURE 7-65. **Buccal mucosa and parotid duct.**

Techniques of Examination. If the patient wears dentures, offer a paper towel and ask the patient to remove them so that you can inspect the underlying mucosa. If you detect any suspicious ulcers or nodules, put on a glove and palpate any lesions, noting any thickening or infiltration of the tissues that might suggest malignancy.

Inspect the following:

The Lips. Observe their color and moisture, and note any lumps, ulcers, cracking, or scaliness.

The Oral Mucosa. Look into the patient's mouth and, with a good light and the help of a tongue blade (Fig. 7-66), inspect the oral mucosa for color, ulcers (Fig. 7-67), white patches, and nodules.

In this patient (Fig. 7-66), the wavy white line on the adjacent buccal mucosa developed where the upper and lower teeth meet, related to irritation from sucking or chewing.

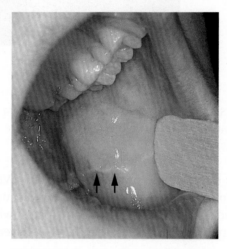

FIGURE 7-66. **Inspect the oral mucosa.**

Bright red edematous mucosa underneath a denture suggests *denture stomatitis* (denture sore mouth). There may be ulcers or papillary granulation tissue.

Watch for central cyanosis or pallor from anemia. See Table 7-22, Abnormalities of the Lips, pp. 290–291.

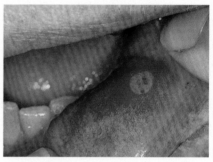

FIGURE 7-67. **Aphthous ulcer on the labial mucosa.**

See Table 7-23, Findings in the Pharynx, Palate, and Oral Mucosa, pp. 292–294.

The Gums and Teeth. Note the color of the gums, which are normally pink. Brown patches may be present, especially but not exclusively in dark-skinned individuals.

Inspect the gum margins and the interdental papillae for swelling or ulceration.

Inspect the teeth. Are any of them missing, discolored, misshapen, or abnormally positioned? To assess tooth, jaw, or facial pain, palpate the teeth for looseness and the gums with your gloved thumb and index finger.

The Roof of the Mouth. Inspect the color and architecture of the hard palate.

Redness of the gingiva suggests *gingivitis,* a black line might indicate *lead poisoning.*

The interdental papillae are swollen in *gingivitis.* See Table 7-24, Findings in the Gums and Teeth, pp. 295–296.

Torus palatinus is a startling but benign midline lump (see p. 293).

The Tongue and the Floor of the Mouth. Ask the patient to put out his or her tongue (Fig. 7-68). Inspect it for symmetry—a test of the hypoglossal nerve (CN XII) (Fig. 7-69).

Note the color and texture of the dorsum of the tongue.

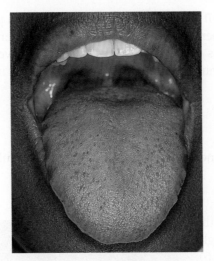

FIGURE 7-68. **Inspect the dorsum of the tongue.**

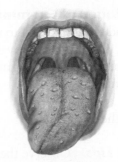

FIGURE 7-69. **Asymmetric protrusion suggests a lesion of CN XII (tongue points toward the side of the lesion).**

Inspect entire oral cavity, especially the sides and undersurface of the tongue and the floor of the mouth, areas where cancer often develops. Note any white or reddened areas, nodules, or ulcerations.

Wearing gloves, palpate any lesions. Ask the patient to protrude the tongue. With your right hand, grasp the tip of the tongue with a square of gauze and gently pull it to the patient's left. Inspect the side of the tongue, and then palpate it with your gloved left hand, feeling for any induration (Figs. 7-70 and 7-71). Reverse the procedure for the other side.

Men aged >50 years, smokers, and heavy users of chewing tobacco and alcohol are at highest risk for cancers of the tongue and oral cavity, usually *squamous cell carcinomas* on the side or base of the tongue. Any persistent nodule or ulcer, red or white, is suspect, especially if indurated. These discolored lesions represent *erythroplakia* and *leukoplakia* and should be biopsied.[72,73]

Note the carcinoma on the left side of the tongue below. Inspection and palpation remain the standard for detection of oral cancers.[74–76]

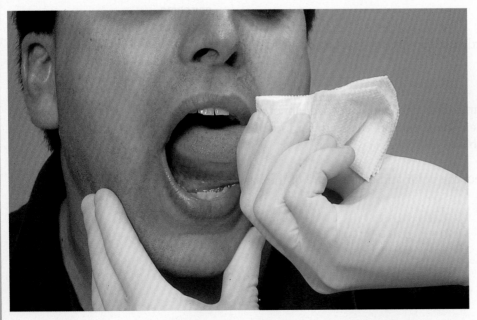

FIGURE 7-70. **Grasp the tongue and inspect the lateral margins.**

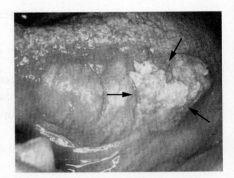

FIGURE 7-71. **Carcinoma on tongue.** (Vokes E, et al. Head and Neck Cancer. *N Engl J Med* 1993;328:184 [arrows added]).

See Table 7-25, Findings in or Under the Tongue, pp. 297–298.

The Pharynx. With the patient's mouth open but the tongue not protruded, ask the patient to say "ah" or yawn. This action helps you see the posterior pharynx well. You can also ask the patient to "open the back of your throat" since many adults have learned to inspect their own posterior pharynx while looking into a mirror.

Alternatively, you can press a tongue blade firmly down on the midpoint of the arched tongue—back far enough to visualize the pharynx but not so far that you cause gagging. Simultaneously, ask for an "ah" or a yawn. Note the rise of the soft palate—a test of CN X (the vagal nerve) (Fig. 7-72).

In CN X paralysis, the soft palate fails to rise and the uvula deviates to the opposite side (points "away from the lesion").

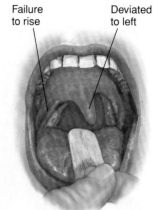

Failure to rise   Deviated to left

FIGURE 7-72. **CN X paralysis.**

Inspect the soft palate, anterior and posterior pillars, uvula, tonsils, and pharynx. Note their color and symmetry and look for exudate, swelling, ulceration, or tonsillar enlargement. If possible, palpate any suspicious area for induration or tenderness. Tonsils have crypts, or deep infoldings of squamous epithelium, where whitish spots of normal exfoliating epithelium may sometimes be seen.

Tonsillar exudates with a beefy red uvula are common in *streptococcal pharyngitis,* but warrant rapid antigen-detection testing or throat culture for diagnosis.[39,77]

Discard your tongue blade after use.

See Table 7-23, Findings in the Pharynx, Palate, and Oral Mucosa, pp. 292–294.

The Neck

Anatomy and Physiology. For descriptive purposes, divide each side of the neck into two triangles bounded by the sternocleidomastoid muscle (Fig. 7-73). Visualize the borders of the two triangles as follows:

■ For the *anterior triangle:* the mandible above, the sternocleidomastoid laterally, and the midline of the neck medially.

■ For the *posterior triangle:* the sternocleidomastoid muscle, the trapezius, and the clavicle. Note that a portion of the omohyoid muscle crosses the lower portion of this triangle and can be mistaken for a lymph node or mass.

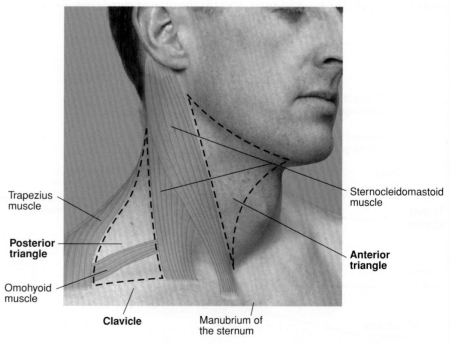

Trapezius muscle

Posterior triangle

Omohyoid muscle

Clavicle

Manubrium of the sternum

Sternocleidomastoid muscle

Anterior triangle

FIGURE 7-73. **Anterior and posterior triangles of the neck.**

Great Vessels. Deep to the sternocleidomastoids run the great vessels of the neck: the *carotid artery* and the *internal jugular vein* (Fig. 7-74). The *external jugular vein* passes diagonally over the surface of the sternocleidomastoid and may be helpful when trying to identify the jugular venous pressure (see pp. 374–378).

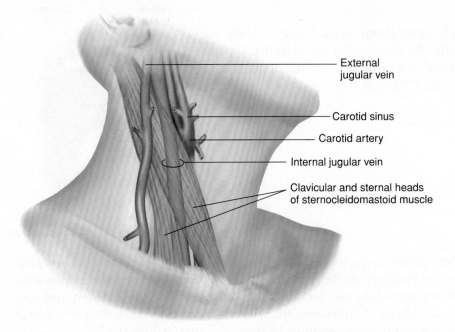

External jugular vein

Carotid sinus

Carotid artery

Internal jugular vein

Clavicular and sternal heads of sternocleidomastoid muscle

FIGURE 7-74. **Great vessels of the neck.**

Midline Structures and Thyroid Gland. Now identify the following midline structures: (1) the mobile *hyoid bone* just below the mandible, (2) the *thyroid cartilage*, readily identified by the notch on its superior edge, (3) the *cricoid cartilage*, (4) the *tracheal rings*, and (5) the *thyroid gland* (Fig. 7-75).

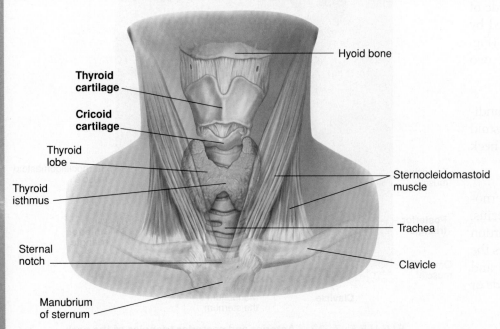

Hyoid bone

Thyroid cartilage

Cricoid cartilage

Thyroid lobe

Thyroid isthmus

Sternocleidomastoid muscle

Trachea

Sternal notch

Clavicle

Manubrium of sternum

FIGURE 7-75. **Midline structures of the neck.**

The thyroid gland is usually located above the suprasternal notch. The thyroid isthmus spans the second, third, and fourth tracheal rings just below the cricoid cartilage. The lateral lobes of the thyroid curve posteriorly around the sides of the trachea and the esophagus; each is about 4 cm to 5 cm in length. Except in the midline, the thyroid gland is covered by thin straplike muscles anchored to the hyoid bone and more laterally by the sternocleidomastoids, which are readily visible.

Lymph Nodes. The *lymph nodes* of the head and neck are variably classified. One classification is shown in Figure 7-76, together with the directions of lymphatic drainage. The deep cervical chain is largely obscured by the overlying sternocleidomastoid muscle, but at its two extremes, the tonsillar node and supraclavicular nodes may be palpable. The submandibular nodes lie superficial to the submandibular gland, and should be differentiated. Nodes are normally round or ovoid, smooth, and smaller than the submandibular gland. The gland is larger and has a lobulated, slightly irregular surface (see p. 254).

Note that the tonsillar, submandibular, and submental nodes drain portions of the mouth and throat as well as the face.

Lymphatic drainage patterns are helpful when assessing possible malignancy or infection: For suspected malignant or inflammatory lesions, look for enlargement of the neighboring regional lymph nodes; when a node is enlarged or tender, look for a source in its nearby drainage area.

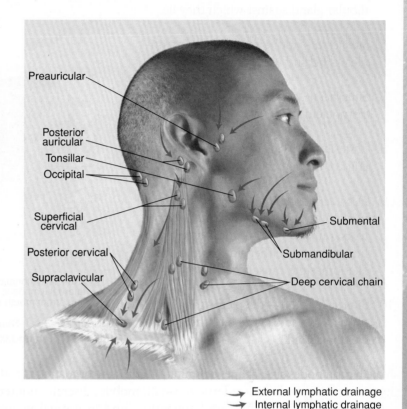

External lymphatic drainage
Internal lymphatic drainage (from mouth and throat)

FIGURE 7-76. Lymph nodes of the neck.

Techniques of Examination. *Inspect the neck,* noting its symmetry and any masses or scars. Look for enlargement of the parotid or submandibular glands, and note any visible lymph nodes.

A scar from past thyroid surgery is a clue to unsuspected thyroid or parathyroid disease.

The Lymph Nodes. *Palpate the lymph nodes.* Using the pads of your index and middle fingers, press gently, moving the skin over the underlying tissues in each area. The patient should be relaxed, with the neck flexed slightly forward and, if needed, turned slightly toward the side being examined. You can usually examine both sides at once, noting both the presence of lymph nodes as well as asymmetry. For the submental node, however, it is helpful to feel with one hand while bracing the top of the head with the other.

Feel in sequence for the following nodes (Fig. 7-77):

1. *Preauricular*—in front of the ear

2. *Posterior auricular*—superficial to the mastoid process

3. *Occipital*—at the base of the skull posteriorly

4. *Tonsillar*—at the angle of the mandible

5. *Submandibular*—midway between the angle and the tip of the mandible. These nodes are usually smaller and smoother than the lobulated submandibular gland against which they lie.

6. *Submental*—in the midline a few centimeters behind the tip of the mandible.

7. *Superficial cervical*—superficial to the sternocleidomastoid.

8. *Posterior cervical*—along the anterior edge of the trapezius.

9. *Deep cervical chain*—deep to the sternocleidomastoid and often inaccessible to examination. Hook your thumb and fingers around either side of the sternocleidomastoid muscle to find them.

10. *Supraclavicular*—deep in the angle formed by the clavicle and the sternocleidomastoid.

A pulsating "tonsillar node" is really the carotid artery. A small hard tender "tonsillar node" high and deep between the mandible and the sternocleidomastoid is probably a styloid process.

> External lymphatic drainage
> Internal lymphatic drainage
(e.g., from mouth and throat)

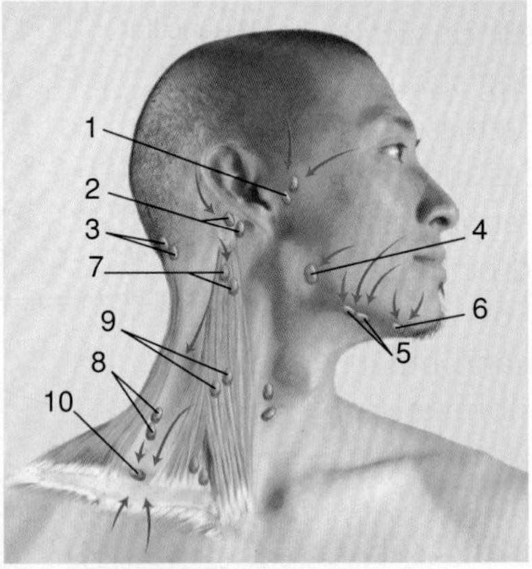

FIGURE 7-77. **Sequence for examining lymph nodes.**

Note lymph nodes size, shape, delimitation (discrete or matted together), mobility, consistency, and any tenderness. Small, mobile, discrete, nontender nodes, sometimes termed "shotty," are frequently found in normal people. Describe enlarged nodes in two dimensions, maximal length and width, for example, 1 cm × 2 cm. Also note any overlying skin changes (erythema, induration, drainage, or breakdown).

Enlargement of a supraclavicular node, especially on the left, suggests possible metastasis from a thoracic or an abdominal malignancy.

Enlarged or tender nodes, if unexplained, call for (1) re-examination of the regions they drain and (2) careful assessment of lymph nodes in other regions to identify regional from generalized lymphadenopathy.

For preauricular and cervical lymph nodes, adopt the techniques to follow.

■ Using the pads of the second and third fingers, palpate the *preauricular nodes* with a gentle rotary motion (Fig. 7-78). Then examine the posterior auricular and occipital lymph nodes.

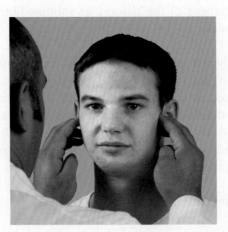

FIGURE 7-78. **Palpate the preauricular nodes.**

Tender nodes suggest inflammation; hard or fixed nodes (fixed to underlying structures and not movable on palpation) suggest malignancy.

- Palpate the *anterior superficial and deep cervical chains*, located anterior and superficial to the sternocleidomastoid. Then palpate the *posterior cervical chain* along the trapezius (anterior edge) and along the sternocleidomastoid (posterior edge). Flex the patient's neck slightly forward toward the side being examined (Fig. 7-79). Examine the supraclavicular nodes in the angle between the clavicle and the sternocleidomastoid (Fig. 7-80). If you feel supraclavicular lymph nodes, a thorough work-up is warranted.

If you palpate supraclavicular lymph nodes, a thorough work-up is warranted.

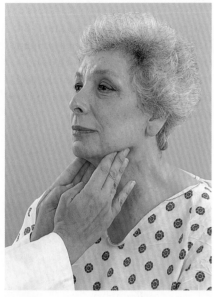

FIGURE 7-79. **Palpate the submandibular nodes.**

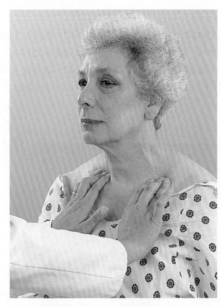

FIGURE 7-80. **Palpate the supraclavicular nodes.**

Enlarged or tender nodes, if unexplained, call for (1) re-examination of the regions they drain and (2) careful assessment of lymph nodes elsewhere so that you can distinguish between regional and generalized lymphadenopathy.

Occasionally, you may mistake a band of muscle or an artery for a lymph node. Unlike a muscle or an artery, you should be able to roll a node in two directions: up and down, and side to side. Neither a muscle nor an artery will pass this test.

Generalized lymphadenopathy is seen in multiple infectious, inflammatory, or malignant conditions such as HIV or AIDS, *infectious mononucleosis, lymphoma, leukemia,* and *sarcoidosis*.

The Trachea and the Thyroid Gland. To orient yourself to the neck, identify the thyroid and cricoid cartilages and the trachea below them.

- *Inspect the trachea* for any deviation from its usual midline position. Then *palpate for any deviation.* Place your finger along one side of the trachea and note the space between it and the sternocleido-mastoid (Fig. 7-81). Compare it with the other side. The spaces should be symmetric.

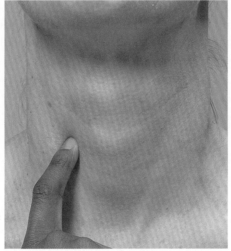

FIGURE 7-81. **Palpate the trachea.**

Masses in the neck may cause tracheal deviation to one side, raising suspicion of conditions in the thorax such as a *mediastinal mass, atelectasis, or a large pneumothorax* (see pp. 339–340).

■ *Auscultate breath sounds over the trachea.* This allows subtle counting of the respiratory rate and establishes a point of reference when assessing upper versus lower airway causes of shortness of breath. When assessing shortness of breath, always remember to listen over the trachea for *stridor* for upper airway etiologies in addition to examining the lungs.

Stridor is an ominous, high-pitched musical sound from severe subglottic or tracheal obstruction that signals a respiratory emergency. Causes include *epiglottitis,*[78] foreign body, goiter, and stenosis from placement of an artificial airway. See also Chapter 8, Thorax and Lungs, pp. 303–342.

■ *Inspect the neck for the thyroid gland.* Tip the patient's head slightly back. Using tangential lighting directed downward from the tip of the patient's chin, *inspect the region below the cricoid cartilage to identify the contours of the gland.* The shadowed lower border of the thyroid glands shown here is outlined by arrows (Fig. 7-82).

The patient in Figures 7-83 and 7-84 has a *goiter,* defined as enlargement of the thyroid gland to twice its normal size. Goiters may be simple, without nodules, or multinodular, and are usually euthyroid.[79–81]

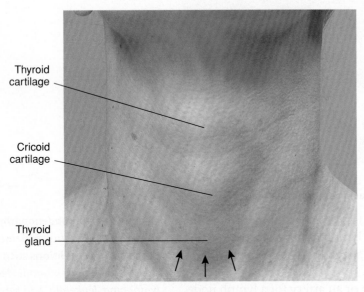

Thyroid cartilage

Cricoid cartilage

Thyroid gland

FIGURE 7-82. Thyroid gland position at rest.

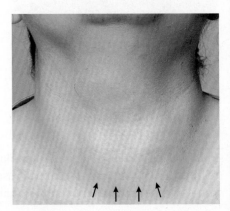

FIGURE 7-83. Thyroid gland with goiter at rest.

■ *Observe the patient swallowing.* Ask the patient to sip some water and to extend the neck again and swallow. Watch for upward movement of the thyroid gland, noting its contour and symmetry. The thyroid cartilage, the cricoid cartilage, and the thyroid gland all rise with swallowing and then fall to their resting positions.

With swallowing, the lower border of this large gland rises and looks less symmetric.

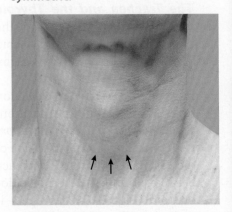

FIGURE 7-84. Thyroid gland with goiter while swallowing.

■ Confirm your visual observations by palpating the gland outlines as you stand facing the patient. This helps prepare you for the more systematic palpation to follow.

■ *Palpate the thyroid gland.* This may seem difficult at first. Use the cues from visual inspection. Find your landmarks—the notched thyroid cartilage and the cricoid cartilage below it (Fig. 7-85). Locate the *thyroid isthmus,* usually overlying the second, third, and fourth tracheal rings.

See Table 7-26, Thyroid Enlargement and Function, p. 299.

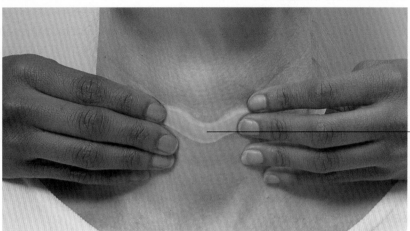

Cricoid cartilage

FIGURE 7-85. **Palpate the thyroid gland.**

Develop good technique by adopting the steps below, which outline the posterior approach to palpation. The anterior approach is similar and yields comparable findings.[81] The thyroid gland is usually easier to palpate in a long slender neck. In shorter necks, hyperextension of the neck may be helpful. If the lower pole of the thyroid gland is not palpable, suspect a retrosternal location. If the thyroid gland is retrosternal, below the suprasternal notch, it is often not palpable.

When the thyroid gland is retrosternal, below the suprasternal notch, it is often not palpable.

Retrosternal goiters can cause hoarseness, shortness of breath, stridor, or dysphagia from tracheal compression; neck hyperextension and arm elevation may cause flushing from compression of the thoracic inlet from the gland itself or from clavicular movement (Pemberton sign). Over 85% are benign.[82,83]

Steps for Palpating the Thyroid Gland (Posterior Approach)

- Ask the patient to flex the neck slightly forward to relax the sternocleidomastoid muscles.
- Place the fingers of both hands on the patient's neck so that your index fingers are just below the cricoid cartilage.
- Ask the patient to sip and swallow water as before. Feel for the thyroid isthmus rising up under your finger pads. It is often, but not always, palpable.
- Displace the trachea to the right with the fingers of the left hand; with the right-hand fingers, palpate laterally for the right lobe of the thyroid in the space between the displaced trachea and the relaxed sternocleidomastoid. Find the lateral margin. In a similar fashion, examine the left lobe.
  The lobes are somewhat harder to feel than the isthmus, so practice is needed. The anterior surface of a lateral lobe is approximately the size of the distal phalanx of the thumb and feels somewhat rubbery.
- Note the *size, shape,* and *consistency* (soft, firm, or hard) of the gland and identify any *nodules* or *tenderness.* In general, benign (or colloid) nodules tend to be more uniform, ovoid structures and are not fixed to surrounding tissue.
- If the thyroid gland is enlarged, listen over the lateral lobes with a stethoscope to detect a *bruit,* a sound similar to a cardiac murmur but of not of cardiac origin.

Although physical characteristics of the thyroid gland, such as size, shape, and consistency, are important, assessment of thyroid function depends on symptoms, signs elsewhere in the body, and laboratory tests.[84–89]

The thyroid is soft in *Graves disease* and may be nodular; it is firm in *Hashimoto thyroiditis* (though not always uniformly) and malignancy.

The thyroid is tender in *thyroiditis.*

A localized systolic or continuous bruit may be heard in *hyperthyroidism* from Graves disease or *toxic multinodular goiter.*

For palpable solitary nodules, ultrasound and possible fine-needle aspiration are advised. Ultrasound usually reveals multiple additional nonpalpable nodules; only 5% of nodules are malignant.[90,91]

The Carotid Arteries and Jugular Veins. Defer a detailed examination of the neck vessels until the cardiovascular examination, when the patient is supine with the head elevated to 30°. For jugular venous distention visible with the patient in the sitting position, assess the heart and lungs promptly. Also be alert to unusually prominent arterial pulsations.

See Chapter 9, Cardiovascular System, pp. 343–417.

Jugular venous distention is a hallmark of *heart failure.*

Note that many clinicians would examine the *CNs* at this point while facing the seated patient.

See Chapter 17, Nervous System, pp. 711–796.

Special Techniques

Eye Protrusion (Proptosis or Exophthalmos). For eyes with *exophthalmos,* or unusual forward protrusion, stand behind the seated patient and inspect from above. Draw the upper lids gently upward, then compare the protrusion of the eyes and the relationship of the corneas to the lower lids. For objective measurement, ophthalmologists use an exophthalmometer. This instrument measures the distance between the lateral angle of the orbit and an imaginary line across the most anterior point of the cornea. The upper limits of normal are 20 to 22 mm.[92–94]

When protrusion exceeds normal, further evaluation by ultrasound or computerized tomography scan often follows.[94]

Exophthalmos is present in approximately 60% of patients with Graves ophthalmopathy and half of patients with Graves disease from autoimmune hyperthyroidism. Common symptoms of Graves ophthalmopathy are diplopia and tearing, grittiness, and pain from corneal exposure. Eyelid retraction (91%), extraocular muscle dysfunction (43%), ocular pain (30%), and lacrimation (23%) are also common.[92–94] See also Table 7-27, Symptoms and Signs of Thyroid Disorders, p. 299.

Nasolacrimal Duct Obstruction. This test helps identify the cause of excessive tearing. Ask the patient to look up. Press on the lower lid close to the medial canthus, just inside the rim of the bony orbit; this compresses the lacrimal sac (Fig. 7-86). Look for fluid regurgitated out of the puncta into the eye. Avoid this test if the area is inflamed and tender.

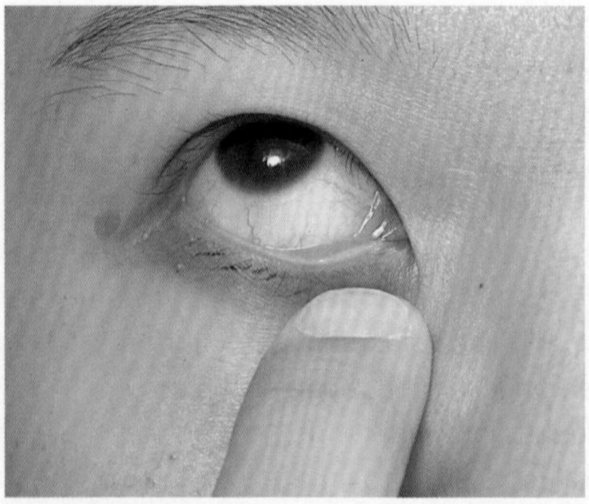

FIGURE 7-86. **Compress the lower lid close to the medial canthus.**

Discharge of mucopurulent fluid from the puncta suggests an obstructed nasolacrimal duct.

A *foreign body* in the eye often involves dust, a speck of sand, a paint chip, an insect, or a dislodged eyelash trapped underneath the lid, causing patients to sense something in their eye. Foreign bodies can be superficial, sticking to the eye surface or beneath the lid, or penetrating—usually a piece of metal that pierces the outer cornea or sclera.

Everting the Upper Eyelid to Search for a Foreign Body. To search thoroughly for a foreign body in the eye, evert the upper lid following the steps below.

■ Ask the patient to look down and relax the eyes. Be reassuring and use gentle deliberate movements. Raise the upper eyelid slightly so that the lashes protrude, then grasp the upper eyelashes and pull them gently down and forward (Fig. 7-87).

- Place a small stick such as a tongue blade or an applicator at least 1 cm above the lid margin at the upper border of the tarsal plate. Push down on the tongue blade as you raise the edge of the lid, thus everting the eyelid or turning it "inside out." Do not press on the eyeball itself (Fig. 7-88).

- Secure the upper lashes against the eyebrow with your thumb and inspect the palpebral conjunctiva (Fig. 7-89). After your inspection, grasp the upper eyelashes and pull them gently forward. Ask the patient to look up. The eyelid will return to its normal position.

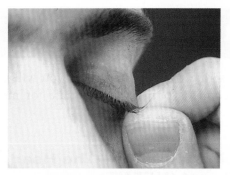

FIGURE 7-87. **To evert eyelid, pull down the upper eyelashes.**

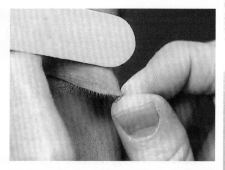

FIGURE 7-88. **Using a tongue blade, evert the edge of the lid.**

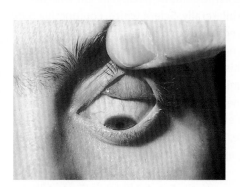

FIGURE 7-89. **Inspect the palpebral conjunctiva.**

This view allows you to see the upper palpebral conjunctiva and look for a *foreign body* that might be lodged there.

Swinging Flashlight Test. The swinging flashlight test is a clinical test for functional impairment of the optic nerves (Fig. 7-90). In dim light, note the size of the pupils. After asking the patient to gaze into the distance, swing the beam of a penlight for 1 to 2 seconds first into one pupil, then into the other. Normally, each illuminated eye constricts promptly. The opposite eye also constricts consensually.

In left-sided optic nerve damage, the pupils usually react as follows: When the light beam shines into the normal right eye, there is brisk constriction of both pupils (direct response on the right and consensual response on the left). When the light swings over to the abnormal left eye, partial dilation of both pupils will occur. The afferent stimulus on the left is reduced, so the efferent signals to both pupils are also reduced and a net dilation occurs. This demonstrates an afferent pupillary defect, sometimes termed a *Marcus Gunn pupil.*

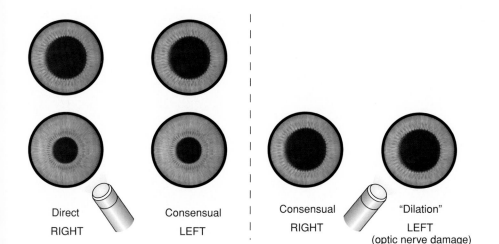

Direct RIGHT   Consensual LEFT

Consensual RIGHT   "Dilation" LEFT (optic nerve damage)

FIGURE 7-90. **Swinging flashlight test.**

Recording Your Findings

Initially you may use sentences to describe your findings; later you will use phrases. The style in the next box contains phrases appropriate for most write-ups.

Recording the Physical Examination—The Head, Eyes, Ears, Nose, and Throat (HEENT)

HEENT: Head—The skull is normocephalic/atraumatic (NC/AT). Hair with average texture. *Eyes*—Visual acuity 20/20 bilaterally. Sclera white, conjunctiva pink. Pupils are 4 mm constricting to 2 mm, equally round and reactive to light and accommodations. Disc margins sharp; no hemorrhages or exudates, no arteriolar narrowing. *Ears*—Acuity good to whispered voice. Tympanic membranes (TMs) with good cone of light. Weber midline. AC > BC. *Nose*—Nasal mucosa pink, septum midline; no sinus tenderness. *Throat (or Mouth)*—Oral mucosa pink, dentition good, pharynx without exudates.

    Neck—Trachea midline. Neck supple; thyroid isthmus palpable, lobes not felt.

    Lymph Nodes—No cervical, axillary, epitrochlear, inguinal adenopathy.

OR

    Head—The skull is normocephalic/atraumatic. Frontal balding. *Eyes*—Visual acuity 20/100 bilaterally. Sclera white; conjunctiva injected. Pupils constrict 3 mm to 2 mm, equally round and reactive to light and accommodation. Disc margins sharp; no hemorrhages or exudates. Arteriolar-to-venous ratio (AV ratio) 2:4; no AV nicking. *Ears*—Acuity diminished to whispered voice; intact to spoken voice. TMs clear. *Nose*—Mucosa swollen with erythema and clear drainage. Septum midline. Tender over maxillary sinuses. *Throat*—Oral mucosa pink, dental caries in lower molars, pharynx erythematous, no exudates.

    Neck—Trachea midline. Neck supple; thyroid isthmus midline, lobes palpable but not enlarged.

    Lymph Nodes—Submandibular and anterior cervical lymph nodes tender, 1 cm × 1 cm, rubbery and mobile; no posterior cervical, epitrochlear, axillary, or inguinal lymphadenopathy.

These findings suggest myopia and mild arteriolar narrowing as well as upper respiratory infection.

Table 7-1 Primary Headaches

Headaches are classified as *primary,* without underlying pathology, or *secondary,* with a serious underlying cause often warranting urgent attention. Secondary headaches are more likely to occur after age 50 years with a sudden severe onset and should be ruled out before making the diagnosis of a primary headache.[3] About 90% of headaches are primary headaches and fall into four categories: tension, migraine, cluster, and chronic daily headache. The features of tension, migraine, and cluster headaches are highlighted below. *Chronic daily headache* is not a diagnosis, but a category containing pre-existing headaches that have been transformed into more pronounced forms of migraines, chronic tension-type headaches, and medication-overuse headaches and last more than 15 days a month for more than 3 months.[16] Risk factors include obesity; more than one headache a week; caffeine ingestion; use of headache medications >10 days a month, such as analgesics, ergots, and triptans; and sleep and mood disorders.

	Tension	Migraines	Cluster
Process	Process unclear—possibly heightened CNS pain sensitivity. Involves pericranial muscle tenderness; etiology also unclear	Neuronal dysfunction, possibly of brainstem origin, involving low serotonin level, spreading cortical depression and trigeminovascular activation; types: with aura, without aura, variants	Process unclear—possibly hypothalamic then trigeminoautonomic activation
Lifetime Prevalence	Most common headache (40%); prevalence about 50%	10% of headaches; prevalence 18% of U.S. adults; affects ~15% of women, 6% of men	<1%, more common in men.
Location	Usually bilateral; may be generalized or localized to the back of the head and upper neck or to the frontotemporal area	Unilateral in ~70%; bifrontal or global in ~30%	Unilateral, usually behind or around the eye or temple
Quality and Severity	Steady; pressing or tightening; nonthrobbing pain; mild to moderate intensity	Throbbing or aching, pain, moderate to severe in intensity; preceded by an aura in up to 30%	Sharp, continuous, intense; severe in intensity
Timing			
Onset	Gradual	Fairly rapid, reaching a peak in 1–2 hours	Abrupt; peaks within minutes
Duration	30 minutes to 7 days	4–72 hours	15 minutes to 3 hours
Course	Episodic; may be chronic	Recurrent—usually monthly, but weekly in ~10%; peak incidence early to mid-adolescence	Episodic, clustered in time, with several each day for 4–8 weeks and then relief for 6–12 months
Associated Symptoms	Sometimes photophobia, phonophobia; scalp tenderness; nausea absent	Prodrome: nausea, vomiting, photophobia, phonophobia; aura in 30%; either visual (flickering, zig-zagging lines), or motor (paresthesias of hand, arm, or face, or language dysfunction)	Unilateral autonomic symptoms: lacrimation, rhinorrhea, miosis, ptosis, eyelid edema, conjunctival infection
Triggers/ Factors That Aggravate or Provoke	Sustained muscle tension, as in driving or typing; stress; sleep disturbances	Alcohol, certain foods, or stress may provoke; also menses, high altitude; aggravated by noise and bright light	During attack, sensitivity to alcohol may increase
Factors That Relieve	Possibly massage, relaxation	Quiet, dark room; sleep; sometimes transient relief from pressure on the involved artery	

Sources: Headache Classification Committee of the International Headache Society (IHS). The International Classification of Headache Disorders, 3rd edition (beta version). *Cephalalgia.* 2013;33:629; Lipton RB, Bigal ME, Steiner TJ, et al. Classification of primary headaches. *Neurology.* 2004;63:427; Sun-Edelstein C, Bigal ME, Rappoport AM. Chronic migraine and medication overuse headache: clarifying the current International Headache Society classification criteria. *Cephalalgia.* 2009;29:445; Lipton RB, Stewart WF, Seymour D, et al. Prevalence and burden of migraine in the United States: data from the American Migraine Study II. *Headache.* 2001;41:646; Fumal A, Schoenen J. Tension-type headache: current research and clinical management. *Lancet Neurol.* 2008;7:70; Nesbitt AD, Goadsby PJ. Cluster headache. *BMJ.* 2012;344:e2407.

Table 7-2 Secondary Headaches and Cranial Neuralgias

Type	Process	Location	Quality and Severity
Secondary Headaches *Analgesic Rebound*	Withdrawal of medication	Previous headache pattern	Variable
Headaches from Eye Disorders *Errors of Refraction (farsightedness and astigmatism, but not nearsightedness)*	Probably the sustained contraction of the extraocular muscles, and possibly of the frontal, temporal, and occipital muscles	Around and over the eyes; may radiate to the occipital area	Steady, aching, dull
Acute Glaucoma	Sudden increase in intraocular pressure (see p. 270)	Pain in and around one eye	Steady, aching, often severe
Headache from Sinusitis	Mucosal inflammation of the paranasal sinuses	Usually frontal sinuses above the eyes or over the maxillary sinus	Aching or throbbing, severity variable; consider possible migraine
Meningitis	Viral or bacterial infection of the meninges surrounding the brain and spinal cord	Generalized	Steady or throbbing, very severe
Subarachnoid Hemorrhage— "Thunderclap Headache"	Bleeding from a ruptured cerebral saccular aneurysm; rarely from AV malformation, mycotic aneurysm	Generalized	Very severe, "the worst of my life"
Brain Tumor	Mass lesion causing displacement of or traction on pain-sensitive arteries and veins or pressure on nerves	Variable, including lobes of brain, cerebellum, brain-stem	Aching, steady, dull pain worse on awakening the better after several hours
Giant Cell (Temporal) Arteritis	Transmural lymphocytic vasculitis often involving multinucleated giant cells that disrupts the internal elastic lamina of large-caliber arteries	Localized near the involved artery, most often the temporal artery in those > age 50, women > men (2:1 ratio)	Throbbing, generalized, persistent; often severe
Postconcussion Headache	Follows mild acceleration-deceleration traumatic brain injury; may involve axonal, cerebrovascular autoregulatory, neurochemical injury	Often but not always localized to the injured area	Dull, aching, constant; may have features of tension and migraine headaches
Cranial Neuralgias *Trigeminal Neuralgia (CN V)*	Vascular compression of CN V, usually near entry to pons leading to focal demyelination, aberrant discharge; 10% with causative intracranial lesion	Cheek, jaws, lips, or gums; trigeminal nerve divisions 2 and 3 > 1	Shock-like, stabbing, burning; severe

Note: Blanks appear in this table when the categories are not applicable or not usually helpful in assessing the problem.

Sources: Headache Classification Committee of the International Headache Society (IHS). The International Classification of Headache Disorders, 3rd ed. (beta version). *Cephalalgia.* 2013;33:629; Schwedt TJ, Matharu MS, Dodick DW. Thunderclap headache. *Lancet Neurol.* 2006;5:621; Van de Beek D, de Gans J, Spanjaard L, et al. Clinical features and prognostic factors in adults with bacterial meningitis. *N Engl J Med.* 2004;351:1849; Salvarini C, Cantini F, Hunder GG. Polymyalgia rheumatica and giant cell arteritis. *Lancet.* 2008;372:234; Smetana GW, Shmerling RH. Does this patient have temporal arteritis? *JAMA.* 2002;287:92; Ropper AH, Gorson KC. Clinical practice. Concussion. *N Engl J Med.* 2007;356:166. American College of Physicians. Neurology—MKSAP 16. Philadelphia, 2012.

Timing			Associated Symptoms	Factors That Aggravate or Provoke	Factors That Relieve
Onset	*Duration*	*Course*			
Variable	Depends on prior headache pattern	Depends on frequency of "mini-withdrawals"	Depends on prior headache pattern	Fever, carbon monoxide, hypoxia, withdrawal of caffeine, other headache triggers	Depends on cause
Gradual	Variable	Variable	Eye fatigue, "sandy" sensations in eyes, redness of conjunctiva	Prolonged use of the eyes, particularly for close work	Rest of the eyes
Often rapid	Variable, may depend on treatment	Variable, may depend on treatment	Blurred vision, nausea and vomiting; halos around lights, reddening of eye	Sometimes provoked by mydriatic drops	
Variable	Often daily several hours at a time, persisting until treatment	Often daily in a repetitive pattern	Local tenderness, nasal congestion, discharge, and fever	May be aggravated by coughing, sneezing, or jarring the head	Nasal decongestants, antibiotics
Fairly rapid, usually <24 hours; may be sudden onset	Variable, usually days	Viral: usually <1 week; bacterial: persistent until treatment	Fever, stiff neck, photophobia, change in mental status		Immediate antibiotics until diagnosis of if bacterial or viral
Sudden onset; can be less than a minute	Variable, usually days	Varies according to presenting severity and level of consciousness; worst if initial coma	Nausea, vomiting, loss of consciousness, neck pain. Possible prior neck symptoms from "sentinel leaks"	Rebleeding, ↑ intracranial pressure, cerebral edema	Subspecialty treatments
Variable	Often brief; depends on location and rate of growth	Intermittent but may progress in intensity over a period of days	Seizures, hemiparesis, field cuts, personality changes. Also nausea, vomiting, vision change, gait change	May be aggravated by coughing, sneezing, or sudden movements of the head	Subspecialty treatments
Gradual or rapid	Variable	Recurrent or persistent over weeks to months	Tenderness over temporal artery, adjacent scalp; fever (in ~50%), fatigue, weight loss; new headache (~60%), jaw claudication (~50%), visual loss or blindness (~15%–20%), polymyalgia rheumatica (~50%)	Movement of neck and shoulders	Often sterioids
Within 7 days of the injury up to 3 months	Weeks to up to a year	Tends to diminish over time	Drowsiness, poor concentration, confusion, memory loss, blurred vision, dizziness, irritability, restlessness, fatigue	Mental and physical exertion, straining, stooping, emotional excitement, alcohol	Rest; medication
Abrupt, paroxysmal	Each jab lasts seconds but recurs at intervals of seconds or minutes	May recur daily for weeks to months then resolve; can be chronic progressive	Exhaustion from recurrent pain	Touching certain areas of the lower face or mouth; chewing, talking, brushing teeth	Medication; neurovascular decompression

Table 7-3 Red Eyes

	Conjunctivitis	**Subconjunctival Hemorrhage**
	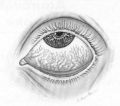	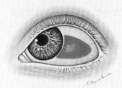
Pattern of Redness	Conjunctival injection: diffuse dilatation of conjunctival vessels with redness that tends to be maximal peripherally	Leakage of blood outside of the vessels, producing a homogeneous, sharply demarcated, red area that resolves over 2 weeks
Pain	Mild discomfort rather than pain	Absent
Vision	Not affected except for temporary mild blurring due to discharge	Not affected
Ocular Discharge	Watery, mucoid, or mucopurulent	Absent
Pupil	Not affected	Not affected
Cornea	Clear	Clear
Significance	Bacterial, viral, and other infections; highly contagious; allergy; irritation	Often none. May result from trauma, bleeding disorders, or sudden increase in venous pressure, as from cough

	Corneal Injury or Infection	**Acute Iritis**	**Acute Angle Closure Glaucoma**
	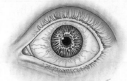	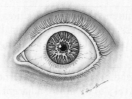	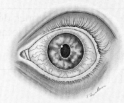
Pattern of Redness	Ciliary injection: The deeper vessels radiating from the limbus are dilated, creating a reddish violet flush. Ciliary injection is an important sign of these three conditions but is not always visible. The eye may be diffusely red instead. Other signs of these serious disorders are pain, decreased vision, unequal pupils, and a clouded cornea.		
Pain	Moderate to severe, superficial	Moderate, aching, deep	Severe, aching, deep
Vision	Usually decreased	Decreased; photophobia	Decreased
Ocular Discharge	Watery or purulent	Absent	Absent
Pupil	Not affected unless iritis develops	Small and irregular	Dilated, fixed
Cornea	Changes depending on cause	Clear or slightly clouded; injection confined to corneal limbus	Steamy, cloudy
Significance	Abrasions, and other injuries; viral and bacterial infections	Associated with systemic infection, Herpes zoster, tuberculosis, or autoimmune diseases; refer promptly	Acute increase in intraocular pressure constitutes an emergency

Source: Leibowitz HM. The red eye. *N Engl J Med.* 2000;342:345.

Table 7-4 Dizziness and Vertigo

"Dizziness" is a nonspecific term used by patients encompassing several disorders that clinicians must carefully sort out. A detailed history usually identifies the primary etiology. It is important to learn the specific meanings of the following terms or conditions:

- *Vertigo*—a spinning sensation accompanied by nystagmus and ataxia; usually from *peripheral vestibular dysfunction* (~40% of "dizzy" patients) but may be from a *central brainstem lesion* (~10%; causes include atherosclerosis, multiple sclerosis, vertebrobasilar migraine, or transient ischemic attack [TIA])

- *Presyncope*—a near faint from "feeling faint or lightheaded"; causes include orthostatic hypotension, especially from medication, arrhythmias, and vasovagal attacks (~5%)

- *Disequilibrium*—unsteadiness or imbalance when walking, especially in older patients, causes include fear of walking, visual loss, weakness from musculoskeletal problems, and peripheral neuropathy (up to 15%)

- *Psychiatric*—causes include anxiety, panic disorder, hyperventilation, depression, somatization disorder, alcohol, and substance abuse (~10%)

- *Multifactorial or unknown*—(up to 20%)

Peripheral and Central Vertigo

	Onset	Duration and Course	Hearing	Tinnitus	Additional Features
Peripheral Vertigo					
Benign Positional Vertigo	Sudden, often when rolling onto the affected side or tilting up the head	Onset a few seconds to <1 minute Lasts a few weeks, may recur	Not affected	Absent	Sometimes nausea, vomiting, nystagmus
Vestibular Neuronitis (Acute Labyrinthitis)	Sudden	Onset hours to up to 2 weeks May recur over 12–18 months	Not affected	Absent	Nausea, vomiting, nystagmus
Ménière Disease	Sudden	Onset several hours to ≥1 day Recurrent	Sensorineural hearing loss—recurs, eventually progresses	Present, fluctuating	Pressure or fullness in affected ear; nausea, vomiting, nystagmus
Drug Toxicity	Insidious or acute—linked to loop diuretics, aminoglycosides, salicylates, alcohol	May or may not be reversible Partial adaptation occurs	May be impaired	May be present	Nausea, vomiting
Acoustic Neuroma	Insidious from CN VIII compression, vestibular branch	Variable	Impaired, one side	Present	May involve CN V and VII
Central Vertigo	Often sudden (see causes above)	Variable but rarely continuous	Not affected	Absent	Usually with other brainstem deficits—dysarthria, ataxia, crossed motor and sensory deficits

Sources: Chan Y. Differential diagnosis of dizziness. *Curr Opin Otolaryngol Head Neck Surg.* 2009;17:200; Kroenke K, Lucas CA, Rosenberg ML, et al. Causes of persistent dizziness: a prospective study of 100 patients in ambulatory care. *Ann Intern Med.* 1992;117:898; Tusa RJ. Vertigo. *Neurol Clin.* 2001;19:23; Lockwood AH, Salvi RJ, Burkard RF. Tinnitus. *N Engl J Med.* 2002;347:904.

Table 7-5 Selected Facies

FACIAL SWELLING

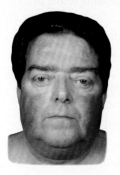

Cushing Syndrome

The increased adrenal cortisol production of Cushing syndrome produces a round or "moon" face with red cheeks. Excessive hair growth may be present in the mustache, sideburn areas, and chin (as well as the chest, abdomen, and thighs).

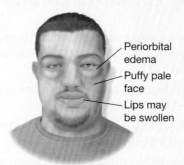

Periorbital edema
Puffy pale face
Lips may be swollen

Nephrotic Syndrome

Glomerular disease causes excess albumin excretion, which reduces intravascular colloid osmotic pressure, causing hypovolemia, then sodium and water retention. The face becomes edematous and often pale. Swelling usually appears first around the eyes and in the morning. When severe, the eyes appear slitlike.

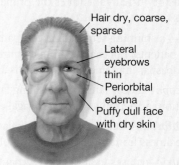

Hair dry, coarse, sparse
Lateral eyebrows thin
Periorbital edema
Puffy dull face with dry skin

Myxedema

In severe hypothyroidism (*myxedema*) mucopolysaccharide deposition in the dermis leads to a dull, puffy facies. The edema, often pronounced around the eyes, does not pit with pressure. The hair and eyebrows are dry, coarse, and thinned, classically with loss of the lateral third of the eyebrows. The skin is dry.

OTHER FACIES

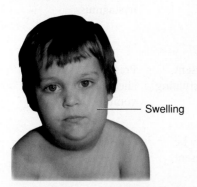

Swelling

Parotid Gland Enlargement

Chronic bilateral asymptomatic parotid gland enlargement may be associated with obesity, diabetes, cirrhosis, and other conditions. Note the swellings anterior to the ear lobes and above the angles of the jaw. Gradual unilateral enlargement suggests neoplasm. Acute enlargement is seen in mumps.

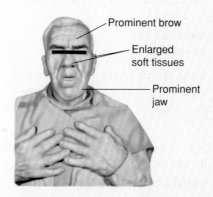

Prominent brow
Enlarged soft tissues
Prominent jaw

Acromegaly

The increased growth hormone of acromegaly produces enlargement of both bone and soft tissues. The head is elongated, with bony prominence of the forehead, nose, and lower jaw. Soft tissues of the nose, lips, and ears also enlarge. The facial features appear generally coarsened.

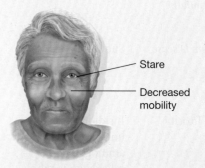

Stare
Decreased mobility

Parkinson Disease

In this neurodegenerative disorder linked to loss of the neurotransmitter dopamine, there is decreased facial mobility and a masklike facies, with decreased blinking and a characteristic stare. Since the neck and upper trunk tend to flex forward, the patient seems to peer upward toward the observer. Facial skin becomes oily, and drooling may occur.

Table 7-6 Visual Field Defects

Visual Field Defects

1. *Horizontal Defect* Occlusion of a branch of the central retinal artery may cause a horizontal (altitudinal) defect. Ischemia of the optic nerve can produce a similar defect.

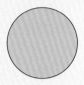

2. *Blind Right Eye (Right Optic Nerve)* A lesion of the optic nerve and, of course, of the eye itself, produces unilateral monocular blindness.

3. *Bitemporal Hemianopsia (Optic Chiasm)* A lesion at the optic chiasm (such as a pituitary tumor), may involve only fibers crossing over to the opposite side. Since these fibers originate in the nasal half of each retina, visual loss involves the temporal half of each field.

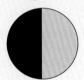

4. *Left Homonymous Hemianopsia (Right Optic Tract)* A lesion of the optic tract, interrupts fibers originating on the same side of both eyes. Visual loss in the eyes is, therefore, similar (homonymous) and involves half of each field (hemianopsia).

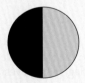 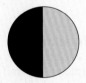

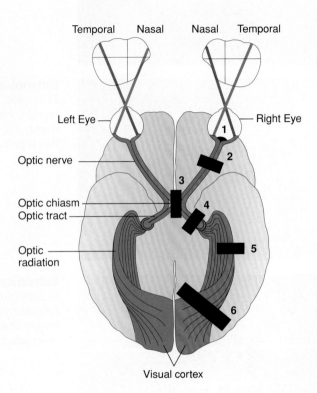

5. *Homonymous Left Superior Quadrantic Defect (Right Optic Radiation, Partial)* A partial lesion of the optic radiation in the temporal lobe, may involve only a portion of the nerve fibers, producing, for example, a homonymous quadrantic ("pie in the sky") defect.

 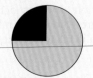

6. *Left Homonymous Hemianopsia (Right Optic Radiation)* A complete interruption of fibers in the optic radiation, produces a visual defect similar to that produced by a lesion of the optic tract.

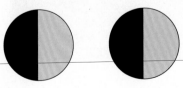

Table 7-7 Variations and Abnormalities of the Eyelids

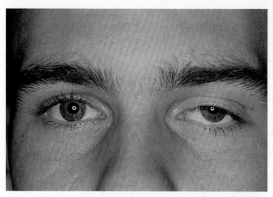

Ptosis

Ptosis is a drooping of the upper lid. Causes include myasthenia gravis, damage to the oculomotor nerve (CN III), and damage to the sympathetic nerve supply (*Horner syndrome*). A weakened muscle, relaxed tissues, and the weight of herniated fat may cause senile ptosis. Ptosis may also be congenital.

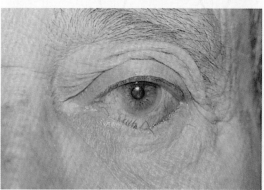

Entropion

Entropion, more common in the elderly, is an inward turning of the lid margin. The lower lashes, which are often invisible when turned inward, irritate the conjunctiva and lower cornea. Ask the patient to squeeze the lids together and then open them; then check for an entropion that is less obvious.

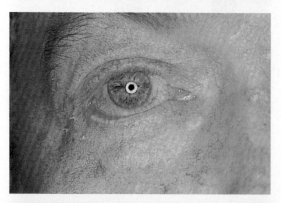

Ectropion

In ectropion, the lower lid margin turns outward, exposing the palpebral conjunctiva. When the punctum of the lower lid turns outward, the eye no longer drains well, and tearing occurs. Ectropion is also more common in older adults.

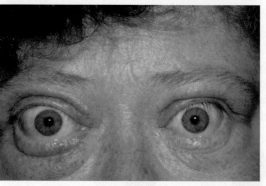

Lid Retraction and Exophthalmos

A wide-eyed stare suggests retracted eyelids. Note the rim of sclera between the upper lid and the iris. Retracted lids and "lid lag" when eyes move from up to down markedly increase the likelihood of hyperthyroidism, especially when accompanied by a fine tremor, moist skin, and heart rate >90 beats per minute.[99]

Exophthalmos describes protrusion of the eyeball, a common feature of Graves ophthalmopathy, triggered by autoreactive T lymphocytes. In this disorder, there is a spectrum of eye changes, ranging from lid retraction to extraocular muscle dysfunction, dry eyes, ocular pain, and lacrimation. Changes do not always progress. In unilateral exophthalmos, consider Graves disease (though usually bilateral), trauma, orbital tumor, and granulomatous disorders.[94]

Source of photos: *Ptosis, Ectropion, Entropion*—Tasman W, Jaeger E, eds. *The Wills Eye Hospital Atlas of Clinical Ophthalmology*, 2nd ed. Philadelphia: Lippincott Williams & Wilkins, 2001.

Table 7-8 Lumps and Swellings in and Around the Eyes

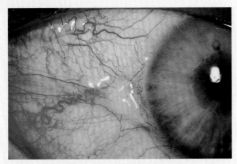

Pinguecula

A harmless yellowish triangular nodule in the bulbar conjunctiva on either side of the iris. Appears frequently with aging, first on the nasal and then on the temporal side.

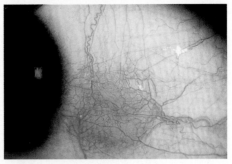

Episcleritis

A localized ocular inflammation of the episcleral vessels. Vessels appear movable over the scleral surface. May be nodular or show only redness and dilated vessels. Seen in rheumatoid arthritis, Sjögren syndrome, and herpes zoster.

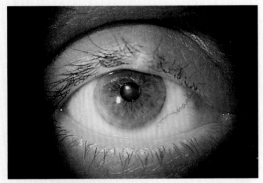

Stye (Hordeolum)

A painful, tender, red infection at the inner or outer margin of the eyelid, usually from *Staphylococcus aureus* (at the inner margin—from an obstructed meibomian gland; at the outer margin—from an obstructed eyelash follicle or tear gland).

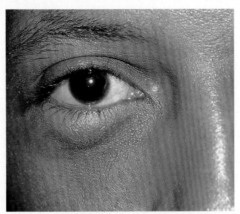

Chalazion

A subacute nontender, usually painless nodule caused by a blocked meibomian gland. May become acutely inflamed but, unlike a stye, usually points inside the lid rather than on the lid margin.

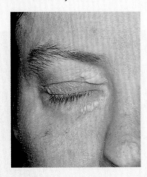

Xanthelasma

Slightly raised, yellowish, well-circumscribed cholesterol-filled plaques that appear along the nasal portions of one or both eyelids. Half of affected patients have *hyperlipidemia*; it is also common in *primary biliary cirrhosis*.

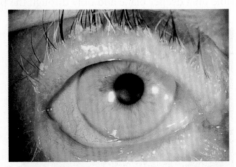

Blepharitis

A chronic inflammation of the eyelids at the base of the hair follicles, often from *S. aureus*. There is also a scaling seborrheic variant.

Source of photos: Tasman W, Jaeger E, eds. *The Wills Eye Hospital Atlas of Clinical Ophthalmology*, 2nd ed. Philadelphia: Lippincott Williams & Wilkins, 2001.

Table 7-9 Opacities of the Cornea and Lens

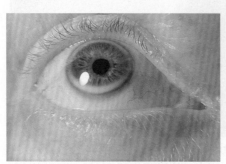

Corneal Arcus. A thin grayish white arc or circle not quite at the edge of the cornea. Accompanies normal aging but also seen in younger adults, especially African Americans. In young adults, suggests possible hyperlipoproteinemia. Usually benign.

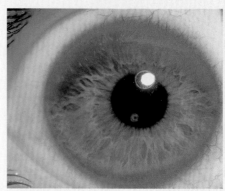

Kayser-Fleischer Ring. A golden to red brown ring, sometimes shading to green or blue, from copper deposition in the periphery of the cornea found in *Wilson disease*. Due to a rare autosomal recessive mutation of the ATO7B gene on chromosome 13 causing abnormal copper transport, reduced biliary copper excretion, and abnormal accumulation of copper in the liver and tissues throughout the body. Patients present with liver disease, renal failure, and neurologic symptoms of tremor, dystonia, and a variety of psychiatric disorders.[95,96]

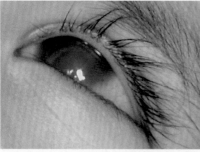

Corneal Scar. A superficial grayish white opacity in the cornea, secondary to an old injury or to inflammation. Size and shape are variable. Do not confuse with the opaque lens of a cataract, visible on a deeper plane and only through the pupil.

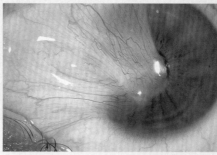

Pterygium. A triangular thickening of the bulbar conjunctiva that grows slowly across the outer surface of the cornea, usually from the nasal side. Reddening may occur. May interfere with vision as it encroaches on the pupil.

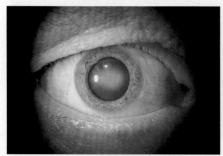

Cataracts. Opacitiy of the lenses visible through the pupil. Risk factors are older age, smoking, diabetes, corticosteroid use.

Nuclear Cataract. A nuclear cataract looks gray when seen by a flashlight. If the pupil is widely dilated, the gray opacity is surrounded by a black rim.

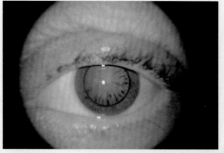

Peripheral Cataract. Produces spokelike shadows that point—gray against black, as seen with a flashlight, or black against red with an ophthalmoscope. A dilated pupil, as shown here, facilitates this observation.

Table 7-10 Pupillary Abnormalities

Unequal Pupils (Anisocoria)—Anisocoria represents a defect in the constriction or dilatation of one pupil. Constriction to light and near effort is mediated by parasympathetic pathways, and pupillary dilatation by sympathetic pathways. The light reaction in bright and dim light identifies the abnormal pupil. When anisocoria is greater in bright light than in dim light, the larger pupil cannot constrict properly. Causes include blunt trauma to the eye, open-angle glaucoma (p. 270), and impaired *parasympathetic* innervation to the iris, as in tonic pupil and oculomotor nerve (CN III) paralysis. When anisocoria is greater in dim light, the smaller pupil cannot dilate properly, as in Horner syndrome, caused by an interruption of the *sympathetic* innervation. Assessing the near reaction is also important in determining the cause. See also Table 17-13, Pupils in Comatose Patients, p. 792.

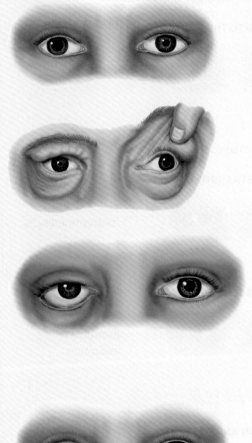

Tonic Pupil (*Adie Pupil*). Pupil is large (dilated), regular, and usually unilateral. Reaction to light is severely reduced and slowed, or even absent. Constriction during the near vision is present, although very slow (tonic). These changes reflect parasympathetic denervation. Slow accommodation causes blurred vision.

Oculomotor Nerve (CN III) Paralysis. The pupil is large and fixed to light and near effort. Ptosis of the upper eyelid (due to impaired CN III innervation of the levator palpebrae muscle) and lateral deviation of the eye downward and outward are almost always present.

Horner Syndrome. The affected pupil is *small,* unilateral, reacts briskly to light and near effort, but *dilates slowly,* especially in dim light. Anisocoria is >1 mm, with ipsilateral ptosis of the eyelid and often loss of sweating on the forehead. These findings reflect the classic triad of *Horner syndrome—miosis, ptosis* and *anhydrosis,* due to a lesion in the sympathetic pathways anywhere from the hypothalamus through the brachial plexus and cervical ganglia into the oculasympathetic fibers of the eye. Causes include ipsilateral brainstem lesions, neck and chest tumors affecting the ipsilateral sympathetic ganglia, and orbital trauma or migraines.[100] In congenital Horner syndrome, the involved iris is lighter in color than its fellow (*heterochromia*).

Small, Irregular Pupils (Argyll Robertson Pupils). The pupils are small, irregular and usually bilateral. They constrict with near vision and dilate with far vision (a normal near reaction) but do not react to light, seen in neurosyphilis and rarely in diabetes.

Equal Pupils and One Blind Eye. Unilateral blindness does not cause anisocoria as long as the sympathetic and parasympathetic innervation to both irises is normal. A light directed into the seeing eye produces a direct reaction in that eye and a consensual reaction in the blind eye. A light directed into the blind eye, however, causes no response in either eye.

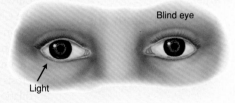

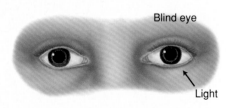

Table 7-11 Dysconjugate Gaze

There are a number of abnormal patterns of gaze related to developmental disorders and cranial nerve abnormalities.

Developmental Disorders

Developmental dysconjugate gaze is caused by an imbalance in ocular muscle tone. This imbalance has many causes, may be hereditary, and usually appears in early childhood. These gaze deviations are classified according to direction:

Esotropia

Exotropia

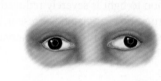

Disorders of Cranial Nerves

New onset of dysconjugate gaze in adults usually results from cranial nerve injuries, lesions, or abnormalities from causes such as trauma, multiple sclerosis, syphilis, and others.

A Left Cranial Nerve VI Paralysis

LOOKING TO THE RIGHT

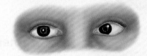

Eyes are conjugate.

Cover–Uncover Test

A cover–uncover test may be helpful. Here is what you would see in the right monocular esotropia illustrated above.

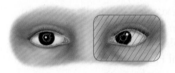

Corneal reflections are asymmetric.

COVER

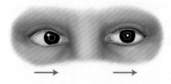

The right eye moves outward to fix on the light. (The left eye is not seen but moves inward to the same degree.)

UNCOVER

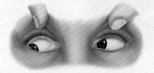

The left eye moves outward to fix on the light. The right eye deviates inward again.

LOOKING STRAIGHT AHEAD

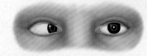

Esotropia appears.

LOOKING TO THE RIGHT

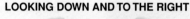

Esotropia is maximum.

A Left Cranial Nerve IV Paralysis

LOOKING DOWN AND TO THE RIGHT

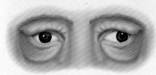

The left eye cannot look down when turned inward. Deviation is maximum in this direction.

A Left Cranial Nerve III Paralysis

LOOKING STRAIGHT AHEAD

The eye is pulled outward by action of the CN VI. Upward, downward, and inward movements are impaired or lost. Ptosis and pupillary dilation may be associated.

Table 7-12 Normal Variations of the Optic Disc

Physiologic Cupping

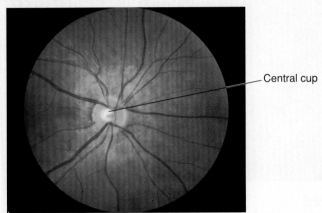

Central cup

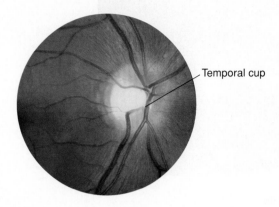

Temporal cup

The physiologic cup is a small whitish depression in the optic disc, the entry point for the retinal vessels. Although sometimes absent, the cup is usually visible either centrally or toward the temporal side of the disc. Grayish spots are often seen at its base.

Rings and Crescents

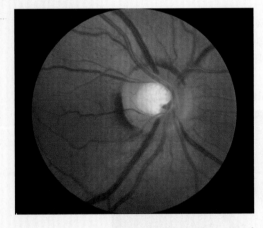

Medullated Nerve Fibers

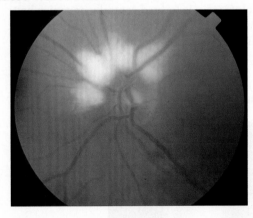

Rings and crescents are often seen around the optic disc. These are developmental variations that appear as either white sclera, black retinal pigment, or both, especially along the temporal border of the disc. Rings and crescents are not part of the disc itself and should not be included in your estimate of the disc diameter.

Medullated or myelinated nerve fibers are a much less common but dramatic finding. Appearing as irregular white patches with feathered margins, they obscure the disc edge and retinal vessels. They have no pathologic significance.

Table 7-13 Abnormalities of the Optic Disc

Normal

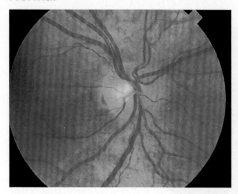

Process
Tiny disc vessels give normal color to the disc.

Appearance
Color yellowish orange to creamy pink
Disc vessels tiny
Disc margins sharp (except perhaps nasally)
The physiologic cup is located centrally or somewhat temporally. It may be conspicuous or absent. Its diameter from side to side is usually less than half that of the disc.

Papilledema

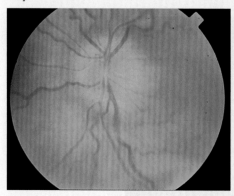

Process
Elevated intracranial pressure causes intraaxonal edema along the optic nerve, leading to engorgement and swelling of the optic disc.

Appearance
Color pink, hyperemic
Often with loss of venous pulsations
Disc vessels more visible, more numerous, curve over the borders of the disc
Disc swollen with margins blurred
The physiologic cup is not visible.
Seen in intracranial mass, lesion, or hemorrhage, meningitis

Glaucomatous Cupping

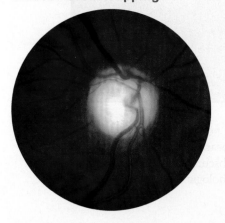

Process
Increased intraocular pressure within the eye leads to increased cupping (backward depression of the disc) and atrophy. The base of the enlarged cup is pale.

Appearance
Death of optic nerve fibers leads to loss of the tiny disc vessels.

Optic Atrophy

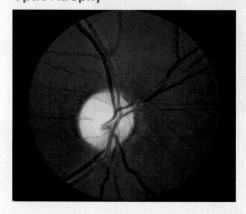

Process
The physiologic cup is enlarged, occupying more than half of the disc's diameter, at times extending to the edge of the disc. Retinal vessels sink in and under the cup, and may be displaced nasally.

Appearance
Color white
Tiny disc vessels absent
Seen in optic neuritis, multiple sclerosis, temporal arteritis

Sources of photos for *Normal*—Tasman W, Jaeger E, eds. *The Wills Eye Hospital Atlas of Clinical Ophthalmology*, 2nd ed. Philadelphia, PA: Lippincott Williams & Wilkins, 2001; *Papilledema, Glaucomatous Cupping, Optic Atrophy*—Courtesy of Ken Freedman, MD.

Normal Retinal Artery and Arteriovenous (AV) Crossing

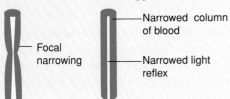

— Arterial wall (invisible)
— Column of blood
— Light reflex

The normal arterial wall is transparent; usually only the column of blood is visible. The normal light reflex is narrow—about one-fourth the diameter of the blood column. Because the arterial wall is transparent, a vein crossing beneath the artery appears right up to the column of blood on either side.

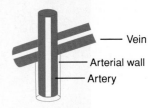

— Vein
— Arterial wall
— Artery

Retinal Arteries in Hypertension

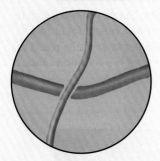

— Focal narrowing

— Narrowed column of blood
— Narrowed light reflex

In hypertension, increased pressure damages the vascular endothelium, leading to deposition of plasma macromolecules and thickening of the arterial wall, causing focal or generalized narrowing of the lumen and the light reflex.

Copper Wiring

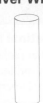

Sometimes the arteries, especially those close to the disc, become full and somewhat tortuous and develop an increased light reflex with a bright coppery luster, called *copper wiring.*

Silver Wiring

Occasionally the wall of a narrowed artery becomes opaque so there is no visible blood, called silver wiring.

AV Crossing

When the arterial walls lose their transparency, changes appear in the arteriovenous crossings. Decreased transparency of the retina probably also contributes to the first two changes shown below.

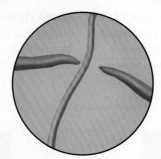

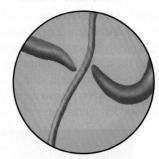

Concealment or AV Nicking. The vein appears to stop abruptly on either side of the artery.

Tapering. The vein appears to taper down on either side of the artery.

Banking. The vein is twisted on the distal side of the artery and forms a dark, wide knuckle

Table 7-15 Red Spots and Streaks in the Fundi

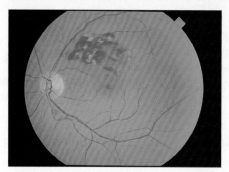
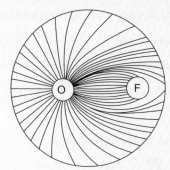

Superficial Retinal Hemorrhages. Small, linear, flame-shaped, red streaks in the fundi, shaped by the superficial bundles of nerve fibers that radiate from the optic disc in the pattern illustrated (O = optic disc; F = fovea). Sometimes the hemorrhages occur in clusters and look like a larger hemorrhage but can be identified by the linear streaking at the edges. These hemorrhages are seen in severe hypertension, papilledema, and occlusion of the retinal vein, among other conditions. An occasional superficial hemorrhage has a white center consisting of fibrin, which has many causes.

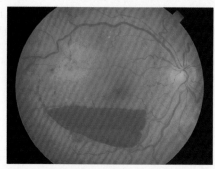
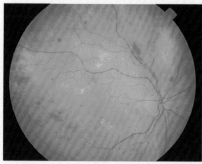

Preretinal Hemorrhage. Develops when blood escapes into the potential space between the retina and vitreous. This hemorrhage is typically larger than retinal hemorrhages. Because it is anterior to the retina, it obscures any underlying retinal vessels. In an erect patient, red cells settle, creating a horizontal line of demarcation between plasma above and cells below. Causes include a sudden increase in intracranial pressure.

Deep Retinal Hemorrhages. Small, rounded, slightly irregular red spots that are sometimes called dot or blot hemorrhages. They occur in a deeper layer of the retina than flame-shaped hemorrhages. Diabetes is a common cause.

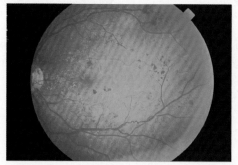
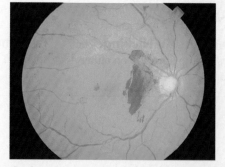

Microaneurysms. Tiny, round, red spots commonly seen in and around the macular area. They are minute dilatations of very small retinal vessels; the vascular connections are too small to be seen with an ophthalmoscope. A hallmark of diabetic retinopathy.

Neovascularization. Refers to the formation of new blood vessels. They are more numerous, more tortuous, and narrower than neighboring blood vessels in the area and form disorderly looking red arcades. A common feature of the proliferative stage of diabetic retinopathy. The vessels may grow into the vitreous, where retinal detachment or hemorrhage may cause loss of vision.

Source of photos: Tasman W, Jaeger E, eds. *The Wills Eye Hospital Atlas of Clinical Ophthalmology*, 2nd ed. Philadelphia: Lippincott Williams & Wilkins, 2001.

Table 7-16 Ocular Fundi: Normal and Hypertensive Retinopathy

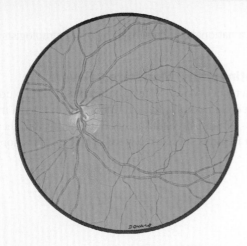

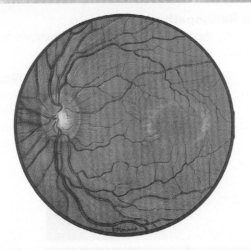

Normal Fundus of a Light-Skinned Person

Inspect the optic disc. Follow the major vessels in four directions, noting their relative sizes and any arteriovenous crossings—both are normal here. Inspect the macular area. The slightly darker fovea is just discernible; no light reflex is visible in this subject. Look for any lesions in the retina. Note the striped, or tessellated, character of the fundus, especially in the lower field, that comes from normal underlying choroidal vessels. The fundus of a light-skinned person with brunette coloring is redder.

Normal Fundus of a Dark-Skinned Person

Again, inspect the disc, vessels, macula, and retina. The ring around the fovea is a normal light reflection. The color of the fundus has a grayish brown, almost purplish cast, which comes from pigment in the retina and the choroid that characteristically obscures the choroidal vessels; no tessellation is visible.

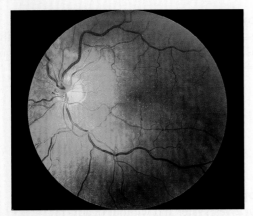

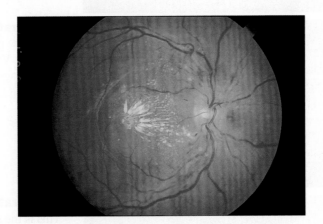

Hypertensive Retinopathy

Marked arteriolar-venous crossing changes are seen, especially along the inferior vessels. Copper wiring of the arterioles is present. A cotton-wool spot is seen just superior to the disc. Incidental disc drusen are also present but are unrelated to hypertension.

Hypertensive Retinopathy with Macular Star

Note the punctate exudates are readily visible: some are scattered; others radiate from the fovea to form a macular star. Note the two small, soft exudates about 1 disc diameter from the disc. Find the flame-shaped hemorrhages sweeping toward 7, 8, and 10 o'clock; a few more may be seen toward 10 o'clock. These two fundi show changes typical of severe hypertensive retinopathy, which is often accompanied by papilledema (p. 241).

Source of photos: *Hypertensive Retinopathy, Hypertensive Retinopathy with Macular Star*—Tasman W, Jaeger E, eds. *The Wills Eye Hospital Atlas of Clinical Ophthalmology*. 2nd ed. Philadelphia, PA: Lippincott Williams & Wilkins, 2001.

Source: Wong TY, Mitchell P. Hypertensive retinopathy. *N Engl J Med*. 2004;351:2310.

Table 7-17 Ocular Fundi: Diabetic Retinopathy

Diabetic Retinopathy

Study carefully the fundi in the series of photographs below. They represent a national standard used by ophthalmologists to assess diabetic retinopathy.[97, 98]

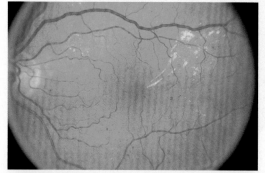

Nonproliferative Retinopathy, Moderately Severe

Note tiny red dots or microaneurysms. Note also the ring of hard exudates (white spots) located superotemporally. Retinal thickening or edema in the area of the hard exudates can impair visual acuity if it extends into the center of the macula. Detection requires specialized stereoscopic examination.

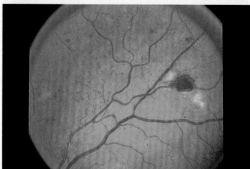

Nonproliferative Retinopathy, Severe

In the superior temporal quadrant, note the large retinal hemorrhage between two cotton-wool patches, beading of the retinal vein just above them, and tiny tortuous retinal vessels above the superior temporal artery.

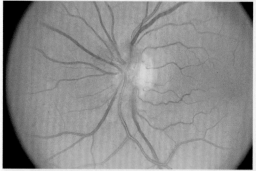

Proliferative Retinopathy, with Neovascularization

Note new preretinal vessels arising on the disc and extending across the disc margins. Visual acuity is still normal, but the risk for visual loss is high. Photocoagulation reduces this risk by >50%.

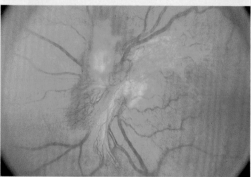

Proliferative Retinopathy, Advanced

This is the same eye, but 2 years later and without treatment. Neovascularization has increased, now with fibrous proliferations, distortion of the macula, and reduced visual acuity.

Source of photos: *Nonproliferative Retinopathy, Moderately Severe; Proliferative Retinopathy, With Neovascularization; Nonproliferative Retinopathy, Severe; Proliferative Retinopathy, Advanced*—Early Treatment Diabetic Retinopathy Study Research Group. Courtesy of MF Davis, MD, University of Wisconsin, Madison.

Source: Frank RB. Diabetic retinopathy. *N Engl J Med.* 2004;350:48.

Table 7-18 Light-Colored Spots in the Fundi

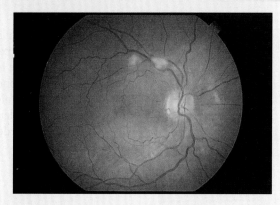

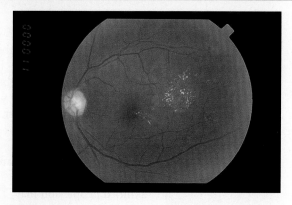

Soft Exudates: Cotton-Wool Patches

Cotton-wool patches are white or grayish, ovoid lesions with irregular "soft" borders. They are moderate in size but usually smaller than the disc. They result from extruded axoplasm from retinal ganglion cells caused by microinfarcts of the retinal nerve fiber layer. Seen in hypertension, diabetes, HIV and other viruses, and numerous other conditions.

Hard Exudates

Hard exudates are creamy or yellowish, often bright, lesions with well-defined "hard" borders. They are small and round but may coalesce into larger irregular spots. They often occur in clusters or in circular, linear, or star-shaped patterns. They are lipid residues of serous leakage from damaged capillaries. Causes include diabetes and vascular dysplasias.

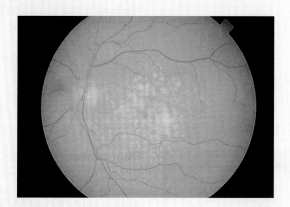

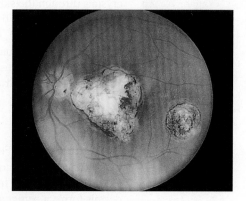

Drusen

Drusen are yellowish round spots that vary from tiny to small. The edges may be soft, as here, or hard (p. 242). They are haphazardly distributed but may concentrate at the posterior pole between the optic disc and the macula. Drusen consist of dead retinal pigment epithelial cells. Seen in normal aging and age-related macular degeneration.

Healed Chorioretinitis

Here inflammation has destroyed the superficial tissues to reveal a well-defined, irregular patch of white sclera marked with dark pigment. Size varies from small to very large. *Toxoplasmosis* is illustrated. Multiple, small, somewhat similar-looking areas may be due to laser treatments. Here there is also a temporal scar near the macula.

Source of photos: *Cotton-Wool Patches, Drusen, Healed Chorioretinitis*—Tasman W, Jaeger E, eds. *The Wills Eye Hospital Atlas of Clinical Ophthalmology*. 2nd ed. Philadelphia, PA: Lippincott Williams & Wilkins, 2001; *Hard Exudates*—Courtesy of Ken Freedman, MD. American Academy of Ophthalmology. Optic fundus signs. At http://www.aao.org/theeyeshaveit/optic-fundus/index.cfm. Accessed March 23, 2015.

Table 7-19 Lumps on or Near the Ear

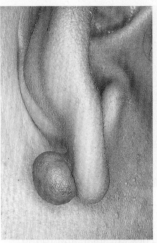

Keloid. A firm, nodular, hypertrophic mass of scar tissue extending beyond the area of injury. It may develop in any scarred area but is most common on the shoulders and upper chest. A keloid on a pierced earlobe may have unwanted cosmetic effects. Keloids are more common in darker-skinned people and may recur following treatment.

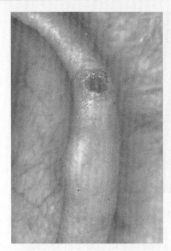

Chondrodermatitis Helicis. This chronic inflammatory lesion starts as a painful, tender papule on the helix or antihelix. Here the upper lesion is at a later stage of ulceration and crusting. Reddening may occur. Biopsy is needed to rule out carcinoma.

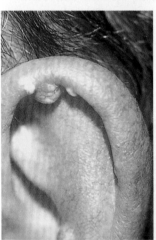

Tophi. A deposit of uric acid crystals characteristic of chronic tophaceous gout. It appears as hard nodules in the helix or antihelix and may discharge chalky white crystals through the skin. It also may appear near the joints, hands (p. 703), feet, and other areas. It usually develops after chronic sustained high blood levels of uric acid.

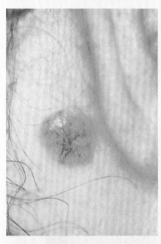

Basal Cell Carcinoma. This raised nodule shows the lustrous surface and telangiectatic vessels of basal cell carcinoma, a common slow-growing malignancy that rarely metastasizes. Growth and ulceration may occur. These are more frequent in fair-skinned people overexposed to sunlight.

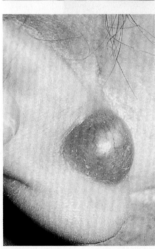

Cutaneous Cyst. Formerly called a *sebaceous cyst,* a dome-shaped lump in the dermis forms a benign closed firm sac attached to the epidermis. A dark dot (blackhead) may be visible on its surface. Histologically, it is usually either (1) an *epidermoid* cyst, common on the face and neck, or (2) a *pilar (trichilemmal)* cyst, common in the scalp. Both may become inflamed.

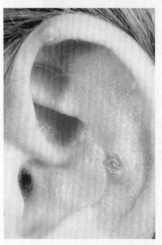

Rheumatoid Nodules. In chronic rheumatoid arthritis, look for small lumps on the helix or antihelix and additional nodules elsewhere on the hands and along the surface of the ulna distal to the elbow (p. 702), and on the knees and heels. Ulceration may result from repeated injuries. These nodules may antedate the arthritis.

Sources of photos: *Keloid*—Sams WM Jr, Lynch PJ, eds. *Principles and Practice of Dermatology.* Edinburgh: Churchill Livingstone, 1990; *Tophi*—du Vivier A. *Atlas of Clinical Dermatology.* 2nd ed. London, UK: Gower Medical Publishing, 1993; *Cutaneous Cyst, Chondrodermatitis Helicis*—Young EM, Newcomer VD, Kligman AM. *Geriatric Dermatology: Color Atlas and Practitioner's Guide.* Philadelphia, PA: Lea & Febiger, 1993; *Basal Cell Carcinoma*—Phillips T, Dover J. Recent Advances in Dermatology. *N Engl J Med.* 326:169–170, 1992; *Rheumatoid Nodules*—Champion RH, Burton JL, Ebling FJG, eds. *Rook/Wilkinson/Ebling Textbook of Dermatology.* 5th ed. Oxford, UK: Blackwell Scientific, 1992.

Table 7-20 Abnormalities of the Eardrum

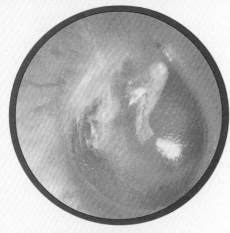

Normal Eardrum (Right)

This normal right eardrum the tympanic membrane, is pinkish gray. Note the malleus lying behind the upper part of the drum. Above the short process lies the *pars flaccida.* The remainder of the drum is the *pars tensa.* From the umbo, the bright cone of light fans anteriorly and downward. Posterior to the malleus, part of the incus is visible behind the drum. The small blood vessels along the handle of the malleus are normal.

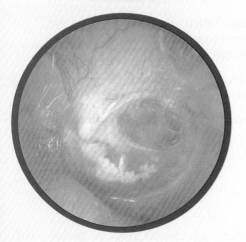

Perforation of the Eardrum

Perforations are holes in the eardrum, usually from purulent infections of the middle ear. They may be *central,* if not involving the margin of the drum, or *marginal,* when the margin is involved. The membrane covering the perforation may be notably thin and transparent.

The more common central perforation is illustrated here. A reddened ring of granulation tissue surrounds the perforation, indicating chronic infection. The eardrum itself is scarred, and no landmarks are visible. Discharge from the infected middle ear may drain out through the perforated opening, which often closes in the healing process, as in the next photo. There may be associated earache or even hearing loss, especially if the perforations are large.

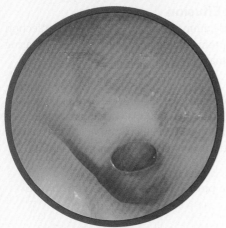

Tympanosclerosis

Tympanosclerosis is a scarring process of the middle ear from otitis media that involves deposition of hyaline and calcium and phosphate crystals in the eardrum and middle ear. When severe it may entrap the ossicles and cause conductive hearing loss.

In the inferior portion of this left eardrum, note the large, chalky white patch with irregular margins. It is typical of tympanosclerosis: a deposition of hyaline material within the layers of the tympanic membrane that sometimes follows a severe episode of otitis media. It does not usually impair hearing and is seldom clinically significant.

Other abnormalities in this eardrum include a *healed perforation* (the large oval area in the upper posterior drum) and signs of a *retracted drum.* A retracted drum is pulled medially, away from the examiner's eye, and the malleolar folds are tightened into sharp outlines. The short process often protrudes sharply, and the handle of the malleus, pulled inward at the umbo, looks foreshortened and more horizontal.

Sources of photos: *Normal Eardrum*—Hawke M, Keene M, Alberti PW. *Clinical Otoscopy: A Text and Colour Atlas.* Edinburgh: Churchill Livingstone, 1984; *Perforation of the Drum, Tympanosclerosis*—Courtesy of Michael Hawke, MD, Toronto, Canada.

(continued)

Table 7-20 Abnormalities of the Eardrum (*Continued*)

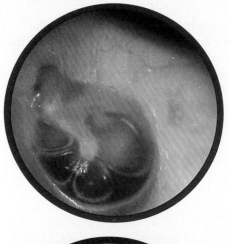

Serous Effusion

Serous effusions are usually caused by viral upper respiratory infections (*otitis media with serous effusion*) or by sudden changes in atmospheric pressure as from flying or diving (*otitic barotrauma*). The eustachian tube cannot equalize the air pressure in the middle ear and outside air. Air is absorbed from the middle ear into the bloodstream, and serous fluid accumulates in the middle ear instead. Symptoms include fullness and popping sensations in the ear, mild conduction hearing loss, and, sometimes, pain.

Amber fluid behind the eardrum is characteristic, as in this patient with otitic barotrauma. A fluid level, a line between air above and amber fluid below, can be seen on either side of the short process. Air bubbles (not always present) can be seen here within the amber fluid.

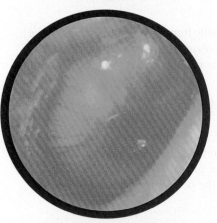

Acute Otitis Media with Purulent Effusion

Acute otitis media with purulent effusion is commonly caused by bacterial infection from *S. pneumoniae* or *H. influenzae*. Symptoms include earache, fever, and hearing loss. The eardrum reddens, loses its landmarks, and bulges laterally, toward the examiner's eye.

Here the eardrum is bulging, and most landmarks are obscured. Redness is most obvious near the umbo, but dilated vessels can be seen in all segments of the drum. A diffuse redness of the entire drum often develops. Spontaneous rupture (perforation) of the drum may follow, with discharge of purulent material into the ear canal.

Hearing loss is the conductive type. Acute purulent otitis media is much more common in children than in adults.

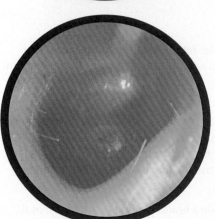

Bullous Myringitis

In bullous myringitis, painful hemorrhagic vesicles appear on the tympanic membrane, the ear canal, or both. Symptoms include earache, blood-tinged discharge from the ear, and conductive hearing loss.

In this right ear, at least two large vesicles (bullae) are discernible on the drum. The drum is reddened, and its landmarks are obscured.

This condition is caused by mycoplasma, viral, and bacterial otitis media.

Sources of photos: *Serous Effusion*—Hawke M, Keene M, Alberti PW. *Clinical Otoscopy: A Text and Colour Atlas*. Edinburgh: Churchill Livingstone, 1984; *Acute Otitis Media, Bullous Myringitis*—The Wellcome Trust, National Medical Slide Bank, London, UK.

Table 7-21 Patterns of Hearing Loss

	Conductive Loss	Sensorineural Loss
	Tympanic membrane / Middle ear / Cochlear nerve	Tympanic membrane / Middle ear / Cochlear nerve
Pathophysiology	External or middle ear disorder impairs sound conduction to inner ear. Causes include foreign body, *otitis media,* perforated eardrum, and otosclerosis of ossicles.	Inner ear disorder involves cochlear nerve and neuronal impulse transmission to the brain. Causes include loud noise exposure, inner ear infections, trauma, acoustic neuroma, congenital and familial disorders, and aging.
Usual Age of Onset	Childhood and young adulthood, up to age 40 years	Middle or later years
Ear Canal and Drum	Abnormality usually visible, except in otosclerosis	Problem not visible
Effects	Little effect on sound Hearing seems to improve in noisy environment Voice remains soft because inner ear and cochlear nerve are intact	Higher registers are lost, so sound may be distorted Hearing worsens in noisy environment Voice may be loud because hearing is difficult
Weber Test (in Unilateral Hearing Loss)	Tuning fork at vertex Sound lateralizes to *impaired ear*—room noise not well heard, so detection of vibrations *improves.*	Tuning fork at vertex Sound lateralizes to *good ear*—inner ear or cochlear nerve damage impairs transmission to affected ear.
Rinne Test	Tuning fork at external auditory meatus; then on mastoid bone BC longer than or equal to AC (BC ≥ AC). While air conduction through the external or middle ear is impaired, vibrations through bone bypass the problem to reach the cochlea.	Tuning fork at external auditory meatus; then on mastoid bone AC longer than BC (AC > BC). The inner ear or cochlear nerve is less able to transmit impulses regardless of how the vibrations reach the cochlea. The normal pattern prevails.

Table 7-22 Abnormalities of the Lips

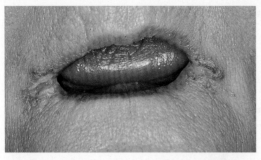

Angular Cheilitis

Angular cheilitis starts with softening of the skin at the angles of the mouth, followed by fissuring. It may be due to nutritional deficiency or, more commonly, to overclosure of the mouth, seen in people with no teeth or with ill-fitting dentures. Saliva wets and macerates the infolded skin, often leading to secondary infection with *Candida,* as seen here.

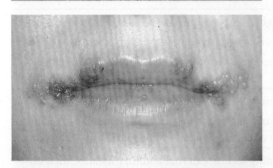

Actinic Cheilitis

Actinic cheilitis is a precancerous condition that results from excessive exposure to sunlight and affects primarily the lower lip. Fair-skinned men who work outdoors are most often affected. The lip loses its normal redness and may become scaly, somewhat thickened, and slightly everted. Solar damage predisposes to squamous cell carcinoma of the lip, so examine these skin lesions carefully.

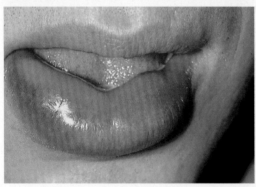

Herpes Simplex (*Cold Sore, Fever Blister*)

The herpes simplex virus (HSV) produces recurrent and painful vesicular eruptions of the lips and surrounding skin. A small cluster of vesicles first develops. As these break, yellow-brown crusts form. Healing takes 10 to 14 days. Both new and erupted vesicles are visible here.

Angioedema

Angioedema is a localized subcutaneous or submucosal swelling caused by leakage of intravascular fluid into interstitial tissue. Two types are common. When vascular permeability is triggered by mast cells in allergic and NSAID reactions, look for associated urticaria and pruritus. These are uncommon in angioedema from bradykinin and complement-derived mediators, the mechanism in ACE-inhibitor reactions. Angioedema is usually benign and resolves within 24 to 48 hours. It can be life threatening when it involves the larynx, tongue, or upper airway or develops into anaphylaxis.

Sources of photos: *Angular Cheilitis, Herpes Simplex, Angioedema*—Neville B, et al. *Color Atlas of Clinical Oral Pathology.* Philadelphia, PA: Lea & Febiger, 1991; Used with permission; *Actinic Cheilitis*—Langlais RP, Miller CS. *Color Atlas of Common Oral Diseases.* Philadelphia, PA: Lea & Febiger, 1992. Used with permission.

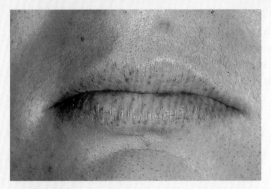

Hereditary Hemorrhagic Telangiectasia (Osler-Weber-Rendu syndrome)

Multiple small red spots on the lips strongly suggest hereditary hemorrhagic telangiectasia, an autosomal dominant endothelial disorder causing vascular fragility and arteriovascular malformations (AVMs). Telangiectasias are also visible on the oral mucosa, nasal septal mucosa, and fingertips. Nosebleeds, gastrointestinal bleeding, and iron deficiency anemia are common. AVMs in the lungs and brain can cause life-threatening hemorrhage and embolic disease.

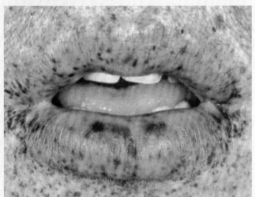

Peutz–Jeghers Syndrome

Look for prominent small brown pigmented spots in the dermal layer of the lips, buccal mucosa, and perioral area. These spots may also appear on the hands and feet. In this autosomal dominant syndrome, these characteristic skin changes accompany numerous intestinal polyps. The risk of gastrointestinal and other cancers ranges from 40% to 90%. Note that these spots rarely appear around the nose and mouth.

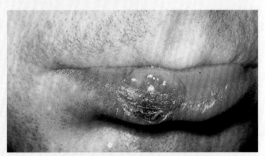

Chancre of Primary Syphilis

This ulcerated papule with an indurated edge usually appears after 3 to 6 weeks of incubating infection from the spirochete *Treponema pallidum*. These lesions may resemble a carcinoma or crusted cold sore. Similar primary lesions are common in the pharynx, anus, and vagina but may escape detection since they are painless, nonsuppurative, and usually heal spontaneously in 3 to 6 weeks. Wear gloves during palpation since these chancres are infectious.

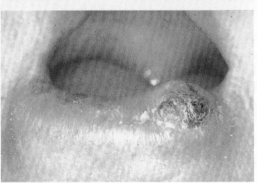

Carcinoma of the Lip

Like actinic cheilitis, squamous cell carcinoma usually affects the lower lip. It may appear as a scaly plaque, as an ulcer with or without a crust, or as a nodular lesion, as illustrated here. Fair skin and prolonged exposure to the sun are common risk factors.

Sources of photos: *Hereditary Hemorrhagic Telangiectasia*—Langlais RP, Miller CS. *Color Atlas of Common Oral Diseases*. Philadelphia, PA: Lea & Febiger, 1992; Used with permission; *Peutz-Jeghers Syndrome*—Robinson HBG, Miller AS. *Colby, Kerr, and Robinson's Color Atlas of Oral Pathology*. Philadelphia, PA: JB Lippincott, 1990; *Chancre of Syphilis*—Wisdom A. *A Colour Atlas of Sexually Transmitted Diseases*. 2nd ed. London: Wolfe Medical Publications, 1989; *Carcinoma of the Lip*—Tyldesley WR. *A Colour Atlas of Orofacial Diseases*. 2nd ed. London: Wolfe Medical Publications, 1991.

Table 7-23 Findings in the Pharynx, Palate, and Oral Mucosa

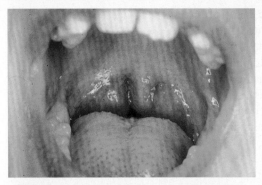

Large Normal Tonsils

Normal tonsils may be large without being infected, especially in children. They may protrude medially beyond the pillars and even to the midline. Here they touch the sides of the uvula and obscure the pharynx. Their color is pink. The white marks are light reflections, not exudate.

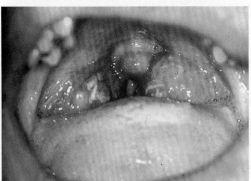

Exudative Tonsillitis

This red throat has a white exudate on the tonsils. This, together with fever and enlarged cervical nodes, increases the probability of *group A streptococcal infection* or *infectious mononucleosis*. Anterior cervical lymph nodes are usually enlarged in the former, posterior nodes in the latter.

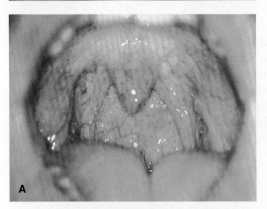

Pharyngitis

These two photos show reddened throats without exudate.
In **A**, redness and vascularity of the pillars and uvula are mild to moderate.

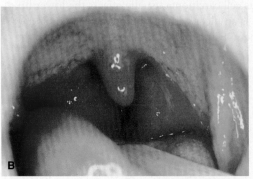

In **B**, redness is diffuse and intense. Each patient would probably complain of a sore throat, or at least a scratchy one. Causes are both viral and bacterial. If the patient has no fever, exudate, or enlargement of cervical lymph nodes, the chances of infection by either of two common causes—*Group A streptococci* and *Epstein-Barr virus* (infectious mononucleosis)—are reduced.

Sources of photos: *Large Normal Tonsils, Exudative Tonsillitis, Pharyngitis [A and B]*—The Wellcome Trust, National Medical Slide Bank, London, UK.

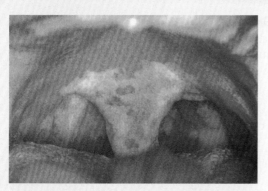

Diphtheria

Diphtheria, an acute infection caused by *Corynebacterium diphtheriae,* is now rare but still important. Prompt diagnosis may lead to life-saving treatment. The throat is dull red, and a gray exudate (pseudomembrane) is present on the uvula, pharynx, and tongue. The airway may become obstructed. Prompt diagnosis may lead to life-saving treatment.

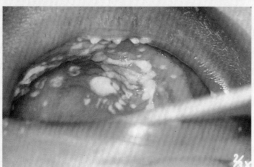

Thrush on the Palate (Candidiasis)

Thrush is a yeast infection from *Candida* species. Shown here on the palate, it may appear elsewhere in the mouth (see p. 297). Thick, white plaques are somewhat adherent to the underlying mucosa. Predisposing factors include (1) prolonged treatment with antibiotics or corticosteroids and (2) AIDS.

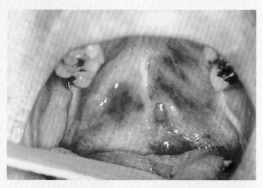

Kaposi Sarcoma in AIDS

The deep purple color of these lesions suggests Kaposi sarcoma, a low-grade vascular tumor associated with human herpesvirus 8. The lesions may be raised or flat. About a third of patients with Kaposi sarcoma have lesions in the oral cavity; other affected sites are the gastrointestinal tract and the lungs. Antiretroviral therapy has markedly reduced the prevalence of this disease.

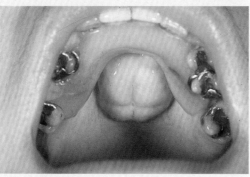

Torus Palatinus

A torus palatinus is a midline bony growth in the hard palate that is fairly common in adults. Its size and lobulation vary. Although alarming at first glance, it is harmless. In this example, an upper denture has been fitted around the torus.

Sources of photos: *Diphtheria*—Harnisch JP, et al. Diphtheria among alcoholic urban adults. *Ann Intern Med.* 1989;111:77; *Thrush on the Palate*—The Wellcome Trust, National Medical Slide Bank, London, UK; *Kaposi's Sarcoma in AIDS*—Ioachim HL. *Textbook and Atlas of Disease Associated with Acquired Immune Deficiency Syndrome.* London: Gower Medical Publishing, 1989.

(continued)

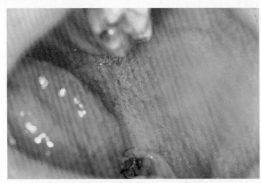

Fordyce Spots (*Fordyce Granules*)

Fordyce spots are normal sebaceous glands that appear as small yellowish spots in the buccal mucosa or on the lips. Here they are seen best anterior to the tongue and lower jaw. These spots are usually not numerous.

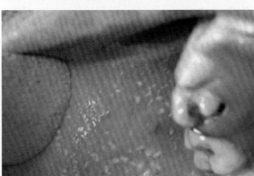

Koplik Spots

Koplik spots are an early sign of measles (rubeola). Search for small white specks that resemble grains of salt on a red background. They usually appear on the buccal mucosa near the first and second molars. In this photo, look also in the upper third of the mucosa. The rash of measles appears within a day.

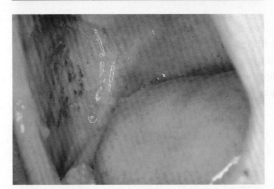

Petechiae

Petechiae are small red spots caused by blood that escapes from capillaries into the tissues. Petechiae in the buccal mucosa, as shown, are often caused by accidentally biting the cheek. Oral petechiae may be due to infection or decreased platelets, and trauma.

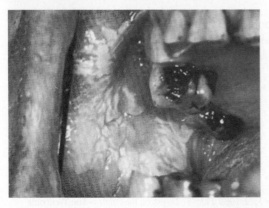

Leukoplakia

A thickened white patch (*leukoplakia*) may occur anywhere in the oral mucosa. The extensive example shown on this buccal mucosa resulted from frequent chewing of tobacco, a local irritant. This benign reactive process of the squamous epithelium may lead to cancer and should be biopsied. Another risk factor is human papillomavirus infection.

Table 7-24 Findings in the Gums and Teeth

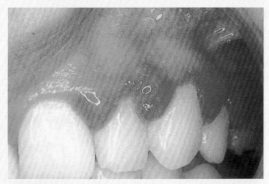

Marginal Gingivitis

Marginal gingivitis is common during adolescence, early adulthood, and pregnancy. The gingival margins are reddened and swollen, and the interdental papillae are blunted, swollen, and red. Brushing the teeth often makes the gums bleed. *Plaque*—the soft white film of salivary salts, protein, and bacteria that covers the teeth and leads to gingivitis—is not readily visible.

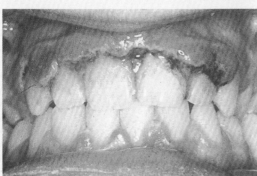

Acute Necrotizing Ulcerative Gingivitis

This uncommon form of gingivitis occurs suddenly in adolescents and young adults and is accompanied by fever, malaise, and enlarged lymph nodes. Ulcers develop in the interdental papillae. Then the destructive (necrotizing) process spreads along the gum margins, where a grayish pseudomembrane develops. The red, painful gums bleed easily; the breath is foul.

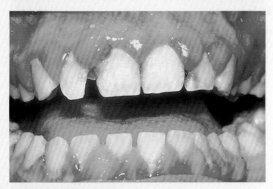

Gingival Hyperplasia

Gums enlarged by hyperplasia are swollen into heaped-up masses that may even cover the teeth. The redness of inflammation may coexist, as in this example. Causes include phenytoin therapy (as in this case), puberty, pregnancy, and leukemia.

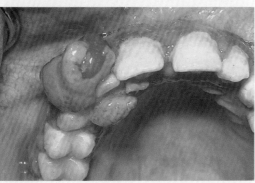

Pregnancy Tumor (*Pregnancy Epulis* or *Pyogenic Granuloma*)

Red purple papules of granulation tissue form in the gingival interdental papillae, in the nasal cavity, and sometimes on the fingers. They are red, soft, painless, and usually bleed easily. They occur in 1% to 5% of pregnancies and usually regress after delivery. Note the accompanying gingivitis.

Sources of photos: *Marginal Gingivitis, Acute Necrotizing Ulcerative Gingivitis*—Tyldesley WR. *A Colour Atlas of Orofacial Diseases.* 2nd ed. London: Wolfe Medical Publications, 1991; *Gingival Hyperplasia*—Courtesy of Dr. James Cottone; *Pregnancy Tumor*—Langlais RP, Miller CS. *Color Atlas of Common Oral Diseases.* Philadelphia, PA: Lea & Febiger, 1992. Used with permission.

(continued)

Table 7-24 Findings in the Gums and Teeth (*Continued*)

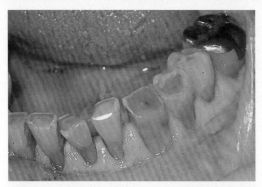

Attrition of Teeth; Recession of Gums

In many elderly people, the chewing surfaces of the teeth are worn down by repetitive use so that the yellow-brown dentin becomes exposed—a process called *attrition*. Note also the *recession of the gums*, which has exposed the roots of the teeth, giving a "long in the tooth" appearance.

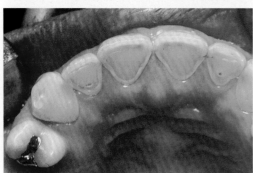

Erosion of Teeth

Teeth may be eroded by chemical action. Note here the erosion of the enamel from the lingual surfaces of the upper incisors, exposing the yellow-brown dentin. This results from recurrent regurgitation of stomach contents, as in bulimia.

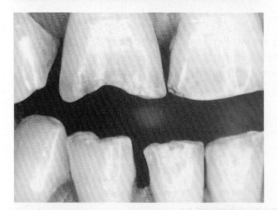

Abrasion of Teeth with Notching

The biting surface of the teeth may become abraded or notched by recurrent trauma, such as holding nails or opening bobby pins between the teeth. Unlike Hutchinson teeth, the sides of these teeth show normal contours; size and spacing of the teeth are unaffected.

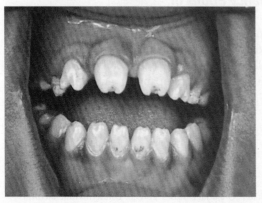

Hutchinson Teeth in Congenital Syphilis

Hutchinson teeth are smaller and more widely spaced than normal and are notched on their biting surfaces. The sides of the teeth taper toward the biting edges. The upper central incisors of the permanent (not the deciduous) teeth are most often affected. These teeth are a sign of congenital syphilis.

Sources of photos: *Attrition of Teeth, Erosion of Teeth*—Langlais RP, Miller CS. *Color Atlas of Common Oral Diseases*. Philadelphia, PA: Lea & Febiger, 1992. Used with permission; *Abrasion of Teeth, Hutchinson Teeth*—Robinson HBG, Miller AS. *Colby, Kerr, and Robinson's Color Atlas of Oral Pathology*. Philadelphia, PA: JB Lippincott, 1990.

Table 7-25 Findings in or Under the Tongue

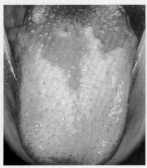

Geographic Tongue. In this benign condition, the dorsum shows scattered smooth red areas denuded of papillae. Together with the normal rough and coated areas, they give a maplike pattern that changes over time.

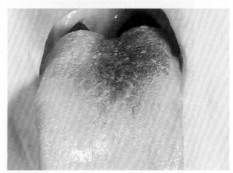

Black Hairy Tongue. Note the "hairy" yellowish to brown and black hypertrophied and elongated papillae on the tongue's dorsum. This benign condition is associated with *Candida* and bacterial overgrowth, antibiotic therapy, and poor dental hygiene. It also may occur spontaneously.

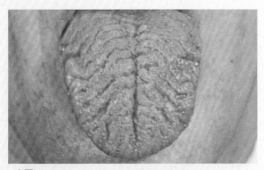

Fissured Tongue. Fissures appear with increasing age, sometimes termed *furrowed tongue*. Food debris may accumulate in the crevices and become irritating, but a fissured tongue is benign.

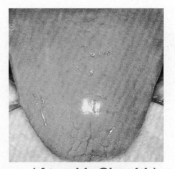

Smooth Tongue (*Atrophic Glossitis*). A smooth and often sore tongue that has lost its papillae, sometimes just in patches, suggests a deficiency in riboflavin, niacin, folic acid, vitamin B_{12}, pyridoxine, or iron, or treatment with chemotherapy.

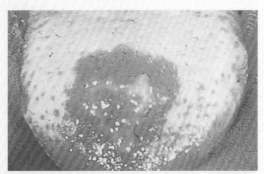

Candidiasis. Note the thick white coating from *Candida* infection. The raw red surface is where the coat was scraped off. Infection may also occur without the white coating. It is seen in immunosuppression from chemotherapy or prednisone therapy.

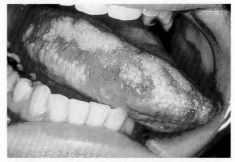

Oral Hairy Leukoplakia. These whitish raised asymptomatic plaques with a feathery or corrugated pattern occur most often on the sides of the tongue. Unlike candidiasis, these areas cannot be scraped off. This condition is caused by Epstein-Barr virus infection and is seen in HIV and AIDS infection.

(continued)

Table 7-25 Findings in or Under the Tongue (*Continued*)

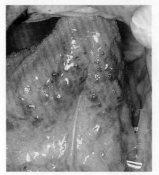

Varicose Veins. Small purplish or blue-black round swellings appear under the tongue with age. These dilatations of the lingual veins have no clinical significance.

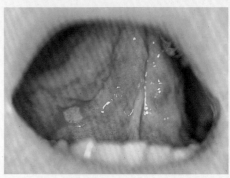

Aphthous Ulcer (*Canker Sore*). A painful, shallow whitish-gray oval ulceration surrounded by a halo of reddened mucosa. It may be single or multiple and may also occur on the gingiva and oral mucosa. It heals in 7–10 days, but may recur, as in Bechet disease.

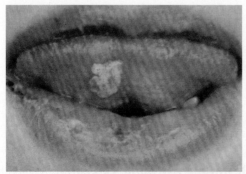

Mucous Patch of Syphilis. This painless lesion of secondary syphilis is highly infectious. It is slightly raised, oval, and covered by a grayish membrane. It may be multiple and occur elsewhere in the mouth.

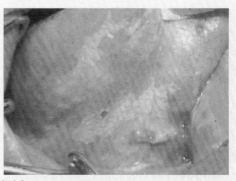

Leukoplakia. With this persisting painless white patch in the oral mucosa, the undersurface of the tongue appears painted white. Patches of any size raise the possibility of squamous cell carcinoma and require biopsy.

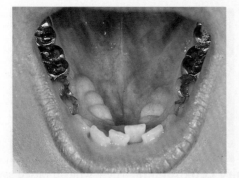

Tori Mandibulares. Rounded bony growths on the inner surfaces of the mandible are typically bilateral, asymptomatic, and harmless.

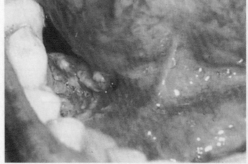

Carcinoma, Floor of the Mouth. This ulcerated lesion is in a common location for carcinoma. Medially, note the reddened area of mucosa, called *erythroplakia*, that is suspicious for malignancy and should be biopsied.

Sources of photos: *Fissured Tongue, Candidiasis, Mucous Patch, Leukoplakia, Carcinoma*—Robinson HBG, Miller AS. *Colby, Kerr, and Robinson's Color Atlas of Oral Pathology.* Philadelphia, PA: JB Lippincott, 1990; *Smooth Tongue*—Courtesy of Dr. R. A. Cawson, from Cawson RA. *Oral Pathology*, 1st ed. London: Gower Medical Publishing, 1987; *Geographic Tongue*—The Wellcome Trust, National Medical Slide Bank, London, UK; *Hairy Leukoplakia*—Ioachim HL. *Textbook and Atlas of Disease Associated With Acquired Immune Deficiency Syndrome.* London: Gower Medical Publishing, 1989; *Varicose Veins*—Neville B, et al. *Color Atlas of Clinical Oral Pathology.* Philadelphia, PA: Lea & Febiger, 1991. Used with permission.

Table 7-26 Thyroid Enlargement and Function

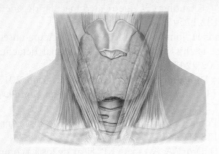

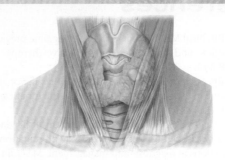

Diffuse Enlargement. Includes the isthmus and lateral lobes; there are no discretely palpable nodules. Causes include Graves disease, Hashimoto thyroiditis, and endemic goiter.

Single Nodule. May be a cyst, a benign tumor, or one nodule within a multinodular gland. It raises the question of malignancy. Risk factors are prior irradiation, hardness, rapid growth, fixation to surrounding tissues, enlarged cervical nodes, and occurrence in men.

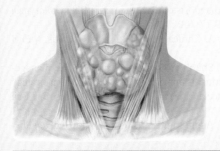

Multinodular Goiter. An enlarged thyroid gland with two or more nodules suggests a metabolic rather than a neoplastic process. Positive family history and continuing nodular enlargement are additional risk factors for malignancy.

Table 7-27 Symptoms and Signs of Thyroid Dysfunction

	Hyperthyroidism	Hypothyroidism
Symptoms	Nervousness	Fatigue, lethargy
	Weight loss despite increased appetite	Modest weight gain with anorexia
	Excessive sweating and heat intolerance	Dry, coarse skin and cold intolerance
	Palpitations	Swelling of face, hands, and legs
	Frequent bowel movements	Constipation
	Tremor and proximal muscle weakness	Weakness, muscle cramps, arthralgias, paresthesias, impaired memory and hearing
Signs	Warm, smooth, moist skin	Dry, coarse, cool skin, sometimes yellowish from carotene, with nonpitting myxedema and loss of hair
	With Graves disease, eye signs such as stare, lid lag, and exophthalmos	Periorbital myxedema
	Increased systolic and decreased diastolic blood pressures	Low-pitched speech
	Tachycardia or atrial fibrillation	Decreased systolic and increased diastolic blood pressures
	Hyperdynamic cardiac pulsations with an accentuated S_1	Bradycardia and, in late stages, hypothermia
	Tremor and proximal muscle weakness	Sometimes decreased intensity of heart sounds
		Prolonged relaxation phase during ankle reflex
		Impaired memory, mixed hearing loss, somnolence, peripheral neuropathy, carpal tunnel syndrome

Sources: Siminoski K. Does this patient have a goiter? *JAMA.* 1995;273:813. McDermott MT. In the clinic: hypothyroidism. *Ann Intern Med.* 2009;151:ITC6–1; McDermott MT. In the clinic: hyperthyroidism. *Ann Intern Med.* 2012;157:ITC1–1. Franklyn JA. Subclinical thyroid disorders—consequences and implications for treatment. *Ann Endocrinol.* 2007;68:229.

References

1. Lipton RB, Bigal ME, Diamond M, et al. Migraine prevalence, disease burden, and the need for preventative therapy. *Neurology.* 2007;68:343.

2. Lipton RB, Stewart WF, Seymour D, et al. Prevalence and burden of migraine in the United States: data from the American Migraine Study II. *Headache.* 2001;41:646.

3. Hale N, Paauw DS. Diagnosis and treatment of headache in the ambulatory care setting: a review of classic presentations and new considerations in diagnosis and management. *Med Clin North Am.* 2014;98:505.

4. Lipton RB, Bigal ME, Steiner TJ, et al. Classification of primary headaches. *Neurology.* 2004;63:427.

5. Headache Classification Committee of the International Headache Society (IHS). The International Classification of Headache Disorders, 3rd edition (beta version). *Cephalalgia.* 2013;33:629.

6. Hainer B, Matheson E. Approach to acute headache in adults. *Am Fam Physician.* 2013;87:682.

7. Sun-Edelstein C, Bigal ME, Rappoport AM. Chronic migraine and medication overuse headache: clarifying the current International Headache Society classification criteria. *Cephalalgia.* 2009;29:445.

8. Fumal A, Schoenen J. Tension-type headache: current research and clinical management. *Lancet Neurol.* 2008;7:70.

9. Olesen J, Steiner T, Bousser MG, et al. Proposals for new standardized general diagnostic criteria for the secondary headaches. *Cephalalgia.* 2009;29:1331.

10. Schwedt TJ, Matharu MS, Dodick DW. Thunderclap headache. *Lancet Neurol.* 2006;5:621.

11. McGregor EA. In the clinic: migraine. *Ann Intern Med.* 2013; 159:ITC5–1.

12. World Health Organization. *Medical Eligibility Criteria For Contraceptive Use.* 4th ed. Geneva: World Health Organization; 2010. Available at: http://www.who.int/reproductivehealth/publications/family_planning/9789241563888/en/. Accessed March 26, 2015.

13. Spector JT, Kahn SR, Jones MR, et al. Migraine headache and ischemic stroke risk: an updated meta-analysis. *Am J Med.* 2010; 123:612.

14. Harris M, Kaneshiro B. An evidence-based approach to hormonal contraception and headaches. *Contraception.* 2009;80:417.

15. Kurth T, Slomke MA, Kase CS, et al. Migraine, headache, and the risk of stroke in women: a prospective study. *Neurology.* 2005;64:1020.

16. Dodick DW. Chronic daily headache. *N Engl J Med.* 2006;354:158.

17. Gardner K. Genetics of migraine: an update. *Headache.* 2006;46:S19.

18. Shingleton BJ, O'Donoghue MW. Blurred vision. *N Engl J Med.* 2000;343:556.

19. Patel K, Patel S. Angle-closure glaucoma. *Dis Mon.* 2014;60:254.

20. Hollands H, Johnson D, Hollands S, et al. Do findings on routine examination identify patients at risk for primary open-angle glaucoma? The rational clinical examination systematic review. *JAMA.* 2013;309:2035.

21. Graves J, Balcer LJ. Eye disorders in patients with multiple sclerosis: natural history and management. *Clin Ophthalmol.* 2010;4:1409.

22. Dooley MC, Foroozan R. Optic neuritis. *J Ophthalmic Vis Res.* 2010;5:182.

23. Balcer LJ. Optic neuritis. *N Engl J Med.* 2006;354:1273.

24. Noble J, Chaudhary V. Age-related macular degeneration. *CMAJ.* 2010;182:1759.

25. Hollands H, Johnson D, Brox AC, et al. Acute-onset floaters and flashes: is this patient at risk for retinal detachment? *JAMA.* 2009;302:2243.

26. Meltzer DI. Painless red eye. *Am Fam Physician.* 2013;88:533.

27. Singh M, Sanborn A. Painful red eye. *Am Fam Physician.* 2013;87:127.

28. Uy J, Forciea MA. In the clinic. Hearing loss. *Ann Intern Med.* 2013;158:ITC4–1.

29. Raviv D, Dror AA, Avraham KB. Hearing loss: a common disorder caused by many rare alleles. *Ann N Y Acad Sci.* 2010;1214:168.

30. Pichichero ME. Otitis media. *Pediatr Clin North Am.* 2013;60:391.

31. Baguley D, McFerran D, Hall D. Tinnitus. *Lancet.* 2013 382(9904):1600.

32. Chan Y. Differential diagnosis of dizziness. *Curr Opin Otolaryngol Head Neck Surg.* 2009;17:200.

33. Wheatley LM, Togias A. Clinical Practice. Allergic rhinitis. *N Engl J Med.* 2015;372:456.

34. Foden N, Burgess C, Shepherd K, et al. A guide to the management of acute rhinosinusitis in primary care: management strategy based on best evidence and recent European guidelines. *Br J Gen Pract.* 2013;63:611.

35. Aring AM, Chan MM. Acute rhinosinusitis in adults. *Am Fam Physician.* 2011;83:1057.

36. Dykewicz MS, Hamilos DL. Rhinitis and sinusitis. *J Allergy Clin Immunol.* 2010;125(2 Suppl 2):S103.

37. McIsaac WJ, Kellner JD, Aufricht P, et al. Empirical validation of guidelines for the management of pharyngitis in children and adults. *JAMA.* 2004;291:1587.

38. Shulman ST, Bisno AL, Clegg HW, et al. Clinical practice guideline for the diagnosis and management of Group A Streptococcal pharyngitis: 2012 Update by the Infectious Diseases Society of America. *Clin Infect Dis.* 2012;55:1279.

39. Wessels MR. Streptococcal pharyngitis. *N Engl J Med.* 2011;364:648.

40. Schwartz SR, Cohen SM, Dailey SH, et al. Clinical practice guideline: hoarseness (dysphonia). *Otolaryngol Head Neck Surg.* 2009;141(3 Suppl 2):S1.

41. Vitale S, Cotch MF, Sperduto RD. Prevalence of visual impairment in the United States. *JAMA.* 2006;295:2158.

42. Chou CF, Cotch MF, Vitale S, et al. Age-related eye diseases and visual impairment among U.S. adults. *Am J Prev Med.* 2013;45:29.

43. U.S. Preventive Services Task Force. Screening for impaired visual acuity in older adults: recommendation statement. *Ann Intern Med.* 2009;151:37, W10.

44. American Academy of Ophthalmology Preferred Practice Patterns Committee. *Preferred Practice Pattern Guideline. Comprehensive Adult Medical Eye Evaluation.* San Francisco, CA: American Academy of Ophthalmology; 2010. Available at http://one.aao.org/preferred-practice-pattern/comprehensive-adult-medical-eye-evaluationoctobe. Accessed March 28, 2015.

45. Vajaranant TS, Wu S, Torres M, et al. The changing face of primary open-angle glaucoma in the United States: demographic and geographic changes from 2011 to 2050. *Am J Ophthalmol.* 2012;154:303.

46. Moyer VA. U.S. Preventive Services Task Force Recommendation Statement: Screening for glaucoma. *Ann Intern Med.* 2013;159:484.

REFERENCES

47. American Academy of Ophthalmology, Screening for Diabetic Retinopathy 2014—Information Statement. November 2006. Updated October 2014. At http://one.aao.org/clinical-statement/screening-diabetic-retinopathy–june-2012. Accessed March 23, 2015.

48. Roberts JE. Ultraviolet radiation as a risk factor for cataract and macular degeneration. *Eye Contact Lens.* 2011;37:246.

49. Ventry IM, Weinstein BE. Identification of elderly people with hearing problems. *ASHA.* 1983;25:37.

50. Moyer VA. U.S. Preventive Services Task Force recommendation statement: Screening for hearing loss in older adults. *Ann Intern Med.* 2012;157:655.

51. Centers for Disease Control and Prevention. Untreated dental caries (cavities) in children ages 2–19, United States. Updated February 2011. Available at http://www.cdc.gov/Features/dsUntreatedCavitiesKids/. Accessed March 28, 2015.

52. Centers for Disease Control and Prevention. Oral health for adults. Updated July 2013. Available at http://www.cdc.gov/oralhealth/children_adults/adults.htm. Accessed March 28, 2015.

53. Eke PI, Dye BA, Wei L, et al. Prevalence of periodontitis in adults in the United States: 2009 and 2010. *J Dent Res.* 2012;91:914.

54. Siegel R, Ma J, Zou Z, Jemal A. Cancer statistics, 2014. *CA Cancer J Clin.* 2014;64:9.

55. Moyer VA. U.S. Preventive Services Task Force recommendation statement: Screening for oral cancer. *Ann Intern Med.* 2014; 160:55.

56. Cleveland JL, Junger ML, Saraiya M, et al. The connection between human papillomavirus and oropharyngeal squamous cell carcinomas in the United States: implications for dentistry. *J Am Dent Assoc.* 2011;142:915.

57. Gillison ML, Broutian T, Pickard RK, et al. Prevalence of oral HPV infection in the United States, 2009–2010. *JAMA.* 2012;307:693.

58. Rethman MP, Carpenter W, Cohen EE, et al. Evidence-based clinical recommendations regarding screening for oral squamous cell carcinomas. *J Am Dent Assoc.* 2010;141:509.

59. Harper RA. *Basic Ophthalmology.* 9th ed. San Francisco, CA: American Academy of Ophthalmology; 2010.

60. Kerr NM, Chew SS, Eady EK, et al. Diagnostic accuracy of confrontation visual field tests. *Neurology.* 2010;74:1184.

61. McGee S. *Evidence Based Physical Diagnosis.* 3rd ed. St. Louis, MO: Elsevier; 2012:516–520.

62. Goodwin D. Homonymous hemianopia: challenges and solutions. *Clin Ophthalmol.* 2014;8:1919.

63. McGee S. *Evidence Based Physical Diagnosis.* 3rd ed. St. Louis, MO: Elsevier; 2012:161.

64. Morgan WH, Lind CR, Kain S. Retinal vein pulsation is in phase with intracranial pressure and not intraocular pressure. *Invest Ophthalmol Vis Sci.* 2012;53:4676.

65. Jacks AS, Miller NR. Spontaneous retinal venous pulsation: aetiology and significance. *J Neurol Neurosurg Psychiatry.* 2004;74:7.

66. Bagai A, Thavendiranathan P, Detsky AS. Does this patient have hearing impairment? *JAMA.* 2006;295:416.

67. McShefferty D, Whitmer WM, Swan IR, et al. The effect of experience on the sensitivity and specificity of the whispered voice test: a diagnostic accuracy study. *BMJ Open.* 2013;3(4). doi: 10.1136/bmjopen-2012–002394.

68. Pirozzo S, Papinczak T, Glasziou P. Whispered voice test for screening for hearing impairment in adults and children: systematic review. *BMJ.* 2003;327:967.

69. Eekhof JA, de Bock GH, de Laat JA, et al. The whispered voice: the best test for screening for hearing impairment in general practice? *Br J Gen Pract.* 1996;46:473.

70. McGee S. *Evidence Based Physical Diagnosis.* 3rd ed. St. Louis, MO: Elsevier; 2012:190.

71. Kaplan A. Canadian guidelines for acute bacterial rhinosinusitis: clinical summary. *Can Fam Physician.* 2014;60:227.

72. Neville BW, Day TA. Oral cancer and precancerous lesions. *CA Cancer J Clin.* 2002;52:195.

73. Brocklehurst P, Kujan O, O'Malley LA, et al. Screening programmes for the early detection and prevention of oral cancer. *Cochrane Database Syst Rev.* 2013;(11):CD004150.

74. Lestón J, Dios DP. Diagnostic clinical aids in oral cancer. *Oral Oncol.* 2010;46:418.

75. Gonsalves WC, Chi AC, Neville BW. Common oral lesions: Part I. Superficial mucosal lesions; Part II: Masses and neoplasia. *Am Fam Physician.* 2007;75:501, 507.

76. Reamy BV, Derby R, Bunt CW. Common tongue conditions in primary care. *Am Fam Physician.* 2010;81(5):627.

77. Kociolek LK, Shulman ST. In the clinic: pharyngitis. *Ann Intern Med.* 2012;157:ITC3–1.

78. Bitner MD, Capes JP, Houry DE. Images in emergency medicine. Adult epiglottitis. *Ann Emerg Med.* 2007;49:560.

79. Bahn RS, Castro MR. Approach to the patient with nontoxic multinodular goiter. *J Clin Endocrinol Metab.* 2011;96:1202.

80. Syrenicz A, Koziołek M, Ciechanowicz A, et al. New insights into the diagnosis of nodular goiter. *Thyroid Res.* 2014;7:6.

81. Siminoski K. Does this patient have a goiter? *JAMA.* 1995;273:813.

82. White ML, Doherty GM, Gauger PG. Evidence-based surgical management of substernal goiter. *World J Surg.* 2008;32:1285.

83. De Filippis EA, Sabet A, Sun MR, et al. Pemberton's sign: explained nearly 70 years later. *J Clin Endocrinol Metab.* 2014;99:1949.

84. Almandoz JP, Gharib H. Hypothyroidism: etiology, diagnosis, and management. *Med Clin North Am.* 2012;96:203.

85. Garber JR, Cobin RH, Gharib H, et al. Clinical practice guidelines for hypothyroidism in adults: cosponsored by the American Association of Clinical Endocrinologists and the American Thyroid Association.; American Association of Clinical Endocrinologists and American Thyroid Association Taskforce on Hypothyroidism in Adults. *Endocr Pract.* 2012;18:988.

86. McDermott MT. In the clinic: hypothyroidism. *Ann Intern Med.* 2009;151:ITC6–1.

87. Bahn RS, Burch HB, Cooper DS, et al. American Thyroid Association; American Association of Clinical Endocrinologists. Hyperthyroidism and other causes of thyrotoxicosis: management guidelines of the American Thyroid Association and American Association of Clinical Endocrinologists. *Endocr Pract.* 2011;17:456.

88. McDermott MT. In the clinic: hyperthyroidism. *Ann Intern Med.* 2012;157:ITC1–1.

89. Franklyn JA. Subclinical thyroid disorders—consequences and implications for treatment. *Ann Endocrinol.* 2007;68:229.

90. Durante C, Costante G, Lucisano G, et al. The natural history of benign thyroid nodules. *JAMA.* 2015;313:926.

91. Popoveniuc G, Jonklaas J. Thyroid nodules. *Med Clin North Am.* 2012;96:329.

92. Bahn RS. Mechanisms of disease: Graves' ophthalmopathy. *N Engl J Med.* 2010;362:726.

93. Phelps PO, Williams K. Thyroid eye disease for the primary care physician. *Dis Mon.* 2014;60:292.

94. Bartalena L, Tanda LM. Graves' ophthalmopathy. *N Engl J Med.* 2009;380:994.

95. Birkholz ES, Oetting TA. Kayser Fleischer Ring: A systems based review of the ophthalmologist's role in the diagnosis of Wilson's disease. EyeRounds.org. July 28 2009. Available at http://webeye.ophth.uiowa.edu/eyeforum/cases/97-kayser-fleischer-ring-wilsons-disease.htm. Accessed March 29, 2015.

96. Sullivan CA, Chopdar A, Shun-Shin GA. Dense Kayser-Fleischer ring in asymptomatic Wilson's disease (hepatolenticular degeneration). *Br J Ophthalmol.* 2002;86:114.

97. Early Treatment Diabetic Retinopathy Study Research Group. Grading diabetic retinopathy from stereoscopic color fundus photographs—an extension of the modified Airlie House classification. *Ophthalmology.* 1991;98:786.

98. Antonetti DA, Klein R, Gardner TW. Diabetic retinopathy—mechanisms of disease. *N Engl J Med.* 2012;366:1237.

99. McGee S. *Evidence Based Physical Diagnosis,* 3rd ed. St. Louis, MO: Elsevier; 2012:208.

100. McGee S. *Evidence Based Physical Diagnosis,* 3rd ed. St. Louis, MO: Elsevier; 2012:163–179

The Thorax and Lungs

The Bates' suite offers these additional resources to enhance learning and facilitate understanding of this chapter:

- Bates' *Pocket Guide to Physical Examination and History Taking*, 8th edition
- Bates' *Visual Guide to Physical Examination* (Vol. 9: Thorax and Lungs)
- thePoint online resources, for students and instructors: http://thepoint.lww.com

Anatomy and Physiology

Study the *anatomy of the chest wall,* identifying the structures illustrated (Fig. 8-1). Note that the number of the intercostal space between two ribs is the same number as the rib above it.

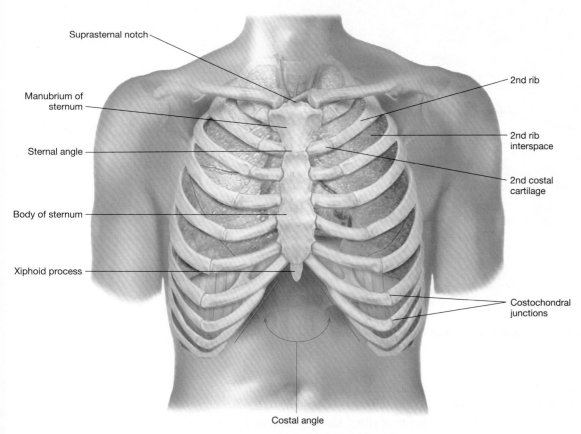

FIGURE 8-1. **Chest wall anatomy.**

Locating Findings on the Chest

Describe chest findings in two dimensions: along the vertical axis and around the circumference of the chest.

Vertical Axis.   To locate findings in the thorax, learn to number the ribs and intercostal spaces (Fig. 8-2). Place your finger in the hollow curve of the suprasternal notch, then move it down approximately 5 cm to the horizontal bony ridge where the manubrium joins the body of the sternum, called the *sternal angle* or the *angle of Louis*. Directly adjacent to the sternal angle is the 2nd rib and its costal cartilage. From here, using two fingers, "walk down" the interspaces *on an oblique line,* illustrated by the red numbers below. (Note that the ribs at the lower edge of the sternum may be too close together to count correctly.) To count the intercostal spaces in a woman, displace the breast laterally or palpate more medially. Avoid pressing too hard on the tender breast tissue.

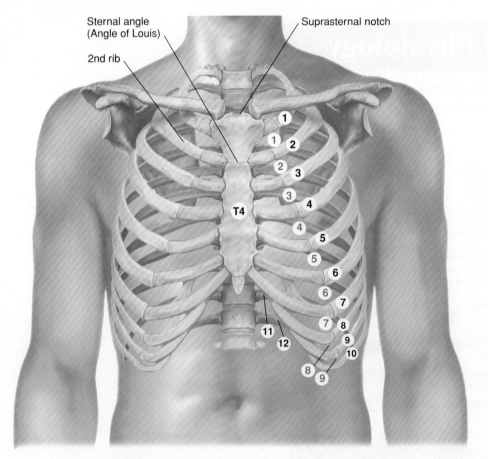

Note special landmarks:

- 2nd intercostal space for needle insertion for tension pneumothorax.
- 4th intercostal space for chest tube insertion.
- T4 for the lower margin of an endotracheal tube on a chest x-ray.

Neurovascular structures run along the inferior margin of each rib, so needles and tubes should be placed just at the superior rib margins.

FIGURE 8-2.   **Anterior ribs and intercostal spaces.**

Note that the costal cartilages of the first seven ribs articulate with the sternum; the cartilages of the 8th, 9th, and 10th ribs articulate with the costal cartilages just above them. The 11th and 12th ribs, the "floating ribs," have no anterior attachments. The cartilaginous tip of the 11th rib usually can be felt laterally, and the 12th rib may be felt posteriorly. When palpated, costal cartilages and ribs feel identical.

Posteriorly, the 12th rib is a starting point for counting ribs and intercostal spaces and provides an alternative to the anterior approach (Fig. 8-3). With the fingers of one hand, press in and up against the lower border of the 12th rib; then "walk up" the intercostal spaces, numbered in red below, or follow a more oblique line up and around to the front of the chest.

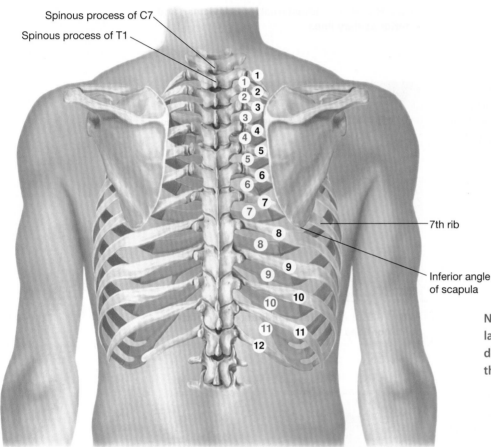

Spinous process of C7
Spinous process of T1

7th rib

Inferior angle of scapula

Note the T7–T8 intercostal space as a landmark for thoracentesis with needle insertion immediately superior to the 8th rib.

FIGURE 8-3. Posterior ribs and intercostal spaces.

The inferior tip of the scapula is another useful bony landmark; it usually lies at the level of the 7th rib or interspace.

The spinous processes of the vertebrae are also useful landmarks. When the neck is flexed forward, the most protruding process is usually the vertebra of C7. If two processes are equally prominent, they are C7 and T1. You can often palpate and count the processes below them, especially when the spine is flexed.

Circumference of the Chest. Visualize a series of vertical lines as shown in Figures 8-4 through 8-6. The *midsternal* and *vertebral lines* are easily demarcated and reproducible; the others are visualized. The *midclavicular line* drops vertically from the midpoint of the clavicle. To find it, accurately identify both ends of the clavicle (see p. 646).

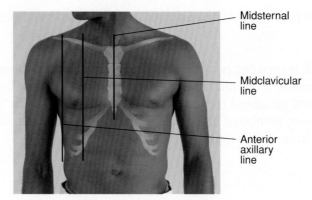

Midsternal line

Midclavicular line

Anterior axillary line

FIGURE 8-4. Midsternal, midclavicular, and anterior axillary lines.

The *anterior* and *posterior axillary lines* drop vertically from the anterior and posterior axillary folds, the muscle masses that border the axilla. The *midaxillary line* drops from the apex of the axilla.

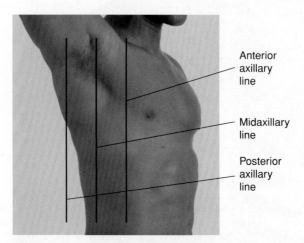

Anterior axillary line

Midaxillary line

Posterior axillary line

FIGURE 8-5. Anterior, midaxillary, and posterior lines.

Posteriorly, the *vertebral line* overlies the spinous processes of the vertebrae. The *scapular line* drops from the inferior angle of the scapula.

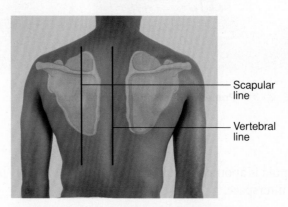

Scapular line

Vertebral line

FIGURE 8-6. Vertebral and scapular lines.

Lungs, Fissures, and Lobes.

Picture the lungs and their fissures and lobes on the chest wall. Anteriorly, the apex of each lung rises approximately 2 to 4 cm above the inner third of the clavicle (Fig. 8-7). The lower border of the lung crosses the 6th rib at the midclavicular line and the 8th rib at the midaxillary line. Posteriorly, the lower border of the lung lies at about the level of the T10 spinous process (Fig. 8-8). On inspiration, it descends in the chest cavity during contraction and descent of the diaphragm.

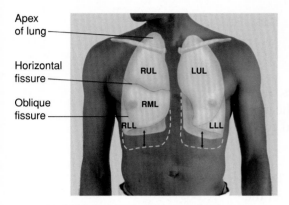

FIGURE 8-7. **The anterior lungs.**

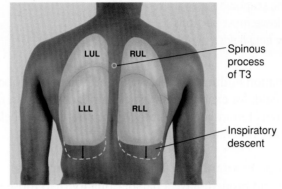

FIGURE 8-8. **The posterior lungs.**

Each lung is divided roughly in half by an *oblique (major) fissure*. This fissure may be approximated by a string that runs from the T3 spinous process obliquely down and around the chest to the 6th rib at the midclavicular line (Fig. 8-9). The right lung is further divided by the *horizontal (minor) fissure*. Anteriorly, this fissure runs close to the 4th rib and meets the oblique fissure in the midaxillary line near the 5th rib. The *right lung* is thus divided into *upper, middle,* and *lower lobes* (*RUL, RML,* and *RLL*). The *left lung* has only *two lobes,* upper and lower (*LUL, LLL*) (Fig. 8-10). Each lung receives deoxygenated blood from its *pulmonary artery.* Oxygenated blood returns from each lung to the left atrium via the *pulmonary veins.*

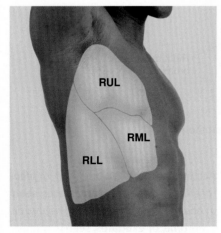

FIGURE 8-9. **Right lung lobes and fissures.**

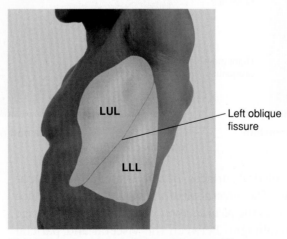

FIGURE 8-10. **Left lung lobes and fissures.**

Locations on the Chest. Learn the general anatomical terms used to locate chest findings.

Anatomic Descriptors of the Chest

Supraclavicular—above the clavicles
Infraclavicular—below the clavicles
Interscapular—between the scapulae
Infrascapular—below the scapulae
Bases of the lungs—the lowermost portions
Upper, middle, and *lower lung fields*

Usually, physical examination findings correlate with the underlying lobes. Signs in the right upper lung field, for example, almost certainly originate in the right upper lobe. However, signs found laterally in the right middle lung field could come from any of the three different lobes.

The Trachea and Major Bronchi (the Tracheobronchial Tree). Breath sounds over the trachea and bronchi have a harsher quality than those over the denser lung parenchyma. Learn the locations of these structures. The trachea bifurcates into its mainstem bronchi at the levels of the sternal angle anteriorly and the T4 spinous process posteriorly (Figs. 8-11 and 8-12). The *right main bronchus* is wider, shorter, and more vertical than the left main bronchus and directly enters the hilum of the lung. The *left main bronchus* extends inferolaterally from below the aortic arch and anterior to the esophagus and thoracic aorta and then enters the lung *hilum.* Each main bronchus then divides into *lobar* then into *segmental bronchi* and *bronchioles,* terminating in the sac-like *pulmonary alveoli,* where gas exchange occurs.

Aspiration pneumonia is more common in the right middle and lower lobe because the right main bronchus is more vertical.

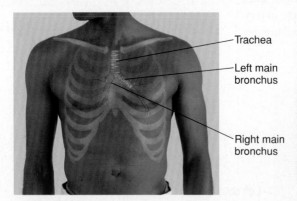

FIGURE 8-11. **Trachea and mainstem bronchi, anterior view.**

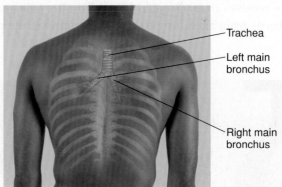

FIGURE 8-12. **Trachea and mainstem bronchi, posterior view.**

The Pleurae. Two continuous pleural surfaces, or serous membranes, separate the lungs from the chest wall. The *visceral pleura* covers the outer surface of the lungs. The *parietal pleura* lines the *pleural cavity* along the inner rib cage and the upper surface of the diaphragm. Between the visceral and parietal pleura is the *pleural space,* containing serous *pleural fluid.* The surface tension of the pleural fluid keeps the lung in contact with the thoracic wall, allowing the lung to expand and contract during respiration. The visceral pleura lacks

Accumulations of pleural fluid, or *pleural effusions,* may be transudates, seen in *heart failure, cirrhosis,* and *nephrotic syndrome,* or exudates, seen in numerous conditions including *pneumonia,* malignancy, *pulmonary embolism, tuberculosis,* and *pancreatitis.*

sensory nerves, but the parietal pleura is richly innervated by the intercostal and phrenic nerves.

Irritation of the parietal pleura produces pleuritic pain with deep inspiration in *viral pleurisy, pneumonia, pulmonary embolism, pericarditis,* and collagen vascular diseases.

Breathing.   Breathing is primarily automatic, controlled by respiratory centers in the brainstem that generate the neuronal drive for the muscles of respiration. The principal muscle of inspiration is the *diaphragm.* During inspiration, the diaphragm contracts, descends in the chest, and expands the thoracic cavity, compressing the abdominal contents and pushing out the abdominal wall. The muscles in the rib cage also expand the thorax, especially the *scalenes,* which run from the cervical vertebrae to the first two ribs, and the parasternal intercostal muscles, or *parasternals,* which cross obliquely from the sternum to the ribs. As the thorax expands, intrathoracic pressure decreases, drawing air through the tracheobronchial tree into the *alveoli,* or distal air sacs, filling the expanding lungs. Oxygen diffuses into the adjacent pulmonary capillaries as carbon dioxide exchanges from the blood into the alveoli.

During expiration, the chest wall and lungs recoil and the diaphragm relaxes and rises passively. Abdominal muscles assist in expiration. As air flows outward, the chest and abdomen return to their resting positions.

Normal breathing is quiet and easy—barely audible near the open mouth as a faint whish. When a healthy person lies supine, the breathing movements of the thorax are relatively slight. By contrast, the abdominal movements are usually easy to see. In the sitting position, movements of the thorax become more prominent.

During exercise and in certain diseases, extra work is required to breathe, and accessory muscles are recruited; the sternocleidomastoids (SCM) and the scalenes may become visible (Fig. 8-13).

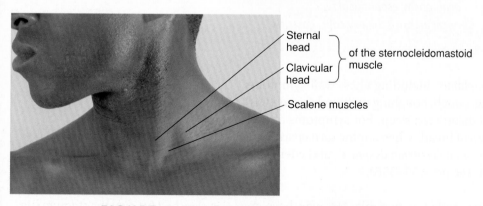

Sternal head ⎫
Clavicular head ⎬ of the sternocleidomastoid muscle

Scalene muscles

FIGURE 8-13. **Accessory muscles in the neck.**

The Health History

Common or Concerning Symptoms

- Chest pain
- Shortness of breath (dyspnea)
- Wheezing
- Cough
- Blood-streaked sputum (hemoptysis)
- Daytime sleepiness or snoring and disordered sleep

Chest Pain. Complaints of *chest pain* or *chest discomfort* raise concerns about the heart but often arise from other structures in the thorax and lungs. To assess this symptom, you must pursue a dual investigation of both thoracic and cardiac causes. Sources of chest pain are listed below. For this important symptom, keep all of these possibilities in mind.

See Table 8-1, Chest Pain, pp. 330–331.

Sources of Chest Pain and Related Causes

The myocardium	*Angina pectoris, myocardial infarction, myocarditis*
The pericardium	*Pericarditis*
The aorta	*Aortic dissection*
The trachea and large bronchi	*Bronchitis*
The parietal pleura	*Pericarditis, pneumonia, pneumothorax, pleural effusion, pulmonary embolus*
The chest wall, including the musculoskeletal and neurologic systems	*Costochondritis, herpes zoster*
The esophagus	*Gastroesophageal reflux disease, esophageal spasm, esophageal tear*
Extrathoracic structures such as the neck, gallbladder, and stomach	*Cervical arthritis, biliary colic, gastritis*

Chest pain is reported in one in four patients with panic and anxiety disorders.[1-3]

This section focuses on *pulmonary complaints*, including chest wall symptoms, difficulty breathing (*dyspnea*), wheezing, cough, coughing up blood (*hemoptysis*), and daytime sleepiness or snoring and disordered sleep. For symptoms of exertional chest pain, palpitations, shortness of breath when supine (*orthopnea*) or at night relieved by sitting upright (*paroxysmal nocturnal dyspnea*), and edema, see Chapter 9, The Cardiovascular System (see pp. 355–358).

Your initial questions should be as open-ended as possible. "Do you have any discomfort or unpleasant feelings in your chest?" Ask the patient to point to the location of the pain in the chest. Watch for any gestures as the patient describes the pain. Elicit all seven attributes of chest pain to distinguish among its various causes (see p. 79).

A clenched fist over the sternum suggests *angina pectoris;* a finger pointing to a tender spot on the chest wall suggests *musculoskeletal pain;* a hand moving from the neck to the epigastrium suggests *heartburn.*

Lung tissue has no pain fibers. Pain in conditions such as pneumonia or pulmonary infarction usually arises from inflammation of the adjacent parietal pleura. Muscle strain from prolonged recurrent coughing or costochondral inflammation may also be responsible. The pericardium also has few pain fibers. The pain of pericarditis stems from inflammation of the adjacent parietal pleura. Extrapulmonary sources of chest pain include gastroesophageal reflux disease and anxiety, but the mechanism remains obscure.[1–4]

Shortness of Breath (Dyspnea) and Wheezing. *Shortness of breath,* or *dyspnea,* is a painless but uncomfortable awareness of breathing that is inappropriate to the level of exertion.[5] Thoroughly assess this telltale symptom of cardiac and pulmonary disease.

The degree of dyspnea, combined with spirometry, is a key component of important *chronic obstructive pulmonary disease (COPD)* classification systems that guide patient management.[6–8]

Ask, "Have you had any difficulty breathing?" Find out if the symptom occurs at rest or with exertion, and how much exertion produces onset. Because of variations in age, body weight, and physical fitness, there is no absolute scale for quantifying shortness of breath. Instead, make every effort to determine its severity based on the patient's daily activities. How many steps or flights of stairs can the patient climb before pausing for breath? What about carrying bags of groceries, vacuuming, or making the bed? Has shortness of breath altered the patient's lifestyle and daily activities? How? Carefully elicit the timing and setting, any associated symptoms, and relieving or aggravating factors.

See Table 8-2, Dyspnea, pp. 332–333.

Most patients relate shortness of breath to their level of activity. Anxious patients present a different picture. They may describe difficulty taking a deep enough breath, a smothering sensation with inability to get enough air, and *paresthesias,* which are sensations of tingling or "pins and needles" around the lips or in the extremities.

Anxious patients may have episodic dyspnea during both rest and exercise and also *hyperventilation,* or rapid shallow breathing.

Wheezes are musical respiratory sounds that may be audible to the patient and to others.

Wheezing occurs in partial lower airway obstruction from secretions and tissue inflammation in *asthma,* or from a foreign body.[9]

Cough. *Cough* is a common symptom that ranges in significance from trivial to ominous. Typically, cough is a reflex response to stimuli that irritate receptors in the larynx, trachea, or large bronchi. These stimuli include mucus, pus, blood, as well as external agents such as allergens, dust, foreign bodies, or even extremely hot or cold air. Other causes include inflammation of the respiratory mucosa, pneumonia, pulmonary edema, and compression of the bronchi or bronchioles from a tumor or enlarged peribronchial lymph nodes. Cough may also be cardiovascular in origin.

See Table 8-3, Cough and Hemoptysis, p. 334.

Cough can signal *left-sided heart failure.*

For complaints of cough, pursue a thorough assessment. Establish the duration. Is the cough *acute,* lasting less than 3 weeks; *subacute,* lasting 3 to 8 weeks; or *chronic,* more than 8 weeks?

The most common cause of *acute cough* is viral upper respiratory infections. Also consider acute bronchitis, pneumonia, left-sided heart failure, asthma, foreign body, smoking, and ace-inhibitor therapy. Postinfectious cough, pertussis, acid reflux, bacterial sinusitis, and asthma can cause *subacute cough. Chronic cough* is seen in postnasal drip, asthma, gastroesophageal reflux, chronic bronchitis, and bronchiectasis.[10–17]

Ask whether the cough is dry or produces sputum, or phlegm.

Mucoid* sputum is translucent, white, or gray and seen in viral infections and *cystic fibrosis; purulent* sputum—yellow or green—often accompanies *bacterial pneumonia.

Ask the patient to describe the volume of any sputum and its color, odor, and consistency.

Foul-smelling sputum is present in anaerobic *lung abscess,* thick tenacious sputum in *cystic fibrosis.*

To help patients quantify volume, try a multiple-choice question. "How much do you think you cough up in 24 hours: a teaspoon, tablespoon, quarter cup, half cup, cupful?" If possible, ask the patient to cough into a tissue; inspect the phlegm, and note its characteristics. The symptoms associated with a cough often lead to its cause.

Large volumes of purulent sputum are present in *bronchiectasis* and *lung abscess.*

Diagnostically helpful symptoms include fever and productive cough in *pneumonia;* wheezing in *asthma;* and chest pain, dyspnea, and orthopnea in *acute coronary syndromes.*

Hemoptysis.   *Hemoptysis* refers to blood coughed up from the lower respiratory tract; it may vary from blood-streaked sputum to frank blood. For patients reporting hemoptysis, quantify the volume of blood produced, the setting and activity, and any associated symptoms. Hemoptysis is rare in infants, children, and adolescents.

See Table 8-3, Cough and Hemoptysis, p. 334. Causes include *bronchitis; malignancy;* and *cystic fibrosis* and, less commonly, *bronchiectasis, mitral stenosis, Goodpasture syndrome,* and *Wegener granulomatosis.* Massive hemoptysis (>200 cm^3) may be life-threatening.[18]

Before using the term "hemoptysis," try to confirm the source of the bleeding. Blood or blood-streaked material may originate in the nose, mouth, pharynx, or gastrointestinal tract and is easily mislabeled. If vomited, it probably originates in the gastrointestinal tract. Occasionally, however, blood from the nasopharynx or the gastrointestinal tract is aspirated and then coughed out.

Blood originating in the stomach is usually darker than blood from the respiratory tract and may be mixed with food particles.

Daytime Sleepiness or Snoring and Disordered Sleep.   Patients may report excessive daytime sleepiness and fatigue. Ask about problems with snoring, witnessed *apneas* (defined as breathing cessation for ≥10 seconds), awakening with a choking sensation, or morning headache.

These symptoms, especially daytime sleepiness and snoring, are hallmarks of *obstructive sleep apnea,* commonly seen in patients with obesity, posterior malocclusion of the jaw (retrognathia), treatment-resistant hypertension, heart failure, atrial fibrillation, stroke, and type 2 diabetes. Mechanisms include instability of the brainstem respiratory center, disordered sleep arousal, disordered contraction of upper airway muscles (genioglossus malfunction), and anatomic changes contributing to airway collapse such as obesity, among others.[19,20]

Health Promotion and Counseling: Evidence and Recommendations

Important Topics for Health Promotion and Counseling

- Tobacco cessation
- Lung cancer
- Immunizations—influenza and streptococcal pneumonia vaccines

Tobacco Cessation.   Despite declining smoking rates over the past several decades, 19% of U.S. adults continue to smoke, although the proportion of heavy smokers (>30 cigarettes per day) has dropped from about 13% to 8%.[21] Nearly 90% of smokers first tried cigarettes by age 18 years.[22] About 23% of high-school students and 7% of middle-school students use tobacco products, most often cigarettes or cigars, and use is higher among males than females. Smokers are more likely than nonsmokers to develop cardiovascular disease, emphysema, and lung cancer. Tobacco use is the leading preventable cause of premature death in the United States, accounting for one in five deaths each year.[23] Half of all long-term smokers die of smoking-related diseases, losing an average of 10 years of life.

Quitting smoking significantly reduces disease risk. The facts below can be motivating when counseling smokers.

- Quitting tobacco reduces the *cardiovascular risk* of heart attack and death from coronary heart disease *by half* after just 1 year.

- *Stroke risk* is reduced within 2 to 5 years to the same level as a nonsmoker.

- *Lung cancer risk* is cut in half after 10 years.

The United States Preventive Services Task Force (USPSTF) has given a grade A recommendation to screening all adults, particularly pregnant women, for tobacco use and providing tobacco cessation interventions to all who are using tobacco.[24]

Adverse Effects of Smoking on Health and Disease

Condition	Increased Risk Compared with Nonsmokers
• Coronary artery disease	2–4 times higher
• Stroke	2–4 times higher
• Peripheral vascular disease	10 times higher
• COPD mortality	12–13 times higher
• Lung cancer	23 times higher mortality in men
	13 times higher mortality in women

Source: Centers for Disease Control and Prevention, DHHS. Smoking and tobacco use. Fact sheet. Health effects of cigarette smoking. Available at: http://www.cdc.gov/tobacco/data_statistics/fact_sheets/health_effects/effects_cig_smoking/index.htm. Accessed March 31, 2015.

In addition to respiratory tract cancers, smoking contributes to cancers of the bladder, cervix, colon and rectum, kidney, oropharynx, larynx, esophagus, stomach, liver, and pancreas as well as acute myeloid leukemia.[25] Smoking increases risk of infertility, preterm birth, low birth weight, and sudden infant death syndrome. Smoking is associated with developing diabetes, cataracts, and rheumatoid arthritis. Nonsmokers exposed to smoke also have increased risk of lung cancer, ear and respiratory infections, and asthma.

Clinicians should focus on prevention and cessation, especially in teenagers and pregnant women.[26] Because most smokers see a health care provider each year and nearly 70% of smokers express interest in quitting, clinicians have an important opportunity to identify and treat tobacco dependence.[27,28] Behavioral support and pharmacotherapy are both effective strategies. Combining these strategies is more effective than either strategy alone as it addresses withdrawal symptom and cravings as well as enhances motivation and skills for quitting. The benefits of even brief counseling interventions are considerable—advising smokers to quit during every visit raises quit rates by 30%.[29] Use the "5 As" framework or the Stages of Change model to assess readiness to quit.[24,30] Motivational interviewing techniques are also helpful for patients who are not yet ready to quit smoking.[27,28]

Assessing Readiness to Quit Smoking: Brief Interventions Models

5 As Model	Stages of Change Model
• Ask about tobacco use	• Precontemplation—"I don't want to quit."
• Advise to quit	• Contemplation—"I am concerned but not ready to quit now."
• Assess willingness to make a quit attempt	• Preparation—"I am ready to quit."
• Assist in quit attempt	• Action—"I just quit."
• Arrange follow-up	• Maintenance—"I quit 6 months ago."

Nicotine is highly addicting, comparable to heroin and cocaine, and quitting is difficult. More than 80% of smokers who try to quit on their own resume smoking within 30 days and only 3% of smokers quit successfully each year.[31] Stimulation of the nicotinic cholinergic receptors in the brain increases release of dopamine, which enhances pleasure and modulates mood. Daily smokers inhale enough nicotine to achieve almost complete receptor saturation. The inhaled nicotine reaches the brain in seconds, causing a powerful and reinforcing rush effect. Use cognitive therapy techniques to help smokers recognize and design strategies to combat the features of addiction: craving, triggers such as stress or environmental cues, and signs of withdrawal like irritability, poor concentration, anxiety, and depressed mood. Quit rates roughly double when counseling is combined with pharmacotherapies such as nicotine replacement, bupropion, and varenicline.[32]

Lung Cancer

Epidemiology. Lung cancer is the second most frequently diagnosed cancer in the United States and the leading cause of cancer death for both men and women.[33] Over 200,000 new cases and nearly 160,000 deaths (accounting for about 27% of all cancer deaths) were expected in 2014. Incidence rates and death rates have been decreasing since 2006.

Risk Factors. Cigarette smoking is by far the leading risk factor for lung cancer, accounting for about 90% of lung cancer deaths.[22] Longer smoking histories and higher numbers of cigarettes smoked are associated with higher risk. Radon, an invisible, odorless, radioactive gas released from soil and rocks in the ground, is the second leading cause of lung cancer in the United States. Other environmental and occupational exposures include second-hand smoke, asbestos, heavy metals, organic chemicals, ionizing radiation, and air pollution. Lung cancer also has a familial risk.

Prevention. The most important strategies aim to prevent people from ever using tobacco products and getting tobacco users to quit. The previous section highlights smoking cessation strategies. Avoiding environmental and occupational exposures can also reduce lung cancer risk.

Screening. Another strategy for addressing the burden of cancer is screening, also known as *secondary prevention,* which targets finding and treating early-stage cancers. This is particularly important for lung cancer; cancers diagnosed at an early stage (before metastasis) have a 54% 5-year relative survival.[34] Meanwhile, the 5-year relative survival is a dismal 4% for cancers diagnosed at later stages (metastatic). Unfortunately, only 15% of lung cancers are diagnosed at an early stage.

Screening Tests and Evidence. Numerous studies conducted over many years have shown that lung cancer screening with chest x-ray or sputum cytology is not effective. Recently, however, the National Lung Screening Trial (NLST) showed that screening with low-dose computed tomography (LDCT) reduced the risk of dying from lung cancer compared to chest x-ray screening.[35] The NLST was a randomized trial that enrolled more than 53,000 adults aged 55 to 74 years at risk for lung cancer due to at least a 30-pack-year smoking history or current smoking or having quit within the past 15 years. Subjects received three annual screenings with LDCT or chest x-rays. After nearly 7 years of follow-up, lung cancer deaths were reduced by 20% with LDCT compared to chest x-ray. However, the absolute benefit was small; >320 subjects needed screening to prevent one lung cancer death. Although about 40% of study subjects had an abnormal LDCT, over 95% of these results were false positives. Screening can lead to harms, including anxiety over false-positive tests, complications from invasive diagnostic procedures, and cancer risks from radiation exposure.

Screening Guidelines from Major Organizations. The USPSTF has given lung cancer screening with LDCT a B rating, meaning that there is a net benefit to offering screening.[36] Annual LDCT screening is recommended for current smokers (or those who have quit within the last 15 years) aged 55 to 79 years. The American Cancer Society also recommends annual screening, although only until age 74 years.[37] Both organizations agree that all current smokers should receive counseling about smoking cessation and should be offered cessation interventions. Before offering screening, clinicians should engage patients in discussions about the potential benefits, limitations, and harms of screening—and emphasize that screening is not a substitute for smoking cessation.

Immunizations (Adults)

Influenza. *Influenza* can cause substantial morbidity and mortality, especially during the late fall and winter, peaking in February.[38] The number of annual deaths related to influenza varies depending on the virus type and subtype, ranging from a few thousand to nearly 50,000 deaths. The Centers for Disease Control (CDC) Advisory Committee on Immunization Practices (ACIP) updates its recommendations for vaccination annually. Two types of vaccine are available: the "flu shot," an inactivated vaccine containing killed virus, and a nasal-spray vaccine containing attenuated live viruses, approved only for healthy people between the ages of 2 and 49 years.[39] Because influenza viruses mutate from year to year, each vaccine contains three to four vaccine strains and is modified yearly. Note that annual vaccination is recommended for everyone aged ≥6 months.

Summary of 2015-2016 CDC Influenza Vaccine Recommendations—Adults

Annual vaccination is recommended for all people aged 6 months and older, especially the groups listed below.[40]

- Adults with chronic pulmonary and cardiovascular conditions (except hypertension) and renal, hepatic, neurologic, hematologic, or metabolic disorders (including diabetes mellitus); adults who are immunosuppressed or morbidly obese
- Adults ≥50 years of age
- Pregnant women and women up to 2 weeks postpartum
- Residents of nursing homes and long-term care facilities
- American Indians and Alaska natives
- Health care personnel
- Household contacts and caregivers of children ≤5 years of age (especially infants ≤age 6 months) and of adults ≥50 years of age with clinical conditions placing them at higher risk for complications of influenza

Streptococcal Pneumonia. *Streptococcal pneumonia* causes pneumonia, bacteremia, and meningitis. In 2009, invasive pneumococcal disease accounted for 43,500 cases and 5,000 deaths.[41] However, the introduction of the 7-valent pneumococcal vaccination for infants and children in 2000 has directly and indirectly (through herd immunity) reduced pneumococcal infections among children and adults.[42] Since 2010, infants younger than age 2 years have routinely been vaccinated with the 13-valent pneumococcal conjugate vaccine (PCV13). In 2014, the ACIP recommended vaccinating adults aged ≥65 years using the PCV13 along with the 23-valent inactivated pneumococcal polysaccharide vaccine (PPSV23). The vaccines should not be coadministered. Adults in this age range who never received the PPSV23 should first receive the PCV13 followed 6 to 12 months later by the PPSV23. Adults aged ≥65 years previously vaccinated with PPSV23 should receive a dose of PCV13 no earlier than 1 year following the most recent PPSV23 vaccination. The ACIP recommends using PCV13 and PPSV23 for the high-risk groups listed below.

Summary of 2015 CDC Pneumococcal Vaccine Recommendations

- Adults ≥65 years
- Children and adults from ages 2 to 64 years with chronic illnesses specifically associated with increased risk of pneumococcal infection (sickle cell disease, cardiovascular and pulmonary disease, diabetes, alcoholism, cirrhosis, cochlear implants, and leaks of cerebrospinal fluid)
- Any adult aged 19 to 64 years who is a smoker or has asthma
- Adults and children older than age 2 years who are immunocompromised (including from HIV infection, AIDS, long-term steroids, Hodgkin disease, lymphoma or leukemia, kidney failure, multiple myeloma, nephrotic syndrome, organ transplant, damaged spleen or no spleen, radiation, or chemotherapy)
- Residents of nursing homes or long-term care facilities

Techniques of Examination

For best results, examine the posterior thorax and lungs while the patient is sitting, and the anterior thorax and lungs with the patient supine. Be considerate when draping the patient's gown. For men, arrange the gown so that you can see the full chest. For women, cover the anterior chest when you examine the back; for the anterior examination, drape the gown over each half of the chest as you examine the other half. Begin with inspection, then palpate, percuss, and auscultate. Try to visualize the underlying lobes and compare the right lung field with the left, carefully noting any asymmetries.

- *With the patient sitting,* examine the posterior thorax and lungs. The patient's arms should be folded across the chest with hands resting, if possible, on the opposite shoulders. This position swings the scapulae laterally and increases access to the lung fields. Then ask the patient to lie down.

■ *With the patient supine,* examine the anterior thorax and lungs. For women, this position allows the breasts to be gently displaced. Some clinicians examine both the posterior and anterior chest with the patient sitting, which is also satisfactory.

■ *For patients who cannot sit up,* ask for assistance so that you can examine the posterior chest in the sitting position. If this is not possible, roll the patient to one side and then to the other. Percuss and auscultate both lungs in each position. Because ventilation is relatively greater in the dependent lung, you are more likely to hear abnormal wheezes or crackles on the dependent side (see p. 325).

Initial Survey of Respiration and the Thorax

Even though the respiratory rate might already be recorded, again carefully *observe the rate, rhythm, depth, and effort of breathing.* A healthy resting adult breathes quietly and regularly about 20 times a minute. Note whether expiration lasts longer than usual.

See Table 8-4, Abnormalities in Rate and Rhythm of Breathing, p. 335, including *bradypnea, tachypnea,* hyperventilation, *Cheyne–Stokes* breathing, and ataxic breathing. Delayed expiration occurs in *COPD.*

Begin by observing the patient for signs of respiratory distress.

Signs of Respiratory Distress

■ Assess the respiratory rate for *tachypnea* (>25 breaths/minute).

Tachypnea increases the likelihood of *pneumonia* and cardiac disease.

■ Inspect the patient's color for *cyanosis or pallor.* Recall earlier relevant findings, such as the shape and color of the fingernails.

Cyanosis in the lips, tongue, and oral mucosa signals hypoxia. Pallor and sweating (*diaphoresis*) are common in heart failure. Clubbing of the nails (see p. 211) occurs in *bronchiectasis, congenital heart disease, pulmonary fibrosis, cystic fibrosis, lung abscess,* and *malignancy.*

■ Listen for *audible sounds of breathing.* Is there audible whistling during inspiration over the neck or lungs?

Audible high-pitched inspiratory whistling, or *stridor,* is an ominous sign of upper airway obstruction in the larynx or trachea that requires urgent airway evaluation. Wheezing is either expiratory or continuous.

■ Inspect the neck. During inspiration, is there *contraction of the accessory muscles,* namely the SCM and scalene muscles, or supraclavicular retraction? During expiration, is there contraction of the intercostal or abdominal oblique muscles? Is the trachea midline?

Accessory muscle use signals difficulty breathing from COPD or respiratory muscle fatigue. Lateral displacement of the trachea occurs in *pneumothorax, pleural effusion,* and *atelectasis.*

Also *observe the shape of the chest,* which is normally wider than it is deep. The ratio of the anteroposterior (AP) diameter to the lateral chest diameter is usually 0.7 to 0.75 up to 0.9 and increases with aging.[43]

This ratio may exceed 0.9 in COPD, producing a *barrel-chest appearance,* although evidence of this correlation is conflicting.

Examination of the Posterior Chest

Inspection. Standing in a midline position behind the patient, note the *shape of the chest* and *how the chest moves*, including the following:

- Deformities or asymmetry in chest expansion

- Abnormal muscle retraction of the intercostal spaces during inspiration, most visible in the lower intercostal spaces.

- Impaired respiratory movement on one or both sides or a unilateral lag (or delay) in movement.

Palpation. As you palpate the chest, focus on areas of tenderness or bruising, respiratory expansion, and fremitus.

- *Identify tender areas.* Carefully palpate any area where the patient reports pain or has visible lesions or bruises. Note any palpable *crepitus*, defined as a crackling or grinding sound over bones, joints, or skin, with or without pain, due to air in the subcutaneous tissue.

- *Assess any skin abnormalities* such as masses or sinus tracts (blind, inflammatory, tube-like structures opening onto the skin).

- *Test chest expansion.* Place your thumbs at about the level of the 10th ribs, with your fingers loosely grasping and parallel to the lateral rib cage (Fig. 8-14). As you position your hands, slide them medially just enough to raise a loose fold of skin between your thumbs over the spine. Ask the patient to inhale deeply. Watch the distance between your thumbs as they move apart during inspiration, and feel for the range and symmetry of the rib cage as it expands and contracts. This movement is sometimes called *lung excursion.*

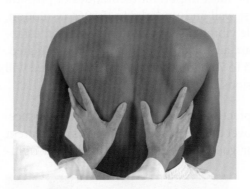

FIGURE 8-14. **Assess lung expansion.**

See Table 8-5, Deformities of the Thorax, p. 336.

Asymmetric expansion occurs in large pleural effusions.

Retraction occurs in severe *asthma, COPD*, or upper airway obstruction.

Unilateral impairment or lagging suggests pleural disease from *asbestosis* or *silicosis*; it is also seen in phrenic nerve damage or trauma.

Intercostal tenderness can develop over inflamed pleurae, costal cartilage tenderness in *costochondritis*.

Tenderness, bruising, and bony "step-offs" are common over a fractured rib. Crepitus may be palpable in overt fractures and arthritic joints; crepitus and chest wall edema are seen in *mediastinitis*.

Although rare, sinus tracts suggest infection of the underlying pleura and lung (as in *tuberculosis* or *actinomycosis*).

Unilateral decrease or delay in chest expansion occurs in chronic fibrosis of the underlying lung or pleura, pleural effusion, lobar pneumonia, pleural pain with associated splinting, unilateral bronchial obstruction, and paralysis of the hemidiaphragm.

■ *Palpate both lungs for symmetric tactile fremitus* (Fig. 8-15). Fremitus refers to the palpable vibrations that are transmitted through the bronchopulmonary tree to the chest wall as the patient is speaking and is normally symmetric. Fremitus is typically more prominent in the interscapular area than in the lower lung fields and easier to detect over the right lung than the left. It disappears below the diaphragm.

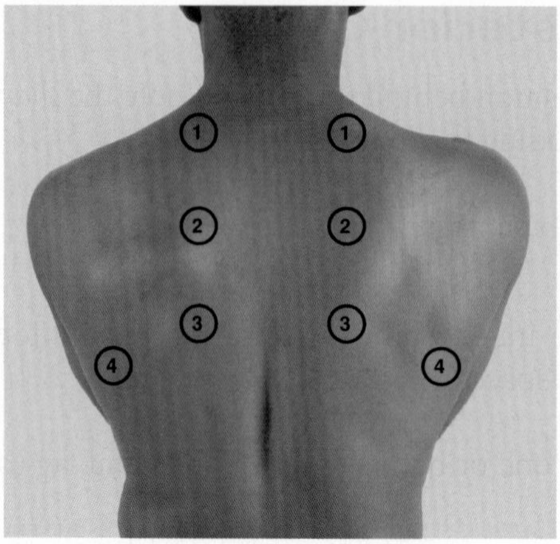

Fremitus is decreased or absent when the voice is higher pitched or soft or when the transmission of vibrations from the larynx to the surface of the chest is impeded by a thick chest wall, an obstructed bronchus, *COPD*, or *pleural effusion*, fibrosis, air (*pneumothorax*), or an infiltrating tumor.

FIGURE 8-15. Locations for palpating fremitus.

To detect fremitus, use either the ball (the bony part of the palm at the base of the fingers) or the ulnar surface of your hand to optimize the vibratory sensitivity of the bones in your hand. Ask the patient to repeat the words "ninety-nine" or "one-one-one." Initially practice with one hand until you feel the transmitted vibrations. Use both hands to palpate and *compare symmetric areas of the lungs* in the pattern shown in the photograph. Identify and locate any areas of increased, decreased, or absent fremitus. If fremitus is faint, ask the patient to speak more loudly or in a deeper voice.

Tactile fremitus is a somewhat imprecise assessment technique, but does direct your attention to possible asymmetries. Confirm any disparities by listening for underlying breath sounds, voice sounds, and whispered voice sounds. All these attributes should increase or decrease together.

Asymmetric decreased fremitus raises the likelihood of unilateral *pleural effusion*, pneumothorax, or neoplasm, which decreases transmission of low-frequency sounds; asymmetric *increased* fremitus occurs in unilateral pneumonia which increases transmission through consolidated tissue.[44]

Percussion. Percussion is one of the most important techniques of physical examination. Percussion sets the chest wall and underlying tissues in motion, producing audible sound and palpable vibrations. Percussion helps you establish whether the underlying tissues are air-filled, fluid-filled, or consolidated. The percussion blow penetrates only 5 to 7 cm into the chest, however, and will not aid in detection of deep-seated lesions.

The technique of percussion can be practiced on any surface. As you practice, listen for changes in percussion notes over different types of materials or different parts of the body. The key points for good technique, described for a right-handed person, are detailed below:

■ Hyperextend the middle finger of your left hand, known as the *pleximeter finger.* Press its distal interphalangeal joint firmly on the lung surface to be percussed (Fig. 8-16). *Avoid surface contact by any other part of the hand because this dampens out vibrations.* Note that the thumb and second, fourth, and fifth fingers are not touching the chest wall.

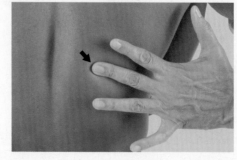

FIGURE 8-16. Press the pleximeter finger firmly on the chest wall.

- Position your right forearm quite close to the surface, with the hand cocked upward. The middle finger should be partially flexed, relaxed, and poised to strike.

- With a *quick, sharp but relaxed wrist motion,* strike the pleximeter finger with the right middle finger, called the *plexor finger* (Fig. 8-17). Aim at your distal interphalangeal joint. Your goal is to transmit vibrations through the bones of this joint to the underlying chest wall. Use the same force for each percussion strike and the same pleximeter pressure to avoid changes in the percussion note due to your technique rather than underlying findings.

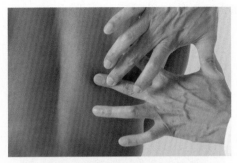

FIGURE 8-17. **Strike the pleximeter finger with the right middle finger.**

- Strike using the *tip of the plexor finger,* not the finger pad. The striking finger should be almost at right angles to the pleximeter. A short fingernail is recommended to avoid injuring your knuckle.

- Withdraw your striking finger quickly to avoid damping the vibrations you have created (Fig. 8-18).

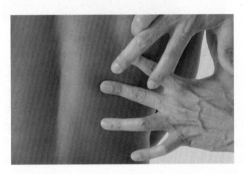

FIGURE 8-18. **Withdraw the striking finger quickly.**

In summary, the movement is at the wrist. It is directed, brisk, yet relaxed and slightly bouncy.

Percussion Notes. With your plexor or striking finger, use the lightest percussion that produces a clear note. A thick chest wall requires a more forceful percussion blow than a thin one. However, if a *louder* note is needed, apply more pressure with the *pleximeter* finger.

When percussing the lower posterior chest, stand somewhat to the side rather than directly behind the patient. In this position it is easier to place your pleximeter finger more firmly on the chest, making your plexor strike more effective by creating a better percussion note.

- *When comparing two areas,* use the same percussion technique in both areas. Percuss or strike twice in each location and listen for differences in the percussion notes at the two locations.

- *Learn to identify five percussion notes.* You can practice four of them on yourself. These notes differ in their basic qualities of sound, intensity, pitch, and duration. Train your ear by concentrating on one quality at a time as you percuss first in one location, then in another. Review the description of percussion notes on p. 323. Healthy lungs are *resonant*.

While the patient keeps both arms crossed in front of the chest, percuss the thorax in symmetric locations on each side from the apex to the base.

■ *Percuss one side of the chest and then the other at each level* in a ladder-like pattern, as shown in Figure 8-19. Omit the areas over the scapulae—the thickness of muscle and bone alters the percussion notes over the lungs. Identify and locate the area and quality of any abnormal percussion note.

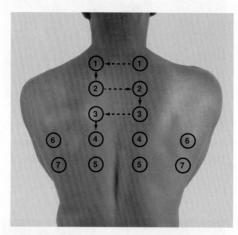

FIGURE 8-19. **Percuss and auscultate in a "ladder" pattern.**

■ *Identify the descent of the diaphragm,* or *diaphragmatic excursion.* First, *determine the level of diaphragmatic dullness* during quiet respiration. Holding the pleximeter finger *above and parallel* to the expected level of dullness, percuss downward in progressive steps until dullness clearly replaces resonance. Confirm this level of change by percussing downward from adjacent areas both medially and laterally (Fig. 8-20).

Dullness replaces resonance when fluid or solid tissue replaces air-containing lung or occupies the pleural space beneath your percussing fingers. Examples include: *lobar pneumonia,* in which the alveoli are filled with fluid and blood cells; and pleural accumulations of serous fluid (*pleural effusion*), blood (*hemothorax*), pus (*empyema*), fibrous tissue, or tumor. Dullness makes pneumonic and pleural effusion three to four times more likely, respectively.[45]

Generalized hyperresonance is common over the hyperinflated lungs of COPD or *asthma. Unilateral hyperresonance* suggests a large pneumothorax or an air-filled bulla.

This technique tends to overestimate actual movements of the diaphragm.[45]

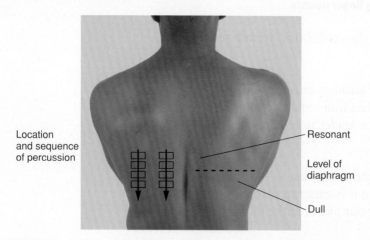

Location and sequence of percussion

Resonant

Level of diaphragm

Dull

FIGURE 8-20. **Identify the extent of diaphragmatic excursion.**

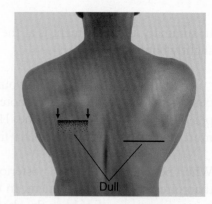

Dull

FIGURE 8-21. **Absent descent of the diaphragm can indicate pleural effusion.**

An abnormally high level suggests a *pleural effusion* or an elevated hemidiaphragm from *atelectasis* or *phrenic nerve paralysis* (Fig. 8-21).

Percussion Notes and Their Characteristics

	Relative Intensity	Relative Pitch	Relative Duration	Example of Location	Pathologic Examples
Flat	Soft	High	Short	Thigh	*Large pleural effusion*
Dull	Medium	Medium	Medium	Liver	*Lobar pneumonia*
Resonant	Loud	Low	Long	Healthy lung	*Simple chronic bronchitis*
Hyperresonant	Very loud	Lower	Longer	Usually none	*COPD, pneumothorax*
Tympanitic	Loud	High[a]	Longer	Gastric air bubble or puffed-out cheek	*Large pneumothorax*

[a]Distinguished mainly by its musical timbre.

Note that with this technique, you are identifying the boundary between the resonant lung tissue and the duller structures below the diaphragm. You are not percussing the diaphragm itself. You can infer the probable location of the diaphragm from the level of dullness.

Now, *estimate the extent of diaphragmatic excursion* by determining the distance between the level of dullness on full expiration and the level of dullness on full inspiration, normally about 3 to 5.5 cm.[46]

Auscultation. Auscultation is the most important examination technique for assessing air flow through the tracheobronchial tree. Auscultation involves (1) listening to the sounds generated by breathing, (2) listening for any adventitious (added) sounds, and (3) if abnormalities are suspected, listening to the sounds of the patient's spoken or whispered voice as they are transmitted through the chest wall. Before beginning auscultation, ask the patient to cough once or twice to clear mild atelectasis or airway mucus that can produce unimportant extra sounds.

Listen to the breath sounds with the diaphragm of your stethoscope after instructing the patient to breathe deeply through an open mouth. Always place the stethoscope directly on the skin. Clothing alters the characteristics of the breath sounds and can introduce friction and added sounds.

Use the ladder pattern suggested for percussion, moving from one side to the other and comparing symmetric areas of the lungs. Listen to at least one full breath in each location. If you hear or suspect abnormal sounds, auscultate adjacent areas to assess the extent of any abnormality. If the patient becomes lightheaded from hyperventilation, allow the patient to take a few normal breaths.

Note the *intensity* of the breath sounds, which reflects the air flow rate at the mouth, and may vary from one area to another. Breath sounds are usually louder in the lower posterior lung fields. If the breath sounds seem faint, ask the patient to breathe more deeply. Shallow breathing or a thick chest wall can both alter breath sound intensity.

Bedclothes, paper gowns, and even chest hair can generate confusing crackling sounds that interfere with auscultation. For chest hair, press harder or moisten the hair.

Air movement through a partially obstructed nose or nasopharynx can also introduce abnormal sounds.

Breath sounds may be decreased when air flow is decreased (as in obstructive lung disease or respiratory muscle weakness) or when the transmission of sound is poor (as in *pleural effusion, pneumothorax,* or *COPD*).

Is there a *silent gap* between the inspiratory and expiratory sounds?

A gap suggests bronchial breath sounds.

Listen for the *pitch, intensity, and duration of the inspiratory and expiratory sounds.* Are vesicular breath sounds distributed normally over the chest wall? Are breath sounds diminished, or are there bronchovesicular or bronchial breath sounds in unexpected places? If so, in what distribution?

Breath Sounds (Lung Sounds). Learn to identify breath sounds by their intensity, their pitch, and the relative duration of their inspiratory and expiratory phases. Normal breath sounds are:

In cold or tense patients, watch for muscle contraction sounds—muffled, low-pitched rumbling, or roaring noises. Changing the patient's position may eliminate this noise. To reproduce these sounds on yourself, do a Valsalva maneuver (straining down) as you listen to your own chest.

- *Vesicular,* or soft and low pitched. They are heard throughout inspiration, continue without pause through expiration, and then fade away about one third of the way through expiration.

- *Bronchovesicular,* with inspiratory and expiratory sounds about equal in length, at times separated by a silent interval. Detecting differences in pitch and intensity is often easier during expiration.

- *Bronchial,* or louder, harsher and higher in pitch, with a short silence between inspiratory and expiratory sounds. Expiratory sounds last longer than inspiratory sounds.

- *Tracheal,* or loud harsh sounds heard over the trachea in the neck.

The characteristics of these four kinds of breath sounds are summarized below.

Characteristics of Breath Sounds

	Duration of Sounds	Intensity of Expiratory Sound	Pitch of Expiratory Sound	Locations Where Heard Normally
Vesicular[a]	Inspiratory sounds last longer than expiratory sounds.	Soft	Relatively low	Over most of both lungs
Broncho-vesicular	Inspiratory and expiratory sounds are almost equal.	Intermediate	Intermediate	Often in the 1st and 2nd interspaces anteriorly and between the scapulae
Bronchial	Expiratory sounds last longer than inspiratory ones.	Loud	Relatively high	Over the manubrium, (larger proximal airways)

If bronchovesicular or bronchial breath sounds are heard in locations distant from those listed, suspect replacement of air-filled lung by fluid-filled or consolidated lung tissue.

See Table 8-6, Normal and Altered Breath and Voice Sounds, p. 337.

(*continued*)

Characteristics of Breath Sounds (continued)

	Duration of Sounds	Intensity of Expiratory Sound	Pitch of Expiratory Sound	Locations Where Heard Normally
Tracheal ⋀	Inspiratory and expiratory sounds are almost equal.	Very loud	Relatively high	Over the trachea in the neck

[a]The thickness of the bars indicates intensity; the steeper their incline, the higher the pitch.

Sources: Loudon R and Murphy LH. Lungs sounds. *Am Rev Respir Dis.* 1994;130:663; Bohadana A, Izbicki G, Kraman SS. Fundamentals of lung auscultation. *N Engl J Med.* 2014;370:744; Wilkins RL, Dexter JR, Murphy RLH, et al. Lung sound nomenclature survey, *Chest.* 1990;98:886; Schreur HJW, Sterk PJ, Vanderschoot JW, et al. Lung sound intensity in patients with emphysema and in normal subjects at standardised airflows. *Thorax.* 1992;47:674; Bettancourt PE, DelBono EA, Speigelman D, et al. Clinical utility of chest auscultation in common pulmonary disease. *Am J Resp Crit Care Med.* 1994;150:1921.

Adventitious (Added) Sounds. Listen for any *added, or adventitious, sounds* that are superimposed on the usual breath sounds. Detection of adventitious sounds—*crackles* (sometimes called *rales*), *wheezes,* and *rhonchi*—is an important focus of your examination, often leading to diagnosis of cardiac and pulmonary conditions. The most common adventitious sounds are described below. Note that the American Thoracic Society describes rhonchi as a low-pitched wheeze (unrelated to airway secretions), so some recommend not using the term "rhonchi."[47,48]

For further discussion and other added sounds, see Table 8-7, Adventitious (Added) Lung Sounds: Causes and Qualities, p. 338.

Adventitious or Added Breath Sounds

Crackles (or Rales)	Wheezes and Rhonchi
Discontinuous	**Continuous**
• Intermittent, *nonmusical,* and brief	• Sinusoidal, *musical,* prolonged (but not necessarily persisting throughout the respiratory cycle)
• Like dots in time	• Like dashes in time
• *Fine crackles:* soft, high-pitched (~650 Hz), very brief (5–10 ms) · · · · ·	• *Wheezes:* relatively high-pitched (≥400 Hz) with hissing or shrill quality (>80 ms) wwwww
• *Coarse crackles:* somewhat louder, lower in pitch (~350 Hz), brief (15–30 ms) · · · · ·	• *Rhonchi:* relatively low-pitched (150–200 Hz) with snoring quality (>80 ms) ∿∿∿

Crackles can arise from abnormalities of the lung parenchyma (*pneumonia, interstitial lung disease, pulmonary fibrosis, atelectasis, heart failure*) or of the airways (*bronchitis, bronchiectasis*).

Wheezes arise in the narrowed airways of *asthma, COPD,* and *bronchitis.*

Many clinicians use the term "rhonchi" to describe sounds from secretions in large airways that may change with coughing.

Source: Loudon R, Murphy LH. Lungs sounds. *Am Rev Respir Dis.* 1994;130:663; Bohadana A, Izbicki G, Kraman SS. Fundamentals of lung auscultation. *N Engl J Med.* 2014;370:744.

If you hear *crackles*, especially those that do not clear after coughing, listen carefully for the following characteristics.[47,49–52] These are clues to the underlying condition:

- Loudness, pitch, and duration, summarized as fine or coarse crackles

- Number, few to many

- Timing in the respiratory cycle

- Location on the chest wall

- Persistence of their pattern from breath to breath

- Any change after a cough or change in the patient's position

Fine late inspiratory crackles that persist from breath to breath suggest abnormal lung tissue.

The crackles of heart failure are usually best heard in the posterior inferior lung fields.

Clearing of crackles, wheezes, or rhonchi after coughing or position change suggests inspissated secretions, seen in *bronchitis* or *atelectasis*.

In some normal people, crackles may be heard at the anterior lung bases after maximal expiration. Crackles in dependent portions of the lungs may also occur after prolonged recumbency.

If you hear *wheezes* or *rhonchi,* note their timing and location. Do they change with deep breathing or coughing? Beware of the silent chest, in which air movement is minimal.

In the advanced airway obstruction of severe asthma, wheezes and breath sounds may be absent due to low respiratory airflow (the "silent chest"), a clinical emergency.

Findings predictive of *COPD* include combinations of symptoms and signs, especially dyspnea and wheezing by self-report or examination, plus >70 pack-years of smoking, history of bronchitis or emphysema, and decreased breath sounds. Diagnosis requires spirometry and, often, further pulmonary testing.[6,53–58]

Note that *tracheal sounds* originating in the neck such as *stridor* and *vocal cord dysfunction* can be transmitted to the chest and mistaken for wheezing, leading to inappropriate or delayed treatment.

Stridor and laryngeal sounds are loudest over the neck, whereas true wheezes and rhonchi are faint or absent over the neck.[47]

Note any *pleural rubs*, which are coarse, grating biphasic sounds heard primarily during expiration.

Pleural rubs may be heard in *pleurisy, pneumonia,* and *pulmonary embolism*.

Transmitted Voice Sounds. If you hear abnormally located bronchovesicular or bronchial breath sounds, assess transmitted voice sounds using three techniques below. With diaphragm of your stethoscope, listen in symmetric areas over the chest wall for abnormal vocal resonances suspicious for pneumonia or pleural effusion.

Increased transmission of voice sounds suggests that embedded airways are blocked by inflammation or secretions.[47] See Table 8-6, Normal and Altered Breath and Voice Sounds, p. 337.

- *Egophony.* Ask the patient to say "ee." You will normally hear a muffled long E sound.

If "ee" sounds like "A" and has a nasal bleating quality, an E-to-A change, or egophony, is present.

- *Bronchophony.* Ask the patient to say "ninety-nine." Normally the sounds transmitted through the chest wall are muffled and indistinct. Louder voice sounds are called *bronchophony.*

Localized bronchophony and egophony are seen in lobar consolidation from pneumonia. In patients with fever and cough, the presence of bronchial breath sounds and egophony more than triples the likelihood of pneumonia.[59]

- *Whispered pectoriloquy.* Ask the patient to whisper "ninety-nine" or "one-two-three." The whispered voice is normally heard faintly and indistinctly, if at all.

Louder, clearer whispered sounds are called whispered pectoriloquy.

Examination of the Anterior Chest

When examined in the supine position, the patient should lie comfortably with arms somewhat abducted. If the patient is having difficulty breathing, raise the head of the examining table or the bed to increase respiratory excursion and ease of breathing.

Persons with severe *COPD* may prefer to sit leaning forward, with lips pursed during exhalation and arms supported on their knees or a table.

Inspection. Observe the shape of the patient's chest and the movement of the chest wall. Note:

- Deformities or asymmetry of the thorax

See Table 8-5, Deformities of the Thorax, p. 336.

- Abnormal retraction of the lower intercostal spaces during inspiration, or any supraclavicular retraction

Abnormal retraction occurs in severe asthma, COPD, or upper airway obstruction.
Lag occurs in underlying diseases of the lung or pleura.

- Local lag or impairment in respiratory movement

Palpation. Palpate the anterior chest wall for the following purposes:

- *Identification of tender areas*

- *Assessment of bruising, sinus tracts, or other skin changes*

Tender pectoral muscles or costal cartilages suggest, but do not prove, that chest pain has a localized musculoskeletal origin.

- *Assessment of chest expansion.* Place your thumbs along each costal margin, your hands along the lateral rib cage (Fig. 8-22). As you position your hands, slide them medially a bit to raise loose skin folds between your thumbs. Ask the patient to inhale deeply. Observe how far your thumbs diverge as the thorax expands, and feel for the extent and symmetry of respiratory movement.

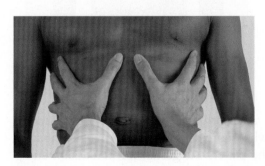

FIGURE 8-22. **Assess chest expansion.**

■ *Assessment of tactile fremitus.* If needed, compare both sides of the chest, using the ball or ulnar surface of your hand. Fremitus is usually decreased or absent over the precordium. When examining a woman, gently displace the breasts as necessary (Fig. 8-23).

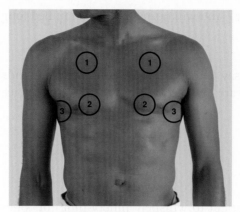

FIGURE 8-23. **Locations for palpating fremitus.**

Percussion. As needed, percuss the anterior and lateral chest, again comparing both sides (Fig. 8-24). The heart normally produces an area of dullness to the left of the sternum from the 3rd to the 5th interspaces.

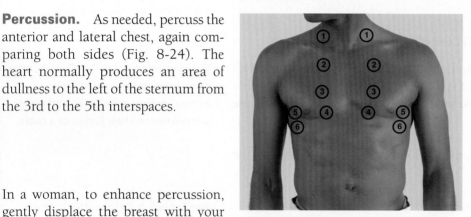

FIGURE 8-24. **Palate and percuss in a "ladder" pattern.**

In a woman, to enhance percussion, gently displace the breast with your left hand while percussing with the right, or ask the patient to move the breast for you.

Dullness represents airway obstruction from inflammation or secretions. Because pleural fluid usually sinks to the lowest part of the pleural space (posteriorly in a supine patient), only a very large effusion can be detected anteriorly.

The hyperresonance of *COPD* may obscure dullness over the heart.

The dullness of *right middle lobe pneumonia* typically occurs behind the right breast. Unless you displace the breast, you may miss the abnormal percussion note.

Identify and locate any area with an abnormal percussion note.

Percuss for liver dullness and gastric tympany. With your pleximeter finger above and parallel to the expected upper border of liver dullness, percuss in progressive steps downward in the right midclavicular line (Fig. 8-25). Identify the upper border of liver dullness. Later, during the abdominal examination, you will use this method to estimate the size of the liver. As you percuss down the chest on the left, the resonance of normal lung usually changes to the tympany of the gastric air bubble.

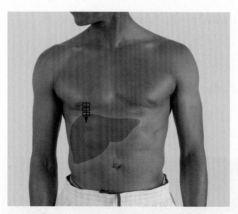

FIGURE 8-25. **Percuss for liver dullness and gastric tympany.**

The hyperinflated lung of *COPD* often displaces the upper border of the liver downward and lowers the level of diaphragmatic dullness posteriorly.

Auscultation. Listen to the chest anteriorly and laterally as the patient breathes with mouth open, and somewhat more deeply than normal. Compare symmetric areas of the lungs, using the pattern suggested for percussion and extending it to adjacent areas, if indicated.

■ *Listen to the breath sounds,* noting their intensity and identifying any variations from normal vesicular breathing. Breath sounds are usually louder in the upper anterior lung fields. Bronchovesicular breath sounds may be heard over the large airways, especially on the right.

■ *Identify any adventitious sounds,* time them in the respiratory cycle, and locate them on the chest wall. Do they clear with deep breathing?

■ If indicated, *listen for transmitted voice sounds.*

See Table 8-7, Adventitious (Added) Lung Sounds: Causes and Qualities, p. 338, and Table 8-8, Physical Findings in Selected Chest Disorders, pp. 339–340.

Special Techniques

Clinical Assessment of Pulmonary Function.   Walk tests are practical, simple ways to assess cardiopulmonary function commonly used in rehabilitation and pre- and postoperative settings. The 2002 American Thoracic Society guidelines that standardize the 6-minute walk test continue to predict clinical outcomes in most patients with COPD.[60,61] The test is easy to administer and requires only a 100-foot hallway. It measures "the distance that a patient can quickly walk on a flat, hard surface in a period of 6 minutes" and provides a global evaluation of the pulmonary and cardiovascular systems, neuromuscular units, and muscle metabolism. Review the specifics of testing, which should be done on two occasions and include taking the clinical history and vital signs. This test as well as shorter tests continue to be evaluated.[58]

Forced Expiratory Time.   This test assesses the expiratory phase of breathing, which is typically slowed in obstructive pulmonary disease. Ask the patient to take a deep breath in and then breathe out as quickly and completely as possible with mouth open. Listen over the trachea with the diaphragm of a stethoscope and time the audible expiration. Try to get three consistent readings, allowing a short rest between efforts, if necessary.

Patients ≥age 60 years with a forced expiratory time of ≥9 seconds are four times more likely to have COPD.[62]

Identification of a Fractured Rib.   Local pain and tenderness of one or more ribs raise the question of fracture. By AP compression of the chest, you can help to distinguish a fracture from soft-tissue injury. With one hand on the sternum and the other on the thoracic spine, squeeze the chest. Is this painful, and where?

An increase in the local pain (distant from your hands) suggests rib fracture rather than just soft-tissue injury.

Recording Your Findings

Note that initially you may use sentences to describe your findings; later you will use phrases.

Recording the Physical Examination—The Thorax and Lungs

"Thorax is symmetric with good expansion. Lungs resonant. Breath sounds vesicular; no crackles, wheezes, or rhonchi. Diaphragms descend 4 cm bilaterally."
OR
"Thorax symmetric with moderate kyphosis and increased AP diameter, decreased expansion. Lungs are hyperresonant. Breath sounds distant with delayed expiratory phase and scattered expiratory wheezes. Fremitus decreased; no bronchophony, egophony, or whispered pectoriloquy. Diaphragms descend 2 cm bilaterally."

These findings suggest *COPD*.

Table 8-1 Chest Pain

Problem	Process	Location	Quality	Severity
Cardiovascular				
Angina Pectoris	Temporary myocardial ischemia, usually secondary to coronary atherosclerosis	Retrosternal or across the anterior chest, often radiates to the shoulders, arms, neck, lower jaw, or upper abdomen	Pressing, squeezing, tight, heavy, occasionally burning	Mild to moderate, sometimes perceived as discomfort rather than pain
Myocardial Infarction	Prolonged myocardial ischemia, resulting in irreversible muscle damage or necrosis	Same as in angina	Same as in angina	Often, but not always, a severe pain
Pericarditis	Irritation of parietal pleura adjacent to the pericardium	Retrosternal or left precordial, may radiate to the tip of left shoulder	Sharp, knifelike	Often severe
Aortic Dissection	A splitting within the layers of the aortic wall, allowing passage of blood to dissect a channel	Anterior or posterior chest, radiating to the neck, back, or abdomen	Ripping, tearing	Very severe
Pulmonary				
Pleuritic Pain	Inflammation of the parietal pleura, as in pleurisy, pneumonia, pulmonary infarction, or neoplasm; rarely, subdiaphragmatic abscess	Chest wall overlying the process	Sharp, knifelike	Often severe
Gastrointestinal and Other				
Gastrointestinal Reflux Disease	Irritation or inflammation of the esophageal mucosa due to reflux of gastric acid from lowered esophageal sphincter tone	Retrosternal, may radiate to the back	Burning, may be squeezing	Mild to severe
Diffuse Esophageal Spasm	Motor dysfunction of the esophageal muscle	Retrosternal, may radiate to the back, arms, and jaw	Usually squeezing	Mild to severe
Chest Wall Pain, Costochondritis	Variable, including trauma, inflammation of costal cartilage	Often below the left breast or along the costal cartilages	Stabbing, sticking, or dull, aching	Variable
Anxiety, Panic Disorder	Unclear	Precordial, below the left breast, or across the anterior chest	Stabbing, sticking, or dull, aching	Variable

Note: Chest pain may be referred from extrathoracic structures in the neck (*arthritis*) and abdomen (*biliary colic, acute cholecystitis*).

Timing	Factors That Aggravate	Factors That Relieve	Associated Symptoms
Usually 1–3 min but up to 10 min. Prolonged episodes up to 20 min	Often exertion, especially in the cold; meals; emotional stress. May occur at rest	Often, but not always, rest, nitroglycerin	Sometimes dyspnea, nausea, sweating
20 min to several hours	Not always triggered by exertion	Not relieved by rest	Dyspnea, nausea, vomiting, sweating, weakness
Persistent	Breathing, changing position, coughing, lying down, sometimes swallowing	Sitting forward may relieve it	Seen in autoimmune disorders, postmyocardial infarction, viral infection, chest irradiation
Abrupt onset, early peak, persistent for hours or more	Hypertension		If thoracic, hoarseness, dysphagia; also syncope, hemiplegia, paraplegia
Persistent	Deep inspiration, coughing, movements of the trunk		Of the underlying illness
Variable	Large meal; bending over, lying down	Antacids, sometimes belching	Sometimes regurgitation, dysphagia; also cough, laryngitis, asthma
Variable	Swallowing of food or cold liquid; emotional stress	Sometimes nitroglycerin	Dysphagia
Fleeting to hours or days	Coughing; movement of chest, trunk, arms		Often local tenderness
Fleeting to hours or days	May follow effort, emotional stress		Breathlessness, palpitations, weakness, anxiety

Table 8-2 Dyspnea

Problem	Process	Timing
Left-Sided Heart Failure *(Left Ventricular Failure or Mitral Stenosis)*	Elevated pressure in pulmonary capillary bed with transudation of fluid into interstitial spaces and alveoli, decreased compliance (increased stiffness) of the lungs, increased work of breathing	Dyspnea may progress slowly, or suddenly as in acute pulmonary edema
Chronic Bronchitis	Excessive mucus production in bronchi, followed by chronic obstruction of airways	Chronic productive cough followed by slowly progressive dyspnea
Chronic Obstructive Pulmonary Disease (COPD)	Overdistention of air spaces distal to terminal bronchioles, with destruction of alveolar septa, alveolar enlargement, and limitation of expiratory air flow	Slowly progressive dyspnea; relatively mild cough later
Asthma	Reversible bronchial hyperresponsiveness involving release of inflammatory mediators, increased airway secretions, and bronchoconstriction	Acute episodes, separated by symptom-free periods. Nocturnal episodes common
Diffuse Interstitial Lung Diseases *(e.g., Sarcoidosis, Widespread Neoplasms, Idiopathic Pulmonary Fibrosis, and Asbestosis)*	Abnormal and widespread infiltration of cells, fluid, and collagen into interstitial spaces between alveoli; many causes	Progressive dyspnea, which varies in its rate of development with the cause
Pneumonia	Infection of lung parenchyma from the respiratory bronchioles to the alveoli	An acute illness, timing varies with the causative agent
Spontaneous Pneumothorax	Leakage of air into pleural space through blebs on visceral pleura, with resulting partial or complete collapse of the lung	Sudden onset of dyspnea
Acute Pulmonary Embolism	Sudden occlusion of part of pulmonary arterial tree by a blood clot that usually originates in deep veins of legs or pelvis	Sudden onset of tachypnea, dyspnea
Anxiety with Hyperventilation	Overbreathing, with resultant respiratory alkalosis and fall in arterial partial pressure of carbon dioxide (pCO_2)	Episodic, often recurrent

Sources: Parshall MB, Schwartzstein RM, Adams L, et al; American Thoracic Society Committee on Dyspnea. An official American Thoracic Society statement: update on the mechanisms, assessment, and management of dyspnea. *Am J Respir Crit Care Med.* 2012;185:435; Wenzel RP, Fowler AA. Acute bronchitis. *N Engl J Med.* 2006;355:2125; Badgett RG, Tanaka DJ, Hunt DK, et al. Can moderate chronic obstructive pulmonary disease be diagnosed by historical and physical findings alone? *Am J Med.* 1993;94:188; Holleman DR, Simel DL. Does the clinical examination predict airflow limitation? *JAMA.* 1995;273:63; Straus SE, McAlister FA, Sackett DL, et al. The accuracy of patient history, wheezing, and laryngeal measurements in diagnosing obstructive airway disease. *JAMA.* 2000;283:1853; Panettieri RA. In the clinic: asthma. *Ann Intern Med.* 2007;146:ITC6–1; Littner M. In the clinic: chronic obstructive

Factors That Aggravate	Factors That Relieve	Associated Symptoms	Setting
Exertion, lying down	Rest, sitting up, though dyspnea may become persistent	Often cough, orthopnea, paroxysmal nocturnal dyspnea; sometimes wheezing	History of heart disease or its predisposing factors
Exertion, inhaled irritants, respiratory infections	Expectoration; rest, though dyspnea may become persistent	Chronic productive cough, recurrent respiratory infections; wheezing may develop	History of smoking, air pollutants, recurrent respiratory infections; often present with COPD
Exertion	Rest, though dyspnea may become persistent	Cough, with scant mucoid sputum	History of smoking, air pollutants, sometimes a familial deficiency in α_1-antitrypsin
Variable, including allergens, irritants, respiratory infections, exercise, cold, and emotion	Separation from aggravating factors	Wheezing, cough, tightness in chest	Environmental conditions
Exertion	Rest, though dyspnea may become persistent	Often weakness, fatigue; cough less common than in other lung diseases	Varied; exposure to trigger substances
Exertion, smoking	Rest, though dyspnea may become persistent	Pleuritic pain, cough, sputum, fever, though not necessarily present	Varied
		Pleuritic pain, cough	Often a previously healthy young adult or adult with emphysema
Exertion	Rest, though dyspnea may become persistent	Often none; retrosternal oppressive pain if massive occlusion; pleuritic pain, cough, syncope, hemoptysis, and/or unilateral leg swelling and pain from instigating deep vein thrombosis; anxiety (see below)	Postpartum or postoperative periods; prolonged bed rest; heart failure, chronic lung disease, and fractures of hip or leg; deep venous thrombosis (often not clinically apparent); also hypercoagulability, hereditary (i.e., protein C, S, factor V Leiden deficiency) or acquired (e.g., cancer, hormonal therapy)
Often occurs at rest; an upsetting event may not be evident	Breathing in and out of a paper or plastic bag may help	Sighing, lightheadedness, numbness or tingling of the hands and feet, palpitations, chest pain	Other manifestations of anxiety may be present, such as chest pain diaphoresis, palpitations

pulmonary disease. *Ann Intern Med.* 2011;154:ITC4–1; Neiwoehner DR. Outpatient management of severe COPD. *N Engl J Med.* 2010;362:1407; Global Initiative for Chronic Obstructive Lung Disease. Global strategy for the diagnosis, management, and prevention of chronic obstructive pulmonary disease. Updated 2015. Available at http://www.goldcopd.org/uploads/users/files/GOLD_Report_2015_Feb18.pdf. Accessed April 6, 2015; Neiderman M. In the clinic: community-acquired pneumonia. *Ann Intern Med.* 2009;151:ITC4–1–ITC4–16; Agnelli G, Becattini C. Acute pulmonary embolism. *N Engl J Med.* 2010;363:266; Katerndahl DA. Chest pain and its importance in patients with panic disorder: an updated literature review. *Prim Care Companion J Clin Psychiatry.* 2008;10:376.

Table 8-3 Cough and Hemoptysis

Problem	Cough and Sputum	Associated Symptoms and Setting
Acute Inflammation		
Laryngitis	Dry cough, may become productive of variable amounts of sputum	Acute fairly minor illness with hoarseness. Often associated with viral rhinosinusitis.
Acute Bronchitis	Cough, may be dry or productive	Acute, often viral, illness generally without fever or dyspnea; at times with burning retrosternal discomfort.
Mycoplasma and Viral Pneumonias	Dry hacking cough, may become productive of mucoid sputum	Acute febrile illness, often with malaise, headache, and possibly dyspnea.
Bacterial Pneumonias	Sputum is mucoid or purulent; may be **blood-streaked, diffusely pinkish, or rusty**	Acute illness with chills, often high fever, dyspnea, and chest pain. Commonly from *Streptococcus pneumonia, Haemophilus influenza, Moraxella catarrhalis; Klebsiella* in alcoholism, especially if underlying smoking, chronic bronchitis and COPD, cardiovascular disease, diabetes.
Chronic Inflammation		
Postnasal Drip	Chronic cough; sputum mucoid or mucopurulent	Postnasal discharge may be seen in posterior pharynx. Associated with allergic rhinitis, with or without sinusitis.
Chronic Bronchitis	Chronic cough; sputum mucoid to purulent, may be **blood-streaked or even bloody**	Often with recurrent wheezing and dyspnea, and prolonged history of tobacco abuse.
Bronchiectasis	Chronic cough; sputum purulent, often copious and foul-smelling; may be **blood-streaked or bloody**	Recurrent bronchopulmonary infections common; sinusitis may coexist.
Pulmonary Tuberculosis	Cough, dry or with mucoid or purulent sputum; may be **blood-streaked or bloody**	Early, no symptoms. Later, anorexia, weight loss, fatigue, fever, and night sweats.
Lung Abscess	Sputum purulent and foul-smelling; may be **bloody**	Usually from aspiration pneumonia with fever and infection from oral anaerobes and poor dental hygiene; often with dysphagia or episode of impaired consciousness.
Asthma	Cough, at times with thick mucoid sputum, especially near end of an attack	Episodic wheezing and dyspnea, but cough may occur alone. Often with a history of allergies.
Gastroesophageal Reflux	Chronic cough, especially at night or early in the morning	Wheezing, especially at night (often mistaken for asthma), early morning hoarseness, and repeated attempts to clear the throat. Often with heartburn and regurgitation.
Neoplasm		
Lung Cancer	Cough, dry to productive; sputum may be **blood-streaked or bloody**	Commonly with dyspnea, weight loss, and history of tobacco abuse.
Cardiovascular Disorders		
Left Ventricular Failure or Mitral Stenosis	Often dry, especially on exertion or at night; may progress to the **pink frothy sputum** of pulmonary edema or to frank hemoptysis	Dyspnea, orthopnea, paroxysmal nocturnal dyspnea.
Pulmonary Embolism	Dry cough, at times with hemoptysis	Tachypnea, chest or pleuritic pain, dyspnea, fever, syncope, anxiety; factors that predispose to deep venous thrombosis.
Irritating Particles, Chemicals, or Gases	Variable. There may be a latent period between exposure and symptoms.	Exposure to irritants. Eyes, nose, and throat may be affected.

Sources: Irwin RS, Madison JM. The diagnosis and treatment of cough. *N Engl J Med.* 2000;343:1715; Metlay JP, Kapoor WN, Fine MJ. Does this patient have community-acquired pneumonia? Diagnosing pneumonia by history and physical examination. *JAMA.* 1997;378:1440; Neiderman M. In the clinic: community-acquired pneumonia. *Ann Intern Med.* 2009;151:ITC4–1; Barker A. Bronchiectasis. *N Engl J Med.* 2002;346:1383; Wenzel RP, Fowler AA. Acute bronchitis. *N Engl J Med.* 2006;355:2125; Kerlin MP. In the clinic. Asthma. *Ann Intern Med.* 2014;160:ITC3–1; Escalante P. In the clinic: tuberculosis. *Ann Intern Med.* 2009;150:ITC6–1; Agnelli G, Becattini C. Acute pulmonary embolism. *N Engl J Med.* 2010;363:266.

Table 8-4 Abnormalities in Rate and Rhythm of Breathing

When observing respiratory patterns, note the rate, depth, and regularity of the patient's breathing. Traditional terms, such as tachypnea, are given below so that you will understand them, but simple descriptions are recommended.

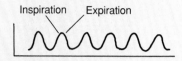

Normal

The respiratory rate is about 14–20 per min in normal adults and up to 44 per min in infants.

Slow Breathing (*Bradypnea*)

Slow breathing with or without an increase in tidal volume that maintains alveolar ventilation. Abnormal alveolar hypoventilation without increased tidal volume can arise from uremia, drug-induced respiratory depression, and increased intracranial pressure.

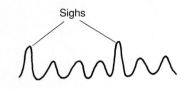

Sighing Respiration

Breathing punctuated by frequent sighs suggests *hyperventilation syndrome*—a common cause of dyspnea and dizziness. Occasional sighs are normal.

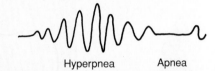

Rapid Shallow Breathing (*Tachypnea*)

Rapid shallow breathing has numerous causes, including salicylate intoxication, restrictive lung disease, pleuritic chest pain, and an elevated diaphragm.

Cheyne–Stokes Breathing

Periods of deep breathing alternate with periods of *apnea* (no breathing). This pattern is normal in children and older adults during sleep. Causes include heart failure, uremia, drug-induced respiratory depression, and brain injury (typically bihemispheric).

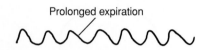

Obstructive Breathing

In obstructive lung disease, expiration is prolonged due to narrowed airways increase the resistance to air flow. Causes include asthma, chronic bronchitis, and COPD.

Rapid Deep Breathing (*Hyperpnea, Hyperventilation*)

In *hyperpnea,* rapid deep breathing occurs in response to metabolic demand from causes such as exercise, high altitude, sepsis, and anemia. In *hyperventilation,* this pattern is independent of metabolic demand, except in respiratory acidosis. Light-headedness and tingling may arise from decreased CO_2 concentration. In the comatose patient, consider hypoxia, or hypoglycemia affecting the midbrain or pons. *Kussmaul breathing* is compensatory overbreathing due to systemic acidosis. The breathing rate may be fast, normal, or slow.

Ataxic Breathing (*Biot Breathing*)

Breathing is irregular—periods of apnea alternate with regular deep breaths which stop suddenly for short intervals. Causes include meningitis, respiratory depression, and brain injury, typically at the medullary level.

Table 8-5 Deformities of the Thorax

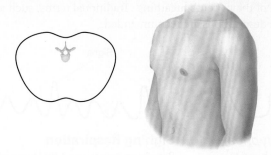

Normal Adult

The lateral diameter of the thorax in the normal adult is greater than its AP diameter. The ratio of its AP diameter to the lateral diameter is normally ~0.7 up to 0.9 and increases with aging.[43]

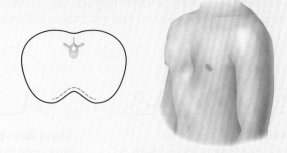

Funnel Chest (*Pectus Excavatum*)

Note depression in the lower portion of the sternum. Compression of the heart and great vessels may cause murmurs.

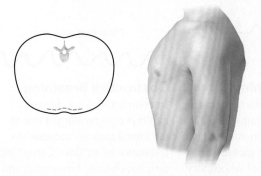

Barrel Chest

There is an increased AP diameter. This shape is normal during infancy, and often accompanies aging and chronic obstructive pulmonary disease.

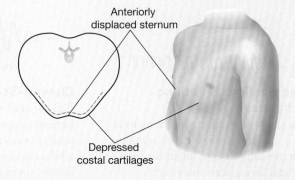

Anteriorly displaced sternum

Depressed costal cartilages

Pigeon Chest (*Pectus Carinatum*)

The sternum is displaced anteriorly, increasing the AP diameter. The costal cartilages adjacent to the protruding sternum are depressed.

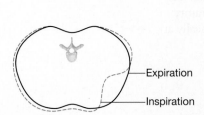

Expiration

Inspiration

Traumatic Flail Chest

Multiple rib fractures may result in paradoxical movements of the thorax. As descent of the diaphragm decreases intrathoracic pressure, on inspiration, the injured area caves inward; on expiration, it moves outward.

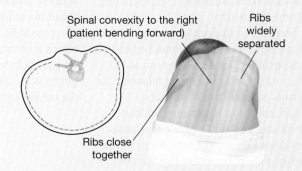

Spinal convexity to the right (patient bending forward)

Ribs widely separated

Ribs close together

Thoracic Kyphoscoliosis

Abnormal spinal curvatures and vertebral rotation deform the chest. Distortion of the underlying lungs may make interpretation of lung findings very difficult.

Table 8-6 Normal and Altered Breath and Voice Sounds

The origins of breath sounds continue to be investigated.[47] Acoustic studies indicate that turbulent air flow in the pharynx, glottis, and subglottic region produce tracheal breath sounds, which are similar to bronchial sounds. The inspiratory component of vesicular breath sounds seems to arise in the lobar and segmental airways; the expiratory component arises in the more central larger airways. Normally, tracheal and bronchial sounds may be heard over the trachea and mainstem bronchi; vesicular breath sounds predominate throughout most of the lungs. When lung tissue loses airflow, there is increased transmission of high-pitched sounds. If the tracheobronchial tree is open, bronchial breath sounds may replace the normal vesicular sounds over airless areas of the lung. This change occurs in lobar pneumonia when the alveoli get filled with fluid and cellular debris—a process called *consolidation.* Other causes include pulmonary edema or, rarely, hemorrhage. Bronchial breath sounds usually correlate with an increase in tactile fremitus and transmitted voice sounds. These findings are summarized below.

	Normal Air-Filled Lung	**Consolidated Airless Lung (Lobar Pneumonia)**
	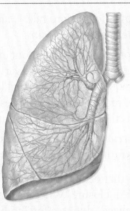 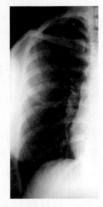	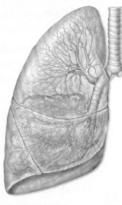 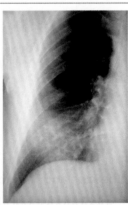
Breath Sounds	Predominantly vesicular	Bronchial or bronchovesicular over the involved area
Transmitted Voice Sounds	Spoken words muffled and indistinct	Spoken "ee" heard as "ay" (*egophony*)
	Spoken "ee" heard as "ee"	Spoken words louder (*bronchophony*)
	Whispered words faint and indistinct, if heard at all	Whispered words louder, clearer (*whispered pectoriloquy*)
Tactile Fremitus	Normal	Increased
	NOTE: In the hyperinflated lung of COPD, breath sounds are decreased (muffled to distant) to absent and transmitted voice sounds and fremitus are decreased.	NOTE: In the dull lung of pleural effusion, breath sounds are decreased to absent (bronchial sounds possible at upper margin of effusion). Transmitted voice sounds are decreased to absent (but may be increased at upper margin of effusion). Fremitus is decreased.

Table 8-7 Adventitious (Added) Lung Sounds: Causes and Qualities

Sound	Causes and Qualities
Crackles	Crackles are discontinuous nonmusical sounds that can be early inspiratory (as in *COPD*), late inspiratory (as in *pulmonary fibrosis*), or biphasic (as in *pneumonia*). They are currently considered to result from a series of tiny explosions when small distal airways, deflated during expiration, pop open during inspiration. With few exceptions, recent acoustic studies indicate that the role of secretions as a cause of crackles is less likely.[47,48]
	Fine crackles are softer, higher pitched, and more frequent per breath than coarse crackles. They are heard from *mid to late inspiration,* especially in the dependent areas of the lung, and change according to body position. They have a shorter duration and higher frequency than coarse crackles. Fine crackles appear to be generated by the "sudden inspiratory opening of small airways held closed by surface forces during the previous expiration."[47]
	Examples include *pulmonary fibrosis* (known for "Velcro rales") and interstitial lung diseases such as *interstitial fibrosis* and *interstitial pneumonitis.*
	Coarse crackles appear in early inspiration and last throughout expiration (*biphasic*), have a popping sound, are heard over any lung region, and do not vary with body position. They have a longer duration and lower frequency than fine crackles, change or disappear with coughing, and are transmitted to the mouth. Coarse crackles appear to result from "boluses of gas passing through airways as they open and close intermittently."[47]
	Examples include *COPD, asthma, bronchiectasis, pneumonia* (crackles may become finer and change from mid to late inspiratory during recovery), and *heart failure.*
Wheezes and Rhonchi	*Wheezes* are continuous musical sounds that occur during rapid airflow when bronchial airways are narrowed almost to the point of closure. Wheezes can be inspiratory, expiratory, or biphasic. They may be localized, due to a foreign body, mucous plug, or tumor, or heard throughout the lung. Although wheezes are typical of asthma, they can occur in a number of pulmonary diseases. Recent studies suggest that as the airways become more narrowed, wheezes become less audible, culminating finally in "the silent chest" of severe asthma requiring immediate intervention.
	Rhonchi are considered by some to be a variant of wheezes, arising from the same mechanism, but lower in pitch. Unlike wheezes, rhonchi may disappear with coughing, so secretions may be involved.[47]
Stridor	*Stridor* is a continuous, high-frequency, high-pitched musical sound produced during airflow through a narrowing in the upper respiratory tract. Stridor is best heard over the neck during inspiration, but can be biphasic. Causes of the underlying airway obstruction include tracheal stenosis from intubation, airway edema after device removal, epiglottitis, foreign body, and anaphylaxis. Immediate intervention is warranted.
Pleural Rub	A *pleural rub* is a discontinuous, low-frequency, grating sound that arises from inflammation and roughening of the visceral pleura as it slides against the parietal pleura. This nonmusical sound is biphasic, heard during inspiration and expiration, and often best heard in the axilla and base of the lungs.
Mediastinal Crunch *(Hamman Sign)*	A *mediastinal crunch* is a series of precordial crackles synchronous with the heartbeat, not with respiration. Best heard in the left lateral position, it arises from air entry into the mediastinum causing mediastinal emphysema (*pneumomediastinum*). It usually produces severe central chest pain and may be spontaneous. It has been reported in cases of tracheobronchial injury, blunt trauma, pulmonary disease, use of recreational drugs, childbirth, and rapid ascent from scuba diving.[63]

Sources: Bohadana A, Izbicki G, Kraman SS. Fundamentals of lung auscultation. *N Engl J Med.* 2014;370:744; McGee S. *Evidence-based Physical Diagnosis,* 3rd ed. Philadelphia, PA: Saunders, 2012; Loudon R, Murphy LH. Lungs sounds. *Am Rev Respir Dis.* 1994;130:663.

Table 8-8 Physical Findings in Selected Chest Disorders

The red boxes in this table provide a framework for the clinical assessment of common chest disorders. Start with the three boxes under percussion. Note resonant, dull, and hyperresonant. Then move from each of these to other boxes that emphasize some of the key differences among various conditions. The changes described vary with the extent and severity of the disorder. Abnormalities deep in the chest usually produce fewer signs than superficial ones, and may cause no signs at all. Use the table for the direction of typical changes, not for absolute distinctions.

Condition	Percussion Note	Trachea	Breath Sounds	Adventitious Sounds	Tactile Fremitus and Transmitted Voice Sounds
Normal The tracheobronchial tree and alveoli are open; pleurae are thin and close together; mobility of the chest wall is unimpaired.	**Resonant**	Midline	Vesicular, except perhaps bronchovesicular and bronchial sounds over the large bronchi and trachea, respectively	None, except a few transient inspiratory crackles at the bases of the lungs	Normal
Left-Sided Heart Failure Increased pressure in the pulmonary veins causes congestion and interstitial edema (around the alveoli); bronchial mucosa may become edematous.	**Resonant**	Midline	Vesicular (normal)	*Late inspiratory crackles* in the dependent portions of the lungs; possibly *wheezes*	Normal
Chronic Bronchitis The bronchi are chronically inflamed and a productive cough is present. Airway obstruction may develop.	**Resonant**	Midline	Vesicular (normal)	None; possible scattered coarse *crackles* in early inspiration and expiration; possible *wheezes* or *rhonchi*	Normal
Lobar Pneumonia (*Consolidation*) Alveoli fill with fluid, as in pneumonia	**Dull** over the airless area	Midline	*Bronchial* over the involved area	*Late inspiratory crackles* over the involved area	*Increased* over the involved area, with *egophony, bronchophony,* and *whispered pectoriloquy*
Partial Lobar Obstruction (*Atelectasis*) When a plug (from mucus or a foreign object) obstructs bronchial air flow, affected alveoli collapse and become airless	**Dull** over the airless area	May be *shifted toward involved side*	*Usually absent* when bronchial plug persists. Exceptions include right upper lobe atelectasis, where adjacent tracheal sounds may be transmitted.	None	*Usually absent* when the bronchial plug persists. In right upper lobe atelectasis may be *increased.*
Pleural Effusion Fluid accumulates in the pleural space and separates air-filled lung from the chest wall, blocking the transmission of breath sounds.	**Dull** to flat over the fluid	*Shifted toward the unaffected side* in a large effusion	*Decreased to absent,* but bronchial breath sounds may be heard near top of large effusion.	None, except a *possible pleural rub*	*Decreased to absent, but may be increased* toward the top of a large effusion

(continued)

Table 8-8 Physical Findings in Selected Chest Disorders (*Continued*)

Condition	Percussion Note	Trachea	Breath Sounds	Adventitious Sounds	Tactile Fremitus and Transmitted Voice Sounds
Pneumothorax When air leaks into the pleural space, usually unilaterally, the lung recoils away from the chest wall. Pleural air blocks transmission of sound.	**Hyperresonant** or tympanitic over the pleural air	*Shifted toward the unaffected side if tension pneumothorax*	*Decreased to absent* over the pleural air	None, except a *possible pleural rub*	*Decreased to absent* over the pleural air
Chronic Obstructive Pulmonary Disease (COPD) Slowly progressive disorder in which the distal air spaces enlarge and lungs become hyperinflated. Chronic bronchitis may precede or follow the development of COPD.	Diffusely **hyperresonant**	Midline	*Decreased to absent,* with delayed expiration	None, or the crackles, wheezes, and rhonchi of associated chronic bronchitis	*Decreased*
Asthma Widespread, usually reversible, airflow obstruction with bronchial hyperresponsiveness and underlying inflammation. During attacks, as air flow decreases lungs hyperinflate.	**Resonant** to diffusely **hyperresonant**	Midline	*Often obscured by wheezes*	*Wheezes, possibly crackles*	*Decreased*

References

1. Huffman JC, Pollack MH, Stern TA. Panic disorder and chest pain: mechanisms, morbidity, and management. *Prim Care Companion J Clin Psychiatry.* 2002;4:54.

2. Demiryoguran NS, Karcioglu O, Topacoglu H, et al. Anxiety disorder in patients with non-specific chest pain in the emergency setting. *Emerg Med J.* 2006;23:99.

3. Katerndahl DA. Chest pain and its importance in patients with panic disorder: an updated literature review. *Prim Care Companion J Clin Psychiatry.* 2008;10:376.

4. McConaghy JR, Oza RS. Outpatient diagnosis of acute chest pain in adults. *Am Fam Physician.* 2013;87:177.

5. Parshall MB, Schwartzstein RM, Adams L, et al; American Thoracic Society Committee on Dyspnea. An official American Thoracic Society statement: update on the mechanisms, assessment, and management of dyspnea. *Am J Respir Crit Care Med.* 2012;185:435.

6. Global Initiative for Chronic Obstructive Lung Disease. Global strategy for the diagnosis, management, and prevention of chronic obstructive pulmonary disease. Updated 2015. Available at http://www.goldcopd.org/uploads/users/files/GOLD_Report_2015_Feb18.pdf. Accessed March 14, 2015.

7. Celli BR, Cote CG, Marin JM, et al. The body-mass index, airflow obstruction, dyspnea, and exercise capacity index in chronic obstructive pulmonary disease. *N Engl J Med.* 2004;350:1005.

8. Bestall JC, Paul EA, Garrod R, et al. Usefulness of the Medical Research Council (MRC) dyspnoea scale as a measure of disability in patients with chronic obstructive pulmonary disease. *Thorax.* 1999;54:581.

9. Kerlin MP. In the clinic. Asthma. *Ann Intern Med.* 2014;160: ITC3–1.

10. Benich JJ 3rd, Carek PJ. Evaluation of the patient with chronic cough. *Am Fam Physician.* 2011;84:887.

11. Canning BJ, Chang AB, Bolser DC, et al. Anatomy and neurophysiology of cough: CHEST Guideline and Expert Panel report. *Chest.* 2014;146:1633.

12. Musher DM, Thorner AR. Community acquired pneumonia. *N Engl J Med.* 2014;371:1619.

13. Wunderink RG, Waterer GW. Clinical practice. Community-acquired pneumonia. *N Engl J Med.* 2014;370:543.

14. Bel EH. Clinical practice. Mild asthma. *N Engl J Med.* 2013;369:549.

15. Braman SS. Chronic cough due to acute bronchitis: ACCP evidence-based clinical practice guidelines. *Chest.* 2006;129(1 Suppl):95S.

16. Novosad SA, Barker AF. Chronic obstructive pulmonary disease and bronchiectasis. *Curr Opin Pulm Med.* 2013;19:133.

17. Moulton BC, Barker AF. Pathogenesis of bronchiectasis. *Clin Chest Med.* 2012;33:211.

18. Lara AR, Schwarz MI. Diffuse alveolar hemorrhage. *Chest.* 2010;137:1164.

19. Jordan AS, McSharry DG, Malhotra A. Adult obstructive sleep apnoea. *Lancet.* 2014;383(9918):736.

20. Balanchandran JS, Patel SR. In the clinic: obstructive sleep apnea. *Ann Intern Med.* 2014;161:ITC1.

21. Vital signs: current cigarette smoking among adults aged ≥18 years—United States, 2005–2010. *MMWR Morb Mortal Wkly Rep.* 2011;60(35):1207.

22. Centers for Disease Control and Prevention. Smoking and tobacco use. Youth and tobacco Use 2014. Available at http://www.cdc.gov/tobacco/data_statistics/fact_sheets/youth_data/tobacco_use./Accessed January 29, 2015.

23. U.S. Department of Health and Human Services. *How Tobacco Smoke Causes Disease: The Biology and Behavioral Basis for Smoking-Attributable Disease: A Report of the Surgeon General.* Atlanta, GA: U.S. Department of Health and Human Services, Centers for Disease Control and Prevention, National Center for Chronic Disease Prevention and Health Promotion, Office on Smoking and Health; 2010. Available at http://www.ncbi.nlm.nih.gov/books/NBK53017/. Accessed January 29, 2015.

24. U.S. Preventive Services Task Force. Counseling and interventions to prevent tobacco use and tobacco-caused disease in adults and pregnant women: reaffirmation recommendation statement. *Ann Intern Med.* 2009;150:551.

25. Centers for Disease Control and Prevention. Fact sheets. Health effects of cigarette smoking. 2014. Available at http://www.cdc.gov/tobacco/data_statistics/fact_sheets/health_effects/effects_cig_smoking/index.htm. Accessed January 29, 2015.

26. Moyer VA. Primary care interventions to prevent tobacco use in children and adolescents: U.S. Preventive Services Task Force recommendation statement. *Ann Intern Med.* 2013;159:552.

27. Rigotti NA. Strategies to help a smoker who is struggling to quit. *JAMA.* 2012;308:1573.

28. Fiore MC, Baker TB. Clinical practice. Treating smokers in the health care setting. *N Engl J Med.* 2011;365:1222.

29. Ranney L, Melvin C, Lux L, et al. Systematic review: smoking cessation intervention strategies for adults and adults in special populations. *Ann Intern Med.* 2006;145:845.

30. Norcross JC, Prochaska JO. Using the stages of change. *Harv Ment Health Lett.* 2002;18:5.

31. Benowitz NL. Nicotine addiction. *N Engl J Med.* 2010;362:2295.

32. Stead LF, Lancaster T. Combined pharmacotherapy and behavioural interventions for smoking cessation. *Cochrane Database Syst Rev.* 2012;10:CD008286.

33. Siegel R, Ma J, Zou Z, et al. Cancer statistics, 2014. *CA Cancer J Clin.* 2014;64:9.

34. Howlader N, Noone AM, Krapcho M, et al. *SEER Cancer Statistics Review, 1975–2011.* Bethesda, MD: National Cancer Institute; 2014.

35. Aberle DR, Adams AM, Berg CD, et al. Reduced lung-cancer mortality with low-dose computed tomographic screening. *N Engl J Med.* 2011;365:395.

36. Moyer VA. Screening for lung cancer: U.S. Preventive Services Task Force recommendation statement. *Ann Intern Med.* 2014;160:330.

37. Wender R, Fontham ET, Barrera E Jr., et al. American Cancer Society lung cancer screening guidelines. *CA Cancer J Clin.* 2013;63:107.

38. Estimates of deaths associated with seasonal influenza—United States, 1976–2007. *MMWR Morb Mortal Wkly Rep.* 2010;59(33):1057.

39. Grohskopf LA, Olsen SJ, Sokolow LZ, et al. Prevention and control of seasonal influenza with vaccines: recommendations of the Advisory Committee on Immunization Practices (ACIP)—United States, 2014–2015 influenza season. *MMWR Morb Mortal Wkly Rep.* 2014;63(32):691.

40. Centers for Disease Control and Prevention. Prevention and control of seasonal influenza with vaccines. Recommendations of the Advisory Committee on Immunization Practices–United States, 2015–2016. Updated August 6, 2015. Available at http://www.cdc.gov/flu/professionals/acip/index.htm. Accessed November 13, 2015.

41. Updated recommendations for prevention of invasive pneumococcal disease among adults using the 23-valent pneumococcal polysaccharide vaccine (PPSV23). *MMWR Morb Mortal Wkly Rep.* 2010;59(34):1102.

42. Tomczyk S, Bennett NM, Stoecker C, et al. Use of 13-valent pneumococcal conjugate vaccine and 23-valent pneumococcal polysaccharide vaccine among adults aged >/= 65 years: recommendations of the Advisory Committee on Immunization Practices (ACIP). *MMWR Morb Mortal Wkly Rep.* 2014;63(37):822. See also Centers for Disease Control and Prevention. Vaccine information statement. Pneumococcal polysaccharide vaccine - What you need to know; April 4, 2015. At http://www.cdc.gov/vaccines/hcp/vis/vis-statements/ppv.pdf. Accessed November 13, 2015.

43. McGee S. *Ch 26, Inspection of the Chest. In Evidence-based Physical Diagnosis.* 3rd ed. Philadelphia, PA: Saunders; 2012:233–234.

44. McGee S. *Ch 27, Palpation and Percussion of the Chest. In Evidence-based Physical Diagnosis.* 3rd ed. Philadelphia, PA: Saunders; 2012:240.

45. McGee S. *Ch 27, Palpation and Percussion of the Chest. In Evidence-Based Physical Diagnosis.* 3rd ed. Philadelphia, PA: Saunders; 2012:248.

46. Wong CL, Holroyd-Leduc J, Straus SE. Does this patient have a pleural effusion? *JAMA.* 2009;301:309.

47. Bohadana A, Izbicki G, Kraman SS. Fundamentals of lung auscultation. *N Engl J Med.* 2014;370:744.

48. McGee S. *Ch 28, Auscultation of the Lungs. In Evidence-Based Physical Diagnosis.* 3rd ed. Philadelphia, PA: Saunders; 2012:260.

49. Loudon R, Murphy LH. Lungs sounds. *Am Rev Respir Dis.* 1994;130:663.

50. Epler GR, Carrrington CB, Gaensler EA. Crackles (rales) in the interstitial pulmonary diseases. *Chest.* 1978;73:333.

51. Nath AR, Capel LH. Inspiratory crackles and mechanical events of breathing. *Thorax.* 1974;29:695.

52. Nath AR, Capel LH. Lung crackles in bronchiectasis. *Thorax.* 1980;35:694.

53. Littner M. In the clinic: chronic obstructive pulmonary disease. *Ann Intern Med.* 2011;154:ITC4–1.

54. Niewoehner DE. Clinical practice. Outpatient management of severe COPD. *N Engl J Med.* 2010;362:1407.

55. Qaseem A, Wilt TJ, Weinberger SE, et al; American College of Physicians; American College of Chest Physicians; American Thoracic Society; European Respiratory Society. Diagnosis and management of stable chronic obstructive pulmonary disease: a clinical practice guideline update from the American College of Physicians, American College of Chest Physicians, American Thoracic Society, and European Respiratory Society. *Ann Intern Med.* 2011;155:179.

56. Holleman DR, Simel DL. Does the clinical examination predict airflow limitation? *JAMA.* 1995;273:63.

57. Straus SE, McAlister FA, Sackett DL, et al. The accuracy of patient history, wheezing, and laryngeal measurements in diagnosing obstructive airway disease. *JAMA.* 2000;283:1853.

58. Spruit MA, Singh SJ, Garvey C, et al; ATS/ERS Task Force on Pulmonary Rehabilitation. An official American Thoracic Society/European Respiratory Society statement: key concepts and advances in pulmonary rehabilitation. *Am J Respir Crit Care Med.* 2013;188:e13.

59. McGee S. *Ch 30, Pneumonia. In Evidence-Based Physical Diagnosis.* 3rd ed. Philadelphia, PA: Saunders; 2012:272.

60. American Thoracic Society Committee on Proficiency Standards for Clinical Pulmonary Function Laboratories. ATS statement: guidelines for the six-minute walk test. *Am J Respir Crit Care Med.* 2002;166:111.

61. Spruit MA, Watkins ML, Edwards LD, et al. Evaluation of COPD longitudinally to identify predictive surrogate endpoints (ECLIPSE) study investigators. Determinants of poor 6-min walking distance in patients with COPD: the ECLIPSE cohort. *Respir Med.* 2010;104:849.

62. McGee S. *Ch 29, Ancillary Tests. In Evidence-Based Physical Diagnosis.* 3rd ed. Philadelphia, PA: Saunders; 2012:267–268.

63. Kouritas VK, Papagiannopoulos K. Pneumomediastinum. *J Thorac Dis.* 2015;7(Suppl 1):S44.

9

The Cardiovascular System

The Bates' suite offers these additional resources to enhance learning and facilitate understanding of this chapter:

- Bates' *Pocket Guide to Physical Examination and History Taking*, 8th edition
- Bates' *Visual Guide to Physical Examination* (Vol. 10: Cardiovascular System)
- thePoint online resources, for students and instructors: http://thepoint.lww.com

Listening to the heart has come to epitomize the art of bedside diagnosis. Mastering the skills of cardiac examination requires patience, practice, and repetition—a process especially vulnerable to evolving technology and the time constraints of clinical practice.[1–4] Many reports attest to the current decline in physical examination skills, well documented for the cardiovascular system at all levels of training.[5–12] As you study this chapter, combining your knowledge of anatomy and physiology with hands-on practice of inspection, palpation, and auscultation brings rewards of proven diagnostic value. Take advantage of the numerous programs for learning cardiac physiology and auscultation that can reinforce your growing clinical acumen, and pursue the emerging literature that compares the effectiveness of different modes of learning these important skills.[13–22]

Anatomy and Physiology

Surface Projections of the Heart and Great Vessels

Visualize the underlying structures of the heart as you inspect the anterior chest. Note that the *right ventricle* (RV) occupies most of the anterior cardiac surface. This chamber and the pulmonary artery form a wedgelike structure behind and to the left of the sternum, outlined in black (Fig. 9-1).

The inferior border of the RV lies below the junction of the sternum and the xiphoid process. The RV narrows superiorly and joins the pulmonary artery at the level of the sternal angle, or "base of the heart," a clinical term that refers to the superior aspect of the heart at the right and left 2nd interspaces adjacent to the sternum.

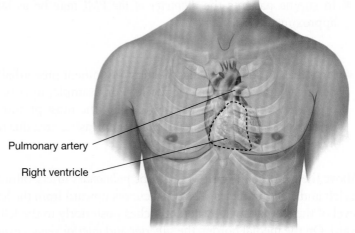

Pulmonary artery

Right ventricle

FIGURE 9-1. Chest wall and cardiac anatomy.

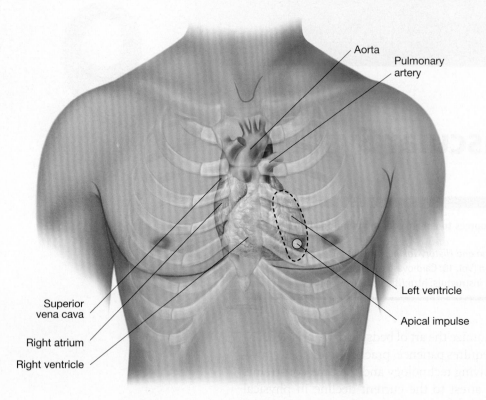

FIGURE 9-2. **Cardiac anatomy—major structures.**

The *left ventricle,* behind the RV and to the left, forms the left lateral margin of the heart (Fig. 9-2). Its tapered inferior tip is often termed the *cardiac apex.* It is clinically important because it produces the apical impulse, identified during palpation of the precordium as the *point of maximal impulse (PMI).* This impulse locates the left border of the heart and is normally found in the 5th intercostal space at or just medial to the left midclavicular line (or 7 to 9 cm lateral to the midsternal line). The PMI is not always palpable, even in a healthy patient with a normal heart. Detection is affected by both the patient's body habitus and position during the examination.

Rarely, in *situs inversus* and *dextrocardia,* the PMI is located on the right side of the chest.

- In supine patients the *diameter of the PMI* may be as large as a quarter, approximately 1 to 2.5 cm.

A PMI >2.5 cm is evidence of *left ventricular hypertrophy (LVH)* from *hypertension* or *aortic stenosis.*

- Note that, in some patients, the most prominent precordial impulse may not be at the apex of the left ventricle. For example, in patients with chronic obstructive pulmonary disease (COPD), the most prominent palpable impulse or PMI may be in the xiphoid or epigastric area due to *right ventricular hypertrophy.*

Displacement of the PMI lateral to the midclavicular line or >10 cm lateral to the midsternal line occurs in *LVH* and also in ventricular dilatation from *myocardial infarction (MI)* or *heart failure.*

Above the heart lie the *great vessels.* The *pulmonary artery* bifurcates quickly into its left and right branches. The *aorta* curves upward from the left ventricle to the level of the sternal angle, where it arches posteriorly to the left and then downward. On the medial border, the *superior* and *inferior venae cavae* channel venous blood from the upper and lower portions of the body into the right atrium.

Cardiac Chambers, Valves, and Circulation

Circulation through the heart is diagrammed below. Identify the cardiac chambers, valves, and direction of blood flow. Because of their location, the *mitral* and *tricuspid valves* are often called *atrioventricular (AV) valves*. The *aortic* and *pulmonic valves* are called *semilunar valves* because the valve leaflets are shaped like half moons.

As the heart valves close, the heart sounds of S_1 and S_2 arise from vibrations emanating from the leaflets, the adjacent cardiac structures, and the flow of blood. Study carefully the opening and closing of the AV and semilunar valves in relation to events in the cardiac cycle to improve your diagnostic accuracy as you auscultate the heart. In Figure 9-3, note that the aortic and pulmonic valves are closed, and the mitral and tricuspid valves are open, as seen in diastole.

In most adults over age 40 years, the diastolic sounds of S_3 and S_4 are pathologic, and are correlated with heart failure and acute myocardial ischemia.[19,23,24] In recent studies, an S_3 corresponds to an abrupt deceleration of inflow across the mitral valve, and an S_4 to increased left ventricular end diastolic stiffness which decreases compliance.[25-27]

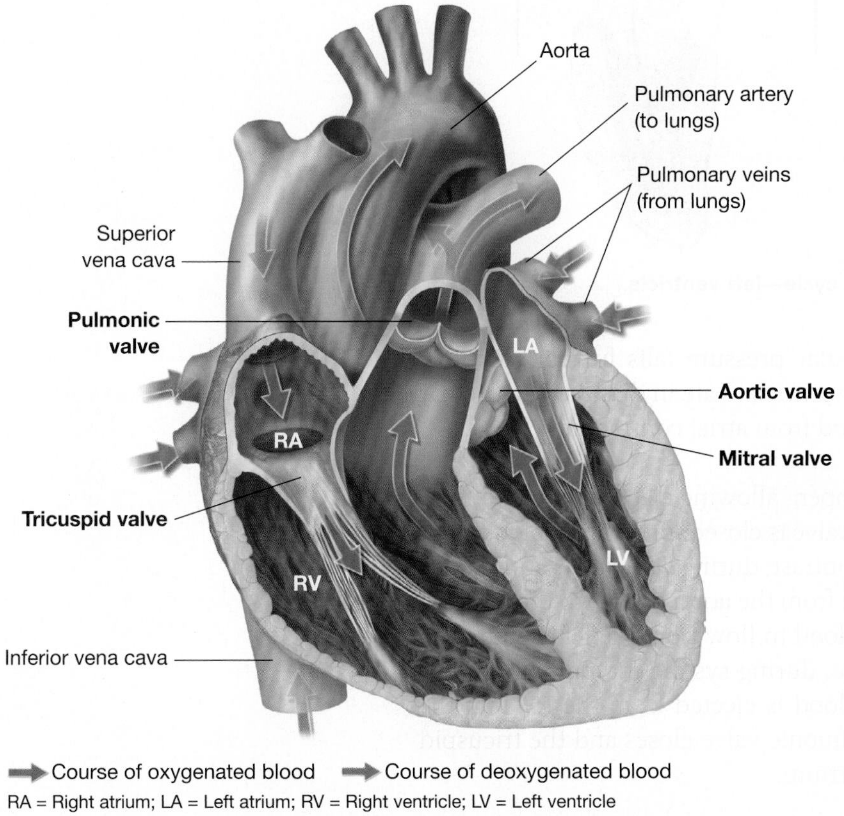

Aorta

Pulmonary artery (to lungs)

Pulmonary veins (from lungs)

Superior vena cava

Pulmonic valve

LA

Aortic valve

RA

Mitral valve

Tricuspid valve

LV

RV

Inferior vena cava

➡ Course of oxygenated blood   ➡ Course of deoxygenated blood

RA = Right atrium; LA = Left atrium; RV = Right ventricle; LV = Left ventricle

FIGURE 9-3. Cardiac chambers, valves, and circulation.

Events in the Cardiac Cycle

The heart serves as a pump that generates varying pressures as its chambers contract and relax. Systole is the period of ventricular contraction. As shown in Figure 9-4, pressure in the left ventricle rises, from less than 5 mm Hg in its resting state, to a normal peak of 120 mm Hg. After the ventricle ejects much of its blood into the aorta, the pressure levels off and starts to fall. Diastole is the

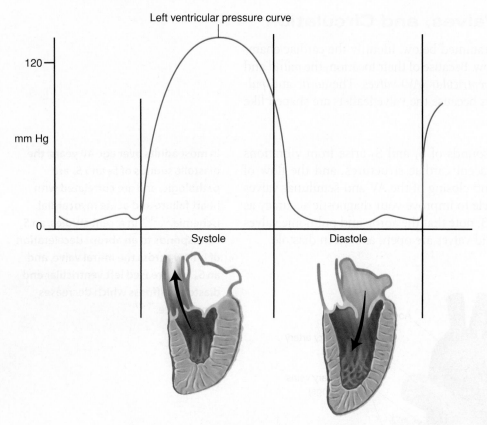

FIGURE 9-4. Cardiac cycle—left ventricle.

period of ventricular relaxation. Ventricular pressure falls further to below 5 mm Hg, and blood flows from atrium to ventricle. Late in diastole, ventricular pressure rises slightly during inflow of blood from atrial contraction.

Note that during *systole* the aortic valve is open, allowing ejection of blood from the left ventricle into the aorta. The mitral valve is closed, preventing blood from regurgitating back into the left atrium. In contrast, during *diastole* the aortic valve is closed, preventing regurgitation of blood from the aorta back into the left ventricle. The mitral valve is open, allowing blood to flow from the left atrium into the relaxed left ventricle. At the same time, during systole the pulmonic valve opens and the tricuspid valve closes as blood is ejected from the RV into the pulmonary artery. During diastole, the pulmonic valve closes and the tricuspid valve opens as blood flows into the right atrium.

Understanding the interrelationships of the pressure gradients in the left heart (the left atrium, left ventricle, and aorta), together with the position and movement of the four heart valves, is fundamental to understanding heart sounds. An extensive literature explores how heart sounds are generated. Possible explanations include closure of the valve leaflets; tensing of related structures, leaflet positions, and pressure gradients at the time of atrial and ventricular systole; and the acoustic effects of moving columns of blood.

Trace the changing left ventricular pressures and sounds through one cardiac cycle. Note that S_1 and S_2 define the duration of systole and diastole. Right heart sounds occur at pressures that are usually lower than those on the left, and are usually less audible. The explanations given here are oversimplified, but retain clinical usefulness.

During *diastole,* pressure in the blood-filled left atrium slightly exceeds that in the relaxed left ventricle, and blood flows from left atrium to left ventricle across the open mitral valve (Fig. 9-5). Just before the onset of ventricular systole, atrial contraction produces a slight pressure rise in both chambers.

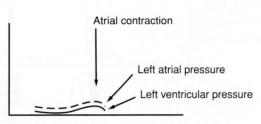

FIGURE 9-5. **Cardiac cycle—diastole.**

During *systole,* the left ventricle starts to contract and ventricular pressure rapidly exceeds left atrial pressure, closing the mitral valve (Fig. 9-6). Closure of the mitral valve produces the first heart sound, S_1.

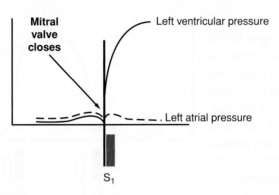

FIGURE 9-6. **Diastole—mitral valve closes.**

As left ventricular pressure continues to rise, it quickly exceeds the pressure in the aorta and forces the aortic valve open (Fig. 9-7). In some pathologic conditions, an early systolic ejection sound (Ej) accompanies the opening of the aortic valve. Normally, maximal left ventricular pressure corresponds to systolic blood pressure.

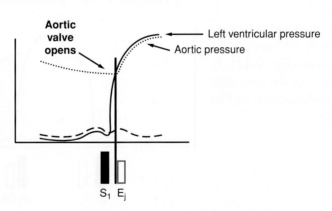

FIGURE 9-7. **Systole—aortic valve opens.**

As the left ventricle ejects most of its blood, ventricular pressure begins to fall. When left ventricular pressure drops below aortic pressure, the aortic valve closes (Fig. 9-8). Aortic valve closure produces the second heart sound, S_2, and another diastole begins.

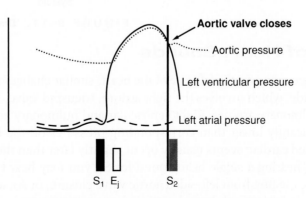

FIGURE 9-8. **Systole—aortic valve closes.**

In *diastole,* left ventricular pressure continues to drop and falls below left atrial pressure. The mitral valve opens (Fig. 9-9). This event is usually silent, but may be audible as a pathologic opening snap (OS) if valve leaflet motion is restricted, as in mitral stenosis.

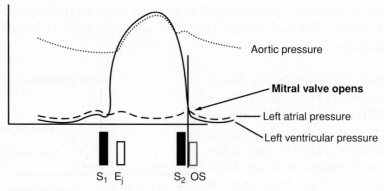

FIGURE 9-9. Diastole—mitral valve opens.

After the mitral valve opens, there is a period of rapid ventricular filling as blood flows early in diastole from left atrium to left ventricle (Fig. 9-10). In children and young adults, a third heart sound, S_3, may arise from rapid deceleration of the column of blood against the ventricular wall. In older adults, an S_3, sometimes termed "an S_3 gallop," usually indicates a pathologic change in ventricular compliance.

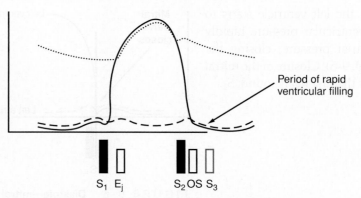

FIGURE 9-10. Diastole—rapid ventricular filling; S_3.

Finally, although not often heard in normal adults, a fourth heart sound, S_4, marks atrial contraction (Fig. 9-11). It immediately precedes S_1 of the next beat and can also reflect a pathologic change in ventricular compliance.

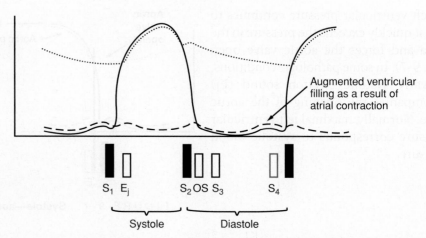

FIGURE 9-11. Diastole—atrial contraction; S_4.

The Splitting of Heart Sounds

While these events are occurring on the left side of the heart, similar changes are occurring on the right side, which involves the right atrium, tricuspid valve, RV, pulmonic valve, and pulmonary arteries. Right ventricular and pulmonary arterial pressures are significantly lower than corresponding pressures on the left side. Note that right-sided cardiac events usually occur slightly later than those on the left. Instead of a hearing a single heart sound for S_2, you may hear two discernible components, the first from left-sided aortic valve closure, or A_2, and the second from right-sided closure of the pulmonic valve, or P_2.

The second heart sound, S_2, and its two components, A_2 and P_2, are caused primarily by closure of the aortic and pulmonic valves, respectively. During inspiration, the right heart filling time is increased, which increases right ventricular stroke volume and the duration of right ventricular ejection compared with the neighboring left ventricle. This delays the closure of the pulmonic valve, P_2, splitting S_2 into its two audible components. During expiration, these two components fuse into a single sound, S_2 (Fig. 9-12). Note that because walls of veins contain less smooth muscle, the venous system has more capacitance than the arterial system and lower systemic pressure. Distensibility and impedance in the pulmonary vascular bed contribute to the "hangout time" that delays P_2.[28]

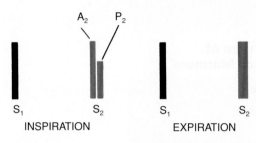

FIGURE 9-12. **Spitting of S_2 during inspiration.**

Of the two components of the S_2, A_2 is normally louder, reflecting the high pressure in the aorta. It is heard throughout the precordium. In contrast, P_2 is relatively soft, reflecting the lower pressure in the pulmonary artery. It is heard best in its own area, the 2nd and 3rd left interspaces close to the sternum. It is here that you should search for the splitting of S_2.

S_1 also has two components, an earlier mitral and a later tricuspid sound. The mitral sound—the principal component of S_1—is much louder, again reflecting the higher pressures on the left side of the heart. It can be heard throughout the precordium and is loudest at the cardiac apex. The softer tricuspid component is heard best at the lower left sternal border; it is here that you may hear a split S_1. The earlier louder mitral component may mask the tricuspid sound, however, and splitting is not always detectable. Splitting of S_1 does not vary with respiration.

Heart Murmurs

Heart murmurs are distinct heart sounds distinguished by their pitch and their longer duration. They are attributed to turbulent blood flow and are usually diagnostic of valvular heart disease. At times, they may also represent "innocent" flow murmurs, especially in young adults. A *stenotic valve* has an abnormally narrowed valvular orifice that obstructs blood flow, as in *aortic stenosis,* and causes a characteristic murmur. So does a valve that fails to fully close, as in *aortic regurgitation.* Such a valve allows blood to leak backward in a retrograde direction and produces a *regurgitant* murmur.

To identify murmurs accurately, you must learn where they are best heard on the chest wall, their timing in systole or diastole, and their descriptive qualities. In the Techniques of Examination section, you will learn to integrate location and timing with the murmur's shape, maximal intensity, direction of radiation, grade of intensity, pitch, and quality (see pp. 373–399).

Relation of Auscultatory Findings to the Chest Wall

The locations on the chest wall where you auscultate heart sounds and murmurs help identify the valve or chamber where they originate.

Chest Wall Location and Origin of Valve Sounds and Murmurs

Chest Wall Location	Typical Origin of Sounds and Murmurs
Right 2nd interspace to the apex	Aortic valve
Left 2nd and 3rd interspaces close to the sternum, but also at higher or lower levels	Pulmonic valve
At or near the lower left sternal border	Tricuspid valve
At and around the cardiac apex	Mitral valve

These areas overlap, as illustrated in Figure 9-13. Integrating the auscultatory location with the timing of the sound or murmur, either systole or diastole, is an important first step in identifying sounds and murmurs correctly, and often leads to accurate bedside diagnosis when integrated with other cardiac findings.

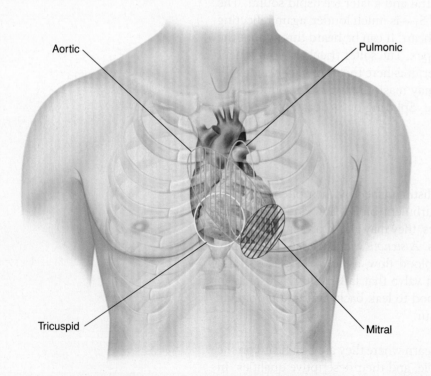

FIGURE 9-13. Listening areas on the chest wall.

The Conduction System

An electrical conduction system stimulates and coordinates the contraction of cardiac muscle.

Normally, each electrical impulse originates in the *sinus node,* a group of specialized cardiac cells located in the right atrium near the junction of the vena cava. The sinus node acts as the cardiac pacemaker and automatically discharges an impulse about 60 to 90 times a minute. This impulse travels through both atria to the *AV node,* a specialized group of cells located low in the atrial septum. Here, the impulse is delayed before passing down the bundle of His and its branches to the ventricular myocardium. Muscular contraction follows: first the atria, then the ventricles. The normal conduction system is diagrammed in Figure 9-14 in simplified form.

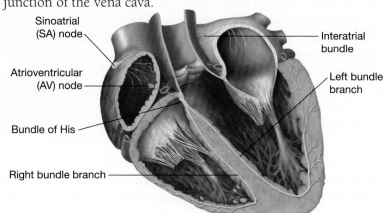

FIGURE 9-14. **Cardiac conduction system.**

The Electrocardiogram. The electrocardiogram, or ECG, records these events. Contraction of cardiac smooth muscle produces electrical activity, resulting in a series of waves on the ECG. The ECG consists of *six limb leads* in the *frontal plane* (Fig. 9-15) and *six chest or precordial leads* in the *transverse plane* (Fig. 9-16).

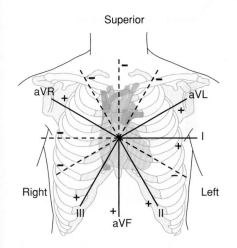

FIGURE 9-15. **Limb leads: frontal plane.**

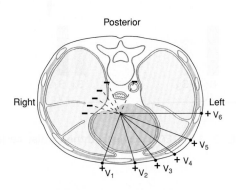

FIGURE 9-16. **Chest leads: transverse plane.**

- Electrical vectors approaching a lead cause a *positive,* or *upward, deflection.*

- Electrical vectors moving away from the lead cause a *negative,* or *downward, deflection.*

- When positive and negative vectors balance, they are *isoelectric* and appear as a straight line.

P, Q, R, S, and T Waves. The deflections of the *normal ECG* and their duration are briefly summarized here and shown in Figure 9-17. You will need further instruction and considerable practice to interpret recordings from patients.

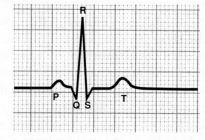

FIGURE 9-17. **ECG deflections.**

- The small *P wave* of atrial depolarization (duration up to 80 milliseconds; *PR interval* 120 to 200 milliseconds)
- The larger *QRS complex* of ventricular depolarization (up to 100 milliseconds), consisting of one or more of the following:
  - the Q *wave*, a downward deflection from septal depolarization
  - the *R wave*, an upward deflection from ventricular depolarization
  - the *S wave*, a downward deflection following an R wave
- A *T wave* of ventricular repolarization, or recovery (duration relates to QRS)

ECG Waves and the Cardiac Cycle. The electrical impulse slightly precedes the myocardial contraction that it stimulates. The relation of electrocardiographic waves to the cardiac cycle is shown in Figure 9-18.

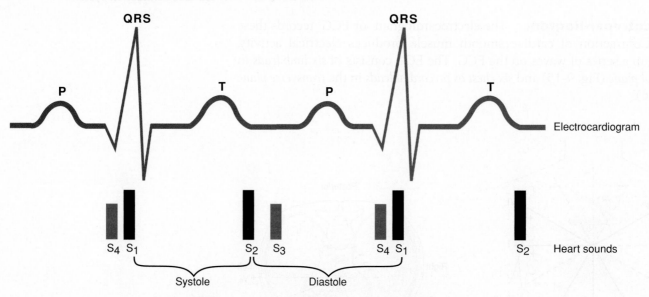

FIGURE 9-18. **ECG waves and the cardiac cycle.**

The Heart as a Pump

The left and right ventricles pump blood into the systemic and pulmonary arterial trees, respectively. *Cardiac output,* the volume of blood ejected from each ventricle during 1 minute, is the product of *heart rate* and *stroke volume*. Stroke volume (the volume of blood ejected with each heartbeat) depends in turn on preload, myocardial contractility, and afterload.

- *Preload* refers to the load that stretches the cardiac muscle before contraction. The volume of blood in the RV at the end of diastole constitutes its preload for the next beat. Right ventricular preload is increased by increasing venous return to the right heart. Physiologic causes include inspiration and the increased volume of blood flow from exercising muscles. The increased blood volume of a dilated RV in heart failure also increases preload. Causes of decreased right ventricular preload include exhalation, decreased left ventricular output, and pooling of blood in the capillary bed or the venous system.

■ *Myocardial contractility* refers to the ability of the cardiac muscle, when given a load, to shorten. Contractility increases when stimulated by action of the sympathetic nervous system and decreases when blood flow or oxygen delivery to the myocardium is impaired.

■ *Afterload* refers to the degree of vascular resistance to ventricular contraction. Sources of resistance to contraction include the tone in the walls of the aorta, the large arteries, and the peripheral vascular tree (primarily the small arteries and arterioles), as well as the volume of blood already in the aorta.

Pathologic increases in preload and afterload, called *volume overload* and *pressure overload,* respectively, produce changes in ventricular function that may be clinically detectable. These changes include alterations in ventricular impulses, detectable by palpation, and in normal heart sounds. Pathologic heart sounds and murmurs may also develop.

The terms *heart failure with preserved ejection fraction (EF)* and *heart failure with reduced EF* are now preferred to "congestive heart failure" because of differences in treatment.[29]

Arterial Pulses and Blood Pressure

With each contraction, the left ventricle ejects a volume of blood into the aorta that then perfuses the arterial tree. As the ensuing pressure wave moves rapidly through the arterial system it generates the *arterial pulse.* Although the pressure wave travels quickly, many times faster than the blood itself, a palpable delay between ventricular contraction and peripheral pulses makes the pulses in the arms and legs unsuitable for timing events in the cardiac cycle.

Blood pressure in the arterial system varies during the cardiac cycle, peaking in systole and falling to its lowest trough in diastole (Fig. 9-19). These are the levels that are measured with the blood pressure cuff, or sphygmomanometer. The difference between systolic and diastolic pressures is known as the *pulse pressure.*

Factors Affecting Blood Pressure

- Left ventricular stroke volume
- Distensibility of the aorta and the large arteries
- Peripheral vascular resistance, particularly at the arteriolar level
- Volume of blood in the arterial system

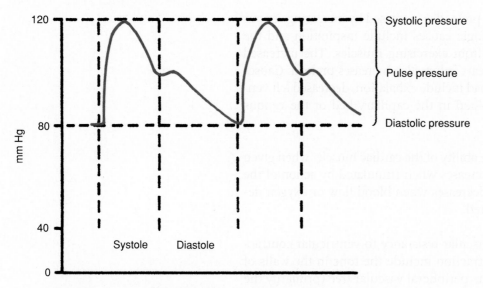

FIGURE 9-19. **Blood pressure and pulse pressure in the cardiac cycle.**

Changes in any of these four factors alter systolic pressure, diastolic pressure, or both. Blood pressure levels fluctuate strikingly throughout any 24-hour period, varying with physical activity, emotional state, pain, noise, environmental temperature, use of coffee, tobacco, and other drugs, and even time of day.

Jugular Venous Pressure and Pulsations

The jugular veins provide an important index of right heart pressures and cardiac function. Jugular venous pressure (JVP) reflects right atrial pressure, which in turn equals central venous pressure and right ventricular end-diastolic pressure. The JVP is best estimated from the right internal jugular vein, which has the most direct channel into the right atrium. Some affirm that the right external jugular vein can also be used.[30] Because the jugular veins lie deep to the sternocleidomastoid (SCM) muscles, learn to identify the pulsations they transmit to the surface of the neck, briefly described below, and measure their highest point of oscillation.

See pp. 374–379 for more detailed discussion of the JVP and techniques for its examination.

Changing pressures in the right atrium during diastole and systole produce oscillations of filling and emptying in the jugular veins, or *jugular venous pulsations* (Fig. 9-20). Atrial contraction produces an *a wave* in the jugular veins just before S_1 and systole, followed by the *x descent* of atrial relaxation. As right atrial pressure begins to rise with inflow from the vena cava during right ventricular systole, there is a second elevation, the *v wave*, followed by the *y descent* as blood passively empties into the RV during early and middiastole.

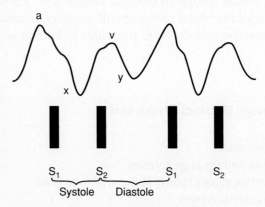

FIGURE 9-20. **Jugular venous pulsations.**

Changes Over the Life Span

Aging may affect the location of the apical impulse, the pitch of heart sounds and murmurs, the stiffness of the arteries, and blood pressure. For example, the *PMI* is usually easily palpated in children and young adults; as the chest deepens in its anteroposterior (AP) diameter, the impulse gets harder to find. For the same reason, *splitting of S$_2$* may be harder to hear in older people as its pulmonic component becomes less audible. Furthermore, at some time during the life span, almost everyone has a *heart murmur.* Most murmurs occur without other evidence of cardiovascular abnormality and are considered normal variants. These common murmurs vary with age, and knowing their patterns helps you to distinguish normal from abnormal.

Turn to Chapter 18, Assessing Children: Infancy Through Adolescence, pp. 799–925, and to Chapter 19, The Pregnant Woman, p. 943, for discussion of these innocent murmurs.

Murmurs may originate in large blood vessels as well as in the heart. The *jugular venous hum,* which is common in children, may still be heard through young adulthood (see pp. 878–879). A second more important example is the *cervical systolic murmur* or *bruit,* which may be innocent in children but suspicious for atherosclerotic disease in adults.

The Health History

Common or Concerning Symptoms

- Chest pain
- Palpitations
- Shortness of breath: dyspnea, orthopnea, or paroxysmal nocturnal dyspnea
- Swelling (edema)
- Fainting (syncope)

Assessing Cardiac Symptoms—Overview and Comparison with Baseline Activity Levels. This section approaches chest symptoms from a *cardiac standpoint,* and includes the important symptoms of chest pain, palpitations, shortness of breath from orthopnea or paroxysmal nocturnal dyspnea (PND), swelling from edema, and fainting. For chest symptoms, be systematic as you think through the range of possible cardiac, pulmonary, and extrathoracic etiologies. Study the various causes of *chest pain, dyspnea, wheezing, cough,* and even *hemoptysis,* because these symptoms can be cardiac as well as pulmonary in origin.

Review the Health History section of Chapter 8, The Thorax and Lungs, pp. 303–342; Table 8-1, Chest Pain, pp. 330–331; and Table 8-2, Dyspnea, pp. 332–333.

When assessing cardiac symptoms, it is important to quantify the patient's baseline level of activity. For example, in patients with chest pain, does the pain occur with climbing stairs? How many flights? How many steps? How about with walking—50 feet, one block, more? What about carrying groceries, making beds, or vacuuming? How does this compare with these activities in the past?

When did the symptoms appear or change? If the patient is short of breath, does this occur at rest, during exercise, or after climbing stairs? Sudden shortness of breath has different implications in an athlete compared to a person who only walks from one room to another. Quantifying the baseline level of activity helps establish both the severity of the patient's symptoms and their significance as you consider the next steps for management.

Chest Pain.   *Chest pain* is one of the most serious of all patient complaints, and accounts for 1% of primary care outpatient visits.[31] It is the most common symptom of coronary heart disease (CHD), which affects over 15 million Americans age ≥20 years.[32] In 2012, the prevalence of MI was 7.6 million people and of angina pectoris, 8.2 million. CHD is the leading killer of both men and women. In 2011, CHD accounted for one in seven U.S. deaths. Death rates remain highest for black men and black women compared to other ethnic groups.

As you evaluate your patient's history of chest pain, always consider life-threatening diagnoses such as angina pectoris, MI, dissecting aortic aneurysm, and pulmonary embolus.[31,34-36] Learn to distinguish cardiovascular causes from disorders of the pericardium, trachea and bronchi, parietal pleura, esophagus, and chest wall, and from extrathoracic causes in the neck, shoulder, gallbladder, and stomach.

Both men and women with acute coronary syndrome usually present with the classic symptoms of exertional angina; however, women, particularly those over age 65, are more likely to report atypical symptoms that may go unrecognized, such as upper back, neck, or jaw pain, shortness of breath, paroxysmal nocturnal dyspnea, nausea or vomiting, and fatigue, making careful history taking especially important.[37-39] Failure to identify cardiac causes of chest pain can have dire consequences. Inappropriate discharge from the emergency room results in a 25% mortality rate.[40]

Begin with open-ended questions… "Please tell me about any symptoms you might be having in your chest." Then elicit more specific details. Ask the patient to *point to the pain* and describe all seven features of the symptom. Clarify "Is the pain related to exertion?" and "What kinds of activities bring on the pain?" Also, "How intense is the pain, on a scale of 1 to 10?"… "Does it radiate into the neck, shoulder, back, or down your arm?"… "Are there any associated symptoms like shortness of breath, sweating, palpitations, or nausea?"… "Does it ever wake you up at night?"… "What do you do to make it better?"

Palpitations.   *Palpitations* involve an unpleasant awareness of the heartbeat. Patients use various terms to describe palpitations such as skipping, racing, fluttering, pounding, or stopping of the heart. Palpitations may be irregular, rapidly slow down or accelerate, or arise from the increased forcefulness of cardiac contraction. Anxious and hyperthyroid patients may report palpitations. Palpitations do not necessarily mean heart disease. In contrast, the most serious dysrhythmias, such as ventricular tachycardia, often do not produce palpitations.

Classic exertional pain, pressure, or discomfort in the chest, shoulder, back, neck, or arm in *angina pectoris*, is seen in 18% of patients with acute MI[32]; atypical descriptors also are common, such as cramping, grinding, pricking or, rarely, tooth or jaw pain.[33]

***Acute coronary syndrome* is increasingly used to describe the clinical syndromes caused by acute myocardial ischemia, which include *unstable angina, non–ST elevation MI,* and *ST elevation infarction*.[32]**

Causes of chest pain in the absence of coronary artery disease on angiogram include *microvascular coronary dysfunction* and *abnormal cardiac nocioception*, which require specialized testing.[37] Roughly half of women with chest pain and normal angiograms have microvascular coronary dysfunction.

Anterior chest pain, often tearing or ripping and radiating into the back or neck, occurs in *acute aortic dissection*.[36,41]

See Table 9-1, Selected Heart Rates and Rhythms, and Table 9-2, Selected Irregular Rhythms, for selected heart rates and rhythms (pp. 400–401).

If there are symptoms or signs of irregular heart action, obtain an ECG. This includes *atrial fibrillation*, which causes an "irregularly irregular" pulse often identified at the bedside.

Reword your questions if needed—"Are you ever aware of your heartbeat? What is it like?" Ask the patient to tap out the rhythm with a hand or finger. Was it fast or slow? Regular or irregular? How long did it last? If there was an episode of rapid heartbeats, did they start and stop suddenly or gradually? For this group of symptoms, an ECG is indicated.

Teach selected patients how to take serial measurements of their pulse rates in case they have further episodes.

Clues in the history include: transient skips and flip-flops (possible *premature contractions*); rapid regular beating of sudden onset and offset (possible *paroxysmal supraventricular tachycardia*); and a rapid regular rate of <120 beats per minute, especially if gradually starting and stopping (possible *sinus tachycardia*).

Shortness of Breath.   *Shortness of breath* is a common patient concern that can represent *dyspnea, orthopnea,* or *PND. Dyspnea* is an uncomfortable awareness of breathing that is inappropriate to a given level of exertion. This complaint is common in patients with cardiac or pulmonary problems.

Sudden dyspnea occurs in *pulmonary embolus, spontaneous pneumothorax,* and anxiety.

See Chapter 8, The Thorax and Lungs, pp. 303–342.

Orthopnea is dyspnea that occurs when the patient is supine and improves when the patient sits up. Classically, it is quantified by the number of pillows the patient uses for sleeping, or by the fact that the patient needs to sleep sitting up. Make sure that the patient is using extra pillows or sleeping upright due to shortness of breath and not other causes.

Orthopnea and PND occur in *left ventricular heart failure* and *mitral stenosis* and also in *obstructive lung disease.*

PND describes episodes of sudden dyspnea and orthopnea that awaken the patient from sleep, usually 1 or 2 hours after going to bed, prompting the patient to sit up, stand up, or go to a window for air. There may be associated wheezing and coughing. The episode usually subsides but may recur at about the same time on subsequent nights.

PND may be mimicked by *nocturnal asthma attacks.*

Swelling (Edema).   Swelling, or *edema,* refers to the accumulation of excessive fluid in the extravascular interstitial space. Interstitial tissue can absorb up to 5 L of fluid, accommodating up to a 10% weight gain, before pitting edema appears.[43,44] Causes vary from systemic to local. Focus on the location, timing, and setting of the swelling, and on associated symptoms. "Have you had any swelling anywhere? Where? … Anywhere else? When does it occur? Is it worse in the morning or at night? Do your shoes get tight?"

Causes are frequently cardiac (right or left ventricular dysfunction; pulmonary hypertension) or pulmonary (obstructive lung disease),[45] but can also be nutritional (*hypoalbuminemia*), and/or positional. *Dependent edema* appears in the lowest body parts: the feet and lower legs when sitting, or the sacrum when bedridden. *Anasarca* is severe generalized edema extending to the sacrum and abdomen.

Continue with "Are the rings tight on your fingers? Are your eyelids puffy or swollen in the morning? Have you had to let out your belt?" Also, "Have your clothes gotten tight around the middle?" Consider asking patients who retain fluid to record daily morning weights because edema may not be obvious until several liters of extra fluid have accumulated.

Look for the periorbital puffiness and tight rings of *nephrotic syndrome* and an enlarged waistline from *ascites* and *liver failure.*

Fainting (Syncope).   Fainting, blacking out, or *syncope,* is a transient loss of consciousness followed by recovery. Since the most common cause is neurocardiogenic (also called neutrally mediated vasodepressor syncope or vasovagal syncope) and of cardiac origin from arrhythmias in only ~20% of cases, please turn to Chapter 17, The Nervous System, p. 724 and Table 17-3, pp. 778–779 for discussion of the symptoms and causes of syncope.

Health Promotion and Counseling: Evidence and Recommendations

Important Topics for Health Promotion and Counseling

- The challenges of cardiovascular disease screening
- Special populations at risk
- Screening for cardiovascular risk factors
  - *Step 1:* Screen for global risk factors
  - *Step 2:* Calculate 10-year and lifetime CVD risk using an online calculator
  - *Step 3:* Track individual risk factors—hypertension, diabetes, dyslipidemias, metabolic syndrome, smoking, family history, and obesity
- Promoting lifestyle changes and risk factor modification

CVD, which consists primarily of hypertension (which accounts for the vast majority of diagnoses), CHD, heart failure, and stroke, affects nearly 84 million U.S. adults.[46] CVD is the leading cause of death in the United States, accounting for almost 800,000 deaths in 2011. CVD death rates have been declining due to both reduction in cardiovascular risk factors, or *primary prevention,* and improvements in *secondary prevention*—treatments following clinical CVD events, such as heart attack and stroke. However, CVD still accounts for about one of every three deaths in the United States, and obesity, diabetes, hypertension, physical inactivity, and tobacco abuse present important challenges to achieving greater reductions in the burden of CVD.[47]

Health promotion to prevent CVD includes screening for and addressing important risk factors, knowledge of evidence-based guidelines and interventions, and acquisition of interviewing and counseling skills that nurture healthier lifestyles and behaviors. As emerging clinicians, your task is threefold:

See discussion of Promoting Lifestyle and Risk Factor Modification, p. 358, and Chapter 3, Interviewing and the Health History, p. 81, for discussion of motivational interviewing.[48]

1. To understand important epidemiologic data about CVD and prevention

2. To identify modifiable cardiovascular risk factors

3. To help patients reduce cardiovascular risk by adopting lifestyle changes and appropriate pharmacologic treatments

The Challenges of Cardiovascular Disease Screening. New studies continually refine our understanding of the epidemiology of CVD and provide evidence-based guidance for preventive interventions. Many cardiovascular diseases share common risk factors, and major professional societies of related disciplines are now issuing joint guidelines. As a result, screening guidelines are becoming more complex as approaches to specific risk groups become more customized. For example, guidelines for prescribing aspirin for primary prevention now differ by gender, age, and risk of CHD versus stroke.[49,50] Increasingly, clinicians are urged to engage patients in shared decision making, helping them make informed personalized decisions about preventive interventions which can have both benefits and harms. As an aid, online calculators are available for rapidly assessing risk for coronary artery disease and stroke.

This section on Health Promotion and Counseling section provides an *approach* to screening and prevention, but you should review the excellent reports listed below for a deeper understanding of the evidence base of recent recommendations.

Key Reports on Cardiovascular Health and Risk Assessment

- Heart disease and stroke statistics—2016 update: a report from the American Heart Association (AHA).[32] *Updated annually.*
- 2013 American College of Cardiology (ACC)/AHA guideline on the assessment of cardiovascular risk: a report of the ACC/AHA Task Force on Practice Guidelines.[51]
- Effectiveness-based guidelines for the prevention of CVD in women—2011 update: a guideline from the AHA.[52]
- Management of high blood pressure in blacks. An update of the International Society on Hypertension in Blacks consensus statement 2010.[53]
- Guidelines for the primary prevention of stroke. A guideline for healthcare professionals from the AHA/American Stroke Association 2014.[54]
- American Diabetes Association. Executive summary: Standards of medical care in diabetes—2015.[55] *Updated annually.*

Screening Early. Heart disease has "a long asymptomatic latent period," and about half of all coronary deaths lack prior warning signs or cardiac diagnoses.[56] Consequently, clinicians are encouraged to assess *lifetime risk* in asymptomatic patients, possibly beginning as early as age 20 years. Earlier risk assessment can lead to more timely interventions to lower the burden of CVD.

The Challenge of Risk Factor Reduction. The 2020 AHA goals promote the concept of "*ideal cardiovascular health,*" defined as:

> The absence of clinically manifest CVD and the simultaneous presence of optimal levels of seven health metrics, including four health behaviors (lean body mass index <25 kg/m², not smoking, being physically active, and following a healthy diet), and three health factors (untreated total cholesterol <200 mg/dL, untreated blood pressure <120/<80 mm Hg, and fasting blood glucose <100 mg/dL).[46]

Figure 9-21, based on data available in 2014, shows that substantial portions of the United States population fail to reach ideal cardiovascular health. Among U.S. adults age ≥20 years, the age-standardized prevalence of ideal levels of cardiovascular health behaviors and factors ranges widely: for the healthy diet score—0.5%; weight—31%; blood pressure—45%; physical activity—41%; cholesterol—47%; fasting glucose—58%; and never smoked or stopped smoking for more than 12 month—76%. *Most U.S. adults, ~68%, have two, three, or four criteria at ideal levels of cardiovascular health.* Approximately 13% of U.S. adults meet five or more criteria, 5% meet six or more criteria, and virtually none meet seven criteria at ideal levels.[32]

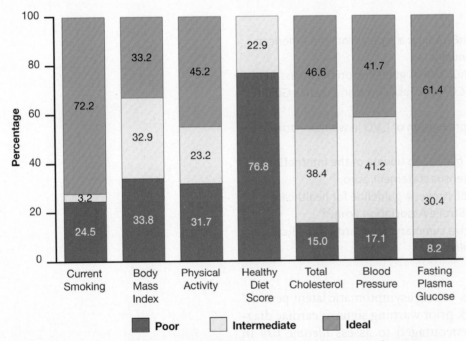

FIGURE 9-21. **American Heart Association Prevalence Estimates for poor, intermediate, and ideal cardiovascular health (U.S. adults, 2014).** Source: Go AS, Mozaffarian D, Roger VL, et al. Heart disease and stroke statistics—2014 update: a report from the American Heart Association. *Circulation.* 2014;129:e28.

The AHA has set the ambitious goals of improving cardiovascular health for all Americans between 2010 and 2020 by 20% and of reducing deaths from CVD and stroke by 20%.[32]

Special Populations at Risk

Women. Women have become increasingly aware that CVD is their leading cause of death.[57] Improved CVD prevention and treatment efforts for women have led to dramatic decreases in the age-adjusted mortality rates for CHD—a decrease of nearly two thirds between 1980 and 2007.[57,58] Nonetheless, in the 2011 Guideline for the Prevention of Cardiovascular Disease in Women, the AHA cautioned that "reversing a trend of the past 4 decades, CHD death rates in U.S. women 35 to 54 years of age now actually appear to be increasing," which the AHA attributed to the effects of obesity.[52] Men's cardiovascular risk scores have improved more than women's in recent years, though the prevalence of diabetes has increased in both sexes.[59] The statistics below illuminate concerning issues for cardiovascular health in women.

Cardiovascular Disease in U.S. Women

- 2013 data indicate that CVD death rates remain significantly higher for black women than white women, 247 versus 184 per 100,000, largely due to disparities in risk factors such as hypertension, diabetes, and obesity.[32] CHD death rates are also higher for black women than white women, 94.7 versus 75.0 per 100,000.
- Women age >65 years have a slightly higher prevalence of *hypertension* than men, but a much higher prevalence of uncontrolled hypertension. Black women have the highest prevalence of hypertension (46%) and uncontrolled hypertension. About two thirds of all U.S. women are now *overweight or obese,* contributing to the epidemic of type 2 diabetes and increasing risks for MI and stroke.
- Women account for nearly 60% of stroke deaths in the United States and have a higher lifetime risk of stroke than men. Stroke risk increases with age, and women have a greater life expectancy than men. Women also have a lower awareness of heart disease and stroke symptoms.
- Women have unique risk factors for stroke: pregnancy, hormone therapy, early menopause, and preeclampsia. Women are more likely than men to have risk factors of atrial fibrillation, migraine with aura, obesity, and metabolic syndrome. Atrial fibrillation, which increases stroke risk fivefold in women, is often asymptomatic and undetected. For these reasons, the 2014 AHA expert panel on stroke prevention highlighted risk stratification and appropriate anticoagulation for women with atrial fibrillation.[60]

In 2011, the AHA, recognizing the special cardiovascular risk faced by women, adopted more specific CVD risk classifications. They recommended placing women into one of three categories: *high risk, at risk,* and *"ideal"* cardiovascular health.[52]

American Heart Association Cardiovascular Risk Categories for Women

High Risk

- ≥1 of the high-risk states, including existing CHD, CVD, peripheral arterial disease, abdominal aortic aneurysm, diabetes mellitus, or end-stage or chronic renal disease
- 10-year predicted risk of >10%

At Risk

- ≥1 major risk factors including smoking, blood pressure ≥120/≥80 or treated hypertension, total cholesterol ≥200 mg/dL, HDL-c <50 mg/dL, or treated dyslipidemia, obesity, poor diet, physical inactivity, or family history of premature CVD
- Evidence of advanced subclinical atherosclerosis (e.g., coronary calcification, carotid plaque, intima-media thickness), metabolic syndrome, or poor exercise capacity on a treadmill test
- Systemic autoimmune collagen vascular disease (e.g., lupus or rheumatoid arthritis)
- History or preeclampsia, gestational diabetes, or pregnancy-induced hypertension

Ideal Cardiovascular Health (All of These)

- Total cholesterol <200 mg/dL (untreated)
- BP <120/<80 (untreated)
- Fasting glucose <100 mg/dL (untreated)
- Body mass index <25 kg/m²
- Abstinence from smoking
- Physical activity at goal: ≥150 minutes/week moderate intensity, ≥75 minutes/week vigorous intensity, or combination
- Healthy diet

Source: Mosca L, Benjamin EJ, Berra K, et al. Effectiveness-based guidelines for the prevention of CVD in women—2011 update: A guideline from the American Heart Association. *Circulation.* 2011; 123:1243.

African Americans. CVD death rates show marked ethnic disparities: in 2013, they were 357 versus 271 per 100,000 for black men compared to white men, and 247 versus 184 per 100,000 for black women compared to white women.[32] Overall, about 40% of white adults have ≥three of the seven AHA cardiovascular health metrics (see above) at ideal levels compared to about 30% of black adults.[32] Selected striking CVD disparities are shown on next page. The high prevalence of high cholesterol, obesity, and diabetes in Mexican Americans places them at similar risk to blacks.

Cardiovascular Diseases and Risk Factors: Prevalence in U.S. White and Black Adults

	Men		Women	
	White	Black	White	Black
Total Cardiovascular Disease	36.1%	46.0%	31.9%	48.3%
Coronary Heart Disease	7.8%	7.2%	4.6%	7.0%
Hypertension	32.9%	44.9%	30.1%	46.1%
Stroke	2.2%	4.2%	2.5%	4.7%
Diabetes (Physician Diagnosed)	7.6%	13.8%	6.1%	14.6%
Overweight/Obesity	72.7%	69.4%	61.2%	81.9%
Cholesterol ≥200 mg/dL	39.9%	37.4%	45.9%	40.7%
Smoking	21.7%	21.1%	18.7%	15.0%
Physical Activity (Meeting Federal Aerobic Guidelines)	57.0%	49.8%	50.0%	34.6%

Sources: Mozaffarian D, Benjamin EJ, Go AS, et al. Heart Disease and Stroke Statistics—2016 Update: A Report From the American Heart Association. *Circulation* 2016;133:e38; Centers for Disease Control and Prevention. Prevalence of coronary heart disease—United States, 2006–2010. *MMWR Morb Mortal Wkly Rep.* 2011;60:1377.

Screening for Cardiovascular Risk Factors

Step 1: Screen for Global Risk Factors. Begin routine screening at 20 years for individual risk factors or "global" risk of CVD and for any family history of premature heart disease (age <55 years in first-degree male relatives and age <65 years in first-degree female relatives). Recommended screening intervals are listed below.

Major Cardiovascular Risk Factors and Screening Frequency

Risk Factor	Screening Frequency	Goal
Family history of premature CVD	Update regularly	
Cigarette smoking	At each visit	Cessation
Poor diet	At each visit	Improved overall eating pattern
Physical inactivity	At each visit	30 minutes moderate intensity daily

(continued)

Major Cardiovascular Risk Factors and Screening Frequency (continued)

Risk Factor	Screening Frequency	Goal
Obesity, especially central adiposity	At each visit	BMI 20–25 kg/m^2; waist circumference: ≤40 inches for men, ≤35 inches for women
Hypertension	At each visit	<140/90 for adults <60 years, adults >60 with diabetes or chronic kidney disease; <150/90 for all other adults age ≥60 years
Dyslipidemias	Every 5 years if low risk Every 2 years if strong risk	Initiate statin therapy if meeting ACC/AHA guidelines
Diabetes	Every 3 years (if normal) beginning at age 45 years; more frequently at any age if risk factors	Prevent/delay diabetes for those with HbA1c of 5.7–6.4%
Pulse	At each visit	Identify and treat atrial fibrillation

Sources: Adapted from: Goff DC, Jr., Lloyd-Jones DM, Bennett G, et al. 2013 ACC/AHA guideline on the assessment of cardiovascular risk: a report of the American College of Cardiology/American Heart Association Task Force on Practice Guidelines. *J Am Coll Cardiol.* 2014;63(25 Pt B):2935; Stone NJ, Robinson JG, Lichtenstein AH, et al. 2013 ACC/AHA guideline on the treatment of blood cholesterol to reduce atherosclerotic cardiovascular risk in adults: a report of the American College of Cardiology/American Heart Association Task Force on Practice Guidelines. *Circulation.* 2014;129:S1; James PA, Oparil S, Carter BL, et al. 2014 evidence-based guideline for the management of high blood pressure in adults: report from the panel members appointed to the Eighth Joint National Committee (JNC 8). *JAMA.* 2014;311:507; Meschia JF, Bushnell C, Boden-Albala B, et al. Guidelines for the primary prevention of stroke: a statement for healthcare professionals from the American Heart Association/American Stroke Association. *Stroke.* 2014;45:3754; Flack JM, Sica DA, Bakris G, et al. Management of high blood pressure in Blacks: an update of the International Society on Hypertension in Blacks consensus statement. *Hypertension.* 2010;56:780; American Diabetes A. Executive summary: Standards of medical care in diabetes—2014. *Diabetes Care.* 2014; 37 Suppl 1:S5.

Step 2: Calculate 10-Year and Lifetime CVD Risk Using an Online Calculator. Use the CVD risk calculators to establish 10-year and lifetime risk for patients ages 40 to 79 years. The most recent ACC/AHA Cholesterol Guideline provides a new risk-assessment calculator.[61]

CVD Risk Calculators

- http://my.americanheart.org/cvriskcalculator
- http://www.acc.org/tools-and-practice-support/mobile-resources/features/2013-prevention-guidelines-ascvd-risk-estimator?w_nav=S.

The risk estimates, which incorporate age, gender, smoking history, total cholesterol level, HDL cholesterol level, systolic blood pressure, antihypertensive therapy, and diabetes, are based on pooled data from population-based studies. The new calculators provide gender and race-specific risk estimates for a first MI, CHD death, or fatal or nonfatal stroke.

Step 3: Track Individual Risk Factors—Hypertension, Diabetes, Dyslipidemias, Metabolic Syndrome, Smoking, Family History, and Obesity

Hypertension. About one third of U.S. adults over the age of 20 years have hypertension (defined as a blood pressure ≥140/90 mm Hg), representing nearly 80 million people.[32] Over 40% of U.S. cardiovascular mortality and 30% of overall mortality is attributed to hypertension, representing an estimated 362,000 deaths in 2010.[47,62]

- *Primary (essential) hypertension* is the most common cause of hypertension: risk factors include age, genetics, black race, obesity and weight gain, excessive salt intake, physical inactivity, and excessive alcohol use.

- *Secondary hypertension* accounts for less than 5% of hypertension cases. Causes include sleep apnea, chronic kidney disease, renal artery stenosis, medications, thyroid disease, parathyroid disease, Cushing syndrome, hyperaldosteronism, pheochromocytoma, and coarctation of the aorta.

While the prevalence of hypertension is similar between men and women, prevalence in blacks is substantially higher than in whites. Most hypertensive adults know of their diagnosis, though only about 75% are taking medications and only half have achieved their target blood pressure goal.[56,63] The U.S. Preventive Services Task Force (USPSTF) has issued a grade A recommendation for hypertension screening among adults 18 years and older.[64] The American Society of Hypertension[68] and Seventh Joint National Committee on Prevention, Detection, and Treatment of High Blood Pressure[69] have suggested categories for classifying blood pressure readings (Table).

In 2014, the Eighth Joint National Committee on Prevention, Detection, Evaluation, and Treatment of High Blood Pressure issued updated guidelines shown with strength of evidence for specific recommendations on the next page.[65] These recommendations have not been universally accepted, even among members of the Joint National Committee.[66–68]

Blood Pressure Classification for Adults—JNC 7, American Society of Hypertension

Category	Systolic (mm Hg)	Diastolic (mm Hg)
Normal	<120	<80
Prehypertension	120–139	80–89
Stage 1 hypertension		
Age ≥18 to <60 yrs	140–159	90–99
Age ≥60 yrs[a]	150–159	90–99
Stage 2 hypertension	≥160	≥100
If diabetes or renal disease (including age ≥60 yrs)	<140	<90

[a]The American Society of Hypertension raises this cutoff to age ≥80 years.

Sources: Weber MA, Schiffrin EL, White WB, et al. Clinical practice guidelines for the management of hypertension in the community: A statement by the American Society of Hypertension and the International Society of Hypertension. *J Clin Hypertens*. 2014;16:14; Chobanian AV, Bakris GL, Black HR, et al. The Seventh Report of the Joint National Committee on Prevention, Detection, Evaluation, and Treatment of High Blood Pressure—The JNC 7 Report. *JAMA*. 2003;289:2560. Available at http://www.nhlbi.nih.gov/health-pro/guidelines/current/

JNC 8: Indications and Strength of Evidence for Initiating Pharmacologic Therapy to Lower Blood Pressure

Age ≥60 years	Systolic blood pressure ≥150 mm Hg or diastolic blood pressure ≥90 mm Hg (strong recommendation)
Age <60 years	Systolic blood pressure ≥140 mm Hg (expert opinion) Diastolic blood pressure ≥90 mm Hg (strong recommendation)
Age >18 years with chronic kidney disease or diabetes	Systolic blood pressure ≥140 mm Hg or diastolic blood pressure ≥90 mm Hg (expert opinion)

Source: James PA, Oparil S, Carter BL, et al. 2014 evidence-based guideline for the management of high blood pressure in adults: report from the panel members appointed to the Eighth Joint National Committee (JNC 8). *JAMA*. 2014;311:507.

See Chapter 4, Beginning the Physical Examination: General Survey, Vital Signs, and Pain, pp. 118–119, for discussion of the benefits of restricting dietary sodium to <2,300 mg/day and increasing physical activity for CVD risk reduction and control of hypertension.[70]

The AHA, ACC, and the American Society of Hypertension issued guidelines in 2015 for treating hypertension in patients with existing coronary artery disease. A blood pressure of <140/90 mm Hg is an appropriate goal for most patients with coronary artery disease, congestive heart failure, or acute coronary syndrome. Lowering blood pressure below 130/80 mm Hg may be appropriate for some patients with coronary artery disease, previous heart attacks, history of stroke or transient ischemic attack, carotid artery disease, peripheral arterial disease, or abdominal aortic aneurysm.[71]

Public health efforts such as the "Million Hearts" initiative have targeted blood pressure control as an important step in reducing cardiovascular morbidity and mortality.[72]

Diabetes.   Diabetes wreaks devastating health consequences in the United States and worldwide. The dramatic increase in obesity coupled with physical inactivity has created an epidemic of diabetes. The CDC estimated that in 2012, diabetes affected over 12% of U.S. adults, or nearly 29 million people.[73] This figure includes over 8 million adults who are undiagnosed. Another 86 million adults (37% of the population) have prediabetes. The total prevalence of diabetes in the United States is expected to double by 2050.

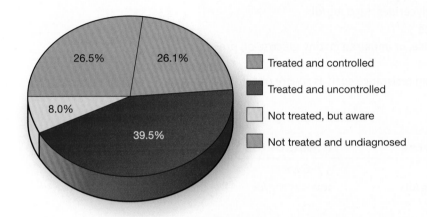

FIGURE 9-22.   Treatment of diabetes. Source: National Health and Nutrition Examination Survey (NHANES) 2011–2012 in Go AS, Mozaffarian D, Roger VL, et al. Heart disease and stroke statistics—2014 update: a report from the American Heart Association. *Circulation.* 2014;129:e28. Available at http://www.ncbi.nlm.nih.gov/pubmed/24352519. Accessed April 5, 2015.

There are striking disparities in the age-adjusted diabetes prevalences among adults: 7% to 9% of whites and Asian Americans compared to ~13% of Hispanics and blacks, rising to 16% of American Indian/Alaska Natives.[73] Unfortunately, as shown in Figure 9-22, only 25% of those affected are treated and controlled, and diabetes is associated with a two-fold increased risk of CVD events and mortality.

Although diabetes unequivocally increases the risk of CVD, early detection and treatment has not been firmly established to improve cardiovascular outcomes. Nonetheless, the 2015 American Diabetes Association guidelines support screening and then diagnosing diabetes if fasting glucose is ≥126 mg/dL and HbA1c values exceed 6.5%.[74] Diagnostic criteria for diabetes and prediabetes, as well as screening guidelines, are shown on the next page. Screening should be initiated at age 45 years and repeated at 3-year intervals. Screening should be initiated at any age for adults having a BMI of ≥25 and additional risk factors.

American Diabetes Association 2015: Classification and Diagnosis of Diabetes

Screening Criteria

Healthy adults with no risk factors: begin at age 45 years, repeat at 3-year intervals

Adults with BMI ≥25 kg/m² and additional risk factors:

- Physical inactivity
- First-degree relative with diabetes
- Members of a high-risk ethnic population—African American, Hispanic/Latino American, Asian American, Pacific Islander
- Mothers of infants ≥4.08 kg (9 lb) at birth or diagnosed with gestational diabetes
- Hypertension ≥140/90 mm Hg or on therapy for hypertension
- HDL cholesterol <35 mg/dL and/or triglycerides >250 mg/dL
- Women with polycystic ovary syndrome
- HbA1c ≥5.7%, impaired glucose tolerance, or impaired fasting glucose on previous testing
- Other conditions associated with insulin resistance such as severe obesity, acanthosis nigricans
- History of CVD

Diagnostic Criteria	Diabetes[a]	Prediabetes
HbA1c	≥6.5%	5.7–6.4%
Fasting plasma glucose (on at least 2 occasions)	≥126 mg/dL	100–125 mg/dL
2-hour plasma glucose (oral glucose tolerance test)	≥200 mg/dL	140–199 mg/dL
Random glucose, if classic symptoms	≥200 mg/dL	

[a]In the absence of classic symptoms, an abnormal test must be repeated to confirm the diagnosis. However, if two different tests are both abnormal then no additional testing is necessary.

Source: American Diabetes Association. Classification and diagnosis of diabetes. *Diabetes Care.* 2015;38(Suppl):S8.

Dyslipidemias. The USPSTF has issued a grade A recommendation for routine lipid screening for all men of age >35 years and women >45 years who are at increased risk for CHD.[75] The Task Force also issued a grade B recommendation to screen for lipid disorders beginning at age 20 years for men and women who have diabetes, hypertension, obesity, tobacco use, noncoronary atherosclerosis, or family history of early CVD. These recommendations are currently being updated.

In 2014, the ACC/AHA published "a guideline on the treatment of blood cholesterol to reduce atherosclerotic cardiovascular risk in adults."[61] This guideline offers evidence-based recommendations on using statins to treat cholesterol in high-risk groups (Fig. 9-23). Persons with clinical atherosclerotic CVD include "those with an acute coronary syndrome and those with a history of MI, stable or unstable, angina, coronary of other arterial revascularization, or stroke, transient ischemic attack, or peripheral arterial disease … of atherosclerotic origin." In addition, the ACC/AHA provides a calculator for clinicians and patients to estimate 10-year and lifetime gender and race-specific risks for CHD and stroke events to guide statin use for primary prevention: ACC/AHA Risk Calculator, *http://tools.cardiosource.org/ASCVD-Risk-Estimator/* (see also p. 365).

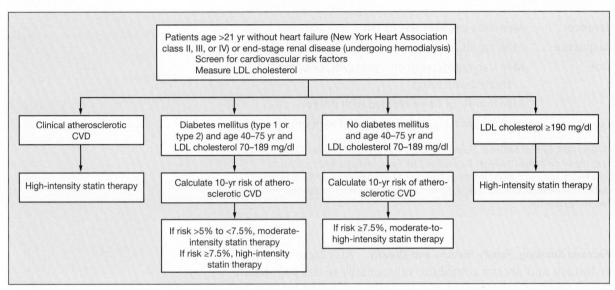

FIGURE 9-23. American College of Cardiology/American Heart Association cholesterol guideline, 2013.[76]

Use the CVD risk calculators to establish 10-year risk. The most recent ACC/AHA Cholesterol Guideline provides evidence-based recommendations for initiating statin therapy based on risk level.[61] The recommendations shown in Figure 9-23 are briefly summarized below. The guideline notes that high-intensity therapy lowers LDL by about 50% and moderate-intensity therapy lowers LDL by 30% to 50%.

- For patients with clinical CVD (secondary prevention) or LDL cholesterol levels >190 mg/dL (primary prevention)—prescribe high-intensity statin therapy.

- For patients with diabetes and/or LDL cholesterol levels from 70 to 189 mg/dL—determine the 10-year risk of atherosclerotic CVD with the new risk calculator (see above). Although the evidence for initiating statins for primary prevention is stronger for adults with 10-year risks above 7.5%, statins can also be considered for risk levels between 5% and <7.5%.

- However, the guideline also states that clinicians and patients should engage in shared decision making, addressing the potential benefits and harms of prescribing statins and eliciting patient preferences before initiating therapy. The guideline firmly emphasizes the importance of encouraging all patients to adhere to a healthy lifestyle.

The Metabolic Syndrome.   The metabolic syndrome consists of a cluster of risk factors that increase risk of both CVD and diabetes. In 2009, the International Diabetes Association, the National Heart Lung Blood Institute, the AHA, and other societies established diagnostic criteria as the presence of ≥three of the five risk factors listed below.[77] The prevalence of this syndrome in U.S. adults ≥20 years of age is approximately 34%.[46]

Metabolic Syndrome: 2009 Diagnostic Criteria— Must Meet ≥3 of 5

Waist circumference	Men ≥102 cm, women ≥88 cm
Fasting plasma glucose	≥100 mg/dL, or being treated for elevated glucose
HDL cholesterol	Men <40 mg/dL, women <50 mg/dL, or being treated with drugs
Triglycerides	≥150 mg/dL, or being treated with drugs
Blood pressure	≥130/≥85 mm Hg, or being treated with drugs

Source: Alberti KG, Eckel RH, Grundy SM, et al. Harmonizing the metabolic syndrome: a joint interim statement of the International Diabetes Federation Task Force on Epidemiology and Prevention; National Heart, Lung, and Blood Institute; American Heart Association; World Heart Federation; International Atherosclerosis Society; and International Association for the Study of Obesity. *Circulation.* 2009;120:1640.

Other Risk Factors: Smoking, Family History, and Obesity.   Risk factors such as smoking, family history, and obesity contribute substantially to the population burden of CVD.[46,78] *Smoking* increases the risk of CHD and stroke by two- to fourfold compared to nonsmokers or past smokers who quit >10 years previously. About 14% of the annual cardiovascular deaths in the population, or over 150,000 deaths, are attributed to smoking. Among adults, 13% report a *family history* of heart attack or angina before age 50 years. Along with a family history of premature revascularization, this risk factor is associated with about a 50% increased lifetime risk for CHD and for CVD mortality. *Obesity,* or BMI over 30 kg/m², contributed to 112,000 excess adult deaths compared to those of normal weight, and was associated with 13% of CVD deaths in 2004.

Promoting Lifestyle Change and Risk Factor Modification. Motivating behavior change is challenging, but it is an essential clinical skill for risk factor reduction. Promoting cardiovascular health is a high priority for *Healthy People 2020*. Objectives include increases in physical activity and reductions in: the prevalence of hypertension, tobacco use, and obesity; consumption of calories from solid fats and added sugars; and CHD deaths.[79] The well-known Prochaska model is a useful tool for assessing patient "readiness to change" and tailoring advice to the patient's level of motivation.[80]

The USPSTF has given a B recommendation for referring adults with cardiovascular risk factors to behavioral counseling interventions that encourage a healthy diet and physical activity.[81] The ACC/AHA recommendations on lifestyle management address diet, physical activity, body weight, and tobacco avoidance, as well as controlling hypertension and diabetes.[82]

See Table 4-4, Obesity: Stages of Change Model and Assessing Readiness, p. 142, and Chapter 8, Thorax and Lungs, pp. 303–342, for examples of how this model can be applied to clinical counseling.

Hypertension. Encourage your patients to adopt the recommendations for pertinent lifestyle modifications listed below.

Lifestyle Modifications to Prevent or Manage Hypertension

- Optimal weight, or BMI of 18.5 to 24.9 kg/m²
- Intake of <6 g of sodium chloride or 2.3 g of sodium per day
- Regular aerobic exercise such as brisk walking three to four times a week, averaging 40 minutes per session
- Moderate alcohol consumption per day of ≤2 drinks for men and ≤1 drink for women (2 drinks = 1 oz ethanol, 24 oz beer, 10 oz wine, or 2 to 3 oz whiskey)
- Diet rich in fruits, vegetables, whole grains, and low-fat dairy products with reduced intake of saturated and total fat, sweets, and red meats

Source: Eckel RH, Jakicic JM, Ard JD, et al. 2013 AHA/ACC guideline on lifestyle management to reduce cardiovascular risk: a report of the American College of Cardiology/American Heart Association Task Force on Practice Guidelines. *Circulation.* 2014;129:S76.

Tobacco Use. Ask every patient "Do you smoke or use tobacco products?" and then ask tobacco users "Do you want to quit?" Use the "5 As" framework and the Stages of Change model described in Chapter 8 to develop strategies for quitting. Encourage patients to use services that increase quit rates like the National Smoking Cessation Hotline: 1-800-QUIT NOW. If the patient is not using tobacco, ask whether they are former users. If so, encourage continued abstinence—and consider interventions to prevent relapse for recent quitters.[83]

See discussion on Tobacco Cessation, Chapter 8, Thorax and Lungs, pp. 313–315.

Obesity: Healthy Eating and Weight Loss. Begin with a dietary history to explore the patient's eating habits, then target the importance of foods low in total fat, especially foods low in saturated and *trans* fats. Foods with mono- and polyunsaturated fats and the omega-3 fatty acids found in fish oils help lower serum cholesterol. A Mediterranean diet (fruits, vegetables, seafood, white meat, wine), supplemented by extra-virgin olive oil and nuts, has been shown to reduce major cardiovascular events among high-risk patients.[84] Review the food sources of these healthy and unhealthy fats in the box below.

See discussion of Optimal Weight, Nutrition, and Diet in Chapter 4, Beginning the Physical Examination: General Survey, Vital Signs, and Pain, pp. 114–118.

Food Sources of Healthy and Unhealthy Fats

Healthy Fats	*Foods high in monounsaturated fat:* nuts, such as almonds, pecans, and peanuts; sesame seeds; avocados; canola, sunflower, high oleic safflower, olive, and peanut oil; peanut butter[85]
	Foods high in polyunsaturated fat: corn, cottonseed, and soybean oil; walnuts; pumpkin or sunflower seeds; soft (tub) margarine; mayonnaise; salad dressings
	Foods high in omega-3 fatty acids: flaxseed, walnuts, tuna, anchovies, herring, mackerel, rainbow trout, salmon, sardines, shrimp

(*continued*)

Food Sources of Healthy and Unhealthy Fats (continued)

Unhealthy Fats	*Foods high in saturated fat:* high-fat dairy products—cream, cheese, ice cream, whole and 2% milk, butter, and sour cream; bacon; chocolate; coconut oil; lard and gravy from meat drippings; high-fat meats like ground beef, bologna, hot dogs, and sausage *Foods high in* trans *fat:* snacks and baked goods with hydrogenated or partially hydrogenated oil, stick margarines, shortening, and fried foods

Source: U.S. Department of Agriculture and U.S. Department of Health and Human Services. *Dietary Guidelines for Americans,* 2010. Washington, D.C., U.S. Government Printing Office. 7th ed. Available at http://www.health.gov/dietaryguidelines/dga2010/DietaryGuidelines2010.pdf. Accessed March 30, 2015.

Less than 1% of the U.S. population meets most healthy dietary goals for fruits and vegetables, fish, sodium, sugar-sweetened drinks, and whole grains. Nearly 35% of adult Americans are obese (BMI ≥30 kg/m^2), an epidemic problem in the United States since 1980.[46] Healthy People 2020 targets reductions in the proportions of obese children and adolescents and in caloric intake from solid fats and added sugars.[79]

You should counsel patients about unhealthy weight. Assess BMI as described in Chapter 4. Discuss the principles of healthy eating. Patients with a high fat intake are more likely to accumulate body fat than those with diets high in protein and carbohydrates. Help the patient to set realistic goals for diet and exercise that promote healthy eating habits *for life.*

Physical Activity. About 12% of the population burden of CVD is attributed to insufficient physical activity.[56] A major goal of Healthy People 2020 is to increase the proportion of people meeting federal physical activity targets for aerobic and muscle strengthening activity.[79]

■ For aerobic activity, adults should perform at least 150 minutes (2 hours and 30 minutes) of moderate-intensity cardiorespiratory activity, such as brisk walking, each week.[86] Markers that help patients recognize the onset of aerobic metabolism include deep breathing, sweating in cool temperatures, and pulse rates exceeding 60% of the maximum normal age-adjusted heart rate (220 minus the person's age).

■ Muscle strengthening activities, which include resistance training and lifting weights, can increase fitness and bone strength. Activities strengthening all the major muscle groups should be performed at least twice weekly.

■ Spur motivation by emphasizing the important benefits to health and well-being, even with just an hour of moderate-intensity activity each week— "some is better than none."

Inactive adults should only gradually increase their activity toward the recommended goals to avoid injuries. Be sure to assess any pulmonary, cardiac, or musculoskeletal conditions that may limit the patient's exercise capacity.

Techniques of Examination

Turn now to the classic techniques for examining the heart and great vessels. A sound knowledge of cardiovascular anatomy and physiology is key to understanding the hemodynamics of this *closed-pump forward-flow system*. It is only through diligent repetition, however, that you will gain confidence in the accuracy of your clinical findings.[22] Examine each patient carefully and methodically. Practice examining normal patients will help you recognize when patients have important cardiac pathology. Knowing how well these findings, by themselves or in concert with others, predict the presence or absence of cardiac disease is vitally important. The "test characteristics" of cardiac findings such as sensitivity, specificity, and likelihood ratios, are provided when pertinent and available. Students can also turn to several excellent resources for more detailed information.[87,88]

As you practice the cardiac examination, be sure you are proficient in the basic objectives listed below.

Cardiac Examination Skills: Objectives for Mastery

- Describe the chest wall anatomy and identify the key listening areas.
- Evaluate the jugular venous pulse, the carotid upstroke, and presence or absence of carotid bruits.
- Palpate and describe the PMI.
- Auscultate S_1 and S_2 in six positions from the base to the apex.
- Recognize the effect of the P-R interval on the intensity of S_1.
- Identify physiologic and paradoxical splitting of S_2.
- Auscultate and recognize abnormal sounds in early diastole, including an S_3 and OS of mitral stenosis.
- Auscultate and recognize an S_4 later in diastole.
- Distinguish systolic and diastolic murmurs, using maneuvers when needed.
- Evaluate and interpret a paradoxical pulse.

BLOOD PRESSURE AND HEART RATE

The general appearance of the patient provides many clues to cardiac illness, so pay special attention to the patient's color, respiratory rate, and level of anxiety, in addition to blood pressure and heart rate. Since auscultation is so important for detecting subtle findings, examine the patient in a quiet comfortable room where distractions and noise are at a minimum.

See Chapter 4, Beginning the Physical Examination: General Survey, Vital Signs, and Pain, especially Blood Pressure, pp. 124–132.

As you begin, review the blood pressure and heart rate recorded at the start of the visit. If you need to repeat these measurements, or if they have not already been done, measure the blood pressure and heart rate using optimal technique.[89,90]

In brief review, after letting the patient rest for at least 5 minutes in a quiet setting with feet on the floor, choose a correctly sized cuff and position the patient's unclothed arm at heart level, either resting on a table if the patient is seated, or supported at midchest level if supine or standing. Heart level is usually at the 4th intercostal space at the sternum. Make sure the bladder of the cuff is centered over the brachial artery. Inflate the cuff approximately 30 mm Hg above the pressure at which the brachial or radial pulse disappears. As you deflate the cuff, listen first for the Korotkoff sounds of at least two consecutive heartbeats; these mark the *systolic* pressure. Then listen for the disappearance point of the heartbeats, which marks the *diastolic* pressure. For *heart rate,* palpate the radial pulse using the pads of your index and middle fingers, or auscultate the apical pulse with your stethoscope.

At higher arm levels, the blood pressure recordings will be lower; at lower levels, the blood pressure recordings will be higher.

A growing literature documents the poor reliability of clinic blood pressure measurements.[91–94] Multiple averaged measurements improve precision, especially when using automated home and ambulatory blood pressure readings, which are more reliable, accurate, and better correlated with cardiovascular outcomes than clinic readings.

JUGULAR VENOUS PRESSURE AND PULSATIONS

Jugular Venous Pressure

Identifying the JVP. Estimating the JVP is one of the most important and frequently used skills of physical examination. The JVP closely parallels pressure in the right atrium, or central venous pressure, related primarily to volume in the venous system.[95] The JVP is best assessed from pulsations in the right internal jugular vein, which is directly in line with the superior vena cava and right atrium.[96–99] The internal jugular veins lie deep to the SCM muscles in the neck and are not directly visible, so you must learn to identify the pulsations of the internal jugular vein that are transmitted to the surface of the neck (Fig. 9-24). Pulsations in the *right external jugular vein* can also be used,[30] but the route from the vena cava is more tortuous, and examination can be impaired by kinking and obstruction at the base of the neck and by obesity.[96,100] Note that the jugular veins and pulsations are difficult to see in children under 12 years of age, so inspection is not useful in this age group.

See discussion of the double peak of the *a* and *v waves* and of the *x* and *y descent* on p. 378.

Although the JVP accurately predicts elevations in fluid volume in heart failure, its prognostic value for heart failure outcomes and mortality is unclear.[101]

Pressure changes from right atrial filling, contraction, and emptying cause fluctuations in the JVP and its waveforms that are visible to the examiner. The dominant movement of the JVP is inward, coinciding with the x descent.[96] In contrast, the dominant movement of the carotid pulse, often confused with the JVP, is outward. Careful observation of the fluctuations of the JVP yields clues about volume status, right and left ventricular function, patency of the tricuspid and pulmonary valves, pressures in the pericardium, and arrhythmias caused by junctional rhythms and AV blocks. For example, JVP falls with loss of blood or decreased venous vascular tone and increases with right or left heart failure, pulmonary hypertension, tricuspid stenosis, AV dissociation, increased venous vascular tone, and pericardial compression or tamponade.

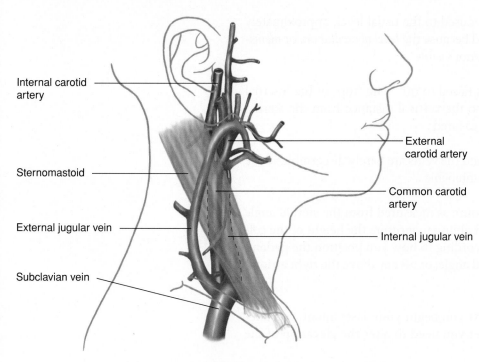

Internal carotid artery

Sternomastoid

External jugular vein

Subclavian vein

External carotid artery

Common carotid artery

Internal jugular vein

FIGURE 9-24. Internal and external jugular veins.

The Oscillation Point of the JPV. To estimate the level of the JVP, learn to find the *highest point of oscillation in the internal jugular vein* or, alternatively, the point above which the external jugular vein appears collapsed. The JVP is usually measured in vertical distance above the *sternal angle* (also called the *angle of Louis*), the bony ridge adjacent to the second rib where the manubrium joins the body of the sternum.

Study carefully the illustrations in Figure 9-25. Note that in the three positions, the sternal angle remains roughly 5 cm above the right midatrium. In this patient, the pressure in the internal jugular vein is somewhat elevated.

Some authors report that at 30° to 45°, the estimated JVP may be 3 cm lower than catheter measurements from the right midatrium.[102,103]

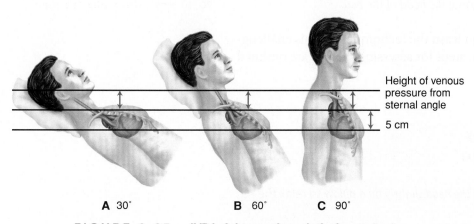

Height of venous pressure from sternal angle

5 cm

A 30°   **B** 60°   **C** 90°

FIGURE 9-25. JVP height remains relatively constant.

■ In *Position A,* the head of the bed is raised to the usual level, approximately 30°, but the JVP cannot be measured because the *level of oscillation,* or *meniscus,* is above the jaw and, therefore, not visible.

■ In *Position B,* the head of the bed is raised to 60°. The "top" of the internal jugular vein is now easily visible, so the vertical distance from the sternal angle or right atrium can now be measured.

■ In *Position C,* the patient is upright and the veins are barely discernible above the clavicle, making measurement untenable.

Note that the height of the venous pressure as measured from the sternal angle is *similar* in all three positions, but your ability to *measure* the height of the column of venous blood, or JVP, differs according to how you position the patient. JVP measured at >3 cm above the sternal angle, or >8 cm above the right atrium, is considered elevated or abnormal.

The JVP and Volume Status.   As you begin your assessment, consider the patient's volume status and whether you need to alter the elevation of the head of the bed or examining table.

■ The usual starting position for the head of the bed or examining table when assessing the JVP is 30°. Turn the patient's head slightly to the left, then the right, and identify the external jugular vein on each side. Then focus on the internal jugular venous pulsations on the right, transmitted from deep in the neck to the overlying soft tissues. The JVP is the highest oscillation point, or meniscus, of the jugular venous pulsations that is usually evident in euvolemic patients.

■ If the patient is *hypovolemic,* you can anticipate that *the JVP will be low,* causing you to *lower the head of the bed,* sometimes even to 0°, to see the point of oscillation best.

■ Likewise, if the patient is volume-overloaded, or *hypervolemic,* anticipate that *the JVP will be high,* causing you to *raise the head of the bed.*

Measuring the JVP.   To help you learn the techniques for this challenging portion of the cardiac examination, steps for assessing the JVP are outlined below.

A hypovolemic or septic patient may have to lie flat before you see the neck veins. In contrast, when there is volume overload, you may need to elevate the patient's head to 60° or even 90° to locate the oscillation point.

Steps for Measuring the Jugular Venous Pressure

1. Make the patient comfortable. *Raise the head slightly on a pillow* to relax the SCM muscles.
2. *Raise the head of the bed or examining table to about 30°. Turn the patient's head slightly away from the side you are inspecting.*

(*continued*)

Steps for Measuring the Jugular Venous Pressure (*continued*)

3. Use *tangential lighting* and examine both sides of the neck. Identify the external jugular vein on each side, then find the internal jugular venous pulsations.
4. *If necessary, raise or lower the head of the bed* until you can see the oscillation point or meniscus of the internal jugular venous pulsations in the lower half of the neck.
5. Focus on the *right internal jugular vein*. Look for pulsations in the suprasternal notch, between the attachments of the SCM muscle on the sternum and clavicle, or just posterior to the SCM. Distinguish the pulsations of the internal jugular vein from those of the carotid artery (see box below).
6. *Identify the highest point of pulsation in the right jugular vein.* Extend a long rectangular object or card horizontally from this point and a centimeter ruler vertically from the sternal angle, making an exact right angle. Measure the vertical distance in centimeters above the sternal angle where the horizontal object crosses the ruler and add to this distance 5 cm, the distance from the sternal angle to the center of the right atrium. *The sum is the JVP.*

Distinguishing Jugular Venous Pulsations from Carotid Pulsations. The following features help to distinguish jugular from carotid artery pulsations.[98]

Distinguishing Internal Jugular and Carotid Pulsations

Internal Jugular Pulsations	Carotid Pulsations
Rarely palpable	Palpable
Soft biphasic undulating quality, usually with two elevations and *characteristic inward deflection* (x descent)	A more vigorous thrust with a *single outward component*
Pulsations eliminated by light pressure on the vein(s) just above the sternal end of the clavicle	Pulsations not eliminated by pressure on veins at sternal end of clavicle
Height of pulsations changes with position, normally dropping as the patient becomes more upright	Height of pulsations unchanged by position
Height of pulsations usually falls with inspiration	Height of pulsations not affected by inspiration

Establishing the true vertical and horizontal lines to measure the JVP is difficult. Place the zero point of your ruler on the sternal angle and line it up with a vertical edge in the room. Then place a card or rectangular object at an exact right angle to the ruler (Fig. 9-26). This constitutes your horizontal line. Move it up or down—still horizontal—so that the lower edge rests at the top of the jugular pulsations, and read the vertical distance on the ruler. Round your measurement off to the nearest centimeter.

An elevated JVP is highly correlated with both acute and chronic heart failure.[102,104–110] It is also seen in *tricuspid stenosis, chronic pulmonary hypertension, superior vena cava obstruction, cardiac tamponade,* and *constrictive pericarditis.*[111–113]

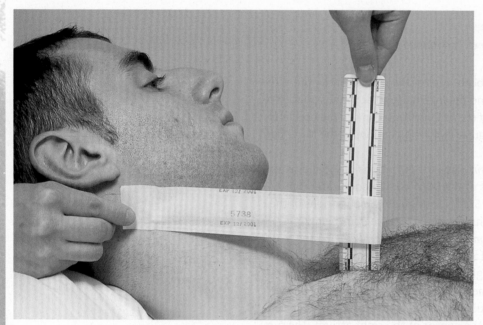

FIGURE 9-26. **Measure the JVP with a horizontal card and vertical ruler.**

JVP measured at >3 cm above the sternal angle, or more than 8 cm in total distance above the right atrium, is considered *elevated above normal*.

The highest point of venous pulsations may lie below the level of the sternal angle. Under these circumstances, venous pressure is not elevated and seldom needs to be measured.

Jugular Venous Pulsations. Oscillations in the right internal jugular vein, and often in the external jugular vein, reflect changing pressures in the right atrium. Careful inspection of these waveforms reveals two quick peaks and two troughs, diagrammed in Figure 9-27. Considerable practice and experience are required to discern these fluctuations.

■ The first elevation, the presystolic *a wave,* reflects the slight rise in atrial pressure that accompanies atrial contraction. It occurs just prior to S_1 and before the carotid upstroke.

■ The following trough, the *x descent,* starts with atrial relaxation. It continues as the RV, contracting during systole, pulls the floor of the atrium downward, and ends just before S_2. During ventricular systole, blood continues to flow into the right atrium from the venae cavae.

■ The tricuspid valve is closed, the chamber begins to fill, and right atrial pressure begins to rise again, creating the second elevation, the *v wave.* When the tricuspid valve opens early in diastole, blood in the right atrium flows passively into the RV, and right atrial pressure falls again, creating the second trough, or *y descent.*

In patients with obstructive lung disease, the JVP can appear elevated on expiration, but the veins collapse on inspiration. This finding does not indicate heart failure.

An elevated JVP is >95% specific for an increased left ventricular end diastolic pressure and low left ventricular EF, although its role as a predictor of hospitalization and death from heart failure is less clear.[102,114]

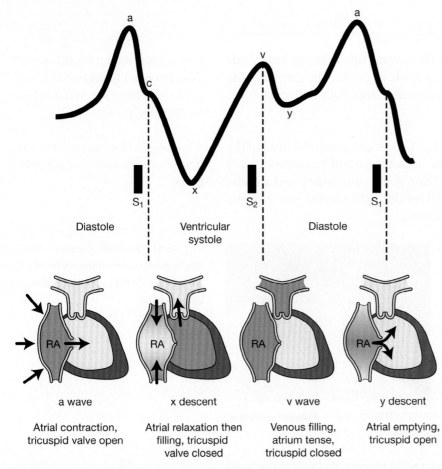

FIGURE 9-27. **Jugular venous pulsations.** (Adapted with permission from Douglas G, Nicol F, Robertson C. *Macleod's Clinical Examination*, 13th ed. London: Elsevier, 2013.)

■ A simplified way to remember the three peaks is: *a* for *a*trial contraction, *c* for *c*arotid transmission (although this may represent closure of the tricuspid valve),[102] and *v* for *v*enous filling. To the naked eye, the two descents, *x* and *y*, are the most visible events in the cycle of atrial contraction, atrial relaxation, atrial filling, and atrial emptying again followed by atrial contraction. Of the two, the sudden collapse of the *x* descent late in systole is more prominent, occurring just before S_2. The *y* descent follows S_2 early in diastole.

Observe the amplitude and timing of the jugular venous pulsations. To time them, feel the left carotid artery with your right thumb or listen to the heart simultaneously. The *a* wave just precedes S_1 and the carotid pulse, the *x* descent can be seen as a systolic collapse, the *v* wave almost coincides with S_2, and the *y* descent follows early in diastole. Look for absent or unusually prominent waves.

Abnormally prominent a waves occur in increased resistance to right atrial contraction, as in *tricuspid stenosis*; also in severe 1st-, 2nd-, and 3rd-degree AV block, supraventricular tachycardia, junctional tachycardia, *pulmonary hypertension*, and *pulmonic stenosis*.

Absent a waves signal atrial fibrillation.

Increased v waves occur in *tricuspid regurgitation, atrial septal defects,* and *constrictive pericarditis.*

THE CAROTID PULSE

Next, examine the *carotid pulse*, including the carotid upstroke, its amplitude and contour, and the presence or absence of *thrills* or *bruits*. The carotid pulse provides valuable information about cardiac function, especially aortic valve stenosis and regurgitation.

For irregular rhythms, see Table 9-1, Selected Heart Rates and Rhythms, p. 400, and Table 9-2, Selected Irregular Rhythms, p. 401.

To assess *amplitude and contour*, the patient should be supine with the head of the bed elevated to about 30°. First inspect the neck for carotid pulsations, often visible just medial to the SCM muscles. Then place your index and middle fingers (Fig. 9-28) or left thumb (Fig. 9-29) on the right carotid artery in the lower third of the neck and palpate for pulsations.

A tortuous and kinked carotid artery may produce a unilateral pulsatile bulge.

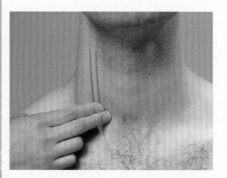

FIGURE 9-28. **Palpate the carotid pulse with index and middle fingers.**

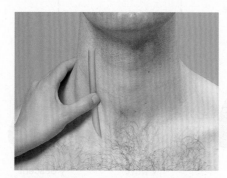

FIGURE 9-29. **Palpate with the thumb.**

Causes of decreased pulsations include decreased stroke volume from shock or MI and local atherosclerotic narrowing or occlusion.

Press just inside the medial border of a relaxed SCM muscle, roughly at the level of the cricoid cartilage. Avoid pressing on the *carotid sinus,* which lies adjacent to the top of the thyroid cartilage. For the left carotid artery, use your right fingers or thumb. Never palpate both carotid arteries at the same time. This may decrease blood flow to the brain and induce syncope.

Pressure on the carotid sinus may cause reflex bradycardia or drop in blood pressure.

Slowly increase pressure until you feel a maximal pulsation; then slowly decrease pressure until you best sense the arterial pressure and contour. Assess the pulse characteristics listed below.

See Table 9-3, Abnormalities of the Arterial Pulse and Pressure Waves, p. 402.

Assessment Characteristics of the Carotid Pulse

- The *amplitude of the pulse.* This correlates reasonably well with the pulse pressure.

The carotid pulse is small, thready, or weak in cardiogenic shock; the pulse is bounding in aortic regurgitation (see p. 411).

- The *contour of the pulse wave,* namely the speed of the upstroke, the duration of its summit, and the speed of the downstroke. The normal upstroke is *brisk;* it is smooth, rapid, and follows S₁ almost immediately. The summit is smooth, rounded, and roughly midsystolic. The downstroke is less abrupt than the upstroke.

The carotid upstroke is *delayed* in *aortic stenosis.*

(continued)

Assessment Characteristics of the Carotid Pulse (*continued*)

- Any *variations in amplitude,* either from beat to beat or with respiration.

- *The timing of the carotid upstroke in relation to* S_1 *and* S_2. Note that the normal carotid upstroke follows S_1 and precedes S_2. This relationship is very helpful in correctly identifying S_1 and S_2, especially when the heart rate is increased and the duration of diastole, normally longer than systole, is shortened and approaches the duration of systole.

Pulsus alternans and a bigeminal pulse vary beat to beat; a *paradoxical pulse* varies with respiration, described below.

Pulsus Alternans. In *pulsus alternans,* the rhythm of the pulse remains *regular,* but the *force* of the arterial pulse alternates because of alternating strong and weak ventricular contractions. *Pulsus alternans* almost always indicates severe left ventricular dysfunction. It is usually best felt by applying light pressure on the radial or femoral arteries. Use a blood pressure cuff to confirm your finding. After raising the cuff pressure, lower it slowly to just below the systolic level. The initial Korotkoff sounds are the strong beats. As you lower the cuff, you will hear the softer sounds of the alternating weak beats, which will eventually disappear, causing the remaining Korotkoff sounds to double.

Alternately loud and soft Korotkoff sounds or a sudden doubling of the apparent heart rate as the cuff pressure declines signals *pulsus alternans* (see p. 402).

Placing the patient in the upright position may accentuate this finding.

Paradoxical Pulse. This is a greater than normal drop in systolic blood pressure during inspiration. If the pulse varies in amplitude with respiration or you suspect cardiac tamponade (because of jugular venous distention, dyspnea, tachycardia, muffled heart tones, and hypotension), use a blood pressure cuff to check for a *paradoxical pulse.* As the patient breathes quietly, lower the cuff pressure to the systolic level. Note the pressure level at which the first sounds can be heard. Then drop the pressure very slowly until sounds can be heard throughout the respiratory cycle. Again note the pressure level. The difference between these two levels is normally no greater than 3 or 4 mm Hg.

The pressure when Korotkoff sounds are first heard is the highest systolic pressure during the respiratory cycle. The pressure when sounds are heard throughout the cycle is the lowest systolic pressure. A difference between these levels of ≥ 10 mm Hg to 12 mm Hg constitutes a *paradoxical pulse,* found most commonly in acute *asthma* and *obstructive pulmonary disease* (see p. 402). It also occurs in *pericardial tamponade* and at times in *constrictive pericarditis* and *acute pulmonary embolism.*

Carotid Artery Thrills and Bruits. As you palpate the carotid artery, you may detect vibrations, or *thrills,* like the throat vibrations of a cat when it purrs. Proceed to auscultation.

Thrills in aortic stenosis are transmitted to the carotid arteries from the suprasternal notch or 2nd right intercostal space.

Auscultate both the carotid arteries to listen for a *bruit,* a murmur-like sound arising from turbulent arterial blood flow. Ask the patient to stop breathing for ~15 seconds, then listen with the diaphragm of the stethoscope, which generally detects the higher frequency sounds of arterial bruits better than the bell.[115] Note that higher-grade stenoses may have lower frequency or even absent sounds, more amenable to detection with the bell. Place the diaphragm near the upper end of the thyroid cartilage below the angle of the jaw, which overlies the bifurcation of the common carotid artery into the external and internal carotid arteries. A bruit in this location is less likely to be confused with a transmitted murmur from the heart or subclavian or vertebral artery bruits.

Although usually caused by atherosclerotic luminal stenosis, bruits are also caused by a tortuous carotid artery, external carotid arterial disease, aortic stenosis, the hypervascularity of hyperthyroidism, and external compression from thoracic outlet syndrome. Bruits do not correlate with clinically significant underlying disease.[116-118]

Listen for bruits in older patients and patients with suspected cerebrovascular disease.

Because auscultation has low sensitivity and specificity for detecting asymptomatic carotid disease (46% to 77% and 71% to 98%) and there are high rates of false positives with ultrasound, the USPSTF recommends against routine screening.[124] Consider further evaluation for high-risk groups.[125-128]

Carotid artery stenosis causes ~10% of ischemic strokes and doubles the risk of CHD.[119-121] The prevalence of asymptomatic carotid stenosis in the United States is ~1% for stenoses occluding 75% to 90% of the lumen, and increases significantly with age.[119,122,123] The 5-year risk of ipsilateral stroke from asymptomatic stenoses of over 70% is ~5%.

The Brachial Artery. In patients with carotid obstruction, kinking, or thrills, assess the pulse in the *brachial artery*, applying the techniques described previously for determining amplitude and contour.

The patient's arm should rest with the elbow extended, palm up. Cup your hand under the patient's elbow or support the forearm. You may need to flex the elbow to a varying degree to get optimal muscular relaxation. Use the index and middle fingers or thumb of your opposite hand for palpation. Feel for the pulse just medial to the biceps tendon (Fig. 9-30).

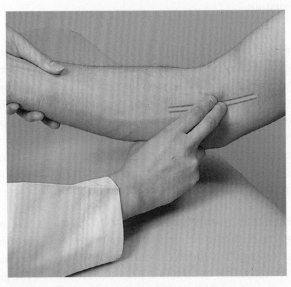

FIGURE 9-30. **Palpate the brachial pulse.**

THE HEART

Positioning the Patient. For the cardiac examination, stand at the patient's right side. The patient should be supine, with the upper body and head of the bed or examining table raised to about 30°. To assess the PMI and extra heart sounds such as S_3 or S_4, ask the patient to turn to the left side, termed the left lateral decubitus position—this brings the ventricular apex closer to the chest wall. To bring the left ventricular outflow tract closer to the chest wall and improve detection of aortic regurgitation, have the patient sit up, lean forward, and exhale. The box on next page summarizes patient positions and a suggested sequence for the examination.

Sequence of the Cardiac Examination

Patient Position	Examination	Accentuated Findings
Supine, with the head elevated 30°	After examining the JVP and carotid pulse, inspect and palpate the precordium: the 2nd right and left interspaces; the RV; and the LV, including the apical impulse (diameter, location, amplitude, duration).	
Left lateral decubitus	Palpate the apical impulse to assess its diameter. Listen at the apex with the *bell* of the stethoscope.	Low-pitched extra sounds such as an S_3, opening snap, diastolic rumble of *mitral stenosis*
Supine, with the head elevated 30°	Listen at the 2nd right and left interspaces, down the left sternal border to the 4th and 5th interspaces, and across to the apex the six listening areas with the *diaphragm*, then the *bell* (see p. 391). As indicated, listen at the lower right sternal border for right-sided murmurs and sounds, often accentuated with inspiration, with the *diaphragm* and *bell*.	
Sitting, leaning forward, after full exhalation	Listen down the left sternal border and at the apex with the *diaphragm*.	Soft decrescendo higher-pitched diastolic murmur of *aortic regurgitation*

Location and Timing of Cardiac Findings. Identify both the anatomical location of impulses, heart sounds, and murmurs and where they fall in the cardiac cycle. Remember to integrate your findings with the characteristics of the patient's JVP and carotid upstroke.

- Identify the *anatomical location* of cardiac findings in terms of interspaces and the distance of the PMI from the midclavicular (or midsternal) line. The midsternal line offers the most reproducible zero point for measurement, but some experts recommend the midclavicular line due to its better correlation with left ventricular pathology, as long as the midpoint between the acromio-clavicular and sternoclavicular joints is carefully identified.[129]

- Identify the *timing of impulses, sounds,* and *murmurs* in relation to the cardiac cycle. Timing of sounds is often possible through auscultation alone, but aided by inspection and palpation as well. In most patients with normal or slow heart rates, it is easy to identify the paired heart sounds of S_1 and S_2 that mark the onset of systole and diastole. The relatively long diastolic interval after S_2 separates one pair from the next (Fig. 9-31).

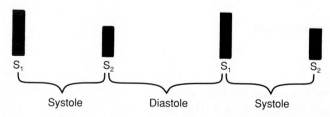

FIGURE 9-31. Diastole (S_2 to S_1) lasts longer than systole (S_1 to S_2).

The relative intensity of S_1 and S_2 is also helpful. S_1 is usually louder than S_2 at the apex; S_2 is usually louder than S_1 at the base.

"Inching" your stethoscope also helps clarify the timing of S_1 and S_2. Return to a place on the chest, typically the base, where it is easy to identify S_1 and S_2. Get their rhythm clearly in mind. Then inch your stethoscope down the left sternal border in steps until you hear changes in the sounds.

At times, the intensities of S_1 and S_2 may be abnormal, or at rapid heart rates the duration of diastole may shorten, making it difficult to distinguish systole from diastole. Palpation of the carotid artery during auscultation is an invaluable aid to the timing of sounds and murmurs. Since the carotid upstroke always occurs in systole immediately after S_1, sounds or murmurs coinciding with the upstroke are systolic; sounds or murmurs following the carotid upstroke are diastolic.

For example, S_1 is diminished in *first-degree heart block;* S_2 is diminished in *aortic stenosis.*

Inspection

Careful inspection of the anterior chest may reveal the location of the *apical impulse* or *PMI,* or less commonly, the ventricular movements of a left-sided S_3 or S_4. Shine a tangential light across the chest wall over the cardiac apex to make these movements more visible. Plan to further characterize these movements as you proceed to palpation. Keep in mind the anatomic locations diagrammed in Figure 9-32.

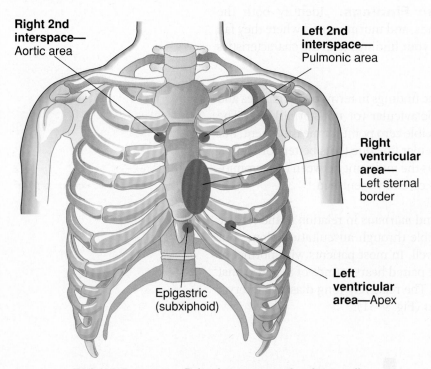

Right 2nd interspace— Aortic area

Left 2nd interspace— Pulmonic area

Right ventricular area— Left sternal border

Left ventricular area—Apex

Epigastric (subxiphoid)

FIGURE 9-32. **Palpation areas on the chest wall.**

Palpation

Begin with general palpation of the chest wall. In women, keeping the right chest draped, gently lift the breast with your left hand or ask the woman to do this to assist you.

Heaves, Lifts, Thrills; S_1 and S_2, S_3 and S_4.   Using the techniques below, palpate in the 2nd right interspace, the 2nd left interspace, along the sternal border, and at the apex for heaves, lifts, thrills, impulses from the RV, and the four heart sounds.

- To palpate *heaves and lifts,* use your palm and/or hold your fingerpads flat or obliquely against the chest. Heaves and lifts are sustained impulses that rhythmically lift your fingers, usually produced by an enlarged right or left ventricle or atrium and occasionally by ventricular aneurysms.

- For *thrills,* press the ball of your hand (the padded area of your palm near the wrist) firmly on the chest to check for a buzzing or vibratory sensation caused by underlying turbulent flow. If present, auscultate the same area for murmurs. Conversely, once a murmur is detected, it is easier to palpate a thrill in the position that accentuates the murmur, such as the leaning forward position after detecting aortic regurgitation.

  The presence of a thrill changes the grading of the murmur, as described in pp. 396.

- Palpate impulses from the *RV* in the right ventricular area, normally at the lower left sternal border and in the subxiphoid area (see p. 375).

  Palpation is less useful in patients with a thickened chest wall or increased AP diameter.

- To palpate S_1 *and* S_2, using firm pressure, place your right hand on the chest wall. With your left index and middle fingers, palpate the carotid upstroke to identify S_1 and S_2 just before and just after the upstroke. With practice, you will succeed in palpating S_1 and S_2. For S_3 *and* S_4, apply lighter pressure at the cardiac apex to detect the presence of any extra movements.

Left Ventricular Area

The Apical Impulse or Point of Maximal Impulse.   The apical impulse represents the brief early pulsation of the left ventricle as it moves anteriorly during contraction and contacts the chest wall. In most examinations the apical impulse is the PMI; however, pathologic conditions such as right ventricular hypertrophy, a dilated pulmonary artery, or an aortic aneurysm may produce a pulsation that is more prominent than the apex beat.

In *dextrocardia,* a rare congenital transposition of the heart, the heart is situated in the right chest cavity and generates a right-sided apical impulse. Use percussion to help locate the heart border, the liver, and stomach. In full *situs inversus,* the heart, trilobed lung, stomach, and spleen are on the right, and the liver and gallbladder are on the left.

If you cannot identify the apical impulse with the patient supine, ask the patient to roll partly onto the left side into the *left lateral decubitus* position. Palpate again, using the palmar surfaces of several fingers (Fig. 9-33). If you cannot find the apical impulse, ask the patient to exhale fully and stop breathing for a few seconds. When examining a woman, it may be helpful to displace the left breast upward or laterally as necessary, or ask her to do this for you.

The apex beat is palpable in 25% to 40% of adults in the supine position and in 50% to 73% of adults in the left lateral decubitus position, especially those who are thin.[129,130] Obesity, a very muscular chest wall, or an increased AP diameter of the chest may obscure detection.

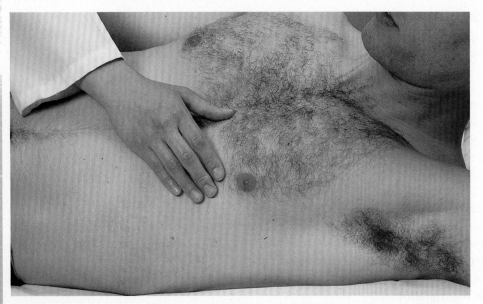

FIGURE 9-33. Palpate the apical impulse in the left lateral decubitus position.

Once you have found the apical impulse, make finer assessments with your fingertips, and then with one finger (Fig. 9-34). With experience, you will learn to palpate the apical impulse in most patients.

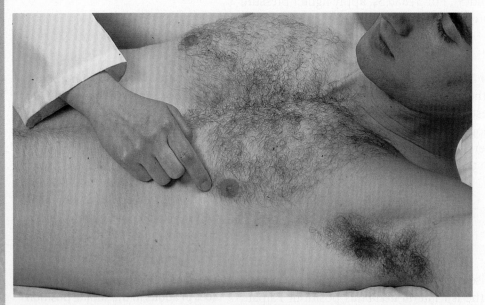

FIGURE 9-34. Palpate the apical impulse with one finger.

Now assess the location, diameter, amplitude, and duration of the apical impulse. You may wish to have the patient breathe out and briefly stop breathing to check your findings.

See Table 9-4, Variations and Abnormalities of the Ventricular Impulses, p. 403, for how to characterize the PMI as tapping, sustained, or diffuse.

- *Location.* Initially try to assess location with the patient *supine,* because the left lateral decubitus position displaces the apical impulse to the left. Locate two points: the interspaces, usually the 5th or possibly the 4th, which give the vertical location; and the distance in centimeters from the *midclavicular line* (or *midsternal line*), which gives the horizontal location (Fig. 9-35). For the midclavicular line, use a ruler to mark the midpoint between the sternoclavicular and acromioclavicular joints so that other clinicians can reproduce your findings.

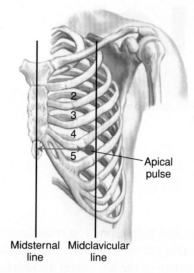

Midsternal line   **Midclavicular line**

FIGURE 9-35. **Locate the apical impulse (PMI).**

Pregnancy or a high left diaphragm may shift the apical impulse upward and to the left.

Lateral displacement toward the axillary line from ventricular dilatation is seen in *heart failure, cardiomyopathy,* and *ischemic heart disease;* and also in thoracic deformities and mediastinal shift.

Lateral displacement from the midclavicular line makes increased left ventricular volume and a low left ventricular EF 5 and 10 times more likely, respectively.[129]

- *Diameter.* Palpate the diameter of the apical impulse. In the supine patient, it usually measures less than 2.5 cm, about the size of a quarter, and occupies only one interspace. It may feel larger in the left lateral decubitus position.

In the left lateral decubitus position, a *diffuse* PMI with a diameter >3 cm signals left ventricular enlargement;[131] a diameter of >4 cm makes left ventricular overload almost 5 times more likely.[129]

- *Amplitude.* Estimate the amplitude of the impulse. Is the PMI brisk and tapping, diffuse, or sustained? These are three important descriptors in clinical practice. Normally, the amplitude of the PMI is small and feels *brisk* and *tapping* (Fig. 9-36). Some young adults have an increased amplitude, or *hyperkinetic* impulse, especially when excited or after exercise; the duration, however, is normal.

A *hyperkinetic* high-amplitude impulse may occur in *hyperthyroidism, severe anemia,* pressure overload of the left ventricle from *hypertension* or *aortic stenosis,* or volume overload of the left ventricle from *aortic regurgitation.*

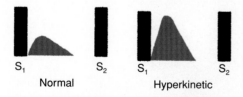

S_1 S_2 S_1 S_2
Normal   Hyperkinetic

FIGURE 9-36. **PMI amplitude— normal and hyperkinetic.**

- *Duration.* Duration is the most useful characteristic of the apical impulse for identifying hypertrophy of the left ventricle. To assess duration, auscultate the heart sounds as you palpate the apical impulse, or watch the movement of your stethoscope as you listen at the apex. Estimate the proportion of systole occupied by the apical impulse. Normally, it lasts through the first two thirds of systole, or often less, but does not continue to the second heart sound (Fig. 9-37).

A *sustained* high-amplitude impulse significantly increases the likelihood of LVH from the pressure overload seen in *hypertension.*[131] If such an impulse is displaced laterally, consider volume overload.

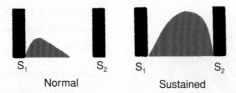

S_1 S_2
Normal

S_1 S_2
Sustained

FIGURE 9-37. PMI duration— normal and sustained.

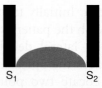

S_1 S_2
Hypokinetic

FIGURE 9-38. Sustained hypokinetic PMI of dilated cardiomyopathy.

A *diffuse* sustained low-amplitude (hypokinetic) impulse is seen in *heart failure* and *dilated cardiomyopathy.*

A brief early to middiastolic impulse represents a palpable S_3; an outward movement just before S_1 signifies a palpable S_4.

Palpable S_3 and S_4. By inspection and palpation, you may detect early and late diastolic ventricular movements that are synchronous with pathologic third and fourth heart sounds. With the patient in the left lateral decubitus position, palpate the apical beat gently with one finger as the patient exhales and briefly stops breathing. By marking an X on the apex, you may be able to palpate these brief diastolic outward movements.

Right Ventricular Area—The Left Sternal Border in the 3rd, 4th, and 5th Interspaces.

With the patient supine and the head elevated to 30°, ask the patient to exhale and briefly stop breathing, then place the tips of your curved fingers in the left 3rd, 4th, and 5th interspaces to palpate for the systolic impulse of the RV (Fig. 9-39). If there is a palpable impulse, assess its location, amplitude, and duration. In thin individuals, you may detect a brief systolic tap, especially when stroke volume is increased by conditions such as anxiety.

A sustained left parasternal movement beginning at S_1 points to pressure overload from *pulmonary hypertension* and *pulmonic stenosis* or the chronic ventricular volume overload of an *atrial septal defect*. A sustained movement later in systole can be seen in *mitral regurgitation*.

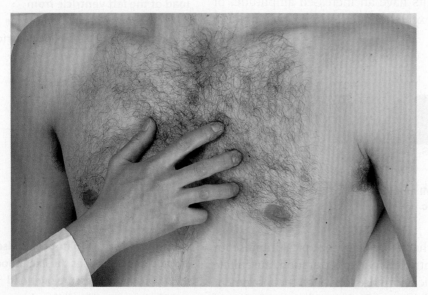

FIGURE 9-39. Palpate right ventricular systolic impulse.

Occasionally, the diastolic movements of *right-sided S_3 and S_4* are palpable in the left 4th and 5th interspaces. Time them by auscultation or palpation of the carotid upstroke.

In patients with an increased AP diameter, ask the patient to inhale and briefly stop breathing. Palpate for the RV in the *epigastric* or *subxiphoid area*. With your hand flattened, press your index finger just under the rib cage and up toward the left shoulder to assess any right ventricular pulsations (Fig. 9-40). The inspiratory position moves your hand well away from the pulsations of the abdominal aorta, which might otherwise confuse your findings.

In obstructive pulmonary disease, hyperinflation of the lungs may prevent palpation of the hypertrophied RV in the left parasternal area. The RV impulse is readily palpated high in the epigastrium where heart sounds are also more audible.

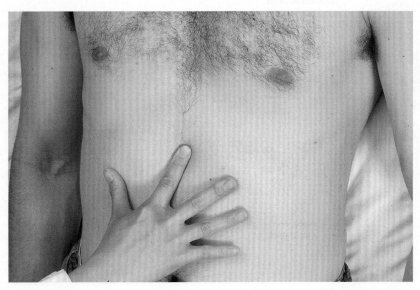

FIGURE 9-40. **Palpate in epigastric area if increased AP diameter.**

Pulmonic Area—The Left 2nd Interspace.
This interspace overlies the *pulmonary artery*. As the patient holds expiration, inspect and palpate for pulmonary artery pulsations and transmitted heart sounds, especially if patients are excited or examined after exercise.

A prominent pulsation here often accompanies dilatation or increased flow in the pulmonary artery. A palpable S₂ points to increased pulmonary artery pressure from *pulmonary hypertension*.

Aortic Area—The Right 2nd Interspace.
This interspace overlies the aortic outflow tract. Search for pulsations and palpable heart sounds.

A pulsation here suggests a dilated or aneurysmal aorta. A palpable S₂ can accompany systemic *hypertension*.

PERCUSSION

Palpation has replaced percussion when estimating cardiac size. If you cannot palpate the apical impulse, percussion may be your only option, but has limited correlation with the cardiac borders. Starting well to the left on the chest, percuss from resonance toward cardiac dullness in the 3rd, 4th, 5th, and, possibly, 6th interspaces.

A markedly dilated failing heart may have a hypokinetic apical impulse displaced far to the left. A large pericardial effusion may make the impulse undetectable.

AUSCULTATION

Auscultation of heart sounds and murmurs is a pre-eminent skill that leads directly to important clinical diagnoses. The ACC and the AHA has deemed cardiac auscultation as "the most widely used method of screening for valvular heart disease."[132] Review the six auscultatory areas in Figure 9-41, with the following caveats: (1) many authorities discourage designations such as "aortic area," because murmurs may be loudest in other areas, and (2) these areas do not apply to patients with cardiac dilatation or hypertrophy, anomalies of the great vessels, or dextrocardia.

Heart sounds and murmurs that originate in the four valves radiate widely, as illustrated in Figure 9-42. Use anatomical location rather than valve area to describe your findings.

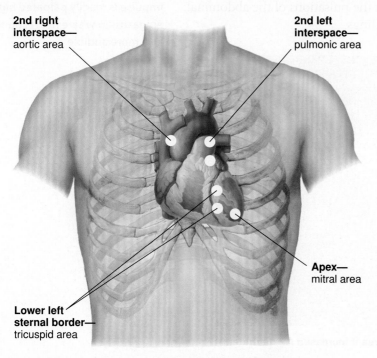

FIGURE 9-41. Auscultatory areas on the chest wall.

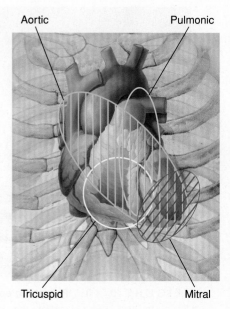

FIGURE 9-42. Radiation of heart sounds and murmurs.

Throughout your examination, take your time at each of the six auscultatory areas. Concentrate on each of the events in the cardiac cycle, listening carefully to S_1, then S_2, then other sounds and murmurs occurring in systole and diastole. Techniques for assessing these events are described in the pages that follow.

Know Your Stethoscope! It is important to understand the uses of both the diaphragm and the bell.

- *The diaphragm.* The diaphragm is better for picking up the relatively high-pitched sounds of S_1 and S_2, the murmurs of aortic and mitral regurgitation, and pericardial friction rubs. *Listen throughout the precordium* with the diaphragm, pressing it firmly against the chest.

- *The bell.* The bell is more sensitive to the low-pitched sounds of S_3 and S_4 and the murmur of mitral stenosis. Apply the bell lightly, with just enough pressure to produce an air seal with its full rim. *Use the bell at the apex, then move medially along the lower sternal border.* Resting the heel of your hand on the chest like a fulcrum may help you to maintain light pressure.

Firm pressure on the bell can stretch the underlying skin and make it function more like the diaphragm. Low-pitched sounds like S_3 and S_4 may then disappear—an observation that can help identify them. In contrast, high-pitched

Many types of stethoscopes are available. Learn about the various options before purchasing this expensive instrument. Some are "tunable," allowing you to vary the pressure on the diaphragm to alter its acoustic characteristics; others are electronic and can amplify and even digitally record auscultatory events.

sounds such as a midsystolic click, an ejection sound, or an OS will persist or get louder.

The Pattern of Auscultation. In a quiet room, auscultate the heart with your stethoscope with the patient's head and upper chest elevated to 30°. Start at either the base or apex, listening first with the diaphragm, then with the bell.

- Some experts recommend *starting at the apex and moving to the base:* Move the stethoscope from the PMI medially to the left sternal border, superiorly to the 2nd interspace, then across the sternum to the 2nd interspace at the right sternal border, stopping at "the 6 listening spots" marked by the white circles in Figure 9-41. To clarify findings, "inch" the stethoscope in smaller increments as needed (see p. 384).

- Alternatively, you can *start at the base and inch your stethoscope to the apex:* with your stethoscope in the right 2nd interspace close to the sternum, move along the left sternal border in each interspace from the 2nd through the 5th, and then toward the apex.

Two Important Maneuvers. For new patients and patients needing a complete cardiac examination, use two additional maneuvers to enhance detection of mitral stenosis and aortic regurgitation.

- *Mitral stenosis.* Ask the patient to *roll into the left lateral decubitus position,* which brings the left ventricle closer to the chest wall. Place the bell of your stethoscope lightly on the apical impulse (Fig. 9-43).

This position accentuates a left-sided S_3 and S_4 and mitral murmurs, especially *mitral stenosis*. Otherwise, you may miss these important findings.

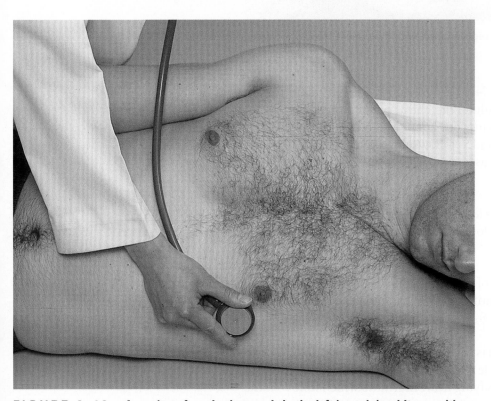

FIGURE 9-43. **Auscultate for mitral stenosis in the left lateral decubitus position.**

■ *Aortic regurgitation.* Ask the patient to *sit up, lean forward, exhale completely, and briefly stop breathing after expiration.* Pressing the diaphragm of your stethoscope on the chest, listen along the left sternal border and at the apex, pausing periodically so the patient may breathe (Fig. 9-44).

You may easily miss the soft diastolic decrescendo murmur of *aortic regurgitation* unless you listen at this position.

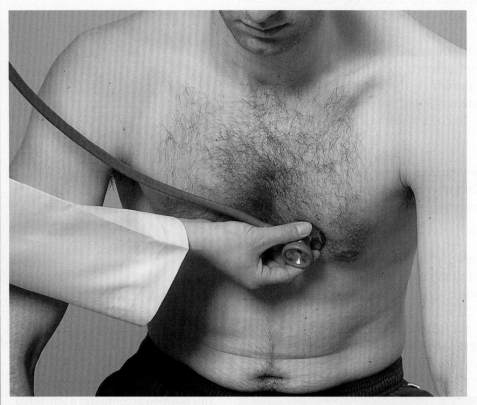

F I G U R E 9 - 4 4 .   **Auscultate for aortic regurgitation with the patient leaning forward.**

Identifying Systole and Diastole.   To facilitate the correct identification of systole and diastole, as you auscultate the chest, palpate the right carotid artery in the lower third of the neck with your left index and middle fingers—S_1 falls just before the carotid upstroke and S_2 follows the carotid upstroke. Be sure to compare the intensities of S_1 and S_2 as you move your stethoscope through the listening areas above.

■ At the base, you will note that S_2 is louder than S_1 and may split with respiration. At the apex, S_1 is usually louder than S_2 unless the PR interval is prolonged.

■ By carefully noting the intensities of S_1 and S_2, you will confirm each of these sounds and thereby correctly identify *systole,* the interval between S_1 and S_2, and *diastole,* the interval between S_2 and S_1.

The correct timing of systole and diastole is the fundamental prerequisite to identifying events in the cardiac cycle. Review the guides to auscultation on next page and learn the tips for identifying heart murmurs which follow in the next section.

Auscultatory Sounds

Heart Sounds	Guides to Auscultation	
S_1	Note its intensity and any apparent splitting. Normal splitting is detectable along the lower left sternal border.	See Table 9-5, Variations in the First Heart Sound—S_1, p. 404. Note that S_1 is louder at more rapid heart rates, and PR intervals are shorter.
S_2	Note its intensity.	
Split S_2	Listen for splitting of this sound in the 2nd and 3rd left interspaces. Ask the patient to breathe quietly, and then slightly more deeply than normal. Does S_2 split into its two components, as it normally does? If not, ask the patient to (1) breathe a little more deeply, or (2) sit up. Listen again. A thick chest wall may make the pulmonic component of S_2 inaudible.	See Table 9-6, Variations in the Second Heart Sound—S_2, p. 405. When either A_2 or P_2 is absent, as in aortic or pulmonic valve disease, S_2 is persistently single.
	Width of split. How wide is the split? It is normally quite narrow.	
	Timing of split. When in the respiratory cycle do you hear the split? It is normally heard late in inspiration.	Expiratory splitting suggests a valvular abnormality (p. 405).
	Does the split disappear as it should, during exhalation? If not, listen again with the patient sitting up.	Persistent splitting results from delayed closure of the pulmonic valve or early closure of the aortic valve.
	Intensity of A_2 and P_2. Compare the intensity of the two components, A_2 and P_2; A_2 is usually louder.	A loud P_2 points to *pulmonary hypertension*.
Extra Sounds in Systole	Such as ejection sounds or systolic clicks Note their location, timing, intensity, and pitch, and variations with respiration	The systolic click of mitral valve prolapse is the most common extra sound. See Table 9-7, Extra Heart Sounds in Systole, p. 406.
Extra Sounds in Diastole	Such as S_3, S_4, or an opening snap Note the location, timing, intensity, and pitch, and variations with respiration. An S_3 or S_4 in athletes is a normal finding.	See Table 9-8, Extra Heart Sounds in Diastole, p. 407.
Systolic and Diastolic Murmurs	Murmurs are differentiated from S_1, S_2, and extra sounds by their longer duration.	See Table 9-9, Midsystolic Murmurs, pp. 408–409; Table 9-10, Pansystolic (Holosystolic) Murmurs, p. 410; and Table 9-11, Diastolic Murmurs, p. 411.

Identifying Heart Murmurs. Correctly identifying heart murmurs is a diagnostic challenge. A systematic approach, thorough understanding of cardiac anatomy and physiology, and, above all, your dedication to the practice and mastery of techniques of examination will lead to your success. Whenever possible, compare your findings with those of an experienced clinician to improve your clinical acumen. Review the tips for identifying heart murmurs, then carefully study the subsequent sections on the timing, shape, location, radiation, intensity, pitch, and quality of heart murmurs for more details.[140] Study the tables at the end of the chapter to further expand your skills. Reinforce your learning by listening to heart sound recordings, which can increase accurate identification of heart murmurs (and generally transfers to actual patients).[15,17–19,21,22]

Tips for Identifying Heart Murmurs

- Time the murmur—is it in systole or diastole? What is its duration?
- Locate where on the precordium the murmur is loudest—at the base, along the sternal border, at the apex? Does it radiate?
- Conduct any necessary maneuvers, such as having the patient lean forward and exhale or turn to the left lateral decubitus position.
- Determine the shape of the murmur—for example, is it crescendo or decrescendo, is it holosystolic?
- Grade the intensity of the murmur from 1 to 6, and determine its pitch and quality.
- Identify associated features such as the quality of S_1 and S_2, the presence of extra sounds such as S_3, S_4, or an OS, or the presence of additional murmurs.
- Be sure you are listening in a quiet room!

Timing. First decide if you are hearing a *systolic murmur,* falling between S_1 and S_2, or a *diastolic murmur,* falling between S_2 and S_1. Palpating the carotid pulse as you listen can help you with timing. Murmurs that coincide with the carotid upstroke are systolic.

Diastolic murmurs usually represent valvular heart disease. Systolic murmurs point to valvular disease but can be physiologic flow murmurs arising from normal heart valves.

Murmurs detected during pregnancy should be promptly evaluated for possible risk to the mother and fetus, especially those of *aortic stenosis* or *pulmonary hypertension.*[154]

Systolic Murmurs

Systolic murmurs are typically *midsystolic* or *pansystolic*. Midsystolic murmurs can be *functional murmurs;* these are typically short midsystolic murmurs that decrease in intensity with maneuvers that reduce left ventricular volume, such as standing, sitting up, and straining during the Valsalva maneuver. These murmurs are often heard in healthy patients and are not pathologic. Early systolic murmurs are uncommon and are not depicted below.

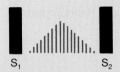

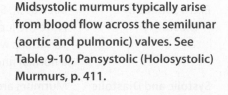

Midsystolic murmur: Begins after S_1 and stops before S_2. Brief gaps are audible between the murmur and the heart sounds. Listen carefully for the gap just before S_2, which is more readily detected and, if present, usually confirms the murmur as midsystolic, not pansystolic.

Midsystolic murmurs typically arise from blood flow across the semilunar (aortic and pulmonic) valves. See Table 9-10, Pansystolic (Holosystolic) Murmurs, p. 411.

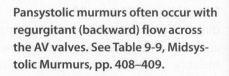

Pansystolic (holosystolic) murmur: Starts with S_1 and stops at S_2, without a gap between murmur and heart sounds.

Pansystolic murmurs often occur with regurgitant (backward) flow across the AV valves. See Table 9-9, Midsystolic Murmurs, pp. 408–409.

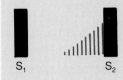

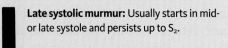

Late systolic murmur: Usually starts in mid- or late systole and persists up to S_2.

This is the murmur of mitral valve prolapse and is often, but not always, preceded by a systolic click (see p. 406); the murmur of mitral regurgitation may also be late systolic.

Diastolic Murmurs

Diastolic murmurs may be early diastolic, middiastolic, or late diastolic.

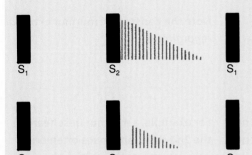

Early diastolic murmur: Starts immediately after S_2, without a discernible gap, then usually fades into silence before the next S_1.

Early diastolic murmurs typically reflect regurgitant flow across incompetent semilunar valves.

Middiastolic murmur: Starts a short time after S_2. It may fade away, as illustrated, or merge into a late diastolic murmur.

Middiastolic and presystolic murmurs reflect turbulent flow across the AV valves. See Table 9-11, Diastolic Murmurs, p. 411.

Late diastolic (presystolic) murmur: Starts late in diastole and typically continues up to S_1.

Continuous Murmurs

Some congenital and clinical conditions produce continuous murmurs.

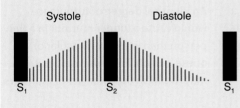

Continuous murmur: Begins in systole and extends into all or part of diastole (but is not necessarily uniform throughout).[140]

Congenital *patent ductus arteriosus* and *AV fistulas,* common in dialysis patients, produce continuous murmurs that are nonvalvular in origin. Venous hums and pericardial friction rubs also have both systolic and diastolic components. See Table 9-12, Cardiovascular Sounds with Both Systolic and Diastolic Components, p. 412.

Shape. The shape or configuration of a murmur is determined by its intensity over time.

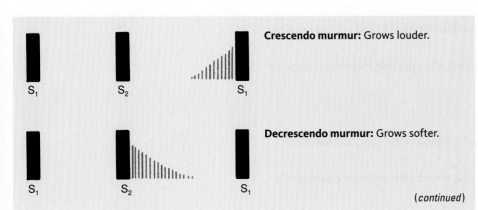

Crescendo murmur: Grows louder.

Note the presystolic murmur of *mitral stenosis* in normal sinus rhythm.

Decrescendo murmur: Grows softer.

Note the early diastolic murmur of *aortic regurgitation.*

(*continued*)

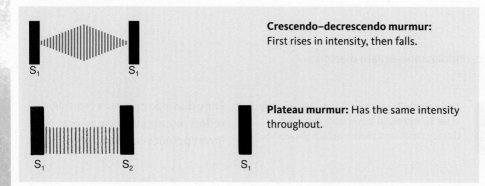

Crescendo–decrescendo murmur: First rises in intensity, then falls.

S_1 S_1

Plateau murmur: Has the same intensity throughout.

S_1 S_2 S_1

Listen for the midsystolic murmur of *aortic stenosis* and *innocent flow murmurs.*

Note the pansystolic murmur of *mitral regurgitation.*

Location of Maximal Intensity. This is determined by the site where the murmur originates. Find the location by exploring the area where you hear the murmur. Describe where you hear it best in terms of the intercostal space and its proximity to the sternum, the apex, or its measured distance from the midclavicular, midsternal, or one of the axillary lines.

For example, a murmur best heard in the 2nd right interspace often originates at or near the aortic valve.

Radiation or Transmission from the Point of Maximal Intensity. This reflects not only the site of origin but also the intensity of the murmur, the direction of blood flow, and bone conduction in the thorax. Explore the area around a murmur and determine where else you can hear it.

The murmur of *aortic stenosis* often radiates to the neck in the direction of arterial flow, especially on the right side. In *mitral regurgitation,* the murmur often radiates to the axilla, supporting transmission by bone conduction.[141,160]

Intensity. This is usually graded on a six-point scale and expressed as a fraction. The numerator describes the intensity of the murmur wherever it is loudest; the denominator indicates the scale you are using. Intensity is influenced by the thickness of the chest wall and the presence of intervening tissue.

An identical degree of turbulence would cause a louder murmur in a thin person than in a very muscular or obese person. Emphysematous lungs may diminish the intensity of murmurs.

Grade murmurs using the six-point scale below (the Levine grading system).[161,162] Note that grades 4 through 6 require the added presence of a palpable thrill.

For maneuvers, see Special Techniques, pp. 397–399.

Gradations of Murmurs

Grade	Description
Grade 1	Very faint, heard only after listener has "tuned in"; may not be heard in all positions
Grade 2	Quiet, but heard immediately after placing the stethoscope on the chest
Grade 3	Moderately loud
Grade 4	Loud, with *palpable thrill*
Grade 5	Very loud, with *thrill.* May be heard when the stethoscope is partly off the chest
Grade 6	Very loud, with *thrill.* May be heard with stethoscope entirely off the chest

Pitch. This is categorized as high, medium, or low.

Quality. This is described in terms such as blowing, harsh, rumbling, and musical.

Other useful characteristics of murmurs and heart sounds include variation with respiration, the position of the patient, and other special maneuvers.

Integrating Cardiovascular Assessment

Cardiovascular assessment requires more than careful examination. You need to correctly identify and interpret individual findings, fit them together in a logical pattern, and correlate your cardiac findings with the patient's blood pressure and heart rate, carotid upstroke and JVP, the arterial pulses, the remainder of your physical examination, and the patient's history. Evaluating systolic murmurs illustrates this point.

Integrated Assessment: Systolic Murmurs

An asymptomatic teenager might have a grade 2/6 midsystolic murmur in the 2nd and 3rd left interspaces. Because this suggests a pulmonic murmur you should assess the RV for hypertrophy by carefully palpating the left parasternal area. Because pulmonic stenosis and atrial septal defects can cause this murmur, auscultate carefully for a split S_2, any ejection sounds, and variation with inspiration. Listen to the murmur after the patient sits up. Look for evidence of anemia, hyperthyroidism, or pregnancy that could cause such a murmur by increasing the flow across the aortic or the pulmonic valve. If all your findings are normal, your patient probably has a *functional murmur*—one with no pathologic significance.

Integrating this information allows you to generate a differential diagnosis about the origin of the murmur and pursue further evaluation.

Special Techniques: Maneuvers to Identify Murmurs and Heart Failure

The maneuvers described below help distinguish mitral valve prolapse and hypertrophic cardiomyopathy from aortic stenosis.

Standing and Squatting. When a person is *standing up,* venous return to the heart decreases, as does peripheral vascular resistance. Arterial blood pressure, stroke volume, and the volume of blood in the left ventricle all decline. With *squatting,* vascular and volume changes occur in the opposite direction. These maneuvers help (1) to identify a prolapsed mitral valve and (2) to distinguish hypertrophic cardiomyopathy from aortic stenosis.

Secure the patient's gown so that it will not interfere with your examination, and prepare for prompt auscultation. Instruct the patient to squat next to the examining table and hold on to it for balance. Listen to the heart with the patient in the squatting position and again in the standing position.

A fully described murmur might be: a "medium-pitched, grade 2/6, blowing decrescendo diastolic murmur, best heard in the 4th left interspace, with radiation to the apex" (*aortic regurgitation*).

Right-sided heart murmurs generally increase with inspiration; left-sided murmurs generally increase with expiration.[132]

A 60-year-old woman with angina might have a harsh 3/6 midsystolic crescendo–decrescendo murmur in the right 2nd interspace radiating to the neck. These findings are consistent with *aortic stenosis* but could arise from *aortic sclerosis* (leaflets are sclerotic but not stenotic), a dilated aorta, or increased flow across a normal valve. Assess any delay in the carotid upstroke and the intensity of A_2 for evidence of *aortic stenosis*. Check the apical impulse for LVH. Listen for *aortic regurgitation* as the patient leans forward and exhales.

Maneuvers to Identify Systolic Murmurs

Maneuver	Cardiovascular Effect	Effect on Systolic Sounds and Murmurs		
		Mitral Valve Prolapse	Hypertrophic Cardiomyopathy	Aortic Stenosis
Squatting; Valsalva: Release Phase	**Increased left ventricular volume** from ↑ venous return to heart	↓ prolapse of mitral valve	↓ outflow obstruction	↑ blood volume ejected into aorta
	Increased vascular tone: ↑ arterial blood pressure; ↑ peripheral vascular resistance	*Delay of click* and *murmur shortens*	↓ **intensity of murmur**	↑ **intensity of murmur**
Standing; Valsalva: Strain Phase	**Decreased left ventricular volume** from ↓ venous return to heart	↑ prolapse of mitral valve	↑ outflow obstruction	↓ blood volume ejected into aorta
	Decreased vascular tone: ↓ arterial blood pressure	*Click moves earlier in systole* and *murmur lengthens*	↑ **intensity of murmur**	↓ **intensity of murmur**

Valsalva Maneuver. The Valsalva maneuver involves forcible exhalation against a closed glottis after full inspiration, causing increased intrathoracic pressure. The normal systolic blood pressure response follows four phases: (1) transient increase during onset of the "strain" phase when the patient bears down, due to increased intrathoracic pressure; (2) sharp decrease to below baseline as the "strain" phase is maintained, due to decreased venous return; (3) further acute drop of both blood pressure and left ventricular volume during the "release" phase, due to decreased intrathoracic pressure; and (4) "overshoot" increased blood pressure, due to reflex sympathetic activation and increased stroke volume.[142,163] This maneuver has several uses at the bedside.

To distinguish the murmur of *hypertrophic cardiomyopathy*, ask the supine patient to "bear down, like straining during a bowel movement." Alternatively, place one hand on the patient's midabdomen and ask the patient to strain against it. With your other hand, place your stethoscope on the patient's chest and listen at the lower left sternal border.

The murmur of *hypertrophic cardiomyopathy* is the only systolic murmur that increases during the "strain phase" of the Valsalva maneuver due to increased outflow tract obstruction.[143]

The Valsalva maneuver can also identify *heart failure* and *pulmonary hypertension*. Inflate the blood pressure cuff to 15 mm Hg greater than the systolic blood pressure and ask the patient to perform the Valsalva maneuver for 10 seconds, then resume normal respiration. Keep the cuff pressure locked at 15 mm Hg above the baseline systolic pressure during the entire maneuver and for 30 seconds afterward. Listen for Korotkoff sounds over the brachial artery throughout. Typically, only phases 2 and 4 are significant, since phases 1 and 3 are too short for clinical detection. *In healthy patients, phase 2, the "strain" phase, is silent; Korotkoff sounds are heard after straining is released during phase 4.*

In patients with *severe heart failure,* blood pressure remains elevated and there are Korotkoff sounds during the phase 2 strain phase, but not during phase 4 release, termed *"the square wave" response.* This response is highly correlated with volume overload and elevated left ventricular end-diastolic pressure and pulmonary capillary wedge pressure, in some studies outperforming brain natriuretic peptide.[142,163]

Isometric Handgrip.   Isometric handgrip increases the systolic murmurs of mitral regurgitation, pulmonic stenosis, and ventricular septal defect, and also the diastolic murmurs of aortic regurgitation and mitral stenosis.[132]

Transient Arterial Occlusion.   Transient compression of both arms by bilateral blood pressure cuff inflation to 20 mm Hg greater than peak systolic blood pressure augments the murmurs of mitral regurgitation, aortic regurgitation, and ventricular septal defect.[132]

Recording Your Findings

Note that initially you may use sentences to describe your findings; later you will use phrases. The style below contains phrases appropriate for most write-ups.

Recording the Cardiovascular Examination

"The JVP is 3 cm above the sternal angle with the head of bed elevated to 30°. Carotid upstrokes are brisk, without bruits. The PMI is tapping, 1 cm lateral to the midclavicular line in the 5th intercostal space. Crisp S_1 and S_2. At the base, S_2 is louder than S_1 with physiologic split of $A_2 > P_2$. At the apex, S_1 is louder than S_2. There are no murmurs or extra sounds."
OR
"The JVP is 5 cm above the sternal angle with the head of bed elevated to 50°. Carotid upstrokes are brisk; a bruit is heard over the left carotid artery. The PMI is diffuse, 3 cm in diameter, palpated at the anterior axillary line in the 5th and 6th intercostal spaces. S_1 and S_2 are soft. S_3 is present at the apex. High-pitched harsh 2/6 holosystolic murmur best heard at the apex, radiating to the axilla."

These findings suggest *heart failure with volume overload* with possible *left carotid occlusion* and *mitral regurgitation*.[104,106,114,164,165]

Table 9-1 Selected Heart Rates and Rhythms

Cardiac rhythms may be classified as *regular or irregular.* When rhythms are irregular or rates are either fast or slow, obtain an ECG to identify the origin of the beats (sinus node, AV node, atrium, or ventricle) and the conduction pattern. The normal range for normal sinus rhythm is reported at 50 to 90 beats/minute.[42] Note that AV nodal rhythms, including AV block, may have a fast, normal, or slow ventricular rate.

	ECG Pattern	Usual Resting Rate

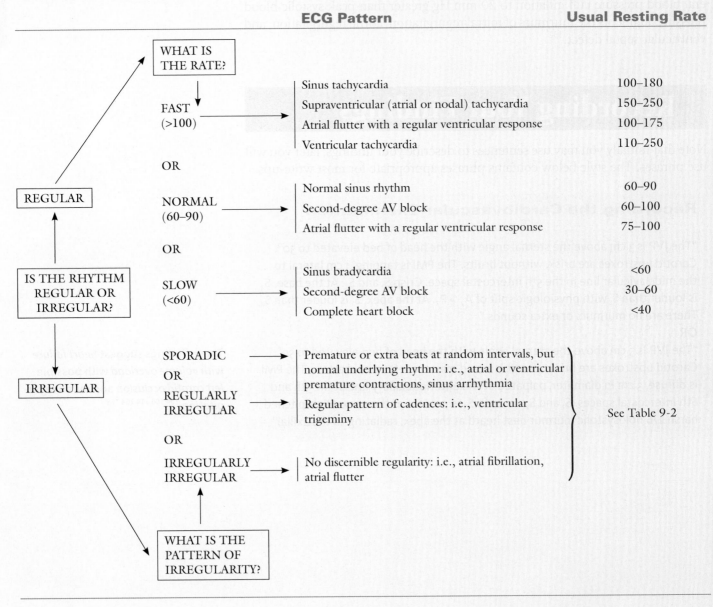

Sinus tachycardia		100–180
Supraventricular (atrial or nodal) tachycardia		150–250
Atrial flutter with a regular ventricular response		100–175
Ventricular tachycardia		110–250
Normal sinus rhythm		60–90
Second-degree AV block		60–100
Atrial flutter with a regular ventricular response		75–100
Sinus bradycardia		<60
Second-degree AV block		30–60
Complete heart block		<40
Premature or extra beats at random intervals, but normal underlying rhythm: i.e., atrial or ventricular premature contractions, sinus arrhythmia		
Regular pattern of cadences: i.e., ventricular trigeminy		See Table 9-2
No discernible regularity: i.e., atrial fibrillation, atrial flutter		

Table 9-2 Selected Irregular Rhythms

Type of Rhythm	ECG Waves and Heart Sounds	

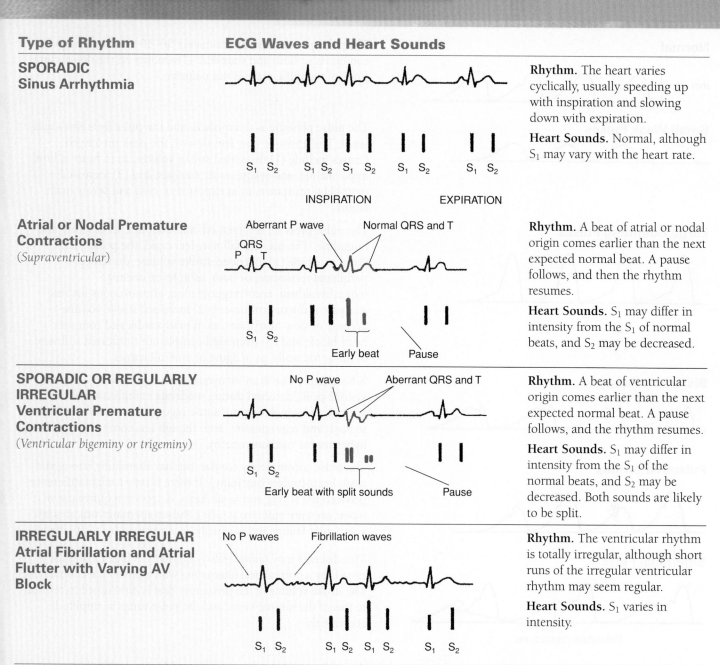

SPORADIC
Sinus Arrhythmia

Rhythm. The heart varies cyclically, usually speeding up with inspiration and slowing down with expiration.

Heart Sounds. Normal, although S_1 may vary with the heart rate.

Atrial or Nodal Premature Contractions
(Supraventricular)

Rhythm. A beat of atrial or nodal origin comes earlier than the next expected normal beat. A pause follows, and then the rhythm resumes.

Heart Sounds. S_1 may differ in intensity from the S_1 of normal beats, and S_2 may be decreased.

SPORADIC OR REGULARLY IRREGULAR
Ventricular Premature Contractions
(Ventricular bigeminy or trigeminy)

Rhythm. A beat of ventricular origin comes earlier than the next expected normal beat. A pause follows, and the rhythm resumes.

Heart Sounds. S_1 may differ in intensity from the S_1 of the normal beats, and S_2 may be decreased. Both sounds are likely to be split.

IRREGULARLY IRREGULAR
Atrial Fibrillation and Atrial Flutter with Varying AV Block

Rhythm. The ventricular rhythm is totally irregular, although short runs of the irregular ventricular rhythm may seem regular.

Heart Sounds. S_1 varies in intensity.

Table 9-3 Abnormalities of the Arterial Pulse and Pressure Waves

Normal

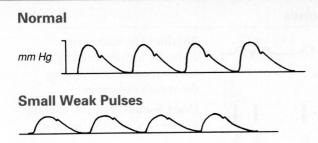

The pulse pressure is approximately 30–40 mm Hg. The pulse contour is smooth and rounded. (The notch on the descending slope of the pulse wave is not palpable.)

Small Weak Pulses

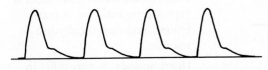

The pulse pressure is diminished, and the pulse feels weak and small. The upstroke may feel slowed, the peak prolonged. Causes include (1) decreased stroke volume, as in heart failure, hypovolemia, and severe aortic stenosis; and (2) increased peripheral resistance, as in exposure to cold and severe heart failure.

Large Bounding Pulses

The pulse pressure is increased, and the pulse feels strong and bounding. The rise and fall may feel rapid, the peak brief. Causes include (1) increased stroke volume, decreased peripheral resistance, or both, as in fever, anemia, hyperthyroidism, aortic regurgitation, arteriovenous fistulas, and patent ductus arteriosus; (2) increased stroke volume because of slow heart rates, as in bradycardia and complete heart block; and (3) decreased compliance (increased stiffness) of the aortic walls, as in aging or atherosclerosis.

Bisferiens Pulse

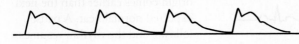

A bisferiens pulse is an increased arterial pulse with a double systolic peak, detected during moderate compression of the artery. Causes include pure aortic regurgitation, combined aortic stenosis and regurgitation, and, though less commonly palpable, hypertrophic cardiomyopathy.

Pulsus Alternans

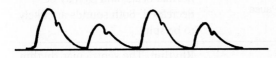

The pulse is completely regular, but has alternating strong and weak beats (unlike bigeminy). If there is only a slight difference between the strong and weak beats, detection requires use of a blood pressure cuff (see p. 381). Pulsus alternans indicates left ventricular failure and is usually accompanied by a left-sided S_3.

Bigeminal Pulse

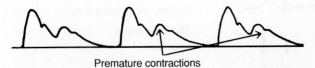

Premature contractions

This disorder may mimic pulsus alternans. A bigeminal pulse is caused by a normal beat alternating with a premature contraction. The stroke volume of the premature beat is diminished in relation to that of the normal beats, and the pulse varies in amplitude accordingly.

Paradoxical Pulse

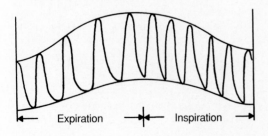

Expiration Inspiration

A paradoxical pulse may be detected by a palpable decrease in the pulse amplitude on quiet inspiration. If the sign is less pronounced, a blood pressure cuff is needed. Systolic pressure decreases by >10–12 mm Hg during inspiration. A paradoxical pulse occurs in pericardial tamponade, exacerbations of asthma and COPD, and constrictive pericarditis.

Table 9-4 Variations and Abnormalities of the Ventricular Impulses

In the healthy heart, the *left ventricular impulse* is usually the *PMI*. This brief impulse is generated by the movement of the ventricular apex against the chest wall during contraction. The *right ventricular impulse* is normally not palpable beyond infancy, and its characteristics are indeterminate. Learn the classical descriptors of the normal left ventricular PMI:

- *Location:* in the 4th or 5th interspace, at the midclavicular line
- *Diameter: discrete,* or ≤2 cm
- *Amplitude: brisk* and *tapping*
- *Duration:* ≤2/3 of systole

Careful examination of the ventricular impulse gives you important clues about underlying cardiovascular hemodynamics. The characteristics of the ventricular impulse change as the left and right ventricles adapt to high-output states (anxiety, hyperthyroidism, and severe anemia) and to the more pathologic conditions of chronic pressure or volume overload. In addition to the normal *brisk tapping* PMI, learn to recognize three additional types of ventricular impulses and their distinguishing features in the table below:

- *Hyperkinetic:* The *hyperkinetic ventricular impulse* from transiently increased stroke volume—this change does not necessarily indicate heart disease.
- *Sustained:* The *sustained* ventricular impulse of ventricular hypertrophy from chronic pressure load, known as *increased afterload* (see p. 387).
- *Diffuse:* The *diffuse* ventricular impulse of ventricular dilation from chronic volume overload, or *increased preload.*

| | Left Ventricular Impulse | | | Right Ventricular Impulse | | |
	Hyperkinetic	Pressure Overload	Volume Overload	Hyperkinetic	Pressure Overload	Volume Overload
Examples of Causes	Anxiety, hyperthyroidism, severe anemia	Aortic stenosis, hypertension	Aortic or mitral regurgitation; cardiomyopathy	Anxiety, hyperthyroidism, severe anemia	Pulmonic stenosis, pulmonary hypertension	Atrial septal defect
Location	Normal	Normal	Displaced to the left and possibly downward	3rd, 4th, or 5th left interspaces	3rd, 4th, or 5th left interspaces, also subxiphoid area	Left sternal border, extending toward the left cardiac border, also subxiphoid area
Diameter	~2 cm, though increased amplitude may make diameter feel larger	>2 cm	>2 cm	Not useful	Not useful	Not useful
Amplitude	More forceful tapping	More forceful tapping	*Diffuse*	Slightly more forceful	More forceful	Slightly to markedly more forceful
Duration	<2/3 systole	*Sustained* (up to S$_2$)	Often slightly sustained	Normal	*Sustained*	Normal to slightly sustained

Table 9-5 Variations in the First Heart Sound—S₁

Normal Variations

S_1 is softer than S_2 at the *base* (right and left 2nd interspaces).

S_1 is often but not always louder than S_2 at the *apex*.

Accentuated S₁

S_1 is accentuated in (1) tachycardia, rhythms with a short PR interval, and high cardiac output states (e.g., exercise, anemia, hyperthyroidism) and (2) mitral stenosis. In these conditions, the mitral valve is still open wide at the onset of ventricular systole and then closes quickly.

Diminished S₁

S_1 is diminished in first-degree heart block, left bundle branch block, and myocardial infarction due to weak ventricular contraction. Early mitral valve closure occurring before ventricular contraction also causes a soft S_1, seen in acute aortic regurgitation.

Varying S₁

S_1 varies in intensity (1) in complete heart block, when atria and ventricles are beating independently of each other and (2) in any totally irregular rhythm (e.g., atrial fibrillation). In these situations, the mitral valve is in varying positions before being shut by ventricular contraction. Its closure sound, therefore, varies in loudness.

Split S₁

Delayed closure of the tricuspid valve increases splitting of S_1, best heard along the lower left sternal border where the tricuspid component, often too faint to be heard, becomes audible. A prominent split S_1 occurs when right ventricular contraction is delayed, as in right bundle branch block and left premature contractions. This split may sometimes be heard at the apex, but must be distinguished from an S_4, an aortic ejection sound, and an early systolic click.

Table 9-6 Variations in the Second Heart Sound—S$_2$

	Inspiration	Expiration	

Physiologic Splitting

Listen for *physiologic splitting* of S$_2$ in the *2nd or 3rd left interspace*. The pulmonic component of S$_2$ is usually too faint to be heard at the apex or aortic area, where S$_2$ is a single sound derived only from aortic valve closure. Normal splitting is *accentuated by inspiration,* which increases the interval between A$_2$ and P$_2$, and *disappears on expiration.* In some patients, especially younger ones, S$_2$ may not become single on expiration until the patient sits up.

Pathologic Splitting
(*Audible splitting occurs during expiration and suggests heart disease.*)

Wide physiologic splitting of S$_2$ refers to an increase in the usual splitting of S$_2$ during inspiration that persists throughout the respiratory cycle. Wide splitting is caused by delayed closure of the pulmonic valve (as in pulmonic stenosis or right bundle branch block) or early closure of the aortic valve (mitral regurgitation). Right bundle branch block is illustrated here.

Fixed splitting refers to wide splitting that does not vary with respiration, often due to prolonged right ventricular systole, seen in atrial septal defect (when the pulse is regular) and in right ventricular failure.

Paradoxical or reversed splitting refers to splitting that appears on expiration and disappears on inspiration. Closure of the aortic valve is abnormally delayed so that A$_2$ follows P$_2$ in expiration. Normal inspiratory delay of P$_2$ makes the split disappear. The most common cause is left bundle branch block.

A$_2$ and P$_2$: 2nd Right Interspace

A$_2$ with Increased Intensity (A$_2$ can usually be heard only in right 2nd interspace): occurs in systemic hypertension because of the increased pressure load. Increased intensity also occurs when the aortic root is dilated, attributed to the increased proximity of the aortic valve to the chest wall.

P$_2$ with Increased Intensity: When P$_2$ is equal to or louder than A$_2$, suspect pulmonary hypertension. Other causes include a dilated pulmonary artery and an atrial septal defect. When a split S$_2$ is heard widely, extending to the apex and the right base, P$_2$ is accentuated.

A$_2$ Decreased or Absent: occurs in calcific aortic stenosis due to valve immobility. If A$_2$ is inaudible, no splitting is heard.

P$_2$ Decreased or Absent: This usually occurs from the increased AP diameter of the chest associated with aging. It can also result from pulmonic stenosis. If P$_2$ is inaudible, no splitting is heard.

Table 9-7 Extra Heart Sounds in Systole

There are two kinds of extra heart sounds in systole: (1) early ejection sounds and (2) clicks, commonly heard in mid- and late systole.

Early Systolic Ejection Sounds

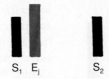

Early systolic ejection sounds occur shortly after S_1, coincident with sudden pathologic halting of the aortic and pulmonic valves as they open in early systole.[133] They are relatively high in pitch, have a sharp clicking quality, and are best heard with the diaphragm. An ejection sound indicates CVD.

Listen for an *aortic ejection sound* at both the base and apex. It may be louder at the apex and usually does not vary with respiration. An aortic ejection sound may accompany a dilated aorta, or aortic valve disease from congenital stenosis or a bicuspid aortic valve.[134,135]

A *pulmonic ejection sound* is heard best in the 2nd and 3rd left interspaces. When S_1, usually relatively soft in this area, appears to be loud, consider a possible pulmonic ejection sound. Its intensity often *decreases with inspiration*. Causes include dilatation of the pulmonary artery, pulmonary hypertension, and pulmonic stenosis.

Systolic Clicks

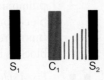

Systolic clicks are usually caused by *mitral valve prolapse*—an abnormal systolic ballooning of part of the mitral valve into the left atrium related to leaflet redundancy and elongation of the chordae tendineae. The clicks are usually mid- or late systolic. Prolapse of the mitral valve is a common cardiac condition, affecting about 2% to 3% of the general population, with equal prevalence in men and women.[136–138] Systolic clicks may also be of extracardiac or mediastinal origin.

Squatting

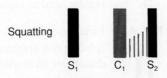

The click is usually single, but there may be more than one, usually at or medial to the apex, but also at the lower left sternal border. The click is high-pitched, so best heard with the diaphragm. It is often followed by a late systolic murmur from mitral regurgitation that crescendos up to S_2. Auscultatory findings are notably variable. Most patients have only a click, some have only a murmur, and some have both.

Standing

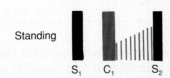

In *mitral valve prolapse*, findings vary from one examination to the next and often change with body position. Several positions are recommended to identify the syndrome: supine, seated, squatting, and standing. *Squatting (and the Valsalva release phase) delays the click and murmur due to increased venous return; standing (and the Valsalva strain phase) moves them closer to S_1 (see p. 398).*

Table 9-8 Extra Heart Sounds in Diastole

Opening Snap

S_1 S_2 OS S_1

The opening snap (*OS*) is a very early diastolic sound caused by abrupt deceleration during the opening of a *stenotic mitral valve*. It is best heard just medial to the apex and along the lower left sternal border. If loud, an OS radiates to the apex and to the pulmonic area, where it may be mistaken for the pulmonic component of a split S_2. Its high pitch and snapping quality help to distinguish it from an S_2, but it becomes less audible as the valve leaflets become more calcified. It is heard better with the *diaphragm*.

S_3

S_1 S_2 S_3 S_1

You will detect *physiologic* S_3 frequently in children and young adults to the age of 35 or 40 years, and often during the last trimester of pregnancy. Occurring early in diastole during rapid ventricular filling, it is later than an OS, dull and low in pitch, and heard best at the apex in the left lateral decubitus position. The *bell* of the stethoscope should be used with very light pressure.

A *pathologic* S_3 or *ventricular gallop* sounds like a physiologic S_3. An S_3 in adults over age 40 years is usually pathologic, arising from high left ventricular filling pressures and abrupt deceleration of inflow across the mitral valve at the end of the rapid filling phase of diastole.[25,27] Causes include decreased myocardial contractility, heart failure, and ventricular volume overload from aortic or mitral regurgitation, and left-to-right shunts. Listen for a *left-sided* S_3 at the apex in the left lateral decubitus position. A *right-sided* S_3 is usually heard along the lower left sternal border or below the xiphoid with the patient supine, and is louder on inspiration. The term *gallop* comes from the cadence of three heart sounds, especially at rapid heart rates, which sounds like "Kentucky."

S_4

S_1 S_2 S_4 S_1

An S_4 (*atrial sound* or *atrial gallop*) occurs just before S_1. It is dull, low in pitch, and best heard at the apex with the bell. Listen at the lower left sternal border for a right ventricular S_4 (or in the subxiphoid area if obstructive lung disease). An S_4 is occasionally normal, especially in trained athletes and older age groups. More commonly, it is due to ventricular hypertrophy or fibrosis causing stiffness and increased resistance (or decreased compliance) during ventricular filling following atrial contraction.[26,139]

Causes of a left-sided S_4 include hypertensive heart disease, aortic stenosis, and ischemic and hypertrophic cardiomyopathy. A *left-sided* S_4 is heard best at the apex in the left lateral decubitus position, with a cadence like "Tennessee." The less common *right-sided* S_4 is heard along the lower left sternal border or below the xiphoid. It often gets louder with inspiration. Causes include pulmonary hypertension and pulmonic stenosis.

An S_4 is also associated with delayed conduction between the atria and ventricles. This delay separates the normally faint atrial sound from the louder S_1 and makes it audible. An S_4 is never heard when there no atrial contraction (absent during atrial fibrillation).

Occasionally, a patient has both an S_3 and an S_4, producing a *quadruple rhythm* of four heart sounds. At rapid heart rates, the S_3 and S_4 may merge into one loud extra heart sound, called a *summation gallop*.

Table 9-9 Midsystolic Murmurs

Midsystolic ejection murmurs are the most common kind of heart murmur. They may be (1) *innocent*—without any detectable physiologic or structural abnormality; (2) *physiologic*—from physiologic changes in body metabolism; or (3) *pathologic*—arising from structural abnormalities in the heart or great vessels.[140–143] Midsystolic murmurs tend to peak near midsystole and usually stop before S_2. The crescendo–decrescendo or "diamond" shape is not always audible, but the gap between the murmur and S_2 helps to distinguish midsystolic from pansystolic murmurs.

	Innocent Murmurs	Physiologic Murmurs
	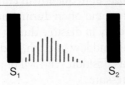	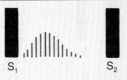
Murmur	*Location.* Left 2nd to 4th interspaces between the left sternal border and the apex	Similar to innocent murmurs
	Radiation. Minimal	
	Intensity. Grade 1 to 2, possibly 3	
	Pitch. Soft to medium	
	Quality. Variable	
	Maneuvers. Usually decreases or disappears on sitting	
Associated Findings	None: normal splitting, no ejection sounds, no diastolic murmurs, and no palpable evidence of ventricular enlargement. Occasionally, both an innocent murmur and pathologic murmur are present.	Signs of physiologic causes (see mechanisms below)
Mechanism	Turbulent blood flow, probably generated by ventricular ejection of blood into the aorta from the left and occasionally the right ventricle. Very common in children and young adults, but may also be present in older adults. There is no underlying CVD.	Turbulence due to a temporary increase in blood flow in predisposing conditions such as anemia, pregnancy, fever, and hyperthyroidism.

Pathologic Murmurs

Aortic Stenosis[135,144,145]	Hypertrophic Cardiomyopathy[146]	Pulmonic Stenosis[147]
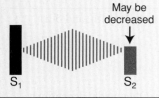	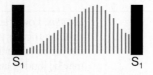	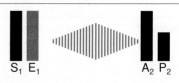
Location. Right 2nd and 3rd interspaces	*Location.* Left 3rd and 4th interspaces	*Location.* Left 2nd and 3rd interspaces
Radiation. Often to the carotids, down the left sternal border, even to the apex. If severe, may radiate to left 2nd and 3rd interspaces	*Radiation.* Down the left sternal border to the apex, possibly to the base, but not to the neck	*Radiation.* If loud, toward the left shoulder and neck
Intensity. Sometimes soft, but often loud, with a thrill (Grade 4/6 and above)	*Intensity.* Variable. See Maneuvers.	*Intensity.* Soft to loud; if loud, associated with a thrill
Pitch. Medium, harsh; crescendo–decrescendo may be higher at the apex	*Pitch.* Medium	*Pitch.* Medium; crescendo–decrescendo
Quality. Often harsh; may be more musical at the apex	*Quality.* Harsh	*Quality.* Often harsh
Maneuvers. Heard best with the patient sitting and leaning forward	*Maneuvers.* Intensity decreases with squatting and Valsalva release phase (increases venous return), increases with standing and Valsalva strain phase (decreases left ventricular volume) (see p. 398)	
As aortic stenosis worsens, the murmur peaks later in systole, and A_2 decreases in intensity. A_2 may be delayed and merged with $P_2 \rightarrow$ single S_2 on expiration or a paradoxical S_2 split. Carotid upstroke may be *delayed,* with a slow rise, small amplitude, and decreased volume. The hypertrophied left ventricle may produce a *sustained* apical impulse and an S_4 due to decreased compliance. After age 40 years there may be a dilated aorta and murmur of aortic regurgitation. Subendocardial ischemia due to poor coronary perfusion distal to the valve causes angina and syncope.	The carotid upstroke rises *quickly,* unlike aortic stenosis. The apical impulse is *sustained.* S_2 may be single. An S_4 is usually present at the apex (unlike mitral regurgitation). Usually benign, but progresses in 25% to syncope, ischemia, atrial fibrillation, dilated cardiomyopathy and heart failure, and stroke, with increased risk of sudden death.	The JVP is usually normal, but may have prominent *a* wave. The right ventricular impulse is often *sustained.* An early pulmonic ejection sound is present in mild to moderate stenosis. In severe stenosis, S_2 is widely split and P_2 softens. May hear a right-sided S_4 over the left sternal border.
Significant stenosis causes turbulent blood flow across the valve, and increases left ventricular afterload. The most common cause is valve calcification in older adults, at times progressing from nonobstructing *sclerosis* (present in 25%) to stenosis. The second most common cause is a congenital *bicuspid aortic valve,* often not recognized until adulthood.	Unexplained diffuse or focal ventricular hypertrophy with myocyte disarray and fibrosis associated with unusually rapid ejection of blood from the left ventricle during systole. Outflow tract obstruction of flow may coexist. Associated distortion of the mitral valve may cause mitral regurgitation.	Primarily a congenital disorder with valvular, supravalvular, or subvalvular stenosis. Stenosis impairs flow across the valve, increasing right ventricular afterload. In an *atrial septal defect,* increased flow across the pulmonic valve may mimic pulmonic stenosis.

Table 9-10 Pansystolic (Holosystolic) Murmurs

Pansystolic (holosystolic) murmurs are pathologic, arising from blood flow from a chamber with high pressure to one of lower pressure, through a valve or other structure that should be closed. The murmur begins immediately with S_1 and continues up to S_2.

	Mitral Regurgitation[137,148–150]	Tricuspid Regurgitation[151–153]	Ventricular Septal Defect
Murmur	*Location.* Apex	*Location.* Lower left sternal border. If right ventricular pressure is high and the ventricle is enlarged, the murmur may be loudest at the apex and confused with mitral regurgitation.	*Location.* Left 3rd, 4th, and 5th interspaces
	Radiation. To the left axilla, less often to the left sternal border	*Radiation.* To the right of the sternum, to the xiphoid area, and at times to the left midclavicular line, but not into the axilla.	*Radiation.* Often wide, depending on the size of the defect.
	Intensity. Soft to loud; if loud, associated with an apical thrill	*Intensity.* Variable	*Intensity.* Often very loud, with a thrill. Smaller defects have louder murmurs.
	Pitch. Medium to high	*Pitch.* Medium	*Pitch.* High, holosystolic. Smaller defects have murmurs with a higher pitch.
	Quality. Harsh, holosystolic	*Quality.* Blowing, holosystolic	*Quality.* Often harsh
	Maneuvers. Unlike tricuspid regurgitation, the intensity of the murmur does not change with inspiration.	*Maneuvers.* Unlike mitral regurgitation, the intensity increases with inspiration.	
Associated Findings	S_1 normal (75%), loud (12%), soft (12%) An apical S_3 reflects volume overload of the left ventricle. The apical impulse may be *diffuse* and laterally displaced. There may be a sustained lower left parasternal impulse from a dilated left atrium.	The right ventricular impulse is increased in amplitude and may be sustained, with a "precordial rock." An S_3 may be audible along the lower left sternal border. The JVP is often elevated, with large *v* waves in the jugular veins, a pulsatile liver, ascites, and edema.	S_2 may be obscured by the loud murmur. Findings and associated findings vary with the size of the defect. Larger defects cause left-to-right shunts, pulmonary hypertension, and right ventricular overload.
Mechanism	When the *mitral valve fails to close fully in systole,* blood regurgitates from left ventricle to left atrium, causing the murmur and increasing left ventricular preload, ultimately leading to left ventricular dilatation. Causes are structural, from mitral valve prolapse, infectious endocarditis, rheumatic heart disease, and collagen vascular disease; and functional, from ventricular dilatation and dilatation of the mitral valve annulus and from leaflet, papillary muscle, or chordae tendinae dysfunction.	When the *tricuspid valve fails to close fully in systole,* blood regurgitates from RV to right atrium, producing a murmur. The most common causes are: right ventricular failure and dilatation, with resulting enlargement of the tricuspid orifice, often induced by pulmonary hypertension or left ventricular failure; and endocarditis—the RV and pulmonary artery pressures are low, so the murmur is early systolic.	A ventricular septal defect is a congenital abnormality classified according to one of four locations in the ventricular septum. The defect is a conduit for *bloodflow from the relatively high-pressure left ventricle into the low-pressure right ventricle.* The defect may be accompanied by aortic regurgitation, tricuspid regurgitation, and aneurysms of the ventricular septum; an uncomplicated lesion is described here.

Table 9-11 Diastolic Murmurs

Diastolic murmurs are almost always pathologic. There are two basic types in adults. *Early decrescendo diastolic murmurs* signify regurgitant flow through an incompetent semilunar valve, usually the aortic. *Rumbling diastolic murmurs in mid- or late diastole* point to stenosis of an AV valve, usually the mitral. Diastolic murmurs are less common than systolic murmurs and more difficult to hear, requiring more meticulous examination (see important *Maneuvers* below).

	Aortic Regurgitation[155–158]	Mitral Stenosis[153,156]
	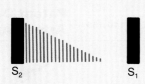	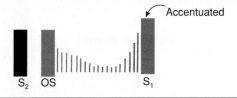
Murmur	*Location.* Left 2nd to 4th interspaces *Radiation.* If loud, to the apex, perhaps to the right sternal border *Intensity.* Grade 1 to 3 *Pitch.* High. *Use the diaphragm.* *Quality.* Blowing decrescendo; may be mistaken for breath sounds *Maneuvers.* The murmur is heard best with the *patient sitting, leaning forward,* with breath held after exhalation.	*Location.* Usually limited to the apex *Radiation.* Little or none *Intensity.* Grade 1 to 4 *Pitch.* Decrescendo low-pitched rumble with pre-systolic accentuation. *Use the bell.* *Maneuvers.* Placing the bell exactly on the apical impulse, turning the patient into a *left lateral position,* and mild exercise like handgrips make the murmur audible. It is heard better in exhalation.
Associated Findings	With advancing severity, the diastolic pressure drops to as low as 50 mm Hg; the pulse pressure can widen by >80 mm Hg. The apical impulse becomes *diffuse,* displaced laterally and downward, and increased in diameter, amplitude, and duration. A systolic ejection sound may be present; S₂ is increased in aortic root dilatation and decreased if leaflets are thickened and calcified; and an S₃ often reflects ventricular dysfunction from both volume and pressure overload. A midsystolic flow murmur or a mitral diastolic (*Austin Flint*) murmur, usually with middiastolic and presystolic components, reflect increased regurgitant flow. The arterial pulse wave collapses suddenly creating bounding arterial pulses with *pistol shot sounds* on light pressure of the diaphragm, especially with arm elevation (Corrigan pulse), a *to–fro murmur* over the brachial or femoral artery with firm pressure (Duroziez sign), and capillary pulsations with nail blanching (Quincke pulses).	S₁ is loud and may be palpable at the apex. An OS often follows S₂ and initiates the murmur. If pulmonary hypertension develops, P₂ is accentuated, the right ventricular parasternal impulse becomes palpable, and the *a* wave of the JVP is more prominent. The apical impulse is small and tapping. Atrial fibrillation occurs in about a third of symptomatic patients, with ensuing risks of thromboembolism.
Mechanism	The aortic valve leaflets fail to close completely during diastole, causing regurgitation from the aorta back into the left ventricle and left ventricular overload. The associated midsystolic flow murmur results from the ejection of this increased stroke volume across the aortic valve. The mitral diastolic (*Austin Flint*) murmur is seen in moderate to severe disease and attributed to diastolic impingement of the regurgitant flow on the anterior leaflet of the mitral valve. Causes include leaflet abnormalities, aortic pathology (Marfan syndrome), and subvalvular abnormalities such as subaortic stenosis or an atrial septal defect.	The stiffened mitral valve leaflets move into the left atrium in midsystole and narrow the valve opening, causing turbulence. The resulting murmur has two components: (1) middiastolic (during rapid ventricular filling) and (2) presystolic accentuation, possibly related to ventricular contraction. The most common cause worldwide is rheumatic fever, which causes fibrosis, calcification, and thickening of the leaflets and commissures, and chordal fusion.

Table 9-12 Cardiovascular Sounds with Both Systolic and Diastolic Components

Some cardiovascular sounds extend beyond one phase of the cardiac cycle. Three examples, all nonvalvular in origin, are: (1) a *venous hum*, a benign sound produced by turbulence of blood in the jugular veins—common in children; (2) a *pericardial friction rub*, produced by inflammation of the pericardial sac; and (3) *patent ductus arteriosus*, a congenital anomaly that persists after birth causing a left-to-right shunt from the aorta to the pulmonary artery. *Continuous murmurs* begin in systole and extend through S_2 into all or part of diastole, as in *patent ductus arteriosus*. Arteriovenous fistulas, common in dialysis patients, also produce continuous murmurs.

	Venous Hum	Pericardial Friction Rub[140,159]	Patent Ductus Arteriosus
Timing	Continuous murmur without a silent interval. Loudest in diastole.	Inflammation of the visceral and parietal pericardium from pericarditis produces a coarse grating sound with one, two, or three components (ventricular systole; ventricular filling and atrial contraction during diastole). Rubs are heard with and without pericardial effusions.	Continuous murmur in both systole and diastole, often with a silent interval late in diastole. Loudest in late systole, obscures S_2, and fades in diastole.
Location	Above the medial third of the clavicles, especially on the right, often when the head is turned in the opposite direction. Best heard when patient in sitting position; disappears when patient supine.	Usually best heard in the left 3rd interspace next to the sternum with the patient sitting and leaning forward with breath held after forced expiration. (In contrast, a pleural rub is heard only during inspiration.) May come and go spontaneously and require auscultation in several positions. Causes include myocardial infarction, uremia, connective tissue disease.	Left 2nd interspace
Radiation	Right or left 1st and 2nd interspaces	Minimal.	Toward the left clavicle
Intensity	Soft to moderate. The hum is obliterated by pressure on the internal jugular vein.	Superficial sound of varying intensity that seems "close to the stethoscope."	Usually loud, sometimes associated with a thrill
Quality	Humming, roaring	Scratchy, scraping, grating	Harsh, machinery-like
Pitch	Low (heard better with the *bell*)	High (heard better with the *diaphragm*)	Medium

References

1. Clark D 3rd, Ahmed MI, Dell'italia LJ, et al. An argument for reviving the disappearing skill of cardiac auscultation. *Cleve Clin J Med.* 2012;79:536.

2. Delora A. The decline of cardiac auscultation: 'the ball of the match point is poised on the net'. *J Cardiovasc Med.* 2008;9:1173.

3. Markel H. The stethoscope and the art of listening. *N Engl J Med.* 2006;354:551.

4. Simel DL. Time, now, to recover the fun in the physical examination rather than abandon it. *Arch Intern Med.* 2006;166:603.

5. Vukanovic-Criley JM, Hovanesyan A, Criley SR, et al. Confidential testing of cardiac examination competency in cardiology and noncardiology faculty and trainees: a multicenter study. *Clin Cardiol.* 2010;33:738.

6. Wayne DB, Butter J, Cohen ER, et al. Setting defensible standards for cardiac auscultation skills in medical students. *Acad Med.* 2009;84(10 Suppl):S94.

7. Marcus G, Vessey J, Jordan MV, et al. Relationship between accurate auscultation of a clinically useful third heart sound and level of experience. *Arch Intern Med.* 2006;166:617.

8. Vukanovic-Criley JM, Criley S, Warde CM, et al. Competency in cardiac examination skills in medical students, trainees, physicians, and faculty. A multicenter study. *Arch Intern Med.* 2006;166:610.

9. March SK, Bedynek JL Jr, Chizner MA. Teaching cardiac auscultation: effectiveness of a patient-centered teaching conference on improving cardiac auscultatory skills. *Mayo Clin Proc.* 2005; 80;1443.

10. RuDusky BM. Auscultation and Don Quixote. *Chest.* 2005;127: 1869.

11. Mangione S. Cardiac auscultatory skills of physicians-in-training: a comparison of three English-speaking countries. *Am J Med.* 2001;110:210.

12. Mangione S. Cardiac auscultatory skills of internal medicine and family practice trainees. A comparison of diagnostic proficiency. *JAMA.* 1997;278:717.

13. McKinney J, Cook DA, Wood D, et al. Simulation-based training for cardiac auscultation skills: systematic review and meta-analysis. *J Gen Intern Med.* 2013;28:283.

14. McGaghie WC, Issenberg SB, Cohen ER, et al. Translational educational research: a necessity for effective health-care improvement. *Chest.* 2012;142:1097.

15. Norman G, Dore K, Grierson L. The minimal relationship between simulation fidelity and transfer of learning. *Med Ed.* 2012;46:636.

16. McGaghie WC, Issenberg SB, Cohen ER, et al. Does simulation-based medical education with deliberate practice yield better results than traditional clinical education? A meta-analytic comparative review of the evidence. *Acad Med.* 2011;86:706.

17. University of Washington Department of Medicine. Introduction: examination for heart sounds & murmurs. Advanced physical diagnosis. Learning and teaching at the bedside. Available at https://depts.washington.edu/physdx/heart/index.html. Accessed June 16, 2015.

18. Butter J, McGaghie WC, Cohen ER, et al. Simulation-based mastery learning improves cardiac auscultation skills in medical students. *J Gen Intern Med.* 2010;25:780.

19. Michaels AD, Khan FU, Moyers B. Experienced clinicians improve detection of third and fourth heart sounds by viewing acoustic cardiography. *Clin Cardiol.* 2010;33:E36.

20. Saxena A, Barrett MJ, Patel AR, et al. Merging old school methods with new technology to improve skills in cardiac auscultation. *Semin Med Pract.* 2008;11:21.

21. Vukanovic-Criley JM, Boker JR, Criley SR, et al. Using virtual patients to improve cardiac examination competency in medical students. *Clin Cardiol.* 2008;31:334.

22. Barrett MJ, Lacey CS, Sekara AE, et al. Mastering cardiac murmurs. The power of repetition. *Chest.* 2004;126:470.

23. Lee E, Michaels AD, Selvester RH, et al. Frequency of diastolic third and fourth heart sounds with myocardial ischemia induced during percutaneous coronary intervention. *J Electrocardiol.* 2009;42:39.

24. Marcus GM, Gerber IL, McKeown BH, et al. Association between phonocardiographic third and four heart sound and objective measure of left ventricular function. *JAMA.* 2005;293:2238.

25. Shah SJ, Marcus GM, Gerber IL, et al. Physiology of the third heart sound: novel insights from tissue Doppler imaging. *J Am Soc Echocardiogr.* 2008;21:394.

26. Shah SJ, Nakamura K, Marcus GM, et al. Association of the fourth heart sound with increased left ventricular end-diastolic stiffness. *J Card Fail.* 2008;14:431.

27. Shah SJ, Michaels AD. Hemodynamic correlates of the third heart sound and systolic time intervals. *Congest Heart Fail.* 2006;12(4 suppl 1):8.

28. O'Rourke RA, Braunwald E. Ch 209, Physical examination of the cardiovascular system. In *Harrison's Principles of Internal Medicine.* 16th ed. New York: McGraw-Hill; 2005:1307.

29. Yancy CW, Jessup M, Bozkurt B, et al. 2013 AACF/AHA Guideline for the Management of Heart Failure. *J Am College Cardiol.* 2013; 62:e148.

30. Vinayak AG, Levitt J, Gehlbach B, et al. Usefulness of the external jugular vein examination in detecting abnormal central venous pressure in critically ill patients. *Arch Int Med.* 2006;166:2132.

31. McConaghy JR, Oza RS. Outpatient diagnosis of acute chest pain in adults. *Am Fam Physician.* 2013;87:177.

32. Mozaffarian D, Benjamin EJ, Go AS, et al. Heart Disease and Stroke Statistics—2016 Update: A Report From the American Heart Association. *Circulation* 2016;133:e38.

33. Abrams J. Chronic stable angina. *N Engl J Med.* 2005;352:2524.

34. Wilson JF. In the clinic. Stable ischemic heart disease. *Ann Intern Med.* 2014;160:ITC1.

35. Ashley KE, Geraci SA. Ischemic heart disease in women. *South Med J.* 2013;106:427.

36. Braverman AC. Aortic dissection: prompt diagnosis and emergency treatment are critical. *Cleve Clin J Med.* 2011;78:685.

37. Crea F, Camici PG, Bairey Merz CN. Coronary microvascular dysfunction: an update. *Eur Heart J.* 2014;35:1101.

38. Canto JG, Rogers WJ, Goldberg RJ, et al. Association of age and sex with myocardial infarction symptom presentation and in-hospital mortality. *JAMA.* 2012;307:813.

39. Nugent L, Mehta PK, Bairey Merz CN. Gender and microvascular angina. *J Thromb Thrombolysis.* 2011;31:37.

40. Goldman L, Kirtane AJ. Triage of patient with acute chest syndrome and possible cardiac ischemia: the elusive search for diagnostic perfection. *Ann Intern Med.* 2003;139:987.

41. Hiratzka LF, Bakris GL, Beckman JA, et al. American College of Cardiology Foundation/American Heart Association Task Force on Practice Guidelines; American Association for Thoracic Surgery; American College of Radiology; American Stroke Association; Society of Cardiovascular Anesthesiologists; Society

for Cardiovascular Angiography and Interventions; Society of Interventional Radiology; Society of Thoracic Surgeons; Society for Vascular Medicine. Guidelines for the management of patients with thoracic aortic disease. *Circulation.* 2010;121:e266.

42. Spodick DH. Normal sinus heart rate: appropriate rate thresholds for sinus tachycardia and bradycardia. *S Med J.* 1996;89: 666.

43. Cho S, Atwood JE. Peripheral edema. *Am J Med.* 2002;113:580.

44. Clark AL, Cleland JG. Causes and treatment of oedema in patients with heart failure. *Nat Rev Cardiol.* 2013;10:156.

45. Shah MG, Cho S, Atwood JE, et al. Peripheral edema due to heart disease: diagnosis and outcome. *Clin Cardiol.* 2006;29:31.

46. Go AS, Mozaffarian D, Roger VL, et al. Heart disease and stroke statistics—2014 update: a report from the American Heart Association. *Circulation.* 2014;129:e28.

47. Yang Q, Cogswell ME, Flanders WD, et al. Trends in cardiovascular health metrics and associations with all-cause and CVD mortality among U.S. adults. *JAMA.* 2012;307:1273.

48. Hettema J, Steele J, Miller WR. Motivational interviewing. *Annu Rev Clin Psychol.* 2005;1:91.

49. U.S. Preventive Services Task Force. Aspirin for the prevention of cardiovascular disease: U.S. Preventive Services Task Force recommendation statement. *Ann Intern Med.* 2009;150:396.

50. Wolff T, Miller T, Ko S. Aspirin for the primary prevention of cardiovascular events: an update of the evidence for the U.S. Preventive Services Task Force. *Ann Intern Med.* 2009;150:405.

51. Goff DC Jr, Lloyd-Jones DM, Bennett G, et al. 2013 ACC/AHA guideline on the assessment of cardiovascular risk: a report of the American College of Cardiology/American Heart Association Task Force on Practice Guidelines. *J Am Coll Cardiol.* 2014;63(25 Pt B): 2935.

52. Mosca L, Benjamin EJ, Berra K, et al. Effectiveness-based guidelines for the prevention of cardiovascular disease in women— 2011 update: a guideline from the American Heart Association. *Circulation.* 2011;123:1243.

53. Flack JM, Sica DA, Bakris G, et al. Management of high blood pressure in Blacks: an update of the International Society on Hypertension in Blacks consensus statement. *Hypertension.* 2010;56:780.

54. Meschia JF, Bushnell C, Boden-Albala B, et al. Guidelines for the primary prevention of stroke: a statement for healthcare professionals from the American Heart Association/American Stroke Association. *Stroke.* 2014;45:3754.

55. American Diabetes Association. Standards of medical care in diabetes—2014. *Diabetes Care.* 2015;38(Suppl 1):S1.

56. Greenland P, Alpert JS, Beller GA, et al. 2010 ACCF/AHA guideline for assessment of cardiovascular risk in asymptomatic adults: executive summary: a report of the American College of Cardiology Foundation/American Heart Association Task Force on Practice Guidelines. *Circulation.* 2010;122:2748.

57. Mosca L, Mochari-Greenberger H, Dolor RJ, et al. Twelve-year follow-up of American women's awareness of cardiovascular disease risk and barriers to heart health. *Circ Cardiovasc Qual Outcomes.* 2010;3:120.

58. Ford ES, Ajani UA, Croft JB, et al. Explaining the decrease in U.S. deaths from coronary disease, 1980–2000. *N Engl J Med.* 2007;356:2388.

59. Towfighi A, Zheng L, Ovbiagele B. Sex-specific trends in midlife coronary heart disease risk and prevalence. *Arch Intern Med.* 2009;169:1762.

60. Bushnell C, McCullough LD, Awad IA, et al. Guidelines for the prevention of stroke in women: a statement for healthcare professionals from the American Heart Association/American Stroke Association. *Stroke.* 2014;45:1545.

61. Stone NJ, Robinson JG, Lichtenstein AH, et al. 2013 ACC/AHA guideline on the treatment of blood cholesterol to reduce atherosclerotic cardiovascular risk in adults: a report of the American College of Cardiology/American Heart Association Task Force on Practice Guidelines. *Circulation.* 2014;129:S1.

62. Piper MA, Evans CV, Burda BU, et al. Screening for high blood pressure in adults: A systematic evidence review for the U.S. Preventive Services Task Force. Rockville (MD); 2014. http://www.ncbi.nlm.nih.gov/pubmed/25632496. Accessed April 19, 2015.

63. Ritchey MD, Wall HK, Gillespie C, et al. Million hearts: prevalence of leading cardiovascular disease risk factors—United States, 2005–2012. *MMWR Morb Mortal Wkly Rep.* 2014;63:462.

64. U.S. Preventive Services Task Force. Screening for high blood pressure: U.S. Preventive Services Task Force reaffirmation recommendation statement. *Ann Intern Med.* 2007;147:783.

65. James PA, Oparil S, Carter BL, et al. 2014 evidence-based guideline for the management of high blood pressure in adults: report from the panel members appointed to the Eighth Joint National Committee (JNC 8). *JAMA.* 2014;311:507.

66. Wright JT Jr, Fine LJ, Lackland DT, et al. Evidence supporting a systolic blood pressure goal of less than 150 mm Hg in patients aged 60 years or older: the minority view. *Ann Intern Med.* 2014; 160:499.

67. Krakoff LR, Gillespie RL, Ferdinand KC, et al. 2014 hypertension recommendations from the eighth joint national committee panel members raise concerns for elderly black and female populations. *J Am Coll Cardiol.* 2014;64:394.

68. Weber MA, Schiffrin EL, White WB, et al. Clinical practice guidelines for the management of hypertension in the community: A statement by the American Society of Hypertension and the International Society of Hypertension. *J Clin Hypertens.* 2014;16:14.

69. Chobanian AV, Bakris GL, Black HR, et al. The Seventh Report of the Joint National Committee on Prevention, Detection, Evaluation, and Treatment of High Blood Pressure—The JNC 7 Report. *JAMA.* 2003;289:2560–2572. Available at http://www.nhlbi.nih.gov/health-pro/guidelines/current/hypertension-jnc-7/complete-report. Accessed January 22, 2015.

70. Institute of Medicine, Committee on the Consequences of Sodium Reduction in Populations; Food and Nutrition Board; Board on Population Health and Public Health Practice. Strom BL, Yaktine AL, Oria M (eds). *Sodium Intake in Populations: Assessment of Evidence.* Washington, DC: National Academies Press, 2013.

71. Rosendorff C, Lackland DT, Allison M, et al. Treatment of hypertension in patients with coronary artery disease: A scientific statement from the American Heart Association, American College of Cardiology, and American Society of Hypertension. *J Am Coll Cardiol.* 2015;65:1998.

72. Frieden TR, Berwick DM. The "Million Hearts" initiative—preventing heart attacks and strokes. *N Engl J Med.* 2011;365:e27.

73. Centers for Disease Control and Prevention. *National Diabetes Statistics Report, Estimates of diabetes and its burden in the United States, 2014.* Atlanta, GA: U.S. Department of Health and Human Services; 2015. http://www.cdc.gov/diabetes/pubs/statsreport14/national-diabetes report-web.pdf. Accessed April 19, 2105.

74. American Diabetes Association. Classification and diagnosis of diabetes. *Diabetes Care.* 2015;38(Suppl):S8.

REFERENCES

75. U.S. Preventive Services Task Force. Final recommendation statement. Lipid disorders in adults (cholesterol, dyslipidemia): Screening. 2014. Available at http://www.uspreventiveservicestaskforce.org/Page/Document/RecommendationStatementFinal/lipid-disorders-in-adults-cholesterol-dyslipidemia-screening. Accessed April 19, 2015.

76. Keaney JF Jr., Curfman GD, Jarcho JA. A pragmatic view of the new cholesterol treatment guidelines. *N Engl J Med.* 2014;370:275.

77. Alberti KG, Eckel RH, Grundy SM, et al. Harmonizing the metabolic syndrome: a joint interim statement of the International Diabetes Federation Task Force on Epidemiology and Prevention; National Heart, Lung, and Blood Institute; American Heart Association; World Heart Federation; International Atherosclerosis Society; and International Association for the Study of Obesity. *Circulation.* 2009;120:1640.

78. Office of the Surgeon General. The health consequences of smoking—50 years of progress. A report of the Surgeon General. Rockville, MD: Public Health Service; 2014. http://www.surgeongeneral.gov/library/reports/50-years-of-progress/full-report.pdf. Accessed April 19, 2015.

79. Institute of Medicine of the National Academies. Leading health indicators for Healthy People 2020. Letter Report. Washington, DC; 2011. Available at http://www.iom.edu/~/media/Files/Report%20Files/2011/Leading-Health-Indicators-for Healthy-People-2020/Leading%20Health%20Indicators%202011%20R. Accessed April 19, 2015.

80. Norcross JC, Prochaska JO. Using the stages of change. *Harv Ment Health Lett.* 2002;18:5.

81. LeFevre ML. Behavioral counseling to promote a healthful diet and physical activity for cardiovascular disease prevention in adults with cardiovascular risk factors: U.S. Preventive Services Task Force Recommendation Statement. *Ann Intern Med.* 2014; 161:587.

82. Eckel RH, Jakicic JM, Ard JD, et al. 2013 AHA/ACC guideline on lifestyle management to reduce cardiovascular risk: a report of the American College of Cardiology/American Heart Association Task Force on Practice Guidelines. *Circulation.* 2014;129:S76.

83. Fiore MC, Jaen CR, Bakder TB. Treating tobacco use and dependence: 2008 Update. Clinical Practice Guideline. Rockville, MD: U.S. Department of Health and Human Services. Public Health Service; 2008. Available at http://www.ncbi.nlm.nih.gov/books/NBK63952/. Accessed April 19, 2015.

84. Estruch R, Ros E, Salas-Salvado J, et al. Primary prevention of cardiovascular disease with a Mediterranean diet. *N Engl J Med.* 2013;368:1279.

85. U.S. Department of Agriculture and U.S. Department of Health and Human Services. *Dietary Guidelines for Americans.* 7th ed. Washington, DC: U.S. Government Printing Office; 2010. Available at http://www.health.gov/dietaryguidelines/dga2010/DietaryGuidelines2010.pdf. Accessed March 30, 2015.

86. U.S. Department of Health and Human Services. *2008 Physical Activity Guidelines for Americans.* Washington, DC: U.S. Department of Health and Human Services; 2008. Available at http://www.health.gov/paguidelines/pdf/paguide.pdf. Accessed April 19, 2015.

87. McGee S. *Evidence-based Physical Diagnosis.* 3rd ed. Philadelphia, PA: Saunders; 2012.

88. The Rational Clinical Examination Series, JAMA. Available at http://jamaevidence.mhmedical.com/book.aspx?bookID = 845. Accessed June 12, 2015.

89. Pickering TG, Hall JE, Appel LJ, et al. Recommendations for blood pressure measurement in humans and experimental animals: part 1: blood pressure measurement in humans: a statement for professionals from the Subcommittee of Professional and Public Education of the American Heart Association Council on High Blood Pressure Research. *Circulation.* 2005;111:697.

90. McAlister FA, Straus SE. Evidence-based treatment of hypertension. Measurement of blood pressure: an evidence based review. *BMJ.* 2001;322:908.

91. Powers BJ, Olsen MK, Smith VA, et al. Measuring blood pressure for decision making and quality reporting: where and how many measures? *Ann Intern Med.* 2011;154:781.

92. Appel LJ, Miller ER 3rd, Charleston J. Improving the measurement of blood pressure: is it time for regulated standards? *Ann Intern Med.* 2011;154;838.

93. Ray GM, Nawarskas JJ, Anderson JR. Blood pressure monitoring technique impacts hypertension treatment. *J Gen Intern Med.* 2012;27:623.

94. Umscheid CA, Townsend RR. Is it time for a blood pressure measurement "bundle"? *J Gen Intern Med.* 2012;27:615.

95. Guarracino F, Ferro B, Forfori F, et al. Jugular vein distensibility predicts fluid responsiveness in septic patients. *Crit Care.* 2014;18:647.

96. Devine PJ, Sullenberger LE, Bellin DA, et al. Jugular venous pulse: window into the right heart. *South Med J.* 2007;100:1022.

97. Drazner MH, Hellkamp AS, Leier CV, et al. Value of clinician assessment of hemodynamics in advanced heart failure: the ESCAPE trial. *Circ Heart Fail.* 2008;1:170.

98. Cook DJ, Simel DL. Does this patient have abnormal central venous pressure? *JAMA.* 1996;275:630.

99. Davison R, Cannon R. Estimation of central venous pressure by examination of jugular veins. *Am Heart J.* 1974;87:279.

100. Constant J. Using internal jugular pulsations as a manometer for right atrial pressure measurements. *Cardiology.* 2000;93:26.

101. Meyer P, Ekundayo OJ, Adamopoulos C, et al. A propensity-matched study of elevated jugular venous pressure and outcomes in chronic heart failure. *Am J Cardiol.* 2009;103:839.

102. McGee S. Ch. 34, Inspection of the neck veins. In *Evidence-based Physical Diagnosis,* 3rd ed. Philadelphia, PA: Saunders; 2012:296.

103. Seth R, Magner P, Matzinger F, et al. How far is the sternal angle from the mid-right atrium? *J Gen Intern Med.* 2002;17:852.

104. Hunt SA, Abraham WT, Chin MH, et al. 2009 focused update incorporated into the ACC/AHA 2005 Guidelines for the Diagnosis and Management of Heart Failure in Adults: a report of the American College of Cardiology Foundation/American Heart Association Task Force on Practice Guidelines: developed in collaboration with the International Society for Heart and Lung Transplantation. *Circulation.* 2009;119:e391.

105. Drazner MH, Prasad A, Ayers C, et al. The relationship of right- and left-sided filling pressures in patients with heart failure and a preserved ejection fraction. *Circ Heart Fail.* 2010;3:202.

106. Goldberg LR. In the clinic. Heart failure. *Ann Intern Med.* 2010; 152:ITC 6–1.

107. Fahey T, Jeyaseelan S, McCowan C, et al. Diagnosis of left ventricular systolic dysfunction (LVSD): development and validation of a clinical prediction rule in primary care. *Fam Pract.* 2007; 24:628.

108. Rame JE, Dries DL, Drazner MH. The prognostic value of the physical examination in patients with chronic heart failure. *Congest Heart Fail.* 2003;9:170.

109. Drazner MH, Rame E, Stevenson LW, et al. Prognostic importance of elevated jugular venous pressure and a third heart sound in patients with heart failure. *N Engl J Med.* 2001;345(8):574.

110. Badgett RG, Lucey CR, Muirow CD. Can the clinical examination diagnose left-sided heart failure in adults? *JAMA.* 1997;277:1712.

111. Shaheen K, Alraies MC. Superior vena cava syndrome. *Cleve Clin J Med.* 2012;79:410.

112. Barst RJ, Ertel SI, Beghetti M, et al. Pulmonary arterial hypertension: a comparison between children and adults. *Eur Respir J.* 2011;37:665.

113. LeWinter MM. Clinical practice. Acute pericarditis. *N Engl J Med.* 2014;371:2410.

114. Meyer T, Shih J, Aurigemma G. In the clinic. Heart failure with preserved ejection fraction (diastolic dysfunction). *Ann Intern Med.* 2013;158:ITC 5–1.

115. Sandercock PA, Kavvadia E. The carotid bruit. *Pract Neurol.* 2002;2:221.

116. Ratchford EV, Jin Z, Di Tullio MR, et al. Carotid bruit for detection of hemodynamically significant carotid stenosis: the Northern Manhattan Study. *Neurol Res.* 2009;31:748.

117. Sauve JS, Laupacis A, Feagan B, et al. Does this patient have a clinically important carotid bruit? *JAMA.* 1993;270:2843.

118. Schorr R, Johnson K, Wan J, et al. The prognostic significance of asymptomatic carotid bruits in the elderly. *J Gen Intern Med.* 1998:13;86.

119. Jonas DE, Feltner C, Amick HR, et al. Screening for asymptomatic carotid artery stenosis: a systematic review and meta-analysis for the U.S. Preventive Services Task Force. *Ann Intern Med.* 2014;161:336.

120. Pickett CA, Jackson JL, Hemann BA, et al. Carotid bruits as a prognostic indicator of cardiovascular death and myocardial infarction: a meta-analysis. *Lancet.* 2008;371:1587.

121. Pickett CA, Jackson JL, Hemann BA, et al. Carotid bruits and cerebrovascular disease risk: A meta-analysis. *Stroke.* 2010;41:2295.

122. de Weerd M, Greving JP, de Jong AW, et al. Prevalence of asymptomatic carotid artery stenosis according to age and sex. *Stroke.* 2009;40:1105.

123. Simel DL, Goldstein L. Update: carotid bruit. In: Simel DL, Rennie D, eds. *The Rational Clinical Examination: Evidence-Based Clinical Diagnosis.* New York: McGraw-Hill; 2009. Available at http://jamaevidence.mhmedical.com/content.aspx?bookid=845&sectionid=61357496. Accessed June 12, 2015.

124. LeFevre ML. U.S. Preventive Services Task Force. Screening for asymptomatic carotid artery stenosis: U.S. Preventive Services Task Force recommendation statement. *Ann Intern Med.* 2014;161:356.

125. de Weerd M, Greving JP, Hedblad B, et al. Prediction of asymptomatic carotid artery stenosis in the general population: identification of high-risk groups. *Stroke.* 2014;45:2366.

126. Raman G, Moorthy D, Hadar N, et al. Management strategies for asymptomatic carotid stenosis. *Ann Intern Med.* 2013;158:676.

127. Paraskevas K, Spence JD, Veith FJ, et al. Identifying which patients with asymptomatic carotid stenosis could benefit from intervention. *Stroke.* 2014;45:3720.

128. Daly C, Rodriguez HE. Carotid artery occlusive disease. *Surg Clin North Am.* 2013;93:813.

129. McGee S. Ch. 36, Palpation of the heart. In: *Evidence-based Physical Diagnosis.* 3rd ed. Philadelphia, PA: Saunders; 2012:311.

130. Ehara S, Okuyama T, Shirai N. Comprehensive evaluation of the apex beat using 64-slice computed tomography: Impact of left ventricular mass and distance to chest wall. *J Cardiol.* 2010;55:256.

131. Logar HB, Medvescek NR, Rakovec P. Standardization of the apex beat in the full left lateral position and its diagnostic value in detecting left ventricular dilatation. *Acta Cardiol.* 2011;66:459.

132. American College of Cardiology/American Heart Association Task Force on Practice Guidelines; Society of Cardiovascular Anesthesiologists; Society for Cardiovascular Angiography and Interventions; Society of Thoracic Surgeons, et al. ACC/AHA 2006 guidelines for the management of patients with valvular heart disease: a report of the American College of Cardiology/American Heart Association Task Force on Practice Guidelines developed in collaboration with the Society of Cardiovascular Anesthesiologists. *Circulation.* 2006;114:e84.

133. McGee S. Ch. 40, Miscellaneous heart sounds. In: *Evidence-based Physical Diagnosis.* 3rd ed. Philadelphia, PA: Saunders; 2012:345.

134. Kari FA, Beyersdorf F, Siepe M. Pathophysiological implications of different bicuspid aortic valve configurations. *Cardiol Res Pract.* 2012;2012:735829.

135. Siu SC, Silversides CK. Bicuspid aortic valve disease. *J Am Coll Cardiol.* 2010;55:2789.

136. Topilsky Y, Michelena H, Bichara V, et al. Mitral valve prolapse with mid-late systolic mitral regurgitation: pitfalls of evaluation and clinical outcome compared with holosystolic regurgitation. *Circulation.* 2012:125:1643.

137. Foster E. Mitral regurgitation due to degenerative mitral-valve disease. *N Engl J Med.* 2010;363:156.

138. Hayek E, Gring CN, Griffin BP. Mitral valve prolapse. *Lancet.* 2005;365:507.

139. McGee S. Ch. 39, The third and fourth heart sounds. In: *Evidence-based Physical Diagnosis.* 3rd ed. Philadelphia, PA: Saunders; 2012:341.

140. Chizner MA. Cardiac auscultation: rediscovering the lost art. *Curr Probl Cardiol.* 2008;33:326.

141. McGee S. Etiology and diagnosis of systolic murmurs in adults. *Am J Med.* 2010;123:913.

142. Felker GM, Cuculich PS, Gheorghiade M. The Valsalva maneuver: a bedside "biomarker" for heart failure. *Am J Med.* 2006;119:117.

143. Lembo NJ, Dell'Italia LJ, Crawford MH, et al. Bedside diagnosis of systolic murmurs. *N Engl J Med.* 1988;318:1572.

144. Otto CM, Prendergast B. Aortic-valve stenosis—from patients at risk to severe valve obstruction. *N Engl J Med.* 2014;371:744.

145. Manning WJ. Asymptomatic aortic stenosis in the elderly: a clinical review. *JAMA.* 2013;310:1490.

146. Ho CY. Hypertrophic cardiomyopathy in 2012. *Circulation.* 2012;125:1432.

147. Fitzgerald KP, Lim MJ. The pulmonary valve. *Cardiol Clin.* 2011;29:223.

148. Asgar AW, Mack MJ, Stone GW. Secondary mitral regurgitation in heart failure: pathophysiology, prognosis, and therapeutic considerations. *J Am Coll Cardiol.* 2015;65:1231.

149. Bonow RO. Chronic mitral regurgitation and aortic regurgitation: have indications for surgery changed? *J Am coll Cardiol.* 2013;61:693.

150. Enriquez-Sarano M, Akins CW, Vahanian A. Mitral regurgitation. *Lancet.* 2009;373(9672):1382.

151. Irwin RB, Luckie M, Khattar RS. Tricuspid regurgitation: contemporary management of a neglected valvular lesion. *Postgrad Med J.* 2010:86:648.

152. Mutlak D, Aronson D, Lessick J, et al. Functional tricuspid regurgitation in patients with pulmonary hypertension: is pulmonary artery pressure the only determinant of regurgitation severity? *Chest.* 2009;135:115.

REFERENCES

153. McGee S. Ch. 44, Miscellaneous heart sounds. In: *Evidence-based Physical Diagnosis*. 3rd ed. Philadelphia, PA: Saunders; 2012:394.

154. Pessel C, Bonanno C. Valve disease in pregnancy. *Semin Perinatol*. 2014;348:273.

155. McGee S. Ch. 43, Aortic regurgitation. In: *Evidence-based Physical Diagnosis*. 3rd ed. Philadelphia, PA: Saunders; 2012:379.

156. Maganti K, Rigolin VH, Sarano ME, et al. Valvular heart disease: diagnosis and management. *Mayo Clin Proc*. 2010;85:483.

157. Enriquez-Serano M, Tajik AJ. Clinical practice. Aortic regurgitation. *N Engl J Med*. 2004:351:1539.

158. Babu AN, Kymes SM, Carpenter Fryer SM. Eponyms and the diagnosis of aortic regurgitation: what says the evidence? *Ann Intern Med*. 2003;138:736.

159. McGee S. Ch. 45, Disorders of the pericardium. In: *Evidence-based Physical Diagnosis*. 3rd ed. Philadelphia, PA: Saunders; 2012:400.

160. McGee S. Ch. 41, Heart murmurs: general principles. In: *Evidence-based Physical Diagnosis*. 3rd ed. Philadelphia, PA: Saunders; 2012:354.

161. Levine SA. Notes on the gradation of the intensity of cardiac murmurs. *JAMA*. 1961:177:261.

162. Freeman RA, Levine SA. The clinical significance of the systolic murmur: a study of 1000 consecutive "non-cardiac" cases. *Ann Intern Med*. 1933;6:1371.

163. Opotowsky AR, Ojeda J, Rogers F, et al. Blood pressure response to the Valsalva maneuver. A simple bedside test to determine the hemodynamic basis of pulmonary hypertension. *Am Coll Cardiol*. 2010;56:1352.

164. Cheng RK, Cox M, Neely ML, et al. Outcomes in patients with heart failure with preserved, borderline, and reduced ejection fraction in the Medicare population. *Am Heart J*. 2014;168:721.

165. Gheorghiade M, Vaduganathan M, Fonarow GC, et al. Rehospitalization for heart failure: problems and perspectives. *J Am Coll Cardiol*. 2013;61:391.

The Breasts and Axillae

Anatomy and Physiology

The Female Breast

The female breast lies against the anterior thoracic wall, extending from the clavicle and 2nd rib down to the 6th rib, and from the sternum across to the midaxillary line. Its surface area is generally rectangular rather than round (Fig. 10-1).

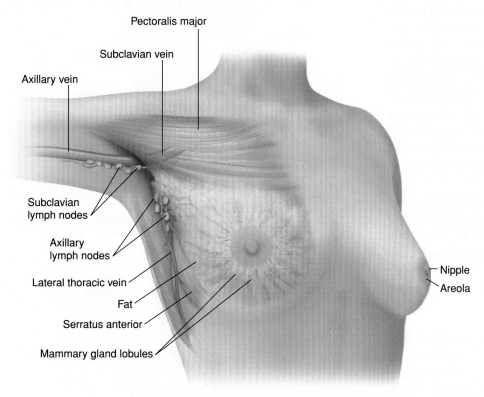

FIGURE 10-1. **The female breast.**

The breast overlies the *pectoralis major* and, at its inferior margin, the *serratus anterior.*

To describe clinical findings, the breast is often divided into four quadrants based on horizontal and vertical lines crossing at the nipple (Fig. 10-2). A fifth area, an axillary tail of breast tissue, sometimes termed the *"tail of Spence,"* extends laterally across the anterior axillary fold. Alternatively, findings can be localized as the time on the face of a clock (e.g., 3 o'clock) and the distance in centimeters from the nipple.

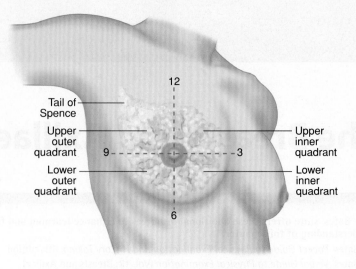

FIGURE 10-2. **Breast quadrants.**

The breast is a hormonally sensitive tissue, responsive to the changes of monthly cycling and aging. *Glandular tissue,* consisting of milk-secreting tubuloalveolar glands and ductules, forms 15 to 20 septated *lobes* radiating around the nipple (Fig. 10-3). Within each lobe are many smaller *lobules.* The glandular tissue within each lobule drains into larger collecting ducts and lactiferous sinuses leading to 5 to 10 porous openings on the surface of the *areola* and the nipple. *Fibrous connective tissue* provides structural support in the form of fibrous bands or suspensory ligaments, also known as Cooper ligaments, connected to both the skin and the underlying fascia. *Adipose tissue,* or fat, surrounds the breast, predominantly in the superficial and peripheral areas. The proportions of these components vary with age, nutritional status, pregnancy, exogenous hormone use, and other factors. After menopause, there is atrophy of glandular tissue, and a notable decrease in the number of lobules.

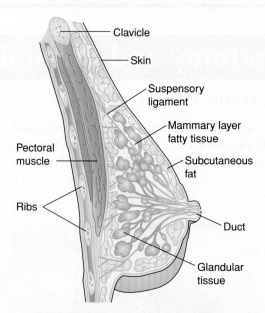

FIGURE 10-3. **Breast anatomy.**

The surface of the areola has small, rounded elevations formed by sebaceous glands, sweat glands, and accessory areolar glands (Fig. 10-4). A few hairs are often seen on the areola. During pregnancy, the sebaceous glands produce an oily secretion that serves as a protective lubricant for the areola and nipple during lactation.

Both the nipple and the areola are supplied with smooth muscle that contracts to express milk from the ductal system during breast-feeding. Rich sensory innervation, especially in the nipple, triggers "milk letdown" following neurohormonal stimulation from

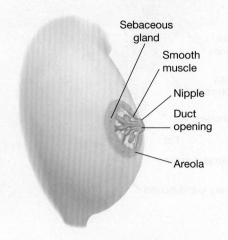

FIGURE 10-4. **Nipple and areola.**

infant sucking. Tactile stimulation of the area, including the breast examination, makes the nipple smaller, firmer, and more erect, whereas the areola puckers and wrinkles. These smooth muscle reflexes are normal and should not be mistaken for signs of breast disease.

The adult breast may be soft, but it often feels granular, nodular, or lumpy. This uneven texture is normal *physiologic nodularity*. It is often bilateral and may occur throughout the breast or only in some areas. The nodularity may increase before menses, a time when breasts often enlarge and become tender or even painful. For breast changes during adolescence and pregnancy, see pp. 896–897 and p. 928.

Occasionally, one or more extra or supernumerary nipples are located along the "milk line," illustrated in Figure 10-5. Usually, only a small nipple and areola are present, often mistaken for a common mole. Those containing glandular tissue occasionally show increased pigmentation, swelling, tenderness, or even lactation during puberty, menstruation, or pregnancy. Possible associations with renal, urogenital, and cardiovascular disorders are under current investigation, but treatment is only needed if there is diagnostic ambiguity, cosmetic concerns, or possible pathology.[1]

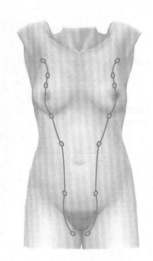

F I G U R E   1 0 - 5 .   **Milk lines.**

The Male Breast

The male breast consists chiefly of a small nipple and areola overlying a thin disc of undeveloped breast tissue consisting primarily of ducts. Lacking estrogen and progesterone stimulation, ductal branching and development of lobules are minimal,[2,3] making it difficult to distinguish male breast tissue from the surrounding muscles of the chest wall. There is a firm button of breast tissue 2 cm or more in diameter in roughly one of three adult men.

Some men develop benign breast enlargement from *gynecomastia,* a proliferation of palpable glandular tissue, or *pseudogynecomastia,* the accumulation of subareolar fat. Causes of gynecomastia include increased estrogen, decreased testosterone, and medication side effects.[4]

Lymphatics

Most lymphatic vessels of the breast drain into the axillary lymph nodes (Fig. 10-6). Of these, the *central nodes* are the most likely to be palpable. They lie along the chest wall, usually high in the axilla and midway between the anterior and posterior axillary folds. Three other groups of lymph nodes drain into the central nodes and are seldom palpable:

- *Pectoral nodes—anterior,* located along the lower border of the pectoralis major inside the anterior axillary fold. These nodes drain the anterior chest wall and much of the breast.

- *Subscapular nodes—posterior,* located along the lateral border of the scapula; palpated deep in the posterior axillary fold. They drain the posterior chest wall and a portion of the arm.

- *Lateral nodes—*located *along the upper humerus.* They drain most of the arm.

Lymph drains from the central axillary nodes to the *infraclavicular* and *supraclavicular* nodes.

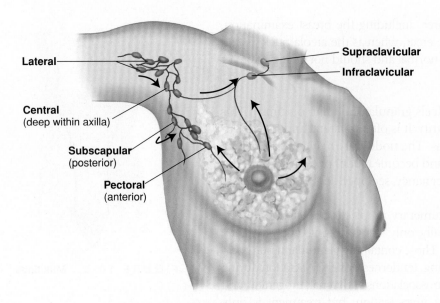

Lateral

Supraclavicular

Infraclavicular

Central
(deep within axilla)

Subscapular
(posterior)

Pectoral
(anterior)

FIGURE 10-6. **Direction of lymph flow.**

Not all the lymphatics of the breast drain into the axilla. Malignant cells from a breast cancer may spread directly to the infraclavicular nodes or into the internal mammary chain of lymph nodes within the chest.

The Health History

Common or Concerning Symptoms

- Breast lump or mass
- Breast discomfort or pain
- Nipple discharge

You can elicit concerns about the breasts during the history or later during the physical examination. Ask if the patient has had any *lumps, discomfort,* or *pain* in her breasts. About 50% of women have palpable lumps or nodularity, and premenstrual enlargement and tenderness are common.[5,6] If your patient reports a lump or mass, identify the precise location, how long it has been present, and any change in size or variation within the menstrual cycle. Ask if there has been any change in breast contour, dimpling, swelling, or puckering of the skin over the breasts.

Breast pain, or *mastalgia,* is the most common breast symptom prompting office visits. Breast pain alone (without mass) is not considered a breast cancer risk factor. Determine if the pain is diffuse or focal, cyclic or noncyclic, and related to medications.

Lumps may be physiologic or pathologic, ranging from cysts and fibroadenomas to breast cancer. See Table 10-1, Common Breast Masses, p. 444, and Table 10-2, Visible Signs of Breast Cancer, p. 445.

Clinical breast examination (CBE) is warranted. Focal breast pain is more likely to merit diagnostic imaging. Medications associated with breast pain include hormonal therapy; psychotropic drugs such as selective serotonin reuptake inhibitors and haloperiodol; spironolactone, and digoxin.[6]

Ask about any *discharge from the nipples* and when it occurs. Does the discharge appear only after compression of the nipple, or is it spontaneous? Physiologic hypersecretion is seen in pregnancy, lactation, chest wall stimulation, sleep, and stress. If spontaneous, what is the color, consistency, and quantity? Is the color milky, brown or greenish, or bloody? Ask if the discharge is unilateral or bilateral. Physiologic discharge is usually bilateral, multiductal, prompted by stimulation, and ranges in color from white to yellowish or green.

Galactorrhea, or the discharge of milk-containing fluid unrelated to pregnancy or lactation, is more likely to be pathologic when it is bloody or serous, unilateral, spontaneous, associated with a mass, and occurring in women aged ≥40 years.[6]

Health Promotion and Counseling: Evidence and Recommendations

Important Topics for Health Promotion and Counseling

- Palpable masses of the breast
- Assessing risk of breast cancer
- Breast cancer screening

Women may experience a wide range of changes in breast tissue and sensation, from cyclic swelling and nodularity to a distinct lump or mass. The examination of the breast is an important opportunity for exploring key concerns for women's health—what to do if a lump or mass is detected, risk factors for breast cancer, and screening measures such as breast self-examination (BSE), the CBE by a skilled clinician, and mammography.

Palpable Masses of the Breast and Breast Symptoms. Breast cancer occurs in up to 4% of women with breast complaints, in approximately 5% of women reporting a nipple discharge, and in up to 11% of women specifically complaining of a breast lump or mass.[3,5] Breast masses show marked variation in etiology, from fibroadenomas and cysts seen in younger women, to abscess or mastitis, to primary breast cancer. On initial assessment, the woman's age and the physical characteristics of the mass provide clues about etiology, as shown below, but definitive diagnosis should be pursued and often requires further evaluation with ultrasound, mammography, or even biopsy.

Palpable Masses of the Breast

Age (in Years)	Common Lesion	Characteristics
15–25	Fibroadenoma	Usually smooth, rubbery, round, mobile, nontender
25–50	Cysts	Usually soft to firm, round, mobile; often tender
	Fibrocystic changes	Nodular, ropelike
	Cancer	Irregular, firm, may be mobile or fixed to surrounding tissue

(continued)

Palpable Masses of the Breast (continued)

Age (in Years)	Common Lesion	Characteristics
Over 50	Cancer until proven otherwise	As above
Pregnancy/ lactation	Lactating adenomas, cysts, mastitis, and cancer	As above

Adapted from Schultz MZ, Ward BA, Reiss M. Breast diseases. In: Noble J, Greene HL, Levinson W, et al. (eds). *Primary Care Medicine*, 2nd ed. St. Louis: MO; 1996; Venet L, Strax P, Venet W, et al. Adequacies and inadequacies of breast examinations by physicians in mass screenings. *Cancer.* 1971;28:1546.

Assessing Risk of Breast Cancer.   Women are increasingly interested in learning about breast cancer. Be familiar with the literature about breast cancer risk factors that support recommendations for screening. Key facts and figures are presented here, but further reading will enhance your counseling of female patients.

Breast Cancer Facts and Figures.   Breast cancer is the most common cause of cancer in women worldwide, accounting for more than 10% of cancers in women. In the United States, a woman born now has a 12%, or 1 in 8, lifetime risk of developing breast cancer.[7] Eighty percent of new breast cancer cases occur after age 50 years, with a median age at diagnosis of age 61 years. The probability of diagnosis increases with each decade.

Age-Specific Probabilities of Developing Invasive Female Breast Cancer[a]

If Current Age is:	The Probability of Developing Breast Cancer in the Next 10 Years is:	Or 1 in:
20	0.1%	1,674
30	0.4%	225
40	1.4%	69
50	2.3%	44
60	3.5%	29
70	3.9%	26
Lifetime Risk	12.3%	8

[a]Among those free of cancer at beginning of age interval. Based on cases diagnosed 2010–2012. Percentages and "1 in" numbers may not be numerically equivalent due to rounding.

Source: American Cancer Society. Breast Cancer Facts and Figures 2013–2014, p 17. Available at http://www.cancer.org/acs/groups/content/@research/documents/document/acspc-042725.pdf. Accessed May 1, 2015. Updated to 2015–2016, © 2015.

Breast cancer is the second leading cause of cancer death in women following lung cancer.[7] Five-year survival rates are 99% for local disease, 84% for regional disease, and 24% for metastatic disease. In its annual report, *Breast Cancer Facts and Figures 2013–2014,* the American Cancer Society highlights important trends in breast cancer statistics.

■ *Relatively stable incidence rates since 2004.* Incidence dropped 7% in 2002–2003, attributed to declining use of hormone replacement therapy (HRT). Subsequent incidence rates have been relatively stable, with a small increase between 2006 and 2010 in both white (0.1%) and African American (0.2%) women.

■ *Declining death rates overall, but more advanced disease and higher mortality in African American women.* Compared to white women, African American women have a higher incidence of breast cancer before age 40 years, are more likely to have larger and estrogen receptor (ER)–negative tumors at the time of diagnosis, and are more likely to die of breast cancer at every age. Although overall breast cancer death rates decreased by 34%, or 1.6% per year, between 1990 and 2010, in 2010 African American women still had a 41% higher mortality rate than white women. This major health disparity is attributed to differences in use of mammography, more aggressive tumor characteristics, access to and response to new treatments, and the presence of coexisting illnesses.

Assessing Risk Factors for Breast Cancer. Be familiar with the breast cancer risk factors and their relative risk, as listed below, and discuss them with your patients.[7,8] The most important risk factor for breast cancer is age. Other *non-modifiable risk factors* are family history of breast and ovarian cancers, inherited genetic mutations, personal history of breast cancer or lobular carcinoma in situ, high levels of endogenous hormones,[9–11] breast tissue density, proliferative lesions with atypia on breast biopsy, and duration of unopposed estrogen exposure related to early menarche, age of first full-term pregnancy, and late menopause. Note that a history of radiation to the chest and diethylstilbestrol (DES) exposure also place women at high risk. *Modifiable risk factors* include: breastfeeding for less than 1 year, postmenopausal obesity, use of HRT, cigarette smoking, alcohol ingestion, physical inactivity, and type of contraception. Nonetheless, over 50% of women with breast cancer have no familial or reproductive risk factors.[12]

Breast Cancer in Women: Factors That Increase Relative Risk

Relative Risk	Factor
>4.0	• Age (65+ vs. <65 years, although risk increases across all ages until age 80)
	• Biopsy-confirmed atypical hyperplasia
	• Certain inherited genetic mutations for breast cancer (*BRCA1* and/or *BRCA2*)
	• Ductal carcinoma in situ
	• Lobular carcinoma in situ
	• Personal history of early-onset (<40 years) breast cancer
	• Two or more first-degree relatives with breast cancer diagnosed at an early age *(continued)*

Breast Cancer in Women: Factors That Increase Relative Risk (continued)

Relative Risk	Factor
2.1–4.0	• High endogenous estrogen or testosterone levels (postmenopausal) • High-dose radiation to chest • Mammographically extremely dense (>50%) breasts compared to less dense (11%–25%) • One first-degree relative with breast cancer
1.1–2.0	• Alcohol consumption • Ashkenazi Jewish heritage • Diethylstilbestrol exposure • Early menarche (<12 years) • Height (>5 feet 3 inches) • High socioeconomic status • Late age at first full-term pregnancy (>30 years) • Late menopause (>55 years) • Mammographically dense (26%–50%) breasts compared to less dense (11%–25%) • Non-atypical ductal hyperplasia or fibroadenoma • Never breastfed a child • No full-term pregnancies • Obesity (postmenopausal)/adult weight gain • Personal history of breast cancer (40+ years) • Personal history of endometrium, ovary, or colon cancer • Recent and long-term use of menopausal hormone therapy containing estrogen and progestin • Recent oral contraceptive use

Source: American Cancer Society. *Breast Cancer Facts & Figures 2015–2016*. Atlanta: American Cancer Society Inc, 2015. Available at http://www.cancer.org/acs/groups/content/@research/documents/document/acspc-046381.pdf. Accessed May 1, 2015.

Male Breast Cancer. Male breast cancer constitutes 1% of breast cancer cases, peaking in frequency between ages 60 and 70 years, although men are at risk at any age.[13] Incidence has been increasing slightly, now at 1.2 cases per 100,000 men, primarily in situ and local-stage tumors.[8,13,14] Incidence increases with age and is higher in African American men compared to white men. Risk factors include radiation exposure, BRCA1 and BRCA2 mutations, Klinefelter syndrome, testicular disorders, family history of male or female breast cancer, alcohol use, cirrhosis, and obesity.

Using Breast Cancer Risk Assessment Tools. In addition to risk factor tables, learn to use several risk assessment tools that clarify breast cancer risk for your patients. The Gail and Claus models estimate absolute lifetime risk of breast cancer and are used the most commonly. They use large population data sets and combinations of risk factors to predict approximate risk, but are less precise at predicting which individual women will get breast cancer.[15–18] The BRCAPRO model is one of several models used for predicting risk of BRCA1 or BRCA2.[19] For more detailed discussion of these and other models, turn to the National Cancer Institute's review of the Genetics of Breast and Ovarian Cancer and reports of the American Cancer Society.[16,20,21] Currently, no single model addresses all of the known risk factors or includes all of the genetic details of personal and family history, so using several tools is advised for individual patients. Devising data-based personalized management strategies remains an ongoing focus for research testing incorporation of biopsy results, breast density, ethnicity, and genetic mutations.[22,23]

The Breast Cancer Risk Assessment Tool (the Gail Model). The *Breast Cancer Risk Assessment Tool,* often called the Gail model, at http://www.cancer.gov/bcrisktool/, updated in 2007, provides 5-year and lifetime estimates of *risk for invasive breast cancer.*[15] It incorporates age, race, first-degree relatives with breast cancer, previous breast biopsies and presence of hyperplasia, age at menarche, and age at first delivery. The Gail model is best used for individuals over age 50 years who have either no family history of breast cancer or one affected first-degree relative, and who have annual screening mammograms. It should not be used for women with a past history of breast cancer or radiation exposure, or those who are 35 years of age or younger. It does not determine risk for noninvasive breast cancer and does not take paternal history or disease in second-degree relatives into account, or age of onset of disease. This model has been updated to include breast density, but depends on use of digital mammography and special software, making it more difficult to use.[24]

The Claus Model. The Claus model assesses risk for high-risk women and incorporates family history for both female and male first- and second-degree relatives, including age of onset.[25] It is based on the woman's current age. It is best used for individuals with no more than two first- or second-degree relatives with breast cancer.[16] An expanded version includes family members with ovarian cancer. This model does not include personal, lifestyle, or reproductive risk factors. Discrepancies in risk assessment between published tables and the computerized program have been reported.[18]

The BRCAPRO Model. The *BRCAPRO model* at http://bcb.dfci.harvard.edu/bayesmendel/software.php is used for high-risk women to assess risk of BRCA1 and BRCA2 mutation in a given family. It incorporates published BRCA1 and BRCA2 mutation frequencies, cancer penetration in affected carriers, and age of onset in first- and second-degree female and male relatives. It does not include nonhereditary risk factors.[26]

Breast Cancer Screening

BRCA1 and BRCA2 Mutations. Begin evaluating a woman's breast cancer risk as early as her 20s by asking about family history, especially the conditions listed below. A pattern of breast or ovarian cancer in maternal or paternal family members is suspicious for autosomal dominant genetic mutations. Be sure to ask about family history of ovarian cancer.

Family History: High-Risk Factors for Familial Breast Cancer

- Age 50 years or younger at diagnosis of breast cancer
- Breast cancer in two or more individuals in the same lineage (paternal or maternal)
- Multiple primary or ovarian tumors in one person
- Breast cancer in a male relative
- Ashkenazi Jewish ancestry
- Family member with a known predisposing gene (including Li–Fraumeni and Cowden syndromes)

The BRCA1 and BRCA2 gene occur in <1% of the population but account for roughly 5% to 10% of female breast cancers.[16] However, these mutations represent only 15% to 20% of the familial breast cancers; they also confer increased risk for ovarian cancer. For BRCA1 mutations, the risk of developing breast cancer by age 70 years is estimated at 44% to 78%, and for BRCA2, the estimated risk is 31% to 51%.[7] If family history is suspect, the next steps for clinicians include using the BRCAPRO calculator, genetic testing, referral for genetic counseling, consideration of mammography as well as magnetic resonance imaging (MRI) for screening, and appropriate specialty referrals.[27] (See p. 431 for recommendations on use of MRI in high-risk women.)

Benign Breast Disease with Proliferative Changes on Biopsy. Since the 1980s, increased mammography screening has resulted in greater detection of benign breast disease, which includes a broad category of diagnoses on biopsy. When biopsy findings are stratified by cell type and pattern, they carry significantly different risks of breast cancer, as shown below. Three categories predominate: nonproliferative changes, proliferative changes without atypia (abnormal cells or patterns of cells), and proliferative changes with atypia.[7,28] Presence of proliferative changes adds small to moderate increases in risk, depending of the absence or presence of atypia.[3,29] Proliferative changes with atypia, or *atypical hyperplasia,* increase relative risk from 2 to 4 times higher, with a cumulative incidence of breast cancer at 25 years of follow-up of 30%.[28,30]

Risk of Breast Cancer and Histology of Benign Breast Lesions

No increased risk, relative risk ~1.3	*Nonproliferative changes:* including cysts and ductal ectasia, mild hyperplasia, simple fibroadenoma, mastitis, granuloma, diabetic mastopathy
Small increased risk, or relative risk 1.5–2.0	*Proliferative without atypia:* including usual ductal hyperplasia, complex fibroadenoma, papilloma
Moderate increased risk, or relative risk >2.0 to ~4.2	*Proliferative with atypia:* including atypical ductal hyperplasia and atypical lobular hyperplasia

Source: Santen RJ, Mansel R. Benign breast disorders. *N Engl J Med.* 2005;353:275; Hartmann LC, Sellers TA, Frost MH, et al. Benign breast disorders and the risk of breast cancer. *N Engl J Med.* 2005;353:229.

Breast Density.   Breast density on mammograms commands increasing importance as a strong independent risk factor for breast cancer—surpassed only by age and BRCA status.[7,31–33] On mammograms, stromal and epithelial fibroglandular tissue appears white or dense, whereas fat tissue appears dark. Studies show that when radiologic density, expressed as a percentage of breast area, reaches 60% to 75% of breast tissue, the relative risk of breast cancer increases four- to sixfold, in part related to the "masking effect" of breast density on smaller cancers, which have the same x-ray attenuation as fibroglandular breast tissue.[32,34] Up to 50% of women undergoing mammography have either heterogeneously dense or extremely dense breasts.[31] Breast density is influenced by a number of variables: inherited genetic factors; reproductive factors such as pregnancy, lactation, and menopause; height; and endogenous hormone exposure. In women with predominantly fatty tissue, mammograms have a sensitivity and specificity of 88% and 96% for detecting breast cancer, compared to 62% and 89% for women with high density.[35]

Centers using digital technology include breast density in their mammography reports. Counseling women about breast density is important because many women are not aware of this risk factor and the need for regular surveillance. Knowledge of breast density may also affect patient decisions about using HRT.

Recommendations for Screening and Chemoprevention.   Mammography combined with the CBE are the most common screening modalities; however, recommendations from professional groups vary about how to screen, when to start screening, and screening intervals, as shown on the next page. The evidence and rationale for decisions about screening bear thoughtful review of the balance of benefits and risks. For mammography, experts commonly raise concerns about *overdiagnosis,* defined as detection of lesions on mammogram that would not otherwise be detected or pathologic during a woman's lifetime. Estimates of overdiagnosis range from 0% to 50%, although some claim that they primarily reflect variations in study follow-up time and adjustment for screening lead time and incidence trends.[36–39] In 2014, the Canadian National Breast Screening study reported the same 25-year cumulative mortality from breast cancer in a screening trial of almost 90,000 women aged 40 to 59 years randomized to either CBE plus five annual mammography screens or CBE and no mammography, with overdiagnosis of 22%, although some have questioned the equivalence of the study and control groups.[38,40] Changes in the recommended guidelines underscore the need for clinicians to be well informed as they counsel individual patients, particularly as more evidence emerges to guide risk-based screening.

Breast Cancer Screening Recommendations

	Mammography	Clinical Breast Examination	Breast Self-Examination
U.S. Preventative Services Task Force—average risk women (2016)	50–74 years—biennially <50 years—individualize screening based on patient specific factors ≥75 years—insufficient evidence to recommend	≥40 years—insufficient evidence to assess additional benefits and harms of CBE beyond screening mammography	Recommends against teaching BSE
American Cancer Society—average risk women (2015)	40–45 years—optional annual screening 45–54 years—annual screening ≥55 years—biennial screening with option to continue annual screens Continue screening if good health and life expectancy ≥10 years	Not recommended due to lack of evidence showing clear benefit	Not recommended due to lack of evidence showing clear benefit
American College of Obstetricians and Gynecologists	≥40 years—annually	20–39 years—every 1–3 years ≥40 years—annually	Encourage breast self-awareness

Sources: U.S. Preventive Services Task Force. Breast Cancer: Screening. January 2016. At http://www.uspreventiveservicestaskforce.org/Page/Document/UpdateSummaryFinal/breast-cancer-screening1?ds=1&s=BREAST CANCER Accessed 2.11.16; Oeffinger KC, Fontham ETH, Etzioni R, et al. Breast cancer screening for women at average risk: 2015 guideline update from the American Cancer Society. *JAMA*. 2015;314:1500. See also http://www.cancer.org/cancer/breastcancer/moreinformation/breastcancerearlydetection/breast-cancer-early-detection-acs-recs. Accessed November 14, 2015. American College of Obstetricians and Gynecologists. Practice bulletin No. 122: breast cancer screening. *Obstet Gynecol*. 2011;118(2 pt 1):372.

Mammography

Women Ages 40 to 50 Years.   Use of screening mammography in this age group has been controversial due to its lower sensitivity and specificity, possibly related to heterogeneous estrogen exposure in women still premenopausal; high numbers of false positives, approaching 9 out of 100 women;[12] and the high rate of resulting invasive procedures. Citing concerns about the net benefit in reduction of mortality, in 2009 and reaffirmed in 2016, the U.S. Preventive Services Task Force (USPSTF) changed its recommendation to *individual decision making,* stating that "the decision to start regular, biennial screening mammography before the age of 50 years should be an individual one and take patient context into account, including the patient's values regarding specific benefits and harms."[39,41] The American College of Physicians makes the same recommendation.[42] The American Cancer Society and the American Medical Association recommend annual mammography beginning at age 40 years.[38] Digital mammography performs better in younger women and women with higher breast density.

Women Ages 50 to 74 Years.   The USFSTF recommends *biennial screening mammograms* for women aged 50 to 74 years, stating that changing to biennial screening would reduce the harms of mammography screening by nearly half. Biennial screening appears to preserve 80% of the benefits of annual screening and averts about 40% of the false-positive results of annual testing, with similar late-stage disease rates at diagnosis and similar 10-year breast cancer-specific survival rates.[12] The American Cancer Society and the American Medical Association recommend annual mammography; the World Health Organization recommends mammography every 1 to 2 years. Mammography screening performs best in the 50–74 year age group, with a sensitivity of 77% to 95% and specificity of 94% to 97%.[42]

Women Ages 75 Years and Older. The USPSTF cites insufficient evidence for a firm recommendation, stating that "no women 75 years or older have been included in the multiple randomized clinical trials of breast cancer screening." The USPSTF, the American Cancer Society, and the American Geriatrics Society support *individual decision making* about continued screening, depending on coexisting conditions and anticipated 5-year survival.

Clinical Breast Examination. The USPSTF states that evidence supporting additional CBE beyond screening mammography is insufficient for establishing the balance of benefits and harms. This is also the position of the World Health Organization and, most recently, the American Cancer Society (2015). The American College of Obstetrics and Gynecology recommends CBE. Standardization of CBE technique would be helpful for both further research and practice. Sensitivity and specificity of CBE are 40% and 88% to 99% and heavily influenced by examiner experience, technique, and duration of the examination.[5,41,43]

Breast Self-Examination. The USPSTF recommends against teaching BSE due to evidence that it does not reduce mortality and may lead to a higher rate of benign breast biopsies.[39] The American Cancer Society (2015) recommends against regular BSE but states that all women should be familiar with how their breasts normally look and feel and should report changes to their health care provider right away. Some advocate BSE as a method for promoting *breast self-awareness,* whereby women report changes in breast appearance or texture promptly in place of routine formal examination, particularly in countries where mammography is not widely available. Some subgroups may be more likely to benefit from BSE, such as women at high risk.[44]

Magnetic Resonance Imaging. Studies of contrast-enhanced MRI for *screening* have focused only on high-risk populations; breast MRI has not yet been evaluated for screening in the general population. Sensitivity is reported at 77%, almost double that of mammograms, but there are twice the number of false positives.[12,41] The American Cancer Society convened an expert panel in 2007, which issued new screening recommendations for use of MRI for women at high risk for breast cancer.[7] The Society recommends annual screening with MRI and mammogram beginning at age 30 years for women at high lifetime risk of breast cancer, or above 20%, as defined by the criteria below. Women at moderate lifetime risk (15% to 20%) are urged to discuss MRI screening with their provider. The USPSTF has concluded that evidence is insufficient to determine the utility of MRI for screening. Expertise in reading MRIs varies across centers and should be considered when making recommendations about this examination, which requires special equipment.

See Patient Instructions for the Breast Self-Examination—American Cancer Society, p. 441.

American Cancer Society Criteria for Adjunct MRI in High-Risk Women

High Lifetime Risk, or ≥20–25%	Moderate Lifetime Risk, or ≥15–20%
• Have a known *BRCA1* or *BRCA2* gene mutation • Have a first-degree relative (mother, father, brother, sister, or child) with a *BRCA1* or *BRCA2* gene mutation, but have not had genetic testing themselves • Had rediation therapy to the chest when they were between 10 and 30 years of age • Have Li-Fraumeni syndrome or Cowden syndrome, or have a first-degree relative with one of these syndromes	• Have a lifetime risk of breast cancer of 15% to 20%, according to risk assessment tools that are based mainly on family history • Have a personal history of breast cancer, ductal carcinoma in situ (DCIS), lobular carcinoma in situ (LCIS), atypical ductal hyperplasia, or atypical lobular hyperplasia • Have extremely dense breasts or unevenly dense breasts when viewed by mammograms

Source: American Cancer Society. *Breast Cancer Facts & Figures 2015–2016.* Atlanta: American Cancer Society Inc, 2015. Available at http://www.cancer.org/acs/groups/content/@research/documents/document/acspc-046381.pdf. Accessed February 5, 2015.

Chemoprevention

Selective Estrogen-receptor Modulators (SERMs). A growing literature documents both the efficacy and the underutilization of the SERMs tamoxifen and raloxifene for *primary prevention of ER-positive breast cancer in breast cancer–free women at high risk,* usually based on a 5-year Gail risk score ≥1.66%.[45,46] A systematic review of clinical trials found that tamoxifen and raloxifene reduce the incidence of ER-positive invasive breast cancer by 7 to 9 events in 1,000 women over 5 years, and that the reduction in incidence was greater with tamoxifen.[47] Studies have shown limited impact on the incidence of ER-negative breast cancers, noninvasive cancers, and mortality.[12,47] Significant side effects are higher with tamoxifen therapy, including thromboembolic events, endometrial cancer, gynecologic and urologic problems, vasomotor symptoms, and cataracts. Since 2002, and reaffirmed in 2014, the USPSTF has recommended discussion of chemoprevention for asymptomatic women aged ≥35 years at increased risk of breast cancer and low risk of adverse events.[48,49] Tamoxifen is approved for use in women of all ages, whereas raloxifene is approved only for postmenopausal women. National Health Survey data from 2010 continue to show that the prevalence of chemoprevention among eligible women in the United States is exceptionally low, perhaps due to clinician and patient concerns about side effects.[50]

Aromatase Inhibitors. Another class of drugs that holds promise for chemoprevention is currently under investigation—the aromatase inhibitors exemestane, anastrazole, and letrozole. In postmenopausal women, these drugs inhibit or inactivate the adrenal enzyme aromatase, which catalyzes the final step in tissue synthesis of estradiol from precursor androgens. Initial studies of exemestane and anastrazole have reported significant reductions in overall breast cancer incidence in high-risk postmenopausal women after 3 and 5 years of follow-up, respectively—0.19% for exemestane compared to 0.55% for placebo, a 65% relative reduction, and 2% for anastrazole compared to 4% for placebo, a hazard ratio of 47%.[51,52] Aromatase inhibitors do not appear to increase the risk of thromboembolic events or endometrial cancers, but do increase the risk of osteoporosis and fractures.

Counseling Women About Breast Cancer

The Challenges of Communicating Risks and Benefits. As breast cancer screening and prevention options become more complex, clinicians should consider how best to express statistics on risks and benefits in terms that patients can easily understand. Framing, or presenting the same information in terms of either increased benefit or decreased harm, is one of several ways of presenting data that can compromise informed consent. For example, Elmore[53] recommends that, instead of reporting a Gail model risk of diagnosis of breast cancer in 5 years as 1.1%, explaining that only 11 out of 1,000 women would get such a diagnosis is easier for patients to grasp. Likewise, using the notion of *absolute risk* may be preferable to using *relative risk* to increase patients' comprehension. For example, relative risk of developing breast cancer among women using combined estrogen and progesterone has been reported as 1.26, or a 26% increased risk in users compared to nonusers.[7,54] Alternatively, among 10,000 users over 5.2 years, the expected number of breast cancers is 38, compared to 30 in 10,000 nonusers. The 26% increased risk results in a total of 8 additional cases of breast cancer over 5.2 years.

Websites for Breast Cancer Information. Encourage your patients to pursue breast cancer–related information from recommended sources to help them make informed choices during shared decision making.

Breast Cancer Websites

Calculators for Assessing Risk of Breast Cancer

- Gail model; updated for African American women: http://www.cancer.gov/bcrisktool/
- BRCAPRO model for probability of BRCA 1 and BRCA2 mutation: http://bcb.dfci.harvard.edu/bayesmendel/software.php
- Centers for Disease Control and Prevention Division of Cancer Prevention and Control—Know BRCA Tool: https://www.knowbrca.org/
- Centers for Disease Control and Prevention Division of Cancer Prevention and Control—Help Women Know: BRCA: https://www.knowbrca.org/Provider

Breast Self-Examination Tutorial

- http://ww5.komen.org/breast-cancer/breatselfawareness.html

National Guidelines for Breast Cancer Screening

- National Guideline Clearinghouse: http://www.guidelines.gov (enter "breast cancer")

Randomized Clinical Trials of New Modalities in Breast Cancer Screening

- National Institutes of Health: https://clinicaltrials.gov/

All websites accessed May 6, 2015.

Techniques of Examination

The Female Breast

Clinical investigation has shown that examiner experience and technique significantly affect the efficacy of the CBE. Clinicians are advised to adopt a more standardized approach, especially for palpation, and to use a systemic up-and-down search pattern, varying palpation pressure, and a circular motion with the fingerpads.[5,41,55] For screening examinations, the length of time spent on palpation is one of the most important factors in detecting suspicious changes, with highest sensitivity when examiners spend 5 to 10 minutes for the examination of both breasts.[56,57] When examination time falls, especially for clinicians in practice compared to trained examiners in clinical trials, sensitivity for detection of breast cancer drops from the 65% range to 28% to 35%, with the attendant hazards of high numbers of false positives.[55,56,58] Experts concur on the importance of the CBE for women with symptoms or a palpable mass, as mammography in women with self-reported or palpable masses may miss up to 13% of invasive cancers.[59]

As you begin the examination, take a courteous gentle approach. Let the patient know that you are about to examine her breasts. This may be a good time to ask if she has noticed any lumps or other breast problems and enhance her awareness of screening guidelines, including techniques for self-examination, if requested. Because breasts tend to swell and become more nodular before menses from increasing estrogen stimulation, the best time for examination is 5 to 7 days *after* the onset of menstruation. Nodules appearing during the premenstrual phase should be re-evaluated at this later time.

Inspection. Adequate inspection initially requires full exposure of the chest, but later in the examination, cover one breast while you are palpating the other. Inspect the breasts and nipples with the patient in the sitting position and disrobed to the waist (Fig. 10-7). A thorough examination of the breasts includes careful inspection for skin changes, symmetry, contours, and retraction in four views—arms at sides, arms over head, arms pressed against hips, and leaning forward. When examining an adolescent girl, assess her breast development according to the Tanner sex maturity ratings described on pages 896–897.

Arms at Sides. Note the clinical features listed below.

■ The *appearance of the skin,* including:

  ■ Color

  ■ Thickening of the skin and unusually prominent pores, which may accompany lymphatic obstruction

---

The most significant risk factors for breast cancer are age, BRCA status, and breast density on mammogram. Personal history of breast cancer, family history, and reproductive factors affecting duration of uninterrupted estrogen exposure are also important. For numerous additional risk factors, see also Breast Cancer in Women: Factors That Increase Relative Risk, pp. 425–426.

See Patient Instructions for the Breast Self-Examination, p. 442.

Redness suggests local infection or inflammatory carcinoma.

Thickening and prominent pores suggest breast cancer.

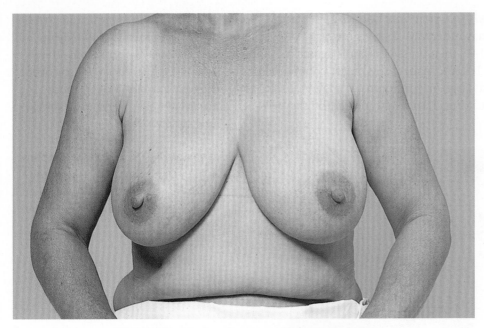

FIGURE 10-7. **Inspect with arms at sides.**

■ *Size and symmetry of the breasts.* Some differences in the size of the breasts and areolae are common and usually normal, as shown in the photograph below.

■ *Contour of the breasts.* Look for changes such as masses, dimpling, or flattening. Compare one side with the other.

Flattening of the normally convex breast suggests cancer. See Table 10-2, Visible Signs of Breast Cancer, p. 445.

■ The characteristics of the nipples, including size and shape, direction in which they point, any rashes or ulceration, or any discharge.

Asymmetry due to change in nipple direction suggests an underlying cancer. Eczematous changes with rash, scaling, or ulceration on the nipple extending to the areola occurs in *Paget disease of the breast,* associated with underlying ductal or lobular carcinoma (see p. 445).[60]

Occasionally, the nipple is *inverted,* or points inward, depressed below the areolar surface. It may be enveloped by folds of areolar skin, as shown in Figure 10-8, but can be moved out from its sulcus. It is usually a normal variant of no clinical consequence, except for possible difficulty when breastfeeding.

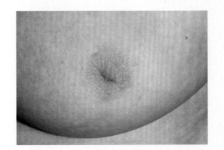

FIGURE 10-8. **Inverted nipple.**

A nipple pulled inward, tethered by underlying ducts signals *nipple retraction* from a possible underlying cancer. The retracted nipple may be depressed, flat, broad, or thickened.

Arms Over Head; Hands Pressed Against Hips; Leaning Forward. To bring out dimpling or retraction that may otherwise be invisible, ask the patient to raise her arms over her head (Fig. 10-9), then press her hands against her hips to contract the pectoral muscles (Fig. 10-10). Inspect the breast contours carefully in each position. If the breasts are large or pendulous, it may be useful to have the patient stand and lean forward (Fig. 10-11), supported by the back of the chair or the examiner's hands.

Breast dimpling or retraction in these positions suggests an underlying cancer. Cancers with fibrous strands attached to the skin and fascia over the pectoral muscles may cause inward dimpling of the skin during muscle contraction.

Occasionally, these signs accompany benign conditions such as posttraumatic fat necrosis or mammary duct ectasia, but should always be further evaluated.

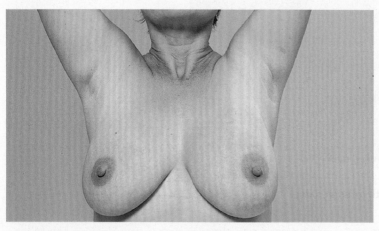

FIGURE 10-9. Inspect with arms over head.

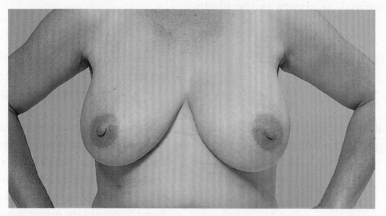

FIGURE 10-10. Inspect with hands pressed against hips.

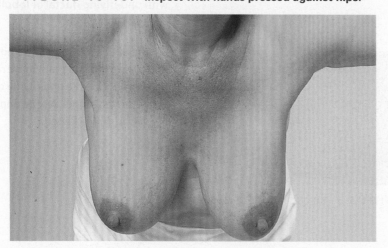

FIGURE 10-11. Inspect while leaning forward.

This position may reveal asymmetry or retraction of the breast, areola, or nipple that is not otherwise visible, suggesting an underlying cancer. See Table10-2, Visible Signs of Breast Cancer, p. 445.

Palpation.   Palpation is best performed when the breast tissue is flattened. The patient should be supine. Palpate the rectangular area extending from the clavicle to the inframammary fold or bra line, and from the midsternal line to the posterior axillary line and well into the axilla to ensure that you examine the tail of the breast.

A thorough examination takes at least 3 minutes for each breast. Use the *pads* of the 2nd, 3rd, and 4th fingers, keeping the fingers slightly flexed. It is important to be *systematic*. The *vertical strip pattern* shown in Figure 10-12 is currently the best validated technique for detecting breast masses.[55] Palpate in *small, concentric circles* applying light, medium, and deep pressure at each examining point. Press more firmly to reach the deeper tissues of a large breast. Examine the entire breast, including the periphery, tail, and axilla.

When pressing deeply on the breast, a normal rib can be mistaken for a hard breast mass.

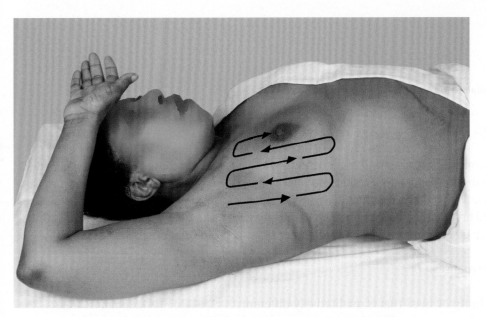

FIGURE 10-12.   **Vertical strip pattern—lateral breast.**

- *Examining the lateral portion of the breast.* To examine *the lateral portion of the breast,* ask the patient to roll onto the opposite hip, placing her hand on her forehead but keeping the shoulders pressed against the bed or examining table. This flattens the lateral breast tissue. Begin palpation in the axilla, moving in a straight line down to the bra line, then move the fingers medially and palpate in a vertical strip up the chest to the clavicle. Continue in vertical overlapping strips until you reach the nipple, then reposition the patient to flatten the medial portion of the breast.

Nodules in the tail of the breast in the axilla (the tail of Spence) are sometimes mistaken for enlarged axillary lymph nodes.

- *Examining the medial portion of the breast.* To examine *the medial portion of the breast,* ask the patient to lie with her shoulders flat against the bed or examining table, placing her hand at her neck and lifting up her elbow until it is even with her shoulder (Fig. 10-13). Palpate in a straight line down from the nipple to the bra line, then back to the clavicle, continuing in vertical overlapping strips to the midsternum.

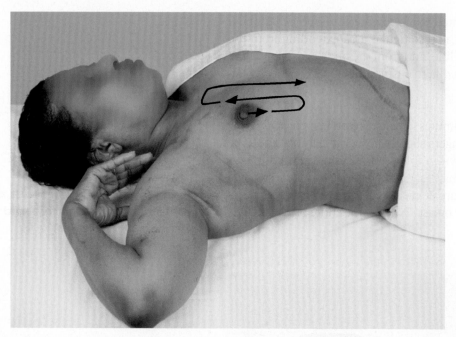

FIGURE 10-13. **Vertical strip pattern—medial breast.**

Examine the breast tissue carefully for:

- *Consistency* of the tissues. Normal consistency varies widely, depending on the proportions of firmer glandular tissue and soft fat. Physiologic nodularity may be present, increasing before menses. Note the firm inframammary ridge, which is the transverse ridge of compressed tissue along the lower margin of the breast, especially in large breasts. This ridge is sometimes mistaken for a tumor.

- *Tenderness* that may occur prior to menses.

- *Nodules.* Palpate carefully for any lump or mass that is qualitatively different from or larger than the rest of the breast tissue. This is sometimes called a *dominant mass* that may be pathologic when evaluated by mammogram, aspiration, or biopsy. Assess and describe the characteristics of any nodule:

  - *Location*—by quadrant or clock, with centimeters from the nipple

  - *Size*—in centimeters

  - *Shape*—round or cystic, disclike, or irregular in contour

  - *Consistency*—soft, firm, or hard

  - *Delimitation*—well circumscribed or not

  - *Tenderness*

  - *Mobility*—in relation to the skin, pectoral fascia, and chest wall. Gently move the breast near the mass and watch for dimpling.

Tender cords suggest mammary duct ectasia, a benign but sometimes painful condition of dilated ducts with surrounding inflammation and, at times, with associated masses.

See Table 10-1, Common Breast Masses, p. 444.

Hard irregular poorly circumscribed nodules, fixed to the skin or underlying tissues, strongly suggest cancer.

Check for cysts and inflamed areas; some cancers may be tender.

Next, try to move the nodule or mass while the patient relaxes her arm and then while she presses her hand against her hip.

A mobile mass that becomes fixed when the arm relaxes is attached to the ribs and intercostal muscles; if fixed when the hand is pressed against the hip, it is attached to the pectoral fascia.

Palpate each nipple, noting its elasticity (Fig. 10-14).

Thickening of the nipple and loss of elasticity suggest an underlying cancer.

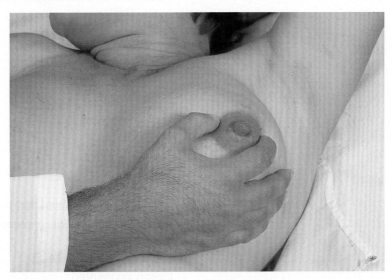

FIGURE 10-14. **Palpate the nipple.**

If there is a history of nipple discharge, try to determine its origin by compressing the areola with your index finger placed in radial positions around the nipple (Fig. 10-15). Watch for discharge expressed from any of the duct openings on the nipple surface. Note the color, consistency, and quantity of any discharge and the exact location where it appears.

Milky discharge unrelated to a prior pregnancy and lactation is *nonpuerperal galactorrhea*. Causes include *hyperthyroidism*, pituitary *prolactinoma*, and dopamine antagonists, including psychotropics and phenothiazines.

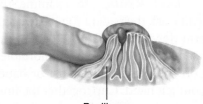

Papilloma

FIGURE 10-16. **Intraductal papilloma.**

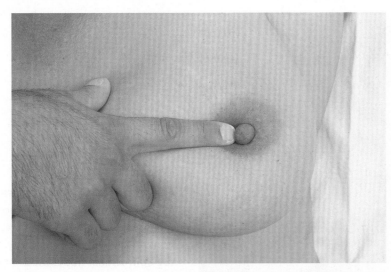

FIGURE 10-15. **Compress the areola for nipple discharge.**

Spontaneous unilateral bloody discharge from one or two ducts warrants further evaluation for *intraductal papilloma,* shown in Figure 10-16, *ductal carcinoma in situ,* or *Paget disease of the breast.* Clear, serous, green, black, or nonbloody discharges that are multiductal are usually benign.[3,6,61]

The Male Breast

Examination of the male breast may be brief, but is important. *Inspect the nipple and areola* for nodules, swelling, or ulceration. *Palpate the areola and breast tissue* for nodules. If the breast appears enlarged (>2 cm), distinguish between the soft fatty enlargement of obesity (*pseudogynecomastia*) and the benign firm disc of glandular enlargement (*gynecomastia*). Breast tissue in gynecomastia is often tender.

Gynecomastia arises from an imbalance of estrogens and androgens, sometimes drug related; it is not a risk factor for male breast cancer. A hard, irregular, eccentric, or ulcerating painless dominant mass suggests *breast cancer.*[4,62,63]

The Axillae

Although the axillae may be examined with the patient lying down, a sitting position is preferable.

Inspection. *Inspect the skin of each axilla, noting evidence of:*

- Rash

- Infection

Sweat gland infection from follicular occlusion (*hidradenitis suppurativa*) may be present.

- Unusual pigmentation

Deeply pigmented velvety axillary skin suggests *acanthosis nigricans*—associated with diabetes; obesity; polycystic ovary syndrome; and, rarely, malignant paraneoplastic disorders.

Palpation

Left Axilla. To examine the left axilla, ask the patient to relax with the left arm down and warn the patient that the examination may be uncomfortable. Support the patient's left wrist or hand with your left hand. Cup together the fingers of your *right hand* and reach as high as you can toward the apex of the axilla (Fig. 10-17). Place your fingers directly behind the pectoral muscles, pointing toward the midclavicle. Now press your fingers in toward the chest wall and slide them downward, trying to palpate the central nodes against the chest wall. Of the axillary nodes, the central nodes are most likely to be palpable. One or more soft, small (<1 cm), nontender nodes are frequently felt.

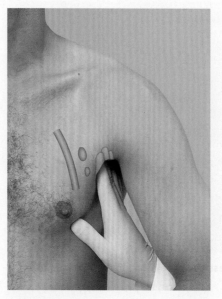

FIGURE 10-17. **Palpate the left axilla.**

Enlarged axillary nodes may result from infection of the hand or arm, recent immunizations or skin tests, or generalized lymphadenopathy. Check the epitrochlear nodes medial to the elbow and other groups of lymph nodes.

Right Axilla. Use your *left hand* to examine the right axilla.

If the central nodes feel large, hard, or tender, or if there is a suspicious lesion in the drainage areas for the axillary nodes, palpate for the other groups of axillary lymph nodes:

- *Pectoral nodes*—grasp the anterior axillary fold between your thumb and fingers, and with your fingers, palpate inside the border of the pectoral muscle.

- *Lateral nodes*—from high in the axilla, feel along the upper humerus.

- *Subscapular nodes*—step behind the patient and, with your fingers, feel inside the muscle of the posterior axillary fold.

- *Infraclavicular and supraclavicular nodes*—Also re-examine the infraclavicular and supraclavicular nodes.

Nodes that are large (≥1 to 2 cm) and firm or hard, matted together, or fixed to the skin or underlying tissues suggest malignancy.

Special Techniques

Examination of the Mastectomy or Breast Augmentation Patient.
The woman with a mastectomy warrants special care on examination.

Inspection. Inspect the mastectomy scar and axilla carefully for any masses, unusual nodularity, or signs of inflammation or infection. Lymphedema may be present in the axilla and upper arm from lymph drainage interrupted by surgery.

Masses, nodularity, and change in color or inflammation, especially in the incision line, suggest recurrence of breast cancer.

Palpation. Palpate gently along the scar—these tissues may be unusually sensitive. Palpate the breast tissue and incision lines bordering breast augmentation or reconstruction. Use a circular motion with two or three fingers. Pay special attention to the upper outer quadrant and axilla. Note any enlarged lymph nodes.

Instructions for the Breast Self-Examination.
For interested or high-risk patients, instruct the patient about how to perform the BSE. A high proportion of breast masses are detected by women examining their own breasts. For screening, the BSE has not been shown to reduce breast cancer mortality, but may promote health awareness and earlier reporting of breast changes or masses, which may reduce unnecessary testing and biopsies compared to monthly self-examination.[7,41] The BSE is best timed 5 to 7 days after menses, when hormonal stimulation of breast tissue is low.

Patient Instructions for the Breast Self-Examination—American Cancer Society

Lying Supine

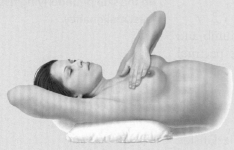

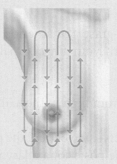

1. Lie down with a pillow under your right shoulder. Place your right arm behind your head.
2. Use the finger pads of the three middle fingers on your left hand to feel for lumps in the right breast. The finger pads are the top third of each finger. Make overlapping, dime-sized circular motions to feel the breast tissue.
3. Apply three levels of pressure in each spot: light, medium, and firm, using firmer pressure for tissue closest to the chest and ribs. A firm ridge in the lower curve of each breast is normal. If you're not sure how hard to press, talk with your health care provider, or try to copy the way the doctor or nurse does it.[a]

4. Examine the breast in an up-and-down or "strip" pattern. Start at an imaginary straight line under the arm, moving up and down across the entire breast, from the ribs to the collarbone, until you reach the middle of the chest bone (the sternum). Remember how your breast feels from month to month.
5. Repeat the examination on your left breast, using the finger pads of the right hand.
6. If you find any masses, lumps, or skin changes, see your clinician right away.

Standing

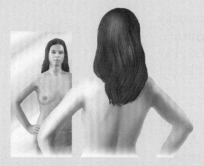

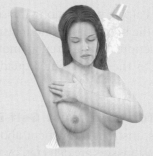

1. While standing in front of a mirror with your hands pressing firmly down on your hips, look at your breasts for any changes of size, shape, contour, or dimpling, or redness or scaliness of the nipple or breast skin. (The pressing down on the hips position contracts the chest wall muscles and enhances any breast changes.)

2. Examine each underarm while sitting up or standing and with your arm only slightly raised so you can easily feel in this area. Raising your arm straight up tightens the tissue in this area and makes it harder to examine.

Adapted from the American Cancer Society. American Cancer Society. Breast awareness and self-exam. Updated April 9, 2015. Available at http://www.cancer.org/cancer/breastcancer/moreinformation/breastcancerearlydetection/breast-cancer-early-detection-acs-recs-bse. Accessed May 7, 2015.

Recording Your Findings

Note that initially you may use sentences to describe your findings; later you will use phrases.

Recording the Breasts and Axillae Examination

"Breasts symmetric and smooth without nodules or masses. Nipples without discharge." (Axillary adenopathy usually included after Neck in section on Lymph Nodes; see p. 266.)
OR
"Breasts pendulous with diffuse fibrocystic changes. Single firm 1 × 1 cm mass, mobile and nontender, with overlying peau d'orange appearance in right breast, upper outer quadrant at 11 o'clock, 2 cm from the nipple."

These findings suggest possible breast cancer.

Table 10-1 Common Breast Masses

The three most common breast masses are *fibroadenoma* (a benign tumor), *cysts,* and *breast cancer.* The clinical characteristics of these masses are listed below. However, any breast mass should be carefully evaluated and usually warrants further investigation by ultrasound, aspiration, mammography, or biopsy. The masses depicted below are large for purposes of illustration. *Fibrocystic changes,* not illustrated, are also commonly palpable as nodular, rope-like densities in women aged 25 to 50 years. They may be tender or painful. They are considered benign and not a risk factor for breast cancer.

	Fibroadenoma	**Cysts**	**Cancer**
Usual Age (in Years)	15–25 years, usually puberty and young adulthood, but up to age 55 years	30–50 years, regress after menopause except with estrogen therapy	30–90 years, most common over age 50 years
Number	Usually single, may be multiple	Single or multiple	Usually single, although may coexist with other nodules
Shape	Round, disclike, or lobular; typically small (1–2 cm)	Round	Irregular or stellate
Consistency	May be soft, usually firm	Soft to firm, usually elastic	Firm or hard
Delimitation	Well delineated	Well delineated	Not clearly delineated from surrounding tissues
Mobility	Very mobile	Mobile	May be fixed to skin or underlying tissues
Tenderness	Usually nontender	Often tender	Usually nontender
Retraction Signs	Absent	Absent	May be present

Table 10-2 Visible Signs of Breast Cancer

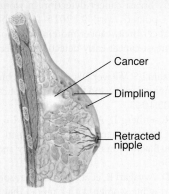

Retraction Signs

As breast cancer advances, it causes fibrosis (scar tissue). Shortening of this tissue produces *dimpling, changes in contour,* and *retraction or deviation of the nipple.* Other causes of retraction include fat necrosis and mammary duct ectasia.

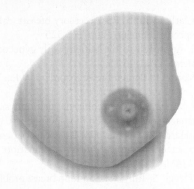

Abnormal Contours

Look for any variation in the normal convexity of each breast, and compare one side with the other. Special positioning may again be useful. Shown here is marked flattening of the lower outer quadrant of the left breast.

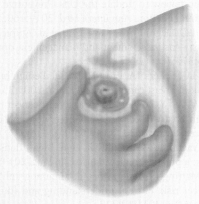

Skin Dimpling

Look for this sign with the patient's arm at rest, during special positioning, and on moving or compressing the breast, as illustrated here.

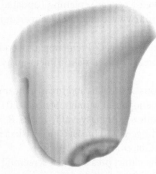

Nipple Retraction and Deviation

A retracted nipple is flattened or pulled inward, as illustrated here. It may also be broadened, and feels thickened. When involvement is radially asymmetric, the nipple may deviate or point in a different direction from its normal counterpart, typically toward the underlying cancer.

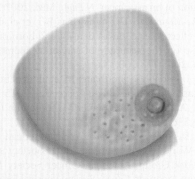

Edema of the Skin

Edema of the skin is produced by lymphatic blockade. It appears as thickened skin with enlarged pores—the so-called *peau d'orange* (orange peel) *sign.* It is often seen first in the lower portion of the breast or areola.

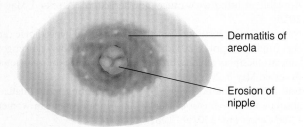

Paget Disease of the Nipple

This uncommon form of breast cancer usually starts as a scaly, eczema-like lesion on the nipple that may weep, crust, or erode. A breast mass may be present. Suspect Paget disease in any persisting dermatitis of the nipple and areola. Often (>60%) presents with an underlying in situ or invasive ductal or lobular carcinoma.

References

1. Loukas M, Clarke P, Tubbs RS. Accessory breasts: A historical and current perspective. *Am Surg.* 2007;73:525.

2. Carlson HE. Approach to the patient with gynecomastia. *J Clin Endocrinol Metab.* 2011;96:15.

3. Santen RJ, Mansel R. Benign breast disorders. *N Engl J Med.* 2005; 353:275.

4. Johnson RE, Murad MH. Gynecomastia: pathophysiology, evaluation, and management. *Mayo Clin Proc.* 2009;84:1010.

5. Barton MB, Harris R, Fletcher SW. Does this patient have breast cancer? The screening clinical breast examination: should it be done? How? *JAMA.* 1999;282:1270.

6. Salzman B, Fleegle S, Tully AS. Common breast problems. *Am Fam Physician.* 2012;86:343.

7. American Cancer Society. *Breast Cancer Facts & Figures 2013–2014.* Atlanta, GA: American Cancer Society Inc; 2013. Available at http://www.cancer.org/acs/groups/content/@research/documents/document/acspc-042725.pdf. Accessed May 1, 2015.

8. National Cancer Institute. Breast Cancer–Breast cancer treatment (updated April 8, 2015). Breast cancer prevention (updated February 27, 2015). Breast cancer screening (updated April 2, 2015). Available at http://www.cancer.gov/cancertopics/types/breast. Accessed May 2, 2015.

9. Walker K, Bratton DJ, Frost C. Premenopausal endogenous oestrogen levels and breast cancer risk: a meta-analysis. *Br J Cancer.* 2011;105:1451.

10. Key TJ. Endogenous oestrogens and breast cancer risk in premenopausal and postmenopausal women. *Steroids.* 2011;76:812.

11. Zeleniuch-Jacquotte A, Afanasyeva Y, Kaaks R, et al. Premenopausal serum androgens and breast cancer risk: a nested case-control study. *Breast Cancer Res.* 2012;14:R32.

12. Nattinger A. In the clinic: breast cancer screening and prevention. *Ann Intern Med.* 2010;152:ITC4.

13. National Cancer Institute. Male breast cancer treatment (updated March 27, 2015). Available at http://www.cancer.gov/cancertopics/pdq/treatment/malebreast/HealthProfessional. Accessed May 2, 2015.

14. Johansen Taber KA, Morisy LR, Osbahr AJ 3rd. Male breast cancer: risk factors, diagnosis, and management (review). *Oncol Rep.* 2010; 24:1115.

15. National Cancer Institute. Breast Cancer Risk Assessment Tool. Available at http://www.cancer.gov/bcrisktool. Accessed May 2, 2015.

16. National Cancer Institute. Genetics of breast and gynecologic cancers (updated April 3, 2015). Available at http://www.cancer.gov/cancertopics/pdq/genetics/breast-and-ovarian/HealthProfessional. Accessed May 3, 2015.

17. Gail MH, Costantino JP, Pee D, et al. Projecting individualized absolute invasive breast cancer risk in African American women. *J Natl Cancer Inst.* 2007;99:1782.

18. Evans DG, Howell A. Review: breast cancer risk-assessment tools. *Breast Cancer Res.* 2007;9:213.

19. Parmigiani G, Chen S, Iversen ES Jr, et al. Validity of models for predicting BRCA1 and BRCA2 mutations. *Ann Intern Med.* 2007; 147:441.

20. Smith RA, Manassaram-Baptiste D, Brooks D, et al. Cancer screening in the United States, 2015: a review of current American cancer society guidelines and current issues in cancer screening. *CA Cancer J Clin.* 2015;65:30.

21. American Cancer Society. American Cancer Society recommendations for early breast cancer detection in women without breast symptoms. Updated April 9, 2015. Available at http://www.cancer.org/cancer/breastcancer/moreinformation/breastcancerearlydetection/breast-cancer-early-detection-acs-recs. Accessed May 3, 2015.

22. Tice JA, O'Meara ES, Weaver DL, et al. Benign breast disease, mammographic breast density, and the risk of breast cancer. *J Natl Cancer Inst.* 2013;105:1043.

23. Boggs DA, Rosenberg L, Adams-Campbell LL, et al. Prospective approach to breast cancer risk prediction in African American women: The Black Women's Health Study model. *J Clin Oncol.* 2015;33:1038.

24. Chen J, Pee D, Ayyagari R, et al. Projecting absolute invasive breast cancer risk in white women with a model that includes mammographic density. *J Natl Cancer Inst.* 2006;98:1215.

25. Claus EB, Risch N, Thompson WD. Autosomal dominant inheritance of early-onset breast cancer. *Cancer.* 1994;73:643.

26. BaysMendel Lab. BRCAPRO. Available at http://bcb.dfci.harvard.edu/bayesmendel/software.php. Accessed May 3, 2015.

27. Nelson HD, Pappas M, Zakher B, et al. Risk assessment, genetic counseling, and genetic testing for BRCA-related cancer in women: a systematic review to update the U.S. Preventive Services Task Force recommendation. *Ann Intern Med.* 2014;160:255.

28. Hartmann LC, Degnim AC, Santen RJ, et al. Atypical hyperplasia of the breast—risk assessment and management options. *N Engl J Med.* 2015;372:78.

29. Hartmann LC, Sellers TA, Frost MH, et al. Benign breast disorders and the risk of breast cancer. *N Engl J Med.* 2005;353:229.

30. Dyrstad SW, Yan Y, Fowler AM, et al. Breast cancer risk associated with benign breast disease: systematic review and meta-analysis. *Breast Cancer Res Treat.* 2015;149:569.

31. Wang AT, Vachon CM, Brandt KR, et al. Breast density and breast cancer risk: a practical review. *Mayo Clin Proc.* 2014;89:548.

32. Boyd NF, Marting LJ, Yaffe MJ, et al. Mammographic density and breast cancer risk: current understanding and future prospects. *Breast Cancer Res.* 2011;13:223.

33. Nelson HD, Zakher B, Cantor A, et al. Risk factors for breast cancer for women aged 40 to 49 years: a systematic review and meta-analysis. *Ann Intern Med.* 2012;156:635.

34. Boyd NF, Guo H, Li M, et al. Mammographic density and the risk and detection of breast cancer. *N Engl J Med.* 2007;356:227.

35. Carney PA, Miglioretti DL, Yankaskas BC, et al. Individual and combined effects of age, breast density, and hormone replacement therapy use on the accuracy of screening mammography. *Ann Intern Med.* 2005;138:168.

36. Loburg M, Lousdal ML, Bretthauer M, et al. Benefits and harms of mammography screening. *Breast Cancer Res.* 2015;17:63.

37. Kalager M, Adami HO, Bretthauer M. Too much mammography. *BMJ.* 2014;348:g1403.

38. Smith RA, Saslow D, Sawyer KA, et al; American Cancer Society High-Risk Work Group; American Cancer Society Screening Older Women Work Group; American Cancer Society Mammography Work Group; American Cancer Society Physical Examination Work Group; American Cancer Society New Technologies Work Group; American Cancer Society Breast Cancer Advisory Group. American Cancer Society guidelines for breast cancer screening: update 2003. *CA Cancer J Clin.* 2003;53:141. Available at http://onlinelibrary.wiley.com/doi/10.3322/canjclin.53.3.141/full. Accessed May 4, 2015.

39. Nelson HD, Tyne K, Haik A, et al. Screening for breast cancer: an update for the U.S. Preventive Services Task Force. *Ann Intern Med.* 2009;151:727.

40. Miller AB, Wall C, Baines CJ, et al. Twenty five year follow-up for breast cancer incidence and mortality of the Canadian National Breast Screening Study: randomized screening trial. *BMJ.* 2014; 348:g366.

41. U.S. Preventive Services Task Force. Screening for breast cancer: U.S. Preventive Services Task Force recommendation statement. *Ann Intern Med.* 2009;151:716.

42. Qaseem A, Snow SV, Aronson M, et al. Screening mammography for women 40 to 49 years of age: a clinical practice guideline from the American College of Physicians. *Ann Intern Med.* 2007;146:511.

43. American College of Obstetricians and Gynecologists. Practice bulletin No. 122: breast cancer screening. *Obstet Gynecol.* 2011; 118(2 pt 1):372.

44. Wilke LG, Broadwater G, Rabiner S, et al. Breast self-examination: defining a cohort still in need. *Am J Surg.* 2009;198:575.

45. Vogel VG, Constantino JP, Wickerham DL, et al. Effects of tamoxifen vs. raloxifene on the risk of developing invasive breast cancer and other disease outcomes: the NSABP study of tamoxifen and raloxifene (STAR) P-2 trial. *JAMA.* 2006;295:2727.

46. Vogel VG, Constantino JP, Wickerham D, et al. Update of the National Surgical Adjuvant Breast and Bowel Project Study of Tamoxifen and Raloxifene (STAR) P-2 Trail. *Cancer Prev Res.* 2010; 3:696.

47. Nelson HD, Smith ME, Griffin JC, et al. Use of medications to reduce risk for primary breast cancer: a systematic review for the U.S. Preventive Services Task Force. *Ann Intern Med.* 2013;158:604.

48. U.S. Preventive Services Task Force. Breast Cancer—Recommendations of the U.S. Preventive Services Task Force. The Guide to Clinical Preventive Services 2014, p. 15. Available at http://www.uspreventiveservicestaskforce.org/Page/Name/tools-and-resources-for-better-preventive-care. Accessed May 6, 2015.

49. Moyer VA, on behalf of the U.S. Preventive Services Task Force. Medications for Risk Reduction of Primary Breast Cancer in Women: U.S. Preventive Services Task Force Recommendation Statement. *Ann Intern Med.* 2013;159:698.

50. Waters EA, McNeel TS, Stevens WM, et al. Use of tamoxifen and raloxifene for breast cancer chemoprevention in 2010. *Breast Cancer Res Treat.* 2012;134:875.

51. Goss PE, Ingle JN, Ales-Martinez JE, et al. Exemestane for breast cancer prevention in postmenopausal women. *N Engl J Med.* 2011; 364:2381.

52. Cuzick J, Sestak I, Forbes JF, et al. Anastrozole for prevention of breast cancer in high-risk postmenopausal women (IBIS-II): an international, double-blind, randomised placebo-controlled trial. *Lancet.* 2014;383(9922):1041.

53. Elmore JG, Gigerenzer G. Benign breast disease: the risks of communicating risk (editorial). *N Engl J Med.* 2005;353:297.

54. Roussouw JE, Anderson GL, Prentice RL, et al. Risks and benefits of estrogen plus progestin in healthy postmenopausal women: principal results from the Women's Health Initiative randomized controlled trial. *JAMA.* 2002;288:321.

55. Barton MB, Elmore JG. Pointing the way to informed medical decision making: test characteristics of clinical breast examination. *J Natl Cancer Inst.* 2009;101:1223.

56. Fenton JJ, Barton MB, Geiger AM, et al. Screening clinical breast examination: how often does it miss lethal breast cancer? *J Natl Cancer Inst Monogr.* 2005;(35):67.

57. Miller AB, Baines CJ. The role of clinical breast examination and breast self-examination. *Prev Med.* 2011;53:118.

58. Chiarelli AM, Majpruz V, Brown P, et al. The contribution of clinical breast examination to the accuracy of breast screening. *J Natl Cancer Inst.* 2009;101:1236.

59. Bryan T, Snyder E. The clinical breast exam: a skill that should not be abandoned. *J Gen Intern Med.* 2013;28:719.

60. Sandoval-Leon AC, Drews-Elger K, Gomez-Fernandez CR, et al. Paget's disease of the nipple. *Breast Cancer Res Treat.* 2013;141:1.

61. Pearlman MD, Griffin JL. Benign breast disease. *Obstet Gynecol.* 2010;116:747.

62. Hines SL, Tan W, Larson JM, et al. A practical approach to guide clinicians in the evaluation of male patients with breast masses. *Geriatrics.* 2008;63:19.

63. Morcos RN, Kizy T. Gynecomastia: when is treatment indicated? *J Fam Pract.* 2012;61:719.

The Abdomen

The Bates' suite offers these additional resources to enhance learning and facilitate understanding of this chapter:

- Bates' *Pocket Guide to Physical Examination and History Taking,* 8th edition
- Bates' *Visual Guide to Physical Examination* (Vol. 13: Abdomen)
- thePoint online resources, for students and instructors: http://thepoint.lww.com

Anatomy and Physiology

Visualize or palpate the bony landmarks of the abdominal wall and pelvis, as shown in Figure 11-1: the *xiphoid process, iliac crest, anterior superior iliac spine, pubic tubercle,* and *symphysis pubis.* The *rectus abdominis muscles* become more prominent when the patient raises the head and shoulders or lifts the legs from the supine position.

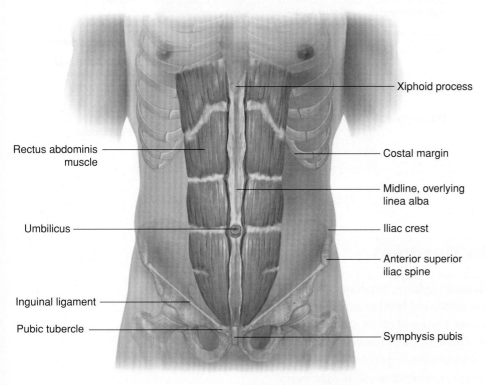

FIGURE 11-1. Landmarks of the abdomen.

Rectus abdominis muscle

Umbilicus

Inguinal ligament

Pubic tubercle

Xiphoid process

Costal margin

Midline, overlying linea alba

Iliac crest

Anterior superior iliac spine

Symphysis pubis

For descriptive purposes, the abdomen is often divided by imaginary lines crossing at the umbilicus, forming the right upper, right lower, left upper, and left lower quadrants (Fig. 11-2). Another system divides the abdomen into nine sections. Terms for three of them are commonly used: epigastric, umbilical, and hypogastric or suprapubic (Fig. 11-3).

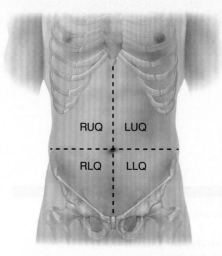

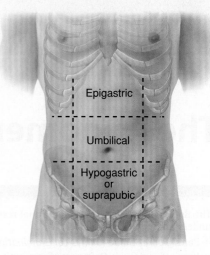

FIGURE 11-2. **Quadrants of the abdomen.**

FIGURE 11-3. **Sections of the abdomen.**

The *abdomen,* or the *abdominopelvic cavity,* lies between the thoracic diaphragm and the pelvic diaphragm and contains two continuous cavities, the abdominal cavity and the pelvic cavity, enclosed by a flexible multilayered wall of muscles and sheet-like tendons. This extended cavity houses most of the digestive organs, the spleen, and parts of the urogenital system (Fig. 11-4). Lining this cavity and folding over viscera such as the stomach and intestines are the *parietal* and *visceral peritoneum.*

Examine the abdomen, moving in a clockwise rotation; several organs are often palpable. Exceptions are the stomach and much of the liver and spleen which lie high in the abdominal cavity close to the diaphragm, where they are protected by the thoracic ribs beyond the reach of the palpating hand. The dome of the diaphragm lies at about the fifth anterior intercostal space.

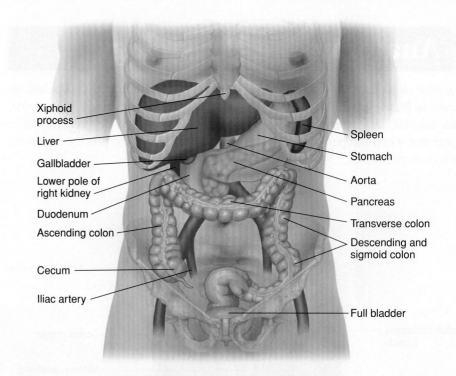

FIGURE 11-4. **Abdominal viscera.**

Abdominal Structures by Quadrant

Right upper quadrant	Liver, gallbladder, pylorus, duodenum, hepatic flexure of colon, and head of pancreas
Left upper quadrant	Spleen, splenic flexure of colon, stomach, body and tail of pancreas, and transverse colon
Left lower quadrant	Sigmoid colon, descending colon, left ovary
Right lower quadrant	Cecum, appendix, ascending colon, right ovary

- In the *right upper quadrant (RUQ),* the soft consistency of the *liver* makes it difficult to palpate through the abdominal wall. The lower margin of the liver, the liver edge, is often palpable at the right costal margin. The *gallbladder,* which rests against the inferior surface of the liver, and the more deeply lying *duodenum* are generally not palpable. Moving medially, the examiner encounters the rib cage with its *xiphoid process,* which protects the stomach. The *abdominal aorta* often has visible pulsations and is usually palpable in the upper abdomen, or *epigastrium.* At a deeper level, the *lower pole of the right kidney* and the tip of the *12th floating rib* may be palpable, especially in children and thin individuals with relaxed abdominal muscles.

- In the *left upper quadrant (LUQ),* the *spleen* is lateral to and behind the stomach, just above the left kidney in the left midaxillary line. Its upper margin rests against the dome of the diaphragm. The 9th, 10th, and 11th ribs protect most of the spleen. The tip of the spleen may be palpable below the left costal margin in a small percentage of adults (in contrast to readily palpable splenic enlargement, or *splenomegaly*). In healthy people the *pancreas* cannot be detected.

- In the *left lower quadrant (LLQ),* you can often palpate the firm, narrow, tubular *sigmoid colon.* Portions of the transverse and descending colon may also be palpable, especially if stool is present. In the lower midline are the *bladder,* the *sacral promontory* consisting of the bony anterior edge of the S1 vertebra (sometimes mistaken for a tumor), and, in women, the *uterus* and *ovaries.*

- In the *right lower quadrant (RLQ)* are bowel loops and the *appendix* at the base of the cecum near the junction of the small and large intestines. In healthy people, these are not palpable.

The *kidneys* are retroperitoneal (posterior) organs. The ribs protect their upper poles (Fig. 11-5). The *costovertebral angle (CVA),* formed by the lower border of the 12th rib and the transverse processes of the upper lumbar vertebrae, defines where to examine for kidney tenderness, called costovertebral angle tenderness (CVAT).

Continuous with the abdominal cavity, but angulated posteriorly, lies the funnel-shaped *pelvic cavity,* which contains the terminal ureters, bladder, pelvic genital organs, and, at times, loops of small and large intestine. These organs are partially protected by the surrounding pelvis.

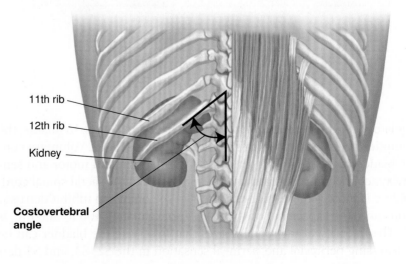

11th rib

12th rib

Kidney

Costovertebral angle

FIGURE 11-5. **Kidneys and costovertebral angle.**

The *bladder* is a hollow reservoir with strong smooth muscle walls composed chiefly of *detrusor muscle*. It accommodates roughly 400 to 500 mL of urine filtered by the kidneys into the renal pelvis and the ureters. Bladder expansion stimulates parasympathetic innervation at relatively low pressures, resulting in detrusor contraction and inhibition (relaxation) of the *internal urethral sphincter*, also under autonomic control. Voiding further requires relaxation of the *external urethral sphincter*, composed of striated muscle under voluntary control. Rising pressure triggers the conscious urge to void, but can be overcome by increased intraurethral pressure that prevents incontinence. Intraurethral pressure is related to smooth muscle tone in the internal urethral sphincter, the thickness of the urethral mucosa, and, in women, sufficient support to the bladder and proximal urethra from pelvic muscles and ligaments to maintain proper anatomical relationships. Striated muscle around the urethra can also contract voluntarily to interrupt voiding (Fig. 11-6).

A distended *bladder* may be palpable above the symphysis pubis.

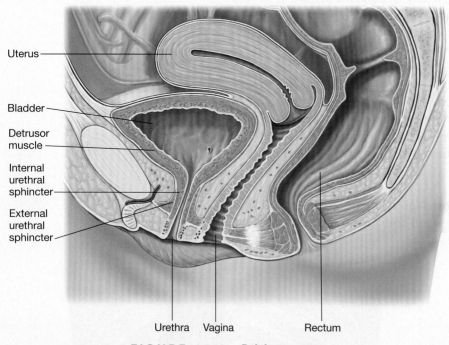

Uterus

Bladder

Detrusor muscle

Internal urethral sphincter

External urethral sphincter

Urethra   Vagina   Rectum

FIGURE 11-6. Pelvic anatomy.

Neuroregulatory control of the bladder functions at several levels. In infants, the bladder empties by reflex mechanisms in the sacral spinal cord. Voluntary control of the bladder depends on higher centers in the brain and motor and sensory pathways connecting the brain and the reflex arcs of the sacral spinal cord. When voiding is inconvenient, higher centers in the brain can inhibit detrusor contractions until the capacity of the bladder, approximately 400 to 500 mL, is exceeded. The integrity of the sacral nerves that innervate the bladder can be tested by assessing perirectal and perineal sensation in the S2, S3, and S4 dermatomes (see p. 764).

The Health History

Common or Concerning Symptoms

Gastrointestinal Disorders	Urinary and Renal Disorders
Abdominal pain, acute and chronic	Suprapubic pain
Indigestion, nausea, vomiting including blood (*hematemesis*), loss of appetite (*anorexia*), early satiety	Difficulty urinating (*dysuria*), urgency, or frequency
	Hesitancy, decreased stream in males
Difficulty swallowing (*dysphagia*) and/or painful swallowing (*odynophagia*)	Excessive urination (*polyuria*) or excess urination at night (*nocturia*)
Change in bowel function	Urinary incontinence
Diarrhea, constipation	Blood in the urine (*hematuria*)
Jaundice	Flank pain and ureteral colic

Gastrointestinal (GI) complaints rank high among reasons for office and emergency room visits. You will encounter a wide variety of upper GI symptoms, including abdominal pain, heartburn, nausea and vomiting, difficulty or pain with swallowing, vomiting of stomach contents or blood, loss of appetite, and jaundice. Abdominal pain alone accounted for more than 1.5 million outpatient visits and 11 million emergency room visits in 2011.[1,2] Lower GI complaints are also common: diarrhea, constipation, change in bowel habits, and blood in the stool, often described as either bright red or dark and tarry.

Numerous symptoms also originate in the *genitourinary tract:* difficulty urinating, urgency and frequency, hesitancy and decreased stream in men, high urine volume, urinating at night, incontinence, blood in the urine, and flank pain and colic from renal stones or infection. These are often accompanied by GI symptoms such as abdominal pain, nausea, and vomiting.

Your skills in history taking and examination, and clustering your findings, are important determinants of sound clinical reasoning and an astute differential diagnosis.

Patterns and Mechanisms of Abdominal Pain

Before exploring common symptoms, review the mechanisms and clinical patterns of abdominal pain. There are three broad categories of abdominal pain:

See Table 11-1, Abdominal Pain, pp. 488–489.

- *Visceral pain* occurs when hollow abdominal organs such as the intestine or biliary tree contract unusually forcefully or are distended or stretched (Fig. 11-7). Solid organs such as the liver can also become painful when their capsules are stretched. Visceral pain may be difficult to localize. It is typically palpable near the midline at levels that vary according to the structure involved, as illustrated on the next page. Ischemia also stimulates visceral pain fibers.

Visceral pain in the RUQ suggests liver distention against its capsule from the various causes of *hepatitis,* including *alcoholic hepatitis.*

Visceral pain varies in quality and may be gnawing, burning, cramping, or aching. When it becomes severe, sweating, pallor, nausea, vomiting, and restlessness may follow.

Visceral periumbilical pain suggests early *acute appendicitis* from distention of an inflamed appendix. It gradually changes to parietal pain in the RLQ from inflammation of the adjacent parietal peritoneum. For pain disproportionate to physical findings, suspect *intestinal mesenteric ischemia.*

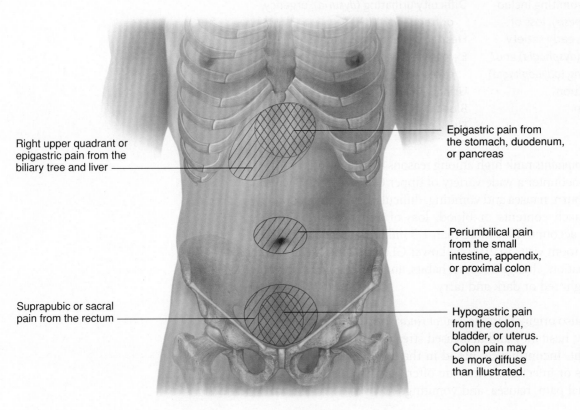

Right upper quadrant or epigastric pain from the biliary tree and liver

Epigastric pain from the stomach, duodenum, or pancreas

Periumbilical pain from the small intestine, appendix, or proximal colon

Suprapubic or sacral pain from the rectum

Hypogastric pain from the colon, bladder, or uterus. Colon pain may be more diffuse than illustrated.

FIGURE 11-7. **Types of visceral pain.**

■ *Parietal pain* originates from inflammation of the parietal peritoneum, called *peritonitis.* It is a steady, aching pain that is usually more severe than visceral pain and more precisely localized over the involved structure. It is typically aggravated by movement or coughing. Patients with parietal pain usually prefer to lie still.

In contrast to *peritonitis,* patients with colicky pain from a renal stone move around frequently trying to find a comfortable position.

■ *Referred pain* is felt in more distant sites which are innervated at approximately the same spinal levels as the disordered structures. Referred pain often develops as the initial pain becomes more intense and seems to radiate or travel from the initial site. It may be palpated superficially or deeply but is usually localized.

Pain of duodenal or pancreatic origin may be referred to the back, pain from the biliary tree, to the right scapular region or the right posterior thorax.

Pain may also be referred to the abdomen from the chest, spine, or pelvis, further complicating the assessment of abdominal pain.

Pain from *pleurisy* or *inferior wall myocardial infarction* may be referred to the epigastric area.

The Gastrointestinal Tract

Upper Abdominal Pain, Discomfort, and Heartburn. The prevalence of recurrent upper abdominal discomfort or pain is approximately 25% in the United States and other Western countries.[3] In recent years, consensus statements from expert societies have clarified the definitions and classification of numerous abdominal symptoms, particularly the 2006 Rome III criteria for functional GI disorders.[4,5] Understanding carefully defined terminology will help you identify the patient's underlying condition.

Acute Upper Abdominal Pain or Discomfort. For patients with abdominal pain, causes range from benign to life threatening, so take the time to conduct a careful history.

- First determine the *timing of the pain.* Is it *acute or chronic?* Acute abdominal pain has many patterns. Did the pain start suddenly or gradually? When did it begin? How long does it last? What is its pattern over a 24-hour period? Over weeks or months? Is the illness acute, or chronic and recurring?

- Ask patients to *describe the pain in their own words.* Pursue important details: "Where does the pain start?" "Does it radiate or travel anywhere?" "What is the pain like?" If the patient has trouble describing the pain, try offering several choices: "Is it aching, burning, gnawing...?"

- Then ask the patient to point to the pain. Patients cannot always clearly describe the location of pain in words. The quadrant where the pain is located helps identify the underlying organs that may be involved. If clothes interfere, repeat the question during the physical examination.

- Ask the patient to rank the *severity of the pain* on a scale of 1 to 10. Note that severity does not always help identify the cause. Sensitivity to abdominal pain varies widely and tends to diminish in older adults, masking acute abdominal conditions. Individual differences in pain thresholds and accommodation to pain during daily activities also affect ratings of severity.

- As you explore *factors that aggravate or relieve the pain,* pay special attention to body position, association with meals, alcohol, medications (including aspirin and aspirin-like drugs and any over-the-counter medications), stress, and use of antacids. Ask if indigestion or discomfort is related to exertion and relieved by rest.

Chronic Upper Abdominal Discomfort or Pain. *Dyspepsia* is defined as chronic or recurrent discomfort or pain centered in the upper abdomen, characterized by postprandial fullness, early satiety, and epigastric pain or burning.[3,5] *Discomfort* is defined as a subjective negative feeling that is nonpainful. It can include various symptoms such as bloating, nausea, upper abdominal fullness, and heartburn.

Studies suggest that neuropeptides such as 5-hydroxytryptophan and substance P mediate interconnected symptoms of pain, bowel dysfunction, and stress.[4]

In emergency rooms, 40% to 45% of patients have nonspecific pain, but 15% to 30% need surgery, usually for *appendicitis,* intestinal obstruction, or *cholecystitis.*[6]

Doubling over with cramping colicky pain signals a *renal stone.* Sudden knife-like epigastric pain often radiating to the back is typical of *pancreatitis.*[7-9]

Epigastric pain occurs with *gastro-esophageal reflux disease (GERD),* *pancreatitis,* and *perforated ulcers.* RUQ and upper abdominal pain are common in *cholecystitis* and *cholangitis.*[10]

Note that angina from inferior wall coronary artery disease may present as "indigestion," but is precipitated by exertion and relieved by rest. See Table 8-1, Chest Pain, pp. 330–331.

■ Note that bloating, nausea, or belching can occur alone but also can accompany other disorders. If these conditions occur alone, they do not meet the criteria for dyspepsia.

■ Many patients with upper abdominal discomfort or pain will have *functional,* or *nonulcer, dyspepsia,* defined as a 3-month history of nonspecific upper abdominal discomfort or nausea not attributable to structural abnormalities or peptic ulcer disease. Symptoms are usually recurring and present for more than 6 months.[5]

Many patients with chronic upper abdominal discomfort or pain complain of *heartburn, dysphagia,* or *regurgitation.* If patients report heartburn and regurgitation together more than once a week, the accuracy of diagnosing *GERD* is over 90%.[3,11,12]

■ *Heartburn* is a rising retrosternal burning pain or discomfort occurring weekly or more often. It is typically aggravated by foods such as alcohol, chocolate, citrus fruits, coffee, onions, and peppermint; or positions like bending over, exercising, lifting, or lying supine.

■ Some patients with GERD have atypical respiratory symptoms such as chest pain, cough, wheezing, and aspiration pneumonia. Others complain of pharyngeal symptoms, such as hoarseness chronic sore throat, and laryngitis.[13]

■ Some patients may have "*alarm symptoms,*" such as

  ■ Difficulty swallowing (*dysphagia*)

  ■ Pain with swallowing (*odynophagia*)

  ■ Recurrent vomiting

  ■ Evidence of GI bleeding

  ■ Early satiety

  ■ Weight loss

  ■ Anemia

  ■ Risk factors for gastric cancer

  ■ Palpable mass

  ■ Painless jaundice.

Bloating may occur with *lactose intolerance, inflammatory bowel disease,* or *ovarian cancer;* belching results from *aerophagia,* or swallowing air.

Multifactorial causes include delayed gastric emptying (20% to 40%), gastritis from *Helicobacter pylori* (20% to 60%), peptic ulcer disease (up to 15% if *H. pylori* is present), *irritable bowel disease,* and psychosocial factors.[3]

These symptoms or mucosal damage on endoscopy are the diagnostic criteria for GERD. Risk factors include reduced salivary flow, which prolongs acid clearance by damping action of the bicarbonate buffer; obesity; delayed gastric emptying; selected medications; and hiatal hernia.

Angina from inferior wall coronary ischemia along the diaphragm may also present as heartburn. See Table 8-1, Chest Pain, pp. 330–331.

A total of 30% to 90% of patients with asthma and 10% with specialty referral for throat conditions have GERD-like symptoms.

Patients who have uncomplicated GERD that fails empiric therapy, age >55 years, and "alarm symptoms" warrant endoscopy to evaluate possible *esophagitis,* peptic strictures, *Barrett esophagus,* or esophageal cancer. Of those with suspected GERD, ~50% to 85% have no disease on endoscopy.[14,15] Approximately 10% of patients with chronic heartburn have Barrett esophagus, a metaplastic change in the esophageal lining from normal squamous to columnar epithelium. In those affected, dysplasia on endoscopy increases the risk of esophageal cancer from 0.1% to 0.5% (no dysplasia) to 6% to 19% per patient year (high-grade dysplasia).[14]

Lower Abdominal Pain and Discomfort. Lower abdominal pain and discomfort may be acute or chronic. Asking the patient to point to the pain and characterize all its features, combined with findings on the physical examination, is key to identifying possible causes. Some acute pain, especially in the suprapubic area or radiating from the flank, originates in the genitourinary tract (see p. 463).

Acute Lower Abdominal Pain. Patients may complain of *acute pain* localized to the *RLQ*. Find out if it is sharp and continuous, or intermittent and cramping, causing them to double over.

RLQ pain or pain that migrates from the periumbilical region, combined with abdominal wall rigidity on palpation, is suspicious for *appendicitis.* In women, consider *pelvic inflammatory disease, ruptured ovarian follicle,* and *ectopic pregnancy.* Combining signs with laboratory inflammatory markers and CT scans markedly reduces misdiagnosis and unnecessary surgery.[16–19]

Cramping pain radiating to the right or LLQ or groin may be a *renal stone.*

When patients report acute pain in the *LLQ* or *diffuse abdominal pain,* investigate associated symptoms such as fever and loss of appetite.

LLQ pain, especially with a palpable mass, signals *diverticulitis.* Diffuse abdominal pain with abdominal distention, hyperactive high-pitched bowel sounds, and tenderness on palpation marks *small* or *large bowel obstruction* (see pp. 488–489); pain with absent bowel sounds, rigidity, percussion tenderness, and guarding points to *peritonitis.*

Chronic Lower Abdominal Pain. If there is *chronic pain* in the quadrants of the lower abdomen, ask about change in bowel habits and alternating diarrhea and constipation.

Change in bowel habits with a mass lesion warns of *colon cancer.* Intermittent pain for 12 weeks of the preceding 12 months with relief from defecation, change in frequency of bowel movements, or change in form of stool (loose, watery, pellet-like), linked to luminal and mucosal irritants that alter motility, secretion, and pain sensitivity suggests *irritable bowel syndrome.*[20]

Abdominal Pain and Associated Gastrointestinal Symptoms. Patients often experience abdominal pain in conjunction with other symptoms. Begin by asking "How is your appetite?" then pursue symptoms such as *indigestion, nausea, vomiting,* and *anorexia. Indigestion* is a general term for distress associated with eating that can have many meanings. Urge your patient to be more specific.

- *Nausea,* often described as "feeling sick to my stomach," may progress to retching and vomiting. *Retching* describes involuntary spasm of the stomach, diaphragm, and esophagus that precedes and culminates in *vomiting,* the forceful expulsion of gastric contents out of the mouth.

Anorexia, nausea, and vomiting accompany many GI disorders, including pregnancy, *diabetic ketoacidosis, adrenal insufficiency, hypercalcemia, uremia,* liver disease, emotional states, and adverse drug reactions. Induced vomiting without nausea is more indicative of *anorexia/bulimia.*

Some patients may not actually vomit but raise esophageal or gastric contents without nausea or retching, called *regurgitation*.

Regurgitation occurs in *GERD*, *esophageal stricture*, and *esophageal cancer*.

Ask about any vomitus or regurgitated material and inspect it if possible, noting the color, odor, and quantity. Help the patient to specify the amount: a teaspoon? Two teaspoons? A cupful?

Vomiting and pain indicate *small bowel obstruction*. Fecal odor occurs with *small bowel obstruction* and *gastrocolic fistula*.

Ask specifically if the vomitus contains any blood, and quantify the amount. Gastric juice is clear and mucoid. Small amounts of yellowish or greenish bile are common and have no special significance. Brownish or blackish vomitus with a "coffee grounds" appearance suggests blood altered by gastric acid. Coffee ground emesis or red blood is called *hematemesis*.

Hematemesis may accompany *esophageal* or *gastric varices*, *Mallory–Weiss tears*, or *peptic ulcer disease*.

Is there any dehydration or electrolyte imbalance from prolonged vomiting or significant blood loss? Do the patient's symptoms suggest any complications of vomiting, such as aspiration into the lungs, seen in debilitated, obtunded, or elderly patients?

Symptoms of blood loss such as light-headedness or syncope depend on the rate and volume of bleeding and are rare until blood loss exceeds 500 cm³.

■ *Anorexia* is loss or lack of appetite. Find out if it arises from intolerance to certain foods, fear of abdominal discomfort (or *"food fear"*), or distortions in self-image. Check for associated nausea and vomiting.

"Food fear" with abdominal pain and a slightly distended soft nontender abdomen are hallmarks of *mesenteric ischemia*.

Patients may complain of unpleasant *abdominal fullness* after light or moderate meals, or *early satiety*, the inability to eat a full meal. A dietary assessment or recall may be warranted (see Chapter 4, General Survey, Vital Signs, and Pain, pp. 117–118).

If fullness or early satiety, consider *diabetic gastroparesis*, anticholinergic medications, *gastric outlet obstruction*, and *gastric cancer*; if early satiety, also consider *hepatitis*.

Other Gastrointestinal Symptoms

Difficulty Swallowing (Dysphagia) and/or Painful Swallowing (Odynophagia). Less commonly, patients may report difficulty swallowing from impaired passage of solid foods or liquids from the mouth to the stomach, or *dysphagia*. Food seems to stick or "not go down right," suggesting motility disorders or structural anomalies. The sensation of a lump or foreign body in the throat unrelated to swallowing, called a *globus* sensation, is not true dysphagia.

For types of dysphagia, see Table 11-2, Dysphagia, p. 490.

Indicators of *oropharyngeal dysphagia* include drooling, nasopharyngeal regurgitation, and cough from aspiration. Gurgling or regurgitation of undigested food occurs in GERD, motility disorders, and structural disorders like *esophageal stricture* and *Zenker diverticulum*. Causes are generally mechanical/obstructive in younger adults and neurologic/muscular in older adults (stroke, Parkinson disease).[21]

Ask the patient to point to where the dysphagia occurs.

Pointing to below the sternoclavicular notch suggests *esophageal dysphagia*.

Pursue which types of foods provoke symptoms: solids, or solids and liquids? Establish the timing. When does the dysphagia start? Is it intermittent or persistent? Is it progressing? If so, over what time period? Are there associated symptoms and clinical conditions?

If solid foods, consider structural causes like *esophageal stricture*, webbing or *Schatzki ring*, and neoplasm; if solids and liquids, a motility disorder like *achalasia* is more likely.

Is there *odynophagia,* or pain on swallowing?

Consider esophageal ulceration from ingestion of aspirin or nonsteroidal anti-inflammatory agents, caustic ingestion, radiation, or infection with *Candida, cytomegalovirus, herpes simplex,* or *HIV.*

Change in Bowel Function.   To assess *bowel function,* start with open-ended questions: "How are your bowel movements?" "How often do they occur in a week?" "Do you have any difficulties?" "Have you noticed any change in stool pattern or appearance?" The range of normal frequency is broad, and can be as low as three bowel movements per week.

Some patients may complain of passing excessive gas, or *flatus,* normally about 600 mL/d.

Causes include aerophagia, ingestion of legumes or other gas-producing foods, *intestinal lactase deficiency,* and *irritable bowel syndrome.*

Diarrhea.   *Diarrhea* is defined as painless loose or watery stools during ≥75% of defecations for the prior 3 months, with symptom onset at least 6 months prior to diagnosis.[22,23] Stool volume may increase to >200 g in 24 hours.

See Table 11-3, Diarrhea, pp. 491–493.

- Ask about the duration. *Acute diarrhea* lasts up to 2 weeks. *Chronic diarrhea* is defined as lasting 4 weeks or more.

Acute diarrhea, especially foodborne, is usually caused by infection.[20] Chronic diarrhea is typically noninfectious in origin, as in *Crohn disease* and *ulcerative colitis.*

- Ask about the characteristics of the diarrhea, including volume, frequency, and consistency.

High-volume frequent watery stools are usually from the small intestine; small-volume stools with tenesmus, or diarrhea with mucus, pus, or blood occur in rectal inflammatory conditions.

- Is there mucus, pus, or blood? Is there associated *tenesmus,* a constant urge to defecate, accompanied by pain, cramping, and involuntary straining?

- Does diarrhea occur at night?

Nocturnal diarrhea is usually pathologic.

- Are the stools greasy or oily? Frothy? Foul-smelling? Floating on the surface because of excessive gas?

Oily residue, sometimes frothy or floating, occurs with *steatorrhea* (fatty diarrheal stools) from malabsorption in *celiac sprue, pancreatic insufficiency,* and *small bowel bacterial overgrowth.*

- Explore associated features that are important in identifying possible causes. These include current and alternative medications, especially antibiotics, recent travel, diet patterns, baseline bowel habits, and risk factors for immunocompromise.

Diarrhea is common with use of penicillins and macrolides, magnesium-based antacids, metformin, and herbal and alternative medicines. If recent hospitalization, consider *Clostridium difficile* infection.[24]

Constipation.   Ask about stool characteristics identified by the Rome III criteria, which stipulate that constipation should be present for the last 3 months

See Table 11-4, Constipation, p. 494.

with symptom onset at least 6 months prior to diagnosis and meet at least two of the following conditions: fewer than three bowel movements per week; 25% or more defecations with either straining or sensation of incomplete evacuation; lumpy or hard stools; or manual facilitation.[22,23]

Types of *primary* or *functional constipation* are normal transit, slow transit, impaired expulsion (from pelvic floor disorders), and constipation-predominant irritable bowel syndrome. Secondary causes include medications and conditions like *amyloidosis, diabetes,* and CNS disorders.[25,26]

- Check if the patient actually looks at the stool and can describe its color and bulk.

Thin, pencil-like stool occurs in an obstructing "apple-core" lesion of the sigmoid colon.

- What remedies has the patient tried? Do medications or stress play a role? Are there associated systemic disorders?

Anticholinergic agents, calcium channel blockers, iron supplements, and opiates can cause constipation. Constipation also occurs with *diabetes, hypothyroidism, hypercalcemia, multiple sclerosis, Parkinson disease,* and *systemic sclerosis.*

- Occasionally, there is no passage of either feces or gas, or *obstipation.*

Obstipation signifies *intestinal obstruction.*

- Inquire about the color of stools. Is there *melena,* or black tarry stools, or *hematochezia,* stools that are red or maroon-colored? Determine the quantity and frequency of any blood.

See Table 11-5, Black and Bloody Stools, p. 495.

Melena may appear with as little as 100 mL of blood from *upper GI bleeding;* hematochezia, if more than 1,000 mL of blood, is usually from *lower GI bleeding,* but if massive can have an upper GI source.

- Is the blood mixed in with stool or on the surface? Does the blood appear as streaks on the toilet paper or is it more copious?

Blood on the surface or toilet paper points to *hemorrhoids.*

Jaundice. *Jaundice* or *icterus,* is a striking yellowish discoloration of the skin and sclerae from increased levels of bilirubin, a bile pigment derived chiefly from the breakdown of hemoglobin. Normally, the hepatocytes conjugate unconjugated bilirubin with other substances, making the bile water soluble, and then excrete the conjugated bilirubin into the bile. The bile passes through the cystic duct into the common bile duct, which also drains the extrahepatic ducts from the liver. More distally, the common bile duct and the pancreatic ducts empty into the duodenum at the ampulla of Vater. Mechanisms of jaundice are listed on next page.

Mechanisms of Jaundice

- Increased production of bilirubin
- Decreased uptake of bilirubin by the hepatocytes
- Decreased ability of the liver to conjugate bilirubin
- Decreased excretion of bilirubin into the bile, resulting in absorption of *conjugated* bilirubin back into the blood

Predominantly unconjugated bilirubin occurs from the first three mechanisms, as in *hemolytic anemia* (increased production) and *Gilbert syndrome.*

Impaired excretion of conjugated bilirubin is seen in *viral hepatitis, cirrhosis, primary biliary cirrhosis,* and drug-induced cholestasis from drugs such as oral contraceptives, methyl testosterone, and chlorpromazine.

Intrahepatic jaundice can be *hepatocellular,* from damage to the hepatocytes, or *cholestatic,* from impaired excretion as a result of damaged hepatocytes or intrahepatic bile ducts. *Extrahepatic* jaundice arises from obstruction of the extrahepatic bile ducts, most commonly the common bile ducts.

Gallstones or *pancreatic, cholangio-, or duodenal carcinoma* may obstruct the common bile duct.

In patients with jaundice, pay special attention to the associated symptoms and setting in which the illness occurred. What was the *color of the urine* as the patient became ill? When the level of conjugated bilirubin increases in the blood, it may be excreted into the urine, turning the urine a dark yellowish brown or tea color. Unconjugated bilirubin is not water-soluble, so it is not excreted into urine. Is there any associated pain?

Dark urine indicates impaired excretion of bilirubin into the GI tract. Painless jaundice points to malignant obstruction of the bile ducts, seen in *duodenal* or *pancreatic carcinoma;* painful jaundice is commonly infectious in origin, as in *hepatitis A* and *cholangitis.*

Ask also about the *color of the stools.* When excretion of bile into the intestine is completely obstructed, the stools become gray or light colored, or *acholic,* without bile.

Acholic stools may occur briefly in *viral hepatitis;* they are common in obstructive jaundice.

Does the skin itch without other obvious explanation? Is there associated pain? What is its pattern? Has it been recurrent in the past?

Itching occurs in cholestatic or obstructive jaundice.

Ask about risk factors for liver diseases, such as the following.

Risk Factors for Liver Disease

- *Hepatitis:* Travel or meals in areas of poor sanitation, ingestion of contaminated water or foodstuffs (*hepatitis A*); parenteral or mucous membrane exposure to infectious body fluids such as blood, serum, semen, and saliva, especially through sexual contact with an infected partner or use of shared needles for injection drug use (*hepatitis B*); illicit injection drug use or blood transfusion (*hepatitis C*)
- *Alcoholic hepatitis* or *alcoholic cirrhosis* (screen patients carefully about alcohol use)
- *Toxic liver damage* from medications, industrial solvents, environmental toxins, or some anesthetic agents
- *Gallbladder disease* or *surgery* that may result in extrahepatic biliary obstruction
- *Hereditary disorders* in the Family History

The Urinary Tract

General questions include: "Do you have any difficulty passing urine?" "How often do you go?" "Do you have to get up at night? How often?" "How much urine do you pass at a time?" "Is there any pain or burning?" "Do you ever rush to urinate in time?" "Do you ever leak any urine? Or find yourself wet unintentionally?" Does the patient sense when the bladder is full and when voiding occurs?

Ask women if sudden coughing, sneezing, or laughing causes loss of urine. Roughly half of young women report this experience even before bearing children. Occasional leakage is not necessarily significant. Ask older men, "Do you have trouble starting your stream?" "Do you have to stand close to the toilet to void?" "Is there a change in the force or size of your stream, or straining to void?" "Do you hesitate or stop in the middle of voiding?" "Is there dribbling when you're through?"

Suprapubic Pain. Disorders in the urinary tract may cause pain in either the abdomen or the back. Bladder disorders may cause *suprapubic pain*. In *bladder infection*, pain in the lower abdomen is typically dull and pressure-like. In sudden overdistention of the bladder, pain is often agonizing; in contrast, chronic bladder distention is usually painless.

Dysuria, Urgency, or Frequency. Infection or irritation of the bladder or urethra frequently leads to *pain on urination*, usually felt as a burning sensation. Some clinicians refer to this as *dysuria*, whereas others use the term *dysuria* to refer to difficulty voiding. Women may report *internal urethral discomfort*, sometimes described as a pressure, or an *external burning* from the flow of urine across irritated or inflamed labia. Men typically feel a burning sensation proximal to the glans penis. In contrast, *prostatic pain* is felt in the perineum and occasionally in the rectum.

Other commonly associated urinary symptoms are *urgency*, an unusually intense and immediate desire to void, sometimes leading to involuntary voiding or *urge incontinence*, and *frequency*, or abnormally frequent voiding. Ask about any related fever or chills, blood in the urine, or any pain in the abdomen, flank, or back (see Fig. 11-8). Men with partial obstruction to urinary outflow often report *hesitancy* in starting the urine stream, *straining to void, reduced caliber and force of the urinary stream,* or *dribbling* as voiding is completed.[27]

Polyuria or Nocturia. Two additional terms describe important changes in patterns of urination. *Polyuria* refers to a significant increase in 24-hour urine volume, roughly defined as exceeding 3 L. It should be distinguished from *urinary frequency,* which can be either the high volume (polyuria) or low volume (infection). *Nocturia* refers to urinary frequency at night, sometimes defined as awakening the patient more than once; urine volumes may be large or small. Clarify the patient's daily total fluid intake and how much occurs in the evening.

See Table 11-6, Frequency, Nocturia, and Polyuria, p. 496.

Involuntary voiding or lack of awareness suggests cognitive or neurosensory deficits.

Stress incontinence arises from decreased intraurethral pressure (see pp. 497–498).

These problems are common in men with partial bladder outlet obstruction from *benign prostatic hyperplasia* or *urethral stricture.*

Pain from sudden overdistention accompanies acute urinary retention.

Painful urination accompanies *cystitis* (bladder infection), *urethritis,* and *urinary tract infections,* bladder stones, tumors, and, in men, *acute prostatitis.* Women report internal burning in *urethritis,* and external burning in *vulvovaginitis.*

Urgency suggests urinary tract infection or irritation from possible urinary calculi. Frequency is common in *urinary tract infection* and *bladder neck obstruction.* In men, painful urination without frequency or urgency suggests *urethritis.* Associated flank or back pain suggests *pyelonephritis.*[28,29]

See Table 15-3, Abnormalities of the Prostate, p. 623.

Causes of polyuria include the high fluid intake of *psychogenic polydipsia* and poorly controlled *diabetes,* the decreased secretion of antidiuretic hormone (ADH) of *central diabetes insipidus,* and the decreased renal sensitivity to ADH of *nephrogenic diabetes insipidus.*

Urinary Incontinence.

Up to 30% of older adults are concerned about *urinary incontinence,* an involuntary loss of urine that can be socially restricting and cause problems with hygiene. If the patient reports incontinence, ask if the patient is leaking small amounts of urine due to increased intra-abdominal pressure from coughing, sneezing, laughing, or lifting. Or following an urge to void, is there an involuntary loss of large amounts of urine? Is there a sensation of bladder fullness, frequent leakage, or voiding of small amounts but difficulty emptying the bladder?

See Table 11-7, Urinary Incontinence, pp. 497–498.

In *stress incontinence,* increased abdominal pressure causes bladder pressure to exceed urethral resistance—there is poor urethral sphincter tone or poor support of bladder neck. In *urge incontinence,* urgency is followed by involuntary leakage due to uncontrolled detrusor contractions that overcome urethral resistance. In *overflow incontinence,* neurologic disorders or anatomic obstruction from pelvic organs or the prostate limit bladder emptying until the bladder becomes overdistended.[30–32]

Bladder control involves complex neuroregulatory and motor mechanisms (see p. 452). Several central or peripheral nerve lesions affecting S2 to S4 can affect normal voiding. Does the patient sense when the bladder is full? And when voiding occurs? There are five broad categories of incontinence, including *functional* and *mixed incontinence.*

Functional incontinence arises from impaired cognition, musculoskeletal problems, or immobility. Combined stress and urge incontinence is *mixed incontinence.*

In addition, the patient's functional status may affect voiding behaviors even when the urinary tract is intact. Is the patient mobile? Alert? Able to respond to voiding cues and reach the bathroom? Is alertness or voiding affected by medications?

Hematuria.

Blood in the urine, or *hematuria,* is a major cause for concern. When visible to the naked eye, it is called *gross hematuria;* the urine may appear obviously bloody. Blood may be detected only during microscopic urinalysis, known as *microscopic hematuria;* smaller amounts of blood may tinge the urine with a pinkish or brownish cast. In women, be sure to distinguish menstrual blood from hematuria. If the urine is reddish, ask about medications that might discolor the urine. Test the urine with a dipstick and microscopic examination before you diagnose *hematuria.*

Myoglobin from *rhabdomyolosis* can also tinge the urine pink in the absence of red cells.

Flank Pain and Ureteral Colic.

Disorders of the urinary tract may also cause kidney pain, often reported as *flank pain,* at or below the posterior costal margin near the CVA. It may radiate anteriorly toward the umbilicus. Kidney pain is a visceral pain usually produced by distention of the renal capsule and typically dull, aching, and steady. *Ureteral colic* is a dramatically different severe colicky pain radiating around the trunk into the lower abdomen and groin, or possibly into the upper thigh, testicle, or labium. Ureteral pain results from sudden distention of the ureter and the renal pelvis. Ask about any associated fever, chills, or hematuria (Fig. 11-8).

Flank pain, fever, and chills signal *acute pyelonephritis.*

Renal or ureteral colic is caused by sudden obstruction of a ureter, for example, from renal or urinary stones or blood clots.

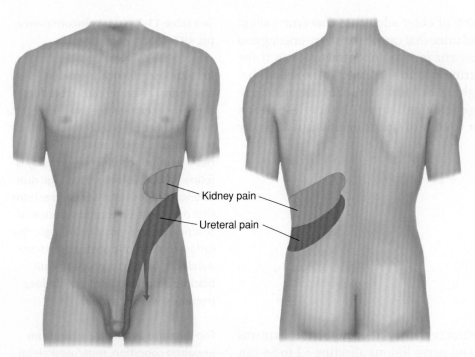

FIGURE 11-8. **Radiation of renal and ureteral pain.**

Health Promotion and Counseling: Evidence and Recommendations

Important Topics for Health Promotion and Counseling

- Screening for alcohol abuse
- Viral hepatitis: risk factors, vaccines, and screening
- Screening for colon cancer

Screening for Alcohol Abuse. The 2013 National Survey on Drug Use and Health (NSDUH) estimated that over 130 million Americans ages 12 years and older, or 52.2%, were current alcohol users based on consumption of alcoholic beverages in the past 30 days; 16.5 million, or 6.3%, were classified as heavy drinkers and 60.1 million, or 22.9%, were classified as binge drinkers.[33] Addictions are increasingly viewed as chronic relapsing behavioral disorders with substance-induced alterations of brain neurotransmitters resulting in tolerance, physical dependence, sensitization, craving, and relapse. The NSDUH data showed that about 17 million persons ages 12 years or older met criteria for alcohol use disorder (dependence or abuse), though only 1.4 million, or 7.9%, underwent treatment at a specialized facility.

Alert clinicians often notice clues of unhealthy alcohol use from social patterns and behavioral issues that are elicited during the history. The patient may report a family history of substance abuse, unstable relationships, difficulty holding jobs, or legal problems related to violent behaviors or driving under the influence.[34,35] Many clinical conditions are associated with chronic excessive alcohol use, including GI diseases, malignancies, cardiovascular diseases, mental health problems, nutritional deficiencies, and neurologic disorders. Excessive alcohol use has numerous short-term health risks, including injuries, violence (homicide, suicide, sexual assault, intimate partner violence), alcohol poisoning, and adverse effects on reproductive health (risky sexual behaviors, miscarriage, and fetal alcohol disorders). The abdominal examination may reveal classic findings of liver disease such as hepatosplenomegaly, ascites, or *caput medusae* (dilated abdominal veins).

See Chapter 3, Interviewing and the Health History, Alcohol and Illicit Drugs, pp. 65–108, and Chapter 5, Behavior and Mental Status, pp. 157–158.

Other classic findings include jaundice, spider angiomas, palmar erythema, Dupuytren contractures, asterixis, and gynecomastia.

Because early detection of at-risk behaviors may be challenging, the U.S. Preventive Services Task Force (USPSTF) recommends screening for risky or hazardous alcohol use and brief behavioral counseling interventions when indicated *for all adults in primary care settings,* including pregnant women (grade B).[36] Learn the approach to identifying problem drinking. If your patient reports drinking alcoholic beverages, ask the initial screening question about heavy drinking (see below) and follow up with the well-validated CAGE questionnaire, the Alcohol Use Disorders Identification Test (AUDIT), or the shorter AUDIT-C questionnaire.[35] Keep in mind cutoffs for problem drinking.

See Chapter 3, Interviewing and the Health History, for the CAGE questions, p. 97.

Screening for Problem Drinking

Standard Drink Equivalents: 1 standard drink is equivalent to 12 oz of regular beer or wine cooler, 8 ounces of malt liquor, 5 ounces of wine, or 1.5 ounces of 80-proof spirits.

Initial Screening Question: "How many times in the past year have you had 4 or more drinks a day (women), or 5 or more drinks a day (men)?"

Definitions of Drinking Levels for Adults—National Institute of Alcohol Abuse and Alcoholism[37]

	Women	Men
Moderate drinking	≤1 drink/d	≤2 drinks/d
Unsafe drinking levels (increased risk for developing an alcohol use disorder)[a]	>3 drinks/d and >7 drinks/wk	>4 drinks/d and >14 drinks/wk
Binge drinking[b]	≥4 drinks on one occasion	≥5 drinks on one occasion

[a]Pregnant women and those with health problems that could be worsened by drinking should not drink any alcohol.

[b]Brings blood alcohol level to 0.08 g%, usually within 2 hrs.

Tailor your recommendations to the severity of the drinking problem, ranging from brief behavioral counseling interventions to clinical therapy and/or long-term rehabilitation programs. Use the helpful National Institute of Alcohol Abuse and Alcoholism publications, "Clinician's Guide for Helping Patients Who Drink Too Much,"[38] and "Prescribing Medications for Alcohol Dependence."[39]

Viral Hepatitis: Risk Factors, Screening, and Vaccination.   The best strategy for preventing infection and transmission of hepatitis A and B is vaccination. Also, educate patients about how the hepatitis viruses spread and behavioral strategies to reduce the risk of infection. Screen high-risk groups for hepatitis B.

Hepatitis A.   Transmission of hepatitis A virus (HAV) is through a fecal–oral route. Fecal shedding followed by poor hand washing contaminates water and foods, leading to infection of household and sexual contacts. Infected children are often asymptomatic, contributing to spread of infection. To reduce transmission, advise hand washing with soap and water after bathroom use or changing diapers, and before preparing or eating food. Diluted bleach can be used to clean environmental surfaces.[40] HAV infection is rarely fatal—fewer than 100 deaths occur each year—and usually only in people with other liver diseases; it does not cause chronic hepatitis.[41]

CDC Recommendations for Hepatitis A Vaccination

- All children at age 1 year
- Individuals with chronic liver disease
- Groups at increased risk of acquiring HAV: travelers to areas with high endemic rates of infection, men who have sex with men, injection and illicit drug users, individuals working with nonhuman primates, and persons who have clotting factor disorders.[42]

The vaccine alone may be administered at any time before traveling to endemic areas.

Postexposure Prophylaxis.   Healthy unvaccinated individuals should receive either a hepatitis A vaccine or a single dose of *immune globulin* (preferred for those ≥age 40 years) within 2 weeks of being exposed to HAV. These recommendations apply to close personal contacts of persons with confirmed HAV, coworkers of infected food handlers, and staff and attendees (and their household members) of child care centers where HAV has been diagnosed in children, staff, or households of attendees.

Hepatitis B.   Hepatitis B virus (HBV) infection is a more serious threat than infection with hepatitis A. The fatality rate for acute infection can be up to 1% and HBV infection can become chronic.[43] Approximately 95% of infections in healthy adults are self-limited, with elimination of the virus and development of immunity. Risk of chronic HBV infection is highest when the immune system is immature—chronic infection occurs in 90% of infected infants and 30% of children infected before age 5 years. About 15% to 25% of those with chronic HBV infection die from cirrhosis or liver cancer, accounting for nearly 3,000 deaths each year in the United States. Most persons with chronic infection are asymptomatic until the onset of advanced liver disease.

Screening. The USPSTF recommends screening for HBV in persons at high risk for infection (grade B), including those born in countries with a high endemic prevalence of HBV infection, persons with HIV, injection drug users, men who have sex with men, and household contacts or sexual partners of HBV-infected persons.[44] The CDC recommends screening all pregnant women, ideally in the first trimester, and universal vaccination for all infants beginning at birth.[43] For adults, vaccine recommendations also target high-risk groups, including those in high-risk settings (see below).

CDC Recommendations for Hepatitis B Vaccination: High-Risk Groups and Settings

- *Sexual contacts,* including sex partners of hepatitis B surface antigen-positive persons, people with more than one sex partner in the prior 6 months, people seeking evaluation and treatment for sexually transmitted infections, and men who have sex with men
- *People with percutaneous or mucosal exposure to blood,* including injection drug users, household contacts of antigen-positive persons, residents and staff of facilities for the developmentally disabled, health care workers, and people on dialysis
- *Others,* including travelers to endemic areas, people with chronic liver disease and HIV infection, and people seeking protection from hepatitis B infection
- *All adults in high-risk settings,* such as sexually transmitted disease (STD) clinics, HIV testing and treatment programs, drug-abuse treatment programs and programs for injection drug users, correctional facilities, programs for men having sex with men, chronic hemodialysis facilities and end-stage renal disease programs, and facilities for people with developmental disabilities

Hepatitis C. There is no vaccination for hepatitis C, so prevention targets counseling to avoid risk factors. Screening should be recommended for high-risk groups.

Hepatitis C virus (HCV), transmitted mainly by percutaneous exposures, is the most prevalent chronic bloodborne pathogen in the United States. Anti-HCV antibody is detectable in just under 2% of the population, though prevalence is markedly increased in high-risk groups, particularly injection drug users.[45] Additional risk factors for HCV infection include blood transfusion or organ transplantation before 1992, transfusion with clotting factors before 1987, hemodialysis, health care workers with needle stick injury or mucosal exposure to HCV-positive blood, HIV infection, and birth from an HCV-positive mother. *Sexual transmission is rare.* Hepatitis C becomes a chronic illness in over 75% of those infected and is a major risk factor for subsequent cirrhosis, hepatocellular carcinoma, and need for liver transplant for end-stage liver disease.[45–47] However, the majority of persons with chronic HCV are unaware of being infected. Response to antiviral therapy (undetectable HCV RNA 24 weeks after completing treatment) ranges from 40% to over 90% depending on the viral genotype and the combination of drugs used for treatment. Consequently, the USPSTF has concluded that screening for hepatitis C infection is of moderate benefit for persons at high risk for infection as well as those born between 1945 and 1965 (grade B).[48]

Screening for Colorectal Cancer

Epidemiology. Colorectal cancer is the third most frequently diagnosed cancer among both men and women (over 140,000 new cases) and the third leading cause of cancer death (nearly 50,000 deaths) each year in the United States.[49] The lifetime risk of diagnosis with colorectal cancer is about 5%, while the lifetime risk for dying from colorectal cancer is about 2%.[50] The good news is that U.S. incidence and mortality rates have been gradually but steadily declining over the past three decades. These trends are attributed to changes in risk factor prevalence, such as decreased tobacco use; increased screening, which both prevents cancers and increases detection of early-stage curable cancers; and improved treatment.[51]

Risk Factors. The strongest risk factors for colorectal cancer are: increasing age; personal history of colorectal cancer, adenomatous polyps, or long-standing inflammatory bowel disease; and family history of colorectal neoplasia—particularly those with affected multiple first-degree relatives, a single first-degree relative diagnosed before age 60 years, or a hereditary colorectal cancer syndrome. Weaker risk factors include male sex, African American race, tobacco use, excessive alcohol use, red meat consumption, and obesity. Aside from age, persons without any strong risk factors are considered average risk—even if they have some of the weak risk factors. Overall, 90% of new cases and 94% of deaths occur after age 50 years[52]; the median age at diagnosis is 68 years and the median age at death is 74 years.[50] While the lifetime risk of colorectal cancer is extremely high in patients with hereditary syndromes, about 75% of colorectal cancers arise in people without any obvious hereditary risk or common exposures among family members.[53]

Prevention. The most effective prevention strategy is to screen for and remove pre-cancerous adenomatous polyps. Screening programs using fecal blood testing or flexible sigmoidoscopy have been shown in randomized trials to reduce the risk of developing colorectal cancer by about 15% to 20%.[54,55] Physical activity, aspirin and nonsteroidal anti-inflammatory drugs (NSAIDs), and postmenopausal combined hormone replacement therapy (estrogen and progestin) are also associated with decreased risk of colorectal cancer.[46–59] However, the USPSTF recommends against routinely using aspirin and NSAIDs for prevention in average-risk persons because the potential harms, including GI bleeding, hemorrhagic stroke, and renal impairment, outweigh the benefits (grade D).[60] Hormone therapy for cancer chemoprevention is not advised; women receiving combined therapy were actually more likely to present with advanced-staged colorectal cancers and appear to have a higher risk for colorectal cancer mortality.[61] Furthermore, hormone therapy is associated with increased risk of breast cancer, cardiovascular events, and venous thromboembolism.[62–64] There has been no convincing evidence that dietary changes or taking supplements can prevent colorectal cancer.[53]

Screening Tests. Screening tests include stool tests that detect occult fecal blood, such as fecal immunochemical tests, high-sensitivity guaiac-based tests, and tests that detect abnormal DNA. Endoscopic tests are also used for screening, including colonoscopy, which visualizes the entire colon and can remove polyps, and flexible sigmoidoscopy, which visualizes the distal 60 cm of the bowel. Imaging tests include the double-contrast barium enema and CT colonography. Any abnormal finding on a stool test, imaging study, or flexible sigmoidoscopy warrants further evaluation with colonoscopy. Screening programs using fecal blood testing or flexible sigmoidoscopy have been shown in randomized trials to reduce the risk colorectal cancer death by about 15% to 30%.[54,55] Although colonoscopy is the gold standard diagnostic test for screening, there is no direct evidence from randomized trials that screening with colonoscopy reduces colorectal cancer incidence or mortality. Complications of colonoscopy include perforation and bleeding;[65] patients are usually sedated during the procedure, but many are averse to the extensive bowel preparation required.

Guidelines. The USPSTF and a collaborative multiorganizational group, consisting of the American Cancer Society, the U.S. Multi-Society Task Force on Colorectal Cancer, and the American College of Radiology, both strongly endorse colorectal cancer screening and have issued screening guidelines.[66,67] The USPSTF, which gives a grade A recommendation for colorectal cancer screening in average-risk adults ages 50 to 75 years, suggests several screening options, and advises that routine screening stop at age 75 years (see below). The multiorganizational group additionally recommends using double-contrast barium enema or CT colonography every 5 years as well as the fecal DNA test. However, there is no evidence that screening with these tests will reduce colorectal cancer incidence or mortality. Performing digital rectal examination is not recommended for colorectal cancer screening.

U.S. Preventive Services Task Force: 2008 Screening Recommendations for Colorectal Cancer

- Adults ages 50 to 75 years—options (grade A recommendation)
  - High-sensitivity fecal occult blood testing (FOBT) annually, either a guaiac-based or fecal immunochemical test
  - Sigmoidoscopy every 5 years with high-sensitivity FOBT every 3 years
  - Screening colonoscopy every 10 years
- Adults ages 76 to 85 years—do not screen routinely (grade C recommendation)
  - Screening not advised because the benefits are small in comparison to the risks
  - Use individual decision making if screening an adult for the first time
- Adults older than age 85 years—do not screen (grade D recommendation)
  - Screening not advised because "competing causes of mortality preclude a mortality benefit that outweighs harms"

Although screening reduces colorectal cancer incidence and mortality, only about two thirds of the adult U.S. population has complied with recommended screening guidelines, and over a quarter has never been screened.[68] Colonoscopy is the most commonly used test, though people may prefer other tests like FOBTs because they are safer and easier to perform.[69] Keep in mind that the best screening test is the one that gets done!

Higher-risk persons, based on personal history of colorectal neoplasia or long-standing inflammatory bowel disease, or a family history of colorectal neoplasia, should begin screening at a younger age, usually with colonoscopy, and get more frequent testing than average-risk adults.[70]

Techniques of Examination

To begin, explain the steps for examining the abdomen to the patient and locate a good light. The patient should have an empty bladder. Pay special attention when draping to expose the abdomen, as pictured and detailed below.

Tips for Examining the Abdomen

- Make the patient comfortable in the supine position, with a pillow under the head and perhaps under the knees. Slide your hand under the low back to see if the patient is relaxed and lying flat on the table.
- Ask the patient to keep the arms at the sides or folded across the chest. When the arms are above the head, the abdominal wall stretches and tightens, which hinders palpation.
- *Draping the patient.* To expose the abdomen, place the drape or sheet at the level of the symphysis pubis, then raise the gown to below the nipple line just above the xiphoid process. The groin should be visible but the genitalia should remain covered. The abdominal muscles should be relaxed to enhance all aspects of the examination, especially palpation.
- Before you begin, ask the patient to point to any areas of pain so that you can examine these areas last.
- Warm your hands and stethoscope. To warm your hands, rub them together or place them under hot water.
- Approach the patient calmly and avoid quick unexpected movements. Avoid having long fingernails which can scratch or scrape the patient's skin.
- Stand at the patient's *right side* and proceed in a systematic fashion with inspection, auscultation, percussion, and palpation. Visualize each organ in the region you are examining. *Watch the patient's face for any signs of pain or discomfort.*
- If necessary, distract the patient with conversation or questions. If the patient is frightened or ticklish, begin palpation with the patient's hand under yours. After a few moments, slip your hand underneath to palpate directly.

Arching the back pushes the abdomen forward and tightens the abdominal muscles.

The Abdomen

Inspection. First, observe the general appearance of the patient—lying quietly, writhing with discomfort, or gripping one side.

From the right side of the bed, inspect the surface, contours, and movements of the abdomen. Watch for bulges or peristalsis. Try to sit or bend down so that you can view the abdomen tangentially (Fig. 11-9).

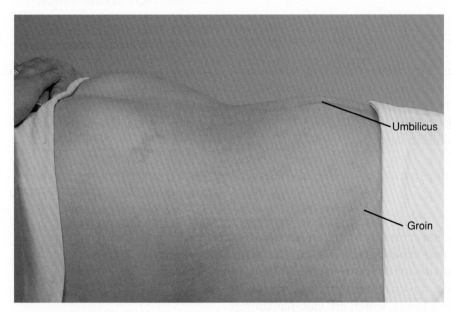

Umbilicus

Groin

FIGURE 11-9. Inspect the contours of the abdomen.

Note especially:

- *The skin*, including:

  - *Temperature.* Check if the skin is warm, or cool and clammy.

  - *Color.* Note any bruises, erythema, or jaundice.

  - *Scars.* Describe or diagram their location.

  - *Striae.* Old silver striae or stretch marks are normal.

    Pink–purple striae are a hallmark of *Cushing syndrome*.

  - *Dilated veins.* A few small veins may be visible normally.

    Dilated veins suggest portal hypertension from *cirrhosis (caput medusae)* or *inferior vena cava obstruction*.

  - *Rashes* or *ecchymoses*

    Ecchymosis of the abdominal wall is seen in intraperitoneal or retroperitoneal hemorrhage.

- *The umbilicus.* Observe its contour and location and any inflammation or bulges suggesting a ventral hernia.

  See Table 11-8, Localized Bulges in the Abdominal Wall, p. 499.

■ *The contour of the abdomen*

   ■ Is it flat, rounded, protuberant, or scaphoid (markedly concave or hollowed)?

See Table 11-9, Protuberant Abdomens, p. 500.

   ■ Do the flanks bulge, or are there any local bulges? Also survey the inguinal and femoral areas.

Observe for the bulging flanks of *ascites,* the suprapubic bulge of a distended bladder or pregnant uterus, and ventral, femoral, or inguinal hernias.

   ■ Is the abdomen symmetric?

Asymmetry suggests a hernia, an enlarged organ, or a mass.

   ■ Are there visible organs or masses? An enlarged liver or spleen may descend below the rib cage.

Inspect for the lower abdominal mass of an ovarian or a uterine cancer.

■ *Peristalsis.* Observe the abdomen for several minutes if you suspect intestinal obstruction. Normally, peristalsis is visible in very thin people.

Inspect for the increased peristaltic waves of *intestinal obstruction.*

■ *Pulsations.* The normal aortic pulsation is frequently visible in the epigastrium.

Inspect for the increased pulsations of an *abdominal aortic aneurysm* (AAA) or *increased pulse pressure.*

Auscultation. Auscultation provides important information about bowel motility. Auscultate the abdomen before performing percussion or palpation, maneuvers which may alter the characteristics of the bowel sounds. Learn to identify variations in normal bowel sounds, the changed sounds suggestive of peritoneal inflammation or obstruction, and *bruits,* which are vascular sounds resembling heart murmurs over the aorta or other arteries in the abdomen.

See Table 11-10, Sounds in the Abdomen, p. 501.

Bruits suggest vascular occlusive disease.

Place the diaphragm of your stethoscope gently on the abdomen. Listen for bowel sounds and note their frequency and character. Normal sounds consist of clicks and gurgles, occurring at an estimated frequency of 5 to 34 per minute. Occasionally you may hear the prolonged gurgles of hyperperistalsis from "stomach growling," called *borborygmi.* Because bowel sounds are widely transmitted through the abdomen, listening in one spot, such as the RLQ, is usually sufficient.

Altered bowel sounds are common in diarrhea, intestinal obstruction, *paralytic ileus,* and *peritonitis.*

   Abdominal Bruits and Friction Rub. If the patient has hypertension, auscultate the epigastrium and in each upper quadrant for *bruits.* Later in the examination, when the patient sits up, listen also in the CVAs.

A bruit in one of these areas that has both systolic and diastolic components strongly suggests *renal artery stenosis* as the cause of hypertension. A total of 4% to 20% of healthy individuals have abdominal bruits.[71]

Auscultate for bruits over the aorta, the iliac arteries, and the femoral arteries (Fig. 11-10).

Bruits with both systolic and diastolic components suggest turbulent blood flow from atherosclerotic arterial disease.

Auscultate over the liver and spleen for *friction rubs.*

Friction rubs are present in hepatoma, gonococcal infection around the liver, splenic infarction, and pancreatic carcinoma.

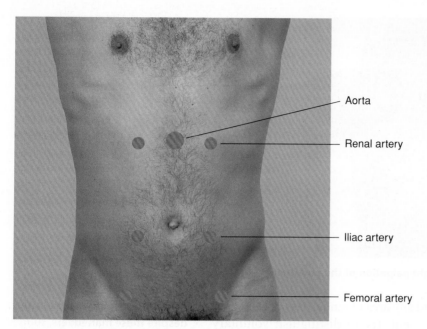

Aorta

Renal artery

Iliac artery

Femoral artery

FIGURE 11-10. Auscultate for bruits.

Percussion. Percussion helps you assess the amount and distribution of gas in the abdomen, viscera and masses that are solid or fluid-filled, and the size of the liver and spleen.

Percuss the abdomen lightly in all four quadrants to determine the distribution of *tympany* and *dullness*. Tympany usually predominates because of gas in the GI tract, but scattered areas of dullness from fluid and feces are also common.

A protuberant abdomen that is tympanitic throughout suggests *intestinal obstruction* or *paralytic ileus*. See Table 11-9, Protuberant Abdomens, p. 500.

- Note any dull areas suggesting an underlying mass or enlarged organ. This observation will guide subsequent palpation.

Dull areas characterize a pregnant uterus, an ovarian tumor, a distended bladder, or a large liver or spleen.

- On each side of a protuberant abdomen, note where abdominal tympany changes to the dullness of solid posterior structures.

Dullness in both flanks prompts further assessment for ascites (see pp. 484–485).

- Briefly percuss the lower anterior chest above the costal margins. On the right, you will usually find the dullness of the liver; on the left, the tympany that overlies the gastric air bubble and the splenic flexure of the colon.

In the rare condition of *situs inversus,* organs are reversed—air bubble on the right, liver dullness on the left.

Palpation

Light Palpation. Gentle palpation aids detection of abdominal tenderness, muscular resistance, and some superficial organs and masses. It also reassures and relaxes the patient.

Keeping your hand and forearm on a horizontal plane, with fingers together and flat on the abdominal wall, palpate the abdomen with a light gentle dipping motion. As you move your hand to different quadrants, raise it just off the skin. Gliding smoothly, palpate in all four quadrants (Fig. 11-11).

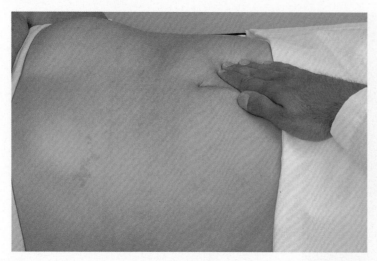

FIGURE 11-11.   **Begin with light palpation of the abdomen.**

Identify any superficial organs or masses and any area of tenderness or increased resistance to palpation. If resistance is present, try to distinguish voluntary guarding from involuntary rigidity or muscular spasm. Voluntary guarding usually decreases with the techniques listed below.

Involuntary rigidity typically persists despite these maneuvers, suggesting *peritoneal inflammation.*

■ Use the methods described earlier to help the patient relax (see p. 470).

■ Palpate after asking the patient to exhale, which usually relaxes the abdominal muscles.

■ Ask the patient to mouth-breathe with the jaws wide open.

Deep Palpation.   Deep palpation is usually required to delineate the liver edge, the kidneys, and abdominal masses. Again using the palmar surfaces of your fingers, press down in all four quadrants (Fig. 11-12). Identify any masses; note their location, size, shape, consistency, tenderness, pulsations, and any mobility with respiration or pressure from the examining hand. Correlate your findings from palpation with their percussion notes.

Abdominal masses may be categorized in several ways: physiologic (pregnant uterus), inflammatory (*diverticulitis*), vascular (an *AAA*), neoplastic (colon cancer), or obstructive (a distended bladder or dilated loop of bowel).

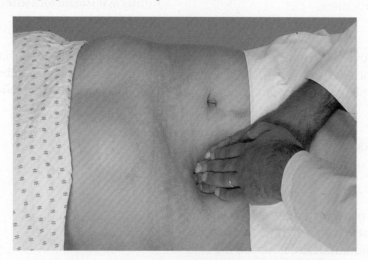

FIGURE 11-12.   **Use two hands for deep palpation.**

Assessing Possible Peritonitis. Inflammation of the parietal peritoneum, or *peritonitis*, signals an *acute abdomen*.[72] Signs of peritonitis include a positive cough test, guarding, rigidity, rebound tenderness, and percussion tenderness. Even before palpation, ask the patient to cough and identify where the cough produces pain. Then palpate gently, starting with one finger then with your hand, to localize the area of pain. As you palpate, check for the peritoneal signs of guarding, rigidity, and rebound tenderness.

When positive, these signs roughly double the likelihood of *peritonitis*; rigidity makes peritonitis almost four times more likely.[73] Causes include *appendicitis, cholecystitis,* and a perforation of the bowel wall.

See also Table 11-11, Tender Abdomens, pp. 502–503.

Signs of Peritonitis

- *Guarding* is a voluntary contraction of the abdominal wall, often accompanied by a grimace that may diminish when the patient is distracted.
- *Rigidity* is an involuntary reflex contraction of the abdominal wall from peritoneal inflammation that persists over several examinations.
- *Rebound tenderness* refers to pain expressed by the patient after the examiner presses down on an area of tenderness and suddenly removes the hand. To assess rebound tenderness, ask the patient "Which hurts more, when I press or let go?" Press down with your fingers firmly and slowly, then withdraw your hand quickly. The maneuver is positive if withdrawal produces pain. Percuss gently to check for percussion tenderness.

The Liver

Because the rib cage shelters most of the liver, direct assessment is limited. Liver size and shape can be estimated by percussion and palpation. Pressure from your palpating hand helps you to evaluate the surface, consistency, and tenderness of the liver.

Percussion. Measure the vertical span of liver dullness in the right midclavicular line after carefully locating the midclavicular line to improve accurate measurement. Use a light to moderate percussion strike, because a heavier strike can lead to underestimates of liver size.[74] Starting at a level well below the umbilicus in the RLQ (in an area of tympany, not dullness), percuss upward toward the liver. Identify the lower border of dullness in the midclavicular line.

Estimates of liver span by percussion have a 60% to 70% correlation with actual span.

Next, identify the upper border of liver dullness. Starting at the nipple line, percuss downward in the midclavicular line until lung resonance shifts to liver dullness. Gently displace a woman's breast as necessary to be sure that you start in a resonant area. The directions of percussion are shown in Figure 11-13.

The span of liver dullness is *increased* when the liver is enlarged.

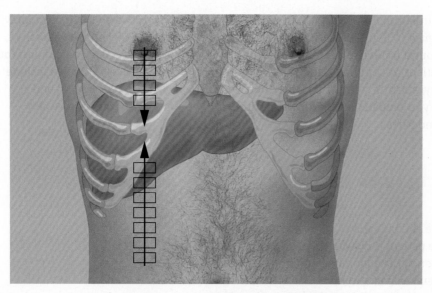

FIGURE 11-13. **Percuss for liver dullness.**

The span of liver dullness is *decreased* when the liver is small, or when there is free air below the diaphragm, as from a *perforated bowel* or *hollow viscus*. Liver span may decrease with resolution of *hepatitis* or *heart failure* or, less commonly, with progression of *fulminant hepatitis*.

Liver dullness may be displaced downward by the low diaphragm of *chronic obstructive pulmonary disease*. Span, however, remains normal.

Now, measure in centimeters the distance between your two points—the vertical span of liver dullness. Normally, the liver span, shown in Figure 11-14, is greater in men than in women and in taller compared to shorter individuals. If the liver seems enlarged, outline the lower edge by percussing medially and laterally.

Dullness from a right pleural effusion or consolidated lung, if adjacent to liver dullness, may *falsely increase* estimated liver size.

Gas in the colon may produce tympany in the RUQ, obscure liver dullness, and *falsely decrease* estimated liver size.

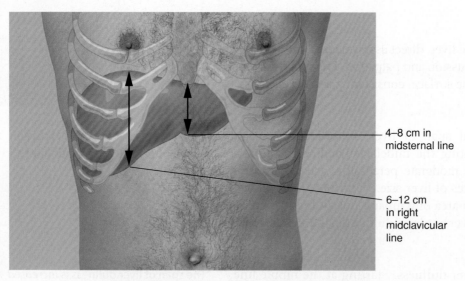

4–8 cm in midsternal line

6–12 cm in right midclavicular line

FIGURE 11-14. **Measure the liver span.**

Measurements of liver span by percussion are more accurate when the liver is enlarged with a palpable edge.[75–77]

In *chronic liver disease,* finding an enlarged palpable liver edge roughly doubles the likelihood of *cirrhosis.*[74]

Palpation. Place your left hand behind the patient, parallel to and supporting the right 11th and 12th ribs and adjacent soft tissues below. Remind the patient to relax on your hand. By pressing your left hand upward, the patient's liver may be felt more easily by your examining hand (Fig. 11-15).

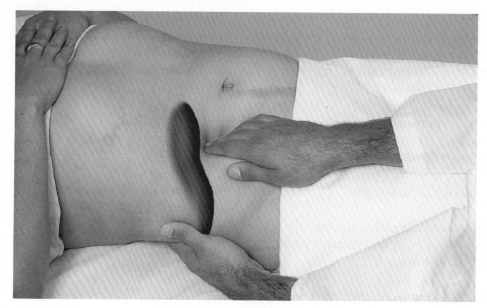

FIGURE 11-15. **Palpate the liver edge.**

Place your right hand on the patient's right abdomen lateral to the rectus muscle, with your fingertips *well below the lower border of liver dullness* (Fig. 11-16). Starting palpation too close to the right costal margin risks missing the lower edge of an enlarged liver that extends into the RLQ (Fig. 11-17). Some examiners point their fingers up toward the patient's head, whereas others prefer a somewhat more oblique position. In either case, press gently in and up.

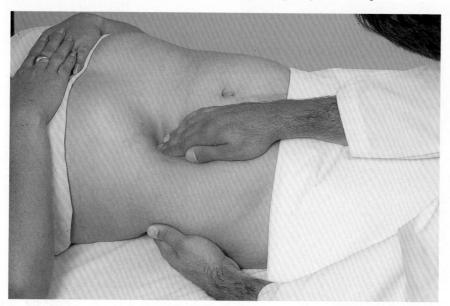

FIGURE 11-16. **Palpate in steps toward the costal margin.**

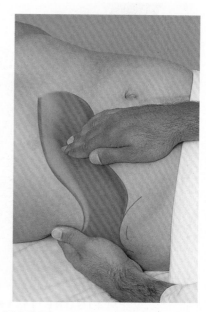

FIGURE 11-17. **Palpating first at the costal margin may miss the liver edge.**

Ask the patient to take a deep breath. Try to feel the liver edge as it slides down to meet your fingertips. When palpable, the normal liver edge is soft, sharp, and regular with a smooth surface. If you feel the edge, slightly lighten the pressure of your palpating hand so that the liver can slip under your finger pads and you can feel its anterior surface. Note any tenderness (the normal liver may be slightly tender).

Firmness or hardness of the liver, bluntness or rounding of its edge, and surface irregularity are suspicious for liver disease.

On inspiration, the liver is palpable about 3 cm below the right costal margin in the midclavicular line. Some patients breathe more with the chest than with the diaphragm. It may be helpful to train such patients to "breathe with the abdomen," which brings the liver, as well as the spleen and kidneys, into a palpable position during inspiration.

To palpate the liver edge, you may have to adapt your examining pressure to the thickness and resistance of the abdominal wall. If you cannot feel the edge, move your palpating hand closer to the costal margin and try again.

A palpable liver edge does not reliably indicate hepatomegaly.

Trace the liver edge both laterally and medially. Palpation through the rectus muscles is especially difficult. Describe the liver edge, and measure its distance from the right costal margin in the midclavicular line.

The "hooking technique". The "hooking technique" may be helpful, especially when the patient is obese. Stand to the right of the patient's chest. Place both hands, side by side, on the right abdomen below the border of liver dullness. Press in with your fingers and up toward the costal margin (Fig. 11-18). Ask the patient to take a deep breath. The liver edge shown in Figure 11-19 is palpable with the fingerpads of both hands.

An obstructed distended gallbladder may merge with the liver, forming a firm oval mass below the liver edge and an area that is dull to percussion.

See Table 11-12, Liver Enlargement: Apparent and Real, p. 504.

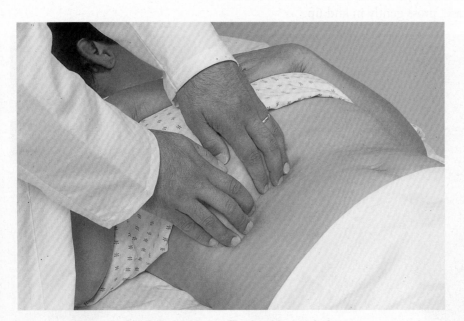

FIGURE 11-18. The hooking technique.

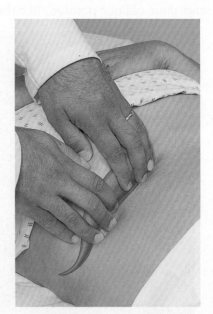

FIGURE 11-19. "Hooking" the liver edge.

Assessing Percussion Tenderness of a Nonpalpable Liver. Place your left hand flat on the lower right rib cage and gently strike your hand with the ulnar surface of your right fist. Ask the patient to compare the sensation with that produced by a similar strike on the left side.

Tenderness over the liver suggests inflammation, found in *hepatitis,* or congestion from *heart failure.*

The Spleen

When a spleen enlarges, it expands anteriorly, downward, and medially, often replacing the tympany of stomach and colon with the dullness of a solid organ. It then becomes palpable below the costal margin. Dullness to percussion suggests splenic enlargement, but may be absent when enlarged spleens lie above the costal margin. Continue to examine the patient from the patient's right side.

Percussion. Two techniques may help you to detect *splenomegaly*, an enlarged spleen:

- *Percuss the left lower anterior chest wall* roughly from the border of cardiac dullness at the 6th rib to the anterior axillary line and down to the costal margin, an area termed *Traube space*. As you percuss along the routes marked by the arrows in the Figures 11-20 and 11-21, note the lateral extent of tympany. Percussion is moderately accurate in detecting splenomegaly (sensitivity, 60% to 80%; specificity, 72% to 94%).[78]

If percussion dullness is present, palpation correctly detects splenomegaly more than 80% of the time.[78]

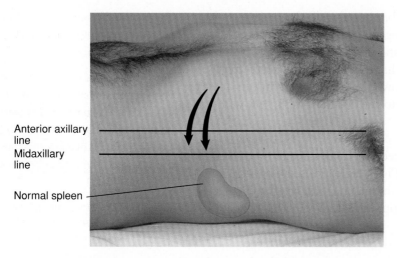

FIGURE 11-20. **Percuss for splenic dullness.**

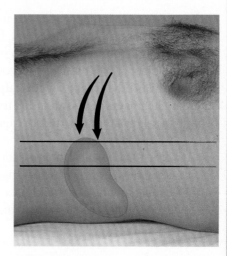

FIGURE 11-21. **Identify splenic enlargement.**

If tympany is prominent, especially laterally, splenomegaly is unlikely. The dullness of a normal spleen is usually masked by the dullness of other posterior tissues.

Fluid or solids in the stomach or colon may also cause dullness in Traube' space.

- *Check for a splenic percussion sign.* Percuss the lowest interspace in the left anterior axillary line (Fig. 11-22). This area is usually tympanitic. Then ask the patient to take a deep breath, and percuss again. When spleen size is normal, the percussion note usually remains tympanitic.

A change in percussion note from tympany to dullness on inspiration is a *positive splenic percussion sign,* but this sign is only moderately useful for detecting splenomegaly (Fig. 11-23).

If either or both of these tests is positive, pay extra attention to palpation of the spleen.

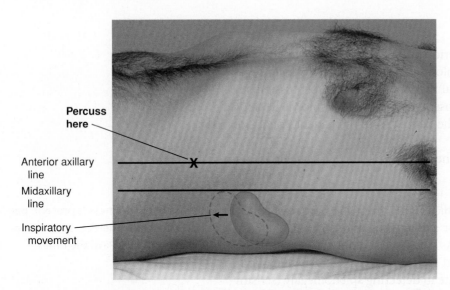

Percuss here

Anterior axillary line

Midaxillary line

Inspiratory movement

FIGURE 11-22. Negative splenic percussion sign.

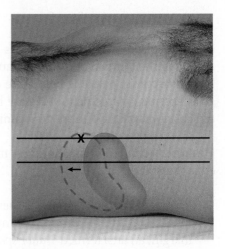

FIGURE 11-23. Positive splenic percussion sign.

Palpation. To enhance relaxation of the abdominal wall, the patient should keep arms at the sides and, if needed, flex the neck and legs. With your left hand, reach over and around the patient to support and press forward the lower left rib cage and adjacent soft tissue. With your right hand below the left costal margin, press in toward the spleen. Begin palpation low enough so that you can detect an enlarged spleen. If your hand is too close to the costal margin, you will not be able to reach up under the rib cage.

■ *Ask the patient to take a deep breath.* Try to feel the tip or edge of the spleen as it comes down to meet your fingertips (Fig. 11-24). Note any tenderness, assess the splenic contour, and measure the distance between the spleen's lowest point and the left costal margin. Approximately 5% of normal adults have a palpable spleen tip.

The examiner may miss an enlarged spleen by starting palpation too high in the abdomen.

Splenomegaly is eight times more likely when the spleen is palpable.[74] Causes include *portal hypertension*, hematologic malignancies, HIV infection, infiltrative diseases like *amyloidosis*, and *splenic infarct* or *hematoma*.

The spleen tip, illustrated in Figure 11-25, is just palpable deep to the left costal margin.

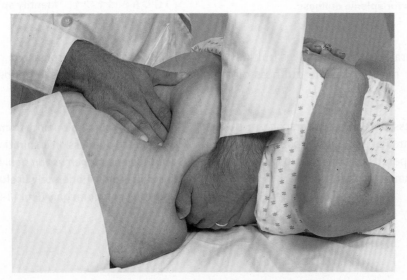

FIGURE 11-24. Palpate for the splenic edge.

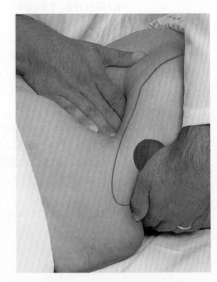

FIGURE 11-25. Spleen tip (purple) palpable below costal margin.

■ Repeat with the patient lying on the right side with legs somewhat flexed at the hips and knees (Fig. 11-26). In this position, gravity may bring the spleen forward and to the right into a palpable location (Fig. 11-27).

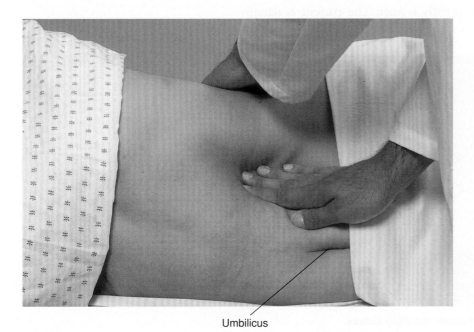

Umbilicus

FIGURE 11-26. Palpate the splenic edge with patient lying on right side.

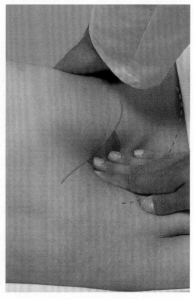

FIGURE 11-27. Edge of enlarged spleen palpable about 2 cm below the left costal margin on deep inspiration.

The Kidneys

Palpation. The kidneys are retroperitoneal and usually not palpable, but learning the techniques for examination helps you distinguish enlarged kidneys from other organs and abdominal masses.

Palpation of the Left Kidney. *Move to the patient's left side.* Place your right hand behind the patient, just below and parallel to the 12th rib, with your fingertips just reaching the CVA. Lift, trying to displace the kidney anteriorly. Place your left hand gently in the LUQ, lateral and parallel to the rectus muscle. Ask the patient to take a deep breath. At the peak of inspiration, press your left hand firmly and deeply into the LUQ, just below the costal margin. Try to "capture" the kidney between your two hands. Ask the patient to breathe out and then to stop breathing briefly. Slowly release the pressure of your left hand, feeling at the same time for the kidney to slide back into its expiratory position. If the kidney is palpable, describe its size, contour, and any tenderness.

A left flank mass can represent either *splenomegaly* or an enlarged left kidney. Suspect *splenomegaly* if there is a palpable notch on medial border, the edge extends beyond the midline, percussion is dull, and your fingers can probe deep to the medial and lateral borders but *not* between the mass and the costal margin. Confirm these findings with further evaluation.

Alternatively, try to palpate the left kidney using the deep palpation technique similar to palpation of the spleen. Standing at the patient's *right side,* with your left hand, reach over and around the patient to lift up beneath the left kidney, and with your right hand, feel deep in the LUQ. Ask the patient to take a deep breath, and feel for a mass. A normal left kidney is rarely palpable.

Suspect an *enlarged kidney* if there is normal tympany in the LUQ and you can probe with your fingers between the mass and the costal margin, but not deep to its medial and lower borders.

Palpation of the Right Kidney. A normal right kidney may be palpable, especially when the patient is thin and the abdominal muscles are relaxed. To capture the right kidney, *return to the patient's right side.* Use your left hand to lift up from the back, and your right hand to feel deep in the RUQ (Fig. 11-28). Proceed as before. The kidney may be slightly tender. The patient is usually aware of a capture and release.

Causes of kidney enlargement include hydronephrosis, cysts, and tumors. Bilateral enlargement suggests *polycystic kidney disease.*

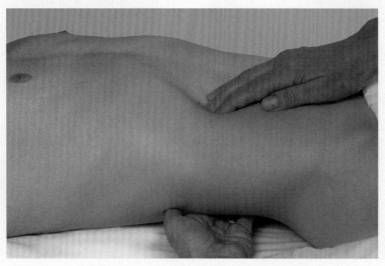

FIGURE 11-28. **Palpate the right kidney.**

Occasionally, a right kidney is more anterior and must be distinguished from the liver. The lower pole of the kidney is rounded, and the liver edge, if palpable, tends to be sharper, and extends farther medially and laterally. The liver itself cannot be captured.

Percussion Tenderness of the Kidneys. If the kidneys are tender to palpation, assess percussion tenderness over the CVAs. Pressure from your fingertips may be enough to elicit tenderness; if not, use fist percussion. Place the ball of one hand in the CVA and strike it with the ulnar surface of your fist (Fig. 11-29). Use enough force to cause a perceptible but painless jar or thud.

To save the patient from repositioning, integrate this assessment into your examination of the posterior lungs or back.

Pain with pressure or fist percussion supports *pyelonephritis* if associated with fever and dysuria, but may also be musculoskeletal.

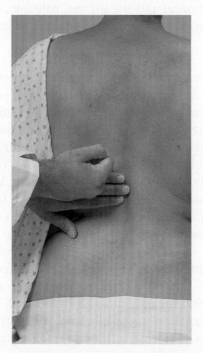

FIGURE 11-29. **Percuss for costovertebral angle tenderness.**

The Bladder

Normally, the bladder is not palpable unless it is distended above the symphysis pubis. Percuss for dullness and the height of the bladder above the symphysis pubis. Bladder volume must be 400 to 600 mL before dullness appears.[74] On palpation, the dome of the distended bladder feels smooth and round. Check for tenderness.

Causes of bladder distention are outlet obstruction from a *urethral stricture* or *prostatic hyperplasia*, medication side effects, and neurologic disorders such as *stroke* or *multiple sclerosis.*

Suprapubic tenderness is common in *bladder infection.*

The Aorta

Press firmly deep in the epigastrium, slightly to the left of the midline, and identify the aortic pulsations. In adults over age 50 years, assess the width of the aorta by pressing deeply in the upper abdomen with one hand on each side of the aorta (Figs. 11-30 to 11-32). In this age group, a normal aorta is not more than 3 cm wide (average, 2.5 cm, excluding the thickness of the skin and abdominal wall). Detection of pulsations is affected by abdominal girth and the diameter of the aorta.

Risk factors for AAA are age ≥65 years, history of smoking, male gender, and a first-degree relative with a history of AAA repair.[79]

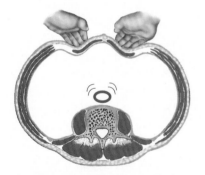 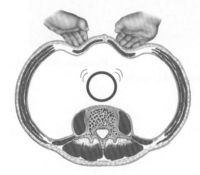

A periumbilical or upper abdominal mass with expansile pulsations that is ≥3 cm in diameter suggests an AAA. Sensitivity of palpation increases as AAAs enlarge: for widths of 3 to 3.9 cm, 29%; 4 to 4.9 cm, 50%; ≥5 cm, 76%.[79,80]

FIGURE 11-30. **Press firmly to detect aortic pulsations.**

FIGURE 11-31. **Identify expanded aortic width.**

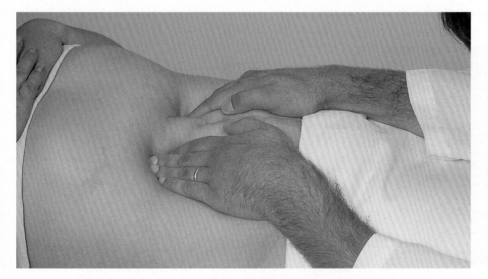

Screening by palpation followed by ultrasound decreases mortality, especially in male smokers 65 years or older. Pain may signal rupture. Rupture is 15 times more likely in AAAs >4 cm than in smaller aneurysms, and carries an 85% to 90% mortality rate.[79,80]

Note that the USPSTF recommends ultrasound screening for men over 65 years who have "ever smoked."[81]

FIGURE 11-32. **Palpate on both sides of the aorta.**

Special Techniques

Assessment Techniques for

- Ascites
- Appendicitis
- Acute cholecystitis
- Ventral hernia
- Mass in abdominal wall

Assessing Possible Ascites. A protuberant abdomen with bulging flanks is suspicious for *ascites*, the most common complication of cirrhosis.[82] Because ascitic fluid characteristically sinks with gravity, whereas gas-filled loops of bowel rise, dullness appears in the dependent areas of the abdomen. Percuss for dullness outward in several directions from the central area of tympany. Map the border between tympany and dullness (Fig. 11-33).

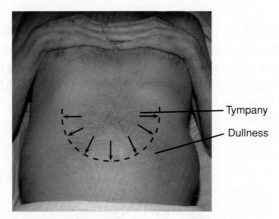

Tympany

Dullness

FIGURE 11-33. Percuss outward to map dullness from ascites.

Ascites reflects the *increased hydrostatic pressure* in cirrhosis (the most common cause of ascites), heart failure, constrictive pericarditis, or inferior vena cava or hepatic vein obstruction. It may signal *decreased osmotic pressure* in nephrotic syndrome, malnutrition, or ovarian cancer.

Two additional techniques help to confirm ascites, although both signs may be misleading.

- *Test for shifting dullness.* Percuss the border of tympany and dullness with the patient supine, then ask the patient to roll onto one side. Percuss and mark the borders again (Fig. 11-34). In a person without ascites, the border between tympany and dullness usually stays relatively constant.

In ascites, dullness shifts to the more dependent side, whereas tympany shifts to the top.

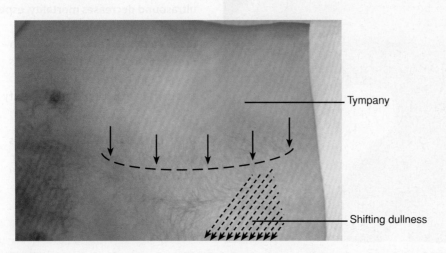

Tympany

Shifting dullness

FIGURE 11-34. Percuss for shifting dullness (here patient turned to right side).

■ *Test for a fluid wave.* Ask the patient or an assistant to press the edges of both hands firmly down the midline of the abdomen. This pressure helps to stop the transmission wave through fat. While you tap one flank sharply with your fingertips, feel on the opposite flank for an impulse transmitted through the fluid (Fig. 11-35). Unfortunately, this sign is often negative until ascites is obvious, and it is sometimes positive in people without ascites.

An easily palpable impulse suggests ascites. A positive fluid wave, shifting dullness, and peripheral edema makes the presence of ascites to three to six times more likely.[83]

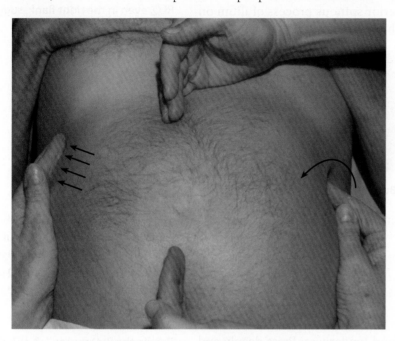

FIGURE 11-35. **Test for a fluid wave.**

Identifying an Organ or a Mass in an Ascitic Abdomen. Try to *ballotte* the organ or mass, exemplified here by an enlarged liver (Fig. 11-36). Straighten and stiffen the fingers of one hand together, place them on the abdominal surface, and make a brief jabbing movement directly toward the anticipated structure. This quick movement often displaces the fluid so that your fingertips can briefly touch the surface of the structure through the abdominal wall (Fig. 11-37).

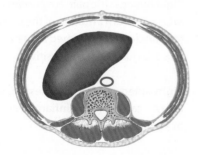

FIGURE 11-36. **Note the enlarged liver.**

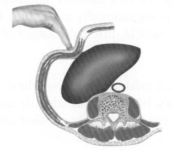

FIGURE 11-37. **Ballotte the liver.**

Assessing Possible Appendicitis.
Appendicitis is a common cause of acute abdominal pain. Assess carefully for the peritoneal signs of acute abdomen and the additional signs of McBurney point tenderness, Rovsing sign, the psoas sign, and the obturator sign described on the next page.

Appendicitis is twice as likely in the presence of RLQ tenderness, Rovsing sign, and the psoas sign; it is three times more likely if there is McBurney point tenderness.[73]

■ Ask the patient to point to where the pain began and where it is now. Ask the patient to cough to see where pain occurs.

The pain of *appendicitis* classically begins near the umbilicus, then migrates to the RLQ. Older adults are less likely to report this pattern.[17]

■ Palpate carefully for an area of local tenderness. Classically, *"McBurney point"* lies 2 inches from the anterior superior spinous process of ilium on a line drawn from that process to the umbilicus (Fig. 11-38).

Localized tenderness anywhere in the RLQ, even in the right flank, suggests *appendicitis*.

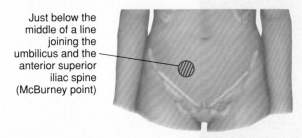

Just below the middle of a line joining the umbilicus and the anterior superior iliac spine (McBurney point)

FIGURE 11-38. McBurney point.

■ Palpate the tender area for guarding, rigidity, and rebound tenderness.

Early voluntary guarding may be replaced by involuntary muscular rigidity and signs of peritoneal inflammation. There may also be RLQ pain on quick withdrawal or deferred rebound tenderness.

■ Palpate for *Rovsing sign* and referred rebound tenderness. Press deeply and evenly in the *LLQ*. Then quickly withdraw your fingers.

Pain in the RLQ during *left*-sided pressure is a *positive Rovsing sign*.

■ Assess the *psoas sign*. Place your hand just above the patient's right knee and ask the patient to raise that thigh against your hand. Alternatively, ask the patient to turn onto the left side. Then extend the patient's right leg at the hip. Flexion of the leg at the hip makes the psoas muscle contract; extension stretches it.

Increased abdominal pain on either maneuver is a *positive psoas sign*, suggesting irritation of the psoas muscle by an inflamed appendix.

■ Though less helpful, assess the *obturator sign*. Flex the patient's right thigh at the hip, with the knee bent, and rotate the leg internally at the hip. This maneuver stretches the internal obturator muscle. Internal rotation of the hip is described on p. 681.

Right hypogastric pain is a *positive obturator sign*, from irritation of the obturator muscle by an inflamed appendix. This sign has very low sensitivity.

■ *Perform a rectal examination and, in women, a pelvic examination.* These maneuvers have low sensitivity and specificity, but they may identify an inflamed appendix atypically located within the pelvic cavity or other causes of the abdominal pain.

Right-sided rectal tenderness may also be caused by an inflamed adnexa or seminal vesicle.

Assessing Possible Acute Cholecystitis. When RUQ pain and tenderness suggest *acute cholecystitis,* assess *Murphy sign*. Hook your left thumb or the fingers of your right hand under the costal margin at the point where the lateral border of the rectus muscle intersects with the costal margin. Alternatively, palpate the RUQ with the fingers of your right hand near the costal margin. If the liver is enlarged, hook your thumb or fingers under the liver edge at a comparable point. Ask the patient to take a deep breath, which forces the liver and gall

A sharp increase in tenderness with inspiratory effort is a *positive Murphy sign*. When positive, Murphy sign triples the likelihood of *acute cholecystitis*.[73]

bladder down toward the examining fingers. Watch the patient's breathing and note the degree of tenderness.

Assessing Ventral Hernias.   Ventral hernias are hernias in the abdominal wall exclusive of groin hernias. If you suspect but do not see an umbilical or incisional hernia, ask the patient to raise both head and shoulders off the table.

The bulge of a hernia will usually appear with this action, but should not be confused with *diastasis recti*, which is a benign 2- to 3-cm gap in the rectus muscles often seen in obese and postpartum patients.

Inguinal and femoral hernias are discussed in Chapter 13, Male Genitalia and Hernias.

Strangulated inguinal, femoral, or scrotal hernias merit prompt surgical evaluation. See discussion of strangulated scrotal hernias on pp. 554–555.

Mass in the Abdominal Wall.   Occasionally, there are masses in the abdominal wall rather than inside the abdominal cavity. Ask the patient either to raise the head and shoulders or to strain down, thus tightening the abdominal muscles. Feel for the mass again.

A mass in the abdominal wall remains palpable; an intra-abdominal mass is obscured by muscular contraction.

Recording Your Findings

Note that initially you may use sentences to describe your findings; later you will use phrases. The style below contains phrases appropriate for most write-ups.

Recording the Abdominal Examination

"Abdomen is protuberant with active bowel sounds. It is soft and nontender; no palpable masses or hepatosplenomegaly. Liver span is 7 cm in the right midclavicular line; edge is smooth and palpable 1 cm below the right costal margin. Spleen and kidneys not felt. No costovertebral angle (CVA) tenderness."
OR
"Abdomen is flat. No bowel sounds heard. It is firm and boardlike, with increased tenderness, guarding, and rebound in the right midquadrant. Liver percusses to 7 cm in the midclavicular line; edge not felt. Spleen and kidneys not felt. No palpable masses. No CVA tenderness.

These findings suggest peritonitis from possible *appendicitis* (see pp. 485–486 and pp. 488–489).

Table 11-1 Abdominal Pain

Problem[84]	Process	Location	Quality
Gastroesophageal Reflux Disease (GERD)[11,14]	Prolonged exposure of esophagus to gastric acid due to impaired esophageal motility or excess relaxations of the lower esophageal sphincter; *Helicobacter pylori* may be present	Chest or epigastric	Heartburn, regurgitation
Peptic Ulcer and Dyspepsia[3,5]	Mucosal ulcer in stomach or duodenum >5 mm, covered with fibrin, extending through the muscularis mucosa; *H. pylori* infection present in 90% of peptic ulcers	Epigastric, may radiate straight to the back	Variable: epigastric gnawing or burning (dyspepsia); may also be boring, aching, or hungerlike No symptoms in up to 20%
Gastric Cancer	Adenocarcinoma in 90%–95%, either intestinal (older adults) or diffuse (younger adults, worse prognosis)	Increasingly in "cardia" and GE junction; also in distal stomach	Variable
Acute Appendicitis[17,18]	Acute inflammation of the appendix with distention or obstruction	Poorly localized *periumbilical pain*, usually migrates to the right lower quadrant	Mild but increasing, possibly cramping Steady and more severe
Acute Cholecystitis[10]	Inflammation of the gallbladder, from obstruction of the cystic duct by gallstone in 90%	Right upper quadrant or epigastrium; may radiate to right shoulder or interscapular area	Steady, aching
Biliary Colic	Sudden obstruction of the cystic duct or common bile duct by a gallstone	Epigastric or right upper quadrant; may radiate to the right scapula and shoulder	Steady, aching; *not* colicky Usually last longer than 3 hrs
Acute Pancreatitis[7,9]	Intrapancreatic trypsinogen activation to trypsin and other enzymes, resulting in autodigestion and inflammation of the pancreas	Epigastric, may radiate straight to the back or other areas of the abdomen; 20% with severe sequelae of organ failure	Usually steady
Chronic Pancreatitis	Irreversible destruction of the pancreatic parenchyma from recurrent inflammation of either large ducts or small ducts	Epigastric, radiating to the back	Severe, persistent, deep
Pancreatic Cancer[85,86]	Predominantly adenocarcinoma (95%); 5% 5-yr survival	If cancer in body or tail, epigastric, in either upper quadrant, often radiates to the back	Steady, deep
Acute Diverticulitis[87]	Acute inflammation of colonic diverticula, outpouchings 5–10 mm in diameter, usually in sigmoid or descending colon	Left lower quadrant	May be cramping at first, then steady
Acute Bowel Obstruction	Obstruction of the bowel lumen, most commonly caused by (1) adhesions or hernias (small bowel), or (2) cancer or diverticulitis (colon)	*Small bowel:* periumbilical or upper abdominal *Colon:* lower abdominal or generalized	Cramping Cramping
Mesenteric Ischemia[88,89]	Occlusion of blood flow to small bowel, from arterial or venous thrombosis (especially superior mesenteric artery), cardiac embolus, or hypoperfusion; can be colonic	May be periumbilical at first, then diffuse; may be postprandial, classically inducing "food fear"	Cramping at first, then steady; pain disproportionate to examination findings

Timing	Aggravating Factors	Relieving Factors	Associated Symptoms and Setting
After meals, especially spicy foods	Lying down, bending over; physical activity; diseases such as scleroderma, gastroparesis; drugs like nicotine that relax the lower esophageal sphincter	Antacids, proton pump inhibitors; avoiding alcohol, smoking, fatty meals, chocolate, selected drugs such as theophylline, calcium channel blockers	Wheezing, chronic cough, shortness of breath, hoarseness, choking sensation, dysphagia, regurgitation, halitosis, sore throat; increases risk of Barrett esophagus and esophageal cancer
Intermittent; duodenal ulcer is more likely than gastric ulcer or dyspepsia to cause pain that (1) wakes the patient at night, and (2) occurs intermittently over a few wks, disappears for months, then recurs	Variable	Food and antacids may bring relief (less likely in gastric ulcers)	Nausea, vomiting, belching, bloating; heartburn (more common in duodenal ulcer); weight loss (more common in gastric ulcer); dyspepsia is more common in the young (20–29 yrs), gastric ulcer in those over 50 yrs, and duodenal ulcer in those 30–60 yrs
Pain is persistent, slowly progressive; duration of pain is typically shorter than in peptic ulcer	Often food; *H. pylori* infection	*Not* relieved by food or antacids	Anorexia, nausea, early satiety, weight loss, and sometimes bleeding; most common in ages 50–70 yrs
Lasts roughly 4–6 hrs, depending on intervention	Movement or cough	If it subsides temporarily, suspect perforation of the appendix.	Anorexia, nausea, possibly vomiting, which typically follow the onset of pain; low fever
Gradual onset; course longer than in biliary colic	Jarring, deep breathing		Anorexia, nausea, vomiting, fever; no jaundice
Rapid onset over a few min, lasts one to several hrs and subsides gradually; often recurrent	Fatty meals but also fasting; often precedes cholecystitis, cholangitis, pancreatitis		Anorexia, nausea, vomiting, restlessness
Acute onset, persistent pain	Lying supine; dyspnea if pleural effusions from capillary leak syndrome; selected medications, high triglycerides may exacerbate	Leaning forward with trunk flexed	Nausea, vomiting, abdominal distention, fever; often recurrent; 80% with history of alcohol abuse or gallstones
Chronic or recurrent course	Alcohol, heavy or fatty meals	Possibly leaning forward with trunk flexed; often intractable	Pancreatic enzyme insufficiency, diarrhea with fatty stools (*steatorrhea*) and *diabetes mellitus*
Persistent pain; relentlessly progressive illness	Smoking, chronic pancreatitis	Possibly leaning forward with trunk flexed; often intractable	Painless jaundice, anorexia, weight loss; glucose intolerance, depression
Often gradual onset		Analgesia, bowel rest, antibiotics	Fever, constipation. Also nausea, vomiting, abdominal mass with rebound tenderness
Paroxysmal; may decrease as bowel mobility is impaired Paroxysmal, though typically milder	Ingestion of food or liquids		Vomiting of bile and mucus (high obstruction) or fecal material (low obstruction); obstipation develops (early); vomiting late if at all; prior symptoms of underlying cause
Usually abrupt in onset, then persistent	Underlying cardiac disease		Vomiting, bloody stool, soft distended abdomen with peritoneal signs, shock; age >50 yrs

Table 11-2 Dysphagia

Process and Problem	Timing	Factors That Aggravate	Factors That Relieve	Associated Symptoms and Conditions
Oropharyngeal Dysphagia	Acute or gradual onset and a variable course, depending on the underlying disorder	Attempts to start the swallowing process		Aspiration into the lungs or regurgitation into the nose with attempts to swallow; from motor disorders affecting the pharyngeal muscles such as stroke, bulbar palsy, or other neuromuscular conditions

Esophageal Dysphagia
Mechanical Narrowing

Process and Problem	Timing	Factors That Aggravate	Factors That Relieve	Associated Symptoms and Conditions
Mucosal rings and webs	Intermittent	Solid foods	Regurgitation of the bolus of food	Usually none
Esophageal stricture	Intermittent; may become slowly progressive	Solid foods	Regurgitation of the bolus of food	A long history of heartburn and regurgitation
Esophageal cancer	May be intermittent at first; progressive over months	Solid foods, with progression to liquids	Regurgitation of the bolus of food	Pain in the chest and back and weight loss, especially late in the course of illness

Motor Disorders

Process and Problem	Timing	Factors That Aggravate	Factors That Relieve	Associated Symptoms and Conditions
Diffuse esophageal spasm	Intermittent	Solids or liquids	Maneuvers described below; sometimes nitroglycerin	Chest pain that mimics angina pectoris or myocardial infarction and lasts min to hrs; possibly heartburn
Scleroderma	Intermittent; may progress slowly	Solids or liquids	Repeated swallowing; movements such as straightening the back, raising the arms, or a Valsalva maneuver (straining down against a closed glottis)	Heartburn; other manifestations of scleroderma
Achalasia	Intermittent; may progress	Solids or liquids		Regurgitation, often at night when lying down, with nocturnal cough; possibly chest pain precipitated by eating

Table 11-3 Diarrhea

Problem	Process	Characteristics of Stool	Timing	Associated Symptoms	Setting, Persons at Risk
Acute Diarrhea[90] (≤14 days)					
Secretory Infection (Noninflammatory)	Infection by viruses, preformed bacterial toxins (such as *Staphylococcus aureus*, *Bacillus cereus*, *Clostridium perfringens*, toxigenic *Escherichia coli*, *Vibrio cholerae*), cryptosporidium, *Giardia lamblia*, rotavirus	Watery, without blood, pus, or mucus	Duration of a few days, possibly longer; lactase deficiency may lead to a longer course	Nausea, vomiting, periumbilical cramping pain; temperature normal or slightly elevated	Often travel, a common food source, or an epidemic
Inflammatory Infection	Colonization or invasion of intestinal mucosa (nontyphoid *Salmonella*, *Shigella*, *Yersinia*, *Campylobacter*, enteropathic *E. coli*, *Entamoeba histolytica*, *C. difficile*)	Loose to watery, often with blood, pus, or mucus	An acute illness of varying duration	Lower abdominal cramping pain and often rectal urgency, tenesmus; fever	Travel, contaminated food or water; frequent anal intercourse
Drug-Induced Diarrhea	Action of many drugs, such as magnesium-containing antacids, antibiotics, antineoplastic agents, and laxatives	Loose to watery	Acute, recurrent, or chronic	Possibly nausea; usually little if any pain	Prescribed or over-the-counter medications
Chronic Diarrhea (≥30 days)					
Diarrheal Syndrome					
Irritable bowel syndrome[20]	Altered motility or secretion from luminal and mucosal irritants that change mucosal permeability, immune activation, and colonic transit, including maldigested carbohydrates, fats, excess bile acids, gluten intolerance, enteroendocrine signaling, and changes in microbiomes	Loose; ~50% with mucus; small to moderate volume. Small, hard stools with constipation. May be mixed pattern.	Worse in the morning; rarely at night.	Crampy lower abdominal pain, abdominal distention, flatulence, nausea; urgency, pain relieved with defecation	Young and middle-aged adults, especially women

(continued)

Table 11-3 Diarrhea (*Continued*)

Problem	Process	Characteristics of Stool	Timing	Associated Symptoms	Setting, Persons at Risk
Chronic Diarrhea (≥30 days) (*continued*)					
Fecal impaction/ motility disorders	Partial obstruction by impacted stool only allowing passage of loose feces	Loose, small volume	Variable	Crampy abdominal pain, incomplete evacuation	Older adults, immobilized and institutionalized patients; ensues from selected medications
Cancer of the sigmoid colon	Partial obstruction by a malignant neoplasm	May be blood-streaked	Variable	Change in usual bowel habits, crampy lower abdominal pain, constipation	Middle-aged and older adults, especially older than 55 yrs
Inflammatory Bowel Disease					
Ulcerative colitis	Mucosal inflammation typically extending proximally from the rectum (*proctitis*) to varying lengths of the colon (*colitis* to *pancolitis*), with microulcerations and, if chronic, inflammatory polyps	Frequent, watery, often containing blood	Onset typically abrupt; often recurrent, persisting, and may awaken at night	Cramping, with urgency, tenesmus; fever, fatigue, weakness; abdominal pain if complicated by toxic megacolon; may include episcleritis, uveitis, arthritis, erythema nodosum	Often young adults, Ashkenazi Jewish descendants; linked to altered CD4+ T-cell Th2 response; increases risk of colon cancer
Crohn disease of the small bowel (*regional enteritis*) or colon (*granulomatous colitis*)	Chronic transmural inflammation of the bowel wall, with skip pattern involving the terminal ileum and/ or proximal colon (and rectal sparing); may cause strictures	Small, soft to loose or watery, with bleeding if *colitis*, obstructive symptoms, if *enteritis*	More insidious onset; chronic or recurrent	Crampy periumbilical, right lower quadrant (*enteritis*) or diffuse (*colitis*) pain, with anorexia, fever, and/ or weight loss; perianal or perirectal abscesses and fistulas; may cause small or large bowel obstruction	Often teens or young adults, but also adults of middle age; more common in Ashkenazi Jewish descendants; linked to altered CD4+ T-cell helper Th1 and 17 response; increases risk of colon cancer

Problem	Process	Characteristics of Stool	Timing	Associated Symptoms	Setting, Persons at Risk
Chronic Diarrhea (≥30 days) (*continued*)					
Voluminous Diarrhea					
Malabsorption syndrome	Defective membrane transport or absorption of intestinal epithelium (*Crohn, celiac disease, surgical resection*); impaired luminal digestion (*pancreatic insufficiency*); epithelial defects at brush border (*lactose intolerance*)	Typically bulky, soft, light yellow to gray, mushy, greasy or oily, and sometimes frothy; particularly foul-smelling; usually floats in toilet (*steatorrhea*)	Onset of illness typically insidious	Anorexia, weight loss, fatigue, abdominal distention, often crampy lower abdominal pain. Symptoms of nutritional deficiencies such as bleeding (vitamin K), bone pain and fractures (vitamin D), glossitis (vitamin B), and edema (protein)	Variable, depending on cause
Osmotic diarrhea					
■ Lactose intolerance	Intestinal lactase deficiency	Watery diarrhea of large volume	Follows the ingestion of milk and milk products; relieved by fasting	Crampy abdominal pain, abdominal distention, flatulence	In >50% of African Americans, Asians, Native Americans, Hispanics; in 5–20% of Caucasians
■ Abuse of osmotic purgatives	Laxative habit, often surreptitious	Watery diarrhea of large volume	Variable	Often none	Persons with anorexia nervosa or bulimia nervosa
Secretory diarrhea	Variable: bacterial infection, secreting villous adenoma, fat or bile salt malabsorption, hormone-mediated conditions (gastrin in *Zollinger–Ellison syndrome*, vasoactive intestinal peptide)	Watery diarrhea of large volume	Variable	Weight loss, dehydration, nausea, vomiting, and cramping abdominal pain	Variable depending on cause

Table 11-4 Constipation

Problem	Process	Associated Symptoms and Setting
Life Activities and Habits		
Inadequate Time or Setting for the Defecation Reflex	Ignoring the sensation of a full rectum inhibits the defecation reflex	Hectic schedules, unfamiliar surroundings, bed rest
False Expectations of Bowel Habits	Expectations of "regularity" or more frequent stools than a person's norm	Beliefs, treatments, and advertisements that promote the use of laxatives
Diet Deficient in Fiber	Decreased fecal bulk	Other factors such as debilitation and constipating drugs may contribute
Irritable Bowel Syndrome[20]	Functional change in frequency or form of bowel movement without known pathology; possibly from change in intestinal bacteria.	Three patterns: diarrhea—predominant, constipation—predominant, or mixed. Symptoms present ≥6 mo and abdominal pain for ≥3 mo plus at least 2 of 3 features (improvement with defecation; onset with change in stool frequency; onset with change in stool form and appearance)
Mechanical Obstruction		
Cancer of the Rectum or Sigmoid Colon	Progressive narrowing of the bowel lumen from adenocarcinoma	Change in bowel habits; often diarrhea, abdominal pain, bleeding, occult blood in stool; in rectal cancer, tenesmus and pencil-shaped stools; weight loss
Fecal Impaction	A large, firm, immovable fecal mass, most often in the rectum	Rectal fullness, abdominal pain, and diarrhea around the impaction; common in debilitated, bedridden, and often elderly and institutionalized patients
Other Obstructing Lesions (such as Diverticulitis, Volvulus, Intussusception, or Hernia)	Narrowing or complete obstruction of the bowel	Colicky abdominal pain, abdominal distention, and in intussusception, often "currant jelly" stools (red blood and mucus)
Painful Anal Lesions	Pain may cause spasm of the external sphincter and voluntary inhibition of the defecation reflex.	Anal fissures, painful hemorrhoids, perirectal abscesses
Drugs	A variety of mechanisms	Opiates, anticholinergics, antacids containing calcium or aluminum, and many others
Depression	A disorder of mood	Fatigue, anhedonia, sleep disturbance, weight loss
Neurologic Disorders	Interference with the autonomic innervation of the bowel	Spinal cord injuries, multiple sclerosis, Hirschsprung disease, and other conditions
Metabolic Conditions	Interference with bowel motility	Pregnancy, hypothyroidism, hypercalcemia

Table 11-5 Black and Bloody Stool

Problem	Selected Causes	Associated Symptoms and Setting
Melena		
Refers to passage of black tarry stool	Gastritis, GERD, peptic ulcer (gastric or duodenal)	Usually epigastric discomfort from heartburn, dysmotility; if peptic ulcer, pain after meals (delay of 2–3 hrs if duodenal ulcer; may be asymptomatic
Fecal blood tests are positive		
Involves loss ≥60 mL of blood into the gastrointestinal tract (less in children), usually from the esophagus, stomach, or duodenum with transit time of 7–14 hrs	Gastritis or stress ulcers	Recent ingestion of alcohol, aspirin, or other anti-inflammatory drugs; recent bodily trauma, severe burns, surgery, or increased intracranial pressure
Less commonly, if slow transit, blood loss originates in the jejunum, ileum, or ascending colon	Esophageal or gastric varices	Cirrhosis of the liver or other causes of portal hypertension
In infants, melena may result from swallowing blood during the birth	Reflux esophagitis, Mallory–Weiss tear in esophageal mucosa due to retching and vomiting	Retching, vomiting, often recent ingestion of alcohol
Black Stool		
Black stool from other causes with negative fecal blood tests; stool change has no pathologic significance	Ingestion of iron, bismuth salts, licorice, or even chocolate cookies	Asymptomatic
Stool with Red Blood (*Hematochezia*)		
Usually originates in the colon, rectum, or anus; much less frequently from the jejunum or ileum	Colon cancer	Often a change in bowel habits, weight loss
	Hyperplasia or adenomatous polyps	Often no other symptoms
Upper gastrointestinal hemorrhage may also cause red stool, usually with large blood loss ≥1 L	Diverticula of the colon	Often no symptoms unless inflammation causes diverticulitis
Rapid transit leaves insufficient time for the blood to turn black from oxidation of iron in hemoglobin	Inflammatory conditions of the colon and rectum	
	Ulcerative colitis, Crohn disease	See Table 11-3, Diarrhea, p. 492
	Infectious diarrhea	See Table 11-3, Diarrhea, p. 491
	Proctitis (various causes including anal intercourse)	Rectal urgency, tenesmus
	Ischemic colitis	Lower abdominal pain, sometimes fever or shock in older adults; abdomen typically soft to palpation
	Hemorrhoids	Blood on the toilet paper, on the surface of the stool, or dripping into the toilet
	Anal fissure	Blood on the toilet paper or on the surface of the stool; anal pain
Reddish but Nonbloody Stool	Ingestion of beets	Pink urine, which usually precedes the reddish stool; from poor metabolism of betacyanin

Table 11-6 Urinary Frequency, Nocturia, and Polyuria

Problem	Mechanisms	Selected Causes	Associated Symptoms
Frequency	Decreased bladder capacity		
	Increased bladder sensitivity to stretch because of inflammation	*Infection,* stones, tumor, or foreign body in the bladder	Burning on urination, urinary urgency, sometimes gross hematuria
	Decreased elasticity of the bladder wall	Infiltration by scar tissue or tumor	Symptoms of associated inflammation (see above) are common
	Decreased cortical inhibition of bladder contractions	Motor disorders of the central nervous system, such as a stroke	Urinary urgency; neurologic symptoms such as weakness and paralysis
	Impaired bladder emptying with residual urine in the bladder		
	Partial mechanical obstruction of the bladder neck or proximal urethra	Most commonly, benign prostatic hyperplasia; also urethral stricture and other obstructive lesions of the bladder or prostate	Prior obstructive symptoms: hesitancy in starting the urinary stream, straining to void, reduced size and force of the stream, and dribbling during or at the end of urination
	Loss of S2–S4 innervation to the bladder	Neurologic disease affecting the sacral nerves or nerve roots, e.g., diabetic neuropathy	Weakness or sensory defects
Nocturia *With High Volumes*	Most types of polyuria (see p. 462)		
	Decreased concentrating ability of the kidney with loss of the normal drop in nocturnal urine output	Chronic renal insufficiency due to a number of diseases	Possibly other symptoms of renal insufficiency
	Excessive fluid intake before bedtime	Habit, especially involving alcohol and coffee	
	Fluid-retaining, edematous states. Daytime accumulation of dependent edema that is excreted at night when the patient is supine	Heart failure, nephrotic syndrome, hepatic cirrhosis with ascites, chronic venous insufficiency	Edema and other symptoms of the underlying disorder; urinary output during the day may be reduced as fluid accumulates in the body tissues (see Table 12-1, Peripheral Causes of Edema, p. 534).
With Low Volumes	Urinary frequency		
	Voiding while up at night without a real urge, a "pseudofrequency"	Insomnia	Variable
Polyuria	Deficiency of antidiuretic hormone (*diabetes insipidus*)	A disorder of the posterior pituitary and hypothalamus	Thirst and polydipsia, often severe and persistent; nocturia
	Renal unresponsiveness to antidiuretic hormone (*nephrogenic diabetes insipidus*)	A number of kidney diseases, including hypercalcemic and hypokalemic nephropathy; drug toxicity, e.g., from lithium	Thirst and polydipsia, often severe and persistent; nocturia
	Solute diuresis		
	Electrolytes, such as sodium salts	Large saline infusions, potent diuretics, certain kidney diseases	Variable
	Nonelectrolytes, such as glucose	Uncontrolled diabetes mellitus	Thirst, polydipsia, and nocturia
	Excessive water intake	Primary polydipsia	Polydipsia tends to be episodic; thirst may not be present; nocturia is usually absent

Table 11-7 Urinary Incontinence[a]

Problem	Mechanisms	Symptoms	Physical Signs
Stress Incontinence The urethral sphincter is weakened so that transient increases in intra-abdominal pressure raise the bladder pressure to levels that exceed urethral resistance.	In women, pelvic floor weakness and inadequate muscular and ligamentous support of the bladder neck and proximal urethra change the angle between the bladder and the urethra (see Chapter 14, pp. 592–593). Causes include childbirth and surgery. Local conditions affecting the internal urethral sphincter, such as postmenopausal atrophy of the mucosa and urethral infection, may also contribute. In men, stress incontinence may follow prostate surgery.	Momentary leakage of small amounts of urine with coughing, laughing, and sneezing while the person is in an upright position. Urine loss is unrelated to a conscious urge to urinate.	Stress incontinence may be demonstrable, especially if the patient is examined before voiding and in a standing position. Atrophic vaginitis may be evident. Bladder distention is absent.
Urge Incontinence Detrusor contractions are stronger than normal and overcome the normal urethral resistance. The bladder is typically *small.*	Decreased cortical inhibition of detrusor contractions from stroke, brain tumor, dementia, and lesions of the spinal cord above the sacral level. Hyperexcitability of sensory pathways, as in bladder infections, tumors, and fecal impaction. Deconditioning of voiding reflexes, as in frequent voluntary voiding at low bladder volumes.	Involuntary urine loss preceded by an urge to void. The volume tends to be moderate. Urgency, frequency, and nocturia with small to moderate volumes. If acute inflammation is present, pain on urination. Possibly "pseudo-stress incontinence"—voiding 10–20 sec after stresses such as a change of position, going up- or downstairs, and possibly coughing, laughing, or sneezing.	The small bladder is not detectable on abdominal examination. When cortical inhibition is decreased, mental deficits or motor signs of central nervous system disease are often present. When sensory pathways are hyperexcitable, signs of local pelvic problems or a fecal impaction may be present.

(continued)

Table 11-7 Urinary Incontinence[a] (*Continued*)

Problem	Mechanisms	Symptoms	Physical Signs
Overflow Incontinence Detrusor contractions are insufficient to overcome urethral resistance, causing urinary retention. The bladder is typically flaccid and *large,* even after an effort to void.	Obstruction of the bladder outlet, as in *benign prostatic hyperplasia* or tumor. Weakness of the detrusor muscle associated with peripheral nerve disease at S2–4 level. Impaired bladder sensation that interrupts the reflex arc, as in diabetic neuropathy.	When intravesicular pressure overcomes urethral resistance, continuous dripping or dribbling incontinence ensues. Decreased force of the urinary stream. Prior symptoms of partial urinary obstruction or other symptoms of peripheral nerve disease may be present.	Examination often reveals an enlarged, sometimes tender, bladder. Other signs include prostatic enlargement, motor signs of peripheral nerve disease, a decrease in sensation (including perineal sensation), and diminished to absent reflexes.
Functional Incontinence The patient is functionally unable to reach the toilet in time because of impaired health or environmental conditions.	Problems in mobility resulting from weakness, arthritis, poor vision, or other conditions. Environmental factors such as an unfamiliar setting, distant bathroom facilities, bed rails, or physical restraints.	Incontinence on the way to the toilet or only in the early morning.	The bladder is not detectable on examination. Look for physical or environmental clues as the likely cause.
Incontinence Secondary to Medications Drugs may contribute to any type of incontinence listed.	Sedatives, tranquilizers, anticholinergics, sympathetic blockers, and potent diuretics.	Variable. A careful history and chart review are important.	Variable.

[a]Patients may have more than one kind of incontinence.

Table 11-8 Localized Bulges in the Abdominal Wall

Localized bulges in the abdominal wall include *ventral hernias* (defects in the wall through which tissue protrudes) and subcutaneous tumors such as *lipomas*. The more common ventral hernias are umbilical, incisional, and epigastric. Hernias and *diastasis recti* usually become more evident when the patient is supine and raises the head and shoulders.

Umbilical Hernia

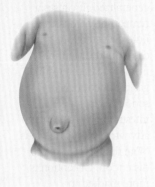

A protrusion through a defective umbilical ring is most common in infants but also occurs in adults. In infants, it usually closes spontaneously within 1–2 yrs.

Diastasis Recti

Separation of the two rectus abdominis muscles, through which abdominal contents form a midline ridge typically extending from the xiphoid to the umbilicus and seen only when the patient raises the head and shoulders. Often present in patients with repeated pregnancies, obesity, and chronic lung disease. It is clinically benign.

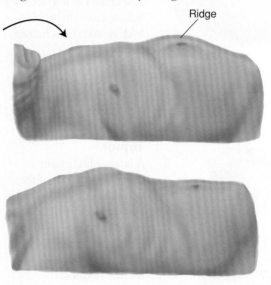

Ridge

Incisional Hernia

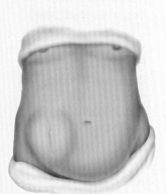

This is a protrusion through an operative scar. Palpate to detect the length and width of the defect in the abdominal wall. A small defect, through which a large hernia has passed, has a greater risk for complications than a large defect.

Epigastric Hernia

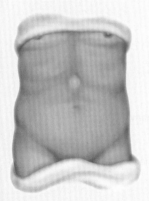

A small midline protrusion through a defect in the linea alba occurs between the xiphoid process and the umbilicus. With the patient coughing or performing a Valsalva maneuver, palpate by running your fingerpad down the linea alba.

Lipoma

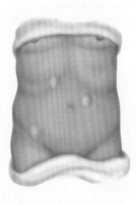

Common, benign, fatty tumors usually in the subcutaneous tissues almost anywhere in the body, including the abdominal wall. Small or large, they are usually soft and often lobulated. Press your finger down on the edge of a lipoma. The tumor typically slips out from under your finger and is well demarcated, nonreducible, and usually nontender.

Table 11-9 Protuberant Abdomens

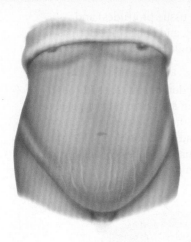

Fat

Fat is the most common cause of a protuberant abdomen. Fat thickens the abdominal wall, the mesentery, and omentum. The umbilicus may appear sunken. A *pannus*, or apron of fatty tissue, may extend below the inguinal ligaments. Lift it to look for inflammation in the skin folds or even for a hidden hernia.

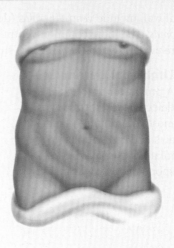

Gas

Gaseous distention may be localized or generalized. It causes a tympanitic percussion note. Selected foods may cause mild distention from increased intestinal gas production. More serious causes are intestinal obstruction and adynamic (paralytic) ileus. Note the location of the distention. Distention is more marked in obstruction in the colon than in the small bowel.

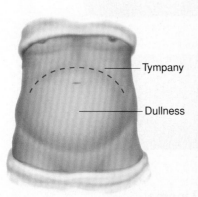

Tumor

A large solid tumor, usually rising out of the pelvis, is dull to percussion. Air-filled bowel is displaced to the periphery. Causes include ovarian tumors and uterine fibroids. Occasionally, a markedly distended bladder is mistaken for such a tumor.

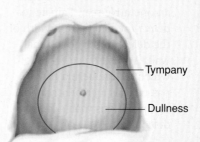

Pregnancy

Pregnancy is a common pelvic "mass." Listen for the fetal heart (see p. 945).

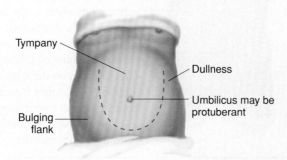

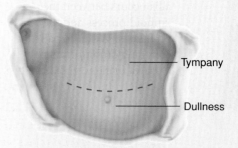

Ascitic Fluid

Ascitic fluid seeks the lowest point in the abdomen, producing bulging flanks that are dull to percussion. The umbilicus may protrude. Turn the patient onto one side to detect the shift in position of the fluid level (shifting dullness). (See pp. 484–485 for the assessment of ascites.)

Table 11-10 Sounds in the Abdomen

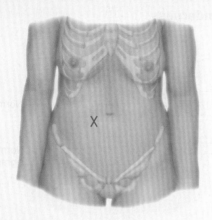

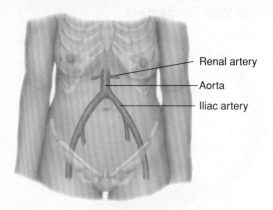

Bowel Sounds

Bowel sounds may be:

- *Increased,* as in diarrhea or *early intestinal obstruction*
- *Decreased,* then absent, as in *adynamic ileus* and *peritonitis.* Before deciding that bowel sounds are absent, sit down and listen where shown for 2 min or even longer.

High-pitched tinkling sounds suggest intestinal fluid and air under tension in a dilated bowel. *Rushes of high-pitched sounds* coinciding with an abdominal cramp signal intestinal obstruction.

Bruits

A *hepatic bruit* suggests carcinoma of the liver or *cirrhosis.* *Arterial bruits* with both systolic and diastolic components suggest partial occlusion of the aorta or large arteries. Such bruits in the epigastrium are suspicious for *renal artery stenosis* or *renovascular hypertension.*

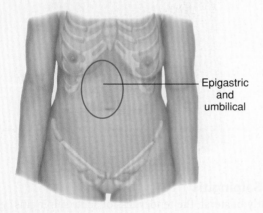

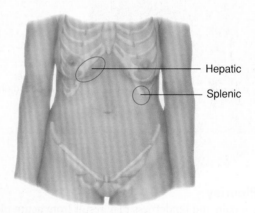

Venous Hum

A venous hum is a rare soft humming noise with both systolic and diastolic components. It points to increased collateral circulation between portal and systemic venous systems, as in *hepatic cirrhosis.*

Friction Rubs

Friction rubs are rare grating sounds with respiratory variation. They indicate inflammation of the peritoneal surface of an organ, as in liver cancer, chlamydial or gonococcal perihepatitis, recent liver biopsy, or splenic infarct. When a systolic bruit accompanies a hepatic friction rub, suspect carcinoma of the liver.

Table 11-11 Tender Abdomens

Abdominal Wall Tenderness

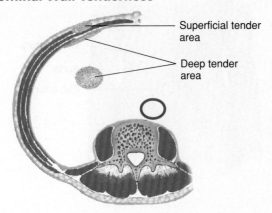

Superficial tender area

Deep tender area

Tenderness may originate in the abdominal wall. When the patient raises the head and shoulders, this tenderness persists, whereas tenderness from a deeper lesion (protected by the tightened muscles) decreases.

Visceral Tenderness

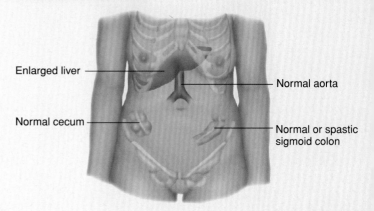

Enlarged liver

Normal aorta

Normal cecum

Normal or spastic sigmoid colon

The structures shown may be tender to deep palpation. Usually the discomfort is dull with no muscular rigidity or rebound tenderness. A reassuring explanation to the patient may prove helpful.

Tenderness from Disease in the Chest and Pelvis

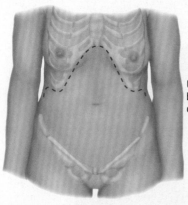

Unilateral or bilateral, upper or lower abdomen

Acute Pleurisy

Abdominal pain and tenderness may result from acute pleural inflammation. When unilateral, it can mimic *acute cholecystitis* or *appendicitis*. Rebound tenderness and rigidity are less common; chest signs are usually present.

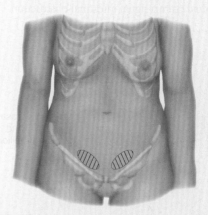

Acute Salpingitis

Frequently bilateral, the tenderness of acute salpingitis (inflammation of the fallopian tubes) is usually maximal just above the inguinal ligaments. Rebound tenderness and rigidity may be present. On pelvic examination, motion of the cervix and uterus causes pain.

Tenderness of Peritoneal Inflammation

Tenderness associated with peritoneal inflammation is more severe than visceral tenderness. Muscular rigidity and rebound tenderness are frequently but not necessarily present. Generalized peritonitis causes exquisite tenderness throughout the abdomen, together with board-like muscular rigidity. These signs on palpation, especially abdominal rigidity, double the likelihood of peritonitis.[73] Local causes of peritoneal inflammation include:

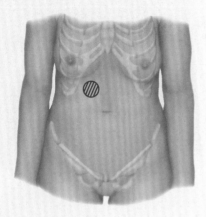

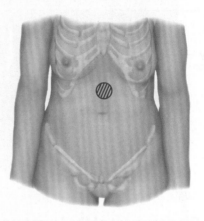

Acute Cholecystitis[10]

Signs are maximal in the right upper quadrant. Check for Murphy sign (see pp. 486–487).

Acute Pancreatitis

In acute pancreatitis, epigastric tenderness and rebound tenderness are usually present, but the abdominal wall may be soft.

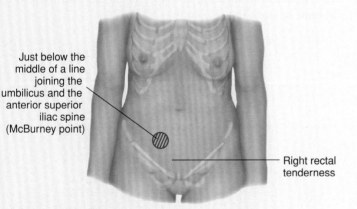

Just below the middle of a line joining the umbilicus and the anterior superior iliac spine (McBurney point)

Right rectal tenderness

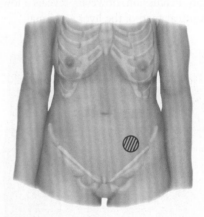

Acute Appendicitis[17,18]

Right lower quadrant signs are typical of acute appendicitis but may be absent early in the course. The typical area of tenderness, McBurney point, is illustrated. Examine other areas of the right lower quadrant as well as the right flank.

Acute Diverticulitis

Acute diverticulitis is a confined inflammatory process, usually in the left lower quadrant, that involves the sigmoid colon. If the sigmoid colon is redundant there may be suprapubic or right-sided pain. Look for localized peritoneal signs and a tender underlying mass. Microperforation, abscess, and obstruction may ensue.

Table 11-12 Liver Enlargement: Apparent and Real

A palpable liver does not necessarily indicate hepatomegaly (an enlarged liver), but more often results from a change in consistency—from the normal softness to an abnormal firmness or hardness, as in cirrhosis. Clinical estimates of liver size should be based on both percussion and palpation, although even these techniques are imperfect compared to ultrasound.

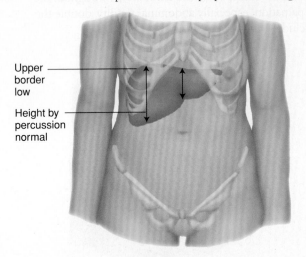

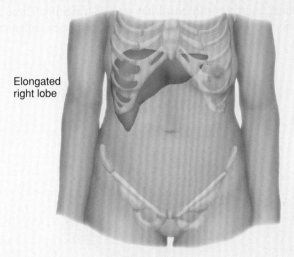

Downward Displacement of the Liver by a Low Diaphragm

This finding is common when the diaphragm is flattened and low, as in COPD. The liver edge may be palpable well below the costal margin. Percussion, however, reveals a low upper edge, and the vertical span of the liver is normal.

Normal Variations in Liver Shape

In some individuals the right lobe of the liver may be elongated and easily palpable as it projects downward toward the iliac crest. Such an elongation, sometimes called *Riedel lobe,* represents a variation in shape, not an increase in liver volume or size.

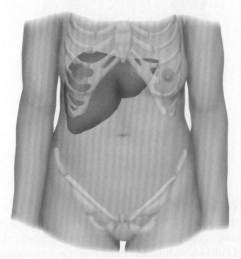

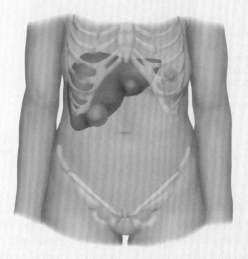

Smooth Large Liver

Cirrhosis may produce an enlarged liver with a firm, *nontender* edge. The cirrhotic liver may also be scarred and contracted. Many other diseases may produce similar findings such as hemochromatosis, amyloidosis, and lymphoma. An enlarged liver with a smooth, *tender* edge suggests inflammation, as in hepatitis, or venous congestion, seen in right-sided heart failure.

Irregular Large Liver

An enlarged liver that is firm or hard with an irregular edge or surface suggests *hepatocellular carcinoma.* There may be one or more nodules. The liver may or may not be tender.

References

1. Centers for Disease Control and Prevention. National Center for Health Statistics. National Hospital Ambulatory Medical Care Survey: 2011 Outpatient Department Summary Tables. Table 7. Twenty leading principal reasons for outpatient department visits: United States, 2011. Available at http://www.cdc.gov/nchs/ahcd.htm. Accessed April 23, 2015.

2. Centers for Disease Control and Prevention. National Center for Health Statistics. National Hospital Ambulatory Medical Care Survey: 2011 Emergency Department Summary Tables. Table 10. Ten leading principal reasons for emergency department visits, by patient age and sex: United States, 2011. Available at http://www.cdc.gov/nchs/ahcd.htm. Accessed April 23, 2015.

3. Talley NJ, Vakil NB, Moayyedi P, et al. American Gastroenterological Association technical review on the evaluation of dyspepsia. *Gastroenterology.* 2005;129:1756.

4. Drossman DA. The functional gastrointestinal disorders and the Rome III process. *Gastroenterology.* 2007;130:1377.

5. Tack J, Talley NJ. Functional dyspepsia—symptoms, definitions and validity of the Rome III criteria. *Nat Rev Gastroenterol Hepatol.* 2013;10:134.

6. Ranji SR, Goldman LE, Simel DL, et al. Do opiates affect the clinical evaluation of patients with acute abdominal pain? *JAMA.* 2006;296:1764.

7. Schneider L, Büchler MW, Werner J. Acute pancreatitis with an emphasis on infection. *Infect Dis Clin North Am.* 2010;24:921.

8. Fogel EL, Sherman S. ERCP for gallstone pancreatitis. *N Engl J Med.* 2014;370:150.

9. Guptak WB. In the clinic: acute pancreatitis. *Ann Intern Med.* 2010;153:ITC5–1.

10. Strasberg S. Acute calculus cholecystitis. *N Engl J Med.* 2008; 358:2804.

11. Wilson J. In the clinic: gastroesophageal reflux disease. *Ann Intern Med.* 2008;149:ITC2–1.

12. DeVault KR, Castell DO. Updated guidelines for the diagnosis and treatment of gastroesophageal reflux disease. *Am J Gastroenterol.* 2005;100:190.

13. Fletcher KC, Goutte M, Slaughter JC, et al. Significance and degree of reflux in patients with primary extraesophageal symptoms. *Laryngoscope.* 2011;121:2561.

14. Shaheen NJ, Weinberg DS, Denberg TD. Upper endoscopy for gastroesophageal reflux disease: best practice advice from the clinical guidelines committee of the American College of Physicians. *Ann Intern Med.* 2012;157:808.

15. Spechler SJ, Souza RF. Barrett's esophagus. *N Engl J Med.* 2014; 371:836.

16. Bao J, Lopez JA, Huerta S. Acute abdominal pain and abnormal CT findings. *JAMA.* 2013;310:848.

17. Howell JM, Eddy OL, Lukens TW, et al. Clinical policy: critical issues in the evaluation and management of emergency department patients with suspected appendicitis. *Ann Emerg Med.* 2010; 55:71.

18. Andersson RE. The natural history and traditional management of appendicitis revisited: spontaneous resolution and predominance of prehospital perforations imply that a correct diagnosis is more important than an early diagnosis. *World J Surg.* 2007;31:86.

19. Andresson RE. Meta-analysis of the clinical and laboratory diagnosis of appendicitis. *Br J Sur.* 2004;91:28.

20. Camilleri M. Peripheral mechanisms in irritable bowel syndrome. *N Engl J Med.* 2012;367:1626.

21. Roden DF, Altman KW. Causes of dysphagia among different age groups: a systematic review of the literature. *Otolaryngol Clin North Am.* 2013;46:965.

22. Rome III Diagnostic Criteria for Functional Gastrointestinal Disorders—Appendix A, pp. 885–898, 2006. Available at http://www.romecriteria.org/criteria./ Accessed April 26, 2015.

23. Longstreth GF, Thompson WG, Chey WD, et al. Functional bowel disorders. *Gastroenterology.* 2006;130:1480.

24. Leffler DA, Lamont JT. Clostridium difficile infection. *N Engl J Med.* 2015;372:1539.

25. Shah BJ, Rughwani N, Rose S. Constipation. In the clinic: constipation. *Ann Intern Med.* 2015;162:ITC-1.

26. Gallegos-Orozco JF, Foxx-Orenstein AE, Sterler SM, et al. Chronic constipation in the elderly. *Am J Gastroenterol.* 2012;107:18.

27. Sarma AV, Wei JT. Benign prostatic hyperplasia and lower urinary tract symptoms. *N Engl J Med.* 2012;367:248.

28. Hooton TM. Uncomplicated urinary tract infection. *N Engl J Med.* 2012;366:1028.

29. Gupta K, Trautner B. In the clinic: urinary tract infection. *Ann Intern Med.* 2012;156:ITC3–1.

30. Bettez M, Tu le M, Carlson K, et al. 2012 update: guidelines for adult urinary incontinence collaborative consensus document for the Canadian Urological Association. *Can Urol Assoc J.* 2012;6:354.

31. Markland AD, Vaughan CP, Johnson TM 2nd, et al. Incontinence. *Med Clin North Am.* 2011;95:539.

32. Holroyd-Leduc JM, Tannenbaum C, Thorpe KE, et al. What type of urinary incontinence does this woman have? *JAMA.* 2008; 299:1446.

33. Substance Abuse and Mental Health Services Administration. *The NSDUH Report: Substance use and mental health estimates from the 2013 National Survey on Drug Use and Health: Overview of findings.* Rockville, MD: Substance Abuse and Mental Health Services Administration; 2014. Available at: http://store.samhsa.gov/shin/content//NSDUH14–0904/NSDUH14–0904.pdf. Accessed March 7, 2015.

34. Centers for Disease Control and Prevention. Fact Sheets—Alcohol Use and Your Health. 2014. Available at http://www.cdc.gov/alcohol/pdfs/alcoholyourhealth.pdf. Accessed March 7, 2015.

35. Wilson JF. In the clinic. Alcohol use. *Ann Intern Med.* 2009; 150:ITC3–1.

36. Moyer VA, U.S. Preventive Services Task Force. Screening and behavioral counseling interventions in primary care to reduce alcohol misuse: U.S. preventive services task force recommendation statement. *Ann Intern Med.* 2013;159:210.

37. National Institute of Alcohol Abuse and Alcoholism. Alcohol Facts and Statistics. 2014. Available at http://pubs.niaaa.nih.gov/publications/AlcoholFacts&Stats/AlcoholFacts&Stats.pdf. Accessed March 7, 2015.

38. National Institute of Alcohol Abuse and Alcoholism. Helping patients who drink too much. A Clinician's Guide. National Institutes of Health, 2005. Available at http://pubs.niaaa.nih.gov/publications/Practitioner/CliniciansGuide2005/guide.pdf. Accessed March 7, 2015.

39. National Institute of Alcohol Abuse and Alcoholism. Prescribing medications for alcohol dependence. National Institutes of Health, 2008. Available at http://pubs.niaaa.nih.gov/publications/Practitioner/CliniciansGuide2005/PrescribingMeds.pdf. Accessed March 7, 2015.

40. Centers for Disease Control and Prevention. Hepatitis A. General information. U.S. Department of Health & Human Services; 2012. Available at http://www.cdc.gov/hepatitis/A/PDFs/HepAGeneral-FactSheet.pdf. Accessed March 7, 2015.

41. Centers for Disease Control and Prevention. Viral Hepatitis Statistics & Surveillance. 2014. Available at http://www.cdc.gov/hepatitis/Statistics/2012Surveillance/Table2.3.htm. Accessed March 7, 2015.

42. Fiore AE, Wasley A, Bell BP. Prevention of hepatitis A through active or passive immunization: recommendations of the Advisory Committee on Immunization Practices (ACIP). *MMWR Recomm Rep.* 2006;55:1.

43. Mast EE, Weinbaum CM, Fiore AE, et al. A comprehensive immunization strategy to eliminate transmission of hepatitis B virus infection in the United States: recommendations of the Advisory Committee on Immunization Practices (ACIP) Part II: immunization of adults. *MMWR Recomm Rep.* 2006;55:1.

44. LeFevre ML. Screening for hepatitis B virus infection in nonpregnant adolescents and adults: U.S. Preventive Services Task Force recommendation statement. *Ann Intern Med.* 2014;161:58.

45. Chou R, Cottrell EB, Wasson N, et al. *Screening for Hepatitis C Virus Infection in Adults.* Rockville, MD: 2012. Available at http://www.ncbi.nlm.nih.gov/pubmed/23304739. Accessed March 7, 2015.

46. Rosen HR. Clinical practice. Chronic hepatitis C infection. *N Engl J Med.* 2011;364:2429.

47. El-Serag HB. Hepatocellular carcinoma. *N Engl J Med.* 2011; 365:1118.

48. Moyer VA. Screening for hepatitis C virus infection in adults: U.S. Preventive Services Task Force recommendation statement. *Ann Intern Med.* 2013;159:349.

49. Siegel RL, Miller KD, Jemal A. Cancer statistics, 2015. *CA Cancer J Clin.* 2015;65:5.

50. Howlader N, Noone AM, Krapcho M, et al. *SEER Cancer Statistics Review, 1975–2011.* Bethesda, MD: National Cancer Institute; 2014. Available at http://seer.cancer.gov/csr/1975_2011. Accessed March 7, 2015.

51. Edwards BK, Ward E, Kohler BA, et al. Annual report to the nation on the status of cancer, 1975–2006, featuring colorectal cancer trends and impact of interventions (risk factors, screening, and treatment) to reduce future rates. *Cancer.* 2010;116:544.

52. American Cancer Society. Colorectal cancer facts & figures 2011–2013, 2011. Available at http://www.cancer.org/acs/groups/content/@epidemiologysurveilance/documents/document/acspc-028312.pdf. Accessed March 7, 2015.

53. National Cancer Institute. Genetics of colorectal cancer (PDQ®). National Institutes of Health; 2015. Available at http://www.cancer.gov/cancertopics/pdq/genetics/colorectal/HealthProfessional. Accessed March 7, 2015.

54. Holme O, Bretthauer M, Fretheim A, et al. Flexible sigmoidoscopy versus faecal occult blood testing for colorectal cancer screening in asymptomatic individuals. *Cochrane Database Syst Rev.* 2013;9: CD009259.

55. Elmunzer BJ, Hayward RA, Schoenfeld PS, et al. Effect of flexible sigmoidoscopy-based screening on incidence and mortality of colorectal cancer: a systematic review and meta-analysis of randomized controlled trials. *PLoS Med.* 2012;9:e1001352.

56. Boyle T, Keegel T, Bull F, et al. Physical activity and risks of proximal and distal colon cancers: a systematic review and meta-analysis. *J Natl Cancer Inst.* 2012;104:1548.

57. Dube C, Rostom A, Lewin G, et al. The use of aspirin for primary prevention of colorectal cancer: a systematic review prepared for the U.S. Preventive Services Task Force. *Ann Intern Med.* 2007; 146:365.

58. Rostom A, Dube C, Lewin G, et al. Nonsteroidal anti-inflammatory drugs and cyclooxygenase-2 inhibitors for primary prevention of colorectal cancer: a systematic review prepared for the U.S. Preventive Services Task Force. *Ann Intern Med.* 2007;146:376.

59. Chlebowski RT, Wactawski-Wende J, Ritenbaugh C, et al. Estrogen plus progestin and colorectal cancer in postmenopausal women. *N Engl J Med.* 2004;350:991.

60. U.S. Preventive Services Task Force. Routine aspirin or nonsteroidal anti-inflammatory drugs for the primary prevention of colorectal cancer: U.S. Preventive Services Task Force recommendation statement. *Ann Intern Med.* 2007;146:361.

61. Simon MS, Chlebowski RT, Wactawski-Wende J, et al. Estrogen plus progestin and colorectal cancer incidence and mortality. *J Clin Oncol.* 2012;30:3983.

62. Chlebowski RT, Hendrix SL, Langer RD, et al. Influence of estrogen plus progestin on breast cancer and mammography in healthy postmenopausal women: the Women's Health Initiative Randomized Trial. *JAMA.* 2003;289:3243.

63. Manson JE, Hsia J, Johnson KC, et al. Estrogen plus progestin and the risk of coronary heart disease. *N Engl J Med.* 2003;349:523.

64. Cushman M, Kuller LH, Prentice R, et al. Estrogen plus progestin and risk of venous thrombosis. *JAMA.* 2004;292:1573.

65. Levin TR, Zhao W, Conell C, et al. Complications of colonoscopy in an integrated health care delivery system. *Ann Intern Med.* 2006; 145:880.

66. U.S. Preventive Services Task Force. Screening for colorectal cancer: U.S. Preventive Services Task Force recommendation statement. *Ann Intern Med.* 2008;149:627.

67. Levin B, Lieberman DA, McFarland B, et al. Screening and surveillance for the early detection of colorectal cancer and adenomatous polyps, 2008: a joint guideline from the American Cancer Society, the U.S. Multi-Society Task Force on Colorectal Cancer, and the American College of Radiology. *CA Cancer J Clin.* 2008;58:130.

68. MMWR Morbidity and Mortality Weekly Report. Vital signs: colorectal cancer screening test use—United States, 2012. *MMWR Morb Mortal Wkly Rep.* 2013;62:881.

69. Inadomi JM, Vijan S, Janz NK, et al. Adherence to colorectal cancer screening: a randomized clinical trial of competing strategies. *Arch Intern Med.* 2012;172:575.

70. Rex DK, Johnson DA, Anderson JC, et al. American College of Gastroenterology guidelines for colorectal cancer screening 2009 [corrected]. *Am J Gastroenterol.* 2009;104:739.

71. McGee S. *Ch 51, Auscultation of the Abdomen, in Evidence-based Physical Diagnosis,* 3rd ed. Philadelphia, PA: Saunders; 2012:453.

72. Cope Z. *The Early Diagnosis Of The Acute Abdomen.* London: Oxford University Press; 1972.

73. McGee S. *Ch 50, Abdominal pain and tenderness, in Evidence-based Physical Diagnosis.* 3rd ed. Philadelphia, PA: Saunders; 2012:441–452.

74. McGee S. *Ch 49, Palpation and percussion of the abdomen, in Evidence-based Physical Diagnosis.* 3rd ed. Philadelphia, PA: Saunders; 2012:428–440.

75. de Bruyn G, Graviss EA. A systematic review of the diagnostic accuracy of physical examination for the detection of cirrhosis. *BMC Med Inform Decis Mak.* 2001;1:6.

REFERENCES

76. Naylor CD. Physical examination of the liver. *JAMA.* 1994;271:1859.

77. Zoli M, Magalotti D, Grimaldi M, et al. Physical examination of the liver: is it still worth it? *Am J Gastroenterol.* 1995;90:1428.

78. Grover SA, Barkun AN, Sackett DL. Does this patient have splenomegaly? *JAMA.* 1993;270:2218.

79. Kent KC. Clinical practice. Abdominal aortic aneurysms. *N Engl J Med.* 2014;371:2101.

80. Lederle F. In the clinic. Abdominal aortic aneurysm. *Ann Intern Med.* 2009;150:ITC5–1.

81. U.S. Preventive Services Task Force. Final Recommendation Statement. Abdominal Aortic Aneurysm: Screening, June 2014. Available at http://www.uspreventiveservicestaskforce.org/Page/Document/RecommendationStatementFinal/abdominal-aortic-aneurysm-screening. Accessed April 28, 2015.

82. Runyon BA, American Association for the Study of Liver Diseases. Introduction to the revised American Association for the Study of Liver Diseases Practice Guideline management of adult patients with ascites due to cirrhosis 2012. *Hepatology.* 2013:1651.

83. Williams JW, Simel DL. Does this patient have ascites? How to divine fluid in the abdomen. *JAMA.* 1992;267:2645.

84. American College of Physicians. *Gastroenterology and Hepatology - Medical Knowledge Self-Assessment Program.* Philadelphia, PA: American College of Physicians; 2013.

85. Ryan DP, Hong TS, Bardeesy N. Pancreatic adenocarcinoma. *N Engl J Med.* 2014;371:1039.

86. Yadav D, Lowenfels AB. The epidemiology of pancreatitis and pancreatic cancer. *Gastroenterology.* 2013;144:1252.

87. Katz LH, Guy DD, Lahat A, et al. Diverticulitis in the young is not more aggressive than in the elderly, but it tends to recur more often: systematic review and meta-analysis. *J Gastroenterol Hepatol.* 2013;28:1274.

88. Acosta S. Mesenteric ischemia. *Curr Opin Crit Care.* 2015;21:171.

89. Sise MJ. Acute mesenteric ischemia. *Surg Clin North Am.* 2014;94:165.

90. DuPont HL. Acute infectious diarrhea in immunocompetent adults. *N Engl J Med.* 2014;370:1532.

The Peripheral Vascular System

Careful assessment is essential for detection of diseases of the peripheral arteries (Fig. 12-1) and veins. *Peripheral artery disease (PAD)* is generally defined as atherosclerotic disease distal to the aortic bifurcation, although some guidelines also include the abdominal aorta.[1,2] PAD affects roughly 8 million Americans, with estimates ranging from 5.8% to 12% of the population older than age 40 years, but is "silent" in 20% to 50% of those affected.[1–3] Prevalence increases with age, rising from 7% of adults aged 60 to 69 years to 23% of adults 80 years of age and older.[4] Detection is doubly important because PAD is both a marker for cardiovascular morbidity and mortality, and a harbinger of functional decline. Risk of death from myocardial infarction and stroke triples in adults with PAD. In 2013, the American College of Cardiology Foundation and the American Heart Association updated their PAD guidelines from 2005 and 2011 to promote improved screening and prevention.[2,5]

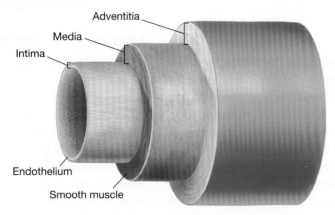

FIGURE 12-1. **Anatomy of arteries.**

Thromboembolic disorders of the *peripheral venous system* in the lower extremities are also common, seen in an estimated 1% of adults aged 60 years and above.[6,7] Roughly two thirds of affected patients present with deep venous thrombosis (DVT), often in hospital settings, and one third with pulmonary thromboembolism (PE).[8,9] Almost one quarter of PE cases present with sudden death.[6] Superficial venous thrombosis also poses risks—one third of those affected are diagnosed with DVT or PE.[10] In addition, DVT in the upper extremity now represents about 10% of the cases of DVT, reflecting complications from increased placement of central venous catheters, cardiac pacemakers, and defibrillators.[11]

Anatomy and Physiology

Arteries

Arteries contain three concentric layers of tissue: the *intima,* the *media,* and the *adventitia* (Figs. 12-1 and 12-2). The *internal elastic membrane* borders the intima and the media; the *external elastic membrane* separates the media from the adventitia.

Atherosclerosis is a chronic inflammatory disease initiated by injury to vascular endothelial cells, provoking atheromatous plaque formation and the vascular lesions of hypertension.

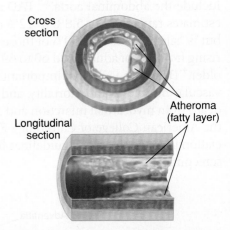

Cross section

Atheroma (fatty layer)

Longitudinal section

FIGURE 12-2. **Arterial atheromas.**

Atheroma formation begins in the intima, where circulating lipoproteins, especially low-density lipoproteins (LDLs), are exposed to proteoglycans from the extracellular matrix, undergo oxidative modification, and trigger a local inflammatory response that attracts mononuclear phagocytes. Once in the intima, phagocytes mature into macrophages, ingest lipids, and become foam cells that develop into fatty streaks.

Intima. Surrounding the lumen of all blood vessels is the *intima,* a single continuous lining of endothelial cells with remarkable metabolic properties.[12] Intact endothelium synthesizes regulators of thrombosis such as prostacyclin, plasminogen activator, and heparin-like molecules. It produces prothrombotic molecules such as von Willebrand factor and plasminogen activator inhibitor. It modulates blood flow and vascular reactivity through synthesis of vasoconstrictors like endothelin and angiotensin-converting enzyme, and vasodilators such as nitric oxide and prostacyclin. The intimal endothelium also regulates immune and inflammatory reactions through elaboration of interleukins, adhesion molecules, and histocompatibility antigens.

Atheroma Formation

- In *complex atheromas*, there is a proliferation of smooth muscle cells and extracellular matrix that breaches the endothelial lining.
- Complex atheromas contain a fibrous cap of smooth muscle cells that overlies a necrotic lipid-rich core, vascular cells, and a wide range of immune cells and prothrombotic molecules.
- Inflammatory mediators that alter collagen repair and cap fibrosis are increasingly implicated in plaque rupture and plaque erosion, which expose thrombogenic factors in the plaque core to coagulation factors in the blood.

Investigators place increasing emphasis on plaque activation, in addition to luminal stenosis, as a major precipitant of ischemia and infarction.[13–15]

Media. The *media* is composed of smooth muscle cells that dilate and constrict to accommodate blood pressure and flow. Its inner and outer boundaries consist of elastic fibers, or *elastin,* and are called *internal* and *external elastic laminae,* or membranes. Small arterioles called the *vasa vasorum* perfuse the media.

Adventitia. The outer layer of the artery is the *adventitia,* the connective tissue containing nerve fibers and the vasa vasorum.

Arterial Branching. Arteries must respond to the variations in cardiac output during systole and diastole. Their anatomy and size vary according to their distance from the heart. The aorta and its immediate branches are *large highly elastic arteries* such as the common carotid and iliac arteries. These arteries course into *medium-sized muscular arteries* such as the coronary and renal arteries. The elastic recoil and smooth muscle contraction and relaxation in the media of large and medium-sized arteries produce arterial pulsatile flow. Medium-sized arteries divide into *small arteries* less than 2 mm in diameter and even smaller *arterioles* with diameters from 20 to 100 μm (sometimes termed "microns"). Resistance to blood flow occurs primarily in the arterioles. Recall that resistance is inversely proportional to the vessel radius, known as the law of Laplace. From the arterioles, blood flows into the vast network of *capillaries,* each the diameter of a single red blood cell, only 7 to 8 μm across. Capillaries have an endothelial cell lining, but no media, facilitating rapid diffusion of oxygen and carbon dioxide.

If a major artery is obstructed, anastomoses between branching networks of smaller arteries can increase in size over time to form *collateral circulation* that perfuses structures distal to the occlusion.

Arterial Pulses. Arterial pulses are palpable in arteries lying close to the body surface.

Pulses in the Arms and Hands.
In the arms, locate pulsations in the arteries shown in Figure 12-3:

- The *brachial artery* at the bend of the elbow just medial to the biceps tendon

- The *radial artery* on the lateral flexor surface

- The *ulnar artery* on the medial flexor surface, although overlying tissues may obscure pulsations in the ulnar artery

Two vascular arches within the hand interconnect the radial and ulnar arteries, doubly protecting circulation to the hand and fingers against possible arterial occlusion.

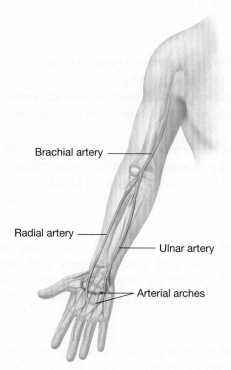

Brachial artery

Radial artery

Ulnar artery

Arterial arches

FIGURE 12-3. **Arteries of the arm.**

Pulses in the Abdomen. In the abdomen, locate the pulsations of the *aorta* in the epigastrium (Fig. 12-4). Not palpable are its three important deeper branches, the celiac trunk and the superior and inferior mesenteric arteries, which perfuse the important organs of the abdominal cavity.

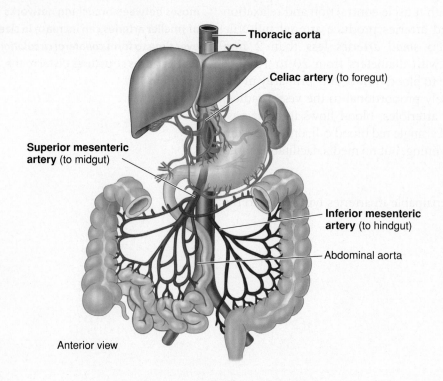

Thoracic aorta

Celiac artery (to foregut)

Superior mesenteric artery (to midgut)

Inferior mesenteric artery (to hindgut)

Abdominal aorta

Anterior view

FIGURE 12-4. **Abdominal aorta and its branches.**

- *Celiac trunk:* esophagus, stomach, proximal duodenum, liver, gallbladder, pancreas, spleen (foregut)

- *Superior mesenteric artery:* small intestine—jejunum, ileum, cecum; large intestine—ascending and transverse colon, right splenic flexure (midgut)

- *Inferior mesenteric artery:* large intestine—descending and sigmoid colon, proximal rectum (hindgut)

Pulses in the Legs. As shown in Figure 12-5, in the legs, palpate pulsations in:

- The *femoral artery* just below the inguinal ligament, midway between the anterior superior iliac spine and the symphysis pubis

- The *popliteal artery,* an extension of the femoral artery that passes medially behind the femur, palpable just behind the knee. The popliteal artery divides into the two arteries perfusing the lower leg and foot, listed below

- The *dorsalis pedis (DP) artery* on the dorsum of the foot just lateral to the extensor tendon of the big toe

- The *posterior tibial (PT) artery* lies behind the medial malleolus of the ankle. An interconnecting arch between its two chief arterial branches protects circulation to the foot.

Veins

Unlike arteries, veins are thin-walled and highly distensible, with a capacity for containing up to two thirds of circulating blood flow. The *venous intima* consists of nonthrombogenic endothelium. Protruding into the lumen are unidirectional valves that promote venous return to the heart. The *media* contains circumferential rings of elastic tissue and smooth muscle that change vein caliber in response to even minor changes in venous pressure. The smallest veins, or *venules,* drain capillary beds and form interconnecting venous plexuses such as the prostatic and the rectal venous plexuses.

Veins from the arms, upper trunk, and head and neck drain into the *superior vena cava,* which empties into the right atrium. Veins from the abdominal viscera, lower trunk, and legs drain into the *inferior vena cava,* except for circulation through the liver. The *portal vein,* at the confluence of the nutrient-rich superior mesenteric and splenic veins, supplies ~75% of the blood flow to the liver, supplemented by oxygenated blood from the hepatic artery. Blood from these vessels flows into the hepatic sinusoids, then drains into three large hepatic veins that empty into the inferior vena cava. Because of their weaker wall structure, the leg veins are susceptible to irregular dilatation, compression, ulceration, and invasion by tumors, and warrant special attention.

Deep and Superficial Venous System of the Legs. The *deep veins* of the legs carry approximately 90% of the venous return from the lower extremities. They are well supported by surrounding tissues.

Despite the rich collateral network that protects the three branches against hypoperfusion, occlusion of the mesenteric arteries can result in bowel ischemia and infarction.

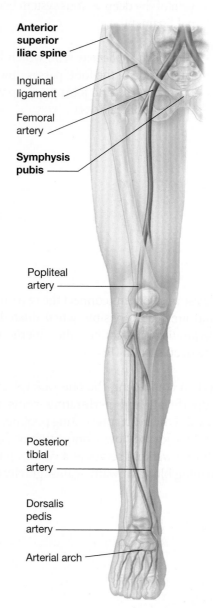

Anterior superior iliac spine

Inguinal ligament

Femoral artery

Symphysis pubis

Popliteal artery

Posterior tibial artery

Dorsalis pedis artery

Arterial arch

FIGURE 12-5. Arteries of the leg.

In contrast, the *superficial veins* are subcutaneous, with relatively poor tissue support (Fig. 12-6). They include:

- The *great saphenous vein,* which originates on the dorsum of the foot, passes just anterior to the medial malleolus, continues up the medial aspect of the leg, and joins the femoral vein of the deep venous system below the inguinal ligament

- The *small saphenous vein,* which begins on the lateral side of the foot, passes upward along the posterior calf, and joins the deep venous system in the popliteal fossa

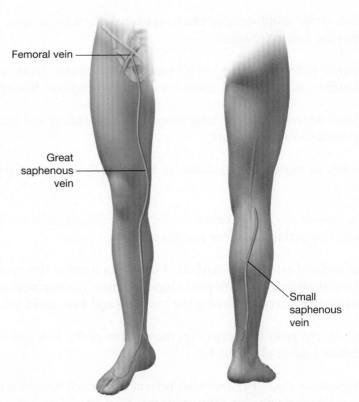

FIGURE 12-6. Superficial veins of the leg.

Anastomotic veins connect the two saphenous veins and are readily visible when dilated. Bridging or *perforating veins* connect the superficial system with the deep system (Fig. 12-7).

When competent, the one-way valves of the deep, superficial, and perforating veins propel blood toward the heart, preventing pooling, venous stasis, and backward flow. Contraction of the calf muscles during walking serves as a venous pump, also propelling blood upward against gravity.

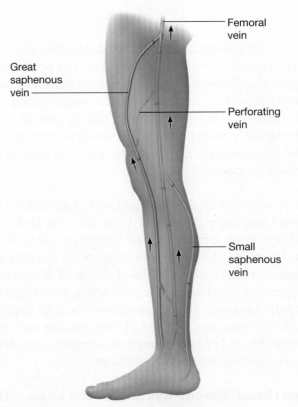

FIGURE 12-7. Deep, superficial, and perforating veins of the leg.

The Lymphatic System

The lymphatic system is an extensive vascular network that drains lymph fluid from body tissues and returns it to the venous circulation. Networks of lymphatic capillaries, the lymphatic plexuses, originate in the extracellular spaces, where the capillaries collect tissue fluid, plasma proteins, cells, and cellular debris via their porous endothelium, which lacks even a basement membrane. The lymphatic capillaries continue centrally as thin vascular channels, then as collecting ducts, and empty into the major veins at the neck. The *right lymphatic duct* drains fluid from the right side of the head, neck, thorax, and right upper limb and empties into the junction of the right internal jugular and the right subclavian veins. The *thoracic duct* collects lymph fluid from the rest of the body and empties into the junction of the left internal jugular and the left subclavian veins. Lymph fluid transported through these channels is filtered through lymph nodes interposed along the way.

Lymph Nodes. Lymph nodes are round, oval, or bean-shaped structures that vary in size according to their location. Some lymph nodes, such as the preauricular nodes, if palpable at all, are typically very small. The inguinal nodes, by contrast, are relatively larger—often 1 cm in diameter and occasionally even 2 cm in an adult.

In addition to its vascular functions, the lymphatic system plays an important role in the body's immune system. Cells within the lymph nodes engulf cellular debris and bacteria and produce antibodies.

Only the superficial lymph nodes are accessible to physical examination. These include the cervical nodes (p. 259), the axillary nodes (p. 421), and nodes in the arms and legs.

Recall that the axillary lymph nodes drain most of the arm (Fig. 12-8). Lymphatics from the ulnar surface of the forearm and hand, the little and ring fingers, and the adjacent surface of the middle finger, however, drain first

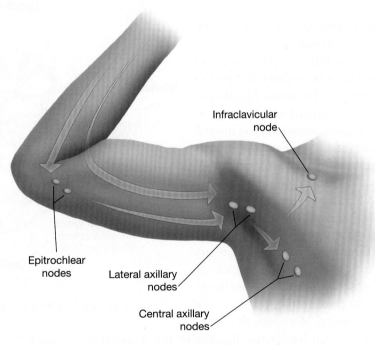

Infraclavicular node

Epitrochlear nodes

Lateral axillary nodes

Central axillary nodes

FIGURE 12-8. **Lymph nodes of the arm.**

into the *epitrochlear nodes.* These are located on the medial surface of the arm approximately 3 cm above the elbow. Lymphatics from the rest of the arm drain primarily into the axillary nodes. Some lymph fluid may go directly to the infraclavicular nodes.

The lymphatics of the lower limb, following the venous supply, consist of both deep and superficial systems (Fig. 12-9). Only the superficial nodes are palpable. The *superficial inguinal nodes* include two groups. The *horizontal group* lies in a chain high in the anterior thigh below the inguinal ligament. It drains the superficial portions of the lower abdomen and buttock, the external genitalia (but not the testes), the anal canal and perianal area, and the lower vagina.

The *vertical group* clusters near the upper part of the saphenous vein and drains a corresponding region of the leg. By contrast, lymphatics from the portion of leg drained by the small saphenous vein (the heel and outer aspect of the foot) join the deep system at the level of the popliteal space. Lesions in this space are not usually associated with palpable inguinal lymph nodes.

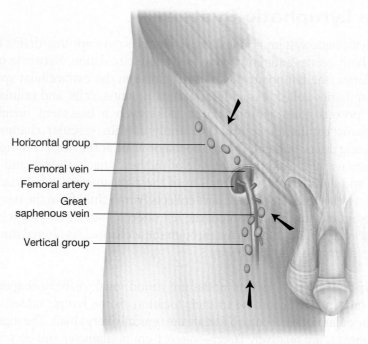

Horizontal group
Femoral vein
Femoral artery
Great saphenous vein
Vertical group

FIGURE 12-9. **Superficial inguinal lymph nodes.**

Transcapillary Fluid Exchange

Blood circulates from arteries to veins through the capillary bed (Fig. 12-10). Traditionally, fluid shifts between the plasma in the intravascular space and tissue interstitial space have been described by the Starling law. Starling proposed outward filtration at the arteriolar end of the capillary (due to hydrostatic and interstitial colloid oncotic pressures) and inward resorption at the venous end of the capillary (due to colloid osmotic pressure from plasma proteins). Recent studies have demonstrated greater complexity in capillary dynamics and the relationships between the endothelial capillary lining, the interstitium, and lymphatic drainage.[16–18] Net filtration appears to continue throughout the capillary, regulated in part by a capillary endothelial glycocalyx layer that affects intravascular volume and net filtration. Interstitial oncotic pressure is notably lower than plasma oncotic pressure. Moreover, the interstitium is more than a reservoir for plasma ultrafiltrate. It is a complex system of fluid containing albumin, a gel consisting of glycosaminoglycan molecules, and collagen. Capillary transendothelial filtration has been found to be significantly less than previously understood. Most filtered fluid returns to the circulation not as fluid resorbed at the venous end of the capillaries, but as lymph. The kidneys also play a role in retention of sodium and water when plasma volume goes down. Much of this fluid enters the interstitial space and appears clinically as edema. Readers are encouraged to review this recent literature, which has implications for use of crystalloid versus colloid fluid resuscitation.

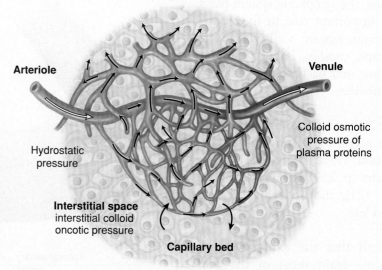

Lymph vessels

Arteriole

Venule

Hydrostatic pressure

Colloid osmotic pressure of plasma proteins

Interstitial space
interstitial colloid oncotic pressure

Capillary bed

FIGURE 12-10. **Capillary fluid exchange.**

Mechanisms for the development of edema include increased plasma volume from sodium retention, altered capillary dynamics resulting in net filtration, inadequate removal of filtered lymph fluid, lymphatic or venous obstruction, and increased capillary permeability.[19,20] See Table 12-1, Types of Peripheral Edema, p. 533.

The Health History

Common or Concerning Symptoms

- Abdominal, flank, or back pain
- Pain or weakness in the arms or legs
- Intermittent claudication
- Cold, numbness, pallor in the legs; hair loss
- Swelling in calves, legs, or feet
- Color change in fingertips or toes in cold weather
- Swelling with redness or tenderness

Peripheral Arterial Disease.   As noted, PAD refers to stenotic, occlusive, and aneurysmal disease of the abdominal aorta, its mesenteric and renal branches, and the arteries of the lower extremities, exclusive of the coronary arteries.[5] Pain in the extremities can also arise from the skin, musculoskeletal system, or nervous system. It may also be referred, like the pain of myocardial infarction that radiates to the left arm.

See Table 12-2, Painful Peripheral Vascular Disorders and Their Mimics, pp. 534–535.

- Ask about abdominal, flank, or back pain, especially in older smokers. Is there unusual constipation or distention? Inquire about for urinary retention, difficulty voiding, or renal colic.

An expanding hematoma from an abdominal aortic aneurysm (AAA) may cause symptoms by compressing the bowel, aortic branch arteries, or the ureters.[21,22]

- If there is persisting abdominal pain, ask about any related "food fear," weight loss, or dark stool.

These symptoms suggest *mesenteric ischemia* from arterial embolism, arterial or venous thrombosis, bowel volvulus or strangulation, or hypoperfusion. Failure to detect acute symptoms can result in bowel necrosis and even death.

- Ask about any pain or cramping in the legs during exertion that is relieved by rest within 10 minutes, called *intermittent claudication*.

Symptomatic limb ischemia with exertion is *atherosclerotic PAD*. Pain with walking or prolonged standing, radiating from the spinal area into the buttocks, thighs, lower legs, or feet, is *neurogenic claudication*. The positive likelihood ratio (LR) of *spinal stenosis* is >6 if the pain is relieved by sitting and bending forward, or if there is bilateral buttock or leg pain.[23]

■ Ask also about *coldness, numbness,* or *pallor* in the legs or *feet* or *loss of hair* over the anterior tibial surfaces.

Hair loss over the anterior tibiae points to decreased arterial perfusion. "Dry" or brown–black ulcers from *gangrene* may ensue.

Because most patients with PAD report minimal symptoms, enquire about two common types of atypical leg pain from PAD that occur prior to critical limb ischemia: *leg pain on exertion and rest* (exertional pain that can begin at rest), and *leg pain/carry on* (exertional pain that does not stop the patient from walking). Ask specifically about the PAD warning signs that follow, particularly in patients aged ≥50 years and those with *PAD risk factors,* especially smoking, but also diabetes, hypertension, elevated cholesterol, African American ethnicity, or coronary artery disease (see pp. 363–364). When the symptoms or risk factors described in the box below are present, pursue careful examination and testing with the ankle–brachial index (ABI) (see also p. 536).

Only 10% of patients have the classic features of leg pain with exertion relieved by rest.[24] Another 30% to 50% have atypical leg pain, and up to 60% are asymptomatic. Asymptomatic patients can have significant functional impairment that limits or slows walking to avoid symptoms as PAD is progressing.

Peripheral Arterial Disease "Warning Signs"

- Fatigue, aching, numbness, or pain that limits walking or exertion in the legs; if present, identify the location. Ask also about erectile dysfunction.
- Any poorly healing or nonhealing wounds of the legs or feet
- Any pain present when at rest in the lower leg or foot and changes when standing or supine

- Abdominal pain after meals and associated "food fear" and weight loss (see Chapter 11)

- Any first-degree relatives with an AAA

Symptom location suggests the site of arterial ischemia:

- buttock, hip: *aortoiliac*
- erectile dysfunction: *iliac–pudendal*
- thigh: *common femoral* or *aortoiliac*
- upper calf: *superficial femoral*
- lower calf: *popliteal*
- foot: *tibial* or *peroneal*

These symptoms suggest intestinal ischemia of the *celiac* or *superior* or *inferior mesenteric arteries.*

Prevalence of AAAs in first-degree relatives is 15% to 28%.[25]

Peripheral Venous Disease (or Venous Thromboembolism).
In patients with central venous catheters, ask about arm discomfort, pain, paresthesias, and weakness.

These symptoms point to upper extremity DVT, most commonly from catheter-associated thrombosis.[11] Most patients are asymptomatic with thrombosis detected on routine screening.

Ask about pain or swelling in the calf or leg.

Because individual clinical features have poor diagnostic value, experts recommend use of well-validated formal clinical scoring systems like the Wells Clinical Score and the Primary Care Rule for all patients with suspected DVT.[8,26]

Health Promotion and Counseling: Evidence and Recommendations

Important Topics for Health Promotion and Counseling

- Screening for lower-extremity peripheral artery disease
- The ankle–brachial index
- Screening for renal artery disease
- Screening for abdominal aortic aneurysm

Screening for Lower-Extremity Peripheral Artery Disease.

Atherosclerotic lower-extremity PAD affects more than 200 million people globally.[27] Prevalence increases with age, ranging from around 5% at ages 40 to 49 years to 15% to 20% in persons aged 80 years and older. Cardiovascular risk factors, particularly smoking and diabetes, increase risk for PAD: an estimated 40% to 60% of PAD patients have coexisting coronary artery disease and/or cerebral artery disease, and the presence of PAD significantly increases the risk for cardiovascular events.[28] Only a minority of PAD patients have classic claudication (exertional calf pain relieved by rest), and many are asymptomatic.[29]

Risk Factors for Lower-Extremity Peripheral Arterial Disease

- Age ≥65 years
- Age ≥50 years with a history of diabetes or smoking
- Leg symptoms with exertion
- Nonhealing wounds

Source: Rooke TW, Hirsch AT, Misra S, et al. Management of patients with peripheral artery disease (compilation of 2005 and 2011 ACCF/AHA Guideline Recommendations): a report of the American College of Cardiology Foundation/American Heart Association Task Force on Practice Guidelines. American College of Cardiology Foundation Task Force, American Heart Association Task Force. *J Am Coll Cardiol.* 2013;61:1555.

The Ankle–Brachial Index.

PAD can be diagnosed noninvasively using the *ABI*. The ABI is the ratio of blood pressure measurements in the foot and arm; values <0.9 are considered abnormal. However, the U.S. Preventive Services Task Force (USPSTF) does not advocate PAD screening due to insufficient evidence for estimating the relative benefits and harms of ABI testing (I statement).[30] Nonetheless, the American College of Cardiology Foundation/American Heart Association (ACCF/AHA) practice guidelines recommend measuring ABI in those at risk, as detailed in the box below, in order to offer therapeutic interventions to reduce the risk of cardiovascular events.[5]

Learn to use the ABI, which is reliable, reproducible, and easy to perform in the office. Although the sensitivity of an abnormal ABI is low (15% to 20%), the specificity is 99%, and the test has high positive and negative predictive values (both >80%).[1] Clinicians or office staff can easily measure systolic blood pressure in the arms using a sphygmomanometer and the pedal pulses using Doppler ultrasound. These values can be entered into calculators available at selected websites (see American College of Physicians, at http://www.sononet.us/abiscore/abiscore.htm).

For patients with PAD and intermittent claudication, the ACCF/AHA guidelines strongly recommend *supervised exercise programs* as the initial treatment.[5] Randomized clinical trials have shown significantly increased pain-free walking distances with supervised exercise programs compared to nonsupervised programs.[31] Other recommendations for managing PAD include: tobacco cessation; treatment of hyperlipidemia; optimal control of diabetes and hypertension; use of antiplatelet agents; meticulous foot care and well-fitting shoes, particularly for diabetic patients; and, in selected cases, revascularization.

Screening for Renal Artery Disease. Atherosclerotic renal artery stenosis (RAS) is present in substantial proportions of patients with end-stage renal disease, congestive heart failure, co-occurring diabetes and hypertension, and other atherosclerotic diseases.[32] Atherosclerotic RAS is associated with markedly increased risks for cardiovascular events.[33] RAS is less commonly caused by fibromuscular dysplasia, usually in women younger than age 40 years. The ACCF/AHA guidelines recommend screening for RAS with either duplex ultrasonography, magnetic resonance angiography, or computed tomographic angiography in patients with the conditions listed in the box below.[5]

See Table 12-3, Using the Ankle–Brachial Index, p. 536.

See Chapter 9, pp. 365–367, for guidelines for assessing blood pressure. The frequency of hypertension arising from RAS is unknown.

Conditions Suspicious for Renal Artery Disease

- Onset of hypertension at age ≤30 years
- Onset of severe hypertension at age ≥55 years
- Accelerated (sudden and persistent worsening of previously controlled hypertension), resistant (not controlled with three drugs), or malignant hypertension (evidence of acute end-organ damage)
- New worsening of renal function or worsening function after use of an angiotensin-converting enzyme inhibitor or an angiotensin-receptor blocking agent
- An unexplained small kidney or size discrepancy of >1.5 cm between the two kidneys
- Sudden unexplained pulmonary edema, especially in the setting of worsening renal function

Screening for Abdominal Aortic Aneurysm. AAA is defined as an infrarenal aortic diameter ≥3 cm. The population prevalence of AAA in adults older than age 50 years ranges from 3.9% to 7.2% in men and from 1% to 1.3% in women.[34,35] The dreaded consequence of AAA is rupture, which is often fatal—most patients die before reaching a hospital. The chances of rupture and mortality increase dramatically when the aortic diameter exceeds 5.5 cm. The strongest *risk factors for AAA* are older age, male sex, smoking, and family history; other potential risk factors include history of other vascular aneurysms, taller height, coronary artery disease, cerebrovascular disease, atherosclerosis, hypertension, and hyperlipidemia.[34]

Because symptoms are uncommon and screening can reduce AAA-related mortality by about 50% over 13 to 15 years, the USPSTF makes a grade B recommendation for one-time ultrasound screening of men aged 65 to 75 years who have smoked more than 100 cigarettes in a lifetime.[36] Clinicians can selectively offer screening to men in this age range who have never smoked (grade C); evidence is insufficient regarding screening women in this age range who have ever smoked (I statement). However, the USPSTF recommends against screening women who have never smoked (grade D). Ultrasound is a noninvasive, inexpensive, and accurate (sensitivity 94% to 100%; specificity 98% to 100%) screening test for diagnosing AAA. Palpation is not sensitive enough to be recommended for screening.

Techniques of Examination

Important Areas of Examination

Arms	Abdomen	Legs
Size, symmetry, skin color	Aortic width and pulsation	Size, symmetry, skin color
Radial pulse, brachial pulse	Inguinal lymph nodes	Femoral, popliteal, dorsalis pedis, and posterior tibial pulses
Epitrochlear lymph nodes		Thighs, calves, and ankles for swelling and peripheral edema

As you intensify your focus on the peripheral vascular system, recall that peripheral arterial disease is often asymptomatic and underdiagnosed, leading to significant morbidity and mortality. Review the techniques for assessing blood pressure, the carotid artery, the aorta, and the renal and femoral arteries on the pages indicated below, which reflect current guidelines.

Summary: Key Components of the Peripheral Arterial Examination

- Measure the blood pressure in both arms (see Chapter 4, p. 130).
- Palpate the carotid upstroke, auscultate for bruits (see Chapter 9, pp. 381–382).

- Auscultate for aortic, renal, and femoral bruits; palpate the aorta and assess its maximal diameter (see Chapter 11, pp. 472, 483).
- Palpate the pulses of the brachial, radial, ulnar, femoral, popliteal, DP, and PT arteries.
- Inspect the ankles and feet for color, temperature, and skin integrity; note any ulcerations; inspect for hair loss, trophic skin changes, hypertrophic nails.

Source: Hirsch AT, Haskal ZJ, Hertzer NR, et al. ACC/AHA 2005 Practice Guidelines for the management of patients with peripheral arterial disease (lower extremity, renal, mesenteric, and abdominal aortic): a collaborative report from the American Association for Vascular Surgery/Society for Vascular Surgery, Society for Cardiovascular Angiography and Interventions, Society for Vascular Medicine and Biology, Society of Interventional Radiology, and the ACC/AHA Task Force on Practice Guidelines (Writing Committee to Develop Guidelines for the Management of Patients With Peripheral Arterial Disease): endorsed by the American Association of Cardiovascular and Pulmonary Rehabilitation; National Heart, Lung, and Blood Institute; Society for Vascular Nursing; TransAtlantic Inter-Society Consensus; and Vascular Disease Foundation. *J Am Coll Cardiol.* 2006;47:1239.

Asymmetric blood pressures are found in *coarctation of the aorta* and *dissecting aortic aneurysm.*

Atherosclerotic disease occurs preferentially in selected arteries—the carotid bifurcation and the proximal renal arteries (and the proximal left anterior descending coronary artery).[14] In the aorta, atherosclerotic disease results in ectasia and the formation of aneurysms.

There are several recommended systems for grading the amplitude of arterial pulses. One system uses a scale of 0 to 3, as shown in the box below.[25] Use the scale adopted by your institution.

If an artery is widely dilated, it is *aneurysmal.*

Recommended Grading of Pulses

3+	Bounding
2+	**Brisk, expected (normal)**
1+	Diminished, weaker than expected
0	Absent, unable to palpate

Bounding carotid, radial, and femoral pulses are present in *aortic regurgitation;* asymmetric diminished pulses point to arterial occlusion from atherosclerosis or embolism.

Arms

Inspection. *Inspect both arms* from the fingertips to the shoulders. Note:

- Their size, symmetry, and any swelling

Swelling from lymphedema of the arm and hand may follow axillary node dissection and radiation therapy.

- The venous pattern

Visible venous collaterals, swelling, edema, and discoloration signal upper extremity DVT.[11]

- The color of the skin and nail beds and the texture of the skin

Palpation. *Palpate the radial pulse* with the pads of your fingers on the flexor surface of the lateral wrist (Fig. 12-11). Partially flexing the patient's wrist may help you feel this pulse. Compare the pulses in both arms.

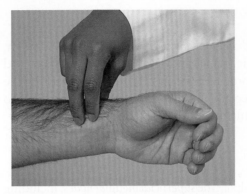

FIGURE 12-11. Palpate the radial pulse.

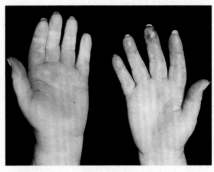

FIGURE 12-12. Raynaud disease.

In *Raynaud disease,* wrist pulses are typically normal, but spasm of more distal arteries causes episodes of sharply demarcated pallor of the fingers, as shown in Figure 12-12 (see Table 12-2, Painful Peripheral Vascular Disorders and Their Mimics, pp. 534–535).

If you suspect arterial insufficiency, palpate the *brachial pulse.* Flex the patient's elbow slightly, and palpate the artery just medial to the biceps tendon at the antecubital crease (Fig. 12-13). The brachial pulse can also be palpated higher in the arm in the groove between the biceps and triceps muscles.

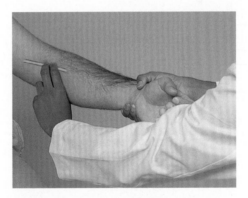

FIGURE 12-13. Palpate the brachial pulse.

Capillary refill time in the digits of >5 seconds has low sensitivity and specificity and is not considered diagnostically helpful.[26]

Palpate one or more *epitrochlear nodes.* With the patient's elbow flexed to about 90° and the forearm supported by your hand, reach around behind the arm and feel in the groove between the biceps and triceps muscles, about 3 cm above the medial epicondyle (Fig. 12-14). If a node is present, note its size, consistency, and tenderness.

Epitrochlear nodes are difficult to identify in most healthy people.

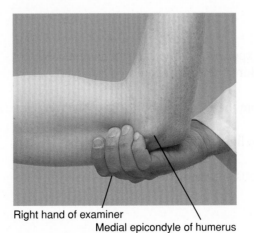

Right hand of examiner

Medial epicondyle of humerus

FIGURE 12-14. Palpate the epitrochlear nodes.

An enlarged epitrochlear node suggests local or distal infection or may be associated with lymphadenopathy from lymphoma or human immunodeficiency virus (HIV).

Abdomen

For techniques of examination of the *abdominal aorta,* see Chapter 11, Abdomen, pp. 472, 483. In brief, listen for aortic, renal, and femoral bruits. Palpate and estimate the width of the abdominal aorta in the epigastric area by measuring the aortic width between two fingers, especially in older adults and smokers due to higher risk of AAA. Assess for a pulsatile mass.

The sensitivity of aortic palpation for AAA ≥4 cm is 60%. Sensitivity for a pulsatile mass, detected in only 50% of diagnosed ruptures, is 40% to 60%. Note that an inguinal mass suspicious for an incarcerated hernia is often diagnosed as an AAA at surgery.[22]

The Inguinal Lymph Nodes.   Palpate the *superficial inguinal nodes,* including both the horizontal and the vertical groups (Fig. 12-15). Note their size, consistency, and discreteness, and note any tenderness. Nontender, discrete inguinal nodes up to 1 cm or even 2 cm in diameter are frequently palpable in normal people.

Lymphadenopathy refers to enlarged lymph nodes, with or without tenderness. Distinguish between local and generalized lymphadenopathy by locating either a causative lesion in the drainage area, or enlarged nodes in at least two other noncontiguous lymph node regions.

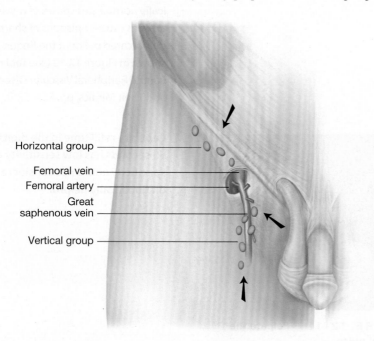

Horizontal group

Femoral vein

Femoral artery

Great saphenous vein

Vertical group

FIGURE 12-15.   **Superficial inguinal lymph nodes.**

Legs

The patient should be supine and draped so that the external genitalia are covered and the legs fully exposed. Stockings or socks should be removed.

Inspection.   Inspect both legs from the groin and buttocks to the feet. Note:

■ Their size, symmetry, and any swelling or edema

■ The venous pattern and any venous enlargement

Individual findings of calf, leg, or ankle swelling or asymmetry; venous dilatation; erythema; or superficial thrombophlebitis have low diagnostic value for DVT compared to combined scoring systems and ultrasound.[8,26] See also Table 12-4, Chronic Insufficiency of Arteries and Veins, p. 537.

■ Any pigmentation, rashes, scars, or ulcers

Ulcers or sores on the feet raise the LR of peripheral vascular disease to 7.[26] See Table 12-5, Common Ulcers of the Ankles and Feet, p. 538.

■ The color and texture of the skin, the color of the nail beds, and the distribution of hair on the lower legs, feet, and toes

Warmth and redness over the calf signal cellulitis. Atrophic and hairless skin is commonly present but not diagnostic of PAD.

Inspect the *color of the skin.*

■ Is there a local area of redness? If so, note its temperature.

Local swelling, redness, warmth, and a subcutaneous cord signal *superficial thrombophlebitis,* an emerging risk factor for DVT.[10]

■ Are there brownish areas near the ankles?

Brownish discoloration or ulcers just above the malleolus suggests *chronic venous insufficiency.*

■ Note any ulcers in the skin. Where are they?

Thickened, brawny skin suggests lymphedema and advanced venous insufficiency.

Inspect the saphenous system for *varicosities.* If present, ask the patient to stand, which allows any varicosities to fill with blood and makes them visible; these changes are easily missed when the patient is supine. Palpate along any varicosities to check for thrombophlebitis.

Varicose veins are dilated and tortuous. Their walls may feel somewhat thickened. Note the many varicose veins along the leg on p. 531.

Inspect and compare the thighs, calves, and ankles for *symmetry.* Note their relative size and the prominence of veins, tendons, and bones. Are the veins unusually prominent (Fig. 12-16)?

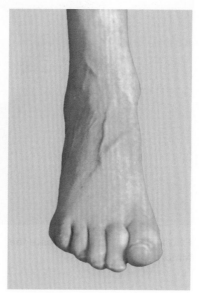

FIGURE 12-16. **Note the prominent veins.**

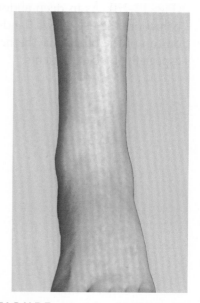

FIGURE 12-17. **Pretibial edema.**

Edema may obscure the veins, tendons, and bony prominences.

Is there swelling or edema (Fig. 12-17)? If so, is it unilateral or bilateral?

Unilateral calf and ankle swelling and edema suggest venous thromboembolic disease (VTE) from DVT, chronic venous insufficiency from prior DVT, or incompetent venous valves; or it may be lymphedema.

Bilateral edema is present in *heart failure, cirrhosis,* and *nephrotic syndrome.* Venous distention suggests a venous cause of edema.

Note the extent of the swelling. How far up the leg does it go?

In DVT, the location of edema suggests the point of occlusion—the popliteal vein if the lower leg or ankle is swollen, the iliofemoral veins if the entire leg is swollen.

If you detect unilateral swelling or edema, *measure the calves* 10 cm below the tibial tuberosity. Normally, the difference in calf circumference is <3 cm. Measure and compare other areas of asymmetry, if needed, including the thighs and ankles.

Calf asymmetry >3 cm increases the LR for DVT to >2.[26] Also consider muscle tear or trauma, Baker cyst (posterior knee), and muscular atrophy.

Palpation: The Peripheral Pulses.

Palpate the femoral, popliteal, and pedal pulses to assess the arterial circulation.

- *The femoral pulse.* Press deeply, below the inguinal ligament and about midway between the anterior superior iliac spine and the symphysis pubis (Fig. 12-18). As in deep abdominal palpation, the use of two hands, one on top of the other, may be helpful, especially in obese patients.

If the femoral pulse is absent, the LR of PAD is >6.[26] If the occlusion is at the aortic or iliac level, all pulses distal to the occlusion are typically affected and may cause postural color changes (see pp. 530–531).

An exaggerated, widened femoral pulse suggests the pathological dilatation of a *femoral aneurysm.*

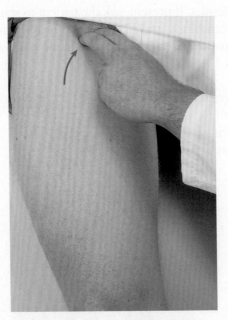

FIGURE 12-18. Palpate the femoral pulse.

■ *The popliteal pulse.* The patient's knee should be somewhat flexed, with the leg relaxed. Place the fingertips of both hands so that they just meet in the midline behind the knee and press them deeply into the popliteal fossa (Fig. 12-19). The popliteal pulse is more difficult to find than other pulses. It is deeper and feels more diffuse.

An exaggerated, widened popliteal pulse suggests a *popliteal artery aneurysm.* Popliteal and femoral aneurysms are uncommon. They are usually from atherosclerosis and occur primarily in men age ≥50 years.

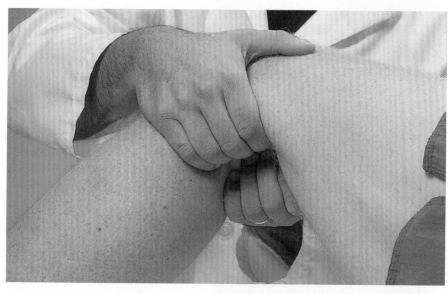

FIGURE 12-19. **Palpate the popliteal pulse.**

If you cannot palpate the popliteal pulse with this approach, try with the patient prone (Fig. 12-20). Flex the patient's knee to about 90°, let the lower leg relax against your shoulder or upper arm, and press your two thumbs deeply into the popliteal fossa (Fig. 12-21).

Atherosclerosis most commonly obstructs arteries in the thigh: The femoral pulse is normal, the popliteal pulse decreased or absent.

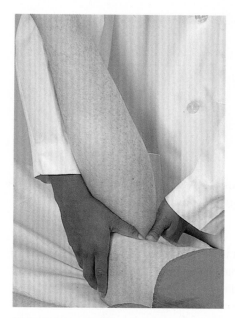

FIGURE 12-20. **Palpate the popliteal pulse, prone position.**

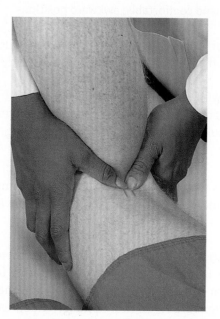

FIGURE 12-21. **Deep palpation in the popliteal fossa.**

- *The DP pulse.* Palpate the dorsum of the foot (not the ankle) just lateral to the extensor tendon of the great toe (Fig. 12-22). The DP artery may be congenitally absent or branch higher in the ankle. If you cannot feel a pulse, explore the dorsum of the foot more laterally.

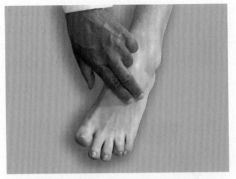

FIGURE 12-22. **Palpate the dorsalis pedis pulse.**

Absent pedal pulses with normal femoral and popliteal pulses raise the LR of PAD to >14.[26]

- *The PT pulse.* Curve your fingers behind and slightly below the medial malleolus of the ankle (Fig. 12-23). This pulse may be hard to feel in a fat or edematous ankle.

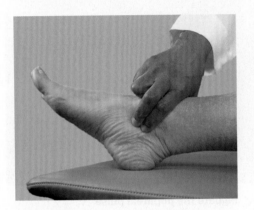

FIGURE 12-23. **Palpate the posterior tibial pulse.**

Acute arterial occlusion from embolism or thrombosis causes pain and numbness or tingling. The limb distal to the occlusion becomes cold, pale, and pulseless. Pursue emergency treatment.

Tips for Palpating Difficult Pulses

- Position your body and examining hand comfortably; awkward positions decrease tactile sensitivity.
- Once your hand is positioned properly, linger and vary the pressure of your fingers to pick up a weak pulsation. If unsuccessful, explore the area gently but more deliberately.
- Do not mistake the patient's pulse with your own pulsating fingertips. If needed, count your own heart rate and compare it to the patient's. The rates are usually different. Your carotid pulse is convenient for this comparison.

Assess the temperature of the feet and legs with the backs of your fingers. Compare one side with the other. Bilateral coldness is usually caused by a cold environment or anxiety.

Asymmetric coolness of the feet has a positive LR of >6 for PAD.[26]

The Peripheral Veins: Swelling and Edema. If swelling or edema is present, *palpate for pitting edema.* Press firmly but gently with your thumb for at least 2 seconds (1) over the dorsum of each foot, (2) behind each medial malleolus, and (3) over the shins (Fig. 12-24). Look for *pitting*—a depression caused by pressure from your thumb. Normally there is none. The severity of edema is graded on a four-point scale, from slight to very marked.

See Table 12-1, Types of Peripheral Edema, p. 533.

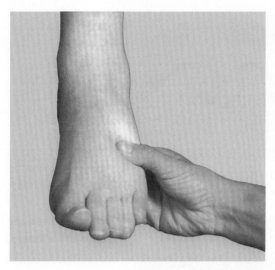

FIGURE 12-24. Palpate for pitting edema.

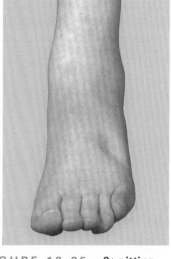

FIGURE 12-25. 3+ pitting edema.

Figure 12-25 shows 3+ pitting edema.

Palpate for any venous tenderness or cords, which can accompany a DVT. DVTs often have no demonstrable signs, so diagnosis often depends on clinical suspicion and testing.

- Palpate the inguinal area just medial to the femoral pulse for tenderness of the femoral vein.

A painful, pale, swollen leg, together with tenderness in the groin over the femoral vein, suggests deep *iliofemoral thrombosis*. Risk of PE in proximal vein thrombosis is 50%.[7]

- Next, with the patient's leg flexed at the knee and relaxed, palpate the calf. With your fingerpads, gently compress the calf muscles against the tibia, and search for any tenderness or cords.

Only half of patients with DVT in the calf have tenderness or venous cords, and absence of calf tenderness does not rule out thrombosis. Note that Homan sign, discomfort behind the knee with forced dorsiflexion on the foot, is neither sensitive nor specific, and discredited by Homan himself.[26]

Special Techniques

Evaluating Arterial Perfusion of the Hand. If you suspect arterial insufficiency in the arm or hand, try to palpate the *ulnar pulse* as well as the radial and brachial pulses. Press deeply on the flexor surface of the medial wrist (Fig. 12-26). Partially flexing the patient's wrist may help you. The pulse of a normal ulnar artery may not be palpable.

The Allen Test. The *Allen test* compares patency of the ulnar and radial arteries. It also ensures patency of the ulnar artery before puncturing the radial artery for blood samples. The patient should rest with hands in lap, palms up.

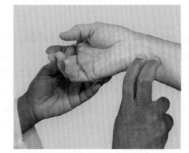

FIGURE 12-26. Palpate the ulnar pulse.

Arterial occlusive disease is much less common in the arms than in the legs. Absent or diminished pulses at the wrist occur in acute embolic occlusion and in *Buerger disease*, or *thromboangiitis obliterans*.

Ask the patient to make a tight fist with one hand; then compress both radial and ulnar arteries firmly between your thumbs and fingers (Fig. 12-27).

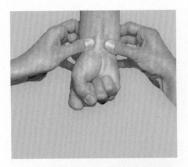

FIGURE 12-27. Compress the radial and ulnar arteries.

Next, ask the patient to open the hand into a relaxed, slightly flexed position (Fig. 12-28). The palm is pale.

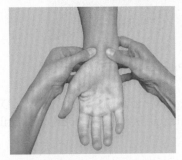

FIGURE 12-28. Pallor when hand relaxed.

Extending the hand fully may cause pallor and a falsely positive test.

Release your pressure over the ulnar artery. If the ulnar artery is patent, the palm flushes within about 3 to 5 seconds (Fig. 12-29).

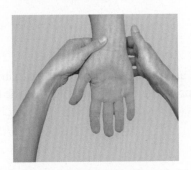

FIGURE 12-29. Palmar flushing—Allen test negative.

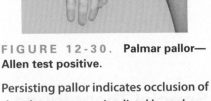

FIGURE 12-30. Palmar pallor—Allen test positive.

Persisting pallor indicates occlusion of the ulnar artery or its distal branches, as shown in Figure 12-30.

Test patency of the radial artery by releasing the radial artery while still compressing the ulnar artery.

Postural Color Changes of Chronic Arterial Insufficiency. If pain or diminished pulses suggest arterial insufficiency, consider looking for postural color changes using the Buerger test (although it has not been studied well).[26] Raise both legs to about 90° for up to 2 minutes until there is maximal pallor of the feet. In light-skinned persons, expect to see normal color, as in this right foot (Fig. 12-31), or slight pallor. In darker-skinned persons, if color changes are difficult to see, inspect the soles of the feet instead, and use tangential lighting to see the veins.

Marked pallor on elevation suggests *arterial insufficiency,* as shown in Figure 12-31, left foot (right side of photo).

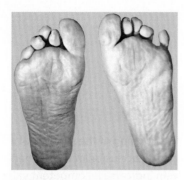

FIGURE 12-31. **The Buerger test—legs elevated.**

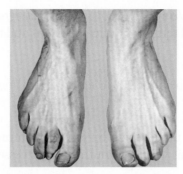

FIGURE 12-32. **The Buerger test—legs when sitting.**

Then ask the patient to sit up with legs dangling down. Compare both feet, noting the time required for:

- Return of pinkness to the skin, normally about 10 seconds or less

- Filling of the veins of the feet and ankles, normally about 15 seconds

This right foot has normal color, and the veins on the foot have filled (Fig. 12-32). These normal responses suggest an adequate circulation.

As shown in Figure 12-32, right side, the left foot is still pale, and the veins are just starting to fill, signs of arterial insufficiency.

Look for any unusual *rubor* (dusky redness) to replace the pallor of the dependent foot. Rubor may take a minute or more to appear.

Normal responses accompanied by diminished arterial pulses point to good collateral circulation around an arterial occlusion.

Persisting dependent rubor suggests arterial insufficiency (see p. 538). If the patient's veins are incompetent, dependent rubor and the timing of color return and venous filling are not reliable tests of arterial insufficiency.

Mapping Varicose Veins. Mapping can demonstrate varicose veins and their origin. With the patient standing, place your palpating fingers gently on a vein and, with your other hand below it, compress the vein sharply (Fig. 12-33). Feel for a pressure wave transmitted to the fingers of your upper hand. A palpable pressure wave indicates that the two parts of the vein are connected.

A wave may also be transmitted downward, but not as easily.

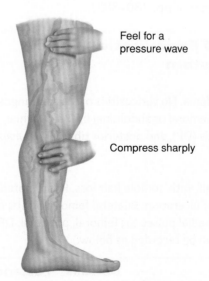

Feel for a pressure wave

Compress sharply

FIGURE 12-33. **Compress with both hands.**

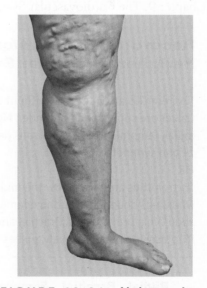

FIGURE 12-34. **Varicose veins.**

Source for Figs. 12-31 and 12-32: Kappert A, Winsor T. *Diagnosis of Peripheral Vascular Disease.* Philadelphia, PA: FA Davis, 1972.

Evaluating the Competency of Venous Valves. Use the *retrograde filling (Trendelenburg) test* to assess the valves of the communicating veins and the saphenous system.

- With the patient supine, elevate one leg to about 90° to empty it of venous blood.

- Occlude the great saphenous vein in the upper thigh by manual compression, using enough pressure to occlude this vein but not the deeper vessels.

- Ask the patient to stand. While you keep the vein occluded, watch for venous filling in the leg. Normally, the saphenous vein fills from below, taking about 35 seconds as blood flows through the capillary bed into the venous system.

- After the patient stands for 20 seconds, release the compression and look for sudden additional venous filling. Normally, slow filling continues because competent valves in the saphenous vein block retrograde flow.

When both steps of this test are normal, the response is termed "negative–negative."

Rapid filling of the superficial veins during occlusion of the saphenous vein indicates incompetent valves in the communicating veins that allow rapid retrograde flow from the deep to the saphenous system.

Sudden additional filling of superficial veins after release of compression indicates incompetent valves in the saphenous vein.

Results can be negative–positive; positive–negative; or, when both steps are abnormal, positive–positive.

Recording Your Findings

Note that initially you may use sentences to describe your findings; later you will use phrases. Written descriptions of lymph nodes appear in Chapter 7, The Head and Neck (see p. 259). Likewise, assessment of the carotid pulse is recorded in Chapter 9, The Cardiovascular System (see pp. 380–382).

Recording the Physical Examination—The Peripheral Vascular System

"Extremities are warm and without edema. No varicosities or stasis changes. Calves are supple and nontender. No femoral or abdominal bruits. Brachial, radial, femoral, popliteal, dorsalis pedis (DP), and posterior tibial (PT) pulses are 2+ and symmetric."

OR

"Extremities are pale below the midcalf, with notable hair loss. Rubor noted when legs dependent but no edema or ulceration. Bilateral femoral bruits; no abdominal bruits heard. Brachial and radial pulses 2+; femoral, popliteal, DP and PT pulses 1+." (Alternatively, pulses can be recorded as below.)

These findings suggest atherosclerotic *peripheral arterial disease*.

	Radial	Brachial	Femoral	Popliteal	Dorsalis Pedis	Posterior Tibial
RT	2+	2+	1+	1+	1+	1+
LT	2+	2+	1+	1+	1+	1+

Table 12-1 Types of Peripheral Edema

Approximately one third of total body water is extracellular fluid, which, in turn, is roughly 25% plasma; the remainder is interstitial fluid. As discussed on p. 516, new evidence has changed the traditional understanding of Starling forces across the capillary bed. Net plasma filtration appears to occur throughout the length of the capillary. Interstitial oncotic pressure is notably lower than plasma oncotic pressure, and lymphatic drainage plays a greater role in returning interstitial fluid to the circulation than previously thought. Several clinical conditions disrupt these forces, resulting in *edema,* which is the clinically evident accumulation of interstitial fluid. Pitting characteristics reflect the viscosity of the edema fluid, based primarily on its protein concentration.[20,26] When protein concentration is low, as in heart failure, pitting and recovery occur within a few seconds. In lymphedema, protein levels are higher and nonpitting is more typical. Not depicted below is *capillary leak syndrome,* in which protein leaks into the interstitial space, seen in burns, angioedema, snake bites, and allergic reactions.

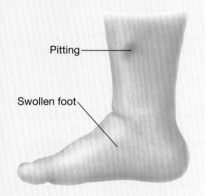

Pitting

Swollen foot

Pitting Edema

Edema is a soft, bilateral palpable swelling from increased interstitial fluid volume and retention of salt and water, demonstrated by pitting after 1 to 2 seconds of thumb pressure on the anterior tibiae and feet. Pitting edema occurs in several conditions: when legs are dependent from prolonged standing or sitting, which leads to increased hydrostatic pressure in the veins and capillaries; heart failure leading to decreased cardiac output; nephrotic syndrome, cirrhosis, or malnutrition leading to low albumin and decreased intravascular colloid oncotic pressure; and with selected medications.

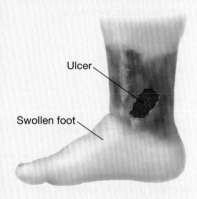

Ulcer

Swollen foot

Chronic Venous Insufficiency

Edema is soft, with pitting on pressure, and occasionally bilateral. Look for brawny changes and skin thickening, especially near the ankle. Ulceration, brownish pigmentation, and edema in the feet are common. It arises from chronic obstruction and incompetent valves in the deep venous system. (See also Table 12-2, Painful Peripheral Vascular Disorders and Their Mimics, pp. 534–535.)

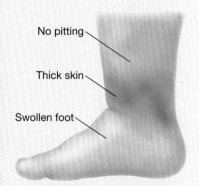

No pitting

Thick skin

Swollen foot

Lymphedema

Edema is initially soft and pitting, then becomes indurated, hard, and nonpitting. Skin is markedly thickened; ulceration is rare. There is no pigmentation. Edema often occurs bilaterally in the feet and toes. Lymphedema arises from interstitial accumulation of protein-rich fluid when lymph channels are infiltrated or obstructed by tumor, fibrosis, or inflammation, or disrupted by axillary node dissection and/or radiation.

Table 12-2 Painful Peripheral Vascular Disorders and Their Mimics

Problem	Process	Location of Pain
Arterial Disorders		
Raynaud Phenomenon: Primary and Secondary[37]	*Raynaud phenomenon, primary:* Episodic reversible vasoconstriction in the fingers and toes, usually triggered by cold temperatures (capillaries are normal); no definable cause	Distal portions of one or more fingers Pain is usually not prominent unless fingertip ulcers develop; numbness and tingling are common
	Raynaud phenomenon, secondary: symptoms/signs related to autoimmune diseases—scleroderma, systemic lupus erythematosus, mixed connective tissue disease; cryoglobulinemia; also to occupational vascular injury; drugs	
Peripheral Arterial Disease	Atherosclerotic disease leading to obstruction of peripheral arteries causing exertional claudication (muscle pain relieved by rest) and atypical leg pain; may progress to ischemic pain at rest	Usually calf muscles, but also occurs in the buttock, hip, thigh, or foot, depending on the level of obstruction; rest pain may be distal in the toes or forefoot
Acute Arterial Occlusion	Embolism or thrombosis	Distal pain, usually involving the foot and leg
Venous Disorders (Lower Extremity)		
Superficial Phlebitis and Superficial Vein Thrombosis	Involves inflammation of a superficial vein (best termed *superficial phlebitis*), at times with venous thrombosis (now termed *superficial vein thrombosis* when clot confirmed by imaging)	Pain and tenderness along the course of a superficial vein, most often in the saphenous system
Deep Venous Thrombosis (DVT)	DVT and PE are disorders of venous thromboembolic disease (VTE); DVTs are distal, limited to the deep calf veins, or proximal, in the popliteal, femoral, or iliac veins	Classically, painful calf swelling with erythema, but can be painless; signs correlate poorly with site of thrombosis
Chronic Venous Insufficiency (Deep)	More severe form of chronic venous disease, with chronic venous engorgement from venous occlusion or incompetent venous valves	Diffuse aching of the leg(s)
Thromboangiitis Obliterans (Buerger Disease)	Inflammatory nonatherosclerotic occlusive disease of small- to medium-sized arteries and veins, especially in smokers; occluding thrombus spares the blood vessel wall	Often digit or toe pain progressing to ischemic ulcerations
Compartment Syndrome	Pressure builds from trauma or bleeding into one of the four major muscle compartments between the knee and ankle; each compartment is enclosed by fascia that limits expansion to accommodate increasing pressure	Tight, bursting pain in calf muscles, usually in the anterior tibial compartment, sometimes with overlying dusky red skin
Acute Lymphangitis	Acute infection, usually from *Streptococcus pyogenes* or *Staphylococcus aureus,* spreading up the lymphatic channels from distal portal of entry such as skin abrasion, ulcer, or dog bite	An arm or a leg
Mimics (Primarily of Acute Superficial Thrombophlebitis)		
Acute Cellulitis	Acute bacterial infection of the skin and subcutaneous tissues, most commonly from *beta-hemolytic streptococci* (erysipelas) and *S. aureus*	In the arms, legs, or elsewhere
Erythema Nodosum	Painful raised, bilateral erythematous lesions from inflammation of subcutaneous fat tissue, seen in systemic conditions such as pregnancy, sarcoidosis, tuberculosis, streptococcal infections, inflammatory bowel disease, drugs (oral contraceptives)	Anterior pretibial surfaces of both lower legs; can also appear on extensor arms, buttocks, and thighs

Timing	Factors That Aggravate	Factors That Relieve	Associated Manifestations
Relatively brief (minutes), but recurrent	Exposure to cold, emotional upset	Warm environment	*Primary:* Distinct digital color changes of pallor, cyanosis, and hyperemia (redness); no necrosis *Secondary:* More severe, with ischemia, necrosis, and loss of digits; capillary loops are distorted
May be brief if relieved by rest; if there is *rest pain,* may be persistent and worse at night	Exercise such as walking; if *rest pain,* leg elevation and bedrest	Rest usually stops the pain in 1–3 min; *rest pain* may be relieved by walking (increases perfusion), sitting with legs dependent	Local fatigue, numbness, progressing to cool dry hairless skin, trophic nail changes, diminished to absent pulses, pallor with elevation, ulceration, gangrene (see p. 538)
Sudden onset; associated symptoms may occur without pain			Coldness, numbness, weakness, absent distal pulses
An acute episode lasting days or longer	Immobility, venous stasis and chronic venous disease, venous procedure, obesity	Supportive care, walking; measures prompted by further testing	Local induration, erythema; if palpable nodules or cords, consider superficial or deep vein thrombosis, both associated with significant risk of DVT and PE
Often hard to determine due to lack of symptoms; one third of untreated calf DVTs extend proximally	Immobilization or recent surgery, lower extremity trauma, pregnancy or postpartum state, hypercoagulable state (e.g., nephrotic syndrome, malignancy)	Antithrombotic and thrombolytic therapy	Asymmetric calf diameters more diagnostic than palpable cord or tenderness over femoral triangle; Homan sign unreliable; high risk of PE (50% with proximal DVT)
Chronic, increasing as the day wears on	Prolonged standing, sitting with legs dependent	Limb elevation, walking	Chronic edema, pigmentation, swelling, and possibly ulceration, especially if advanced age, pregnancy, increased weight, prior history, or trauma (see p. 538)
Ranges from brief recurrent to chronic persistent pain	Exercise	Rest; smoking cessation	May progress to gangrene at tips of digits; can move proximally, with migratory phlebitis and tender nodules along blood vessels; usually involves at least two limbs
Several hours if *acute* (pressure must be relieved to avert necrosis); during exercise if *chronic*	*Acute:* Anabolic steroids; surgical complication; crush injury *Chronic:* Occurs with exercise	*Acute:* Surgical incision to relieve pressure *Chronic:* Avoiding exercise; ice, elevation	Tingling, burning sensations in calf; muscles may feel tight, full; numbness, paralysis if unrelieved
An acute episode lasting days or longer			Red streak(s) on the skin, with tenderness, enlarged, tender lymph nodes, and fever
An acute episode lasting days or longer			Erythema, edema, and warmth *Erysipelas:* Lesion raised and demarcated from skin; involves upper dermis, lymphatics *Cellulitis:* Involves deeper dermis, adipose tissue; may include enlarged, tender lymph nodes and fever
Pain associated with a series of lesions over 2 to 8 wks			2–5-cm lesions, initially elevated, bright red then fade to violet or red-brown; do not ulcerate; often with polyarthralgia, fever, malaise

Table 12-3 Using the Ankle–Brachial Index

Instructions for Measuring the Ankle–Brachial Index (ABI)

1. Patient should rest supine in a warm room for at least 10 min before testing.
2. Place blood pressure cuffs on both arms and ankles as illustrated, then apply ultrasound gel over brachial, dorsalis pedis, and posterior tibial arteries.
3. Measure systolic pressures in the arms
   - Use vascular Doppler to locate brachial pulse
   - Inflate cuff 20 mm Hg above last audible pulse
   - Deflate cuff slowly and record pressure at which pulse becomes audible
   - Obtain 2 measures in each arm and record the average as the brachial pressure in that arm
4. Measure systolic pressures in ankles
   - Use vascular Doppler to locate dorsalis pedis pulse
   - Inflate cuff 20 mm Hg above last audible pulse
   - Deflate cuff slowly and record pressure at which pulse becomes audible
   - Obtain 2 measures in each ankle and record the average as the dorsalis pedis pressure in that leg
   - Repeat above steps for posterior tibial arteries
5. Calculate ABI

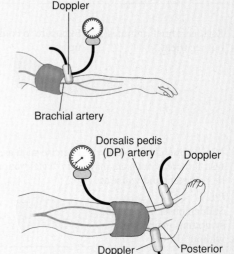

$$\text{Right ABI} = \frac{\text{highest right average ankle pressure (DP or PT)}}{\text{highest average arm pressure (right or left)}}$$

$$\text{Left ABI} = \frac{\text{highest left average ankle pressure (DP or PT)}}{\text{highest average arm pressure (right or left)}}$$

Site	1st reading	2nd reading	Average	Site	1st reading	2nd reading	Average
Left brachial				Right brachial			
Left dorsalis pedis				Right dorsalis pedis			
Left posterior tibial				Right posterior tibial			

Ankle–Brachial Index Calculator

$$A - BI = S_A \div S_B$$

Enter values for systolic pressure at:

The ankle: ☐ mm/Hg

The brachial artery: ☐ mm/Hg

Ankle–brachial index: ☐

Interpretation of Ankle–Brachial Index

>0.90 (with a range of 0.90 to 1.30) = Normal lower extremity blood flow

<0.89 to >0.60 = Mid PAD

<0.59 to >0.40 = Moderate PAD

<0.39 = Severe PAD

Sources: *Ankle–Brachial Calculator*—American College of Physicians. Available at: http://www.sononet.us/abiscore/abiscore.htm. Accessed February 28, 2015; Wilson JF, Laine C, Goldman D. In the clinic: peripheral arterial disease. *Ann Int Med.* 2007;146:ITC 3.

Table 12-4 Chronic Insufficiency of Arteries and Veins

Chronic Arterial Insufficiency (*Advanced*)	Chronic Venous Insufficiency (*Advanced*)

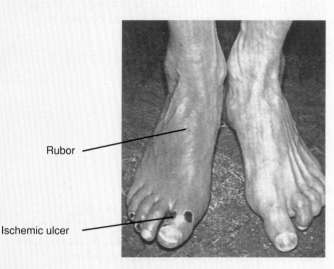

Rubor

Ischemic ulcer

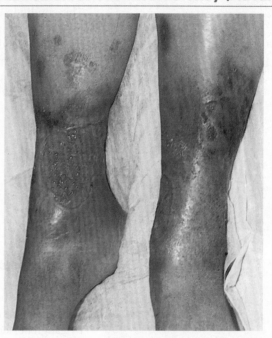

	Chronic Arterial Insufficiency (*Advanced*)	Chronic Venous Insufficiency (*Advanced*)
Pain	Intermittent claudication, progressing to pain at rest	Often painful
Mechanism	Tissue ischemia	Venous stasis and hypertension
Pulses	Decreased or absent	Normal, though may be difficult to feel through edema
Color	Pale, especially on elevation; dusky red on dependency	Normal, or cyanotic on dependency Petechiae and then brown pigmentation appear with chronicity
Temperature	Cool	Normal
Edema	Absent or mild; may develop as the patient tries to relieve rest pain by lowering the leg	Present, often marked
Skin Changes	Trophic changes: thin, shiny, atrophic skin; loss of hair over the foot and toes; nails thickened and ridged	Often brown pigmentation around the ankle, stasis dermatitis, and possible thickening of the skin and narrowing of the leg as scarring develops
Ulceration	If present, involves toes or points of trauma on feet	If present, develops at sides of ankle, especially medially
Gangrene	May develop	Does not develop

Sources of photos: *Arterial Insufficiency*—Kappert A, Winsor T. *Diagnosis of Peripheral Vascular Disease*. Philadelphia, PA: FA Davis, 1972; *Venous Insufficiency*—Marks R: *Skin Disease in Old Age*. London, UK: Martin Dunitz, 1987.

Table 12-5 Common Ulcers of the Ankles and Feet

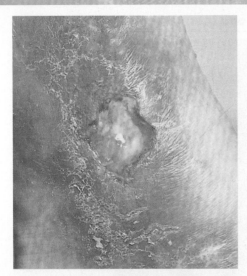

Chronic Venous Insufficiency

This condition usually appears over the medial and sometimes the lateral malleolus. The ulcer contains small, painful granulation tissue and fibrin; necrosis or exposed tendons are rare. Borders are irregular, flat, or slightly steep. Pain affects quality of life in 75% of patients. Associated findings include edema, reddish pigmentation and purpura, venous varicosities, the eczematous changes of stasis dermatitis (redness, scaling, and pruritus), and at times cyanosis of the foot when dependent. Gangrene is rare.

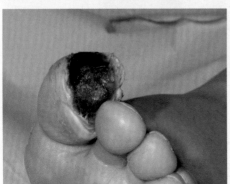

Arterial Insufficiency

This condition occurs in the toes, feet, or possibly areas of trauma (e.g., the shins). Surrounding skin shows no callus or excess pigment, although it may be atrophic. Pain often is severe unless masked by neuropathy. May be accompanied by gangrene, along with decreased pulses, trophic changes, foot pallor on elevation, and dusky rubor on dependency.

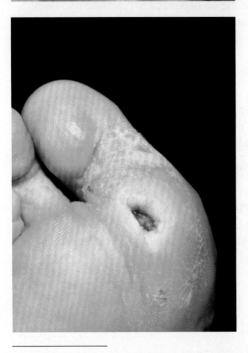

Neuropathic Ulcer

This condition develops in pressure points of areas with diminished sensation; seen in diabetic neuropathy, neurologic disorders, and Hansen disease. The surrounding skin is calloused. There is no pain, so the ulcer may go unnoticed. In uncomplicated cases, there is no gangrene. Associated signs include decreased sensation and absent ankle jerks.

Source of photos: Marks R. *Skin Disease in Old Age*. London, UK: Martin Dunitz, 1987.

References

1. Lin JS, Olson CM, Johnson ES, et al. The ankle-brachial index for peripheral artery disease screening and cardiovascular disease prediction among asymptomatic adults: a systematic evidence review for the U.S. Preventive Services Task Force. *Ann Intern Med.* 2013; 159:333.

2. Olin JW, Allie DE, Belkin M, et al. ACCF/AHA/ACR/SCAI/SIR/SVM/SVN/SVS 2010 performance measures for adults with peripheral artery disease: a report of the American College of Cardiology Foundation/American Heart Association Task Force on performance measures, the American College of Radiology, the Society for Cardiac Angiography and Interventions, the Society for Interventional Radiology, the Society for Vascular Medicine, the Society for Vascular Nursing, and the Society for Vascular Surgery (Writing Committee to Develop Clinical Performance Measures for Peripheral Artery Disease). *Circulation.* 2010;122:2583.

3. Allison MA, Ho E, Denenberg JO, et al. Ethnic-specific prevalence of peripheral arterial disease in the United States. *Am J Prev Med.* 2007;32:328.

4. Ostchega Y, Paulose-Ram R, Dillon CF, et al. Prevalence of peripheral arterial disease and risk factors in persons aged 60 or older: data from the National Health and Nutrition Examination Survey 1999–2004. *J am Geriatir Soc.* 2007;55:583.

5. Rooke TW, Hirsch AT, Misra S, et al. Management of patients with peripheral artery disease (compilation of 2005 and 2011 ACCF/AHA Guideline Recommendations): a report of the American College of Cardiology Foundation/American Heart Association Task Force on Practice Guidelines. American College of Cardiology Foundation Task Force, American Heart Association Task Force. *J Am Coll Cardiol.* 2013;61:1555.

6. Heit JA. The epidemiology of venous thromboembolism in the community. *Arterioscler Thromb Vasc Biol.* 2008;28:370.

7. Bates SM, Ginsberg JS. Treatment of deep-vein thrombosis. *N Engl J Med.* 2004;351:268.

8. Spandorfer J, Galanis T. In the clinic. Deep vein thrombosis. *Ann Intern Med.* 2015;162:ITC-1.

9. Goodacre S, Sutton AJ, Sampson FC. Meta-analysis: The value of clinical assessment in the diagnosis of deep venous thrombosis. *Ann Intern Med.* 2005;143:129.

10. Decousus H, Frappé P, Accassat S, et al. Epidemiology, diagnosis, treatment and management of superficial-vein thrombosis of the legs. *Best Pract Res Clin Haematol.* 2012;25:275.

11. Kucher N. Clinical practice. Deep-vein thrombosis of the upper extremities. *N Engl J Med* .2011;364:861.

12. Mitchell RN. Ch. 11. Blood vessels. In: Kumar VK, Abbas AK, Aster JC, (eds). *In Robbins and Cotran Pathologic Basis of Disease.* 9th ed. Philadelphia, PA: Saunders/Elsevier; 2015.

13. Libby P. Mechanisms of disease: Mechanisms of acute coronary syndromes and their implications for therapy. *N Engl J Med.* 2013;368:2004.

14. Libby P. Ch. 291e. The pathogenesis, prevention, and treatment of atherosclerosis. In: Kasper DL, Fauci AS, Hauser SL, et al (eds). *Harrison's Principles of Internal Medicine.* 19th ed. New York: McGraw-Hill Education; 2015.

15. Ketelhuth DF, Hansson GK. Modulation of autoimmunity and atherosclerosis-common targets and promising translational approaches against disease. *Circ J.* 2015;79:924.

16. Levick JR, Michel CC. Microvascular fluid exchange and the revised Starling principle. *Cardiovasc Res.* 2010;87(2):198.

17. Woodcock TE, Woodcock TM. Revised Starling equation and the glycocalyx model of transvascular fluid exchange: an improved paradigm for prescribing intravenous fluid therapy. *Br J Anaesth.* 2012;108(3):384.

18. Reed RK, Rubin K. Transcapillary exchange: role and importance of the interstitial fluid pressure and the extracellular matrix. *Cardiovasc Res.* 2010;87(2):211.

19. Braunwald E, Loscalzo J. Ch. 50 Edema. In: Kasper DL, Fauci AS, Hauser SL, et al (eds). *Harrison's Principles of Internal Medicine.* 19th ed. New York: McGraw-Hill Education; 2015.

20. Lawenda BD, Mondry TE, Johnstone PA. Lymphedema: a primer on the identification and management of a chronic condition in oncologic treatment. *CA Cancer J Clin.* 2009;59:8.

21. Kent KC. Clinical practice. Abdominal aortic aneurysms. *N Engl J Med.* 2014;371:2101.

22. Lederle FA. In the clinic. Abdominal aortic aneurysm. *Ann Intern Med.* 2009;150:ITC5–1.

23. Suri P, Rainville J, Kalichman L, et al. Does this older adult with lower extremity pain have the clinical syndrome of lumbar spinal stenosis? *JAMA.* 2010;304:2628.

24. McDermott MM. Lower extremity manifestations of peripheral artery disease: the pathophysiologic and functional implications of leg ischemia. *Circ Res.* 2015;116:1540.

25. Hirsch AT, Haskal ZJ, Hertzer NR, et al. ACC/AHA 2005 Practice Guidelines for the management of patients with peripheral arterial disease (lower extremity, renal, mesenteric, and abdominal aortic): a collaborative report from the American Association for Vascular Surgery/Society for Vascular Surgery, Society for Cardiovascular Angiography and Interventions, Society for Vascular Medicine and Biology, Society of Interventional Radiology, and the ACC/AHA Task Force on Practice Guidelines (Writing Committee to Develop Guidelines for the Management of Patients With Peripheral Arterial Disease): endorsed by the American Association of Cardiovascular and Pulmonary Rehabilitation; National Heart, Lung, and Blood Institute; Society for Vascular Nursing; TransAtlantic Inter-Society Consensus; and Vascular Disease Foundation. *J Am Coll Cardiol.* 2005;47:1239.

26. McGee S. Ch. 52 Peripheral Vascular Disease; Ch. 54, Edema and Deep Vein Thrombosis. *Evidence-based Physical Diagnosis.* 3rd ed. Philadelphia, PA: Elsevier; 2012, pp. 459–465; pp. 470–476.

27. Fowkes FG, Rudan D, Rudan I, et al. Comparison of global estimates of prevalence and risk factors for peripheral artery disease in 2000 and 2010: a systematic review and analysis. *Lancet.* 2013;382:1329.

28. Norgren L, Hiatt WR, Dormandy JA, et al. Inter-Society Consensus for the Management of Peripheral Arterial Disease (TASC II). *J Vasc Surg.* 2007;45(Suppl S):S5.

29. McDermott MM. Ankle-brachial index screening to improve health outcomes: where is the evidence? *Ann Intern Med.* 2013;159:362.

30. Moyer VA. Screening for peripheral artery disease and cardiovascular disease risk assessment with the ankle-brachial index in adults: U.S. Preventive Services Task Force recommendation statement. *Ann Intern Med.* 2013;159:342.

31. Fokkenrood HJ, Bendermacher BL, Lauret GJ, et al. Supervised exercise therapy versus non-supervised exercise therapy for intermittent claudication. *Cochrane Database Syst Rev.* 2013;8:CD005263.

32. de Mast Q, Beutler JJ. The prevalence of atherosclerotic renal artery stenosis in risk groups: a systematic literature review. *J Hypertens.* 2009;27:1333.

33. Dworkin LD, Cooper CJ. Clinical practice. Renal-artery stenosis. *N Engl J Med.* 2009;361:1972.

34. Guirguis-Blake JM, Beil TL, Sun X, et al. Primary care screening for abdominal aortic aneurysm: A systematic evidence review for the U.S. Preventive Services Task Force. Rockville, MD; 2014.

35. LeFevre ML. Screening for abdominal aortic aneurysm: U.S. Preventive Services Task Force recommendation statement. *Ann Intern Med.* 2014;161:281.

36. Guirguis-Blake JM, Beil TL, Senger CA, et al. Ultrasonography screening for abdominal aortic aneurysms: a systematic evidence review for the U.S. Preventive Services Task Force. *Ann Intern Med.* 2014;160:321.

37. Varga J. Ch. 382. Systemic sclerosis (scleroderma) and related disorders. In: Kasper DL, Fauci AS, Hauser SL, et al (eds). *Harrison's Principles of Internal Medicine.* 19th ed. New York: McGraw-Hill Education; 2015.

Male Genitalia and Hernias

Anatomy and Physiology

Review the anatomy of the male genitalia (Fig. 13-1). The *shaft of the penis* is formed by three columns of vascular erectile tissue: the *corpus spongiosum,* containing the urethra, and two *corpora cavernosa.* The corpus spongiosum extends from the bulb of the penis to the cone-shaped *glans* with its expanded base, or

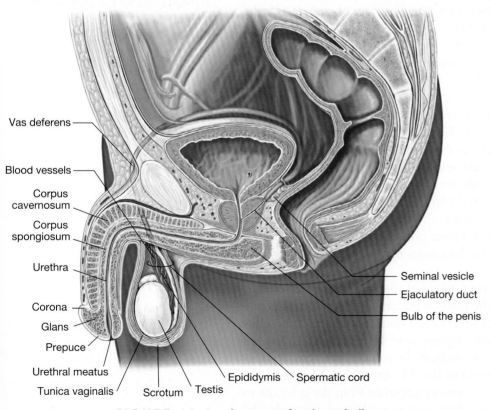

FIGURE 13-1. **Anatomy of male genitalia.**

corona. In uncircumcised men, the glans is covered by a loose, hoodlike fold of skin called the *prepuce* or *foreskin* where *smegma,* or secretions of the glans, may collect. The urethra is located in the ventral midline of the shaft of the penis; urethral abnormalities may sometimes be felt there. The urethra opens into the vertical slit-like *urethral meatus,* located somewhat ventrally at the tip of the glans.

The *testes* are paired ovoid glands consisting primarily of seminiferous tubules and interstitial tissue, covered by a fibrous outer coating, the *tunica albuginea.* The testes are normally 1.5 to 2 cm in length for prepubertal boys and 4 to 5 cm post puberty. Gonadotropin-releasing hormone (GRH) from the hypothalamus stimulates pituitary secretion of luteinizing hormone (LH) and follicle-stimulating hormone (FSH). LH acts on the interstitial Leydig cells to promote synthesis of testosterone, which is converted in target tissues to 5α-dihydrotestosterone. It is 5α-dihydrotestosterone that triggers pubertal growth of the male genitalia, prostate, seminal vesicles, and secondary sex characteristics such as facial and body hair, musculoskeletal growth, and enlargement of the larynx with its associated low-pitched voice. FSH regulates sperm production by the germ cells and Sertoli cells of the seminiferous tubules.

Surrounding or appended to the testes are several structures. The *scrotum* is a loose, wrinkled pouch of skin and underlying dartos muscle. The scrotum is divided into two compartments, each containing a testis or testicle. Covering the testis, except posteriorly, is the serous membrane of the *tunica vaginalis,* derived from the peritoneum of the abdomen and brought down into the scrotum during testicular descent through the deep internal inguinal ring. The parietal layer of the tunica vaginalis cloaks the anterior two thirds of the testis, and the visceral layer lines the adjacent scrotum. On the posterolateral surface of each testis is the softer, comma-shaped *epididymis,* consisting of tightly coiled tubules emanating from the testis that become the *vas deferens.* The epididymis is normally separated from the testis by a palpable sulcus, and provides a reservoir for storage, maturation, and transport of sperm.

If the peritoneal lining remains an open channel to the scrotum it can give rise to an *indirect inguinal hernia.*

The parietal and visceral layers form a potential space for the abnormal fluid accumulation of a *hydrocele.*

During ejaculation, the *vas deferens,* a firm muscular cord-like structure, transports sperm from the tail of the epididymis along a somewhat circular route to the urethra. The *vas* ascends from the scrotal sac into the pelvic cavity through the *inguinal canal,* then loops anteriorly over the ureter to the prostate behind the bladder. There, it merges with the *seminal vesicle* to form the *ejaculatory duct,* which traverses the prostate and empties into the urethra. Secretions from the *vasa deferentia,* the seminal vesicles, and the prostate all contribute to the seminal fluid. Within the scrotum, each vas is closely associated with blood vessels, nerves, and muscle fibers. These structures make up the *spermatic cord.*

Male sexual function depends on normal levels of testosterone, arterial blood flow from the internal iliac artery to the internal pudendal artery and its penile artery and branches, and intact neural innervation from α-adrenergic and cholinergic pathways. Erection from venous engorgement of the corpora cavernosa results from two types of stimuli. Visual, auditory, or erotic cues trigger sympathetic outflow from higher brain centers to the T11 through L2 levels of the spinal cord. Tactile stimulation initiates sensory impulses from the genitalia to the S_2 to S_4 reflex arcs and the parasympathetic pathways through the pudendal nerve. Both sets of stimuli appear to increase levels of nitric oxide and cyclic guanosine monophosphate, resulting in local vasodilation.

Lymphatics

Lymph drainage from the *penis* passes primarily to the deep inguinal and external inguinal nodes. Lymph vessels from the *scrotum* drain into the superficial inguinal lymph nodes. When you find an inflammatory or possibly malignant lesion on these surfaces, assess the inguinal nodes especially carefully for enlargement or tenderness. Lymphatic drainage from the *testes* parallels their venous drainage: the left testicular vein empties into the left renal vein, and the right testicular vein empties into the inferior vena cava. The connecting lumbar and preaortic lymph nodes in the abdomen are clinically undetectable.

See pp. 515–516 for further discussion of the inguinal nodes.

Anatomy of the Groin

Because hernias are relatively common, it is important to understand the anatomy of the groin (Fig. 13-2). The basic landmarks are the anterior superior iliac spine, the pubic tubercle, and the inguinal ligament that runs between them, which are readily identified.

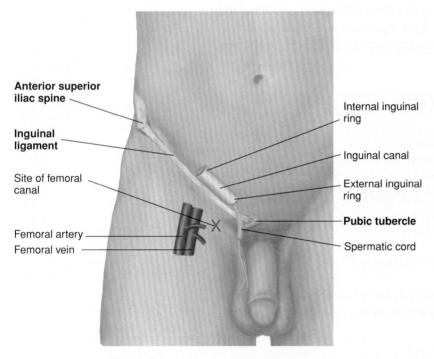

Anterior superior iliac spine

Inguinal ligament

Site of femoral canal

Femoral artery

Femoral vein

Internal inguinal ring

Inguinal canal

External inguinal ring

Pubic tubercle

Spermatic cord

FIGURE 13-2. Anatomy of the groin.

Indirect inguinal hernias develop at the internal inguinal ring, where the spermatic cord exits the abdomen. *Direct inguinal hernias* arise more medially due to weakness in the floor of the inguinal canal and are associated with straining and heavy lifting.

The *inguinal canal,* which lies medial to and roughly parallel to the inguinal ligament, forms a tunnel for the vas deferens as it passes through the abdominal muscles. The internal opening of the canal, the *internal inguinal ring,* is approximately 1 cm above the midpoint of the inguinal ligament. Neither the canal nor the internal ring is palpable through the abdominal wall. The exterior opening of the tunnel, the *external inguinal ring,* is a triangular slit-like structure palpable just above and lateral to the pubic tubercle. When loops of bowel force their way through the inguinal canal, they produce *inguinal hernias,* as illustrated on p. 561.

Another route for a herniating mass is the *femoral canal,* below the inguinal ligament. Although this canal is not visible, you can estimate its location by placing your right index finger, from below, on the right femoral artery. Your middle finger will then overlie the femoral vein; your ring finger, the femoral canal. Femoral hernias protrude at this location.

Femoral hernias are more likely to present as emergencies with bowel incarceration or strangulation.

The Health History

Common or Concerning Symptoms

- Sexual health
- Penile discharge or lesions
- Scrotal pain, swelling, or lesions
- Sexually transmitted infections (STIs)

Sexual Health.   Clinicians and educators recognize the importance of a robust education in sexual health, yet training and clinical expertise remain limited.[1-5] Learn to obtain the sexual history in a respectful and nonjudgmental manner. Your skill and comfort will grow with repetition and practice. To put your patients at ease as you explore the sexual history, adopt the tips in the box below.

See also Chapter 3, The Sexual History, pp. 94–95.

Tips for Taking the Sexual History

- Explain why you are taking the sexual history.
- Convey that you understand that this information is highly personal, and encourage the patient to be open and direct.
- Relate that you gather this history from all your patients.
- Affirm that your conversation is confidential.

For example, you can begin with a general statement such as:

"To provide good care, I need to review your sexual health and see if you are at risk for any sexually transmitted infections. I know this is a sensitive area. Any information you share is confidential and only between us."

Do not overlook patient groups that are often underevaluated, such as those with disabilities, mental illness, traumatic brain injury, and the elderly, and modify your approach as indicated.[6-9] Avoid assumptions about your patients' sexual health or concerns unless they are based on inquiry first.

Sexual Orientation and Gender Identity. Discussing sexual orientation and gender identity touches a vital and multifaceted core of your patients' lives. Reflect on any biases you may have so that they do not interfere with professional responses to your patients' disclosures and concerns. A neutral supportive approach is essential for exploring your patients' health and well-being.[10]

Pose neutral questions about *sexual orientation* and *gender identity* such as:

- "Are you currently dating, sexually active, or in a relationship?" "How would you identify your sexual orientation?" The range of responses includes heterosexual or straight, lesbian, gay, women who have sex with women, men who have sex with men, bisexual, transsexual, and questioning, among others.

- Continue with "How would you describe your gender identity?" Responses include male, female, transsexual, transgendered, intersex, female-to-male, male-to-female, unsure or questioning, or even "prefer not to answer."

Lesbian, Gay, Bisexual, and Transgender Health Care. Several recent surveys provide some of the first national data sets on the lesbian, gay, bisexual, and transgender (LGBT) population. For the first time, in 2013, the National Health Interview Survey included a measure of sexual orientation: in a sample of more than 34,000 adults, 1.6% identified as gay or lesbian, 0.7% identified as bisexual, and 1.1% responded either other or did not know. Most gay and lesbian respondents were between the ages of 18 and 64 years, with a higher percentage of bisexual respondents between 18 and 44 years.[11] In 2012, the Gallup Daily Tracking Survey initiated the largest single study of the distribution of the LGBT population in the United States.[12,13] The Survey added an LGBT identity question that generated 120,000 responses: 3.4% answered "yes" when asked if they identify as LGBT. Of those identifying as LGBT, 53% were women and 6.4% were ages 18 to 29 years. Nearly 13% were in a domestic partnership or living with a partner. Non-whites were more likely to identify as LGBT: African American 4.6%; Asians 4.3%; Hispanics 4.9%; and non-Hispanic white 3.2%. The 2013 American Community Survey of the U.S. Census Bureau reported more than 726,000 households with same-sex couples; 34% had same-sex spouses.[14] In its 2011 report on LGBT health disparities, the Institute of Medicine called for better measures of health care disparities among the diverse LGBT subpopulations to elucidate their differing health behaviors and health care needs.[15]

LGBT patients have higher rates of depression, suicide, anxiety, drug use, sexual victimization, and risk of infection with HIV and STIs.[16–19] The Institute of Medicine has stated that barriers to accessing quality health care for LGBT adults are "a lack of providers who are knowledgeable about LGBT health needs as well as a fear of discrimination in health care settings."[15] The American College of Physicians has called for "enhancing physician understanding of how to provide culturally and clinically competent care for LGBT individuals, addressing environmental and social factors that can affect their mental and physical well-being," in addition to supporting further research into understanding their health needs.[20]

During clinical encounters, LGBT and sexual minority patients often experience significant anxiety related to fears of being accepted; they may be uncomfortable disclosing their sexual behaviors and still fluctuating in their sexual identity. When they experience bias or discrimination, they are unlikely to reveal their sexual identity or concerns.[21–23] Furthermore, reports indicate that clinicians are often unprepared to respond to questions about fertility and transgender issues like hormonal therapy and surgery. Expand your knowledge and clinical skills about gay, lesbian, and transgender health as you talk with your patients and pursue the many resources available.[24–26]

Sexual Response.   Explore the patient's *sexual response.* "How is your current relationship?" "Are you satisfied with your relationship and your sexual activity?" "What about your ability to perform sexually?" If the patient expresses relational or sexual concerns, explore both their psychological and physiologic dimensions. Ask about the meaning of the relationship in the patient's life. Are there any changes in desire or frequency of sexual activity? What is the patient's view of the cause, what responses has the patient tried, and what are the patient's hopes?

Direct questions help you assess each phase of the sexual response. To assess *libido,* or desire, ask "How is your desire for sex?" For the *arousal phase,* ask "Can you achieve and maintain an erection?" Explore the timing, severity, setting, and any other factors that may contribute to the patient's concerns. What about related changes in the relationship with his partner or in his life circumstances? Are there circumstances when erection is normal? On awakening in the early morning or during the night? With other partners? With masturbation?

> Low libido may arise from depression, endocrine dysfunction, or side effects of medications.
>
> *Erectile dysfunction* may be from psychogenic causes, especially if early morning erection is preserved; it may also reflect decreased testosterone, decreased blood flow in the hypogastric arterial system, impaired neural innervation, and diabetes.[27]

To learn about the phase of *orgasm* and *ejaculation* of semen, if ejaculation is premature, or early and out of control, ask "About how long does intercourse last?" "Do you climax too soon?" "Do you feel you have control over climaxing?" "Do you think your partner would like intercourse to last longer?" For reduced or absent ejaculation, "Do you find you cannot reach orgasm even though you can have an erection?" Try to determine whether the problem involves the pleasurable sensation of orgasm, the ejaculation of seminal fluid, or both. Review the frequency and setting of the symptoms, medications, surgery, and neurologic causes.

> Premature ejaculation is common, especially in young men. Less common is reduced or absent ejaculation affecting middle-aged or older men. Possible causes are medications, surgery, neurologic deficits, or lack of androgen. Lack of orgasm with ejaculation is usually psychogenic.

Penile Discharge or Lesions, Scrotal Swelling or Pain, and STIs. Ask about any discharge from the penis, dripping, or staining of underwear. If penile discharge is present, clarify the amount, color, and any fever, chills, rash, or associated symptoms. Note that for men born between 1940 and 1989, the median age of sexual initiation is 16.1 years and the median number of lifetime partners is 8.8, underscoring the importance of screening for STIs.[28]

> Look for yellow penile discharge in *gonorrhea;* white discharge in *nongonococcal urethritis* from *Chlamydia.* See Table 13-1, Sexually Transmitted Infections of the Male Genitalia (p. 557).
>
> Rash, tenosynovitis, monoarticular arthritis, even meningitis, not always with urogenital symptoms, occur in *disseminated gonorrhea.*

Inquire about sores or growths on the penis. Ask about swelling or pain in the scrotum.

Look for an ulcer in syphilitic *chancre* and *herpes;* warts from *human papillomavirus (HPV);* swelling in *mumps orchitis,* scrotal edema, and testicular cancer; pain in *testicular torsion, epididymitis,* and *orchitis.*

See Table 13-2, Abnormalities of the Penis and Scrotum, p. 558, and Table 13-3, Abnormalities of the Testis, p. 559.

Review any previous genital symptoms or past history of infection from *herpes, gonorrhea,* or *syphilis.* Men with multiple or same sex partners, illicit drug use, or prior history of STIs are at increased risk of HIV infection and other new STIs.

Because STIs may involve other areas of the body, explain that "Sexually transmitted infections can involve any body opening where you have sex. It's important for you to tell me if you have oral or anal sex." Ask about symptoms such as sore throat, diarrhea, rectal bleeding, and anal itching or pain.

Infections from oral–penile transmission include *gonorrhea, chlamydia, syphilis,* and *herpes.* Symptomatic or asymptomatic *proctitis* may follow anal intercourse.

Because many infected individuals do not have symptoms or risk factors, ask all patients, "Do you have any concerns about HIV infection?" and discuss the need for *universal testing for HIV.*[29–33]

Health Promotion and Counseling: Evidence and Recommendations

Important Topics for Health Promotion and Counseling

- Screening for STIs and HPV
- Screening for HIV infection and AIDS
- Counseling about sexual practices
- Screening for testicular cancer and testicular self-examination

Prevention of Sexually Transmitted Infections and Human Papillomavirus. The Institute of Medicine has called STIs a "hidden epidemic of enormous health and economic consequence in the United States."[34] Clinicians play a vital role in educating patients about prevention, as well as in detecting and treating STIs. The growing burden of STIs affects the health of all segments of the population, but especially adolescents and young adults.

Facts about STIs

- The Centers for Disease Control and Prevention (CDC) recently estimated that nearly 20 million new STIs occur each year, with almost half in between the ages of 15 and 24 years; the associated health care costs are nearly $16 billion.[35,36]
- Of the nearly 1.8 million new STI cases reported in 2013, nearly 80% were infections from chlamydia, 18% from gonorrhea, and 3% from syphilis (all stages). In recent years, rates of gonorrhea and syphilis infections have been increasing, and chlamydia infections have been declining.
- The CDC notes that these figures underestimate the "true national burden" of STIs; many cases of gonorrhea, chlamydia, and syphilis are unreported, and mandatory reporting is not required for infections such as HPV, trichomoniasis, and genital herpes.

The U.S. Preventive Services Task Force (USPSTF) has given a grade B recommendation for chlamydia and gonorrhea screening in sexually active women age 24 years and younger; the evidence is insufficient to make a recommendation for sexually active men.[37] However, substantial proportions of those with high-risk sexual behaviors are not being tested for STIs (or HIV).

HPV Vaccination. The Advisory Committee on Immunization Practices (ACIP) recommends routine quadrivalent *HPV vaccination in males age 11 or 12 years and through age 21 years if not vaccinated previously* (age 26 years if immunocompromised or having sex with other men).[38] The vaccine can prevent HPV-related diseases in males (genital warts, anal cancer, and penile cancer) and possibly reduce HPV transmission to female sex partners and lower the risk of oropharyngeal cancers. (See also Chapter 14, pp. 577–578.)

Screening for HIV Infection and AIDS. Despite advances in detection and treatment, HIV and AIDS remain significant threats to health, particularly for younger Americans, men who have sex with men, and injection drug users.

Facts about HIV and AIDS

- The CDC estimates that more than 1.2 million Americans ≥age 13 years are currently infected with HIV, with approximately 50,000 new infections annually.[35,39,40]
- More than 600,000 Americans have died with an AIDS diagnosis. At highest risk are men who have sex with men (78% of new infections among males), African Americans (44% of new infections), and Hispanics/Latinos (21% of new infections); injection drug users represent 8% of new HIV infections.
- In 2011, an estimated 14% of infected individuals were unaware of their infected status and only 37% were prescribed antiretroviral therapy (ART).[41]

Identifying early HIV infection and initiating combined ART decreases the risk of progressing to AIDS. Treatment also reduces the risk of transmitting HIV to uninfected heterosexual partners and from a pregnant mother to her child.[42] Current screening recommendations are summarized below.

Summary: Screening Recommendations for HIV

- The USPSTF gives a grade A recommendation for HIV screening of adolescents and adults from age 15 to 65 years and for screening all pregnant women.[42]
- The CDC recommends universal HIV testing for adolescents and adults ages 13 to 64 years in health care settings and prenatal testing of all pregnant women.[43]
- The CDC recommends an opt-out approach to HIV testing—verbally notifying the patient that testing will be performed unless the patient declines. Separate written consent is not required.
- The American College of Physicians recommends extending the upper age for screening to 75 years.[44] The proportion of adults who have ever been tested for HIV increased from 37% in 2000 to 45% in 2010.[45]
- One-time testing for low-risk patients is reasonable, but at least annual testing is recommended for high-risk groups (including adolescents younger than 15 years and older adults), defined as men with male sex partners, individuals with multiple sexual partners, past or present injection drug users, persons who exchange sex for money or drugs, and sex partners of persons who are HIV-infected, bisexual, or injection-drug users.[43] The presence of any STI, or requests for STI testing, warrants testing for coinfection with HIV.

Counseling about Sexual Practices. Clinicians must master the skills of eliciting the sexual history and asking frank but tactful questions about sexual practices. Key information includes the patient's sexual orientation, the number of partners in the past month, and any history of past STIs (see also pp. 94–95). Carefully screen for alcohol and drug use, especially injection drugs. Patient counseling should be interactive and combine information about general risk reduction with personalized messages based on the patient's personal risk behaviors. Implementing this approach, termed *client-centered counseling,* can reduce the frequency of high-risk behaviors and lower the acquisition rates for STIs.[46]

See discussions of the sexual history on pp. 94–95 and pp. 544–547.

As you counsel patients, encourage them to seek prompt attention for any genital lesions or penile discharge. Address preventive behaviors such as using condoms, limiting the number of sexual partners, and establishing regular health care for treatment of STIs and HIV. *Correct use of male condoms* is highly effective in preventing the transmission of HIV, HPV, and other STIs.[47] Key instructions should include:

- Using a new condom with each sex act

- Applying the condom before any sexual contact occurs

- Adding only water-based lubricants

- Immediately withdraw if the condom breaks during sexual activity, and holding the condom during withdrawal to keep it from slipping off.

Screening for Testicular Cancer and Testicular Self-Examination

Epidemiology. In 2015, an estimated 8,430 cases of testicular cancer will be diagnosed in the United States though fewer than 400 males are expected to die from this cancer.[48] While testicular cancer is rare, it is highly treatable when detected early. It is the most commonly diagnosed cancer in white men from ages 20 to 34 years; the risk of diagnosis is five times more common in white men compared to black men.[49] Risk factors are family history, HIV infection, and a history of cryptorchidism (undescended testicle). Cryptorchidism, present in 7% to 10% of men with testicular cancer, confers a 3- to 17-fold increased risk for testicular cancer.[50] About 70% of testicular cancers are localized; most are curable even when diagnosed at advanced stage.

Screening Recommendations. In 2011, the USPSTF concluded that there is inadequate evidence for the benefit of screening, either by clinical examination or self-examination, and advised against screening for testicular cancer in asymptomatic adolescent or adult males (grade D recommendation).[51] In contrast, the American Cancer Society recommends that a testicular examination should be part of a general physical examination.[52] The American Cancer Society does not have a recommendation for regular *testicular self-examinations* (*TSEs*), but does advise men to seek clinical attention for any of the following: a painless lump, swelling, or enlargement in either testicle; pain or discomfort in a testicle or the scrotum; a feeling of heaviness or a sudden fluid collection in the scrotum; or a dull ache in the lower abdomen or the groin.

See pp. 555–556 for patient instructions for TSE.

Techniques of Examination

Many students feel uneasy about examining the male genitalia. "How will the patient react?" "Will he let me examine him?" "Will he have an erection?" Explain what is involved and review each step of the examination so that the patient feels reassured and knows what to expect. When needed, request an assistant to accompany you. Occasionally, if the patient has an erection, explain that this is a normal response, finish your examination, and proceed with a calm demeanor. If the patient refuses the examination, respect the patient's wishes.

For a good genital examination the gowned patient can be either standing or supine. To check for varicoceles, however, the patient should stand, and you should sit comfortably on a chair or stool. The gown should cover the patient's chest and abdomen. Place a drawsheet at the midthigh. *Wear gloves* throughout the examination. Expose the genitalia and inguinal areas. For younger patients, review the sexual maturity ratings on p. 899.

The Penis

Inspection.   Inspect the penis, including:

See Table 13-2, Abnormalities of the Penis and Scrotum, p. 558.

- The *skin*. Inspect the skin on the ventral and dorsal surfaces and the base of the penis for excoriations or inflammation, lifting the penis when necessary.

  Pubic or genital excoriations suggest lice (crabs) or sometimes scabies in the pubic hair.

- The *prepuce* (foreskin). If present, retract the prepuce or ask the patient to retract it. This step is essential for the detection of chancres and carcinomas. Smegma, a cheesy, whitish material, may accumulate normally under the foreskin.

  Phimosis is a tight prepuce that cannot be retracted over the glans. *Paraphimosis* is a tight prepuce that, once retracted, cannot be returned. Edema ensues.

- The *glans*. Look for any ulcers, scars, nodules, or signs of inflammation.

  Balanitis is inflammation of the glans; *balanoposthitis* is inflammation of the glans and prepuce.

- The *urethral meatus*. Inspect the location of the urethral meatus.

  Hypospadias is a congenital ventral displacement of the meatus on the penis (see p. 558).

Compress the glans gently between your index finger above and your thumb below (Fig. 13-3). This maneuver should open the urethral meatus and allow you to inspect it for discharge. Normally, there is none.

If the patient has reported a discharge that you are unable to see, ask him to strip, or milk, the shaft of the penis from its base to the glans. Alternatively, do this yourself. This maneuver may expel some discharge from the urethral meatus for appropriate examination. Have a glass slide and culture materials ready.

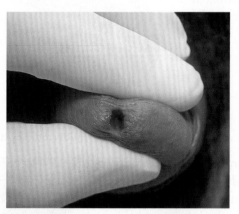

FIGURE 13-3. **Gently compress the glans to inspect the urethral meatus.**

Profuse yellow discharge signals *gonococcal urethritis;* scanty white or clear discharge signals *nongonococcal urethritis.* Definitive diagnosis requires Gram stain and culture.

Palpation.   Palpate the shaft of the penis between your thumb and first two fingers, noting any induration. (This may be omitted in a young asymptomatic male patient.) Palpate any abnormality of the penis, noting any induration or tenderness.

Induration along the ventral surface of the penis suggests a *urethral stricture* or possibly a *carcinoma.* Tenderness in the indurated area suggests periurethral inflammation from a urethral stricture.

If you retract the foreskin, replace it before proceeding on to examine the scrotum.

The Scrotum and its Contents

Inspection. Inspect the scrotum, including:

See Table 13-2, Abnormalities of the Penis and Scrotum, p. 558.

- The *skin.* Lift up the scrotum so that you can inspect its posterior surface. Note any lesions or scars. Inspect the pubic hair distribution.

Inspection may reveal scrotal nevi, hemangiomas, or telangiectasias as well as STIs including condyloma or ulcers from *herpes* and *chancroid* (painful) and *syphilis* and *lymphogranuloma venereum* (painless), with associated inguinal lymphadenopathy.[53]

- The *scrotal contours.* Inspect for swelling, lumps, veins, bulging masses, or asymmetry of the left and right hemiscrotum.

A poorly developed scrotum on one or both sides suggests *cryptorchidism* (an undescended testicle). Common scrotal swellings include indirect *inguinal hernias, hydroceles, scrotal edema,* and, rarely, *testicular carcinoma.*

- The *inguinal areas.* Note any erythema, excoriation, or visible adenopathy.

Erythema and mild excoriation point to fungal infection, not uncommon in this moist area.

There may be dome-shaped white or yellow papules or nodules formed by occluded follicles filled with keratin debris of desquamated follicular epithelium. Such *epidermoid cysts* are common, frequently multiple, and benign (Fig. 13-4).

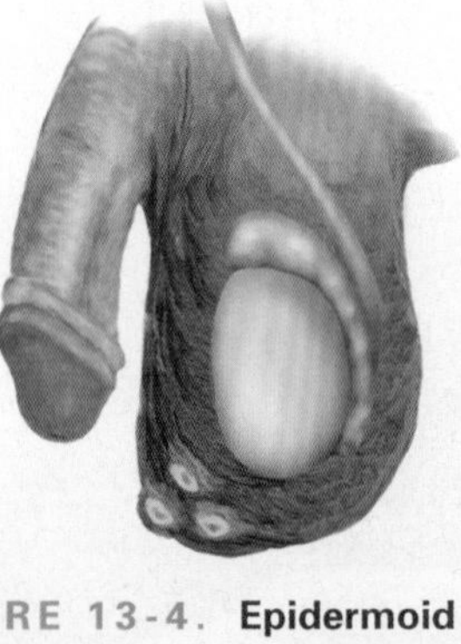

FIGURE 13-4. Epidermoid cysts.

Palpation. If using a one-handed technique, *palpate each testis and epididymis* between your thumb and first two fingers (Fig. 13-5). If using two hands, cradle the testis at both poles in the thumb and fingertips of both hands. Palpate the scrotal contents as you gently slide them back and forth from the fingertips of one hand to the other, without changing the position of your hands as they cup the scrotum. This technique is comfortable for the patient and allows a subtle controlled and accurate examination. The testes should be firm but not hard, descended, symmetric, nontender, and without masses.[53]

See Table 13-3, Abnormalities of the Testis, p. 559, and Table 13-4, Abnormalities of the Epididymis and Spermatic Cord, p. 560.

Tender painful scrotal swelling is present in *acute epididymitis, acute orchitis, torsion of the spermatic cord,* or a *strangulated inguinal hernia.*

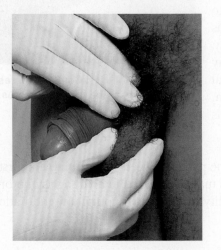

FIGURE 13-5. Palpate the testis and epididymis.

- For each testis, assess size, shape, consistency, and tenderness; feel for any nodules. Pressure on the testis normally produces a deep visceral pain.

- Palpate the epididymis on the posterior surface of each testicle without applying excess pressure, which can cause discomfort. The epididymis feels nodular and cord-like and should not be confused with an abnormal lump. Normally, it should not be tender.

- *Palpate each spermatic cord*, including the vas deferens, between your thumb and fingers, from the epididymis to the external inguinal ring (Fig. 13-6). The vas feels slightly stiff and tubular and is distinct from the accompanying vessels of the spermatic cord.

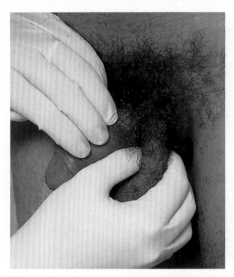

FIGURE 13-6. **Palpate the spermatic cord.**

- Palpate any nodules or swellings.

Swelling in the scrotum apart from the testicles can be evaluated by transillumination. After darkening the room, shine the beam of a strong flashlight from behind the scrotum through the mass. Look for transmission of the light as a red glow.

Hernias

During the examination for hernias, the patient can be either supine or standing. The techniques for examination and examiner hand placement are the same for both positions. The techniques which follow apply to the standing position, but can be replicated for the supine position depending on examiner preference.

Any painless nodule on the testis raises the possibility of *testicular cancer,* a potentially curable cancer with a peak incidence between the ages 15 to 34 years. Recall that lymph drainage from the testes parallels retroperitoneal venous flow from the renal vein and inferior vena cava, the primary site of lymph node involvement in testicular cancer (see p. 516).

To check for a *varicocele,* with the patient standing, palpate the spermatic cord about 2 cm above the testis. Have the patient hold his breath and "bear down" against a closed glottis for about 4 seconds (the Valsalva maneuver).

During this maneuver, a temporary increase in the diameter of the spermatic cord indicates filling of abnormally dilated spermatic veins draining the testis.

The vas deferens, if chronically infected, may feel thickened or beaded. A cystic structure in the spermatic cord suggests a *hydrocele of the cord.*

Swellings containing serous fluid, such as *hydroceles,* light up with a red glow, or transilluminate. Those containing blood or tissue, such as a normal testis, a tumor, or most hernias, do not.

Inspection. Sitting comfortably in front of the patient, with the patient standing and an assistant present, if indicated, *inspect the inguinal regions and genitalia* for bulging areas and asymmetry.

A bulge suggests a *hernia.*

Palpation. *Palpate for an inguinal hernia,* using the techniques below. Continue to face the patient, who should still be standing.

See Table 13-5, Course, Presentation, and Differentiation of Hernias in the Groin, p. 561.

- To examine for an inguinal hernia on either side (the right is illustrated in Fig. 13-7), place the tip of your dominant index finger at the anterior inferior margin of the scrotum, staying superficial to the testicle, then move your finger and hand upward toward the *external inguinal ring,* invaginating the scrotal skin beneath the peripubic fat pad next to the base of the penis.

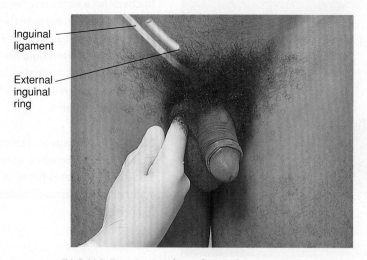

Inguinal ligament

External inguinal ring

FIGURE 13-7. Invaginate the scrotum.

- Follow the spermatic cord upward to the inguinal ligament. Find the triangular slit-like opening of the *external inguinal ring* just above and lateral to the pubic tubercle. Palpate the external inguinal ring and its floor. Ask the patient to cough. Palpate for a distinct bulge or mass that moves against your stationary finger during the cough.

- The external ring may be large enough for you to gently palpate obliquely along the inguinal canal toward the *internal inguinal ring.* Again ask the patient to cough. Check for a bulge that slides down the inguinal canal and taps against the fingertip.

- Use the same techniques with the same dominant finger to examine both sides.

A bulge near the external inguinal ring suggests a *direct inguinal hernia.* A bulge near the internal inguinal ring suggests an *indirect inguinal hernia.* Experts note that distinguishing the type of hernia is difficult, with sensitivity and specificity of 74% to 92%, and 93%. Hernias warrant surgical evaluation, especially when symptomatic or incarcerated. Chance of incarceration is low, estimated at 0.3% to 3% per year, and is 10 times more common with indirect hernias.[54–57]

Palpate for a femoral hernia by placing your fingers on the anterior thigh in the region of the femoral canal. Ask the patient to strain down again or cough. Note any swelling or tenderness.

Evaluating a Possible Scrotal Hernia. To assess a scrotal mass and possible hernia, ask the patient to lie down. The mass may return to the abdomen by itself. If so, it is a hernia. If not:

- Can you get your fingers above the mass in the scrotum?

> If you can place your fingers above the mass, suspect a *hydrocele*.

- Listen to the mass with a stethoscope for bowel sounds, but note that bowel sounds may be transmitted from the abdomen through a hydrocele in the scrotum.

> Transillumination of the scrotal mass may help identify a hydrocele from an intestine-containing hernia.

If your findings suggest a hernia, gently try to reduce it (return it to the abdominal cavity) by sustained pressure with your fingers. Do not attempt this maneuver if the mass is tender or the patient reports nausea and vomiting.

The history may be helpful. The patient can usually tell you what happens to his swelling when lying down and may be able to demonstrate how he reduces it himself.

> A hernia is *incarcerated* when its contents cannot be returned to the abdominal cavity. A hernia is *strangulated* when the blood supply to the entrapped contents is compromised. Suspect strangulation in the presence of tenderness, nausea, and vomiting, and consider surgical intervention. See Table 13-5, Course, Presentation, and Differentiation of Hernias in the Groin, p. 561.

Special Techniques

The Testicular Self-Examination.   The incidence of testicular cancer is low, about 5 per 100,000 men, but it is the most common solid cancer of young men between ages 15 and 34 years, with an estimated lifetime risk of 1:260.[58] Although the USPSTF and the American Cancer Society have not recommended routine TSE for screening, the clinician and patient may wish to teach the TSE to enhance health awareness and self-care. For high-risk patients, review the risk factors for testicular carcinoma, which has an excellent prognosis when detected early: cryptorchidism, which confers a high risk for testicular carcinoma in the undescended testicle; a history of carcinoma in the contralateral testicle; mumps orchitis; an inguinal hernia; a hydrocele in childhood; and a positive family history.

Patient Instructions for the Testicular Self-Examination

This examination is best performed after a warm bath or shower.[59,60] This way, the scrotal skin is warm and relaxed. It is best to do the test while standing.

- Standing in front of a mirror, check for any swelling on the skin of the scrotum.
- With the penis out of the way, gently feel your scrotal sac to locate a testicle. Examine each testicle separately.
- Use one hand to stabilize the testicle. Using the fingers and thumb of your other hand, firmly but gently feel or roll the testicle between your fingers. Feel the entire surface. Find the epididymis. This is a soft, tube-like

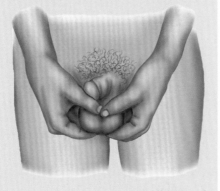

(continued)

Patient Instructions for the Testicular Self-Examination (*continued*)

structure at the back of the testicle that collects and carries sperm, and is not an abnormal lump. Check the other testicle and epididymis the same way.

- If you find a hard lump, an absent or enlarged testicle, a painful swollen scrotum, or any other differences that do not seem normal, do not wait. See your health care provider right away.

As noted by the American Cancer Society, "It's normal for one testicle to be slightly larger than the other, and for one to hang lower than the other. You should also know that each normal testicle has a small, coiled tube (epididymis) that can feel like a small bump on the upper or middle outer side of the testicle. Normal testicles also have blood vessels, supporting tissues, and tubes that carry sperm. Some men may confuse these with abnormal lumps at first. If you have any concerns, ask your doctor or clinician."

Recording Your Findings

Note that initially you may use sentences to describe your findings; later you will use phrases. The style below contains phrases appropriate for most write-ups.

Recording the Male Genitalia Examination

"Circumcised male. No penile discharge or lesions. No scrotal swelling or discoloration. Testes descended bilaterally, smooth, without masses. Epididymis is nontender. No inguinal or femoral hernias."
OR
"Uncircumcised male; prepuce easily retractible. No penile discharge or lesions. No scrotal swelling or discoloration. Testes descended bilaterally; right testicle smooth; 1 × 1 cm firm nodule on left lateral testicle. It is fixed and nontender. Epididymis nontender. No inguinal or femoral hernias."

These findings are suspicious for *testicular carcinoma,* the most common form of cancer in men between the ages of 15 and 34 years.

Table 13-1 Sexually Transmitted Infections of Male Genitalia

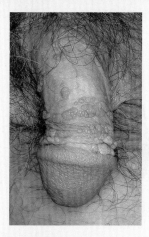

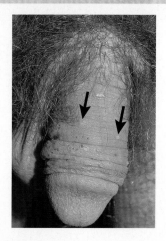

Genital Warts (Condylomata Acuminata)

- *Appearance:* Single or multiple papules or plaques of variable shapes; may be round, acuminate (pointed), or thin and slender. May be raised, flat, or cauliflower-like (verrucous).
- *Causative organism:* HPV, usually subtypes 6, 11; carcinogenic subtypes rare, approximately 5–10% of all anogenital warts. *Incubation:* weeks to months; infected contact may have no visible warts.
- Can arise on penis, scrotum, groin, thighs, anus; usually asymptomatic, occasionally cause itching and pain.
- May disappear without treatment.

Genital Herpes Simplex

- *Appearance:* Small scattered or grouped vesicles, 1 to 3 mm in size, on glans or shaft of penis. Appear as erosions if vesicular membrane breaks.
- *Causative organism:* Usually *Herpes simplex virus 2* (90%), a double-stranded DNA virus. *Incubation:* 2 to 7 days after exposure.
- Primary episode may be asymptomatic; recurrence usually less painful, of shorter duration.
- Associated with fever, malaise, headache, arthralgias; local pain and edema, lymphadenopathy.
- Need to distinguish from genital herpes zoster (usually in older patients with dermatomal distribution) and candidiasis.

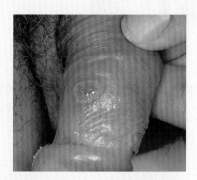

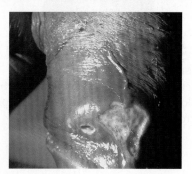

Primary Syphilis

- *Appearance:* Small red papule that becomes a *chancre*, a *painless* erosion up to 2 cm in diameter. Base of chancre is clean, red, smooth, and glistening; borders are raised and indurated. Chancre heals within 3 to 8 wks.
- *Causative organism: Treponema pallidum,* a spirochete. *Incubation:* 9–90 d after exposure.
- May develop inguinal lymphadenopathy within 7 d; lymph nodes are rubbery, nontender, mobile.
- 20%–30% of patients develop secondary syphilis while chancre still present (suggests coinfection with HIV).
- Distinguish from: genital herpes simplex; chancroid; granuloma inguinale from *Klebsiella granulomatis* (rare in the United States; four variants, so difficult to identify).

Chancroid

- *Appearance:* Red papule or pustule initially, then forms a *painful* deep ulcer with ragged nonindurated margins; contains necrotic exudate, has a friable base.
- *Causative organism: Haemophilus ducreyi,* an anaerobic bacillus. *Incubation:* 3–7 d after exposure.
- Painful inguinal adenopathy; suppurative buboes in 25% of patients.
- Need to distinguish from: primary syphilis; genital herpes simplex; lymphogranuloma venereum, granuloma inguinale from *Klebsiella granulomatis* (both rare in the United States).

Table 13-2 Abnormalities of the Penis and Scrotum

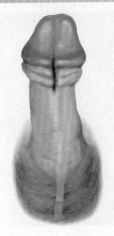

Hypospadias

A congenital displacement of the urethral meatus to the inferior surface of the penis. The meatus may be subcoronal, midshaft, or at the junction of the penis and scrotum (penoscrotal).

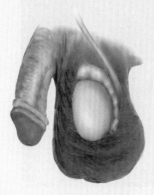

Scrotal Edema

Pitting edema may make the scrotal skin taut; seen in heart failure or nephrotic syndrome.

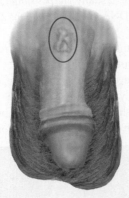

Peyronie Disease

Palpable, nontender, hard plaques are found just beneath the skin, usually along the dorsum of the penis. The patient complains of crooked, painful erections.

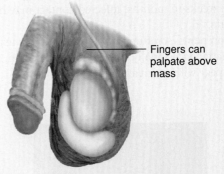

Fingers can palpate above mass

Hydrocele

A nontender, fluid-filled mass within the tunica vaginalis. It transilluminates, and the examining fingers can palpate above the mass within the scrotum.

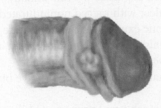

Carcinoma of the Penis

An indurated nodule or ulcer that is usually nontender. Limited almost completely to men who are not circumcised, it may be masked by the prepuce. Any persistent penile sore is suspicious.

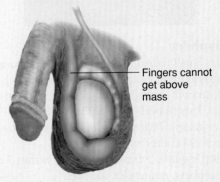

Fingers cannot get above mass

Scrotal Hernia

Usually an *indirect inguinal hernia* that comes through the external inguinal ring, so the examining fingers cannot get above it within the scrotum.

Table 13-3 Abnormalities of the Testis

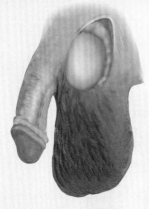

Cryptorchidism

The testis is atrophied and lies outside the scrotum in the inguinal canal, abdomen, or near the pubic tubercle; it may also be congenitally absent. There is no palpable left testis or epididymis in the unfilled scrotum. Cryptorchidism, even with surgical correction, markedly raises the risk of testicular cancer.[61]

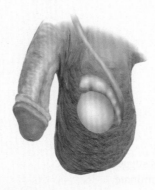

Small Testis

In adults, testicular length is usually ≤3.5 cm. Small firm testes usually ≤2 cm suggest *Klinefelter syndrome*. Small soft testes suggesting atrophy are seen in cirrhosis, myotonic dystrophy, use of estrogens, and hypopituitarism; may also follow orchitis.

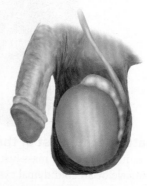

Acute Orchitis

The testis is acutely inflamed, painful, tender, and swollen. It may be difficult to distinguish from the epididymis. The scrotum may be reddened. Seen in mumps and other viral infections; usually unilateral.

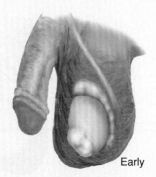

Early

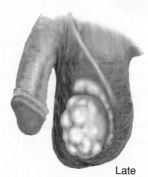

Late

Tumor of the Testis

Usually appears as a painless nodule. Any nodule within the testis warrants investigation for malignancy.

As a testicular neoplasm grows and spreads, it may seem to replace the entire organ. The testicle characteristically feels heavier than normal.

Table 13-4 Abnormalities of the Epididymis and Spermatic Cord

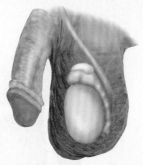

Spermatocele and Cyst of the Epididymis

A painless, movable cystic mass just above the testis suggests a spermatocele or an epididymal cyst. Both transilluminate. The former contains sperm, and the latter does not, but they are clinically indistinguishable.

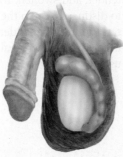

Acute Epididymitis

An acutely inflamed epididymis is indurated, swollen, and notably tender, making it difficult to distinguish from the testis. The scrotum may be reddened and the vas deferens inflamed. Causes include infection from *Neisseria gonorrheae*, *Chlamydia trachomatis* (younger adults), *Escherichia coli*, and *Pseudomonas* (older adults); trauma; and autoimmune disease. Barring urinary symptoms, urinalysis is often negative.

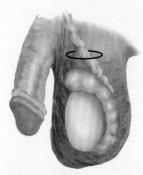

Tuberculous Epididymitis

The chronic inflammation of tuberculosis produces a firm enlargement of the epididymis, which is sometimes tender, with thickening or beading of the vas deferens.

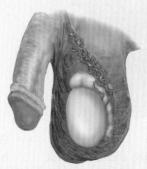

Varicocele of the Spermatic Cord

Varicocele refers to gravity-mediated varicose veins of the spermatic cord, usually found on the left. It feels like a soft "bag of worms" in the spermatic cord above the testis, and if prominent, appears to distort the contours of the scrotal skin. A varicocele collapses in the supine position, so examination should be both supine and standing. If the varicocele does not collapse when the patient is supine, suspect a left spermatic vein obstruction within the abdomen.

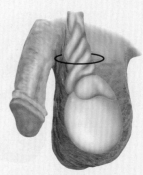

Torsion of the Spermatic Cord

Torsion, or twisting, of the testicle on its spermatic cord produces an acutely painful, tender, and swollen organ that is often retracted upward in the scrotum. The cremasteric reflex is nearly always absent on the affected side in boys or men with testicular torsion. If the presentation is delayed, the scrotum becomes red and edematous. There is no associated urinary infection. Torsion is most common in neonates and adolescents, but can occur at any age. It is a surgical emergency because of obstructed circulation.

Table 13-5 Course, Presentation, and Differentiation of Hernias in the Groin

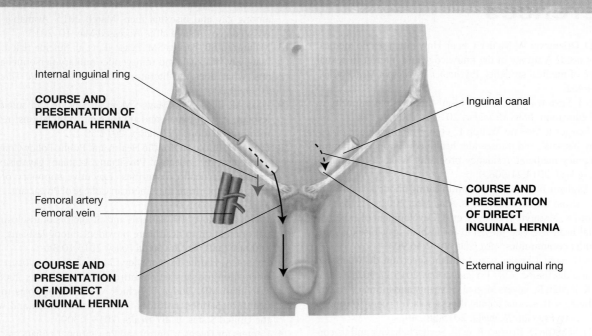

Internal inguinal ring

COURSE AND PRESENTATION OF FEMORAL HERNIA

Femoral artery

Femoral vein

COURSE AND PRESENTATION OF INDIRECT INGUINAL HERNIA

Inguinal canal

COURSE AND PRESENTATION OF DIRECT INGUINAL HERNIA

External inguinal ring

Inguinal Hernias

	Indirect	Direct	Femoral Hernias
Frequency, Age, and Sex	Most common, all ages, both sexes. Often in children; may occur in adults.	Less common. Usually in men older than 40 yrs; rare in women.	Least common. More common in women than in men.
Point of Origin	Above inguinal ligament, near its midpoint (the internal inguinal ring).	Above inguinal ligament, close to the pubic tubercle (near the external inguinal ring).	Below the inguinal ligament; appears more lateral than an inguinal hernia. Can be hard to differentiate from lymph nodes.
Course *(Examining finger in inguinal canal during coughing or straining)*	Often into the scrotum. The hernia comes down the inguinal canal and touches the fingertip.	Rarely into the scrotum. The hernia bulges anteriorly and pushes the side of the finger forward.	Never into the scrotum. The inguinal canal is empty.

References

1. Turner D, Driemeyer W, Nieder T, et al. How much sex do medical students need? A survey of the knowledge and interest in sexual medicine of medical students. *Psychother Psychosom Med Psychol.* 2014;64:452.

2. Lapinski J, Sexton P. Still in the closet: the invisible minority in medical education. *BMC Med Educ.* 2014;14:171.

3. Moll J, Krieger P, Moreno-Walton L, et al. The prevalence of lesbian, gay, bisexual, and transgender health education and training in emergency medicine residency programs: what do we know? *Acad Merg Med.* 2014;21:608.

4. Sack S, Drabant B, Perrin E. Communicating about sexuality: an initiative across the core clerkships. *Acad Med.* 2002;77:1159.

5. Rutherford K, McIntyre J, Daley A, et al. Development of expertise in mental health service provision for lesbian, gay, bisexual and transgender communities. *Med Educ.* 2012;46:903.

6. Kellaher D. Sexual behavior and autism spectrum disorders: an update and discussion. *Curr Psychiatry Rep.* 2015;17:562.

7. Bonfils K, Firmin R, Salyers M, et al. Sexuality and intimacy among people living with serious mental illnesses: factors contributing to sexual activity. *Psychiatr Rehabil J.* 2015;38:249.

8. Turner D, Schottle D, Krueger R, et al. Sexual behavior and its correlates after traumatic brain injury. *Curr Opin Psychiatry.* 2015; 28:180.

9. Lee D, Nazroo J, O'Connor D, et al. Sexual health and well-being among older men and women in England: finding from the English longitudinal study of ageing. *Arch Sex Behav.* 2016;45:133. 2015 January 27. Epub ahead of print.

10. Barbara AM, Doctor F, Chaim G. Asking the right questions 2. Talking with clients about sexual orientation and gender identity in mental health, counselling and addiction settings. Toronto Canada: Centre for Addiction and Mental Health; 2007. Available at http://knowledgex.camh.net/amhspecialists/Screening_Assessment/assessment/ARQ2/Pages/default.aspx. Accessed May 20, 2015.

11. Centers for Disease Control and Prevention. Sexual orientation and health among U.S. adults. National Health Interview Survey, 2013. Available at http://www.cdc.gov/lgbthealth/. Accessed May 10, 2015.

12. Gates GJ, Newport F. Gallup Special Report: The US LGBT adult population. Washington, DC: Gallup, Inc; 2013. See also Gates GJ, Newport F. Special Report: 3.4% of U.S. Adults Identify as LGBT. October 18, 2012. Available at http://www.gallup.com/poll/158066/special-report-adults-identify-lgbt.aspx. Accessed May 11, 2015.

13. Gates GJ. Demographics and LGBT health. *J Health Soc Behav.* 2013;54:72.

14. U.S. Census Bureau. Same sex couples. 2013. Available at http://www.census.gov/hhes/samesex./ Accessed May 10, 2015.

15. Institute of Medicine. *The Health of Lesbian, Gay, Bisexual, and Transgender People: Building a Foundation for Better Understanding.* Washington, DC: National Institutes of Health; 2011. See also Report at https://www.iom.edu/Reports/2011/The-Health-of-Lesbian-Gay-Bisexual-and-Transgender-People.aspx March 31 2011. Accessed May 11, 2015.

16. Centers for Disease Control and Prevention. Lesbian and bisexual women. Updated March 25, 2014. Available at http://www.cdc.gov/lgbthealth/women.htm. Gay and bisexual men. Updated March 25, 2014. Available at http://www.cdc.gov/lgbthealth/msm.htm. Accessed May 10, 2015.

17. Centers for Disease Prevention and Control. CDC fact sheet. HIV among gay and bisexual men. March 2015. Available at http://www.cdc.gov/msmhealth/. Accessed May 10, 2015.

18. Matarazzo BB, Barnes SM, Pease JL, et al. Suicide risk among lesbian, gay, bisexual, and transgender military personnel and veterans: what does the literature tell us? *Suicide Life Threat Behav.* 2014;44:200.

19. Haas AP, Eliason M, Mays VM, et al. Suicide and suicide risk in lesbian, gay, bisexual, and transgender populations: review and recommendations. *J Homosex.* 2011;58:10.

20. Daniel H, Butkus R, for the Health and Public Policy Committee of the American College of Physicians. Lesbian, gay, bisexual, and transgender health disparities: Executive summary of a policy position paper from the American College of Physicians. *Ann Intern Med.* 2015;163:135.

21. Durso LE, Meyer IH. Patterns and predictors of disclosure of sexual orientation to healthcare providers among lesbians, gay men, and bisexuals. *Sex Res Social Policy.* 2013;10:35.

22. Polek CA, Hardie TL, Crowley EM. Lesbians' disclosure of sexual orientation and satisfaction with care. *J Transcult Nurs.* 2008;19:243.

23. Friedman MR, Dodge B, Schick V, et al. From bias to bisexual health disparities: attitudes toward bisexual men and women in the United States. *LGBT Health.* 2014;1:309.

24. Centers for Disease Control and Prevention. Lesbian, gay, bisexual, and transgender health. Updates July 22 2014. Available at http://www.cdc.gov/lgbthealth./ Accessed May 11, 2015.

25. National LGBT Health Education Center. Suggested resources and readings, 2015. Available at http://www.lgbthealtheducation.org/publications/lgbt-health-resources./ Accessed May 11, 2015.

26. Strutz KL, Herring AH, Halpern CT. Health disparities among young adult sexual minorities in the U.S. *Am J Prev Med.* 2015; 48:76.

27. Gareri P, Castagna A, Francomano D. Erectile dysfunction in the elderly: an old widespread issue with novel treatment perspectives. *Int J Endocrin.* 2014;2014:878670.

28. Liu G, Hariri S, Bradley H, et al. Trends and patterns of sexual behaviors among adolescents and adults aged 14 to 59 years, United States. *Sex Transm Dis.* 2015;42:20.

29. Centers for Disease Control and Prevention. Sexually transmitted diseases. Draft for Public Comment Version: Sexually Transmitted Diseases Treatment Guidelines, 2014. Updated November 12, 2014. Available at http://www.cdc.gov/std/treatment/update.htm. Accessed May 11, 2015.

30. U.S. Preventive Services Task Force. USPSTF recommendations for STI screening. February 2014. Available at http://www.uspreventiveservicestaskforce.org/Page/Name/uspstf-recommendations-for-sti-screening. Accessed May 11, 2015.

31. U.S. Preventive Services Task Force. Human immunodeficiency virus (HIV) infection: Screening. April 2013. Available at http://www.uspreventiveservicestaskforce.org/Page/Topic/recommendation-summary/human-immunodeficiency-virus-hiv-infection-screening?ds=1&s=HIV. Accessed May 11, 2015.

32. Skarbinski J, Rosenberg E, Paz-Bailey G, et al. Human Immunodeficiency virus transmission at each step of the care continuum in the United States. *JAMA Intern Med.* 2015;175:588.

33. Meanley S, Gale A, Harmell C, et al. The role of provider interactions on comprehensive sexual healthcare among young men who have sex with men. *AIDS Educ Prev.* 2015;27:15.

34. Institute of Medicine, Eng TR, Butler WT, eds. *The Hidden Epidemic: Confronting Sexually Transmitted Diseases: Summary.*

Washington, DC: National Academies Press (US); 1997. Available at http://www.ncbi.nlm.nih.gov/pubmed/25165803. Accessed May 12, 2015.

35. Centers for Disease Control and Prevention. *Sexually Transmitted Disease Surveillance 2013.* Atlanta: U.S. Department of Health and Human Services; 2014. Available at http://www.cdc.gov/std/stats13/default.htm. Accessed May 11, 2015.

36. Centers for Disease Control and Prevention. CDC Fact Sheet. Reported STDs in the United States. 2013 National Data for Chlamydia, Gonorrhea, and Syphilis, 2014. Available at: http://www.cdc.gov/nchhstp/newsroom/docs/std-trends-508.pdf. Accessed May 11, 2015.

37. LeFevre ML. Screening for Chlamydia and gonorrhea: U.S. Preventive Services Task Force recommendation statement. *Ann Intern Med.* 2014;161:902.

38. Markowitz LE, Dunne EF, Saraiya M, et al. Human papillomavirus vaccination: recommendations of the Advisory Committee on Immunization Practices (ACIP). *MMWR Recomm Rep.* 2014;63(RR-05):1.

39. Centers for Disease Control and Prevention. CDC Fact Sheet. Reported STDs in the United States. 2013 National Data for Chlamydia, Gonorrhea, and Syphilis, 2014. Available at: http://www.cdc.gov/nchhstp/newsroom/docs/std-trends-508.pdf. Accessed May 11, 2015.

40. Centers for Disease Control and Prevention. HIV in the United States: At a Glance, March 2015. Available at: http://www.cdc.gov/hiv/pdf/statistics_basics_ataglance_factsheet.pdf. Accessed May 12, 2015.

41. Bradley H, Hall HI, Wolitski RJ, et al. Vital Signs: HIV diagnosis, care, and treatment among persons living with HIV—United States, 2011. *MMWR Morb Mortal Wkly Rep.* 2014;63:1113.

42. Moyer VA. Screening for HIV: U.S. Preventive Services Task Force Recommendation Statement. *Ann Intern Med.* 2013;159:51.

43. Branson BM, Handsfield HH, Lampe MA, et al. Revised recommendations for HIV testing of adults, adolescents, and pregnant women in health-care settings. *MMWR Recomm Rep.* 2006;55(RR-14):1.

44. Qaseem A, Snow V, Shekelle P, et al. Screening for HIV in health care settings: a guidance statement from the American College of Physicians and HIV Medicine Association. *Ann Intern Med.* 2009;150:125.

45. Centers for Disease Control and Prevention. CDC Fact Sheet. HIV Testing in the United States, 2014. Available at http://www.cdc.gov/nchhstp/newsroom/docs/HIV-Testing-US-508.pdf. Accessed May 12, 2015.

46. Workowski KA, Berman S. Sexually transmitted diseases treatment guidelines, 2010. *MMWR Recomm Rep.* 2010;59(RR-12):1.

47. Centers for Disease Control and Prevention. Condom Effectiveness. Condom Fact Sheet in Brief, 2013. Available at: http://www.cdc.gov/condomeffectiveness/brief.html. Accessed May 12, 2015.

48. Siegel RL, Miller KD, Jemal A. Cancer statistics, 2015. *CA Cancer J Clin.* 2015;65:5.

49. Howlader N, Noone AM, Krapcho M, et al. *SEER Cancer Statistics Review, 1975–2011.* Bethesda, MD: National Cancer Institute; 2014. Available at http://seer.cancer.gov/csr/1975_2011./ Accessed May 12, 2015.

50. National Cancer Institute. Testicular Cancer Screening (PDQ®). Description of the evidence; 2014. Available at http://www.cancer.gov/cancertopics/pdq/screening/testicular/HealthProfessional/page2. Accessed May 12, 2015.

51. U.S. Preventive Services Task Force. Screening for testicular cancer: U.S. Preventive Services Task Force reaffirmation recommendation statement. *Ann Intern Med.* 2011;154:483.

52. American Cancer Society. Testicular Cancer Overview, 2014. Available at http://www.cancer.org/cancer/testicularcancer/overviewguide./ Accessed May 2, 2015.

53. Montgomery JS, Bloom DA. The diagnosis and management of scrotal masses. *Med Clin North Am.* 2011;95:235.

54. Simons MP, Aufenacker T, Bay-Nielsen M, et al. European Hernia Society guidelines on the treatment of inguinal hernia in adult patients. *Hernia.* 2009;13:343.

55. Miserez M, Peeters E, Aufenacker T, et al. Update with level 1 studies of the European Hernia Society guidelines on the treatment of inguinal hernia in adult patients. *Hernia.* 2014;18:151.

56. Kraft BM, Kolb H, Kuckuk B, et al. Diagnosis and classification of inguinal hernias. *Surg Endosc.* 2003;17:2021.

57. Van den Berg JC, de Valois JC, Go PM, et al. Detection of groin hernia with physical examination, ultrasound, and MRI compared with laparoscopic findings. *Invest Radiol.* 1999;34:739.

58. Aberger M, Wilson B, Holzbeierlein JM, et al. Testicular self-examination and testicular cancer: a cost-utility analysis. *Cancer Med.* 2014;3:1629.

59. American Cancer Society. Testicular self-exam. Updated January 21, 2015. Available at http://www.cancer.org/cancer/testicularcancer/moreinformation/doihavetesticularcancer/do-i-have-testicular-cancer-self-exam. Accessed May 13, 2015.

60. U.S. National Library of Medicine, National Institutes of Health. MedlinePlus—Testicular self-exam. Updated December 27 2013. Available at http://www.nlm.nih.gov/medlineplus/ency/article/003909.htm. Accessed May 13, 2015.

61. Kolon TF, Herndon CD, Baker LA, et al; American Urological Association. Evaluation and treatment of cryptorchidism: AUA guideline. *J Urol.* 2014;192:337.

Female Genitalia

The Bates' suite offers these additional resources to enhance learning and facilitate understanding of this chapter:

■ Bates' *Pocket Guide to Physical Examination and History Taking*, 8th edition
■ Bates' *Visual Guide to Physical Examination* (Vol. 15: Female Genitalia, Anus, and Rectum)
■ thePoint online resources, for students and instructors: http://thepoint.lww.com

Anatomy and Physiology

Knowing the basics of pelvic anatomy will enhance your examination skills and improve your detection of abnormal findings. Begin by reviewing the anatomy of the external female genitalia, or *vulva* (Fig. 14-1). Note the *mons pubis*, a hair-covered fat pad overlying the symphysis pubis; the *labia majora*, rounded folds of adipose tissue forming the outer lips of the vagina; the *labia minora*, the thinner pinkish-red folds or inner lips that extend anteriorly to form the *prepuce*; and the *clitoris*. The *vestibule*

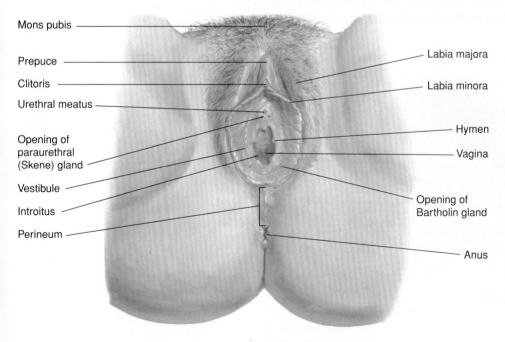

Mons pubis

Prepuce

Clitoris

Urethral meatus

Opening of paraurethral (Skene) gland

Vestibule

Introitus

Perineum

Labia majora

Labia minora

Hymen

Vagina

Opening of Bartholin gland

Anus

FIGURE 14-1. **External female genitalia.**

is the boat-shaped fossa between the labia minora. In its posterior portion lies the vaginal opening, the *introitus*, which in virgins may be hidden by the *hymen*. The term *perineum* refers to the tissue between the introitus and the anus.

The *urethral meatus* opens into the vestibule between the clitoris and the vagina. Just posterior and adjacent to the meatus on either side lie the openings of the *paraurethral (Skene) glands*.

The openings of *Bartholin glands* are located posteriorly on both sides of the vaginal opening but are not usually visible (Fig. 14-2). The glands themselves are situated more deeply.

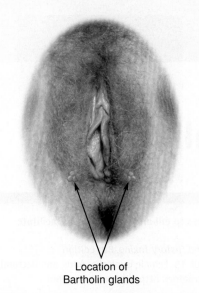

Location of
Bartholin glands

FIGURE 14-2. **Bartholin glands.**

See Table 14-1, Lesions of the Vulva, p. 596, and Table 14-2, Bulges and Swelling of the Vulva, Vagina, and Urethra, p. 597.

The *vagina* is a musculomembranous tube extending upward and posteriorly between the urinary bladder and urethra and the rectum. Its upper third lies at a horizontal plane and terminates in the cup-shaped *fornix*. The vaginal mucosa lies in transverse folds, or rugae.

The vagina lies at almost a right angle to the *uterus*, a thick-walled fibromuscular structure shaped like an inverted pear (Fig. 14-3). Its convex upper surface is the uterine *fundus*. The body of the uterus, or *corpus*, and the cylindrical *cervix* are joined inferiorly at the *isthmus*. The uterine walls contain three layers: the *perimetrium*, with its serosal coating from the perineum; the *myometrium* of distensible smooth muscle; and the *endometrium*, the adherent inner coating. The

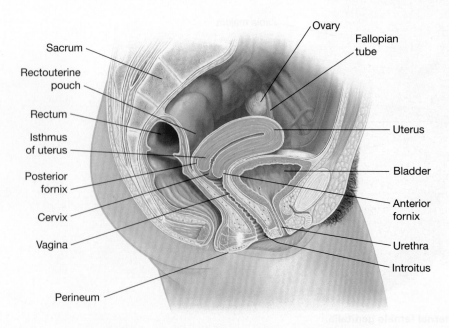

FIGURE 14-3. **Pelvic anatomy—sagittal view.**

cervix protrudes into the vagina, dividing the upper vagina into three recesses, the *anterior, posterior,* and *lateral fornices.*

The vaginal surface of the cervix, the *ectocervix,* is seen easily with the help of a speculum (Fig. 14-4). At its center is a round, oval, or slit-like depression, the *external os* of the cervix, which marks the opening into the endocervical canal. The ectocervix is covered by plushy red *columnar epithelium* that surrounds the os and lines the endocervical canal, and by shiny pink *squamous epithelium* continuous with the vaginal lining. The *squamocolumnar junction* forms the boundary between these two types of epithelium. During puberty, the broad band of columnar epithelium encircling the os, called *ectropion,* is gradually replaced by squamous epithelium. The squamocolumnar junction migrates toward the os, creating the *transformation zone.* This is the area at risk for later dysplasia which is sampled by the Papanicolaou, or Pap, smear.

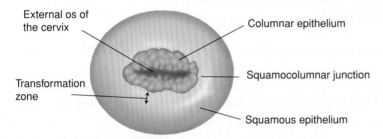

External os of the cervix

Columnar epithelium

Transformation zone

Squamocolumnar junction

Squamous epithelium

FIGURE 14-4. **Cervical epithelia and transformation zone.**

A *fallopian tube* with a fanlike tip, the *fimbria,* extends from the *ovary* to each side of the uterus, and conducts the oocyte from the periovarian peritoneal cavity to the uterine cavity (Fig. 14-5). The two ovaries are almond-shaped glands that vary considerably in size but average approximately $3.5 \times 2 \times 1.5$ cm from adulthood through menopause. The ovaries are palpable on pelvic examination in roughly half of women during the reproductive years. Normally, the fallopian tubes are not palpable. The term *adnexa,* a plural Latin word meaning "appendages," refers to the ovaries, tubes, and supporting tissues.

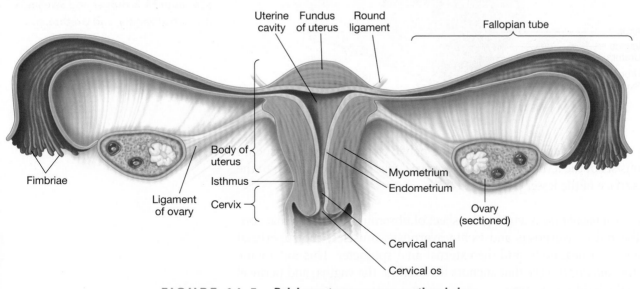

Uterine cavity | Fundus of uterus | Round ligament | Fallopian tube

Fimbriae

Ligament of ovary

Body of uterus

Isthmus

Cervix

Myometrium

Endometrium

Ovary (sectioned)

Cervical canal

Cervical os

FIGURE 14-5. **Pelvic anatomy—cross-sectional view.**

The ovaries have two primary functions: the production of oocytes and the secretion of hormones, including estrogen, progesterone, and testosterone. Increased hormonal secretion during puberty stimulates the growth of the uterus and its endometrial lining, enlargement of the vagina, thickening of the vaginal epithelium, and the development of secondary sex characteristics, including the breasts and pubic hair.

The parietal peritoneum extends downward behind the uterus into a cul-de-sac called the *rectouterine pouch* (pouch of Douglas). You can just reach this area on rectovaginal examination.

The greater pelvis, protected by the bony wings of the ilia, contains the lower abdominal viscera, then narrows inferiorly at the lesser pelvis, which surrounds the pelvic cavity and the perineum. The anatomy and innervation of the pelvis and pelvic organs are complex, but involve several common symptoms and disorders, so review the following text and figures carefully.[1,2]

The pelvic organs are supported by a sling of tissues composed of muscle, ligaments, and endopelvic fascia called the *pelvic floor,* which helps support the pelvic organs above the outlet of the lesser pelvis (Fig. 14-6). Pelvic floor muscles also aid in sexual function (orgasm), urinary and fecal continence, and stabilization of connecting joints. The pelvic floor consists of the pelvic diaphragm and the perineal membrane.

Weakness of the pelvic floor muscles may cause pain; urinary incontinence; fecal incontinence; and prolapse of the pelvic organs that can produce a *cystocele, rectocele,* or *enterocele*. Risk factors are advancing age; prior pelvic surgery or trauma; parity and childbirth; clinical conditions (obesity, diabetes, multiple sclerosis, Parkinson disease); medications (anticholinergics, α-adrenergic blockers); and chronically increased intra-abdominal pressure from chronic obstructive pulmonary disease (COPD), chronic constipation, or obesity.[1]

See Table 14-2, Bulges and Swelling of the Vulva, Vagina, and Urethra, p. 597.

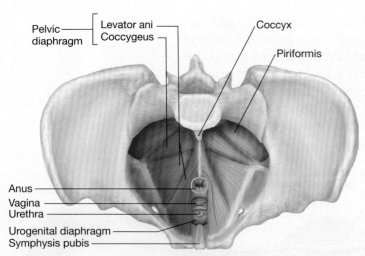

Pelvic diaphragm — Levator ani, Coccygeus; Coccyx; Piriformis; Anus; Vagina; Urethra; Urogenital diaphragm; Symphysis pubis

FIGURE 14-6. Pelvic floor.

- Briefly, the *pelvic diaphragm* separates the pelvic cavity from the perineum and consists of the *levator ani* and the *coccygeal muscles,* which attach to the inner surface of the lesser pelvis.

- The *perineal membrane* is a triangular sheet of fibromuscular tissue that contains the bulbocavernosus and ischiocavernosus muscles, the superficial transverse perineal body, and the external anal sphincter. This membrane spans the *anterior triangle* that anchors the urethra, the vagina, and perineal body to the ischiopubic rami.

- The urethra, vagina, and anorectum pass through the key-like opening in the center of the pelvic diaphragm, the *urogenital (levator) hiatus.*

- Inferior to the pelvic diaphragm is the third supporting structure, the *deep urogenital diaphragm.* This diaphragm includes the external urethral sphincter; the urethra; and the supporting deep transverse perineal muscle, which runs from the inferior ischium to the midline. Note the structures of the *posterior triangle,* principally the external anal sphincter muscle that encircles the rectum and the internal anal sphincter.

- The pelvic diaphragm is innervated by the sacral nerve roots S3 to S5. The perineal membrane and the urogenital diaphragm are innervated by the pudendal nerve.

Loss of urethral support contributes to *stress incontinence.* Weakness of the perineal body from childbirth predisposes to *rectoceles* and *enteroceles.*

In most women, pubic hair spreads downward in a triangular pattern, pointing toward the vagina. In 10% of women, it may form an inverted triangle, pointing toward the umbilicus. This growth is usually not completed until the middle 20s or later. The growth of pubic hair along with breast development are the main components of sexual maturity assessment in girls.

See the Tanner stages of sexual maturity in Chapter 18, Assessing Children: Infancy Through Adolescence, pp. 897–901.

Just before menarche, there is a physiologic increase in vaginal secretions—a normal change that sometimes worries a girl or her mother. As menses become more regular, these increased secretions, or *leukorrhea,* coincide with ovulation. They also accompany sexual arousal. These normal discharges must be differentiated from the discharges of cervical and vaginal infections.

See Table 14-3, Vaginal Discharge, p. 598, and Table 14-6, Abnormalities of the Cervix, p. 600.

Lymphatics. Lymph from the vulva and lower vagina drains into the inguinal nodes. Lymph from the internal genitalia, including the upper vagina, flows into the pelvic and abdominal lymph nodes, which are not palpable.

The Health History

Common and Concerning Symptoms

- Menarche, menstruation, menopause, postmenopausal bleeding
- Pregnancy
- Vulvovaginal symptoms
- Sexual health
- Pelvic pain—acute and chronic
- Sexually transmitted infections (STIs)

Menarche, Menstruation, Menopause. Questions about *menarche, menstruation,* and *menopause* provide an opportunity to explore the patient's concerns and her attitude about her body. Learn to describe menstrual patterns, using the terms on the next page.

The Menstrual History—Helpful Definitions

- *Menarche*—age at onset of menses
- *Dysmenorrhea*—pain with menses, often with bearing down, aching, or cramping sensation in the lower abdomen or pelvis
- *Premenstrual syndrome (PMS)*—a cluster of emotional, behavioral, and physical symptoms occurring 5 days before menses for three consecutive cycles
- *Amenorrhea*—absence of menses
- *Abnormal uterine bleeding*—bleeding between menses; includes infrequent, excessive, prolonged, or postmenopausal bleeding
- *Menopause*—absence of menses for 12 consecutive months, usually occurring between ages 48 and 55 years
- *Postmenopausal bleeding*—bleeding occurring 6 months or more after cessation of menses

Menarche and Menses. When talking with an adolescent girl about menarche, opening questions might include: "How did you first learn about monthly periods? How did you feel when they started? Many girls worry when their periods aren't regular or come late. Has anything like that bothered you?" Explain that girls in the United States usually begin menstruation between ages 9 and 16 years, and that often it takes ≥1 year for menstrual cycles to settle into a regular pattern. Age at menarche is variable, depending on genetic endowment, socioeconomic status, and nutrition. The interval between periods ranges roughly from 24 to 32 days; flow lasts from 3 to 7 days.

For the menstrual history, ask the patient her age when menses began, or *age at menarche*. When did her *last menstrual period (LMP)* start, and, if possible, the one before that, called the *prior menstrual period (PMP)*. How often does she have periods, as measured by the interval between the first day of two successive periods? How regular or irregular are they? How long do they last? How heavy is the flow? What color is it? Flow can be assessed roughly by the number of pads or tampons used daily. Because women differ in their definitions of heavy, moderate, or light flow, ask the patient whether she usually soaks a pad or tampon, or spots it lightly. Further, does she use a pad and tampon at the same time? Does she have any bleeding between periods? Or after intercourse?

The dates of previous periods provide clues to possible pregnancy or menstrual irregularities.

Unlike the normal dark red menstrual discharge, excessive flow tends to be bright red and may include "clots" (not true fibrin clots).

Dysmenorrhea. Dysmenorrhea or pain with menses, is reported by almost half of women patients. Ask if the patient has any discomfort or pain before or during her periods. If so, what is it like, how long does it last, and does it interfere with usual activities? Are there other associated symptoms? Dysmenorrhea may be *primary,* without an organic cause, or *secondary,* with an organic cause.

Primary dysmenorrhea results from increased prostaglandin production during the luteal phase of the menstrual cycle, when estrogen and progesterone levels decline.

Causes of *secondary dysmenorrhea* include endometriosis, adenomyosis (endometriosis in the muscular layers of the uterus), pelvic inflammatory disease (PID), and endometrial polyps.

Premenstrual Syndrome. PMS includes emotional and behavioral symptoms such as depression, angry outbursts, irritability, anxiety, confusion, crying spells, sleep disturbance, poor concentration, and social withdrawal.[3] Ask about signs such as bloating and weight gain, swelling of the hands and feet, and generalized aches and pains. *Criteria for diagnosis* are symptoms and signs in the 5 days prior to menses for at least three consecutive cycles; cessation of symptoms and signs within 4 days after onset of menses; and interference with daily activities.

Amenorrhea. *Amenorrhea* refers to the absence of periods. Absence of ever initiating periods is *primary amenorrhea;* cessation of periods after they have been established is *secondary amenorrhea.* Pregnancy, lactation, and menopause are physiologic causes of secondary amenorrhea.

Other causes of *secondary amenorrhea* include low body weight from any condition, including malnutrition and anorexia nervosa, stress, chronic illness, and hypothalamic–pituitary–ovarian dysfunction.

Abnormal Bleeding. Ask about any *abnormal bleeding.* The term *abnormal uterine bleeding* encompasses several patterns.

Patterns of Abnormal Bleeding

- *Polymenorrhea*, or less than 21-day intervals between menses
- *Oligomenorrhea*, or infrequent bleeding
- *Menorrhagia*, or excessive flow
- *Metrorrhagia*, or intermenstrual bleeding
- Postcoital bleeding

Causes vary by age group and include pregnancy, cervical or vaginal infection or cancer, cervical or endometrial polyps or hyperplasia, fibroids, bleeding disorders, and hormonal contraception or replacement therapy.

Postcoital bleeding suggests cervical polyps or cancer or, in an older woman, atrophic vaginitis.

Menopause. *Menopause* typically occurs between ages 48 and 55 years, peaking at a median age of 51 years. It is defined retrospectively as cessation of menses for 12 months, progressing through several stages of erratic cyclical bleeding. These stages of variable cycle length, often with vasomotor symptoms like hot flashes, flushing, and sweating, represent *perimenopause.* The ovaries stop producing estradiol or progesterone and estrogen levels drop significantly, although some testosterone synthesis persists.[4] Pituitary secretion of luteinizing hormone and follicle-stimulating hormone gradually becomes markedly elevated. Low levels of estradiol remain detectable due to conversion of adrenal steroids in peripheral adipose tissue. During the menopausal transition, women may experience mood shifts; changes in self-image; hot flashes from vasomotor changes; accelerated bone loss; increases in total and low-density lipoprotein cholesterol; and vulvovaginal atrophy with vaginal drying, dysuria, or dyspareunia. Studies suggest that only vasomotor symptoms, vaginal symptoms, and trouble sleeping are consistently linked to menopause. Urinary symptoms may occur in the absence of infection, due to atrophy of the urethra and urinary trigone.

Women may ask about alternative compounds and botanicals for relief of menopause-related symptoms. Most are poorly studied and not proven to be beneficial. Estrogen replacement relieves symptoms, but poses other health hazards.[5] Relatively few medications have been shown to affect symptoms (see p. 582).

Ask a middle-aged or older woman if she has stopped menstruating. When? Continue with "How do (did) you feel about not having your periods anymore?" "Has this affected your life in either a positive or negative way?" Did any symptoms accompany her transition to menopause? Always be sure to ask about any bleeding or spotting after menopause as this may be an early sign of cancer.

Causes of *postmenopausal bleeding* include endometrial cancer, hormone replacement therapy (HRT), and uterine and cervical polyps.

Pregnancy. The health history includes such questions as, "Have you ever been pregnant? How many times?…How many living children do you have?… Have you ever had a miscarriage or an abortion? How many times?" Ask about any difficulties during pregnancy and the timing and circumstances of any abortion, whether spontaneous or induced. How did the woman experience these losses? Obstetricians commonly record the pregnancy history using the "gravida para" system.

See Chapter 19, The Pregnant Woman, pp. 927–954 for further discussion.

The Gravida Para Notation

- G = gravida, or total number of pregnancies
- P = para, or outcomes of pregnancies. After P, you will often see the notations F (full-term), P (premature), A (abortion), and L (living child).

Inquire about methods of contraception used by the patient and her partner. Is the patient satisfied with the method chosen? Are there any questions about the options available?

If amenorrhea suggests a *current pregnancy,* inquire about the date of last intercourse and *common early symptoms:* tenderness, tingling, or increased size of the breasts; urinary frequency; nausea and vomiting; easy fatigability; and sensations that the baby is moving, usually present at about 20 weeks. Be sensitive to the patient's feelings about these topics; explore them when the patient has special concerns. (See also Chapter 19, The Pregnant Woman, p. 927.)

Amenorrhea followed by heavy bleeding suggests a *threatened abortion* or *dysfunctional uterine bleeding* related to lack of ovulation.

Vulvovaginal Symptoms. The most common vulvovaginal symptoms are *vaginal discharge* and *itching.* If the patient reports a discharge, inquire about its amount, color, consistency, and odor. Ask about any local *sores* or *lumps* in the vulvar area. Are they painful? Because patients vary in their understanding of anatomical terms, be prepared to try alternative phrasing such as "Any itching (or other symptoms) near your vagina?…between your legs?…where you urinate?"

See Table 14-1, Lesions of the Vulva, p. 596; and Table 14-3, Vaginal Discharge, p. 598.

Sexual Health. Sexual health plays an important and natural role in overall well-being, yet many clinicians feel ill-equipped to address sexual health issues.[6,7] Patients immediately sense your receptiveness to their concerns in this sensitive and vital area. Maintaining a neutral, nonjudgmental tone helps your patients feel safe and trust you with their concerns. Many patients have strong beliefs about sexual behavior related to their upbringing, faith, ethnicity, educational level, and past experiences. Reassure them that sex in a mature consensual relationship is healthy, and that you explore sexual health with all your patients. Be aware of your own body language, facial expressions, and tone of voice, so that you create an open environment for discussion. In younger patients and adolescents, consider asking the parents to leave the room so that the patients feel free to answer questions without fear of parental disapproval or repercussions, especially when discussing possible sexual abuse.

Sexual Orientation and Gender Identity. Recent surveys indicate 1.6% to 3.4% of Americans' self-identify as lesbian, gay, bisexual, or transgender (LGBT).[8–10] Many are apprehensive about health care encounters, and clinicians are generally underprepared for providing LGBT care. Both the Institute of Medicine (2011) and the American College of Physicians (2015) have called for policies to reduce significant disparities in LGBT health care, including increased risk of suicide, depression, and STIs.[11,12] Listen closely to your patients and probe existing resources to learn about LGBT health issues.[13–15] As you talk with patients, begin with neutral questions about *sexual orientation* and *gender identity*, listed below.[16]

See also The Sexual History, Chapter 3, pp. 94–95; and Tips for Taking a Sexual History and the discussion of gay, lesbian, bisexual and transgender health care in Chapter 13, Male Genitalia and Hernias, pp. 545–546.

- "Are you currently dating, sexually active, or in a relationship?" "How would you identify your sexual orientation?" The range of responses includes heterosexual or straight, lesbian, gay, women who have sex with women, men who have sex with men (MSM), bisexual, transsexual, and questioning, among others.

- "How would you describe your gender identity?" Responses include male, female, transsexual, transgendered, intersex, female-to-male, male-to-female, unsure or questioning, and even "prefer not to answer."

- Continue with, "Do you use protection such as birth control or condoms?… Has anyone ever tried to touch or have sex with you without your consent?"

Sexual Response. Start with general questions such as "How is sex for you?" or "Are you having any problems with sex? This includes sexual intercourse and anal and oral sex." Alternatively, you can ask, "Are you satisfied with your sex life as it is now? Has there been any significant change in the last few years? Are you satisfied with your ability to perform sexually? How does your partner feel?" Studies show that patients are often uncomfortable bringing up these topics. Many prefer to have them initiated by their providers, and most welcome information about sexual health.[17–19]

If the patient has concerns about her response to sex, consider direct questions to help you assess each phase of the sexual response: desire, arousal, and orgasm. "Do you have an interest in (appetite for) sex?" inquires about desire, or *libido*. If indicated, follow up with, "Has your interest in sex increased or decreased?… Can you describe why you think it has changed? Are you and your partners having any difficulties or problems, or any new stress?" Often, stressors like relationship changes, job changes, or even moving affect sexual drive and enjoyment. For *arousal*, ask, "Do you get sexually aroused? Do you lubricate easily (get wet or slippery)? Do you stay too dry?" Continue with, "Do you use lubricants to help with dryness?" For *orgasm*, ask, "Are you able to reach climax (have an orgasm, or 'come')?" "Is it important for you to reach climax?" "Do you enjoy sex if you do not reach orgasm?"

Sexual dysfunction is classified by the phase of sexual response. A woman may lack desire; she may fail to become aroused and attain adequate vaginal lubrication; or, despite adequate arousal, she may be unable to reach orgasm. Causes include lack of estrogen, clinical illness, trauma or abuse, surgery, pelvic anatomy, and psychological and psychiatric conditions.

Ask also about *dyspareunia*, or pain with intercourse. If present, try to localize where the pain occurs. Is it near the outside, at the start of intercourse, or does she feel it farther in, when her partner is pushing deeper? *Vaginismus* refers to an involuntary spasm of the muscles surrounding the vaginal orifice that makes penetration during intercourse painful or impossible.

In addition to identifying and understanding sexual problems, ask about onset, severity (persistent or sporadic), setting, and factors, if any, that make them better or worse. What does the patient think is the source of the problem, what has she tried to do about it, and what does she hope for? The causes of sexual dysfunction are complex and include the patient's general health; medications and drugs, including use of alcohol; knowledge of sexual practices and techniques; her attitudes, values, and fears; the relationship and communication between partners; and the setting in which sexual activity takes place.

Pelvic Pain—Acute and Chronic.

Many women volunteer a history of pelvic pain. *Acute pelvic pain* in menstruating girls and women warrants immediate attention. The differential diagnosis is broad but includes life-threatening conditions such as *ectopic pregnancy, ovarian torsion,* and *appendicitis.* As you identify onset, timing, features of the pain, and associated symptoms, you will need to consider infectious, gastrointestinal (GI), and urinary causes. Be sure to ask about STIs, recent insertion of an intrauterine device (IUD), and any symptoms in the sexual partner. A careful pelvic examination, with attention to vital signs, and testing for pregnancy will help narrow your diagnosis and guide further testing.

Chronic pelvic pain refers to pain that lasts for more than 6 months and does not respond to treatment.[23] It accounts for approximately 10% of ambulatory referrals to gynecologists and 20% of hysterectomies.[24,25] Risk factors are advancing age, prior pelvic surgery or trauma, parity and childbirth, clinical conditions (obesity, diabetes, multiple sclerosis, Parkinson disease), medications (anticholinergics, α-adrenergic blockers), and chronically increased intra-abdominal pressure (COPD, chronic constipation, obesity).[1] Explore gynecologic, urologic, GI, musculoskeletal, and neurological causes.[24] The Pelvic Pain Assessment Form of the International Pelvic Pain Society, which includes screening questions for depression and physical and sexual abuse, as well as a pain map that women complete, is a helpful resource.[26] Asking the woman to keep a daily pain journal, noting any changes in situational, dietary, or seasonal conditions, may also be useful.

Sexually Transmitted Infections.

Local symptoms or findings on physical examination may raise the possibility of *STIs* (also referred to as *sexually transmitted diseases [STDs]*). After establishing the seven attributes of any symptoms, elicit the patient's sexual history. Inquire about sexual contacts and establish the number of sexual partners in the past 3 to 6 months. Ask if the patient has concerns about human immunodeficiency virus (HIV) infection,

---

Superficial pain suggests local inflammation, atrophic vaginitis, or inadequate lubrication; deeper pain may arise from pelvic disorders or pressure on a normal ovary. Causes of *vaginismus* may be physical or psychological.

Commonly, sexual problems are related to situational and psychosocial factors.

The most common cause of acute pelvic pain is *PID*, followed by *ruptured ovarian cyst,* and *appendicitis.*[20] STIs and recent IUD insertion are red flags for PID. Always rule out *ectopic pregnancy* first with serum or urine testing and possible ultrasound.[21,22]

Also consider *mittelschmerz,* which is typically a mild unilateral pain lasting for a few hours to a few days arising at midcycle from ovulation, *ruptured ovarian cyst,* and *tubo-ovarian abscess.*

Endometriosis, from retrograde menstrual flow and extension of the uterine lining outside the uterus, affects 50% to 60% of women and girls with pelvic pain.[27] Other causes include *PID* and *adenosis* and *fibroids,* which are tumors in the uterine wall or submucosal or subserosal surfaces arising from the smooth muscle cells of the myometrium.

Chronic pelvic pain is a red flag for a history of *sexual abuse.* Also consider *pelvic floor spasm* from myofascial pain with trigger points on examination (see pp. 592–593).

desires HIV testing, or has current or past partners at risk. Also ask about oral and anal sex and, if indicated, about symptoms involving the mouth, throat, anus, and rectum. Review the past history of STIs. "Have you ever had herpes?… any other problems such as gonorrhea?…syphilis?…pelvic infections?" Continue with the more general questions suggested on pp. 94–95.

Health Promotion and Counseling: Evidence and Recommendations

Important Topics for Health Promotion and Counseling

- Cervical cancer screening
- Ovarian cancer: risk factors and screening
- Sexually transmitted infections
- Options for family planning
- Menopause and hormone replacement therapy

Cervical Cancer Screening: The Pap Smear and Human Papilloma-virus Infection. Widespread screening with the *Papanicolaou (Pap) smear* has contributed to a significant decline in cervical cancer incidence and mortality. In 2014, an estimated 12,900 women were diagnosed with cervical cancer, with 4,100 deaths.[28] The current estimated incidence rate is 7.8 cases per 100,000 women per year. Most cases of cervical cancer occur in women who have not had appropriate screening.

HPV infection with high-risk oncogenic subtypes is found in virtually all cervical cancers.[29] Roughly 90% of HPV infections are asymptomatic and resolve within 2 years. The most important risk factor for cervical cancer is persistent infection with high-risk HPV subtypes, especially HPV 16 or HPV 18. These two subtypes cause roughly 70% of cervical cancers worldwide. Even the 10% of women with persistent infection rarely progress to cervical cancer if they undergo regular screening, insofar as the average estimated time for a high-grade HPV lesion to progress to cervical cancer is 10 years, allowing a long interval for detection and treatment.[28] Genital infection with low-risk subtypes, such as HPV 6 and HPV 11, is associated with genital warts.

Two notable risk factors for cervical cancer include failure to undergo screening, which accounts for roughly half of women diagnosed with cervical cancer, and multiple sexual partners. Other risk factors include smoking, immunosuppression from any cause including HIV infection, long-term use of oral contraception, coinfection with *Chlamydia trachomatis*, parity, prior cervical cancer, and genetic polymorphisms affecting the entry of HPV DNA into cervical cells.[30]

Cervical Cancer Screening Guidelines, 2015. For the first time, in 2012, the U.S. Preventive Services Task Force (USPSTF), the American College of

Obstetricians and Gynecologists (ACOG), and the American Cancer Society (ACS), in collaboration with the American Society for Colposcopy and Cervical Pathology (ASCCP) and the American Society for Clinical Pathology (ASCP), released guidelines that agree on cervical cancer screening for average-risk women, summarized below, which contain the important definition of average risk.[28,30–32] Note that in 2014, the American College of Physicians found no evidence supporting screening with routine pelvic examinations alone in average-risk, asymptomatic adult women (as distinct from cervical cancer screening or symptom-based examination).[33,34]

Current Cervical Cancer Screening Guidelines for Average-Risk Women: USPSTF, ACS/ASCCP/ ASCP, and ACOG

Variable[a]	Recommendation
Age at which to begin screening	21 yrs
Screening method and interval	Ages 21–65 yrs: cytology every 3 yrs OR
	Ages 21–29 yrs: cytology every 3 yrs
	Ages 30–65 yrs: cytology plus HPV testing (for high-risk or oncogenic HPV types) every 5 yrs
Age at which to end screening	Age >65 yrs, assuming three consecutive negative results on cytology or two consecutive negative results on cytology plus HPV testing within 10 yrs before cessation of screening, with the most recent test performed within 5 yrs
Screening after hysterectomy with removal of the cervix	Not recommended

HPV, human papillomavirus.

[a]Definition of Average Risk: No history of high-grade, precancerous cervical lesion (cervical intraepithelial neoplasia grade 2 or a more severe lesion) or cervical cancer; not immunocompromised (including being HIV-infected); and no in utero exposure to diethylstilbestrol.

Source: Sawaya GF, Kulasingam S, Denberg T, et al. Cervical cancer screening in average-risk women: Best practice advice from the Clinical Guidelines Committee of the American College of Physicians. *Ann Intern Med* 2015;162:851.

Rationale for Screening Recommendations. All three sets of guidelines concur that screening should begin at age 21 years, and that there is no need for annual screening for average-risk women at any age.

■ *Women age <21 years:* Although cytologic abnormalities on Pap smear are common, most HPV infections clear spontaneously within 1 to 2 years. Pap smears in this age group have often led to unnecessary procedures that could affect cervical competency, pregnancy, and childbirth.

■ *Women ages 21 to 65 years:* All three guidelines, including a grade A recommendation from the USPSTF, recommend Pap smear cytology every 3 years or, alternatively, cotesting with cytology plus HPV testing for high-risk subtypes every 5 years. Women with normal cytology but negative high-risk

HPV testing have an estimated risk of cervical intraepithelial neoplasia (CIN) grade 2 or higher at 5 years of only 0.34%.[28] The guidelines agree that testing for HPV alone or cotesting should only begin *after age 30 years,* because the prevalence of self-limited HPV in women age <30 years is still high.

■ *Women age ≥65 years:* All concur that screening can stop if women have had three consecutive negative results on cytology or two consecutive negative results with cotesting within 10 years of cessation of screening (with the most recent test performed within 5 years), as the risk of cervical cancer is low, and risk factors decrease with age.

■ *Women with hysterectomy:* Average-risk women with a hysterectomy and removal of the cervix and no history of high-grade precancer or cervical cancer do not need screening. Screening guidelines for women with a subtotal (supracervical) hysterectomy are the same as for average risk women.[35]

Note that to follow these guidelines, women and clinicians need to have an accurate history of past Pap smear testing and results.

Take the time to understand how Pap smear results are reported. Current classification and management guidelines are based on the Bethesda System of the National Cancer Institute (NCI), revised in 2001.[36,37] The principal categories are provided below. Management depends on the cervical cancer risk and often involves repeat cytology, colposcopy, and DNA testing for HPV.

Conventional Pap smears have a sensitivity and specificity for detecting cervical cancer of 30% to 87% and 86% to 100%, respectively. For liquid-based cytology, these figures are 61% to 95% and 78% to 82%. The sensitivity of Pap smear and HPV DNA testing is 74.6% to 100%.[38–40]

Classification of Pap Smear Cytology: The Bethesda System (2001)

- *Negative for intraepithelial lesion or malignancy:* No cellular evidence of neoplasia is present, although other organisms like *Trichomonas, Candida,* or *Actinomyces* may be reported in this category. Shifts in flora consistent with bacterial vaginosis or cellular changes from herpes simplex may also be reported.
- *Epithelial cell abnormalities:* These include precancerous and cancerous lesions such as:
  - *Squamous cells,* including *atypical squamous cells* (*ASC*), which may be of undetermined significance (ASC-US); *low-grade squamous intraepithelial lesions* (*LSIL*), including mild dysplasia; *high-grade squamous intraepithelial lesions* (*HSIL*), including moderate and severe dysplasia with features suspicious for invasion; and invasive *squamous cell carcinoma.*
  - *Glandular cells,* including *atypical endocervical cells* or *atypical endometrial cells,* specified or not otherwise specified (NOS); *atypical endocervical cells* or *atypical glandular cells, favor neoplasia; endocervical adenocarcinoma in situ;* and *adenocarcinoma.*
- *Other malignant neoplasms,* such as sarcomas or lymphomas, are rare.

The HPV Vaccine

■ *Routine vaccination for girls ages 11 and 12:* The Advisory Committee on Immunization Practices of the Centers for Disease Control (CDC) and the American Academy of Pediatrics recommend a three-dose vaccination series over 6 months with either the quadrivalent or bivalent vaccine for girls and boys at ages 11 or 12, before their first sexual encounter; the series can begin as early as age 9 years.[41,42] The quadrivalent vaccine prevents infection from HPV subtypes 16 and 18, as well as 6 and 11, which cause 90% of genital warts. The bivalent vaccine prevents infection from subtypes 16 and 18. Vaccination with the quadrivalent HPV vaccine is also recommended for the prevention of cervical, vulvar, and vaginal cancers and precancers in females, as well as anal cancers and precancers and genital warts in both females and males.

Starting HPV vaccination early is important. In American adolescents, the prevalence of sexual intercourse in 2013 was 5.6% before age 13 years; 30% by ninth grade, and 64% by the end of high school.[43] Vaccinated women should still get cervical cancer screening because the vaccines do not prevent all HPV subtypes. Also, consistent use of condoms does not eliminate the risk of cervical HPV infection.[44,45]

■ *Catch-up vaccination:* is recommended for females ages 13 through 26 years who have not had prior vaccination or completed the three-dose series. If females reach age 27 years before completing the series, the second and/or third vaccine doses can be administered after age 26 years to complete the series. Prevaccination assessments to establish the need for Pap or high-risk HPV DNA testing are not recommended.

■ The HPV vaccine is recommended for persons with compromised immune systems, including infection with HIV, through age 26 years if they have not been fully vaccinated when younger.

Ovarian Cancer: Risk Factors and Screening.   Many women are fearful of ovarian cancer. Although ovarian cancer is relatively rare, it is the fifth leading cause of cancer-related death for women.[46] Two thirds of women affected are older than age 55 years; most are diagnosed when the disease is already metastatic to the peritoneal cavity or other organs. Overall 5-year survival is only 40%,[47] compared to 94% for the 15% of women who present with local early-stage disease. Currently, there are no effective screening tests, so clinicians face the challenge of improving identification of symptoms. In women older than age 50 years, *three symptoms merit special attention*: abdominal distention, abdominal bloating, and urinary frequency; however, these are usually reported within 3 months of diagnosis and frequently occur in other conditions. The USPSTF reviewed current evidence in 2012 and continued to recommend against screening for ovarian cancer, a grade D recommendation based on findings that there is moderate or high certainty that screening has no net benefit, or that the harms outweigh the benefits.[46]

Risk factors for ovarian cancer include family history and presence of the BRCA1 or BRCA2 gene mutation. Risk is tripled if there is a first-degree relative with breast or ovarian cancer. Carriers of BRCA1 and BRCA2 have a lifetime risk of 40% to 50% and 20% to 30%, respectively.[48] Other risk factors include obesity and nulliparity, with growing evidence of increased risk from use of postmenopausal HRT, especially long-time users and users of sequential estrogen–progesterone schedules.[49,50] More than 90% of ovarian cancers appear to be random. Risk is decreased by use of oral contraceptives, multiple pregnancies, breastfeeding, and tubal ligation. Recent investigations show that in high-risk women (BRCA positive; positive family history), some ovarian cancer cells may arise in the fallopian tubes, creating the option of risk-reducing salpingo-oophorectomy.[51]

Women frequently ask about *CA-125* testing. The CA-125 level is neither sensitive nor specific. Recent studies are investigating additional biomarkers and stratification of CA-125 cutoff points for demographic and clinical subgroups to reduce the high false-positive rate.[47,52] Although CA-125 is elevated in more than 80% of women with ovarian cancer and helps predict relapse after treatment, it is also elevated in many other conditions and cancers, including pregnancy; endometriosis; uterine fibroids; PID; benign cysts; and pancreatic, breast, lung, gastric, and colon cancer. Current investigations of combined screening with CA-125, transvaginal ultrasound, and selected tumor markers have not demonstrated benefits that improve survival.

Sexually Transmitted Infections.   U.S. rates of STIs are the highest in the industrialized world. *Chlamydia trachomatis* is the most commonly reported STI in the United States and the most common STI in women, with an estimated 2.8 million cases annually (although HPV is more prevalent and the most common STI).[53] Often, symptoms are subtle and the infection remains undiagnosed. If untreated, 10% to 15% of women will develop PID, a polymicrobial infection with an 8% to 40% risk of tubal infertility depending on the number of episodes; a third to a half of cases are attributed to coinfection of *C. trachomatis* with *Neisseria gonorrhoeae*.[54,55] *Chlamydia* infection rates are highest in women ages 20 to 24 years, closely followed by women ages 15 to 19 years. African American women and American Indian/Alaskan natives are at highest risk for infection. As with other STIs, risk factors are age younger than 24 years and sexually active; prior infection with *chlamydia* or other STIs, new or multiple partners, inconsistent condom use, and occupational sex work. Detection, groups most affected, and consequences of underdiagnosis and treatment are similar for *gonorrhea*. Infection with *syphilis* is less common, but increasing in men.[56]

To improve detection and treatment, the CDC and the USPSTF[57] strongly recommend screening for STIs, summarized below.

Chlamydial infection is a cause of urethritis, cervicitis, PID, ectopic pregnancy, infertility, and chronic pelvic pain. Risk factors include age younger than 26 years, multiple partners, and prior history of STIs.

CDC STI and HIV Screening Recommendations 2014

- Chlamydia and gonorrhea screening annually for all sexually active women ages <25 years and older women with risk factors such as new or multiple sex partners, or a sex partner infected with an STI.
- Chlamydia, syphilis, hepatitis B, and HIV screening for all pregnant women and gonorrhea screening for at-risk pregnant women starting early in pregnancy, with repeat testing as needed to protect the health of mothers and their infants.
- Chlamydia, gonorrhea, and syphilis screening at least once a year for all sexually active gay, bisexual, and other MSM. MSM who have multiple or anonymous partners should be screened more frequently for STIs (i.e., at 3- to 6-month intervals).
- HIV testing at least once for all adults and adolescents from ages 13 to 64 years.
- HIV testing at least once a year for anyone having unsafe sex or using injection drug equipment. Sexually active gay and bisexual men may benefit from testing every 3 to 6 months.

Source: Centers for Disease Control and Prevention. Sexually transmitted diseases. STD and HIV screening recommendations. Updated December 16, 2014. Available at http://www.cdc.gov/std/prevention/screeningreccs.htm. Accessed May 20, 2015.

HIV Infection. More than 1.2 million Americans are infected with HIV, and one in seven (14%) is unaware of their infection.[58] The number of infected individuals continues to increase, although the number of new infections has remained stable. In 2013, an estimated 47,352 people were diagnosed with HIV infection and an estimated 26,688 people were diagnosed with acquired immune deficiency syndrome (AIDS), bringing the estimated total number of Americans diagnosed with AIDS to 1,194,039. At highest risk, are gay, bisexual, and other MSM of all ethnicities, but especially, young black/African American MSM ages 13 to 24 years. In 2010, MSM represented 4% of the United States male population and 63% of all new infections. White MSM had the largest total number of new infections. Blacks/African Americans and Hispanics/Latinos remain disproportionately affected.

In the United States, 20% of new infections occur in women, primarily through heterosexual contact (84% in 2010) and injection drug use (14%). Women represent 23% of those living with HIV infection. Among infected women, 64% are African American, 18% are white, and 15% are Hispanic/Latinos. The CDC reports that women are not accessing health care and are undertreated: "in 2011, only 45% were engaged in care, and only 32% had achieved viral suppression."[59] Heterosexual transmission is more likely in the following settings: vaginal or anal intercourse without a condom, sex exchanged for drugs, sex with multiple partners, infection with other STIs, women who have been sexually abused, sex with an infected partner with a high viral load of HIV-1, cervical ectopy, sex during menstruation, and sex with a male partner without circumcision. Recurrent vulvocandidiasis, concurrent STIs, abnormal Pap smears (occurring in 40% of HIV-positive women), and HPV infection are warning indications for HIV testing. As shown above, the CDC recommends universal HIV testing for everyone in the age range of 13 to 64 years due to the prevalence of infections in people without known risk factors and underreporting.

Clinician Counseling for Prevention of STIs and HIV. The USPSTF recommends intensive behavioral counseling for all sexually active adolescents and for adults who are at increased risk for STIs, a grade B recommendation.[60] High-intensity counseling with more than 2 hours of intervention contact is the most successful, although this may be challenging for primary care offices compared to integrated practice settings.[61] The USPSTF evidence review notes that successful counseling includes: "prevalence, transmission, and details on how to reduce the risk for transmission; help in identifying personal risk for STIs; training in common behavior change processes, such as problem solving, decision making, and goal-setting; training in communication surrounding condom use and safe sex; and hands-on practice with condoms. Many successful interventions were also specifically tailored to the gender and race/ethnicity of the participants."

Key to effective clinician counseling are respect, compassion, a nonjudgmental attitude, and use of open-ended and understandable questions, such as, "Tell me about any new sex partners" and "Have you ever had anal sex, meaning 'penis in rectum/anus sex'?" The CDC recommends interactive client-centered counseling, tailored to the person's specific risk factors and situation.[62]

See Chapter 3, Interviewing and the Health History, pp. 94–95, on eliciting the sexual history, and Chapter 13, Male Genitalia and Hernias, pp. 548–549, on risk factors for HIV infection.

Training in prevention counseling improves effectiveness. Consult the excellent websites recommended by the CDC such as:

- Effective interventions. HIV prevention that works—at http://effectiveinterventions.org

- Project Respect—at http://depts.washington.edu/nnptc/

Options for Family Planning.   The CDC notes that "Teen pregnancy has declined to the lowest rates in seven decades, yet still ranks highest among the developed countries."[63] Significant health disparities remain: In 2013, non-Hispanic black, Hispanic, and American Indian/Alaska Native teen birth rates were still one and a half to two times higher than the rate for non-Hispanic white teens. Almost half of U.S. pregnancies are unintended. Among pregnancies in teens ages 15 to 19 years and younger than age 15 years, the percentage of unintended pregnancy climbs to over 80% and 98%, respectively. It is important to counsel girls and women about the timing of ovulation in the menstrual cycle and how to plan or prevent pregnancy. Be familiar with the numerous options for contraception and their effectiveness listed below.[64]

Types of Family Planning Methods

Methods	Types of Contraception
Natural	Fertility awareness/periodic abstinence, withdrawal, lactation
Barrier	Male condom, female condom, diaphragm, cervical cap, sponge
Implantable	IUD, subdermal implant of levonorgestrel
Pharmacologic/hormonal	Spermicide, oral contraceptives (estrogen and progesterone; progestin only), estrogen/progesterone injectables and patch, hormonal vaginal contraceptive ring, emergency contraception
Surgery (permanent)	Tubal ligation; transcervical sterilization; vasectomy

Source: Centers for Disease Control and Prevention. Reproductive health. Contraception. Updated April 22, 2015. Available at http://www.cdc.gov/reproductivehealth/UnintendedPregnancy/Contraception.htm. Accessed May 21, 2015.

Failure rates are lowest for the subdermal implant, IUD, female sterilization, and vasectomy at less than 0.8% per year (<1 pregnancy/100 women/yr) and highest for male and female condoms, withdrawal, sponge in parous women, fertility awareness methods, and spermicides at more than 18% per year (or ≥18 pregnancies/100 women/yr). Failure rates for injectables, oral contraceptives, the patch, vaginal ring, and diaphragm range from 6% to 12% per year (or 6 to 12 pregnancies/100 women/yr).

Take the time to understand the patient or couple's concerns and preferences, and respect these preferences whenever possible. Continued use of a preferred method is superior to a more effective method that is abandoned. For teenagers, a confidential setting eases discussion of topics that may seem private and difficult to explore.

Menopause and Hormone Replacement Therapy. For many women, menopause is a profound transition that brings psychological and physiologic changes ranging from mood shifts to hot flashes to vaginal drying and bone loss. Be well informed about the *risks and benefits of HRT* with estrogen and progesterone, a topic women ask about frequently. Following publication of the Women's Health Initiative trials investigating use of postmenopausal estrogen plus progesterone in 2002 and estrogen alone in 2004,[65,66] the USPSTF, ACOG, the American Heart Association, and the North American Menopause Society (NAMS), among others, issued recommendations against using HRT for chronic conditions in postmenopausal women. In 2012, the USPSTF reaffirmed its recommendation against the use of combined estrogen and progestin for the primary prevention of chronic clinical conditions in postmenopausal women, including women with hysterectomies, citing grade D evidence that "there is moderate or high certainty that the service has no net benefit or that the harms outweigh the benefits."[67,68] In its 2012 evidence review of nine randomized controlled trials from 2002 to 2012, the USPSTF concluded that "estrogen plus progestin and estrogen alone decreased risk for fractures but increased risk for stroke, thromboembolic events, gallbladder disease, and urinary incontinence. Estrogen plus progestin increased risk for breast cancer and probable dementia, whereas estrogen alone decreased risk for breast cancer." The American Heart Association, ACOG, and NAMS recommend against the use of postmenopausal hormone therapy for primary or secondary prevention of cardiovascular disease.[69–71] ACOG notes that there is some evidence that transdermal estrogen therapy may have thrombosis-sparing properties and also finds insufficient evidence for recent claims that compounded bioidentical hormones are superior to conventional menopausal HRT. The USPSTF, ACOG, and NAMS advise that use of HRT for menopausal vasomotor symptoms be individualized, low dose, and for the shortest acceptable duration, usually in the range of 1 to 2 years.

Website Resources for Clinicians and Patients

The websites below provide updated information on health promotion and counseling for cervical and ovarian cancer, STIs and HIV, options for family planning, and menopause. More specific references are listed in the References on pp. 604–606.

- American Cancer Society—cervical and ovarian cancer at http://www.cancer.org/
- American College of Physicians—clinical practice guidelines at https://www.acponline.org/clinical_information/guidelines/
- American Congress of Obstetricians and Gynecologists—clinical guidelines at http://www.acog.org/About-ACOG/ACOG-Departments/Deliveries-Before-39-Weeks/ACOG-Clinical-Guidelines
- Centers for Disease Control and Prevention—STIs and HIV at http://www.cdc.gov/std/
- National Cancer Institute—cervical and ovarian cancer at http://www.cancer.gov/
- North American Menopause Society—for professionals at http://www.menopause.org/for-professionals
- U.S. Preventive Services Task Force—recommendations for primary care practice at http://www.uspreventiveservicestaskforce.org/Page/Name/recommendations

Techniques of Examination

Important Areas of Examination

External Examination	Internal Examination
Mons pubis	Vagina, vaginal walls
Labia majora and minora	Cervix
Urethral meatus, clitoris	Uterus, ovaries
Vaginal introitus	Pelvic muscles
Perineum	Rectovaginal wall

Approach to the Pelvic Examination. Many students feel uneasy during their first pelvic examinations. This is normal. At the same time, patients have their own concerns. Some women have had painful, embarrassing, or even demeaning experiences during previous pelvic examinations; others may be facing a pelvic examination for the first time. Some women fear what the clinician may find, and how findings may affect their lives. Asking the patient's permission to perform the examination shows courtesy, respect, and the expectation that the examination is collaborative. Explaining the steps of what you are about to do will also be greatly appreciated. If a Pap smear is to be collected using the glass-slide technique, time the examination so that it does not occur during menses, because blood can interfere with interpretation.

In liquid-based cytology, blood cells can be filtered out.

Take steps to help a woman having her first pelvic examination know what to expect. Use three-dimensional models, show her the equipment, let her handle the speculum, and explain each step both in advance and during the examination to help her learn about her body and feel comfortable. A careful, gentle technique is especially important for minimizing any pain or discomfort.

The woman's response to the pelvic examination may reveal clues about her feelings about the examination and her sexuality. If she pulls away, adducts her thighs, or reacts negatively to the examination, you can gently comment, "I notice you are having some trouble relaxing. Is it just being here, or are you troubled by the examination?…Is anything worrying you?" Behaviors that seem to present an obstacle may lead you to a better understanding of your patient's concerns. Adverse reactions may signal prior physical or sexual abuse and should be explored.[72]

Pelvic examinations during adolescence should respond to indications such as menstrual abnormalities (amenorrhea, excessive bleeding, or dysmenorrhea); unexplained abdominal pain; vaginal discharge; the prescription of contraceptives; bacteriologic and cytologic studies in a sexually active girl; and the patient's request for assessment.

See Chapter 18, Assessing Children: Infancy Through Adolescence, pp. 900–901.

Tips for the Successful Pelvic Examination

The Patient	The Examiner
Avoids intercourse, douching, or use of vaginal suppositories for 24 to 48 hrs before examination	Obtains permission; selects chaperone
	Explains each step of the examination in advance
Empties her bladder before the examination	Drapes the patient from midabdomen to knees; depresses the drape between the knees to provide eye contact with patient
Lies supine, with head and shoulders elevated, arms at her sides or folded across the chest to enhance eye contact and reduce tightening of abdominal muscles	Avoids unexpected or sudden movements
	Chooses a speculum that is the correct size
	Warms the speculum with tap water
	Monitors the comfort of the examination by watching the patient's face
	Uses excellent but gentle technique, especially when inserting the speculum (see pp. 587–588)

Helping the patient to relax is essential for an adequate examination. Adopting the tips recommended helps enhance the patient's comfort. *Always wear gloves,* both during the examination and when handling equipment and specimens. Plan ahead, so that any needed equipment and culture media are readily at hand.

Male examiners should be accompanied by female chaperones. Female examiners should also be assisted if the patient is physically or emotionally disturbed, or if help is needed with the examination.

Sexual Assault.   Cases of *sexual assault* merit special evaluation. Sexual assault includes rape, unwanted genital touching, and forced exposure to pornography. *Rape* is a legal term; in the United States, rape refers to "any penetration of a body orifice (mouth, vagina, or anus) involving force or the threat of force or incapacity (i.e., associated with young or old age, cognitive or physical disability, or drug or alcohol intoxication) and nonconsent."[73] The lifetime prevalence of sexual assault ranges from 13% to 39% among women and 3% among men. The National Intimate Partner and Sexual Violence Survey report of 2011 revealed that 19.3% of women and 1.7% of men have been raped during their lifetimes.[74] Only two thirds of rape victims report the assault to their primary care provider, only 20% to 40% present for clinical evaluation, and less than 40% report rape to law enforcement. Optimally, rape victims should receive care from a trained team at a rape crisis center or emergency room that can provide support, treatment of injuries, and documentation of evidence. Trauma may be extensive, and the time limit for evidence collection is usually 72 to 120 hours. Evidence collection requires patient permission at each step and involves multistep protocols that can take up to 6 hours to perform. Emotional support and prevention of STIs and pregnancy should be addressed.

Seek supervision and consultation as you learn the complex psychological, clinical, and legal dimensions of caring for these patients, and review guidelines and recommendations from the World Health Organization, ACOG, and the CDC.[75–77]

Choosing Equipment.   Assemble the equipment below, and review the supplies and procedures of your own facility before taking cultures and other samples. You will need:

- A movable source of good light

- A vaginal speculum of appropriate size

- Water-soluble lubricant

- Equipment for taking Pap smears, bacteriologic cultures and DNA probes, or other diagnostic testing materials, such as potassium hydroxide and normal saline

Specula are either metal or plastic and come in two basic shapes, named for Pedersen and Graves (Fig. 14-7). Both are available in small, medium, and large sizes. The medium Pedersen speculum is usually most comfortable for sexually active women. The narrow-bladed Pedersen speculum is best for the patient with a small introitus, such as a virgin or an elderly woman. The Graves specula are best for parous women with vaginal prolapse.

Before using a speculum, practice opening and closing its blades, locking the blades in an open position, and releasing them again. The instructions in this chapter apply to a metal speculum; you can easily adapt them to a plastic speculum by handling it before use.

When using a plastic speculum, warn the patient that it typically makes a loud click and may pinch when locked or released, causing discomfort.

Positioning the Patient.   *Drape the patient appropriately* and then assist her into the lithotomy position. Place one heel, then the other into the stirrups. She may be more comfortable in socks or shoes than bare feet. Then

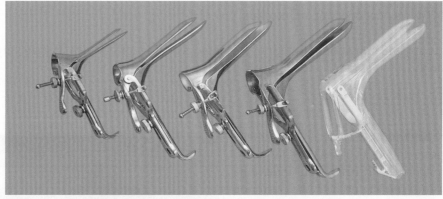

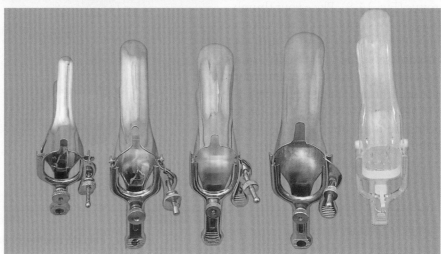

FIGURE 14-7.   Specula, from left to right: small metal Pedersen, medium metal Pedersen, medium metal Graves, large metal Graves, and large plastic Pedersen.

ask her to slide all the way down the examining table until her buttocks extend slightly beyond the edge. Her thighs should be flexed, abducted, and externally rotated at the hips. Make sure her head is supported with a pillow.

External Examination

Assess the Sexual Maturity of an Adolescent Patient. You can assess pubic hair during either the abdominal or the pelvic examination. Note its characteristics and distribution, and rate it according to the Tanner stages, described on p. 901.

Delayed puberty is often familial or related to chronic illness. It may also reflect disorders of the hypothalamus, anterior pituitary gland, or ovaries.

Examine the External Genitalia. Seat yourself comfortably and warn the patient that you will be touching her genital area. Inspect the mons pubis, labia, and perineum. Separate the labia and inspect:

Excoriations or itchy, small, red maculo-papules suggest *pediculosis pubis* (lice or "crabs"), often found at the bases of the pubic hairs.

- The labia minora

- The clitoris

An enlarged clitoris is seen in masculinizing endocrine disorders.

- The urethral meatus

- The vaginal opening, or introitus

Inspect for urethral caruncle, prolapse of the urethral mucosa (p. 597), and tenderness in interstitial cystitis.

Note any inflammation, ulceration, discharge, swelling, or nodules. Palpate any lesions.

For descriptions of *herpes simplex, Behçet disease, syphilitic chancre,* and *epidermoid cyst,* see Table 14-1, Lesions of the Vulva, p. 596.

Bartholin Glands. If the patient reports labial swelling, examine the *Bartholin glands.* Insert your index finger into the vagina near the posterior introitus (Fig. 14-8). Place your thumb outside the posterior part of the labium majus. Palpate each side in turn, at approximately the "4-o'clock" and "8-o'clock" positions, between your finger and thumb, checking for swelling or tenderness. Note any discharge exuding from the duct opening of the gland. If any is present, culture it.

A *Bartholin gland* may become acutely or chronically infected, resulting in swelling. See Table 14-2, Bulges and Swelling of the Vulva, Vagina, and Urethra, p. 597.

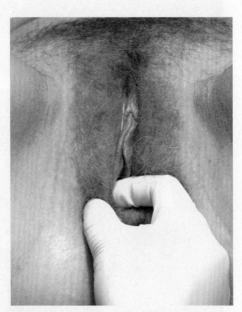

FIGURE 14-8. Palpate the Bartholin gland.

Internal Examination

Insert the Speculum.   Select a speculum of appropriate size and shape, and moisten it with warm water. (Lubricants or gels may interfere with cytologic studies and bacterial or viral cultures.) *Let the patient know you are about to insert the speculum and apply downward pressure.* Some clinicians carefully enlarge the vaginal introitus by lubricating one finger with water and applying downward pressure at its lower margin, then palpate the location of the cervix in order to angle the speculum more accurately. Enlarging the introitus can ease insertion of the speculum and the patient's comfort. With your other hand (usually the left), introduce the closed speculum past your fingers at a downward slope (Fig. 14-9). Avoid pulling on the pubic hair or pinching the labia as you open and close the speculum. Separating the labia majora with your right hand helps to avoid this.

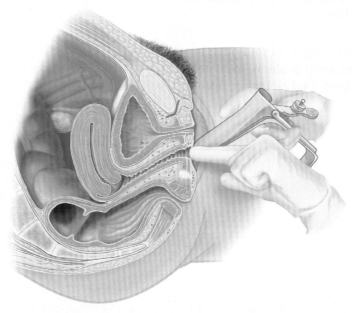

FIGURE 14-9.   **Gently insert the speculum.**

The Small Introitus

Many virginal vaginal orifices admit only a single examining finger. Modify your technique so that you insert only your index finger. Using a small Pedersen speculum may allow limited inspection. When the vaginal orifice is even smaller, an adequate bimanual examination can be performed by placing one finger in the rectum rather than in the vagina, but warn the patient first.

Similar techniques may be indicated for an older woman if the introitus has become atrophied and tight.

An *imperforate hymen* occasionally delays menarche. Check for this possibility when menarche seems unduly late in relation to the development of a girl's breasts and pubic hair.

Two methods help you to avoid placing pressure on the sensitive urethra: (1) when inserting the speculum, hold it at an angle (Fig. 14-10), and then

(2) slide the speculum inward along the posterior wall of the vagina (Fig. 14-11), applying downward pressure to keep the vaginal introitus relaxed.

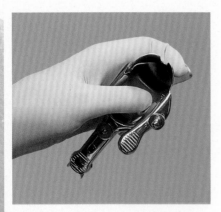

FIGURE 14-10. Entry angle.

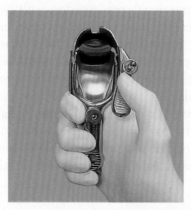

FIGURE 14-11. Angle at full insertion.

After placing the speculum in the vagina, remove your fingers of your other hand from the introitus. Rotate the speculum into a horizontal position, maintaining pressure posteriorly, and insert it to its full length (Fig. 14-12). Do not open the blades of the speculum prematurely.

See Table 14-4, Variations in the Cervical Surface, p. 599; Table 14-5, Shapes of the Cervical Os, p. 600; and Table 14-6, Abnormalities of the Cervix, p. 600.

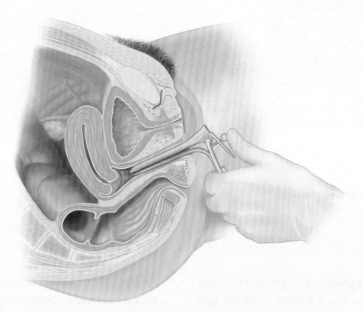

FIGURE 14-12. Insert the speculum to full length.

Inspect the Cervix. Open the speculum carefully. Rotate and adjust the speculum until it cups the cervix and brings it into full view (Fig. 14-13). Fix the speculum in its open position by tightening the thumbscrew. Position the light until you can see the cervix well. When the uterus is retroverted, the cervix points more anteriorly than illustrated. If you have difficulty finding the cervix, withdraw the speculum slightly and reposition it on a different slope. If a discharge obscures your view, wipe it away gently with a large cotton swab.

See retroversion of the uterus, p. 601.

Note the color of the cervix; its position and surface characteristics; and any ulcerations, nodules, masses, bleeding, or discharge. Inspect the cervical os for discharge.

Look for lateral displacement of the cervix in *endometriosis* involving the uterosacral ligaments.

A yellowish discharge on the endocervical swab commonly represents mucopurulent cervicitis from *C. trachomatis, N. gonorrhoeae,* or *herpes simplex* (p. 572). Raised, friable, or lobed wart-like lesions are seen with *condylomata* or *cervical cancer.*

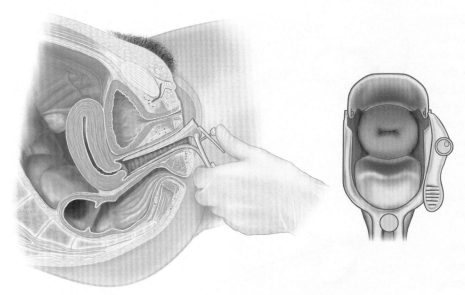

FIGURE 14-13. **Gently open and fix the speculum.**

Obtain Specimens for Cervical Cytology (Pap Smears). Obtain one specimen from the endocervix and another from the ectocervix, or a combination specimen using the cervical brush ("broom"). For best results the patient should not be menstruating. She should avoid intercourse and use of douches, tampons, contraceptive foams or creams, or vaginal suppositories for 48 hours before the examination. For sexually active women ages 26 years or younger, and for other asymptomatic women at increased risk of infection, plan to culture the cervix routinely for *chlamydia.*[78]

Obtaining the Pap Smear: Options for Specimen Collection

Cervical Broom

Many clinicians use a plastic brush tipped with a broom-like fringe to collect a single specimen containing both squamous and columnar epithelial cells. Rotate the tip of the brush in the cervical os, in a full clockwise direction, then place the sample directly into preservative so that the laboratory can prepare the slide (liquid-based cytology).

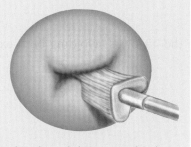

Use of the cervical broom and liquid-based cytology is increasingly common and can also be used to test for *chlamydia* and *gonorrhea.*

   Alternatively, stroke each side of the brush on the glass slide. Promptly place the slide in solution or spray with a fixative as described on the next page.

(*continued*)

Obtaining the Pap Smear: Options for Specimen Collection (*continued*)

Cervical Scrape

Place the longer end of the scraper in the cervical os. Press, turn, and scrape in a full circle, making sure to include the *transformation zone* and the *squamocolumnar junction*. Smear the specimen on a glass slide. Set the slide in a safe spot that is easy to reach. Note that doing the cervical scrape first reduces the presence of red blood cells, which sometimes appear after rotating the endocervical brush.

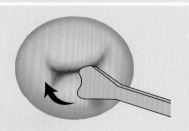

Endocervical Brush

Place the endocervical brush in the cervical os. Roll it between your thumb and index finger, clockwise and counterclockwise. Remove the brush and smear the glass slide using a gentle painting motion to avoid destroying any cells. Place the slide into an ether–alcohol solution at once, or spray it promptly with a special fixative.

Note that for pregnant women, a cotton-tipped applicator, moistened with saline, is advised in place of the endocervical brush.

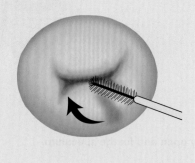

Inspect the Vagina. Withdraw the speculum slowly while observing the vaginal walls. As the speculum clears the cervix, release the thumbscrew and maintain the open position of the speculum with your thumb. During withdrawal, inspect the vaginal mucosa, noting its color and any inflammation, discharge, ulcers, or masses.

Check for bulging in the vaginal wall. Remove either the upper or lower blade of the speculum (or use a single-blade speculum) and ask the woman to bear down so that you can assess the location of vaginal wall relaxation or the degree of uterine prolapse.

Close the speculum as it emerges from the introitus, avoiding both excessive stretching or pinching of the mucosa.

See Table 14-3, Vaginal Discharge, p. 598.

Vaginal discharge often accompanies infection from *Candida, Trichomonas vaginalis,* and bacterial vaginosis. Diagnosis depends on laboratory tests because the sensitivity and specificity of discharge characteristics are low.[79,80] *Vaginal cancer* is rare; diethylstilbestrol (DES) exposure in utero and HPV infection are risk factors.

Use of the lower blade as a retractor during bearing down helps expose anterior vaginal wall defects such as *cystoceles;* likewise, use of the upper blade helps expose *rectoceles.* The standardized Pelvic Organ Quantification (POP-Q) system and diagram is widely used.[81] See Table 14-2, Bulges and Swelling of the Vulva, Vagina, and Urethra, p. 597.

Perform a Bimanual Examination. Lubricate the index and middle fingers of one of your gloved hands, and *from a standing position, insert your lubricated fingers into the vagina,* again exerting pressure primarily posteriorly. Your thumb should be abducted, your ring and little fingers flexed into your palm. Pressing inward on the perineum with your flexed fingers causes little, if any, discomfort and allows you to position your palpating fingers correctly. Note any nodularity or tenderness in the vaginal wall, including the region of the urethra and the bladder anteriorly.

- *Palpate the cervix,* noting its position, shape, consistency, regularity, mobility, and tenderness. Normally, the cervix can be moved somewhat without pain. Feel the fornices around the cervix.

- *Palpate the uterus.* Place your other hand on the abdomen about midway between the umbilicus and the symphysis pubis. While you elevate the cervix and uterus with your pelvic hand, press your abdominal hand in and down, trying to grasp the uterus between your two hands (Fig. 14-14). Note its size, shape, consistency, and mobility, and identify any tenderness or masses.

Stool in the rectum may simulate a rectovaginal mass, but unlike a malignant mass, it can usually be dented by digital pressure. Rectovaginal examination confirms the distinction.

Cervical motion tenderness and/or adnexal tenderness are hallmarks of *PID,* ectopic pregnancy, and appendicitis.

See Table 14-7, Positions of the Uterus, p. 601, and Table 14-8, Abnormalities of the Uterus, p. 602.

Uterine enlargement suggests pregnancy, uterine myomas (fibroids), or malignancy.

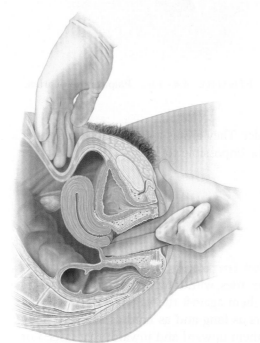

FIGURE 14-14. **Palpate the uterus.**

Now slide the fingers of your pelvic hand into the anterior fornix and palpate the body of the uterus between your hands. In this position, your pelvic fingers can feel the anterior surface of the uterus, and your abdominal hand can feel part of the posterior surface.

Nodules on the uterine surfaces suggest *myomas,* or fibroids (see p. 602).

If you cannot feel the uterus with either of these maneuvers, it may be tipped posteriorly (retrodisplaced). Slide your pelvic fingers into the posterior fornix and feel for the uterus butting against your fingertips. An obese or poorly relaxed abdominal wall may also prevent you from feeling the uterus even when it is located anteriorly.

See *retroversion* and *retroflexion of the uterus* (p. 601).

■ *Palpate each ovary.* Place your abdominal hand on the right lower quadrant, and your pelvic hand in the right lateral fornix (Fig. 14-15). Press your abdominal hand in and down, trying to push the adnexal structures toward your pelvic hand. Try to identify the right ovary or any adjacent adnexal masses. By moving your hands slightly, slide the adnexal structures between your fingers, if possible, and note their size, shape, consistency, mobility, and tenderness. Repeat the procedure on the left side.

Within 3 to 5 years after menopause, the ovaries become atrophic and usually nonpalpable. In postmenopausal women, investigate a palpable ovary for possible *ovarian cyst* or *ovarian cancer.* Pelvic pain, bloating, increased abdominal size, and urinary tract symptoms are more common in women with ovarian cancer.[47]

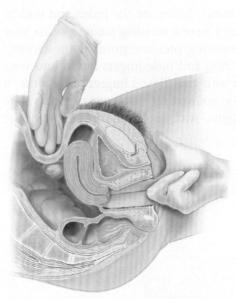

FIGURE 14-15. **Palpate the ovaries.**

Normal ovaries are somewhat tender. They are usually palpable in slender relaxed women, but are difficult or impossible to feel in women who are obese or tense.

Adnexal masses can also arise from a *tubo-ovarian abscess, salpingitis* or inflammation of the fallopian tubes from PID, or *ectopic pregnancy.* Distinguish such a mass from a uterine myoma. See Table 14-9, Adnexal Masses, p. 603.

Assess the Pelvic Floor Muscles for Strength and Tenderness.
After palpating the cervix, uterus, and ovaries, withdraw your examining fingers just clear of the cervix. Then spread them against the vaginal walls. Ask the patient to squeeze around your fingers as long and as hard as she can. Snug compression of your fingers, moving them upward and inward, that lasts 3 or more seconds is full strength. Check for strength, tenderness during contraction, appropriate relaxation after contraction, and endurance in all four vaginal quadrants. Then, with your fingers still placed against the vaginal walls inferiorly, ask the patient to cough several times or to bear down (*Valsalva maneuver*). Look for any urinary leakage during increased abdominal pressure. Watch for abdominal muscle overrecruitment or tightening of the adductor or gluteal muscles.

Muscle weakness arises from aging, vaginal deliveries, and neurologic conditions, and contributes to the urine leakage of *stress incontinence* during increased abdominal pressure. Overrecruitment with tightening, vaginal wall tenderness, and referred pain signal pelvic pain from *pelvic floor spasm, interstitial cystitis, vulvodynia,* and *urethral spasm.*

In patients with pelvic pain or vaginal wall tenderness, palpate the external pelvic floor muscles in a clockwise rotation to identify trigger points (Fig. 14-16).

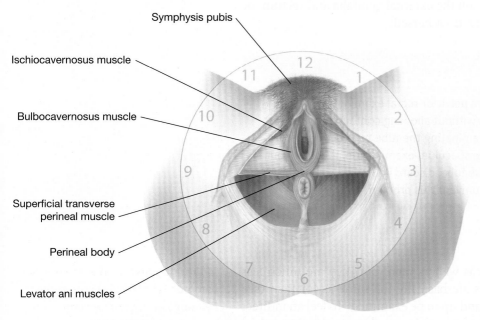

Symphysis pubis

Ischiocavernosus muscle

Bulbocavernosus muscle

Superficial transverse
perineal muscle

Perineal body

Levator ani muscles

FIGURE 14-16. **Palpate the pelvic floor muscles.**

Trigger point tenderness in these muscles accompanies *pelvic floor spasm* and *pelvic floor dysfunction* from trauma, interstitial cystitis, or fibromyalgia. Pelvic floor disorders, present in ~25% of all women and ≥30% of older women, include urinary and fecal incontinence, pelvic organ prolapse, and other sensory and emptying abnormalities of the lower urinary and GI tracts.[2]

Recall that the ischiocavernosus and bulbocavernosus muscles are innervated by the pudendal nerve, so pain may be referred to the perineum and urogenital structures. Trigger-point pain over the levator ani, innervated by the sacral nerve roots S3 to S5, may be referred to the vagina. See also p. 569.

Perform a Rectovaginal Examination if Indicated. The rectovaginal examination (Fig. 14-17) has three primary purposes: to palpate a retroverted uterus, the uterosacral ligaments, cul-de-sac, and adnexa; to screen for colorectal cancer in women ages 50 years or older; and to assess pelvic pathology.

Nodularity and thickening of the uterosacral ligaments occur in endometriosis, also pain with uterine movement.

After withdrawing your fingers from the bimanual examination, change your gloves and lubricate your fingers as needed (see note below on lubricants). Slowly reintroduce your index finger into the vagina and your middle finger into the rectum. Ask the patient to strain down as you do this to relax her anal sphincter. Mention that this may stimulate an urge to move her bowels, but this will not occur. Apply pressure against the anterior and lateral walls with the examining fingers, and downward pressure with the hand on the abdomen.

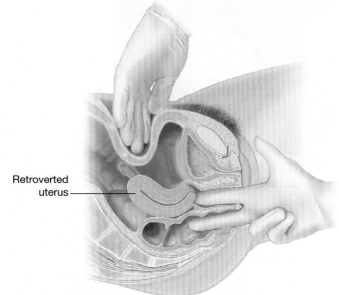

Retroverted
uterus

FIGURE 14-17. **Examine the rectovaginal area.**

Check the rectal vault for masses. If fecal blood testing is planned, change gloves to avoid contaminating fecal material with any blood provoked by collecting the Pap smear. After the examination, wipe off the external genitalia and rectum, or offer tissues to the patient so that she can do it herself.

See Chapter 15, The Anus, Rectum, and Prostate, pp. 621–623.

Using Lubricants

If you handle a tube of lubricant during a pelvic or rectal examination, let the lubricant drop onto your gloved fingers without allowing contact between the tube and the gloves. This prevents contaminating the tube by touching it with your gloved fingers after completing the speculum examination. If you or your assistant inadvertently contaminates the tube, discard it. Small disposable tubes for use with only one patient circumvent this problem.

Hernias

Hernias of the groin occur in women as well as men, but they are much less common. The examination techniques are basically the same as for men (see pp. 553–555). A woman should also stand up to be examined. To feel an indirect inguinal hernia, however, palpate in the labia majora and upward to just lateral to the pubic tubercles.

Indirect inguinal hernias are the most common type of hernias in women. Femoral hernias rank second.

Special Techniques

Assessing Urethritis. To evaluate possible urethritis or inflammation of the paraurethral glands, insert your index finger into the vagina and milk the urethra gently outward from the inside (Fig. 14-18). Note any discharge from or about the urethral meatus. If present, culture it.

Causes of urethritis include infection from *C. trachomatis* and *N. gonorrhoeae*.

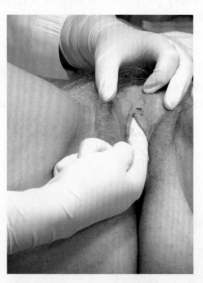

FIGURE 14-18. **Milk the urethra.**

Recording Your Findings

Note that initially you may use sentences to describe your findings; later you will use phrases.

Recording the Physical Examination—Female Genitalia

"No inguinal adenopathy. External genitalia without erythema, lesions, or masses. Vaginal mucosa pink. Cervix parous, pink, and without discharge. Uterus anterior, midline, smooth, and not enlarged. No adnexal tenderness. Pap smear obtained. Rectovaginal wall intact. Rectal vault without masses. Stool brown and negative for fecal blood."

OR

"Bilateral shotty inguinal adenopathy. External genitalia without erythema or lesions. Vaginal mucosa and cervix coated with thin white homogeneous discharge with mild fishy odor. After swabbing cervix, no discharge visible in the cervical os. Uterus midline; no adnexal masses. Rectal vault without masses. Stool brown and negative for fecal blood. pH of vaginal discharge >4.5"

These findings are consistent with *bacterial vaginosis.*

Table 14-1 Lesions of the Vulva

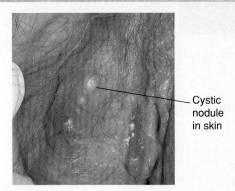

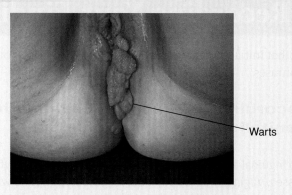

Epidermoid Cyst

A small firm round cystic nodule in the labia suggests an epidermoid cyst. These are yellowish in color. Look for the dark punctum marking the blocked opening of the gland.

Venereal Wart (*Condyloma Acuminatum*)

Warty lesions on the labia and within the vestibule are often condyloma acuminata from infection with *human papillomavirus.*

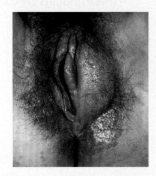

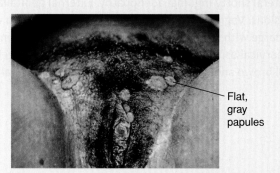

Syphilitic Chancre

This firm painless ulcer from primary syphilis forms ~21 d after exposure to *Treponema pallidum.* It may remain hidden and undetected in the vagina and heals regardless of treatment in 3–6 wks.

Secondary Syphilis (*Condyloma Latum*)

Large raised, round or oval, flat-topped gray or white lesions point to condylomata lata. These are contagious and, along with rash and mucous membrane sores in the mouth, vagina, or anus, are manifestations of secondary syphilis.

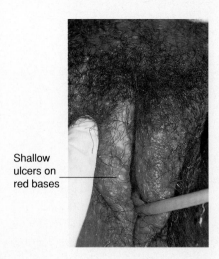

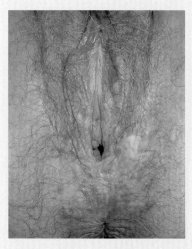

Genital Herpes

Shallow small painful ulcers on red bases are suspicious for infection from genital herpes simplex virus 1 or 2. Ulcers may take 2–4 wks to heal. Recurrent outbreaks of localized vesicles, then ulcers are common.

Carcinoma of the Vulva

An ulcerated or raised red vulvar lesion in an elderly woman may be a vulvar carcinoma, usually a squamous cell carcinoma arising on the labia.

Table 14-2 Bulges and Swelling of the Vulva, Vagina, and Urethra

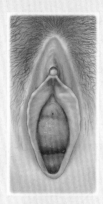

Cystocele

A cystocele is a bulge of the upper two thirds of the anterior vaginal wall, together with the bladder above it. It results from weakened anterior supporting tissues.

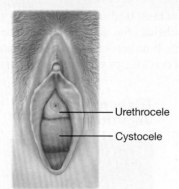

Cystourethrocele

When the entire anterior vaginal wall, together with the bladder and urethra, produces the bulge, a cystourethrocele is present. A groove sometimes defines the border between the urethrocele and cystocele, but is not always present.

— Urethrocele

— Cystocele

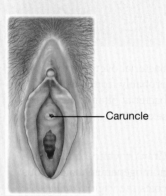

— Caruncle

Urethral Caruncle

A urethral caruncle is a small red benign tumor visible at the posterior urethral meatus. It occurs chiefly in postmenopausal women and usually causes no symptoms. Occasionally, a carcinoma of the urethra is mistaken for a caruncle. To check, palpate the urethra through the vagina for thickening, nodularity, or tenderness, and palpate for inguinal lymphadenopathy.

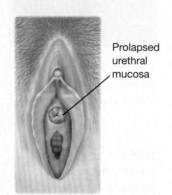

Prolapsed urethral mucosa

Prolapse of the Urethral Mucosa

Prolapsed urethral mucosa forms a swollen red ring around the urethral meatus. It usually occurs before menarche or after menopause. Identify the urethral meatus at the center of the swelling to make this diagnosis.

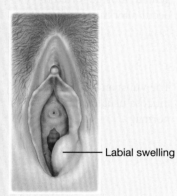

— Labial swelling

Bartholin Gland Infection

Causes of a Bartholin gland infection include trauma, gonococci, anaerobes like bacteroides and peptostreptococci, and *C. trachomatis*. Acutely, the gland appears as a tense, hot, very tender abscess. Look for pus emerging from the duct or erythema around the duct opening. Chronically, a nontender cyst is felt that may be large or small.

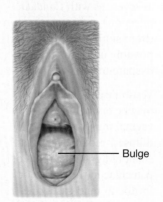

— Bulge

Rectocele

A rectocele is a herniation of the rectum into the posterior wall of the vagina, resulting from a weakness or defect in the endopelvic fascia.

Table 14-3 Vaginal Discharge

Discharge from a vaginal infection must be distinguished from a physiologic discharge. A physiologic discharge is clear or white, may contain white clumps of epithelial cells, and is not malodorous. To distinguish vaginal from cervical discharges, use a large cotton swab to wipe off the cervix. If no cervical discharge is present in the os, suspect a vaginal origin and consider the causes below. Note that the diagnosis of cervicitis or vaginitis hinges on careful collection and analysis of the appropriate laboratory specimens.[79,80]

	Trichomonal Vaginitis	Candidal Vaginitis	Bacterial Vaginosis
Cause	*Trichomonas vaginalis*, a protozoan; often but not always acquired sexually	*Candida albicans*, a yeast (normal overgrowth of vaginal flora); many factors predispose, including antibiotic therapy	Bacterial overgrowth probably from anaerobic bacteria; often transmitted sexually
Discharge	Yellowish green or gray, possibly frothy; often profuse and pooled in the vaginal fornix; may be malodorous	White and curdy; may be thin but typically thick; not as profuse as in trichomonal infection; not malodorous	Gray or white, thin, homogeneous, malodorous; coats the vaginal walls; usually not profuse, may be minimal
Other Symptoms	Pruritus (though not usually as severe as with *Candida* infection); pain on urination (from skin inflammation or possibly urethritis); dyspareunia	Pruritus; vaginal soreness; pain on urination (from skin inflammation); dyspareunia	Unpleasant fishy or musty genital odor; reported to occur after intercourse
Vulva and Vaginal Mucosa	Vestibule and labia minora may be erythematous; the vaginal mucosa may be diffusely reddened, with small red granular spots or petechiae in the posterior fornix; in mild cases, the mucosa looks normal	The vulva and even the surrounding skin are often inflamed and sometimes swollen to a variable extent; the vaginal mucosa is often reddened, with white tenacious patches of discharge; the mucosa may bleed when these patches are scraped off; in mild cases, the mucosa looks normal	The vulva and vaginal mucosa usually appear normal
Laboratory Evaluation	Scan saline wet mount for trichomonads	Scan potassium hydroxide (KOH) preparation for the branching hyphae of *Candida*	Scan saline wet mount for *clue cells* (epithelial cells with stippled borders); sniff for fishy odor after applying KOH ("whiff test"); test the vaginal secretions for pH > 4.5

Table 14-4 Variations in the Cervical Surface

Two kinds of epithelia cover the cervix: (1) shiny pink *squamous epithelium*, which resembles the vaginal epithelium, and (2) deep red, plushy *columnar epithelium,* which is continuous with the endocervical lining. These meet at the *squamocolumnar junction.* When this junction is at or inside the cervical os, only squamous epithelium is seen. A ring of columnar epithelium is often visible to a varying extent around the os—the result of a normal process that accompanies fetal development, menarche, and the first pregnancy.[a]

Squamous epithelium

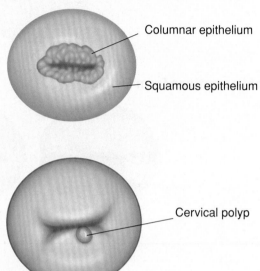

Columnar epithelium

Squamous epithelium

Retention cyst

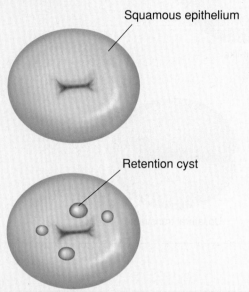

Cervical polyp

As estrogen stimulation increases during adolescence, all or part of this columnar epithelium is transformed into squamous epithelium by a process termed *metaplasia.* This change may block the secretions of columnar epithelium and cause *retention cysts,* also called *nabothian cysts.* These appear as translucent nodules on the cervical surface and have no pathologic significance.

A cervical polyp usually arises from the endocervical canal, becoming visible when it protrudes through the cervical os. It is bright red, soft, and rather fragile. When only the tip is seen, it cannot be differentiated clinically from a polyp originating in the endometrium. Polyps are benign but may bleed.

---

[a]Terminology is in flux. Other terms for the columnar epithelium visible on the ectocervix are *ectropion, ectopy,* and *eversion.*

Table 14-5 Shapes of the Cervical Os

Normal

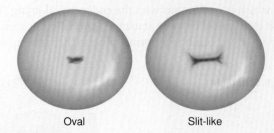

Oval   Slit-like

Types of Lacerations from Delivery

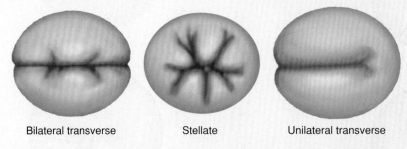

Bilateral transverse   Stellate   Unilateral transverse

Table 14-6 Abnormalities of the Cervix

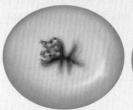

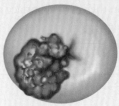

Mucopurulent Cervicitis

Mucopurulent cervicitis produces purulent yellow drainage from the cervical os, usually from *Chlamydia trachomatis, Neisseria gonorrhoeae,* or herpes infection. These infections are sexually transmitted and may occur without symptoms or signs.

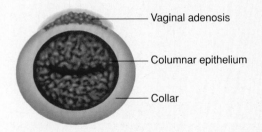

— Vaginal adenosis

— Columnar epithelium

— Collar

Carcinoma of the Cervix

Carcinoma of the cervix begins in an area of metaplasia. In its earliest stages, it cannot be distinguished from a normal cervix. In later stages, an extensive, irregular, cauliflower-like growth may develop. Early frequent intercourse, multiple partners, smoking, and infection with human papillomavirus increase the risk for cervical cancer.

Fetal Exposure to Diethylstilbestrol (DES)

Daughters of women who took DES during pregnancy are at greatly increased risk for several abnormalities, including (1) columnar epithelium that covers most or all of the cervix, (2) vaginal adenosis, i.e., extension of this epithelium to the vaginal wall, and (3) a circular collar or ridge of tissue, of varying shapes, between the cervix and vagina. Much less common is an otherwise rare carcinoma of the upper vagina.

Table 14-7 Positions of the Uterus

Retroversion and retroflexion are usually normal variants.

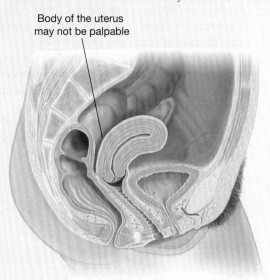

Body of the uterus may not be palpable

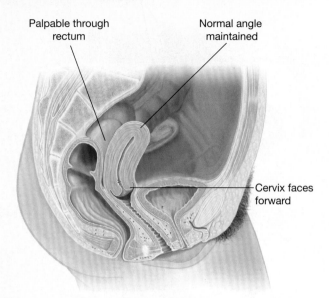

Palpable through rectum

Normal angle maintained

Cervix faces forward

Retroversion of the Uterus

Retroversion of the uterus refers to a tilting backward of the entire uterus, including both the body and the cervix. It is a common variant occurring in approximately 20% of women. Early clues on pelvic examination are a cervix that faces forward and a uterine body that cannot be felt by the abdominal hand. In *moderate retroversion*, the body may not be palpable with either hand. In *marked retroversion*, the body can be felt posteriorly, either through the posterior fornix or through the rectum. A retroverted uterus is usually both mobile and asymptomatic. Occasionally, such a uterus is fixed and immobile, held in place by conditions such as endometriosis or PID.

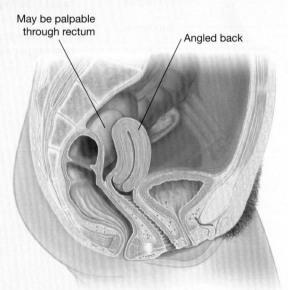

May be palpable through rectum

Angled back

Retroflexion of the Uterus

Retroflexion of the uterus refers to a backward angulation of the body of the uterus in relation to the cervix. The cervix maintains its usual position. The body of the uterus is often palpable through the posterior fornix or through the rectum.

Table 14-8 Abnormalities of the Uterus

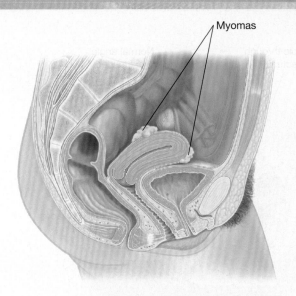

Myomas

Myomas of the Uterus (Fibroids)

Myomas are very common benign uterine tumors. They may be single or multiple and vary greatly in size, occasionally reaching large proportions. They feel like firm irregular nodules that are continuous with the uterine surface. Occasionally, a myoma projecting laterally is confused with an ovarian mass; a nodule projecting posteriorly can be mistaken for a retroflexed uterus. Submucosal myomas project toward the endometrial cavity and are not palpable, although they may be suspected because of an enlarged uterus.

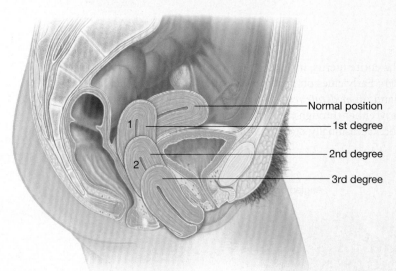

Normal position
1st degree
2nd degree
3rd degree

Prolapse of the Uterus

Prolapse of the uterus results from weakness of the supporting structures of the pelvic floor and is often associated with a cystocele and rectocele. In progressive stages, the uterus becomes retroverted and descends down the vaginal canal to the outside:

- In *first-degree prolapse*, the cervix is still well within the vagina.
- In *second-degree prolapse,* it is at the introitus.
- In *third-degree prolapse* (procidentia), the cervix and vagina are outside the introitus.

Table 14-9 Adnexal Masses

Adnexal masses typically result from disorders of the fallopian tubes or ovaries. Three examples—often hard to differentiate—are described. Note that inflammatory disease of the bowel (such as diverticulitis), carcinoma of the colon, and a pedunculated myoma of the uterus may simulate an adnexal mass.

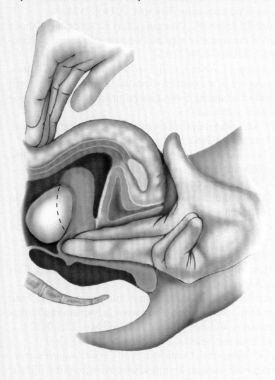

Ovarian Cysts and Ovarian Cancer

Ovarian cysts and tumors may cause adnexal masses on one or both sides. Later, they may extend out of the pelvis. Cysts tend to be smooth and compressible, tumors more solid and often nodular. Uncomplicated cysts are not usually tender.

Small (≤6 cm in diameter), mobile, cystic masses in a young woman are usually benign and often disappear after the next menstrual period. Diagnosis of *polycystic ovary syndrome* rests on exclusion of several endocrine disorders and two of the three features listed: ovulatory dysfunction, androgen excess (hirsutism, acne, alopecia, elevated serum testosterone), and confirmation of polycystic ovaries on ultrasound. Roughly half of affected women are obese, more than 40% have metabolic syndrome, and ~40% have impaired glucose tolerance or diabetes.[82,83]

Ovarian cancer is relatively rare and usually presents at an advanced stage. Symptoms include pelvic pain, bloating, increased abdominal size, and urinary tract symptoms; often there is a palpable ovarian mass.[47] Currently, there are no reliable screening tests. A strong family history of breast or ovarian cancer is an important risk factor but occurs in only 5% of cases.

Ectopic Pregnancy, Including Rupture

Ectopic pregnancy results from implantation of the fertilized ovum outside the endometrial cavity, primarily in the fallopian tube (90% of cases).[21,22] Ectopic pregnancy occurs in 1% to 2% of pregnancies worldwide and remains an important cause of maternal morbidity and mortality. Clinical presentation ranges from subacute, in ~80–90% of cases, to shock from rupture and intraperitoneal hemorrhage (10–30% of cases). Abdominal pain, adnexal tenderness, and abnormal uterine bleeding are the most common clinical features. In more than half of ectopic pregnancies, there is a palpable adnexal mass that is typically large, fixed, and ill-defined, at times with adherent omentum or small or large bowel. In milder cases, there may be a prior history of amenorrhea or other symptoms of a pregnancy.

Risk factors include tubal damage from PID, prior ectopic pregnancy, prior tubal surgery, age older than 35 yrs, presence of an IUD, subfertility (has altered tubal integrity), and assisted reproductive techniques.

Pelvic Inflammatory Disease

PID is due to "spontaneous ascension of microbes from the cervix or vagina to the endometrium, fallopian tubes, and adjacent structures."[84] 85% of cases involve STIs or bacterial vaginosis affecting the fallopian tubes (*salpingitis*) or the tubes and ovaries (*salpingo-oophoritis*), primarily *N. gonorrhoeae* and *C. trachomatis*. Hallmarks of acute disease are adnexal, cervical, and uterine compression tenderness. The diagnosis is imprecise, however—only 75% have confirmed pathogens on tubal laparoscopy. If not treated, a *tubo-ovarian abscess* may ensue; 18% of treated patients report infertility after 3 years. Infection of the fallopian tubes and ovaries may also follow childbirth or gynecologic surgery.

References

1. Johnson CT, Hallock JL, Bienstock JL, et al. (eds). Chapter 26, Anatomy of the female pelvis. *Johns Hopkins Manual of Gynecology and Obstetrics*. 5th ed. Philadelphia, PA: Wolters Kluwer/Lippincott Williams and Wilkins; 2015:338.

2. Tarney CM. Ch.42, Urinary incontinence and pelvic floor disorders. Tarnay C.M. Tarnay, Christopher M. In: DeCherney AH, Nathan L, Laufer N, et al., eds. *Current Diagnosis & Treatment: Obstetrics & Gynecology, 11e*. New York, NY: McGraw-Hill; 2013. Available at http://accessmedicine.mhmedical.com.libproxy.unm.edu/content.aspx?bookid=498&Sectionid=41008634. Accessed May 16, 2015.

3. Freeman EW, Sammel MD, Lin H, et al. Clinical subtypes of premenstrual syndrome and responses to sertraline treatment. *Obstet Gynecol*. 2011;118:1293.

4. Pachman DR, Jones JM, Loprinzi CL. Management of menopause-associated vasomotor symptoms: Current treatment options, challenges and future directions. *Int J Womens Health*. 2010;2:123.

5. North American Menopause Society. Estrogen and progestogen use in postmenopausal women: 2010 position statement of the North American menopause society. *Menopause*. 2010;17:242.

6. Coverdale JH, Balon R, Roberts LW. Teaching sexual history-taking: a systematic review of educational programs. *Acad Med*. 2011;86:1590.

7. Pancholy AB, Goldenhar L, Fellner AN, et al. Resident education and training in female sexuality: results of a national survey. *Sex Med*. 2011;8:361.

8. Centers for Disease Control and Prevention. Sexual orientation and health among U.S. adults. National Health Interview Survey, 2013. Available at http://www.cdc.gov/lgbthealth/. Accessed May 10, 2015.

9. Gates GJ, Newport F. *Gallup Special Report: The US LGBT adult population*. Washington, DC: Gallup, Inc; 2013. See also Gates GJ, Newport F. Special Report: 3.4% of U.S. Adults Identify as LGBT. October 18, 2012. Available at http://www.gallup.com/poll/158066/special-report-adults-identify-lgbt.aspx. Accessed May 11, 2015.

10. Gates GJ. Demographics and LGBT health. *J Health Soc Behav*. 2013;54:72.

11. Institute of Medicine. *The Health of Lesbian, Gay, Bisexual, and Transgender People: Building a Foundation for Better Understanding*. Washington, DC: National Institutes of Health; 2011. See also Report at https://www.iom.edu/Reports/2011/The-Health-of-Lesbian-Gay-Bisexual-and-Transgender-People.aspx March 31, 2011. Accessed May 11, 2015.

12. Daniel H, Butkus R, for the Health and Public Policy Committee of the American College of Physicians. Lesbian, gay, bisexual, and transgender health disparities: Executive summary of a policy position paper from the American College of Physicians. *Ann Intern Med*. 2015;163:135.

13. National LGBT Education Center. Available at http://www.lgbthealtheducation.org./ Accessed May 24, 2015.

14. Centers for Disease Control and Prevention. Lesbian, gay, bisexual, and transgender health. Updated July 15, 2014. Available at http://www.cdc.gov/lgbthealth./ Accessed May 24, 2015.

15. Williams Institute, UCLA. Available at http://williamsinstitute.law.ucla.edu./ Accessed May 24, 2015.

16. Barbara AM, Doctor F, Chaim G. Asking the right questions 2. Talking with clients about sexual orientation and gender identity in mental health, counselling and addiction settings. Toronto Canada: Centre for Addiction and Mental Health, 2007. Available at http://knowledgex.camh.net/amhspecialists/Screening_Assessment/assessment/ARQ2/Pages/default.aspx. Accessed May 16, 2015.

17. Clark RD, Williams AA. Patient preferences in discussing sexual dysfunctions in primary care. *Fam Med*. 2014;46:124.

18. Hatzichristou D, Rosen RC, Derogatis LR, et al. Recommendations for the clinical evaluation of men and women with sexual dysfunction. *J Sex Med*. 2010;7(1 Pt 2):337.

19. Platano G, Margraf J, Alder J, et al. Psychosocial factors and therapeutic approaches in the context of sexual history taking in men: a study conducted among Swiss general practitioners and urologists. *J Sex Med*. 2008;5:2533.

20. Kruszka PS, Kruszka SJ. Evaluation of acute pelvic pain in women. *Am Fam Physician*. 2010;82:141.

21. Orazulike NC, Konje JC. Diagnosis and management of ectopic pregnancy. *Women's Health (London)*. 2013;9:373.

22. Barnhart KT. Ectopic pregnancy. *N Engl J Med*. 2009;361:379.

23. Karnath BM, Breitkopf DM. Acute and chronic pelvic pain in women. *Hospital Physician*. 2007;43:41.

24. Origoni M, Maggiore RMU, Salvatore S, et al. Neurobiological mechanisms of pelvic pain. *Biomed Res Int*. 2014. Available at http://www.hindawi.com/journals/bmri/2014/903848/cta/

25. Shin JH, Howard FM. Management of chronic pelvic pain. *Curr Pain Headache Rep*. 2011;15:377.

26. International Pelvic Pain Society. History and physical. Pelvic pain assessment form. Available at http://www.pelvicpain.org/Professional/Documents-and-Forms.aspx. Accessed May 23, 2015.

27. Giudice LC. Endometriosis. *N Engl J Med*. 2010;362:2389.

28. Sawaya GF, Kulasingam S, Denberg T, et al. Cervical cancer screening in average-risk women: Best practice advice from the Clinical Guidelines Committee of the American College of Physicians. *Ann Intern Med*. 2015;162:851.

29. Centers for Disease Control and Surveillance. 2013 sexually transmitted disease surveillance. Human papillomavirus. Available at http://www.cdc.gov/std/stats13/other.htm#hpv. Accessed May 17, 2015.

30. Moyer A, on behalf of the U.S. Preventive Services Task Force. Screening for cervical cancer: U.S. Preventive Services Task Force recommendation statement. *Ann Intern Med*. 2012;150:880.

31. American Congress of Obstetrician and Gynecologists. ACOG Committee on Practice Bulletins–Gynecology. ACOG Practice Bulletin No. 131: Screening for cervical cancer. Cervical cytology screening. *Obstet Gynecol*. 2012;120:1222.

32. Saslow D, Solomon D, Lawson HW, et al. American Cancer Society, American Society for Colposcopy and Cervical Pathology, and American Society for Clinical Pathology screening guidelines for the prevention and early detection of cervical cancer. *CA Cancer J Clin*. 2012;62:147.

33. Bloomfield HE, Olson A, Greer N, et al. Screening pelvic examinations in asymptomatic, average-risk adult women: An evidence report for a clinical practice guideline from the American College of Physicians. *Ann Intern Med*. 2014;161:46.

34. Qaseem A, Humphrey LL, Harris R, et al. Screening pelvic examination in adult women: a clinical practice guideline from the American College of Physicians. *Ann Intern Med*. 2014;161:67.

35. Smith RA, Manassaram-Baptiste D, Brooks D, et al. Cancer screening in the United States, 2015: a review of current American cancer society guidelines and current issues in cancer screening. *CA Cancer J Clin*. 2015;65:30.

REFERENCES

36. Solomon D, Davey D, Kurman R, et al. The 2001 Bethesda system: terminology for reporting results of cervical cytology. *JAMA*. 2004;291:2990.

37. Wright TC, Cox JT, Massad JS. 2001 consensus guidelines for the management of women with cervical cytologic abnormalities. *JAMA*. 2002;287:2120.

38. Centers for Disease Control and Prevention. Human papillomavirus: HPV information for clinicians, April 2007, p. 18. Cached–pdf available under public.health.oregon.gov https://www.google.com /#q=cdc+human+papillomavirus+hpv+information+for+clinicians+april+2007. Accessed May 19, 2015.

39. Baseman JG, Kulasingam SL, Harris TG, et al. Evaluation of primary cervical cancer screening with an oncogenic human papillomavirus DNA test and cervical cytologic findings among women who attended family planning clinics in the United States. *Am J Obstet Gynecol*. 2008;199:26.e1–8.

40. Kulasingam SL, Hughes JP, Kiviat NB, et al. Evaluation of human papillomavirus testing in primary screening for cervical abnormalities: comparison of sensitivity, specificity, and frequency of referral. *JAMA*. 2002;288:1749.

41. Advisory Committee on Immunization Practices, Centers for Disease Control and Prevention. Human papillomavirus vaccination. Recommendations of the Advisory Committee on Immunization Practices. *MMWR*. 2014;63(RR #5):1–30.

42. Centers for Disease Control and Prevention. Human papillomavirus. HPV Vaccine Information for Clinicians–Fact Sheet. July 8, 2012. Available at http://www.cdc.gov/std/hpv/STDFact-HPV-vaccine-hcp.htm. Accessed May 18, 2015.

43. Centers for Disease Control and Prevention. Youth risk behavior surveillance–United States 2013. Available at http://www.cdc.gov/healthyyouth/data/yrbs/results.htm. Accessed May 19, 2015.

44. Centers for Disease Control and Prevention. Condom effectiveness. Fact sheet for public health personnel. Updated March 25, 2013. Available at http://www.cdc.gov/condomeffectiveness/latex.html. Accessed May 19, 2015.

45. Pierce Campbell CM, Lin HY, Fulp W, et al. Consistent condom use reduces the genital human papillomavirus burden among high-risk men: the HPV infection in men study. *J Infect Dis*. 2012;208:373.

46. U.S. Preventive Services Task Force. Addendum to Screening for ovarian cancer: Evidence update for the U.S. Preventive Services Task Force reaffirmation recommendation statement. Other supporting document for ovarian cancer: screening, September 2012. Available at http://www.uspreventiveservicestaskforce.org/Page/Document/addendum-to-screening-for-ovarian-cancer-evidence-update-for-the-us-preventive-services-task-force-reaffirmation-recommendation-statement/ovarian-cancer-screening#conclusions. Accessed May 19, 2015.

47. Jayson GC, Kohn EC, Kitchener HC, et al. Ovarian cancer. *Lancet*. 2014;384(9951):1376.

48. Rauh-Hain JA, Krivak TC, del Carmen MG, et al. Ovarian cancer screening and early detection in the general population. *Rev Obstet Gyneco*. 2011;4:15.

49. National Cancer Institute. Genetics of breast and gynecologic cancers–for health professionals (PDQ®). Updated April 3, 2015. Available at http://www.cancer.gov/types/breast/hp/breast-ovarian-genetics-pdq. Accessed May 19, 2015.

50. National Cancer Institute. Ovarian, Fallopian Tube, and Primary Peritoneal Cancer Prevention–for health professionals (PDQ®). Who is at risk? Updated May 15, 2015. Available at http://www.cancer.gov/types/ovarian/hp/ovarian-prevention-pdq. Accessed May 19, 2015.

51. Sherman ME, Piedmonte M, Mai PL, et al. Pathologic findings at risk-reducing salpingo-oophorectomy: primary results from Gynecologic Oncology Group Trial GOG-0199. *J Clin Oncol*. 2014;32: 3275.

52. Dorigo O, Berek JS. Personalizing CA125 levels for ovarian cancer screening. *Cancer Prev Res (Phila)*. 2011;4:1356.

53. Centers for Disease Control and Prevention. 2013 Sexually transmitted disease surveillance. Chlamydia. Updated December 16, 2014. Available at http://www.cdc.gov/std/stats13/chlamydia.htm. Accessed May 19, 2015.

54. Centers for Disease Control and Prevention. Pelvic inflammatory disease–CDC fact sheet. Updated May 4, 2015. Available at http://www.cdc.gov/std/pid/stdfact-pid-detailed.htm. Accessed May 20, 2015.

55. Centers for Disease Control and Prevention. Sexually transmitted diseases. STDs and infertility. Updated December 16, 2014. Available at http://www.cdc.gov/std/infertility/default.htm. Accessed May 19, 2015.

56. Centers for Disease Control and Prevention. Sexually transmitted diseases. Updated May 15, 2015. Available at http://www.cdc.gov/std/default.htm. Accessed May 19, 2015.

57. U.S. Preventive Services Task Force. Recommendations (search "Category – Infectious diseases"). Page current May 2015. Available at http://www.uspreventiveservicestaskforce.org/Search. Accessed May 25, 2015.

58. Centers for Disease Control and Prevention. HIV in the United States: At a glance. Updated May 11, 2015. Available at http://www.cdc.gov/hiv/statistics/basics/ataglance.html. Accessed May 25, 2015.

59. Centers for Disease Control and Prevention. HIV/AIDS. HIV among women. Updated March 6, 2015. Available at http://www.cdc.gov/hiv/risk/gender/women/facts/index.html. Accessed May 20, 2015.

60. U.S. Preventive Services Task Force. September 2014. Sexually transmitted infections. Behavioral counseling. Current as of March 2015. Available at http://www.uspreventiveservicestaskforce.org/Page/Topic/recommendation-summary/sexually-transmitted-infections-behavioral-counseling1?ds=1&s=Counseling. Accessed May 20, 2015.

61. O'Connor EA, Lin JS, Burda BU, et al. Behavioral sexual risk-reduction counseling in primary care to prevent sexually transmitted infections: a systematic review for the U.S. Preventive Services Task Force. *Ann Intern Med*. 2014;161:874.

62. Centers for Disease Control and Prevention. 2010 STD treatment guidelines. Clinical prevention guidance. Updated January 28, 2011. Available at http://www.cdc.gov/std/treatment/2010/clinical.htm. Accessed May 20, 2015.

63. Centers for Disease Control and Prevention. Reproductive health. Teen pregnancy–About teen pregnancy. Updated May 19, 2015. Available at http://www.cdc.gov/teenpregnancy/about/index.htm. See also Unintended pregnancy prevention. Available at http://www.cdc.gov/reproductivehealth/UnintendedPregnancy/index.htm. Accessed May 20, 2015.

64. Centers for Disease Control and Prevention. Reproductive health. Contraception. Updated April 22, 2015. Available at http://www.cdc.gov/reproductivehealth/UnintendedPregnancy/Contraception.htm. Accessed May 21, 2015.

65. Rossouw JE, Anderson GL, Prentice RL, et al; Writing Group for the Women's Health Initiative Investigators. Risks and benefits of estrogen plus progestin in healthy postmenopausal women: principal results from the Women's Health Initiative randomized controlled trial. *JAMA*. 2002;288:321.

66. Anderson GL, Limacher M, Assaf AR, et al; Women's Health Initiative Steering Committee. Effects of conjugated equine estrogen in postmenopausal women with hysterectomy: the Women's Health Initiative randomized controlled trial. *JAMA*. 2004;291:1701.

67. U.S. Preventive Services Task Force. Menopausal hormone therapy: preventive medication. October 2012. Available at http://www.uspreventiveservicestaskforce.org/Page/Topic/recommendation-summary/menopausal-hormone-therapy-preventive-medication?ds=1&s=hormone replacement therapy. Accessed May 21, 2015.

68. Nelson HD, Walker M, Zakher B, et al. Menopausal hormone therapy for the primary prevention of chronic conditions: a systematic review to update the U.S. Preventive Services Task Force recommendations. *Ann Intern Med*. 2012;157:104.

69. Mosca L, Benjamin EJ, Berra K, et al. Effectiveness-based guidelines for the prevention of cardiovascular disease in women—2011 update: a guideline from the American Heart Association. *Circulation*. 2011;123:1243.

70. American College of Obstetricians and Gynecologists. Postmenopausal estrogen therapy: Route of administration and risk of venous thromboembolism. Bulletin 556; April 2013. Available at http://www.acog.org/Resources-And-Publications/Committee-Opinions/Committee-on-Gynecologic-Practice/Postmenopausal-Estrogen-Therapy. Hormone therapy and heart disease. Bulletin 565; June 2013. Compounded bioidentical menopausal hormone therapy. Bulletin 532; August 2012. Available at http://www.acog.org/Resources-And-Publications/Committee-Opinions/Committee-on-Gynecologic-Practice/Compounded-Bioidentical-Menopausal-Hormone-Therapy. Accessed May 21, 2015.

71. North American Menopause Society. The 2012 hormone therapy position statement of: The North American Menopause Society. *Menopause*. 2012;19:257.

72. Weitlauf JC, Frayne SM, Finney JW, et al. Sexual violence, post-traumatic stress disorder, and the pelvic examination: how do beliefs about the safety, necessity, and utility of the examination influence patient experiences? *J Women's Health*. 2010;19:1271.

73. Linden JA. Care of the adult patient after sexual assault. *N Engl J Med*. 2011;365:834.

74. Breiding MJ, Smith SG, Basile KC, et al. Prevalence and characteristics of sexual violence, stalking, and intimate partner violence victimization–national intimate partner and sexual violence survey, United States, 2011. *MMWR Surveill Summ*. 2014;63:1.

75. World Health Organization. Sexual and reproductive health. Sexual violence. Available at http://www.who.int/reproductivehealth/topics/violence/sexual_violence/en/. See also Violence and injury prevention. Guidelines for medico-legal care for victims of sexual violence. Available at http://www.who.int/violence_injury_prevention/pu. Accessed May 22, 2015.

76. American Congress of Obstetricians and Gynecologists. Sexual assault. Bulletin 592. April 2014. Available at http://www.acog.org/Resources-And-Publications/Committee-Opinions/Committee-on-Health-Care-for-Underserved-Women/Sexual-Assault. Accessed May 22, 2015.

77. Centers for Disease Control and Prevention. 2010 STD treatment guidelines. Available at http://www.cdc.gov/std/treatment/2010/default.htm. Accessed May 22, 2015.

78. Centers for Disease Control and Prevention. Sexually transmitted diseases. STD and HIV screening recommendations. Updated December 16, 2014. Available at http://www.cdc.gov/std/prevention/screeningreccs.htm. Accessed May 20, 2015.

79. Wilson JF. In the clinic: vaginitis and cervicitis. *Ann Intern Med*. 2009;151:ITC3–1.

80. Eckhert LO. Acute vulvovaginitis. *N Engl J Med*. 2006;355:1244.

81. Bump RC, Mattiasson A, Bo K, et al. The standardization of terminology of female pelvic organ prolapse and pelvic floor dysfunction. *Am J Obstet Gynecol*. 1996;175:10.

82. Legro RS, Arslanian SA, Ehrmann DA, et al. Diagnosis and treatment of polycystic ovary syndrome: an Endocrine Society clinical practice guideline. *J Clin Endocrinol Metab*. 20(1398):4565.

83. Ehrmann LA. Polycystic ovary syndrome. *N Engl J Med*. 2005; 96:593.

84. Brunham RC, Gottleib SL, Paavonen J. Pelvic inflammatory disease. *N Engl J Med*. 2015;372:2039.

The Anus, Rectum, and Prostate

Anatomy and Physiology

The sigmoid colon terminates at the *rectum*, which lies against the sacrum and coccyx, then merges with the short segment of the *anal canal* (Fig. 15-1). The rectum extends from the rectosigmoid junction, anterior to the S3 vertebra, to the anorectal junction at the tip of the coccyx. The external margin of the anal canal is poorly

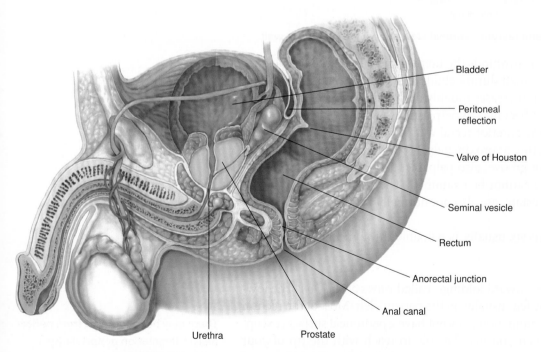

FIGURE 15-1. Anus and rectum—sagittal view.

demarcated, but its moist hairless appearance usually distinguishes it from the surrounding perianal skin. The muscle actions of the voluntary *external anal sphincter* and the involuntary *internal anal sphincter* normally hold the anal canal closed. The internal anal sphincter is an extension of the muscular coat of the rectal wall.

Note carefully the angle of the anal canal, on a line roughly between the anus and umbilicus. Unlike the rectum, the canal is liberally supplied by somatic sensory nerves, and a poorly directed finger or instrument will produce pain.

A serrated line marking the change from skin to mucous membrane demarcates the anal canal from the rectum (Fig. 15-2). This anorectal junction, often called the *pectinate* or *dentate line,* is also the boundary between somatic and visceral nerve supplies. It is easily visible on anoscopic or endoscopic examination, but is not palpable.

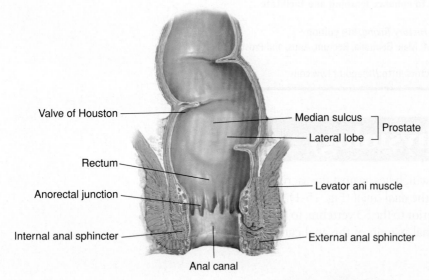

FIGURE 15-2. **Anus and rectum—coronal view showing the anterior wall.**

In the male, the *prostate gland* surrounds the urethra and lies next to the bladder outlet. The prostate gland is small during childhood, but between puberty and approximately age 20 years, it increases roughly fivefold in size. Prostate volume further expands as the gland becomes hyperplastic (see p. 623). The right and left lateral lobes lie against the anterior rectal wall, where they are palpable as a rounded, heart-shaped structure approximately 2.5 cm long. They are separated by a shallow *median sulcus* or groove, also palpable. Note that the anterior and central areas of the prostate cannot be examined. The *seminal vesicles,* shaped like rabbit ears above the prostate, are also not normally palpable.

In the female, the uterine *cervix* usually is palpable through the anterior wall of the rectum.

The rectal wall contains three inward foldings, called *valves of Houston.* The lowest of these can sometimes be felt, usually on the patient's left. Most of the rectum that is accessible to digital examination does not have a peritoneal surface, except for the anterior rectum, which you may be able to reach with the tip of your examining finger.

There may be tenderness from peritoneal inflammation or nodularity if there are peritoneal metastases.

The Health History

Common or Concerning Symptoms and Signs

- Change in bowel habits
- Blood in the stool
- Pain with defecation; rectal bleeding or tenderness
- Anal warts or fissures
- Weak urinary stream
- Burning with urination
- Blood in the urine

Other chapters have addressed many of the symptoms and signs related to the anorectal area and the prostate. To review briefly, ask about any change in the frequency of bowel function, the size or caliber of the stools, diarrhea or constipation, or any abnormal color of the stools. Return to the discussion on pp. 459–460 of these symptoms as well as queries about *blood in the stool*, ranging from black tarry stools (*melena*), to bloody stools (*hematochezia*), to *bright-red blood per rectum*. Also ask about the presence of mucus in the stool.

- Be sure to ask about any personal or family history of colonic polyps or colorectal cancer. Is there any personal history of IBD?

- Is there any pain on defecation? Any itching? Any extreme tenderness in the anus or rectum? Is there mucopurulent discharge or bleeding? Any ulcerations? Does the patient have anal intercourse?

- Is there any history of anal warts or anal fissures?

See Table 11-4, Constipation, p. 494 and Table 11-5, Black and Bloody Stool, p. 495.

Change in stool caliber, especially pencil-thin stools, may warn of *colon cancer*. Blood in the stool may be from polyps, carcinoma, gastrointestinal bleeding, or hemorrhoids; mucus may accompany *villous adenoma, intestinal infections, inflammatory bowel disease (IBD)*, or *irritable bowel syndrome (IBS)*.

Positive answers to these questions indicate increased risk for colorectal cancer and need for further testing. (See Screening Recommendations, Chapter 11, pp. 468–470.)

Anorectal pain, itching, tenesmus, or discharge or bleeding from infection or *rectal abscess* suggest *proctitis*. Causes include *gonorrhea, chlamydia, lymphogranuloma venereum*, receptive anal intercourse, ulcerations of *herpes simplex*, or chancres of *primary syphilis* (see Table 13-1, Sexually Transmitted Infections of Male Genitalia, p. 557). Itching in younger patients may be from pinworms.

Genital warts may arise from *human papillomavirus (HPV)* or *condylomata lata* in secondary syphilis. Anal fissures are seen in *proctitis* and *Crohn disease*.

■ In men, review the pattern of urination (see p. 462). Does the patient have difficulty starting or holding back the urine stream? Is the flow weak? What about frequent urination, especially at night? Is there any blood in the urine or semen or pain with ejaculation?

These genitourinary symptoms suggest *benign prostatic hyperplasia (BPH)* or *prostate cancer,* especially in men older than 70 years.[1]

The American Urological Association (AUA) Symptom Score helps quantify BPH severity and guide management decisions.[2] See Table 15-1, BPH Symptom Score: American Urological Association, p. 620.

■ Also, in men, has there been sudden onset of irritative urinary tract symptoms (frequency, urgency, pain with urination), perineal and low back pain, malaise, fever, or chills?

These symptoms suggest possible *acute prostatitis.*

Health Promotion and Counseling: Evidence and Recommendations

Important Topics for Health Promotion and Counseling

- Prostate cancer prevention and screening
- Colorectal cancer prevention and screening
- Counseling for sexually transmitted infections

Prostate Cancer Prevention and Screening.   Prostate cancer is the most frequently diagnosed nonskin cancer in the United States and the second leading cause of cancer death in men (Fig. 15-3).[3] The advent of prostate-specific antigen (PSA) testing in the late 1980s has been strongly associated with an increasing number of men diagnosed with prostate cancer: by 2000, nearly 60% of American men reported PSA testing[4]; and the lifetime risk of diagnosis with prostate cancer increased from 9% in 1985[5] to 15% in 2011.[6] However, the lifetime risk of dying from prostate cancer has remained around 3%.[6] Figure 15-4 shows age-adjusted cancer incidence and mortality rates based on data from the National Cancer Institute's Surveillance, Epidemiology, and End Results (SEER) program.[6]

Risk Factors.   Age, ethnicity, and family history are the strongest risk factors for prostate cancer. Several guidelines suggest targeting these high-risk men for early screening.[7,8]

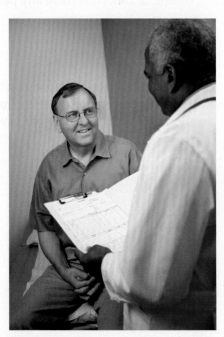

FIGURE 15-3. **Discuss prostate cancer screening.**

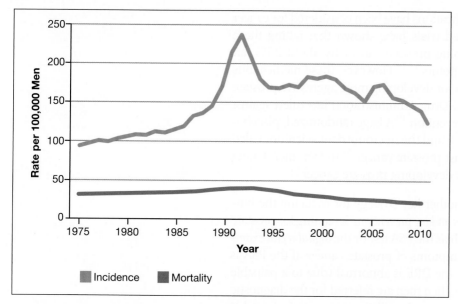

FIGURE 15-4. Prostate cancer age-adjusted incidence and mortality rates, United States, 1975 to 2012.

Risk Factors for Prostate Cancer

- *Age.* Prostate cancer is rare before age 40 years; however, incidence rates begin increasing rapidly after age 50 years.[6] The median age at diagnosis is 66 years.
- *Ethnicity.* African American men have the highest incidence and mortality rates from prostate cancer in the United States and among the highest in the world.[6,9] Compared to white men, a higher percentage of African American men are diagnosed with prostate cancer before age 50 years. They are also more likely to present with an advanced-stage cancer, even after adjusting for access to care.[10,11]
- *Family history.* Genetics appear to play an important role in prostate cancer risk. For men with one affected first-degree relative, namely, a father or brother, risk of developing prostate cancer increases twofold; for men with two or three affected first-degree relatives, risk increases 5- to 11-fold.[12] The BRCA1 and BRCA2 mutations also appear to confer increased risk of prostate cancer.[13]
- *Other risk factors.* Although the evidence is less convincing, other potential risk factors include Agent Orange exposure among Vietnam veterans, diets high in animal fat, obesity, and cigarette smoking.[14–16] However, BPH, a common finding in older men, is not a risk factor for prostate cancer.

Prevention. *Primary prevention* aims to reduce the burden of disease through interventions that prevent cancer from developing. There is no convincing evidence that any lifestyle modification, such as consuming diets high in fruits and vegetables or increasing physical activity, can prevent prostate cancer. Several large studies have evaluated *chemoprevention*—giving a medication or dietary supplement—to prevent prostate cancer from developing. The 5α-reductase inhibitors (5-ARIs) finasteride and dutasteride block the conversion of testosterone to the more potent dihydrotestosterone, shrink prostate tissue, and are routinely used to treat men with BPH.[1] Because male hormones are associated with developing prostate cancer, the 5-ARI medications have been considered for cancer chemoprevention. Randomized controlled trials have shown that taking these medications reduced the risk of developing prostate cancer by about 25%, an absolute decrease of about 5 percentage points.[17,18] However, these medications were also associated with an increased risk for developing more aggressive prostate cancers. Consequently, the U.S. Food and Drug Administration has ruled against marketing these medications for cancer prevention.[19] A large randomized, placebo-controlled trial of the antioxidant vitamin E and the micronutrient selenium failed to show that these agents protected against prostate cancer.[20] In fact, men taking vitamin E had a slightly increased risk for developing prostate cancer.[21]

Prostate Cancer Screening. Another key strategy for reducing the burden of cancer is *screening,* also known as *secondary prevention.* Screening for prostate cancer means offering diagnostic tests such as the *PSA te*st or the *digital rectal examination (DRE)* to men with no signs or symptoms of prostate cancer. If the PSA is abnormal (usually a level >4.0 ng/mL) or the DRE is abnormal (due to a palpable nodule, area of induration, or asymmetry), then men are referred for the diagnostic gold standard—the prostate biopsy. Ideally, screening allows cancers to be found at an early stage so that men can be offered curative aggressive treatments like surgery or radiation. However, prostate cancer screening tests are not very accurate, so screening programs have been controversial.

Prostate Cancer Screening Tests: Prostate-Specific Antigen and the Digital Rectal Examination

PSA. PSA is a glycoprotein produced by prostatic epithelial cells that can be elevated by cancer, but also by BPH, prostate infections, or ejaculation, causing results that are false positives. About 12 in 100 men have a PSA screening test above the level of 4 ng/mL, but only 30% of these men will have prostate cancer on biopsy (the positive predictive value).[7] Overall, using a PSA level of 4 ng/mL to define abnormal detects only 21% of prostate cancers (sensitivity), but 51% of aggressive cancers, based on the microscopic appearance of cancer cells. The associated specificity is 91%, which is the proportion of men without prostate cancer with a normal test. Numerous modifications of PSA have been proposed to increase its accuracy, including measuring changes over time (velocity), the proportion of PSA that is not bound to protein (free), and the PSA density (based on the prostate volume) as well as adjusting the cut-off for abnormal based on the patient's age or race. However, none of these strategies has been shown to improve outcomes, and guidelines recommend against them.

DRE. The *DRE* explores for palpable abnormalities such as nodules, induration, or asymmetry in the peripheral posterior and lateral areas of the prostate gland closest to the examining finger; the DRE is unable to detect cancers in the anterior and central areas of the gland. The sensitivity of DRE is 59%, and the specificity is 94%.[22] An estimated 28% of men with an abnormal DRE will have prostate cancer on biopsy (positive predictive value). However, the majority of prostate cancers detected by DRE have already spread beyond the prostate gland, making them more difficult to cure.[23] Furthermore, the DRE is not very reproducible (low kappa score)—even urologists have problems agreeing with each other whether the DRE is abnormal.[24]

Evidence about Screening. Prostate cancer screening has been very controversial. Some professional organizations began recommending routine screening with the PSA in the early 1990s,[25,26] even though, as noted by the U.S. Preventive Services Task Force (USPSTF), there was insufficient evidence that screening reduces prostate cancer mortality.[27]

The strongest evidence supporting screening comes from studies that randomize subjects to screening or no screening, then follow these groups for many years to determine if screening reduces prostate cancer mortality. Two major studies, the European Randomized Study of Screening for Prostate Cancer (ERSPC)[28] and the Prostate, Lung Colorectal, and Ovarian Cancer Screening Trial (PLCO),[29] were conducted to evaluate the effectiveness of screening. However, the study results, first reported in 2009, were conflicting.

The ERSPC, which randomized over 160,000 men ages 55 to 69 years in seven European countries to receive either PSA screening alone every 2 to 4 years or no screening, found that screening reduced death from prostate cancer by about 20%.[28] The absolute risk reduction, however, was 0.7 in 1,000—meaning that 1,400 men would need to be screened twice in 9 years—and 48 cancers detected—to prevent one prostate cancer death. A recent update after 13 years of follow-up reported that the number of men needing screening and the number of cancers to be detected to prevent one prostate cancer death had dropped to 800 and 27, respectively.[30] However, the ERSPC screening group also had a 70% higher risk of diagnosis with prostate cancer. This is concerning because evidence suggests that 42% to 66% of PSA-detected cancers are overdiagnosed—meaning that they would never cause problems during a man's lifetime.[31] Nonetheless, most men with screen-detected cancers undergo aggressive treatment with surgery or radiation,[32] which frequently leads to complications such as erectile dysfunction, urinary incontinence, and bowel problems that adversely affect quality of life.[33]

The PLCO randomized over 75,000 American men ages 50 to 74 years to either screening with PSA and DRE or a control group with no screening.[29] The PLCO found no survival benefit for screening after 13 years of follow-up, although the screening arm had a 12% increased risk for cancer diagnosis.[34] However, the validity of the PLCO results has been questioned because many of the men enrolled had already been screened before the study began, a substantial proportion of the men in the control group were also being screened during the study, and only a fraction of men with abnormal PSA tests underwent biopsy.[35]

Screening Guidelines from Major Organizations. Major professional organizations, including the USPSTF,[33] the American Cancer Society (ACS),[7] and the AUA,[8] have all issued guidelines in recent years, summarized below. The USPSTF has issued a grade D rating for prostate cancer screening, recommending against screening for asymptomatic men regardless of age, race, or family history. The USPSTF concluded that the harms of screening outweigh the benefits. The other organizations encourage providers to address screening average-risk patients beginning at ages 50 or 55 years. Providers are encouraged to support shared decision making because cancer-screening decisions are complex and very sensitive to patient preferences regarding the potential benefit and harms of screening. If the patient agrees to screening, PSA testing is recommended every 1 to 2 years; the DRE is considered optional. Providers should stop offering screening when patients reach age 70 years, or whenever their life expectancy drops below 10 years. Providers can consider offering screening beginning at age 40 or 45 years to men at high risk for cancer—African Americans and those with a family history of prostate cancer.

Prostate Cancer Screening Guidelines

	American Urological Association[8]	American Cancer Society[7]	United States Preventive Services Task Force[33]
Shared decision making	Yes	Yes (consider using decision aid)	Yes (when patient requests screening)
Age to begin offering screening			No recommendation
Average-risk	40 yrs	50 yrs	
High-risk	40 yrs	40–45 yrs	
Age to stop offering screening	Life expectancy <10 yrs	Life expectancy <10 yrs	No recommendation
Screening tests	PSA DRE (optional)	PSA DRE (optional)	No recommendation
Frequency of screening	Annual	Annual (biennial when PSA < 2.5 ng/mL)	No recommendation
Biopsy referral criteria		PSA ≥ 4 ng/mL Abnormal DRE Individualized risk assessment for PSA levels 2.5–4 ng/mL	No recommendation

Abbreviations: PSA, prostate-specific antigen; DRE, digital rectal examination.

Shared Decision Making. Helping patients make informed decisions about screening can be challenging because of limited provider time for discussion of these issues. One strategy, recommended by the ACS, is to use patient prostate cancer screening decision aids, which can be provided in advance of a clinic visit.[7] Decision aids are educational tools that present facts about prostate cancer, discuss the options for screening and treatment, elicit patient values for the outcomes, and provide guidance for discussing screening with a provider. Studies have shown that using decision aids increases knowledge, reduces uncertainty about making decisions, and increases engagement in the decision-making process, although the effect on getting tested has been variable.[36] A list of decision aids for prostate cancer screening available online is below. When providers discuss prostate cancer with patients, the American College of Physicians recommends eliciting the patient's preferences and documenting them in the clinical record.[37]

Resources for Prostate Cancer Information. Encourage men to take advantage of the many resources available to help them make decisions about prostate cancer screening.

Decision Aids for Prostate Cancer Screening

- Testing for Prostate Cancer, American Cancer Society, 2010: http://www.cancer.org/acs/groups/content/@editorial/documents/document/acspc-024618.pdf
- Prostate Cancer Screening: Take Time to Decide, Centers for Disease Control and Prevention 2013 (see also websites for African Americans and Hispanic Americans): http://www.cdc.gov/cancer/prostate/basic_info/infographic.htm
- Prostate Cancer Screening: Should you get a PSA test?, Mayo Clinic: http://www.mayoclinic.org/diseases-conditions/prostate-cancer/in-depth/prostate-cancer/art-20048087
- PROSDEX: A PSA Decision Aid, University of Cardiff: http://prosdex.cf.ac.uk/index_content.htm
- Decision Aid Tool: Cancer Screening with PSA Testing, American Society of Clinical Oncology: http://www.asco.org/sites/www.asco.org/files/psa_pco_decision_aid_71612.pdf

All websites accessed February 24, 2015.

Colorectal Cancer Prevention and Screening.   In 2008, both the USPSTF and a collaborative multiorganizational group, consisting of the ACS Colorectal Cancer Advisory Group, the U.S. Multi-Society Task Force on Colorectal Cancer, and the American College of Radiology Colon Cancer Committee, issued updated guidelines for colorectal cancer screening.[38,39] These guidelines are reviewed in Chapter 11, The Abdomen, on pp. 469–470. An abbreviated summary is provided below.

See also further review of colorectal screening guidelines in Chapter 11, The Abdomen, pp. 469–470.

- *Offer patients at average risk for colorectal cancer a range of screening options beginning at age 50 years:* annual screening with high-sensitivity fecal occult blood tests (including guaiac-based hemoccult tests and fecal immunochemical tests), colonoscopy every 10 years, or sigmoidoscopy every 5 years (which can be combined with high-sensitivity fecal occult blood testing performed every 3 years). The multiorganizational group also endorsed the options of double-contrast barium enema or computed tomography colonography every 5 years and periodic fecal DNA testing.[39] Guidelines recommend against screening with fecal occult blood testing following a DRE. Routine screening should continue until age 75 years.

- *Identify higher-risk persons* based on a personal history of colorectal neoplasia or long-standing IBD—or a family history of colorectal neoplasia, including hereditary syndromes. These individuals will require intensive screening and surveillance testing with colonoscopy; screening will begin at a younger age and be repeated at shorter intervals than for those at average risk.

Counseling for Sexually Transmitted Infections.   Anal intercourse places men and women at risk for perianal and rectal abrasions and transmission of human immunodeficiency virus (HIV) and other sexually transmitted infections (STIs). Protective measures include abstinence from high-risk behaviors (see pp. 547–550), use of condoms, vaccinations for hepatitis B and HPV, and good hygiene.

Techniques of Examination

For many patients and clinicians, the rectal examination is an unwelcome part of the physical examination. Although it may cause patient discomfort, it is rarely painful. You may choose to omit the rectal examination in adolescents who have no relevant complaints. In middle-aged or older adults, it is important for assessing concerning symptoms and may be part of prostate cancer screening. Be sure to warn the patient about what he or she may feel—including pressure, possible discomfort, and the slow gentle movement of your examining finger.

For suspicion of a colorectal cancer consider lower endoscopy.

The Male Patient

Patient Positioning.   Choose one of several suitable patient positions for conducting the examination, with input from the patient when needed. Usually, the side-lying position (Fig. 15-5) is satisfactory and allows good visualization of the perianal and sacrococcygeal areas. Some clinicians ask the patient to stand and lean forward with his upper body resting across the examining table and hips flexed, although this can seem less dignified. In either position, your examining finger cannot reach the full length of the rectum.

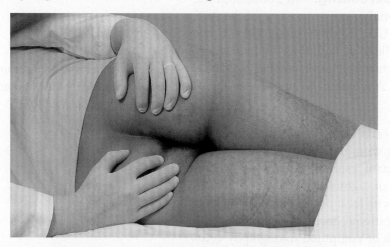

FIGURE 15-5.   **Position the patient on the left side.**

Ask the patient to lie on his left side with his buttocks close to the edge of the examining table near you. Flexing the patient's hips and knees, especially in the upper leg, stabilizes his position and improves visibility. Drape the patient appropriately and adjust the light to ensure good visualization of the perirectal and anal area. Glove your hands and spread the buttocks apart.

■ *Inspect the sacrococcygeal and perianal areas* for lumps, ulcers, inflammation, rashes, or excoriations. Adult perianal skin is normally more pigmented and somewhat coarser than the skin over the buttocks. Palpate any abnormal areas, noting lumps or tenderness.

Anal and perianal lesions include hemorrhoids, venereal warts, herpes, syphilitic chancre, and carcinoma. A linear crack or tear suggests *anal fissure* from large, hard stools, IBD, or STIs. Consider *pruritus ani* if there is swollen, thickened, fissured perianal skin with excoriations.

■ *Examine the anus and rectum.* Lubricate your gloved index finger, explain to the patient what you are going to do, and tell him that the examination may trigger an urge to move his bowels but this will not occur. Ask him to bear down as if having a bowel movement. Inspect the anus, noting any lesions.

■ *Palpate the anal canal.* As the patient bears down, place the pad of your gloved and lubricated index finger over the anus (Fig. 15-6A). As the sphincter relaxes, gently insert your fingertip into the anal canal in the direction pointing toward the umbilicus (Fig. 15-6B). If you feel the sphincter tighten, pause and reassure the patient. When, in a moment, the sphincter relaxes, proceed.

A tender purulent reddened mass with fever or chills suggests an *anal abscess.* Abscesses tunneling to the skin surface from the anus or rectum may form a clogged or draining *anorectal fistula.* Fistulas may ooze blood, pus, or feculent mucus. Consider anoscopy or sigmoidoscopy for better visualization.

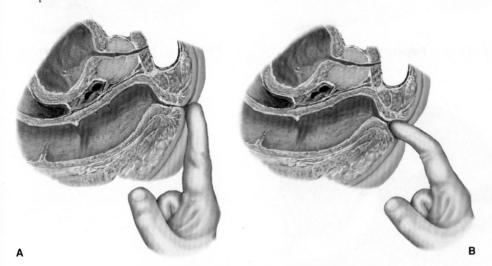

A   B

FIGURE 15-6. **Gently examine the anal canal.**

Occasionally, severe tenderness prevents entry and internal examination. Do not apply force. Instead, place your fingers on both sides of the anus, gently spread the orifice, and ask the patient to bear down.

Look for a lesion, such as an anal fissure, that might explain tenderness.

If you can proceed without undue discomfort to the patient, note:

■ The sphincter tone of the anus. Normally, the muscles of the anal sphincter close snugly around your finger. Initial resting tone reflects the integrity of the internal anal sphincter. To check external sphincter tone, ask the patient to squeeze your finger with the rectal muscles.

■ Tenderness, if any

Sphincter tightness may occur with anxiety, inflammation, or scarring. Sphincter laxity occurs in neurologic diseases, such as S2–S4 cord lesions, and signals possible changes in the urinary sphincter and detrusor muscle. Consider testing perianal sensation.

■ Induration

Induration may be caused by inflammation, scarring, or malignancy.

■ Irregularities or nodules

■ *Palpate the rectal surface.* Insert your finger into the rectum as far as possible. Rotate your hand clockwise to palpate as much of the rectal surface as possible on the patient's right side, then counterclockwise to palpate the surface posteriorly and on the patient's left side (Fig. 15-7).

See Table 15-2, Abnormalities of the Anus, Surrounding Skin, and Rectum, pp. 621–622.

Note any nodules, irregularities, or induration. To bring a possible lesion into reach, take your finger off the rectal surface, ask the patient to bear down, and palpate again.

Note any masses with irregular borders suspicious for *rectal cancer* (Fig. 15-8).

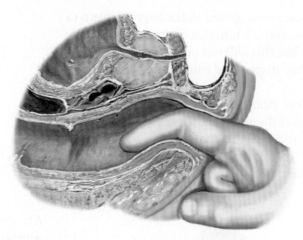

FIGURE 15-7. Palpate the rectal surface.

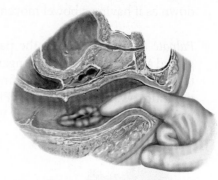

FIGURE 15-8. Rectal cancer.

■ *Palpate the prostate gland.* Then rotate your hand further counterclockwise so that your finger can examine the *posterior surface of the prostate gland* (Fig. 15-9). By turning your body slightly away from the patient, you can feel this area more easily. Tell the patient that examining his prostate gland may prompt an urge to urinate.

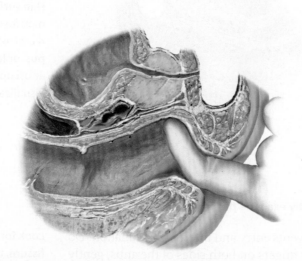

FIGURE 15-9. Palpate the prostate gland.

Sweep your finger carefully over the prostate gland, identifying its *lateral lobes* and the groove of the *median sulcus* between them (Fig. 15-10). Note the size, shape, mobility, and consistency of the prostate, and identify any nodules or tenderness. The normal prostate is rubbery and nontender, with no evidence of fixity to the surrounding tissues.

See Table 15-3, Abnormalities of the Prostate, p. 623.

If possible, *extend your finger above the prostate* to the region of the seminal vesicles and the peritoneal cavity and sweep the anterior wall. Note any nodules or tenderness.

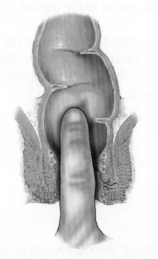

Findings include a rectal "shelf" of peritoneal metastases (see p. 615) or the tenderness of peritoneal inflammation.

Gently withdraw your finger, and wipe the anus or give the patient tissues. Note the appearance of any fecal matter on your glove.

FIGURE 15-10. Palpate the prostate lobes and median sulcus.

The Female Patient

The rectum is usually examined after examining the female genitalia while the woman is in the lithotomy position. This position allows you to conduct the bimanual examination, delineate a possible adnexal or pelvic mass, test the integrity of the rectovaginal wall, and may help you to palpate a cancer high in the rectum.

If only a rectal examination is needed, the lateral position is satisfactory and affords a better view to the perianal and sacrococcygeal areas. Use the same techniques for examination that you use for men. Note that the cervix is readily palpated through the anterior rectal wall. Sometimes, a retroverted uterus is also palpable. Do not mistake either of these, or a vaginal tampon, for a suspicious mass.

Recording Your Findings

Note that initially you may use sentences to describe your findings; later you will use phrases.

Recording the Anus, Rectum, and Prostate Examination

"No perirectal lesions or fissures. External sphincter tone intact. Rectal vault without masses. Prostate smooth and nontender with palpable median sulcus. (Or in a female, uterine cervix nontender.) Stool brown; no fecal blood."
OR
"Perirectal area inflamed; no ulcerations, warts, or discharge. Unable to examine external sphincter, rectal vault, or prostate because of spasm of external sphincter and marked inflammation and tenderness of anal canal."
OR
"No perirectal lesions or fissures. External sphincter tone intact. Rectal vault without masses. Left lateral prostate lobe with 1 × 1 cm firm, hard nodule; right lateral lobe smooth; median sulcus obscured. Stool brown; no fecal blood."

These findings suggest *proctitis* from infectious cause.

These findings are suspicious for *prostate cancer.*

Table 15-1 BPH Symptom Score: American Urological Association

Score or ask the patient to score each of the questions below. Higher scores (maximum 35) indicate more severe symptoms; scores ≤7 are considered mild and generally do not warrant treatment.

PART A	Not at All	Less Than 1 Time in 5	Less Than Half the Time	About Half the Time	More Than Half the Time	Almost Always	Total Points for Each Row
1. Incomplete emptying: Over the past month, how often have you had a sensation of not emptying your bladder completely after you finished urinating?	0	1	2	3	4	5	
2. Frequency: Over the past month, how often have you had to urinate again <2 hours after you finished urinating?	0	1	2	3	4	5	
3. Intermittency: Over the past month, how often have you stopped and started again several times when you urinated?	0	1	2	3	4	5	
4. Urgency: Over the past month, how often have you found it difficult to postpone urination?	0	1	2	3	4	5	
5. Weak stream: Over the past month, how often have you had a weak urinary stream?	0	1	2	3	4	5	
6. Straining: Over the past month, how often have you had to push or strain to begin urination?	0	1	2	3	4	5	
PART B	None	1 Time	2 Times	3 Times	4 Times	5 Times	Points for Part B
7. Nocturia: Over the past month, how many times did you most typically get up to urinate from the time you went to bed at night until the time you got up in the morning?	0	1	2	3	4	5	

TOTAL PARTS A and B (maximum 35)_____

Adapted from: Madsen FA, Bruskewitz RC. Clinical manifestations of benign prostatic hyperplasia. *Urol Clin North Am.* 1995:22:291.

Table 15-2 Abnormalities of the Anus, Surrounding Skin, and Rectum

Pilonidal Cyst and Sinus

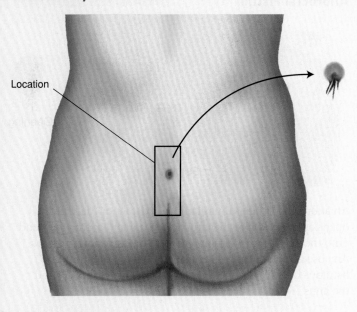

Location

A pilonidal cyst is a fairly common, probably congenital, abnormality located in the midline superficial to the coccyx or the lower sacrum. Look for the opening of a sinus tract, sometimes with a small tuft of hair surrounded by a halo of erythema. Pilonidal cysts are generally asymptomatic, except for slight drainage, but abscess formation and secondary sinus tracts may occur.

External Hemorrhoids (*Thrombosed*)

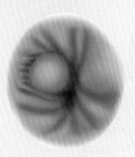

External hemorrhoids are dilated hemorrhoidal veins that originate below the pectinate line that are covered with skin. They seldom produce symptoms unless thrombosis occurs. Thrombosis causes acute local pain that increases with defecation and sitting. A tender, swollen, bluish, ovoid mass is visible at the anal margin.

Internal Hemorrhoids (*Prolapsed*)

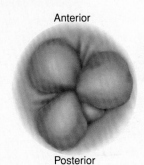

Anterior

Posterior

Internal hemorrhoids are enlargements of the normal vascular cushions located above the pectinate line, usually not palpable. Internal hemorrhoids may cause bright-red bleeding, especially during defecation. They may also prolapse through the anal canal and appear as reddish, moist, protruding masses, typically located in one or more of the positions illustrated.

Prolapse of the Rectum

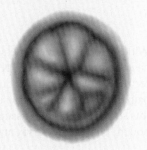

On straining for a bowel movement, the rectal mucosa, with or without its muscular wall, may prolapse through the anus, appearing as a doughnut or rosette of red tissue. A prolapse involving only mucosa is relatively small and shows radiating folds, as illustrated. When the entire bowel wall is involved, the prolapse is larger and covered by concentrically circular folds.

(continued)

Anal Fissure

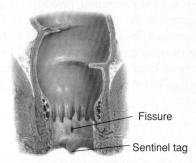

Fissure

Sentinel tag

An anal fissure is a very painful oval ulceration of the anal canal, found most commonly in the midline posteriorly, less commonly in the midline anteriorly. Its long axis lies longitudinally. There may be a swollen "sentinel" skin tag just below it. Gentle separation of the anal margins may reveal the lower edge of the fissure. The sphincter is spastic; the examination is painful. Local anesthesia may be required.

Anorectal Fistula

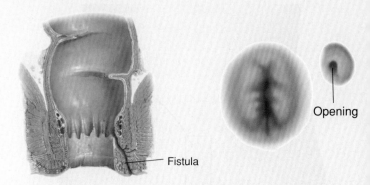

Opening

Fistula

An anorectal fistula is an inflammatory tract or tube that opens at one end into the anus or rectum and at the other end onto the skin surface (as shown here) or into another viscus. An abscess usually antedates such a fistula. Look for the fistulous opening or openings anywhere in the skin around the anus.

Polyps of the Rectum

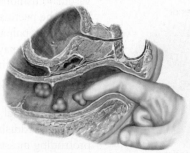

Polyps of the rectum are fairly common. Variable in size and number, they can develop on a stalk (*pedunculated*) or lie on the mucosal surface (*sessile*). They are soft and may be difficult or impossible to feel even when in reach of the examining finger. Endoscopy and biopsy are needed for differentiation of benign from malignant lesions.

Cancer of the Rectum

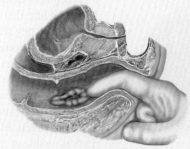

Illustrated here is the firm, nodular, rolled edge of an ulcerated cancer.

Rectal Shelf

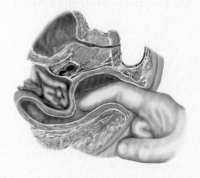

Widespread peritoneal metastases from any source may develop in the area of the peritoneal reflection anterior to the rectum. A firm to hard nodular rectal "shelf" may be just palpable with the tip of the examining finger. In a woman, this shelf of metastatic tissue develops in the rectouterine pouch, behind the cervix and the uterus.

Table 15-3 Abnormalities of the Prostate

Normal Prostate Gland

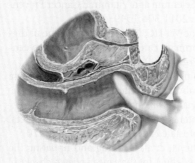

As palpated through the anterior rectal wall, the normal prostate is a rounded, heart-shaped structure approximately 2.5 cm long. The median sulcus can be palpated between the two lateral lobes. Only the posterior surface of the prostate is palpable. Anterior and central lesions, including those that obstruct the urethra, are not detectable by physical examination.

Prostatitis

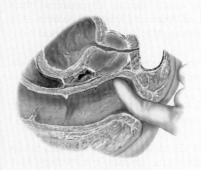

Acute bacterial prostatitis, illustrated here, presents with fever and urinary tract symptoms such as frequency, urgency, dysuria, incomplete voiding, and sometimes low back pain. The gland feels tender, swollen, "boggy," and warm. Examine it gently. More than 80% of infections are caused by gram-negative aerobes such as *Escherichia coli, Enterococcus,* and *Proteus.* In men younger than age 35 yrs, consider sexual transmission of *Neisseria gonorrhea* and *Chlamydia trachomatis.*

Chronic bacterial prostatitis is associated with recurrent urinary tract infections, usually from the same organism. Men may be asymptomatic or have symptoms of dysuria or mild pelvic pain. The prostate gland may feel normal, without tenderness or swelling. Cultures of prostatic fluid usually show infection with *E. coli.*

It may be challenging to distinguish these conditions from the more common *chronic pelvic pain syndrome,* seen in up to 80% of symptomatic men who report obstructive or irritative symptoms on voiding but show no evidence of prostate or urinary tract infection. Physical examination findings are not predictable, but examination is needed to assess any prostate induration or asymmetry suggestive of carcinoma.

Benign Prostatic Hyperplasia

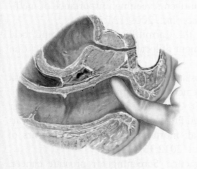

BPH is a nonmalignant enlargement of the prostate gland that increases with age, present in more than 50% of men by age 50 yrs. Symptoms arise both from smooth-muscle contraction in the prostate and bladder neck and from compression of the urethra. They may be irritative (urgency, frequency, nocturia), obstructive (decreased stream, incomplete emptying, straining), or both, and are seen in more than one third of men by age 65 yrs. The affected gland may be normal in size, or may feel symmetrically enlarged, smooth, and firm, though slightly elastic; there may be obliteration of the median sulcus and more notable protrusion into the rectal lumen.

Prostate Cancer

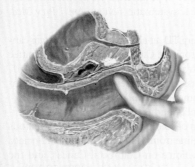

Prostate cancer is suggested by an area of hardness in the gland. A distinct hard nodule that alters the contour of the gland may or may not be palpable. As the cancer enlarges, it feels irregular and may extend beyond the confines of the gland. The median sulcus may be obscured. Hard areas in the prostate are not always malignant. They may also result from prostatic stones, chronic inflammation, and other conditions.

References

1. McVary, KT. BPH: epidemiology and comorbidities. *Am J Manag Care* 2006;12(5 Suppl):S122.

2. Barry MJ, Fowler FJ Jr., O'Leary MP, et al. The American Urological Association symptom index for benign prostatic hyperplasia. The Measurement Committee of the American Urological Association. *J Urol.* 1992;148:1549.

3. Siegel RL, Miller KD, Jemal A. Cancer statistics, 2015. *CA Cancer J Clin.* 2015;65:5.

4. Ross LE, Coates RJ, Breen N, et al. Prostate-specific antigen test use reported in the 2000 National Health Interview Survey. *Prev Med.* 2004;38:732.

5. Seidman H, Mushinski MH, Gelb SK, et al. Probabilities of eventually developing or dying of cancer–United States, 1985. *CA Cancer J Clin.* 1985;35:36.

6. Howlader N, Noone AM, Krapcho M, et al. (eds). *SEER Cancer Statistics Review, 1975–2012.* Bethesda, MD: National Cancer Institute. http://seer.cancer.gov/csr/1975_2012/, based on November 2014 SEER data submission, posted to the SEER website, April 2015.

7. Wolf AM, Wender RC, Etzioni RB, et al. American Cancer Society guideline for the early detection of prostate cancer: update 2010. *CA Cancer J Clin.* 2010;60:70.

8. Carter HB, Albertsen PC, Barry MJ, et al. Early detection of prostate cancer: AUA Guideline. *J Urol.* 2013;190:419.

9. Jemal A, Center MM, DeSantis C, et al. Global patterns of cancer incidence and mortality rates and trends. *Cancer Epidemiol Biomarkers Prev.* 2010;19:1893.

10. Parker PM, Rice KR, Sterbis JR, et al. Prostate cancer in men less than the age of 50: a comparison of race and outcomes. *Urology.* 2011;78:110.

11. Hoffman RM, Gilliland FD, Eley JW, et al. Racial and ethnic differences in advanced-stage prostate cancer: the Prostate Cancer Outcomes Study. *J Natl Cancer Inst.* 2001;93:388.

12. Steinberg GD, Carter BS, Beaty TH, et al. Family history and the risk of prostate cancer. *Prostate.* 1990;17:337.

13. Bancroft EK, Page EC, Castro E, et al. Targeted Prostate Cancer Screening in BRCA1 and BRCA2 Mutation Carriers: Results from the Initial Screening Round of the IMPACT Study. *Eur Urol.* 2014; 66(3):489–499.

14. Chamie K, DeVere White RW, Lee D, et al. Agent Orange exposure, Vietnam War veterans, and the risk of prostate cancer. *Cancer.* 2008;113:2464.

15. Sinha R, Park Y, Graubard BI, et al. Meat and meat-related compounds and risk of prostate cancer in a large prospective cohort study in the United States. *Am J Epidemiol.* 2009;170:1165.

16. Huncharek M, Haddock KS, Reid R, et al. Smoking as a risk factor for prostate cancer: a meta-analysis of 24 prospective cohort studies. *Am J Public Health.* 2010;100:693.

17. Thompson IM, Goodman PJ, Tangen CM, et al. The influence of finasteride on the development of prostate cancer. *N Engl J Med.* 2003;349:215.

18. Andriole GL, Bostwick DG, Brawley OW, et al. Effect of dutasteride on the risk of prostate cancer. *N Engl J Med.* 2010;362:1192.

19. Theoret MR, Ning YM, Zhang JJ, et al. The risks and benefits of 5alpha-reductase inhibitors for prostate-cancer prevention. *N Engl J Med.* 2011;365:97.

20. Lippman SM, Klein EA, Goodman PJ, et al. Effect of selenium and vitamin E on risk of prostate cancer and other cancers: the Selenium and Vitamin E Cancer Prevention Trial (SELECT). *JAMA.* 2009;301:39.

21. Klein EA, Thompson IM Jr., Tangen CM, et al. Vitamin E and the risk of prostate cancer: the Selenium and Vitamin E Cancer Prevention Trial (SELECT). *JAMA.* 2011;306:1549.

22. Hoogendam A, Buntinx F, de Vet HC. The diagnostic value of digital rectal examination in primary care screening for prostate cancer: a meta-analysis. *Fam Pract.* 1999;16:621.

23. Coley CM, Barry MJ, Fleming C, et al. Early detection of prostate cancer. Part I: Prior probability and effectiveness of tests. The American College of Physicians. *Ann Intern Med.* 1997;126:394.

24. Smith DS, Catalona WJ. Interexaminer variability of digital rectal examination in detecting prostate cancer. *Urology.* 1995;45:70.

25. Mettlin C, Jones G, Averette H, et al. Defining and updating the American Cancer Society guidelines for the cancer-related checkup: prostate and endometrial cancers. *CA Cancer J Clin.* 1993;43:42.

26. Early detection of prostate cancer and use of transrectal ultrasound. In: Association AU, ed. *American Urological Association 1992 Policy Statement Book.* Baltimore, MA: American Urological Association; 1992.

27. Harris R, Lohr KN. Screening for prostate cancer: an update of the evidence for the U.S. Preventive Services Task Force. *Ann Intern Med.* 2002;137:917.

28. Schroder FH, Hugosson J, Roobol MJ, et al. Screening and prostate-cancer mortality in a randomized European study. *N Engl J Med.* 2009;360:1320.

29. Andriole GL, Crawford ED, Grubb RL 3rd, et al. Mortality results from a randomized prostate-cancer screening trial. *N Engl J Med.* 2009;360:1310.

30. Schroder FH, Hugosson J, Roobol MJ, et al. Screening and prostate cancer mortality: results of the European Randomised Study of Screening for Prostate Cancer (ERSPC) at 13 years of follow-up. *Lancet.* 2014;384:2027.

31. Draisma G, Etzioni R, Tsodikov A, et al. Lead time and overdiagnosis in prostate-specific antigen screening: importance of methods and context. *J Natl Cancer Inst.* 2009;101:374.

32. Cooperberg MR, Broering JM, Carroll PR. Time trends and local variation in primary treatment of localized prostate cancer. *J Clin Oncol.* 2010;28:1117.

33. Moyer VA. Screening for prostate cancer: U.S. Preventive Services Task Force recommendation statement. *Ann Intern Med.* 2012;157:120.

34. Andriole GL, Crawford ED, Grubb RL, 3rd, et al. Prostate cancer screening in the randomized Prostate, Lung, Colorectal, and Ovarian Cancer Screening Trial: mortality results after 13 years of follow-up. *J Natl Cancer Inst.* 2012;104:125.

35. Hoffman RM. Clinical practice. Screening for prostate cancer. *N Engl J Med.* 2011;365:2013.

36. Volk RJ, Hawley ST, Kneuper S, et al. Trials of decision aids for prostate cancer screening: a systematic review. *Am J Prev Med.* 2007;33:428.

37. Qaseem A, Barry MJ, Denberg TD, et al. Screening for prostate cancer: a guidance statement from the Clinical Guidelines Committee of the American College of Physicians. *Ann Intern Med.* 2013;158:761.

38. U.S. Preventive Services Task Force. Screening for colorectal cancer. Recommendation statement. *Ann Intern Med.* 2008;149:627.

39. Levin B, Lieberman DA, McFarland B, et al. Screening and surveillance for the early detection of colorectal cancer and adenomatous polyps, 2008: a joint guideline from the American Cancer Society, the US Multi-Society Task Force on Colorectal Cancer, and the American College of Radiology. *CA Cancer J Clin.* 2008;58:130.

The Musculoskeletal System

The Bates' suite offers these additional resources to enhance learning and facilitate understanding of this chapter:

- Bates' *Pocket Guide to Physical Examination and History Taking*, 8th edition
- Bates' *Visual Guide to Physical Examination* (Vol. 16: Musculoskeletal System)
- thePoint online resources, for students and instructors: http://thepoint.lww.com

Musculoskeletal disorders are the leading primary diagnosis during office visits in the United States.[1] In 2012, these disorders totaled 93 million visits, or 10% of all ambulatory care visits, highlighting the need for competent office examinations. Arthritis affects one in five Americans, or 22% of the adult population, and is the leading cause of disability, costing well above $128 billion a year.[2] Spinal disorders are the fourth highest diagnostic group for office visits. In 2010, 29% of Americans reported low back pain alone.[3] Low back symptoms, one of the top 20 reasons for office visits, represent a continuing clinical challenge;[1] many cases are "nonspecific," yet they are one of the most common and expensive causes of work-related disability.[4]

Each of the major joints has unique anatomy and directional movement. In this chapter, the Anatomy and Physiology section and Techniques for Examination are *combined* to help students apply their knowledge of the anatomy and function of each joint to the specific examination techniques needed. These sections follow a head-to-toe sequence, beginning with the jaw and joints of the upper extremities and ending with the ankles and feet. For each joint, look for sections on: Joint Overview, which describes the distinguishing anatomical and functional characteristics of the joint; Bony Structures and Joints; Muscle Groups and Additional Structures; and Techniques of Examination, which presents examination techniques specific to that joint—inspection, palpation of bony and soft tissue structures, range of motion (the arc of measurable joint movement in a single plane), and maneuvers for testing joint function and stability. Sharpen your skills of inspection as you examine the surface structures and contours of each joint. Learn to visualize the joint's underlying anatomy. Visualization helps trigger the examination techniques and maneuvers you will need to perform next.

Prevalence for most conditions varies by gender. *Osteoarthritis (OA),* **for example, is more common in women, especially in the knee.**

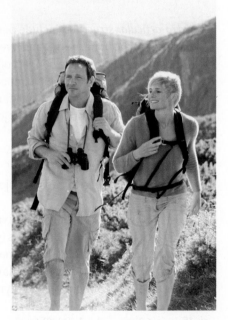

FIGURE 16-1. **Exercise is key to health.**

Approach to Musculoskeletal Disorders

The first goal of your evaluation of musculoskeletal disorders is to characterize the patient's complaint in terms of four key features. Is the joint problem:

- Articular or extra-articular

- Acute (usually <6 weeks) or chronic (usually >12 weeks)

- Inflammatory or noninflammatory

- Localized (monoarticular) or diffuse (polyarticular)

Review the anatomical terminology that pertains to the joints and the useful algorithm in Figure 16-2. The authors note that, "This approach is remarkably effective and relies on clinical and historic features, rather than laboratory testing, to diagnose many common...disorders."[5]

Joint Anatomy—Important Terms

- *Articular structures* include the *joint capsule* and *articular cartilage*, the *synovium* and *synovial fluid, intra-articular ligaments*, and *juxta-articular bone*. Articular cartilage is composed of a collagen matrix containing charged ions and water, allowing the cartilage to change shape in response to pressure or load, acting as a cushion for underlying bone. Synovial fluid provides nutrition to the adjacent relatively avascular articular cartilage.

- *Extra-articular structures* include periarticular ligaments, tendons, bursae, muscle, fascia, bone, nerve, and overlying skin.
  - *Ligaments* are rope-like bundles of collagen fibrils that connect bone to bone.
  - *Tendons* are collagen fibers connecting muscle to bone.
  - *Bursae* are pouches of synovial fluid that cushion the movement of tendons and muscles over bone or other joint structures.

Articular disease typically involves swelling and tenderness of the entire joint, crepitus, instability, "locking," or deformity, and limits both *active and passive range of motion* due to either stiffness or pain.[5]

Extra-articular disease typically involves "point or focal tenderness in regions adjacent to articular structures" and limits *active range of motion*. Extra-articular disease rarely causes swelling, instability, or joint deformity.

Age also provides clues to causes of joint pain.[5]

- If *age <60 years,* consider repetitive strain or overuse syndromes like tendinitis or bursitis, crystalline arthritis (gout; crystalline pyrophosphate deposition disease [CPPD]) (males), rheumatoid arthritis (RA), psoriatic arthritis and reactive (Reiter) arthritis (in inflammatory bowel disease [IBD]), and infectious arthritis from gonorrhea, Lyme disease, or viral or bacterial infections.

- If *age >60 years,* look for OA, gout and pseudogout, polymyalgia rheumatica (PMR), osteoporotic fracture, and septic bacterial arthritis.

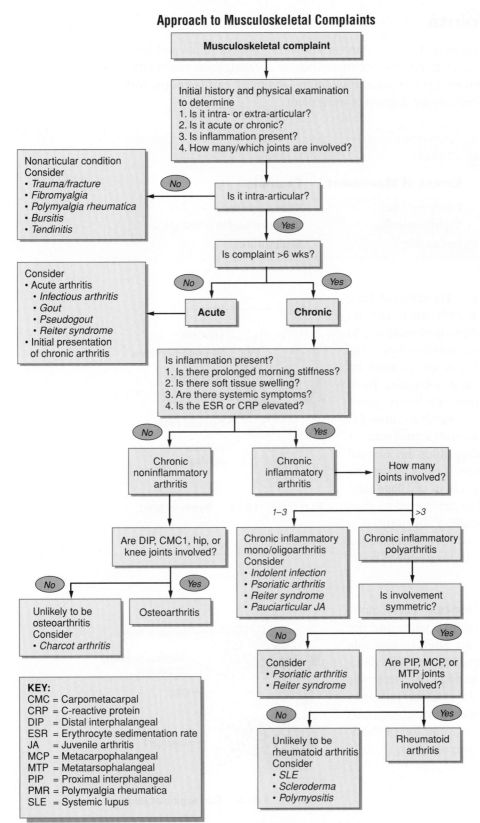

Approach to Musculoskeletal Complaints

FIGURE 16-2. Algorithm for diagnosis of musculoskeletal complaints. SOURCE: Cush JJ, Lipsky PE. In: Longo DL, Fauci AS, Kasper DL, et al. (eds). *Chapter 331,* Approach to Articular and Musculoskeletal Disorders, *in Harrison's Principles of Internal Medicine.* 18th ed. New York, NY: McGraw-Hill; 2012.

Adapted from: Kasper DL, Braunwald E, Fauci AS, et al., eds. Harrison's Principles of Internal Medicine, 16th ed. New York: McGraw-Hill, 2005.

Types of Joints

To evaluate joint function, it is important to know the types of joints and how they articulate, or interconnect, and the role of bursae in easing joint movement. There are three primary types of joint articulation—synovial, cartilaginous, and fibrous—which allow varying degrees of movement.

Joints

Type of Joint	Extent of Movement	Example
Synovial	Freely movable	Knee, shoulder
Cartilaginous	Slightly movable	Vertebral bodies of the spine
Fibrous	Immovable	Skull sutures

Synovial Joints. The bones of these joints do not touch each other, and the joint articulations are *freely movable* within the limits of the surrounding ligaments (Fig. 16-3). The bones are covered by *articular cartilage* and separated by a *synovial cavity* that cushions joint movement. A *synovial membrane* lines the synovial cavity and secretes a small amount of viscous lubricating fluid, the *synovial fluid*. The membrane is attached at the margins of the articular cartilage and pouched or folded to accommodate joint movement. Surrounding the joint is a fibrous *joint capsule*, which is strengthened by ligaments extending from bone to bone.

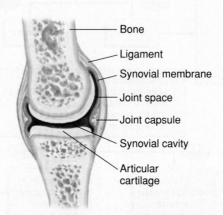

- Bone
- Ligament
- Synovial membrane
- Joint space
- Joint capsule
- Synovial cavity
- Articular cartilage

FIGURE 16-3. **Synovial joint.**

Cartilaginous Joints. These joints, such as the intervertebral joints and the symphysis pubis, are slightly movable (Fig. 16-4). Fibrocartilaginous discs separate the bony surfaces. At the center of each disc is the *nucleus pulposus*, somewhat gelatinous fibrocartilaginous material that serves as a cushion or shock absorber between bony surfaces.

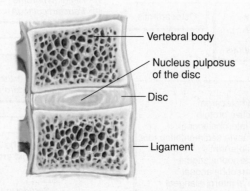

- Vertebral body
- Nucleus pulposus of the disc
- Disc
- Ligament

FIGURE 16-4. **Cartilaginous joint.**

Fibrous Joints. In these joints, such as the sutures of the skull, intervening layers of fibrous tissue or cartilage hold the bones together (Fig. 16-5). The bones are almost in direct contact, which allows *no appreciable movement.*

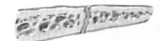

FIGURE 16-5. **Fibrous joint.**

Synovial Joints and Bursae

As you learn to examine the musculoskeletal system, focus on relating the anatomy of the joint to its movement.

Synovial Joints

Type of Joint	Articular Shape	Movement	Example
Spheroidal (ball and socket)	Convex surface in concave cavity	Wide-ranging–flexion, extension, abduction, adduction, rotation, circumduction	Shoulder, hip
Hinge	Flat, planar	Motion in one plane; flexion, extension	Interphalangeal joints of hand and foot; elbow
Condylar	Convex or concave	Movement of two articulating surfaces not dissociable	Knee; temporomandibular joint

Many of the joints we examine are *synovial,* or movable, *joints.* The shape of the articulating surfaces of synovial joints, as well as the surrounding soft tissues, determines the direction and extent of joint motion. Younger people and women tend to have increased soft tissue laxity, leading to increased range of motion ("double-jointed").

Spheroidal Joints. Spheroidal joints have a ball-and-socket configuration—a rounded, convex surface articulating with a concave cuplike cavity, allowing a wide range of rotatory movement, as in the shoulder and hip (Fig. 16-6).

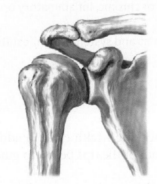

FIGURE 16-6. **Spheroidal joint (ball and socket).**

Hinge Joints. Hinge joints are flat, planar, or slightly curved, allowing only a gliding motion in a single plane, as in flexion and extension of the digits (Fig. 16-7).

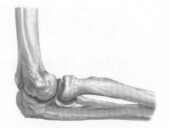

FIGURE 16-7. **Hinge joint.**

Condylar Joints. Condylar joints, such as the knee, have articulating surfaces that are convex or concave (Fig. 16-8). These joints allow flexion, extension, rotation, and motion in the coronal plane.

Bursae. Bursae are roughly disc-shaped synovial sacs that ease joint action and allow adjacent muscles or muscles and tendons to glide over each other during movement. They lie between the skin and the convex surface of a bone or joint, as in the prepatellar bursa of the knee (p. 684) or in areas where tendons or muscles rub against bone, ligaments, or other tendons or muscles, as in the subacromial bursa of the shoulder (pp. 648–652).

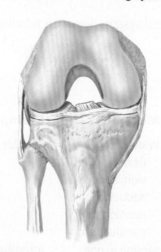

FIGURE 16-8. **Condylar joint.**

As you examine joints, knowing the underlying joint anatomy and allowable movement will help you assess degenerative disorders and trauma. Your knowledge of the soft tissue structures, ligaments, tendons, and bursae will help you evaluate inflammatory disorders and overuse syndromes.

The Health History

Common or Concerning Symptoms

- Joint pain: articular or extra-articular, acute or chronic, inflammatory or noninflammatory, localized or diffuse
- Joint pain: associated constitutional symptoms and systemic manifestations from other organ systems
- Neck pain
- Low back pain

Joint pain is a leading complaint of patients seeking health care. In addition to eliciting the seven features of any joint pain, adopt the tips below to guide your subsequent examination and diagnosis:

See Chapter 3, Interviewing and the Health History, for the seven features of pain, pp. 79–80.

Tips for Assessing Joint Pain

- Ask the patient to *"point to the pain."* This may save considerable time because many patients have trouble pinpointing pain location in words.
- Clarify and record when the pain started and the *mechanism of injury*, particularly if there is a history of trauma.
- Determine whether the pain is *articular* or *extra-articular*, *acute* or *chronic*, *inflammatory* or *noninflammatory*, and *localized (monoarticular)* or *diffuse (polyarticular)*.

Joint Pain: Identifying Important Characteristics

Articular or Extra-articular.   Begin by asking "Do you have any pains in your joints?" Joint pain may be articular or extra-articular. Ask the patient to point to the pain.

- If pain is localized to only one joint, it is *monoarticular.* Pain originating in the small joints of the hands and feet is more sharply localized than pain in larger joints. Pain from the hip joint is especially deceptive. True pain from the hip joint is typically described in the groin. Sacral/sacroiliac pain is often in the buttock, and trochanteric pain from bursitis occurs on the lateral thigh.

  Pain in a single joint suggests injury, monoarticular arthritis, or extra-articular causes like tendinitis or bursitis. Lateral hip pain with focal tenderness over the greater trochanter is typical of *trochanteric bursitis.*

- Joint pain may be *polyarticular,* involving several joints, typically four or more. If polyarticular, what is the *pattern of involvement* . . . migrating from joint to joint or steadily spreading from one joint to multiple joints? Is the involvement *symmetric,* affecting similar joints on both sides of the body?

  In *rheumatic fever* or *gonococcal arthritis,* there is a migratory pattern of spread; in *RA,* the pattern is additive and progressive with symmetric involvement. Inflammatory arthritides are more common in women.

- Joint pain may also be *extra-articular,* involving bones, muscles, and tissues around the joint such as the tendons, bursae, or even overlying skin. Generalized "aches and pains" are called *myalgias* if in muscles, and *arthralgias* if there is pain but no evidence of arthritis.

  Extra-articular pain occurs in inflammation of bursae (*bursitis*), tendons (*tendinitis*), or tendon sheaths (*tenosynovitis*) as well as in *sprains* from stretching or tearing of ligaments.

Note that the symptoms of *decreased joint movement* and *stiffness* can help you decide if the pain is *articular.*

- To assess *decreased* or *limited movement,* ask about changes in activity due to problems with the involved joint, for example, in the ability to walk, stand, lean over, sit or sit up, rise from a sitting position, pinch, grasp, turn a page, or open a door handle or jar. Common activities like combing hair, brushing teeth, eating, dressing, and bathing may also be affected.

  In articular joint pain there is decreased active and passive range or motion and morning stiffness or "gelling" (see page 633); in nonarticular joint pain, there is periarticular tenderness and only passive range of motion remains intact.

- Musculoskeletal *stiffness* refers to a perceived tightness or resistance to movement, in contrast to normal movement that is limber.

Acute or Chronic. *Acute joint pain* typically lasts up to 6 weeks; *chronic pain lasts >12 weeks.*

Assess the onset, duration, quality, and severity of the joint symptoms. Onset is especially important. Did the pain or discomfort develop rapidly over the course of a few hours or insidiously over weeks or even months? Has the pain progressed slowly or fluctuated, with periods of improvement and worsening? How long has the pain lasted? What is it like over the course of a day?... In the morning?... As the day wears on?

If more rapid in onset, how did the pain arise? Was there an acute injury or overuse from repetitive motion of the same part of the body? If the pain comes from trauma, what was the *mechanism of injury* or the specific series of events that caused the joint pain? Furthermore, what aggravates or relieves the pain? What are the effects of exercise, rest, and therapy?

Inflammatory or Noninflammatory. Try to determine whether the joint pain is *inflammatory* or *noninflammatory*. Different mechanisms appear to be involved—interleukins and tumor necrosis factor in inflammatory joint pain, and prostaglandins, chemokines, and growth factors in noninflammatory pain.[8]

Ask about the four cardinal features of inflammation—*swelling, warmth,* and *redness,* in addition to *pain.* Several of these features are best assessed on examination, but patients can often guide you to points of inflammation and pain. Also ask about fever or chills.

Elicit any pattern of *stiffness.* Is it worse in the morning but gradually better with activity? Or is there an intermittent "gel phenomenon," namely brief periods of daytime stiffness following inactivity that usually last from 30 to 60 minutes then get worse again with movement?

Localized or Diffuse. Ask the patient which joints are painful. Joint pain can be *monoarticular, oligoarticular* involving two to four joints, or *polyarticular.* If there is pain in more than one joint, is the pattern of involvement symmetric or asymmetric?

Severe pain of rapid onset in a red swollen joint suggests *acute septic arthritis* or *crystalline arthritis* (gout; CPPD).[6,7] In children, consider *osteomyelitis* in a bone contiguous to a joint.

See Table 16-1, Patterns of Pain in and Around the Joints, pp. 696–697.

Inflammatory disorders have many causes[5]: infectious (*Neisseria gonorrhoeae* or *Mycobacterium tuberculosis*), crystal-induced (*gout, pseudogout*), immune-related (*RA, systemic lupus erythematosus* [*SLE*]), reactive (rheumatic fever, reactive arthritis), or idiopathic.

In noninflammatory disorders, consider trauma (rotator cuff tear), repetitive use (bursitis, tendinitis), degenerative changes (OA), or fibromyalgia.

Inflammation with fever and chills is seen in *septic arthritis;* also consider *crystalline arthritis.*

Morning stiffness that gradually improves with activity is more common in inflammatory disorders like *RA* and *PMR*[9–11]; intermittent stiffness and gelling are seen in *OA*.[12]

***Monoarticular arthritis* can be traumatic, crystalline, or septic. *Oligoarticular arthritis* occurs in infection from gonorrhea or rheumatic fever, connective tissue disease, and OA. *Polyarthritis* may be viral or inflammatory from RA, SLE, or psoriasis.[8]**

Involvement is usually *symmetric* in RA, SLE, and ankylosing spondylitis and *asymmetric* in psoriatic, reactive (Reiter), and IBD-associated arthritis.

Joint Pain: Associated Constitutional Symptoms and Systemic Manifestations from Other Organ Systems. Some joint problems have associated *constitutional symptoms* such as fever, chills, rash, fatigue, anorexia, weight loss, and weakness.

Constitutional symptoms are common in RA, SLE, PMR, and other inflammatory arthritides. High fever and chills suggest an infectious cause.

In inflammatory conditions, initial laboratory tests such as the erythrocyte sedimentation rate, C-reactive protein, platelet count, and hematocrit are helpful.

Leukemia can infiltrate the synovium; chemotherapy can also cause joint pain.

Some joint disorders have systemic manifestations in other organ systems that provide important clues to diagnosis. Ask about any family history of joint or muscle disorders. Watch for the symptoms, signs, and disorders below.

Joint Pain and Systemic Disorders

- Skin conditions
  - Butterfly (malar) rash on the cheeks

    Systemic lupus erythematosus
  - Scaly plaques, especially on extensor surfaces, and pitted nails

    Psoriatic arthritis
  - Heliotrope rash on the upper eyelid

    Dermatomyositis
  - Papules, pustules, or vesicles with reddened bases on the distal extremities

    Gonococcal arthritis
  - Expanding erythematous "target" or "bull's eye" patch early in an illness

    Lyme disease (erythema chronicum migrans)
  - Painful subcutaneous nodules especially in pretibial area

    Sarcoidosis, Behçet disease (erythema nodosum)[13,14]
  - Palpable purpura

    Vasculitis
  - Hives

    Serum sickness, drug reaction
  - Erosions or scaling on the penis and crusted scaling papules on the soles and palms

    Reactive (Reiter) arthritis (with urethritis, uveitis)
  - The maculopapular rash of rubella

    Arthritis of rubella
  - Nailfold capillary changes

    Dermatomyositis, systemic sclerosis
  - Clubbing of the fingernails (see p. 211)

    Hypertrophic osteoarthropathy
- Red, burning, and itchy eyes (conjunctivitis), eye pain and blurred vision (uveitis)

  Reactive (Reiter) arthritis, Behçet syndrome,[13,14] ankylosing spondylitis
- Scleritis

  RA, IBD, vasculitis
- Preceding sore throat

  Acute rheumatic fever or gonococcal arthritis

(*continued*)

Joint Pain and Systemic Disorders (*continued*)

• Oral ulcerations	RA (usually painless); Behçet disease
• Pneumonitis; interstitial lung disease	RA; systemic sclerosis
• Diarrhea, abdominal pain, cramping	IBD, reactive arthritis from Salmonella, Shigella, Yersinia, Campylobacter; scleroderma
• Urethritis	Reactive (Reiter) arthritis, gonococcal arthritis
• Mental status change, facial or other weakness, stiff neck	Lyme disease with central nervous system involvement

Neck Pain. Neck pain is also common. If the patient reports neck trauma, common in motor vehicle accidents, ask about neck tenderness and consider clinical decision rules that identify risk of cervical cord injury. The NEXUS criteria and the Canadian C-Spine Rule are highly sensitive and specific for establishing a low probability of cervical spine injury.[15–17] Persistent pain after blunt trauma or a collision warrants further evaluation.

The NEXUS criteria are normal alertness, no posterior midline cervical spine tenderness, no focal neurologic deficits, no evidence of intoxication, and no painful distracting injury. The Canadian C-Spine Rule includes age, mechanism of injury, low risk factors allowing assessment of range of motion, and testing of neck rotation.

Neck pain is usually self-limited, but it is important to ask about radiation into the arm or scapular area, arm weakness, numbness, or paresthesias.[18] Elicit any of the "red flag" symptoms listed below.

See Table 16-2, Pains in the Neck, p. 698.

Radicular pain signals spinal nerve compression and/or irritation, most commonly at C7 or C6. Unlike low back pain, the principal cause is foraminal impingement from degenerative joint changes (70% to 75%), rather than disc herniation (20% to 25%).[19]

Low Back Pain. Begin by asking "Do you have any back pain?,"—at least 40% of adults have low back pain at least once during their lifetime, usually between the ages of 30 and 50 years, and low back pain is one of the most common reasons for office visits. There are numerous clinical guidelines, but most categorize low back pain into three groups: nonspecific (>90%), nerve root entrapment with radiculopathy or spinal stenosis (~5%), and pain from a specific underlying disease (1% to 2%).[4,20] Note that the term "nonspecific low back pain" is preferred to "sprain" or "strain." Using open-ended questions, get a clear and complete picture of the problem, especially the location and radiation of the pain and any prior history of trauma.

See Table 16-3, Low Back Pain, p. 699.

Nonspecific low back pain is usually from musculoligamentous injuries and age-related degenerative processes of the intervertebral discs and facet joints.

Determine if the pain is *on the midline,* over the vertebrae, or *off the midline.*

For *midline back pain,* diagnoses include musculoligamentous injury; disc herniation; vertebral collapse; spinal cord metastases; and, rarely, epidural abscess. For *pain off the midline,* assess for muscle strain, sacroiliitis, trochanteric bursitis, sciatica, and hip arthritis as well as for renal conditions like pyelonephritis or stones.

Is there radiation into the buttock or lower extremity? Is there any associated numbness or paresthesias?

Sciatica is radicular gluteal and posterior leg pain in the S1 distribution that increases with cough or Valsalva (see pp. 765–766 for related neurologic findings); 85% of cases are associated with a disc disorder, usually at L4–L5 or L5–S1.[21] Leg pain that resolves with rest and/or lumbar forward flexion occurs in *spinal stenosis.*

Importantly, is there any associated bladder or bowel dysfunction?

Consider *cauda equina syndrome* from an S2–S4 midline disc or tumor if there is bowel or bladder dysfunction (usually urinary retention with overflow incontinence), especially if there is saddle anesthesia or perineal numbness. Pursue immediate imaging and surgical evaluation.[4]

Elicit any key warning signs or "red flags" for serious underlying systemic disease.[20]

In cases of low back pain plus another indicator, there is a pretest probability of serious systemic disease of ~10%.[22]

Red Flags for Low Back Pain from Underlying Systemic Disease

- Age <20 years or >50 years
- History of cancer
- Unexplained weight loss, fever, or decline in general health
- Pain lasting more than 1 month or not responding to treatment
- Pain at night or present at rest
- History of intravenous drug use, addiction, or immunosuppression
- Presence of active infection or human immunodeficiency virus (HIV) infection
- Long-term steroid therapy
- Saddle anesthesia, bladder or bowel incontinence
- Neurologic symptoms or progressive neurologic deficit

Health Promotion and Counseling: Evidence and Recommendations

Important Topics for Health Promotion and Counseling

- Nutrition, weight, and physical activity
- Low back pain
- Osteoporosis: risk factors, screening, and assessing fracture risk
- Treating osteoporosis and preventing falls

The integrity of the musculoskeletal system brings many features of a healthy lifestyle into play—nutrition, fitness, optimal weight, and prevention of injury. Each joint has specific vulnerabilities to trauma and wear. Proper lifting, avoiding falls, household safety measures, and a balanced physical activity program protect and preserve well-functioning joints and muscles and prevent or delay the onset of arthritis, chronic back pain, and osteoporosis, all important targets for Healthy People 2020.[25]

Nutrition, Weight, and Physical Activity. Healthy habits directly benefit the skeleton and muscles. Good nutrition supplies calcium for bone mineralization and bone density. A healthy weight reduces excess mechanical stress on weight-bearing joints like the hips and knees.

See Chapter 4, Beginning the Physical Examination: General Survey, Vital Signs, and Pain, pp. 114–118, for further discussion of nutrition and weight.

The Healthy People 2020 objectives set goals for physical activity aimed at increasing the proportion of adults meeting guidelines for aerobic and muscle-strengthening physical activity (Fig. 16-9).[26] These goals are based on the 2008 *Physical Activity Guidelines for Americans,*[27] an evidence-based report that highlights the benefits of physical activity, including risk reduction for early death, cardiovascular disease, hypertension, type 2 diabetes, breast and colon cancer, obesity, osteoporosis, falls, and depression. Physical activity also helps improve sleep quality and cognitive function in older adults.

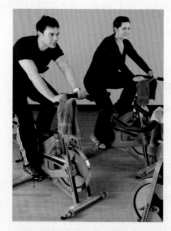

FIGURE 16-9. Encourage physical activity.

Physical Activity Guidelines for Americans

- At least 2 hours and 30 minutes a week of moderate-intensity, or 1 hour and 15 minutes a week of vigorous-intensity, *aerobic physical activity,* or an equivalent combination
- Moderate- or high-intensity *muscle-strengthening activity* that involves all major muscle groups on 2 or more days a week

The report includes guidelines to help sedentary people gradually build up their activity level, starting with 10 minutes of exercise a day. Guided exercise regimens help reduce sports and exercise injuries, which are a significant source of musculoskeletal disorders.

Low Back Pain. The estimated lifetime prevalence of low back pain in the United States population is over 80%.[28] Spinal disorders are among the most frequent reasons for adult outpatient visits,[29] and the annual U.S. economic costs attributed to diagnosing and managing low back pain and lost productivity exceed $100 billion.[27] Most patients with acute low back pain get better within 6 weeks; for patients with nonspecific symptoms, clinical guidelines emphasize reassurance, staying active, analgesics, muscle relaxants, and spinal manipulation therapy.[30] Overall, about 10% to 15% of patients with acute low back pain develop chronic symptoms, often associated with long-term disability.[28] Factors associated with poor outcomes include inappropriate beliefs that low back pain is a serious clinical condition, maladaptive pain-coping behaviors (avoiding work, movement, or other activities for fear of causing back damage), multiple nonorganic physical examination findings, psychiatric disorders, poor general health, high levels of baseline functional impairment, and low work satisfaction.[4,24] Review the nonorganic physical findings (the Waddell signs) on p. 674.[31] Appropriate treatments for chronic low back pain include treatments for acute low back pain as well as back exercises and behavioral therapy.[30] Opioids should be used cautiously, given their adverse effects and risks for abuse.[32]

See Table 16-3, Low Back Pain, p. 699, for serious causes of low back pain, including back pain with sciatica or neurogenic claudication, *compression fracture, malignancy, ankylosing spondylitis,* and infection including *osteomyelitis.*

Studies show that psychosocial factors, now called "yellow flags," strongly affect the course of low back pain.[20,23,24] Ask about anxiety, depression, and work stress. Assess any maladaptive coping, inappropriate fears or beliefs, or tendency to somatization.

Osteoporosis: Risk Factors, Screening, and Assessing Fracture Risk. Osteoporosis is a common U.S. health problem—9% of adults over age 50 years have osteoporosis at the femoral neck or lumbar spine, including 16% of women and 4% of men.[33] Half of all postmenopausal women sustain an osteoporosis-related fracture during their lifetime; 25% develop vertebral deformities; and 15% suffer hip fractures that increase risk of chronic pain, disability, loss of independence, and increased mortality.[34] Although mortality rates are declining, about 3 in 10 patients die in the year following a hip fracture.[35] Men are also at risk: the lifetime risk for an osteoporotic fracture in men over age 50 years is 1 in 4, and men are more likely than women to die in the year following a hip fracture. Nearly half of adults age ≥50 years has osteopenia, representing well over 30 million people, including about 12 million men.[36] The majority of fragility fractures actually occur among osteopenic adults.

Risk Factors for Osteoporosis

- Postmenopausal status in women
- Age ≥50 years
- Prior fragility fracture
- Low body mass index
- Low dietary calcium
- Vitamin D deficiency
- Tobacco and excessive alcohol use
- Immobilization
- Inadequate physical activity
- Osteoporosis in a first-degree relative, particularly with history of fragility fracture
- Clinical conditions such as thyrotoxicosis, celiac sprue, IBD, cirrhosis, chronic renal disease, organ transplantation, diabetes, HIV, hypogonadism, multiple myeloma, anorexia nervosa, and rheumatologic and autoimmune disorders
- Medications such as oral and high-dose inhaled corticosteroids, anticoagulants (long-term use), aromatase inhibitors for breast cancer, methotrexate, selected antiseizure medications, immunosuppressive agents, proton-pump inhibitors (long-term use), and antigonadal therapy for prostate cancer

Screening Recommendations. The U.S. Preventive Services Task Force (USPSTF) gives a grade B recommendation supporting osteoporosis screening for women age ≥65 years and for younger women whose 10-year fracture risk equals or exceeds that of an average-risk 65-year-old white woman.[34] The USPSTF finds that evidence about risks and benefits for men is insufficient (I statement) for recommending routine screening. However, the American College of Physicians recommends that clinicians periodically assess older men for osteoporosis risk and measure bone density for those at increased risk who are candidates for drug therapy.[37] Screen your patients for the many risk factors listed on the preceding page, and proceed to further assessment.

Measuring Bone Density. Bone strength depends on bone quality, bone density, and overall bone size. Because there is no direct measure of bone strength, bone mineral density (BMD)—which provides roughly 70% of bone strength—is used as a reasonable surrogate. Dual energy x-ray absorptiometry (DEXA) scanning of the lumbar spine and femoral neck is the optimal standard for measuring bone density, diagnosing osteoporosis, and guiding treatment decisions. DEXA measurement of bone density at the femoral neck is considered the best predictor of hip fracture.

Bone mass peaks by age 30 years. Bone loss from age-related declines in estrogen and testosterone is initially rapid, then slows and becomes continuous.

The World Health Organization (WHO) scoring criteria for *T scores* and *Z scores,* measured in standard deviations (SDs), are used worldwide. A 1.0 SD decrease in BMD is associated with a twofold increased risk for a fragility fracture.

World Health Organization Bone Density Criteria

- **Osteoporosis:** T score < −2.5 (>2.5 SDs below the young adult mean)
- **Osteopenia:** T score between −1.0 and −2.5 (1.0 to 2.5 SDs below the young adult mean)

Bone densitometry scoring also includes Z scores representing comparisons with age-matched controls. These measurements are useful for determining whether bone loss is caused by an underlying disease or condition.

Assessing Fracture Risk. The USPSTF recommends using WHO's Fracture Risk Assessment (FRAX) calculator. The FRAX calculator generates a 10-year osteoporotic fracture risk based on age; gender; weight; height; parental fracture history; use of glucocorticoids; presence of RA or conditions associated with secondary osteoporosis; tobacco and heavy alcohol use; and, when available, femoral neck BMD. The FRAX calculator also provides a 10-year hip fracture risk. The website for the FRAX Calculator for Assessing Fracture Risk for the United States is http://www.shef.ac.uk/FRAX/tool.jsp?country=9.

FRAX has been validated for African American, Hispanic, and Asian women in the United States and has calculators that are continent- and country-specific.

The USPSTF recommends using a *10-year osteoporotic fracture risk threshold of 9.3%* when considering bone density screening in women ages 50 to 64 years. Screening decisions for women in this age range should account for menopausal status, clinical judgment, and patient preferences and values.

Treating Osteoporosis and Preventing Falls

Calcium and Vitamin D. *Calcium,* the most abundant mineral in the body, is essential for bone health, muscle function, nerve transmission, vascular function, and intracellular signaling and hormonal secretion.[38] Less than 1% of total body calcium supports these metabolic functions; the remaining 99% is stored in teeth and bones. Serum calcium is tightly regulated. The body relies on bone tissue, and not dietary calcium, to maintain stable concentrations in blood, muscle, and intracellular fluid. Bone is subject to constant remodeling from calcium deposition and resorption; the balance between these processes varies during the different stages of life.

Humans acquire *vitamin D* from sunlight, food, and dietary supplements.[38] Vitamin D from the skin and diet is metabolized in the liver to 25-hydroxyvitamin D (25[OH]D), the best determinant of vitamin D status. Serum 25[OH]D is then metabolized in the kidneys to 1,25-dihydroxyvitamin D (1,25[OH]$_2$D), the most active form of vitamin D. Without vitamin D, less than 25% of dietary calcium is absorbed. Parathyroid hormone (PTH) enhances renal tubular absorption of calcium and stimulates the conversion of 25[OH]D to 1,25[OH]$_2$D. PTH also activates osteoblasts, which lay down new bone matrix, and indirectly stimulates osteoclasts, which dissolve bone matrix.

A previous low-impact fracture from standing height or lower is the greatest risk factor for subsequent fracture.

In 2010, the Institute of Medicine (IOM) issued dietary intake recommendations for calcium and vitamin D (see below).[39] The IOM report concluded that serum 25[OH]D levels of 20 ng/mL are sufficient to maintain bone health and warned of potential adverse effects with levels above 50 ng/mL. The IOM reported insufficient evidence to establish nutritional requirements based on studies of the benefits of vitamin D relating to cardiovascular disease, cancer, diabetes, infections, immune disorders, and other extraskeletal conditions. The USPSTF also cited insufficient evidence for determining whether benefits outweighed the harms of screening for vitamin D deficiency in asymptomatic adults (I statement).[40]

Based on review of randomized controlled trial data, the USPSTF also made recommendations about vitamin D and calcium supplementation for the *primary prevention of fractures*. They concluded that evidence was insufficient to recommend supplementation in premenopausal women or men (I statement). Although evidence for supplementation in postmenopausal women was similarly insufficient, the USPSTF did advise against daily supplements <400 International Units of vitamin D_3 and <1,000 mg of calcium (grade D).[41]

Meta-analyses have suggested that *calcium supplements for osteoporosis* are associated with an increased risk for cardiovascular disease events, especially myocardial infarctions.[42] However, several subsequent expert reviews concluded that available evidence did not support a causal association between calcium supplements and cardiovascular disease risk; authors advised that individuals with inadequate dietary calcium intake should use supplements to promote bone health.[43,44] Combined calcium and vitamin D supplementation is associated with a slightly increased risk for kidney stones.[41] No studies have reported harm associated with calcium intake from dietary sources.

Recommended Dietary Intakes of Calcium and Vitamin D for Adults (Institute of Medicine 2010)

Age Group	Calcium (Elemental) mg/d	Vitamin D IU/d
19–50 yrs	1,000	600
51–70 yrs		
Women	1,200	600
Men	1,000	600
71 and older	1,200	800

Source: Ross AC, Manson JE, Abrams SA, et al. The 2011 report on dietary reference intakes for calcium and vitamin D from the Institute of Medicine: what clinicians need to know. *J Clin Endocrinol Metab.* 2011;96:53.

There are two main forms of calcium supplements, calcium carbonate and calcium citrate. Supplements contain variable amounts of elemental calcium.[38] Patients can read these amounts on the Supplement Facts panel. Calcium carbonate is less expensive and should be consumed with food. Calcium citrate is absorbed more easily in individuals with reduced levels of stomach acid and can be taken with or without food. Calcium absorption depends on the total amount consumed at one time—absorption diminishes at higher doses. Counsel patients to take doses of 500 mg at two separate times each day. Vitamin D supplements

See Table 4-5, Nutrition Counseling: Sources of Nutrients, p. 143, for food sources of calcium and vitamin D.

are available in two forms, D_2 (ergocalciferol) and D_3 (cholecalciferol); D_3 increases serum 25(OH)D levels more effectively than D_2.[45]

Antiresorptive and Anabolic Agents. Antiresorptive agents inhibit osteoclast activity and slow bone remodeling, allowing better mineralization of bone matrix and stabilization of the trabecular microarchitecture. These agents include bisphosphonates, selective estrogen-receptor modulators (SERMs), calcitonin, and postmenopausal estrogen. Bisphosphonates are considered the first-line therapy for osteoporosis. Randomized placebo-controlled trials have shown that bisphosphonates, SERMs, estrogen, calcitonin, and PTH significantly reduce risks for vertebral fractures in postmenopausal women; evidence is less conclusive for nonvertebral fractures, and there are no trial data for treating men.[46] Estrogen therapy is now contraindicated due to associated risks of breast cancer and vascular thrombosis.[47] Bisphosphonates have been linked to rare risks of osteonecrosis of the jaw and atypical femur fractures, and SERMs increase the risk for thromboembolic events.[46]

Anabolic agents such as PTH stimulate bone formation by acting primarily on osteoblasts but require subcutaneous administration and monitoring for hypercalcemia. PTH is reserved for patients with severe osteoporosis (T scores < −3.5 or < −2.5 with a fragility fracture) or those who have failed or not tolerated other therapies.[48]

Preventing Falls. More than one in three adults over age 65 years fall each year. Falls are the leading cause of fatal and nonfatal injuries among older adults and account for over $20 billion in direct clinical costs.[49,50] Falls can result in loss of independence in up to 30% of those suffering injuries that limit their mobility. One third of community-dwelling adults will remain in a nursing home for at least 1 year following a hip fracture. Risk factors for falls include increasing age, impaired gait and balance, postural hypotension, loss of strength, medication use, comorbid illness, depression, cognitive impairment, and visual deficits.

The USPSTF gives a grade B recommendation for providing exercise or physical therapy and/or vitamin D supplementation to prevent falls among at-risk community-dwelling adults ages ≥65 years.[51] Effective exercise interventions target balance, gait, and strength training. The USPSTF also recommends daily vitamin D supplementation of 600 to 800 International Units; it found insufficient evidence for or against interventions such as vision correction, discontinuing medications, education or counseling, and home hazard modifications. However, poor lighting, stairs, chairs at awkward heights, slippery or irregular surfaces, and ill-fitting shoes are environmental hazards that are readily corrected. Work with your patients and their families to modify such risks whenever possible, and request home health assessments to target needed home safety measures.

See Chapter 14, Female Genitalia, p. 582, for discussion of hormone replacement therapy.

See also Chapter 20, Assessing Older Adults, for Further Assessment for Preventing Falls, pp. 987–989.

Once injured, articular cartilage is replaced by less resilient fibrocartilage, increasing risk of pain and OA.

Examination of Specific Joints: Anatomy and Physiology and Techniques of Examination

Steps for Examining the Joints

1. Inspect for joint symmetry, alignment, bony deformities, and swelling
2. Inspect and palpate surrounding tissues for skin changes, nodules, muscle atrophy, tenderness
3. Assess range of motion and maneuvers to test joint function and stability and the integrity of ligaments, tendons, bursae, especially if pain or trauma
4. Assess any areas of inflammation, especially tenderness, swelling, warmth, redness

During the interview, the patient has shared his or her ability to carry out normal activities of daily living. Keep the patient's baseline level of function in mind as you perform the musculoskeletal examination.

During the general survey, you have assessed the patient's general appearance, body proportions, and ease of movement. Now visualize the underlying anatomy of the joints and recall pertinent elements of the history, for example, the mechanism of injury if there is trauma, or the time course of symptoms and limitations in function in arthritis.

Your examination should be systematic. Include inspection, palpation of bony structures and related joint and soft tissue structures, assessment of range of motion, and *special maneuvers* to test specific movements. Recall that the anatomical shape of each joint determines its range of motion. There are two phases to *range of motion: active* (by the patient) and *passive* (by the examiner).

If patients have painful joints, move them gently, or let the patients demonstrate the movements themselves, showing you how they manage. For injured joints, consider an x-ray before attempting movement.

Tips for Successful Examination of the Musculoskeletal System

- During inspection, look for *symmetry* of involvement. Is the change in joints symmetric on both sides of the body, or is the change only in one or two joints?

  Acute involvement of only one joint suggests trauma, septic arthritis, or crystalline arthritis. *RA* is typically polyarticular and symmetrical.[10,52–54]

  Note any *deformities* or *malalignment of bones or joints.*

  Malalignment occurs in *Dupuytren contracture* (p. 704), bow-legs (*genu varum*) or knock-knees (*genu valgum*).

  (continued)

Tips for Successful Examination of the Musculoskeletal System (*continued*)

- Use inspection and palpation to assess the *surrounding tissues*, noting skin changes, subcutaneous nodules, and muscle atrophy. Note any *crepitus*, an audible or palpable crunching during movement of tendons or ligaments over bone or areas of cartilage loss. This may occur in joints without pain but is more significant when associated with symptoms or signs.

- Test range of motion and maneuvers (described for each joint) to demonstrate *limitations in range of motion* or *joint instability* from excess mobility of joint ligaments, called *ligamentous laxity*.

- Finally, test *muscle strength* to aid in the assessment of joint function (for these techniques, see Chapter 17, pp. 743–748).

Look for subcutaneous nodules in *RA* or *rheumatic fever;* effusion in trauma; crepitus over inflamed joints in *OA* or over the inflamed tendon sheaths of *tenosynovitis.*

Decreased range of motion is present in arthritis, joints with tissue inflammation or surrounding fibrosis, or bony fixation (*ankylosis*). Anterior cruciate ligament (ACL) laxity occurs in knee trauma; muscle atrophy and weakness is seen in *RA.*

The detail needed for examining joints varies widely. This section presents examination techniques for both comprehensive and targeted assessment of joint function. Patients with extensive or severe musculoskeletal problems will require more time.

See briefer examination techniques for patients without joint symptoms in Chapter 1, Overview: Physical Examination and History Taking, pp. 12–13, and Chapter 4, Beginning the Examination: General Survey, Vital Signs, and Pain, p. 122.

Review the flowchart showing the Approach to Musculoskeletal Complaints (Fig. 16-2, p. 627) to help organize your approach to the examination. Inspect and palpate any joints with signs of inflammation.

Assessing the Four Signs of Inflammation

- *Swelling.* Palpable swelling may involve: (1) the synovial membrane, which can feel boggy or doughy; (2) effusion from excess synovial fluid within the joint space; or (3) soft tissue structures, such as bursae, tendons, and tendon sheaths.

Palpable bogginess or doughiness of the synovial membrane indicates *synovitis,* which is often accompanied by effusion. Palpable joint fluid is present in effusion, tenderness over the tendon sheaths in *tendinitis.*

- *Warmth.* Use the backs of your fingers to compare the involved joint with its unaffected contralateral joint, or with nearby tissues if both joints are involved.

Increased warmth is seen in arthritis, tendinitis, bursitis, and *osteomyelitis.*

- *Redness.* Redness of the overlying skin is the least common sign of inflammation near the joints and is usually seen in more superficial joints like fingers, toes, and knees.

Redness over a tender joint suggests septic or crystalline arthritis, or possibly RA.

- *Pain or tenderness.* Try to identify the specific anatomic structure that is tender.

Diffuse tenderness and warmth over a thickened synovium suggest arthritis or infection; focal tenderness suggests injury and trauma.

Temporomandibular Joint

Overview, Bony Structures, and Joints. The temporomandibular joint (TMJ) is the most active joint in the body, opening and closing up to 2,000 times a day (Figs. 16-10 and 16-11). It is formed by the fossa and articular tubercle of the temporal bone and the condyle of the mandible. It lies midway between the external acoustic meatus and the zygomatic arch.

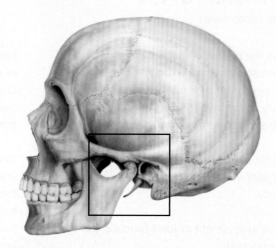

FIGURE 16-10. Temporomandibular joint.

A fibrocartilaginous disc cushions the action of the condyle of the mandible against the synovial membrane and capsule of the articulating surfaces of the temporal bone. Therefore, it is a *condylar synovial joint.*

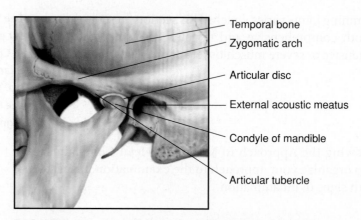

Temporal bone
Zygomatic arch
Articular disc
External acoustic meatus
Condyle of mandible
Articular tubercle

FIGURE 16-11. Temporomandibular joint, inset.

Muscle Groups and Additional Structures. The principal muscles opening the mouth are the *external pterygoids* (Fig. 16-12). Closing the mouth are the muscles innervated by cranial nerve V, the trigeminal nerve— the *masseter,* the *temporalis,* and the *internal pterygoids* (see p. 716).

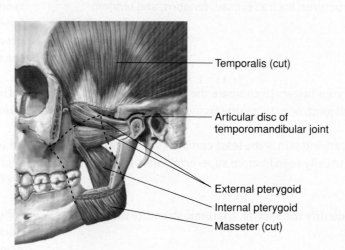

Temporalis (cut)
Articular disc of temporomandibular joint
External pterygoid
Internal pterygoid
Masseter (cut)

FIGURE 16-12. TMJ muscles.

Techniques of Examination

Inspection and Palpation.   Inspect the face for symmetry. Inspect the TMJ for swelling or redness. Swelling may appear as a rounded bulge approximately 0.5 cm anterior to the external auditory meatus.

To locate and palpate the joint, place the tips of your index fingers just in front of the tragus of each ear and ask the patient to open his or her mouth (Fig. 16-13). The fingertips should drop into the joint spaces as the mouth opens. Check for smooth range of motion; note any swelling or tenderness. Snapping or clicking may be felt or heard in normal people.

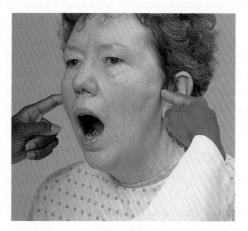

FIGURE 16-13.   **Palpate the TMJ.**

Palpate the muscles of mastication:

■ The *masseters,* externally at the angle of the mandible

■ The *temporal muscles,* externally during clenching and relaxation of the jaw

■ The *pterygoid muscles,* internally between the tonsillar pillars at the mandible

Range of Motion and Maneuvers.   The TMJ has glide and hinge motions in its upper and lower portions, respectively. Grinding or chewing consists primarily of gliding movements in the upper compartments.

Range of motion is threefold: ask the patient to demonstrate opening and closing, protrusion and retraction (by jutting the mandible forward), and lateral, or side-to-side, motion. Normally, as the mouth is opened wide, three fingers can be inserted between the incisors. During normal protrusion of the jaw, the bottom teeth can be placed in front of the upper teeth.

The Shoulder

Overview.   The glenohumeral joint of the shoulder is distinguished by wide-ranging movement in all directions. This joint is largely uninhibited by bony structures. The humeral head contacts less than one third of the surface area of the glenoid fossa and essentially dangles from the scapula, attached by the joint

Facial asymmetry is seen in *TMJ disorders,* a category of orofacial pain with multifactorial etiologies; typically, there is unilateral chronic pain with chewing, jaw clenching, or teeth grinding, often associated with stress and accompanied by headache.[55,56] Pain with chewing also occurs in *trigeminal neuralgia* and *temporal arteritis.*

Swelling, tenderness, and decreased range of motion signal TMJ inflammation or arthritis.

TMJ dislocation can be caused by trauma.

Palpable crepitus or clicking is present in poor occlusion, meniscus injury, or synovial swelling from trauma.

In *TMJ syndrome,* there is pain and tenderness with palpation.

capsule, the intra-articular capsular ligaments, the glenoid labrum, and a meshwork of muscles and tendons.

The shoulder derives its mobility from a complex interconnected structure of three joints, three large bones, and three principal muscle groups, often referred to as the *shoulder girdle*. These structures are viewed as *dynamic stabilizers*, which are capable of movement, or *static stabilizers*, which are incapable of movement.

■ *Dynamic stabilizers:* These consist of the *SITS muscles of the rotator cuff* (**S**upraspinatus, **I**nfraspinatus, **T**eres minor, and **S**ubscapularis), which move the humerus and compress and stabilize the humeral head within the glenoid cavity.

■ *Static stabilizers:* These are the bony structures of the shoulder girdle, the labrum, the articular capsule, and the glenohumeral ligaments. The *labrum* is a fibrocartilaginous ring that surrounds the glenoid and deepens its socket, providing greater stability to the humeral head. The joint capsule is strengthened by tendons of the rotator cuff and glenohumeral ligaments, adding to joint stability.

Bony Structures. The bony structures of the shoulder include the humerus, the clavicle, and the scapula (Fig. 16-14). The scapula is anchored to the axial skeleton only by the sternoclavicular joint and inserting muscles, often called the *scapulothoracic articulation* because it is not a true joint.

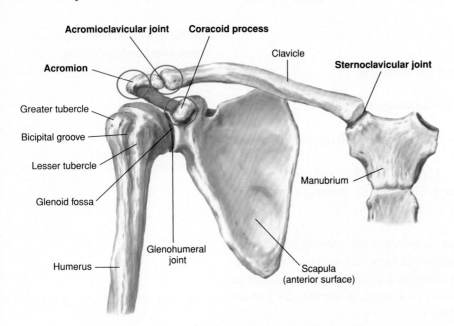

FIGURE 16-14. **Bony anatomy of the shoulder.**

Identify the *manubrium,* the *sternoclavicular joint,* and the *clavicle.* Also identify the *tip of the acromion,* the *greater tubercle of the humerus,* and the *coracoid process,* which are important landmarks of shoulder anatomy.

This muscular meshwork can make it difficult to distinguish shoulder from neck disorders.

Joints. Three different joints articulate at the shoulder:

■ The *glenohumeral joint*. In this joint, the head of the humerus articulates with the shallow glenoid fossa of the scapula. This joint is deeply situated and normally not palpable. It is a ball-and-socket joint, allowing the arm its wide arc of movement—*flexion, extension, abduction* (movement away from the trunk), *adduction* (movement toward the trunk), *rotation*, and *circumduction*.

■ The *sternoclavicular joint*. The convex medial end of the clavicle articulates with the concave hollow in the upper sternum.

■ The *acromioclavicular joint*. The lateral end of the clavicle articulates with the acromion process of the scapula.

Muscle Groups. Three groups of muscles attach at the shoulder:

The Scapulohumeral Group.   This group extends from the scapula to the humerus and includes the muscles inserting directly on the humerus, namely the SITS muscles of the rotator cuff:

■ *Supraspinatus*—runs above the glenohumeral joint; inserts on the greater tubercle

■ *Infraspinatus* and *teres minor*—cross the glenohumeral joint posteriorly; insert on the greater tubercle

■ *Subscapularis* (not illustrated)—originates on the anterior surface of the scapula and crosses the joint anteriorly; inserts on the lesser tubercle

The scapulohumeral group rotates the shoulder laterally (the *rotator cuff*) and depresses and rotates the head of the humerus (Fig. 16-15). See pp. 653–654 for discussion of rotator cuff injuries.

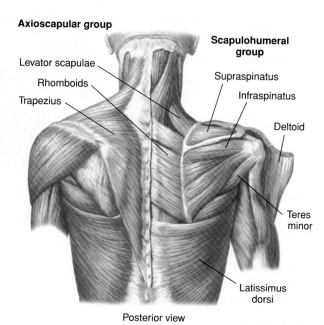

FIGURE 16-15. **Scapulohumeral and axioscapular groups.**

The Axioscapular Group. This group attaches the scapula to the trunk and includes the trapezius, rhomboids, serratus anterior, and levator scapulae (Fig. 16-15). These muscles rotate the scapula and pull the shoulder posteriorly.

The Axiohumeral Group. This group attaches the humerus to the trunk and includes the pectoralis major and minor and the latissimus dorsi (Fig. 16-16). These muscles rotate the shoulder internally.

The biceps and triceps, which connect the scapula to the bones of the forearm, are also involved in shoulder movement, especially forward flexion (biceps) and extension (triceps).

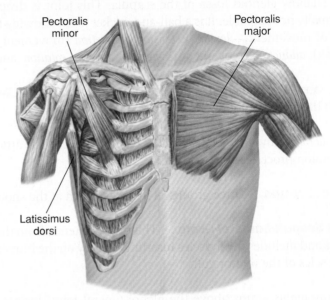

Anterior view

FIGURE 16-16. **Axiohumeral group.**

Additional Structures. Also important to shoulder movement are the *articular capsule* and *bursae.* Surrounding the glenohumeral joint is a fibrous articular capsule formed by the tendon insertions of the rotator cuff and other capsular structures. The loose fit of the capsule allows the shoulder bones to separate, and contributes to the shoulder's wide range of movement. The capsule is lined by a synovial membrane with two outpouchings—the *subscapular bursa* and the *synovial sheath of the tendon of the long head of the biceps.*

To locate the biceps tendon, rotate your arm externally and find the tendinous cord that runs just medial to the greater tubercle (Fig. 16-17). Roll it under your fingers. This is the tendon of the long head of the biceps. It runs in the bicipital groove between the greater and lesser tubercles.

The principal bursa of the shoulder is the *subacromial bursa,* positioned between the acromion and the head of the humerus and overlying the supraspinatus tendon. Abduction of the shoulder compresses this bursa. Normally, the supraspinatus tendon and the subacromial bursa are not palpable. However, if the bursal surfaces are inflamed (*subacromial bursitis*), there may be tenderness just below the tip of the acromion, pain with abduction and rotation, and loss of smooth movement.

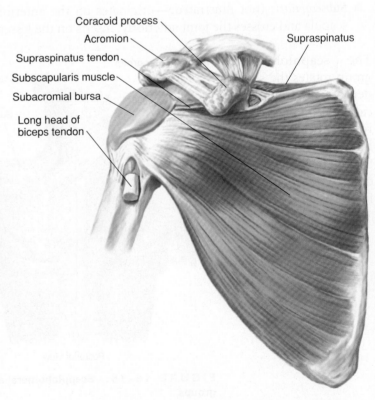

FIGURE 16-17. **Anterior view of the shoulder.**

Techniques of Examination

Inspection. Inspect the shoulder and shoulder girdle anteriorly, then the scapulae and related muscles posteriorly.

Note any swelling, deformity, muscle atrophy or *fasciculations* (fine tremors of the muscles), or abnormal positioning.

Look for swelling of the joint capsule anteriorly or a bulge in the subacromial bursa under the deltoid muscle. Survey the entire upper extremity for color change, skin alteration, or unusual bony contours.

Palpation. Begin by palpating the bony contours and structures of the shoulder, then palpate any area of pain.

- Beginning medially, at the *sternoclavicular joint,* trace the clavicle laterally with your fingers.

- From behind, follow the bony spine of the scapula laterally and upward until it becomes the acromion (**A**), the summit of the shoulder (Fig. 16-18). Its upper surface is rough and slightly convex. Identify the anterior tip of the acromion.

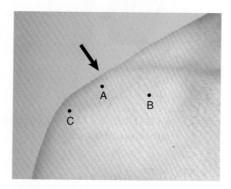

FIGURE 16-18. **Bony landmarks of the shoulder.**

- With your index finger on top of the acromion, just behind its tip, press medially with your thumb to find the slightly elevated ridge that marks the distal end of the clavicle at the *acromioclavicular joint* (shown by the *arrow*). Move your thumb medially and down a short step to the next bony prominence, the *coracoid process* (**B**) of the scapula.

- With your thumb on the coracoid process, allow your fingers to fall on and grasp the lateral aspect of the humerus to palpate the *greater tubercle* (**C**), where the SITS muscles insert.

- Next, to palpate the *biceps tendon* in the intertubercular bicipital groove, keep your thumb on the coracoid process and your fingers on the lateral aspect of the humerus (Fig. 16-19). Remove your index finger and place it halfway between the coracoid process and the greater tubercle on the anterior surface of the arm. As you check for tendon tenderness, rolling the tendon under the fingertips may be helpful. You can also rotate the glenohumeral joint externally, locate the muscle distally near the elbow, and track the muscle and its tendon proximally into the intertubercular groove.

See also Bicipital Tendinitis in Table 16-4, Painful Shoulders, pp. 700–701.

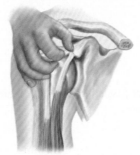

FIGURE 16-19. **Palpate the bicipital groove and tendon.**

- To examine the *subacromial* and *subdeltoid bursae* and the *SITS muscles*, first passively extend the humerus by lifting the elbow posteriorly, which rotates these structures so that they are anterior to the acromion. Palpate carefully over the subacromial and subdeltoid bursae (Figs. 16-20 and 16-21). The underlying palpable SITS muscles are:

Localized tenderness points to *subacromial* or *subdeltoid bursitis,* degenerative changes, or calcific deposits in the rotator cuff. Swelling suggests a *bursal tear* that communicates with the articular cavity.

Tenderness over the SITS muscle insertions and inability to abduct the arm above shoulder level occurs in sprains, tears, and tendon rupture of the rotator cuff, most commonly the *supraspinatus.* See Table 16-4, Painful Shoulders, pp. 700–701.

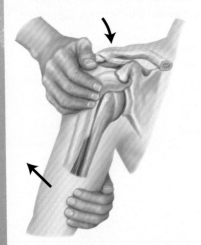

FIGURE 16-20. **Extend the humerus posteriorly.**

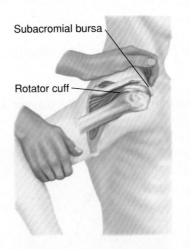

Subacromial bursa

Rotator cuff

FIGURE 16-21. **Palpate the subacromial bursa.**

- Supraspinatus—directly under the acromion

- Infraspinatus—posterior to supraspinatus

- Teres minor—posterior and inferior to the supraspinatus

- Subscapularis—inserts anteriorly and is not palpable

- The fibrous articular capsule and the broad flat tendons of the rotator cuff are so closely associated that they must be examined simultaneously. Swelling in the capsule and synovial membrane is often best detected by looking down on the shoulder from above. Palpate the capsule and synovial membrane beneath the anterior and posterior acromion to check for injury or arthritis.

Tenderness and effusion suggest glenohumeral joint synovitis. If the margins of the capsule and synovial membrane are palpable, a moderate to large effusion is present; minimal synovitis cannot be detected on palpation.

Range of Motion and Maneuvers

Range of Motion. The six motions of the shoulder girdle are flexion, extension, abduction, adduction, and internal and external rotation.

Standing in front of the patient, watch for smooth fluid movement as the patient performs the motions listed in the table below. Learn the specific muscles responsible for each motion. Note the clear simple instructions that prompt the requested patient response. Test muscle strength.

Restricted range of motion occurs in *bursitis, capsulitis, rotator cuff tears* or *sprains,* and *tendinitis.*

Shoulder Girdle Range of Motion

Flexion

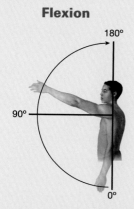

Principal Muscles Affecting Movement
Anterior deltoid, pectoralis major (clavicular head), coracobrachialis, biceps brachii

Patient Instructions
"Raise your arms in front of you and overhead."

Extension

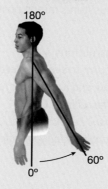

Principal Muscles Affecting Movement
Latissimus dorsi, teres major, posterior deltoid, triceps brachii (long head)

Patient Instructions
"Raise your arms behind you."

Abduction

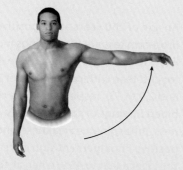

Principal Muscles Affecting Movement
Supraspinatus, middle deltoid, serratus anterior (via upward rotation of the scapula)

Patient Instructions
"Raise your arms out to the side and overhead."

Adduction

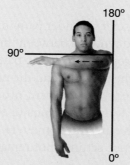

Principal Muscles Affecting Movement
Pectoralis major, coracobrachialis, latissimus dorsi, teres major, subscapularis

Patient Instructions
"Cross your arm in front of your body."

(*continued*)

Note that to test *pure glenohumeral motion,* the patient should raise the arms to shoulder level at 90°, with palms facing down. To test *scapulothoracic motion,* the patient should turn the palms up and raise the arms an additional 60°. The final 30° tests combined glenohumeral and scapulothoracic motion.

Shoulder Girdle Range of Motion (continued)

Internal Rotation

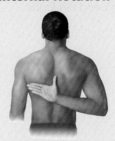

External Rotation

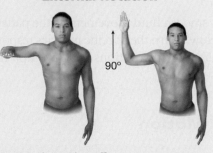

90°

Principal Muscles Affecting Movement

Subscapularis, anterior deltoid, pectoralis major, teres major, latissimus dorsi

Patient Instructions

"Place one hand behind your back and touch your shoulder blade."

Identify the highest midline spinous process the patient is able to reach.

Principal Muscles Affecting Movement

Infraspinatus, teres minor, posterior deltoid

Patient Instructions

"Raise your arm to shoulder level; bend your elbow and rotate your forearm toward the ceiling." OR

"Place one hand behind your neck or head as if you are brushing your hair."

Maneuvers.   The examination of the shoulder often requires evaluation of specific motions and structures. There are more than 150 different maneuvers for testing shoulder function, but few are well studied. Common recommended maneuvers based on available evidence and analyses from three recent reviews[58–60] are described on pp. 653–655. Although performing these maneuvers takes supervision and practice, they increase the likelihood of identifying shoulder pathology.

Rotator cuff disorders are the most common cause of shoulder pain in primary care. Compression of the rotator cuff muscles and tendons between the head of the humerus and the acromion causes "impingement signs" or pain during shoulder movement. Five maneuvers that have the best LRs and the narrowest confidence intervals are currently recommended:[58–60] one pain provocation test, three strength tests, and one composite test. In composite tests, the patient experiences either pain or weakness during the maneuver. Most of the data on these tests come from specialty practice settings but remain useful for general care.

An age of ≥60 years and a positive drop-arm test are the findings most likely to identify a degenerative rotator cuff tear, with positive LRs of 3.2 and 2.9 to 5.0, respectively. The combined findings of supraspinatus weakness, infraspinatus weakness, and a positive impingement sign increase the LR of a tear to 48.0; when all three are absent, the LR falls to 0.02, virtually ruling out the diagnosis.[57,61]

- ■ *Pain provocation test: painful arc test (subacromial bursa and rotator cuff).* This test has a positive LR of 3.7, which is the highest of all the rotator cuff maneuvers. It also has the best negative LR, 0.36, for ruling out rotator cuff disorders. Other common pain provocation tests are the Neer and Hawkins tests, also included in the box on next page, although their positive LRs are <2, so they are less diagnostic.

■ *Strength tests:* internal rotation lag test *(subscapularis),* external rotation lag test *(supraspinatus and infraspinatus),* and drop arm test *(supraspinatus).* These tests have positive LRs of 7.2, 5.6, and 3.3, respectively.

■ *Composite test:* external rotation resistance test *(infraspinatus).* This test has a positive LR of 2.6. Another common composite test is the empty can test.

Maneuvers for Examining the Shoulder

Structure[57–60]	Maneuver/ Type of Test		
Acromioclavicular Joint	*Crossover* or *crossed body adduction test.* Adduct the patient's arm across the chest.	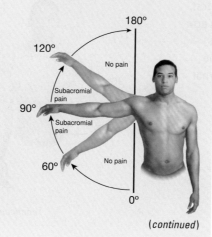	Pain with adduction is a positive test, with a positive LR of 3.7. Acromioclavicular joint tenderness and compression tenderness have low LRs so are not diagnostically helpful.[57]
Overall Shoulder Rotation	*Apley scratch test.* Ask the patient to touch the opposite scapula using the two motions shown below.		Pain during these maneuvers suggests a rotator cuff disorder or adhesive capsulitis.

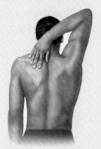 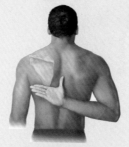

Tests abduction and external rotation.

Tests adduction and internal rotation.

Rotator Cuff *Pain Provocation Tests*	*Painful arc test.* Fully adduct the patient's arm from 0° to 180°.		Shoulder pain from 60° to 120° is a *positive test* for a subacromial impingement/rotator cuff tendinitis disorder, with a positive LR 3.7 and a helpful negative LR of 0.36.

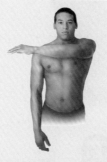

180°
No pain
120°
Subacromial pain
90°
Subacromial pain
60°
No pain
0°

(continued)

Maneuvers for Examining the Shoulder (*continued*)

Structure[57–60]	Maneuver/ Type of Test		

Neer impingement sign. Press on the scapula to prevent scapular motion with one hand, and raise the patient's arm with the other. This compresses the greater tuberosity of the humerus against the acromion.

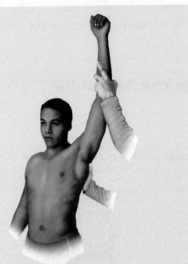

Pain during this maneuver is a *positive test* for a subacromial impingement/ rotator cuff tendinitis disorder, with a positive LR ~1.0 to 1.6.

Hawkins impingement sign. Flex the patient's shoulder and elbow to 90° with the palm facing down. Then, with one hand on the forearm and one on the arm, rotate the arm internally. This compresses the greater tuberosity against the supraspinatus tendon and coracoacromial ligament.

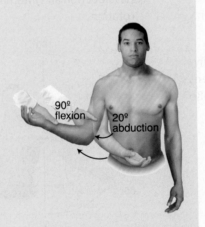

Pain during this maneuver is a *positive test* for supraspinatus impingement/ rotator cuff tendinitis, with a positive LR of ~1.5. When both the Hawkins and Neer signs are absent, the negative LR is helpful at 0.1.

Strength Tests

External rotation lag test. With the patient's arm flexed to 90° with palm up, rotate the arm into full external rotation.

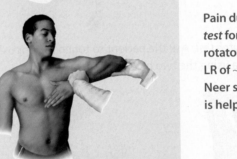

90º flexion

20º abduction

Inability of the patient to maintain external rotation is a *positive test* for supraspinatus and infraspinatus disorders, with a positive LR of 7.2.

(*continued*)

Maneuvers for Examining the Shoulder (*continued*)

Structure[57–60]	Maneuver/ Type of Test		
	Internal rotation lag test. Ask the patient to place the dorsum of the hand on the low back with the elbow flexed to 90°. Then you lift the hand off the back, which further internally rotates the shoulder. Ask the patient to keep the hand in this position.	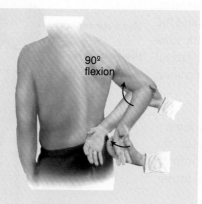 90° flexion	Inability of the patient to hold the hand in this position is *positive test* for a subscapularis disorder, with a positive LR of 5.6 to 6.2 and an excellent negative LR of 0.04.
	Drop-arm test. Ask the patient to fully abduct the arm to shoulder level, up to 90°, and lower it slowly. Note that abduction above shoulder level, from 90° to 120°, reflects action of the deltoid muscle.	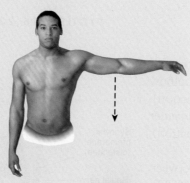	Weakness during this maneuver is a *positive test* for a supraspinatus rotator cuff tear or bicipital tendinitis, with a positive LR of 3.3.
Composite tests	*External rotation resistance test.* Ask the patient to adduct and flex the arm to 90°, with the thumbs turned up. Stabilize the elbow with one hand and apply pressure proximal to the patient's wrist as the patient presses the wrist outward in external rotation.	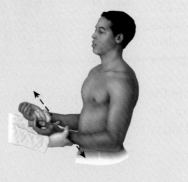	Pain or weakness during this maneuver is a *positive test* for an infraspinatus disorder, with a positive LR of 2.6 and negative LR of 0.49. Limited external rotation points to glenohumeral disease or adhesive capsulitis.
	Empty can test. Elevate the arms to 90° and internally rotate the arms with the thumbs pointing down, as if emptying a can. Ask the patient to resist as you place downward pressure on the arms.	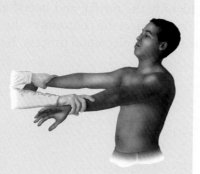	Inability of the patient to hold the arm fully abducted at shoulder level or control lowering the arm is a *positive test* for a suprasinatus rotator cuff tear, with a positive LR of 1.3.

The Elbow

Overview, Bony Structures, and Joints. The elbow helps position the hand in space and stabilizes the lever action of the forearm. The elbow joint is formed by the humerus and the two bones of the forearm, the radius and the ulna (Fig. 16-22). Identify the medial and lateral epicondyles of the humerus and the olecranon process of the ulna.

These bones have three articulations: the *humeroulnar joint,* the *radiohumeral joint,* and the *radioulnar joint.* All three share a large common articular cavity and an extensive synovial lining.

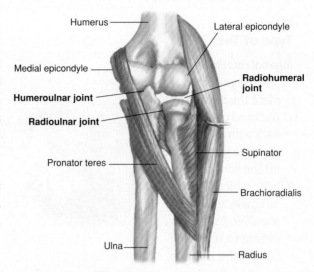

FIGURE 16-22. Left anterior elbow.

Muscle Groups and Additional Structures. Muscles traversing the elbow include the *biceps* and *brachioradialis* (flexion), the *brachialis,* the *triceps* (extension), the *pronator teres* (pronation), and the *supinator* (supination).

Note the location of the *olecranon bursa* between the olecranon process and the skin (Fig. 16-23). The bursa is not normally palpable but swells and becomes tender when inflamed. The *ulnar nerve* runs posteriorly in the ulnar groove between the medial epicondyle and the olecranon process. The radial nerve is adjacent to the lateral epicondyle. On the ventral forearm, the *median nerve* is just medial to the brachial artery in the antecubital fossa.

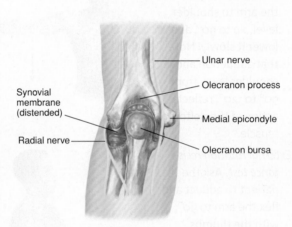

FIGURE 16-23. Left posterior elbow.

Techniques of Examination

Inspection. Support the patient's forearm with your opposite hand so that the elbow is flexed to about 70°. Identify the medial and lateral epicondyles and the olecranon process of the ulna. Inspect the contours of the elbow, including the extensor surface of the ulna and the olecranon process. Note any nodules or swelling.

See Table 16-5, Swollen or Tender Elbows, p. 702.

Swelling over the olecranon process is suspicious for *olecranon bursitis* (see p. 702); inflammation or synovial fluid suggests arthritis.

Palpation. Palpate the olecranon process and press over the epicondyles for tenderness (Fig. 16-24).

Palpate the grooves between the epicondyles and the olecranon process, where the synovium is most easily examined. Normally the synovium and olecranon bursae are not palpable.

The sensitive ulnar nerve can be palpated posteriorly between the olecranon process and the medial epicondyle.

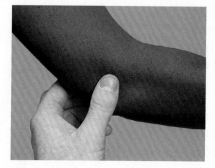

FIGURE 16-24. **Palpate the epicondyles.**

Tenderness distal to the epicondyle is common in *lateral epicondylitis* (tennis elbow) and less common in *medial epicondylitis* (pitcher's or golfer's elbow).

Note any displacement of the olecranon process (Figs. 16-25 and 16-26).

The olecranon is displaced posteriorly in *posterior dislocation of the elbow* and *supracondylar fracture.*

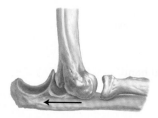

FIGURE 16-25. **Posterior dislocation of the elbow.**

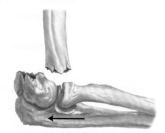

FIGURE 16-26. **Supracondylar fracture of the elbow.**

Range of Motion and Maneuvers. Range of motion includes flexion and extension at the elbow and pronation and supination of the forearm, which also move the wrist and hand (Fig. 16-27). In the box below, note the specific muscles responsible for each motion and the instructions to the patient.

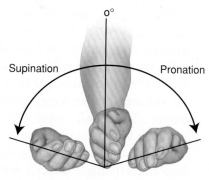

FIGURE 16-27. **Elbow supination and pronation.**

Elbow Range of Motion

Elbow Movement	Primary Muscles Affecting Movement	Patient Instructions
Flexion	Biceps brachii, brachialis, brachioradialis	*"Bend your elbow."*
Extension	Triceps brachii, anconeus	*"Straighten your elbow."*
Supination	Biceps brachii, supinator	*"Turn your palms up, as if carrying a bowl of soup."*
Pronation	Pronator teres, pronator quadratus	*"Turn your palms down."*

After injury, preservation of active range of motion and full elbow extension makes fracture highly unlikely. Full elbow extension has a sensitivity of 84% to >98% and specificity of 48% to >97% for absence of fracture.[62,63] Tenderness over the radial head, olecranon, or medial epicondyle and bruising, plus absent elbow extension, may improve these test characteristics.[64] Full elbow extension also makes intra-articular effusion or hemarthrosis unlikely.

The Wrist and Hands

Overview. The wrist and hands form a complex unit of small highly active joints used almost continuously during waking hours. There is little protection from overlying soft tissue, increasing vulnerability to trauma and disability.

Bony Structures. The wrist includes the distal radius and ulna and eight small carpal bones (Fig. 16-28). At the wrist, identify the bony tips of the radius and the ulna.

Identify the carpal bones distal to the wrist joint, each of the five metacarpals, and the proximal, middle, and distal phalanges. Note that the thumb has only two phalanges.

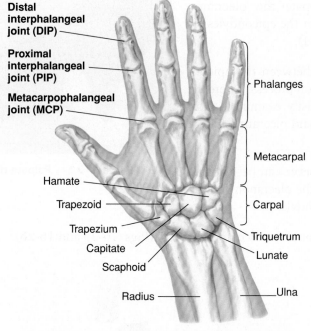

FIGURE 16-28. **Bones of the wrist and hand.**

Joints. The numerous joints of the wrist and hand make the hands unusually dextrous.

- *Wrist joints.* The wrist joints include the *radiocarpal* or *wrist joint,* the *distal radioulnar joint,* and the *intercarpal joints* (Fig. 16-29). The joint capsule, articular disc, and synovial membrane of the wrist join the radius to the ulna and to the proximal carpal bones. On the dorsum of the wrist, locate the groove of the *radiocarpal joint.* This joint provides most of the flexion and extension at the wrist because the ulna does not articulate directly with the carpal bones.

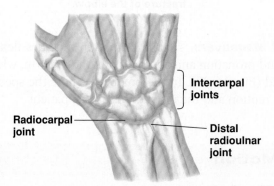

FIGURE 16-29. **Joints of the wrist.**

- *Hand joints.* The joints of the hand include the *metacarpophalangeal joints* (MCPs), the *proximal interphalangeal joints* (PIPs), and the *distal interphalangeal joints* (DIPs). Flex the hand and find the groove marking the MCP joint of each finger (Fig. 16-30). It is distal to the knuckle and is best felt on either side of the extensor tendon.

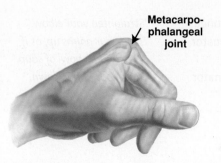

FIGURE 16-30. **Metacarpophalangeal joint.**

Degenerative changes at the first carpometacarpal joint of the thumb are more common in women.

Muscle Groups.   Wrist flexion arises from the two carpal muscles, located on the radial and ulnar surfaces. Two radial and one ulnar muscle provide wrist extension. Supination and pronation are powered by muscle contraction in the forearm.

The thumb is powered by three muscles that form the thenar eminence and provide flexion, abduction, and opposition. The muscles of extension are at the base of the thumb along the radial margin. Movement in the digits depends on action of the flexor and extensor tendons of muscles in the forearm and wrist.

The intrinsic muscles of the hand attaching to the metacarpal bones are involved in flexion (*lumbricals*), abduction (*dorsal interossei*), and adduction (*palmar interossei*) of the fingers.

Additional Structures.   Soft tissue structures, especially tendons and tendon sheaths, are especially important to movement of the wrist and hand. Six extensor tendons and two flexor tendons pass across the wrist and hand to insert on the fingers. Through much of their course these tendons travel in tunnel-like sheaths, generally palpable only when swollen or inflamed.

Be familiar with the structures of the *carpal tunnel,* a channel beneath the palmar surface of the wrist and proximal hand (Fig. 16-31). The channel contains the sheath and flexor tendons of the forearm muscles and the *median nerve.*

Holding the tendons and tendon sheath in place is a transverse ligament, the *flexor retinaculum.* The median nerve lies between the flexor retinaculum and the tendon sheath. The median nerve provides sensation to the palm and the palmar surface of most of the thumb, the second and third digits, and half of the fourth digit. It also innervates the thumb muscles of flexion, abduction, and opposition.

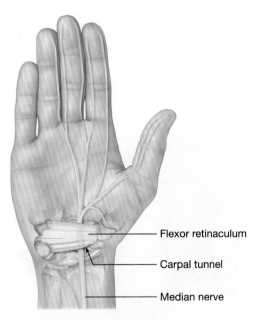

Flexor retinaculum

Carpal tunnel

Median nerve

FIGURE 16-31.   **The carpal tunnel.**

Techniques of Examination

Inspection.   Inspect the position of the hands in motion for smooth natural movement. When the fingers are relaxed they should be slightly flexed; the fingernail edges should be in parallel.

Guarded movement suggests injury. Flexor tendon damage causes abnormal finger alignment.

Inspect the palmar and dorsal surfaces of the wrist and hand carefully for swelling over the joints or signs of trauma.

Diffuse swelling is common in arthritis or infection; local swelling suggests a ganglion. Laceration, puncture, injection marks, burn, or erythema result from trauma. See Table 16-6, Arthritis in the Hands, p. 703, and Table 16-7, Swellings and Deformities of the Hands, p. 704.

Note any deformities of the wrist, hand, or finger bones, as well as any angulation.

Heberden nodes (DIP joints) and Bouchard nodes (PIP joints) are common findings in *OA*. In *RA*, inspect for symmetric deformity in the PIP, MCP, and wrist joints; later, there is MCP subluxation and ulnar deviation.

Observe the contours of the palm, namely the thenar and hypothenar eminences.

Thenar atrophy occurs in median nerve compression from *carpal tunnel syndrome* (sensitivity <50%; specificity >82% to 99%)[65]; in *ulnar nerve compression,* there is hypothenar atrophy.

Note any thickening of the flexor tendons or flexion contractures in the fingers.

Dupuytren flexion contractures in the third, ring, and fifth fingers, arise from thickening of the palmar fascia (see p. 704). Trigger digits are caused by *stenosing tenosynovitis.*[66]

Palpation. At the wrist, palpate the distal radius and ulna on the lateral and medial surfaces (Fig. 16-32). Palpate the groove of each wrist joint with your thumbs on the dorsum of the wrist, your fingers beneath it. Note any swelling, bogginess, or tenderness.

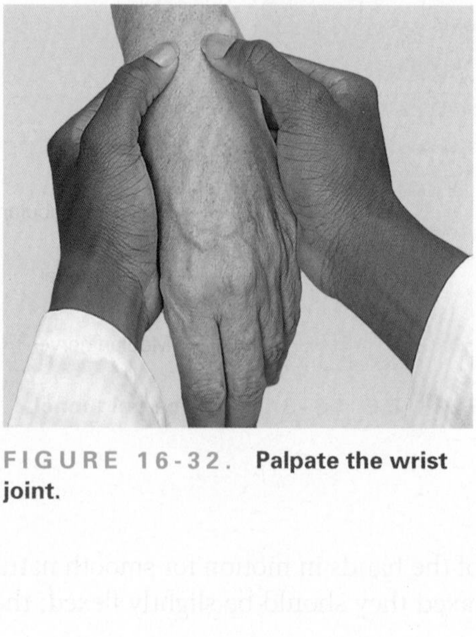

Tenderness over the distal radius after a fall is suspicious for a *Colles fracture.* Bony step-offs also suggest fracture.

In *RA,* there is persisting bilateral swelling and/or tenderness.

FIGURE 16-32. **Palpate the wrist joint.**

Palpate the radial styloid bone and the *anatomic snuffbox,* a hollowed depression just distal to the radial styloid process formed by the abductor and extensor muscles of the thumb (Fig. 16-33). The "snuffbox" is more visible with lateral extension of the thumb away from the hand (abduction).

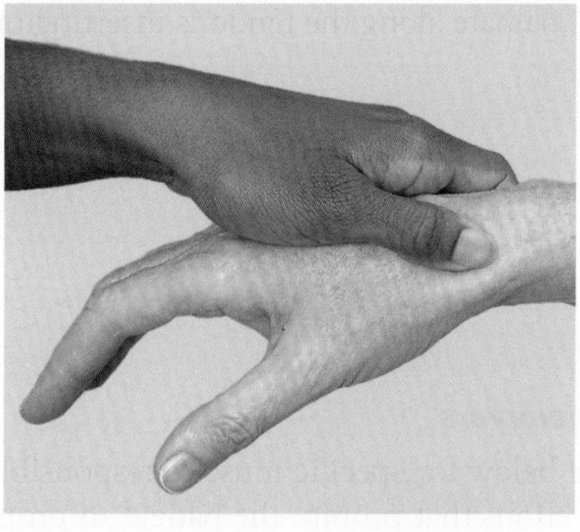

FIGURE 16-33. **Palpate the anatomic snuffbox.**

Tenderness over the extensor and abductor tendons of the thumb at the radial styloid occurs in *de Quervain tenosynovitis* and *gonococcal tenosynovitis.* See Table 16-8, Tendon Sheath, Palmar Space, and Finger Infections, p. 705.

"Snuffbox" tenderness with the wrist in ulnar deviation and pain at the scaphoid tubercle are suspicious for occult *scaphoid fracture,* a common injury.[67] Poor blood supply increases risk of scaphoid bone *avascular necrosis.*

Palpate the eight carpal bones lying distal to the wrist joint, and then each of the five metacarpals and the proximal, middle, and distal phalanges (Fig. 16-34).

Palpate any other area where you suspect an abnormality.

Compress the MCP joints by squeezing the hand from each side between the thumb and fingers. Alternatively, use your thumb to palpate each MCP joint just distal to and on each side of the extensor tendons as your index finger feels the head of the metacarpal in the palm. Note any swelling, bogginess, or tenderness.

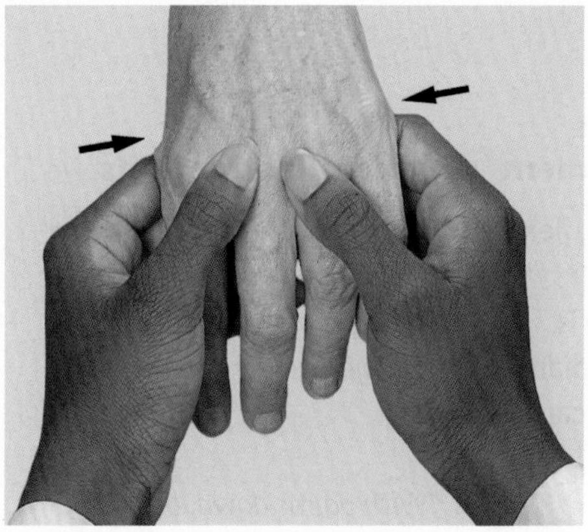

FIGURE 16-34. **Palpate the MCP joints.**

The MCPs are often boggy or tender in *RA,* but are rarely involved in *OA.* Pain with compression also occurs in *posttraumatic arthritis.*

Now examine the fingers and thumb. Palpate the medial and lateral aspects of each PIP joint between your thumb and index finger, again checking for swelling, bogginess, bony enlargement, or tenderness.

There are PIP changes in *RA;* Bouchard nodes in *OA.* Pain at the base of the thumb occurs in *carpometacarpal arthritis.*

Using the same techniques, examine the DIP joints (Fig. 16-36).

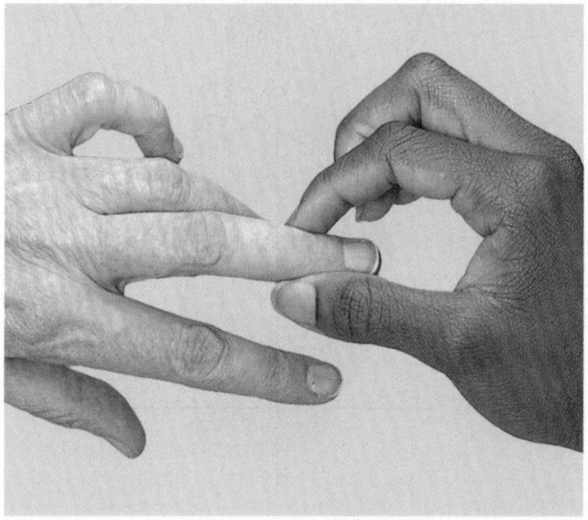

FIGURE 16-35. **Heberden nodes.**

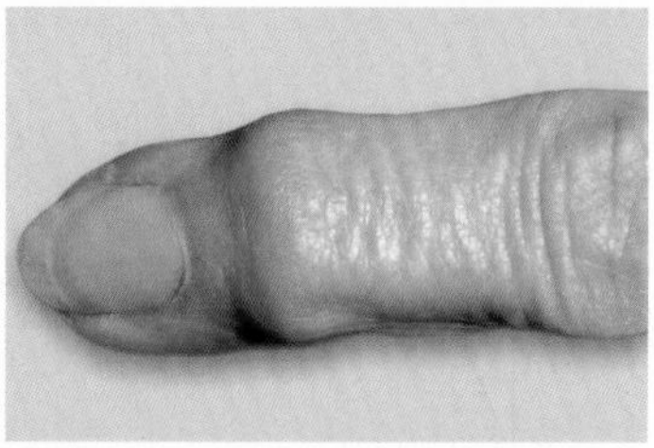

FIGURE 16-36. **Palpate the DIP joints.**

Hard dorsolateral nodules on the DIP joints, or *Heberden nodes* (Fig. 16-35), are common in *OA;* the DIP joints are also involved in *psoriatic arthritis.*

In any area of swelling or inflammation, palpate along the tendons inserting on the thumb and fingers.

Tenderness and swelling occur in *tenosynovitis,* or inflammation of the tendon sheaths. *De Quervain tenosynovitis* involves the extensor and abductor tendons of the thumb as they cross the radial styloid. See Table 16-8, Tendon Sheath, Palmar Space, and Finger Infections, p. 706.

Wrists: Range of Motion and Maneuvers

Range of Motion. Refer to the table below for specific muscles responsible for each movement and use clear instructions that prompt the patient to properly follow your directions. For techniques of testing wrist muscle strength, turn to Chapter 17, The Nervous System, pp. 743–746.

Wrist Range of Motion

Wrist Movement	Primary Muscles Affecting Movement	Patient Instructions
Flexion	Flexor carpi radialis, flexor carpi ulnaris	*"With palms down, point your fingers toward the floor."*
Extension	Extensor carpi ulnaris, extensor carpi radialis longus, extensor carpi radialis brevis	*"With palms down, point your fingers toward the ceiling."*
Adduction (radial deviation)	Flexor carpi ulnaris	*"With palms down, bring your fingers toward the midline."*
Abduction (ulnar deviation)	Flexor carpi radialis	*"With palms down, bring your fingers away from the midline."*

Arthritis, tenosynovitis, and *Dupuytren contracture* all impair range of motion (Figs. 16-37 and 16-38). See Table 16-7, Swellings and Deformities of the Hands, p. 704.

See p. 659 for discussion of pronation and supination, which also involve the wrist and hand.

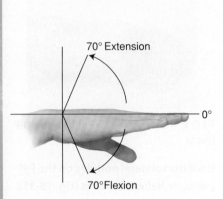

FIGURE 16-37. **Hand flexion and extension.**

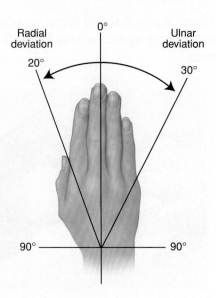

FIGURE 16-38. **Radial and ulnar deviation.**

Maneuvers. Maneuvers for assessing conditions at the wrist are listed on the next page. For complaints of nocturnal hand or arm numbness (*paresthesias*), dropping objects, inability to twist lids off jars, aching at the wrist or even the forearm, and numbness of the first three digits, test for *carpal tunnel syndrome,* the most common entrapment neuropathy, involving compression of the median nerve. Learn the distribution of the median, radial, and ulnar nerve innervations of the wrist and hand (Figs. 16-39 and 16-40). Remember to assess more proximal causes of wrist and hand pain arising from cervical radiculopathy.

Forceful repetitive handwork with wrist flexion such as keyboarding or mail sorting, vibration, cold environments, wrist anatomy, pregnancy, RA, diabetes, and hypothyroidism are risk factors for *carpal tunnel syndrome.*

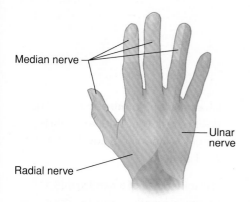

Median nerve

Ulnar nerve

Radial nerve

FIGURE 16-39. **Dorsal surface.**

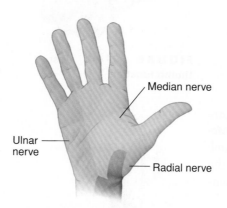

Median nerve

Ulnar nerve

Radial nerve

FIGURE 16-40. **Volar surface.**

You can test sensation as follows:

- Pulp of the index finger—median nerve

- Pulp of the fifth finger—ulnar nerve

- Dorsal web space of the thumb and index finger—radial nerve

Decreased sensation in the median nerve territory is a common sign of *carpal tunnel syndrome* (sensitivity to pinprick and two-point discrimination <50%; specificity >85%; positive LR of hypalgesia is 3.1).[67,68]

Hand Grip. Test *hand grip strength* by asking the patient to grasp your second and third fingers (Fig. 16-41). This tests function of wrist joints, the finger flexors, and the intrinsic muscles and joints of the hand.

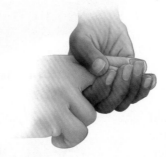

FIGURE 16-41. **Test grip strength.**

Decreased grip strength is a *positive test* for weakness of the finger flexors and/or intrinsic muscles of the hand. It also results from inflammatory or degenerative arthritis, *carpal tunnel syndrome,* epicondylitis, and *cervical radiculopathy.* Grip weakness plus wrist pain are often present in *de Quervain tenosynovitis.*

Thumb Movement. To test thumb function, ask the patient to grasp the thumb against the palm and then move the wrist toward the midline in ulnar deviation (sometimes called the *Finkelstein test*), as shown in Figure 16-42.

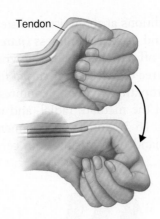

Tendon

FIGURE 16-42. Test thumb function.

Pain during this maneuver identifies *de Quervain tenosynovitis* from inflammation of the abductor pollicis longus and extensor pollicis brevis tendons and tendon sheaths.

Carpal Tunnel Syndrome—Thumb Abduction, Tinel Test, and Phalen Test for Median Nerve Compression. To test *thumb abduction*, ask the patient to raise the thumb straight up as you apply downward resistance (Fig. 16-43).

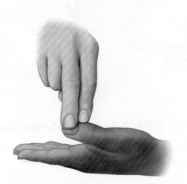

FIGURE 16-43. Test thumb abduction.

Weakness on thumb abduction is a *positive test*. The abductor pollicis longus is innervated only by the median nerve.

Combined use of a hand symptom diagram, median nerve territory hypalgesia, and thumb abduction weakness are most consistent with nerve conduction diagnoses of *carpal tunnel syndrome*.[67,69]

Test *Tinel sign* by tapping lightly over the course of the median nerve in the carpal tunnel as shown in Figure 16-44.

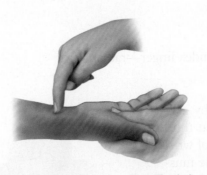

FIGURE 16-44. Test Tinel sign.

Aching and numbness in the median nerve distribution is a *positive test* (sensitivity 23% to 60%; specificity 64% to 91%; LR ≤1.5).[68]

To test *Phalen sign*, ask the patient to hold the wrists in flexion for 60 seconds with the elbows fully extended (Fig. 16-45). Alternatively, ask the patient to press the backs of both hands together to form right angles. These maneuvers compress the median nerve.

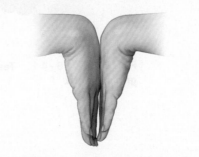

FIGURE 16-45. Test Phalen sign.

Numbness and tingling in the median nerve distribution within 60 seconds is a *positive test* (sensitivity 10% to 91%; specificity 33% to 86%; LR ≤1.5).[68]

Tinel and Phalen signs do not reliably predict positive electrodiagnosis of carpal tunnel disease.[69]

Fingers and Thumbs: Range of Motion and Maneuvers

Range of Motion—Fingers. Assess flexion, extension, abduction, and adduction of the fingers.

- *Flexion and extension* (Fig. 16-46). For *flexion,* to test the lumbricals and finger flexor muscles, ask the patient to *"Make a tight fist with each hand, thumb across the knuckles."* For *extension,* to test the finger extensor muscles, ask the patient to *"Extend and spread the fingers."* At the MCPs, the fingers may extend beyond the neutral position.

  Test the flexion and extension of the PIP and DIP joints (lumbrical muscles). The fingers should open and close easily.

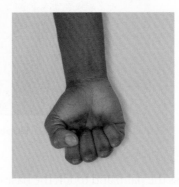

FIGURE 16-46. **Test finger flexion.**

- *Abduction and adduction* (Fig. 16-47). Ask the patient to spread the fingers apart (abduction from dorsal interossei) and back together (adduction from palmar interossei). Check for smooth, coordinated movement.

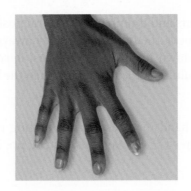

FIGURE 16-47. **Test finger abduction.**

Inspect for impaired hand movement in arthritis, trigger finger, and Dupuytren contracture.

Thumbs. At the *thumb,* assess *flexion, extension, abduction, adduction,* and *opposition* (Figs. 16-48 to 16-51). Each of these movements is powered by a related muscle of the thumb.

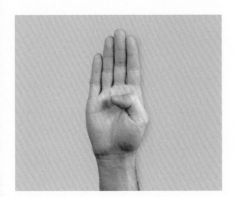

FIGURE 16-48. **Flexion.**

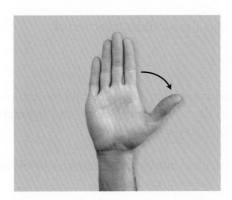

FIGURE 16-49. **Extension.**

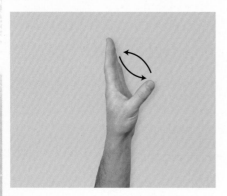

FIGURE 16-50. **Abduction and adduction.**

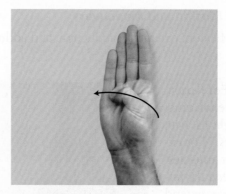

FIGURE 16-51. **Opposition.**

Ask the patient to move the thumb across the palm and touch the base of the fifth finger to test *flexion,* and then to move the thumb back across the palm and away from the fingers to test *extension.*

Next, ask the patient to place the fingers and thumb in the neutral position with the palm up, then have the patient move the thumb anteriorly away from the palm to assess abduction and back down for *adduction.* To test *opposition,* or movements of the thumb across the palm, ask the patient to touch the thumb to each of the other fingertips.

A full examination of the wrist and hand involves detailed testing of muscle strength and sensation, found in Chapter 17, The Nervous System, pp. 743–748.

The Spine

Overview. The vertebral column, or spine, is the central supporting structure of the trunk and back. The *concave curves* of the cervical and lumbar spine and the *convex curves* of the thoracic and sacrococcygeal spine help distribute upper body weight to the pelvis and lower extremities and cushion the concussive impact of walking or running.

The complex mechanics of the back reflect the coordinated action of:

- The vertebrae and intervertebral discs

- An interconnecting system of ligaments between anterior vertebrae and posterior vertebrae, ligaments between the spinous processes, and ligaments between the lamina of two adjacent vertebrae

- Large superficial muscles, deeper intrinsic muscles, and muscles of the abdominal wall

Bony Structures. The vertebral column contains 24 vertebrae stacked on the sacrum and coccyx. A typical vertebra contains sites for joint articulations, weight bearing, and muscle attachments, as well as foramina for the spinal nerve roots and peripheral nerves. Anteriorly, the *vertebral body* supports weight bearing. The posterior *vertebral arch* encloses the spinal cord. Review the location of the vertebral processes and foramina, with particular attention to:

■ The *spinous process* projecting posteriorly in the midline and the two transverse processes at the junction of the *pedicle* and the *lamina*. Muscles attach at these processes.

■ The *articular processes*—two on each side of the vertebra, one facing up and one facing down, at the junction of the pedicles and laminae, often called *articular facets*.

■ The *vertebral foramen*, which encloses the spinal cord, the *intervertebral foramen*, formed by the inferior and superior articulating process of adjacent vertebrae, creating a channel for the spinal nerve roots; and in the cervical vertebrae, the *transverse foramen* for the vertebral artery.

Representative Cervical and Lumbar Vertebrae

C4–C5 Coronal and Lateral Views

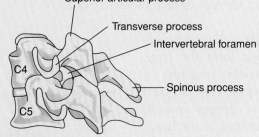

T12–L1 Coronal and Lateral Views

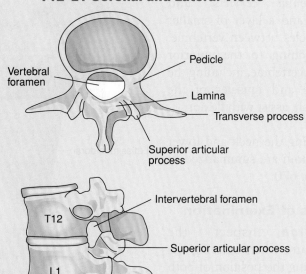

The proximity of the spinal cord and spinal nerve roots to their bony vertebral casing and the intervertebral discs makes them especially vulnerable to disc herniation, impingement from degenerative changes in the vertebrae and facets, and trauma.

Joints. The spine has slightly movable cartilaginous joints between the vertebral bodies and between the articular facets. Between the vertebral bodies are the *intervertebral discs,* each consisting of a soft mucoid central core, the *nucleus pulposus,* rimmed by the tough fibrous tissue of the *annulus fibrosis.* The intervertebral discs cushion movement between vertebrae and allow the vertebral column to curve, flex, and bend. The flexibility of the spine is largely determined by the angle of the articular facet joints relative to the plane of the vertebral body, and varies at different levels of the spine. Note that the vertebral column angles sharply posterior at the *lumbosacral junction* and becomes immovable. The mechanical stress at this angulation contributes to the risk for disc herniation and subluxation, or slippage (*spondylolisthesis*), of L5 on S1.

Muscle Groups. The *trapezius* and *latissimus dorsi* form the large outer layer of muscles attaching to each side of the spine (Fig. 16-52). They overlie two deeper muscle layers—a layer attaching to the head, neck, and spinous processes (*splenius capitis, splenius cervicis,* and *sacrospinalis*) and a layer of smaller intrinsic muscles between vertebrae. Muscles attaching to the anterior surface of the vertebrae, including the *psoas* muscle and muscles of the abdominal wall, assist with flexion.

Muscles moving the neck and lower vertebral column are summarized in the table on p. 670.

Techniques of Examination

Inspection. Inspect the patient's posture when entering the room, including the position of both the neck and trunk.

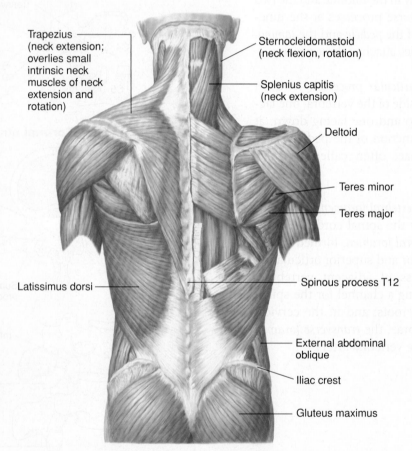

Trapezius (neck extension; overlies small intrinsic neck muscles of neck extension and rotation)

Latissimus dorsi

Sternocleidomastoid (neck flexion, rotation)

Splenius capitis (neck extension)

Deltoid

Teres minor

Teres major

Spinous process T12

External abdominal oblique

Iliac crest

Gluteus maximus

FIGURE 16-52. **Muscles of the back.**

Assess the patient for erect position of the head, neck, and back; for smooth, coordinated neck movement; and for ease of gait.

Neck stiffness signals arthritis, muscle strain, or other underlying pathology that should be pursued; headache may be present.

Drape or gown the patient to expose the entire back for complete inspection. If possible, the patient should be upright in the natural standing position, with feet together and arms at the sides. The head should be midline in the same plane as the sacrum, and the shoulders and pelvis should be level.

Viewing the patient from behind, identify the following (Fig. 16-53):

- Spinous processes, usually more prominent at C7 and T1 and more evident on forward flexion

- Paravertebral muscles on either side of the midline

- Iliac crests

- Posterior superior iliac spines, usually marked by skin dimples.

A line drawn above the posterior iliac crests crosses the spinous process of L4.

Inspect the patient from the side and from behind. Evaluate the spinal curvatures and the features in the display on the next page.

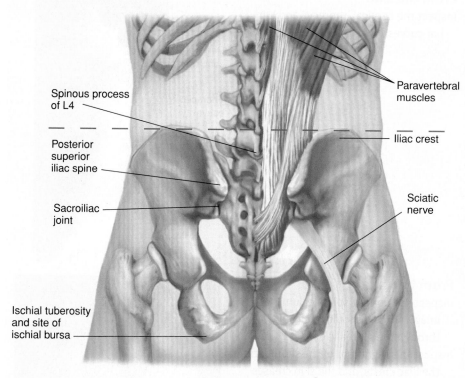

Spinous process of L4

Posterior superior iliac spine

Sacroiliac joint

Ischial tuberosity and site of ischial bursa

Paravertebral muscles

Iliac crest

Sciatic nerve

FIGURE 16-53. **Important anatomy of the back.**

Palpation. From a sitting or standing position, palpate the spinous processes of each vertebra with your thumb.

Vertebral tenderness raises concerns for fracture, dislocation, underlying infection, or arthritis.

In the neck, palpate the *facet joints* that lie between the cervical vertebrae 1 to 2 cm lateral to the spinous processes of C2 to C7. These joints lie deep to the trapezius muscle and may not be palpable unless the neck muscles are relaxed.

Tenderness occurs in arthritis, especially at the facet joints between C5 and C6.

In the lower lumbar area, palpate carefully for vertebral "step-offs" to see if one spinous process seems unusually prominent (or recessed) in relation to the one above it. Identify any tenderness.

Step-offs occur in *spondylolisthesis,* or forward slippage of one vertebra, which may compress the spinal cord.

Palpate over the *sacroiliac joint,* often identified by the dimple overlying the posterior superior iliac spine.

Tenderness over the sacroiliac joint is common in *sacroiliitis* and *ankylosing spondylitis.*[70]

You may wish to percuss the spine for tenderness by thumping, but not too roughly, with the ulnar surface of your fist.

Pain with percussion occurs in vertebral osteoporotic fractures, infection, and malignancy.

Inspection of the Spine

View of Patient

From the side
Inspect the cervical, thoracic, and lumbar curves.

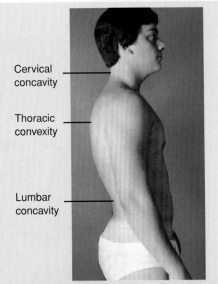

Cervical concavity

Thoracic convexity

Lumbar concavity

Increased *thoracic kyphosis* occurs with aging.

From behind
Inspect the upright spinal column (an imaginary line should fall from C7 through the gluteal cleft).

Inspect the alignment of the shoulders, the iliac crests, and the skin creases below the buttocks (gluteal folds).

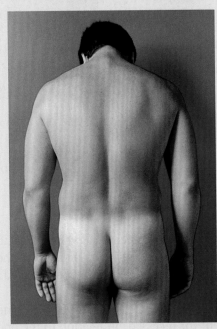

In *scoliosis,* lateral and rotatory curvature of the spine brings the head back to midline. Scoliosis often becomes evident during adolescence, before symptoms appear.

Unequal shoulder heights occur in *scoliosis, the Sprengel deformity of the scapula* from the attachment of an extra bone or band between the upper scapula and C7, *"winging" of the scapula* from loss of long thoracic nerve innervation to the serratus anterior muscle, and contralateral weakness of the trapezius.

Unequal heights of the iliac crests, or *pelvic tilt,* occur in unequal leg lengths, scoliosis, and hip abduction or adduction. Check if unequal leg lengths disappear when a block is placed under the shorter limb. "Listing" of the trunk to one side is seen with a herniated lumbar disc.

Inspect any skin markings, tags, or masses.

Birthmarks, port-wine stains, hairy patches, and lipomas often overlie bony defects such as *spina bifida.*

Café-au-lait spots (discolored patches of skin), skin tags, and fibrous tumors are common in *neurofibromatosis.*

Inspect and palpate the *paravertebral muscles* for tenderness and spasm. Muscles in spasm feel firm and knotted and may be visible.

With the patient's hip flexed and the patient lying on the opposite side, palpate the *sciatic nerve,* the largest nerve in the body, consisting of nerve roots from L4, L5, S1, S2, and S3 (Fig. 16-54). The sciatic nerve lies midway between the greater trochanter and the ischial tuberosity as it runs through the sciatic notch. It is difficult to palpate in most patients.

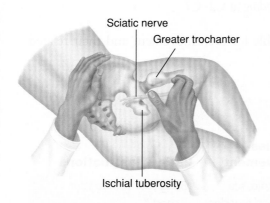

Sciatic nerve
Greater trochanter
Ischial tuberosity

FIGURE 16-54. Palpate the sciatic nerve.

Palpate for tenderness in any other areas suggested by the patient's symptoms. Check for pain radiation into the buttocks, perineum, or legs.

Assess all low back pain for possible *cauda equina compression,* the most serious cause of pain, due to risk of limb paralysis or bladder/bowel dysfunction.

Spasm occurs in degenerative and inflammatory muscle disorders, overuse, prolonged contraction from abnormal posture, and anxiety.

Sciatic nerve tenderness is seen with a herniated disc or nerve root impingement from a mass lesion.

Herniated intervertebral discs, most common at L5–S1 or L4–L5, may cause tenderness of the spinous processes, intervertebral joints, paravertebral muscles, sacrosciatic notch, and sciatic nerve (Fig. 16-55).

See Table 16-3, Low Back Pain, p. 699.

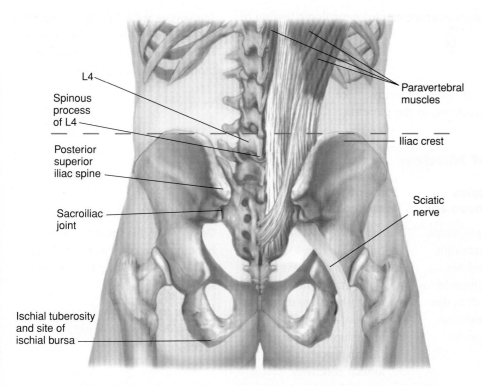

L4
Spinous process of L4
Posterior superior iliac spine
Sacroiliac joint
Ischial tuberosity and site of ischial bursa
Paravertebral muscles
Iliac crest
Sciatic nerve

FIGURE 16-55. Palpate the bony landmarks and muscles of the back.

Range of Motion and Maneuvers

Range of Motion: Neck.   The neck is the most mobile portion of the spine, remarkable for its seven fragile vertebrae supporting the 10- to 15-pound head. *Flexion* and *extension* occur primarily between the skull and C1, the atlas; *rotation* at C1–C2, the axis; and *lateral bending* at C2–C7.

Review the specific muscles responsible for each movement and their related patient instructions in the inset below.

Limited range of motion is caused by stiffness from arthritis, pain from trauma, overuse, and muscle spasm from *torticollis*.

Assess any complaints or findings of neck, shoulder, or arm pain, numbness, or weakness for possible cervical cord or nerve root compression. See Table 16-2, Pains in the Neck, p. 698.

Neck Range of Motion

Neck Movement	Primary Muscles Affecting Movement	Patient Instructions
Flexion	Sternocleidomastoid, scalene, prevertebral muscles	*"Bring your chin to your chest."*
Extension	Splenius capitis and cervicis, small intrinsic neck muscles	*"Look up at the ceiling."*
Rotation	Sternocleidomastoid, small intrinsic neck muscles	*"Look over one shoulder, and then the other."*
Lateral Bending	Scalenes and small intrinsic neck muscles	*"Bring your ear to your shoulder."*

Tenderness, loss of sensation, or weakness warrant careful neurologic testing of the neck and upper extremities.

Tenderness at C1–C2 in *RA* is suspicious for possible subluxation and high cervical cord compression and warrants prompt additional assessment.

Range of Motion: Spinal Column.   In the inset below, note the muscles responsible for each movement and instructions to the patient.

Spinal Column Range of Motion

Back Movement	Primary Muscles Affecting Movement	Patient Instructions
Flexion	Psoas major, psoas minor, quadratus lumborum; abdominal muscles attaching to the anterior vertebrae, such as the internal and external obliques and rectus abdominis	*"Bend forward and try to touch your toes."* Note the smoothness and symmetry of movement, the range of motion, and the curve in the lumbar area. As flexion proceeds, the lumbar concavity should flatten out.

Deformity of the thorax on forward bending, especially when the height of the scapulae is unequal, suggests *scoliosis*.

Persistence of lumbar lordosis suggests muscle spasm or *ankylosing spondylitis*.[70]

(continued)

Spinal Column Range of Motion (continued)

Back Movement	Primary Muscles Affecting Movement	Patient Instructions	
Extension 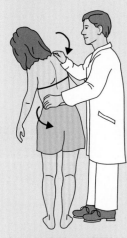	Deep intrinsic muscles of the back, such as the erector spinae and transversospinalis groups	*"Bend back as far as possible."* Support the patient by placing your hand on the posterior superior iliac spine, with your fingers pointing toward the midline.	Decreased *spinal mobility* is common in *OA* and *ankylosing spondylitis*.
Rotation 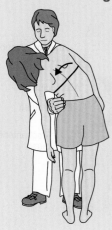	Abdominal muscles, intrinsic muscles of the back	*"Rotate from side to side."* Stabilize the patient's pelvis by placing one hand on the patient's hip and the other on the opposite shoulder. Then rotate the trunk by pulling the shoulder anteriorly and then the hip posteriorly. Repeat these maneuvers for the opposite side.	
Lateral Bending	Abdominal muscles, intrinsic muscles of the back	*"Bend to the side from the waist."* Stabilize the patient's pelvis by placing your hand on the patient's hip. Repeat for the opposite side.	

If these maneuvers provoke pain or tenderness, particularly with radiation into the leg, proceed to careful neurologic testing of the lower extremities.

Consider lumbosacral cord or nerve root compression; arthritis, mass lesion, or infection in the hip, rectum, or pelvis may also cause symptoms. See Table 16-3, Low Back Pain, p. 699.

See Chapter 17, The Nervous System, for the Straight Leg Raise Test, pp. 765–766. Although helpful, this test is not diagnostic of disc herniation.[71–73]

Non-organic physical findings (Waddell signs) include superficial or nonanatomic tenderness, pain on axial loading or simulated rotation, nonreproducibility of pain when the patient is distracted, regional weakness or sensory change, and overreaction to stimuli that should not cause back pain.[24,31]

The Hip

Overview.   The hip joint is deeply embedded in the pelvis and is notable for its strength, stability, and wide range of motion. The stability of the hip joint, essential for weight bearing, arises from the deep fit of the head of the femur into the acetabulum, its strong fibrous articular capsule, and the powerful muscles crossing the joint and inserting below the femoral head, providing leverage for movement of the femur.

Bony Structures and Joints.   The hip joint lies below the middle third of the inguinal ligament but in a deeper plane. It is a ball-and-socket joint; note how the rounded head of the femur articulates with the cup-like cavity of the acetabulum. Because of its overlying muscles and depth, the hip joint is not readily palpable. Review the bones of the pelvis—the *acetabulum,* the *ilium,* and the *ischium*—and the connection inferiorly at the *symphysis pubis* and posteriorly with the sacroiliac bone.

On the *anterior surface of the hip,* locate the following bony structures (Fig. 16-56):

■ The iliac crest at the level of L4

■ The iliac tubercle

■ The anterior superior iliac spine

■ The greater trochanter

■ The pubic tubercle

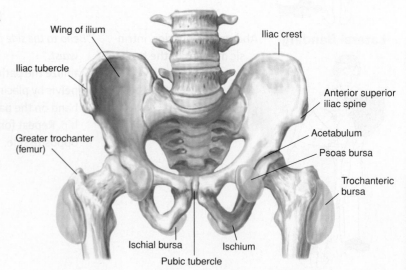

Wing of ilium

Iliac tubercle

Greater trochanter (femur)

Iliac crest

Anterior superior iliac spine

Acetabulum

Psoas bursa

Trochanteric bursa

Ischial bursa

Ischium

Pubic tubercle

FIGURE 16-56.   **Anterior view of the pelvis.**

On the *posterior surface of the hip,* locate the following (Fig. 16-57):

- The posterior superior iliac spine

- The greater trochanter

- The ischial tuberosity

- The sacroiliac joint

Note that you can locate S2 by envisioning an imaginary line across the posterior superior iliac spines.

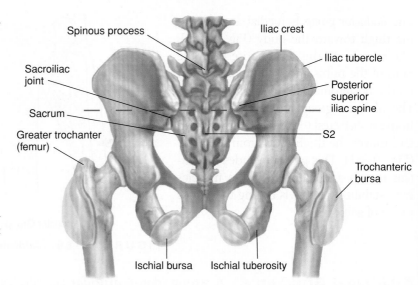

FIGURE 16-57. Posterior view of the pelvis.

Muscle Groups.   Four powerful muscle groups move the hip. Picture these groups as you examine patients, and remember that to move the femur or any bone in a given direction, the muscle must cross the joint line.

The *flexor group* lies anteriorly and flexes the thigh (Fig. 16-58). The primary hip flexor is the *iliopsoas,* extending from above the iliac crest to the lesser trochanter. The *extensor group* lies posteriorly and extends the thigh (Fig. 16-59). The *gluteus maximus* is the primary extensor of the hip. It forms a band crossing from its origin along the medial pelvis to its insertion below the trochanter.

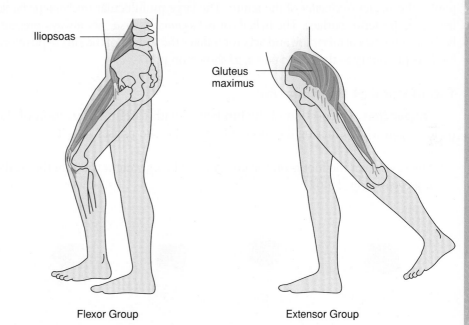

Flexor Group

Extensor Group

FIGURE 16-58. Flexor group.   **FIGURE 16-59.** Extensor group.

The *adductor group* is medial and swings the thigh toward the body (Fig. 16-60). The muscles in this group arise from the rami of the pubis and ischium and insert on the posteromedial aspect of the femur. The *abductor group* is lateral, extending from the iliac crest to the greater trochanter, and moves the thigh away from the body (Fig. 16-61). This group includes the *gluteus medius* and *minimus*. These muscles help stabilize the pelvis during the stance phase of gait.

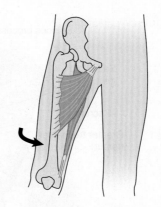

Adductor Group

FIGURE 16-60. **Adductor group.**

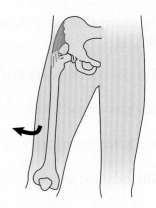

Abductor Group

FIGURE 16-61. **Abductor group.**

Additional Structures. A strong, dense *articular capsule,* extending from the acetabulum to the femoral neck, encases and strengthens the hip joint. The capsule is reinforced by three overlying ligaments and lined with synovial membrane. There are three principal bursae at the hip. Anterior to the joint is the *psoas* (also termed *iliopectineal* or *iliopsoas*) *bursa,* overlying the articular capsule and the psoas muscle. Find the bony prominence lateral to the hip joint—the *greater trochanter* of the femur. The large multilocular *trochanteric bursa* lies on its posterior surface. The *ischial* (or *ischiogluteal*) *bursa,* not always present, lies under the *ischial tuberosity,* and accommodates the weight of the sitting position. Note its proximity to the sciatic nerve, as shown on p. 679.

Techniques of Examination

Inspection. Inspection of the hip begins with careful observation of the patient's gait when entering the room. Observe the two phases of gait:

■ *Stance*—when the foot is on the ground and bears weight (60% of the walking cycle) (Fig. 16-62)

Most hip problems appear during the weight-bearing stance phase.

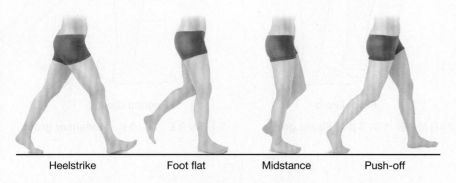

Heelstrike   Foot flat   Midstance   Push-off

THE STANCE PHASE OF GAIT

FIGURE 16-62. **Stance phase of gait.**

■ *Swing*—when the foot moves forward and does not bear weight (40% of the cycle)

Inspect the gait for the width of the base, the shift of the pelvis, and flexion of the knee (Fig. 16-63). The width of the base should be 2 to 4 inches from heel to heel. Normal gait has a smooth, continuous rhythm, achieved in part by contraction of the abductors of the weight-bearing limb. Abductor contraction stabilizes the pelvis and helps maintain balance, raising the opposite hip. The knee should be flexed throughout the stance phase, except when the heel strikes the ground to counteract motion at the ankle.

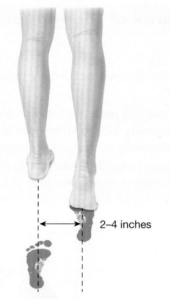

2–4 inches

FIGURE 16-63. Inspect base of gait width.

A wide base suggests cerebellar disease or foot problems. Pain during weight bearing or examiner strike on the heel occurs in *femoral neck stress fractures.*[74,75]

Hip dislocation, arthritis, unequal leg lengths, or abductor weakness can cause the pelvis to drop on the opposite side, producing a waddling gait.

Lack of knee flexion, which makes the leg functionally longer, interrupts the smooth pattern of gait, causing circumduction (swinging the leg out to the side).

Inspect the lumbar portion of the spine for the degree of lordosis and, with the patient supine, assess the length of the legs for symmetry. (To measure leg length, see Special Techniques, p. 694.)

Loss of lordosis occurs with *paravertebral spasm;* excess lordosis suggests a *flexion deformity* of the hip.

Disparities in leg length occur in abduction or adduction deformities and *scoliosis.* Leg shortening and external rotation are common in *hip fracture.*

Inspect the anterior and posterior surfaces of the hip for any areas of muscle atrophy or bruising. The joint is too deeply situated to detect swelling.

Palpation

Bony Landmarks. Palpate the surface landmarks of the hip, identified on p. 674. On the anterior aspect of the hips, these can be located as follows.

Palpation of Bony Landmarks of the Hip

Anterior Landmarks
- Identify the *iliac crest* at the upper margin of the pelvis at the level of L4.
- Follow the downward anterior curve and locate the *iliac tubercle,* marking the widest point of the crest, and continue tracking downward to the *anterior–superior iliac spine.*
- Place your thumbs on the anterior–superior spines and move your fingers downward and laterally from the iliac tubercles to the *greater trochanter* of the femur.
- Then move your thumbs medially and obliquely to the *pubic tubercle,* which lies at the same level as the greater trochanter.

(continued)

Palpation of Bony Landmarks of the Hip (*continued*)

Posterior Landmarks

- Palpate the *posterior–superior iliac spine* directly underneath the visible dimples just above the buttocks.
- Placing your left thumb and index finger over the posterior superior iliac spine, next locate the *greater trochanter* laterally with your fingers at the level of the gluteal fold, and place your thumb medially on the *ischial tuberosity*. The *sacroiliac joint* is not always palpable but may be tender. Note that an imaginary line along the posterior–superior iliac spines crosses the joint at S2.

Inguinal Structures. With the patient supine, ask the patient to place the heel of the leg being examined on the opposite knee. Then palpate along the inguinal ligament, which extends from the anterior–superior iliac spine to the pubic tubercle (Fig. 16-64).

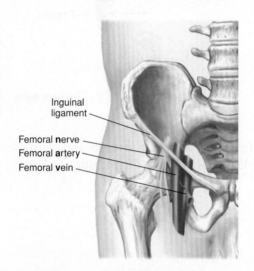

Inguinal ligament
Femoral nerve
Femoral artery
Femoral vein

FIGURE 16-64. The inguinal ligament and N-A-V-E-L.

The femoral nerve, artery, and vein bisect the overlying inguinal ligament; lymph nodes lie medially. The mnemonic **NAVEL** may help you remember the lateral-to-medial sequence of **N**erve–**A**rtery–**V**ein–**E**mpty space–**L**ymph node.

Anterior or inguinal pain, typically deep within the hip joint and radiating to the knee, points to intra-articular pathology; pain radiating to the buttocks or posterior trochanteric region points to extra-articular causes.[75]

Bursae. If the hip is painful, palpate the (psoas) bursa, below the inguinal ligament but on a deeper plane.

Sacroiliac joint tenderness suggests *sacroiliitis.*

Bulges along the ligament suggest an *inguinal hernia* or, at times, an *aneurysm.*

Enlarged lymph nodes point to infection in the pelvis or lower extremity.

Causes of groin tenderness are *synovitis* of the hip joint, *arthritis; bursitis;* or possible *psoas abscess.*

Focal tenderness over the trochanter confirms *trochanteric bursitis.* Tenderness over the posterolateral surface of the greater trochanter occurs in localized tendinitis, muscle spasm from referred hip pain, and *iliotibial band tendinitis.*

Intra-articular causes include *OA, osteonecrosis* of the femoral head, *acetabular labral tears,* and *femoral neck stress fracture.* Extra-articular causes include *trochanteric bursitis,* muscle strain, sacroiliac disorders, and *lumbar radiculopathy.*[74–76]

With the patient resting on one side and the hip flexed and internally rotated, palpate the *trochanteric bursa* lying over the greater trochanter (Fig. 16-65). Normally, the *ischiogluteal bursa,* over the ischial tuberosity, is not palpable unless inflamed (Fig. 16-66).

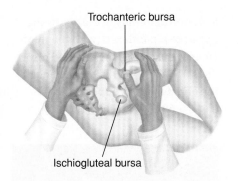

Trochanteric bursa

Ischiogluteal bursa

FIGURE 16-65. Palpate the trochanteric bursa.

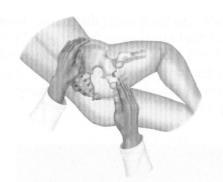

FIGURE 16-66. Palpate the ischiogluteal bursa.

Look for tenderness in *ischiogluteal bursitis* or "weaver's bottom"; because of the adjacent sciatic nerve, this may mimic sciatica.

Range of Motion and Maneuvers

Range of Motion. Assess hip range of motion and the specific muscles responsible for each movement. Review the instructions to the patient. Normal values for hip flexion, abduction, and adduction are 120°, 45°, and 20° respectively.

Hip Range of Motion

Hip Movement	Primary Muscles Affecting Movement	Patient Instructions
Flexion	Iliopsoas	*"Bend your knee to your chest and pull it against your abdomen."*
Extension (actually hyperextension)	Gluteus maximus	*"Lie face down, then bend your knee and lift it up."* OR *"Lying flat, move your lower leg away from the midline and down over the side of the table."*
Abduction	Gluteus medius and minimus	*"Lying flat, move your lower leg away from the midline."*
Adduction	Adductor brevis, adductor longus, adductor magnus, pectineus, gracilis	*"Lying flat, bend your knee and move your lower leg toward the midline."*
External Rotation	Internal and external obturators, quadratus femoris, superior and inferior gemelli	*"Lying flat, bend your knee and turn your lower leg and foot across the midline."*
Internal Rotation	Iliopsoas	*"Lying flat, bend your knee and turn your lower leg and foot away from the midline."*

Maneuvers.   Often, the examiner must assist the patient with movements of the hip, so further detail is provided below for flexion, abduction, adduction, and external and internal rotation. Meta-analyses suggest that no single test discriminates specific hip pathology.[75,77,78]

- *Flexion.* With the patient supine, place your hand under the patient's lumbar spine. Ask the patient to bend each knee in turn up to the chest and pull it firmly against the abdomen (Fig. 16-67). Note that the hip can flex further when the knee is flexed because the hamstrings are relaxed. When the back touches your hand, indicating normal flattening of the lumbar lordosis, further flexion must arise from the hip joint itself.

In *flexion deformity of the hip,* as the opposite hip is flexed (with the thigh against the chest), the affected hip does not allow full hip extension and the affected thigh appears flexed (Fig. 16-68).

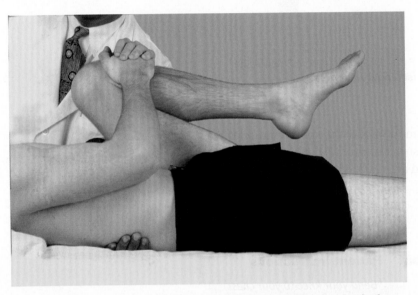

FIGURE 16-67. Hip flexion and flattening of lumbar lordosis.

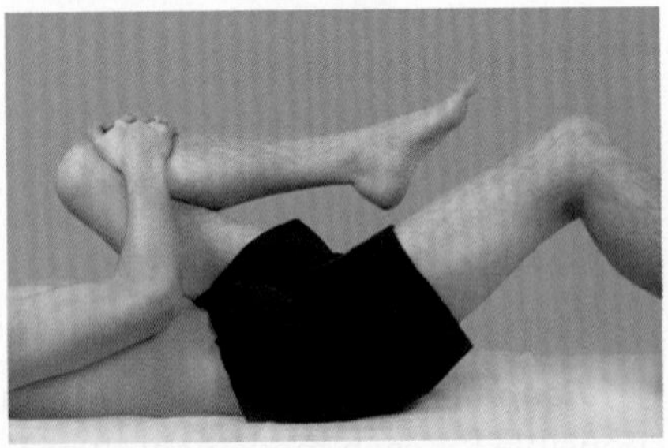

FIGURE 16-68. Flexion deformity of the hip.

As the thigh is held against the abdomen, inspect the degree of flexion at the hip and knee. Normally, the anterior portion of the thigh can almost touch the chest wall. Note whether the opposite thigh remains fully extended, resting on the table.

Flexion deformity may be masked by an increase, rather than flattening, in lumbar lordosis and an anterior pelvic tilt.

- *Extension.* With the patient lying face down, extend the thigh toward you in a posterior direction. Alternatively, carefully position the supine patient near the edge of the table and extend the leg posteriorly.

- *Abduction.* Stabilize the pelvis by pressing down on the opposite anterior–superior iliac spine with one hand. With the other hand, grasp the ankle and abduct the extended leg until you feel the iliac spine move (Fig. 16-69). This movement marks the limit of hip abduction.

Restricted abduction and internal and external rotation are common in hip OA. The LR for resisted external rotation due to pain is as high as 32.6.[12,77]

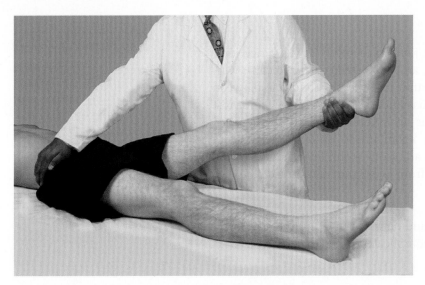

FIGURE 16-69. **Abduct the leg.**

■ *Adduction.* With the patient supine, stabilize the pelvis, hold one ankle, and move the leg medially across the body and over the opposite extremity (Fig. 16-70).

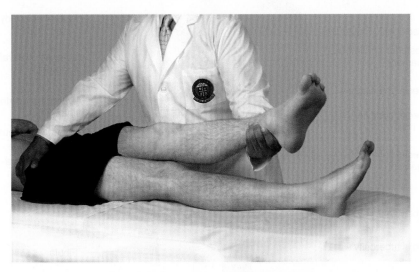

FIGURE 16-70. **Adduct the leg.**

■ *External and internal rotation.* Flex the leg to 90° at hip and knee, stabilize the thigh with one hand, grasp the ankle with the other, and swing the lower leg—medially for external rotation at the hip, and laterally for internal rotation (Fig. 16-71). Although confusing at first, it is the motion of the head of the femur in the acetabulum that identifies these movements.

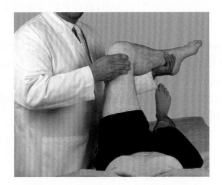

FIGURE 16-71. **Test internal and external rotation of the hip.**

Pain with maximal flexion and adduction and internal rotation or with abduction and external rotation with full extension signals *acetabular labral tear.*[74,75]

The Knee

Overview.   The knee joint is the largest joint in the body. It is a hinge joint involving three bones: the femur, the tibia, and the patella (or knee cap), with three articular surfaces, two between the femur and the tibia and one between the femur and the patella. Note how the two rounded condyles of the femur rest on the relatively flat tibial plateau. There is no inherent stability in the knee joint itself, making it dependent on four ligaments to hold its articulating femur and tibia in place. This feature, in addition to the lever action of the femur on the tibia and the lack of padding from overlying fat or muscle, makes the knee highly vulnerable to injury.

Bony Structures.   Learn the bony landmarks in and around the knee. These will guide your examination of this complicated joint (Fig. 16-72).

- On the *medial surface,* identify the *adductor tubercle,* the *medial epicondyle* of the femur, and the *medial condyle* of the tibia.

- On the *anterior surface,* identify the patella, which rests on the anterior articulating surface of the femur midway between the epicondyles, embedded in the tendon of the quadriceps muscle. This tendon continues below the knee joint as the *patellar tendon,* which inserts distally on the *tibial tuberosity.*

- On the *lateral surface,* find the *lateral epicondyle* of the femur, the *lateral condyle* of the tibia, and the head of the *fibula.*

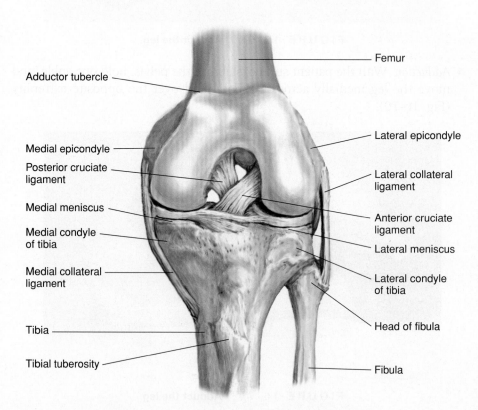

FIGURE 16-72.   Anterior view of the knee.

Labels: Adductor tubercle — Medial epicondyle — Posterior cruciate ligament — Medial meniscus — Medial condyle of tibia — Medial collateral ligament — Tibia — Tibial tuberosity — Femur — Lateral epicondyle — Lateral collateral ligament — Anterior cruciate ligament — Lateral meniscus — Lateral condyle of tibia — Head of fibula — Fibula

Joints.   Two condylar *tibiofemoral joints* are formed by the convex curves of the medial and lateral condyles of the femur as they articulate with the concave condyles of the tibia. The third articular surface is the *patellofemoral joint.* The patella slides on the groove of the anterior aspect of the distal femur, called the *trochlear groove,* during flexion and extension of the knee.

Problems with patellar tracking, for example, in patients with shallower grooves, especially women, can lead to arthritis, anterior knee pain, and patellar dislocation.

Muscle Groups. Powerful muscles move and support the knee. The *quadriceps femoris* extends the knee, covering the anterior, medial, and lateral aspects of the thigh (Figs. 16-73 and 16-74). The *hamstring muscles* lie on the posterior aspect of the thigh and flex the knee.

In women, quadriceps contraction often exerts a more lateral pull (Q angle) that alters patellar tracking, contributing to anterior knee pain.

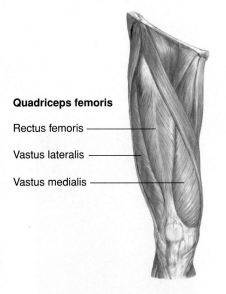

FIGURE 16-73. Quadriceps femoris—anterior view.

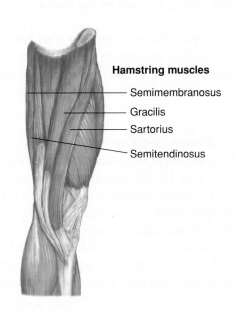

FIGURE 16-74. Hamstring muscles—medial view.

Additional Structures

Menisci and Ligaments. The menisci and two important pairs of ligaments, the collaterals and the cruciates, are crucial to stability of the knee. Learn the location of these structures from the illustrations on p. 682 and below (Fig. 16-75).

■ The *medial and lateral menisci* cushion the action of the femur on the tibia. These crescent-shaped fibrocartilaginous discs add a cup-like surface to the otherwise flat tibial plateau.

■ The *medial collateral ligament (MCL)*, not easily palpable, is a broad, flat ligament connecting the medial femoral epicondyle to the medial condyle of the tibia. The medial portion of the MCL also attaches to the medial meniscus.

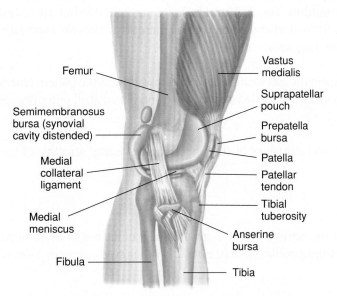

FIGURE 16-75. Left knee—medial view.

■ The *lateral collateral ligament (LCL)* connects the lateral femoral epicondyle and the head of the fibula. The MCL and LCL provide medial and lateral stability to the knee joint.

■ The *ACL* crosses obliquely from the anterior medial tibia to the lateral femoral condyle, preventing the tibia from sliding forward on the femur.

■ The *posterior cruciate ligament (PCL)* crosses from the *posterior* tibia and lateral meniscus to the medial femoral condyle, preventing the tibia from slipping backward on the femur. Although the ACL and PCL lie within the knee joint so are not palpable, they are nonetheless crucial to the anteroposterior stability of the knee.

Negative Infrapatellar Space and Suprapatellar Pouch. Inspect the concavities that are usually evident adjacent and superior to each side of the patella, known as the "negative infrapatellar space" (Fig. 16-76). Occupying these areas is the synovial cavity of the knee, one of the largest joint cavities in the body. This cavity includes an extension 6 cm above the upper border of the patella, lying upward and deep to the quadriceps muscle, called the *suprapatellar pouch.* The joint cavity covers the anterior, medial, and lateral surfaces of the knee, as well as the condyles of the femur and tibia posteriorly. Although the synovium is not normally palpable, these areas may become swollen and tender when the joint is inflamed or injured.

Bursae. Several bursae lie near the knee. The *prepatellar bursa* lies between the patella and the overlying skin. The *anserine bursa* lies 1 to 2 cm below the knee joint on the medial surface, proximal and medial to the attachments of the medial hamstring muscles on the proximal tibia. It cannot be palpated due to these overlying tendons. Now identify the large *semimembranosus bursa* that communicates with the joint cavity, also on the posterior and medial surfaces of the knee.

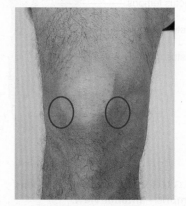

FIGURE 16-76. Normal negative infrapatellar spaces.

Techniques of Examination. Learn to examine "the seven structures of the knee": the medial and lateral menisci, the LCL and MCL, the ACL and PCL, and the patellar tendon. The ACL and PCL are not palpable but are tested by specific maneuvers. Palpation and maneuvers of these structures are especially helpful in primary care diagnosis.

Inspection. Inspect the gait for a smooth rhythmic flow as the patient enters the room. The knee should be extended at heel strike and flexed at all other phases of swing and stance.

Check the alignment and contours of the knees. Observe any atrophy of the quadriceps muscles.

Inspect for any loss of the normal hollows around the patella, a sign of swelling in the knee joint and suprapatellar pouch; note any other swelling in or around the knee.

Stumbling or "giving way" of the knee during heel strike suggests *quadriceps weakness* or abnormal patellar tracking.

Bow-legs (*genu varum*) and knock-knees (*genu valgum*) are common. Quadriceps atrophy signals hip girdle weakness in older adults.

Swelling over the patella occurs in *prepatellar bursitis* (housemaid's knee). Swelling over the tibial tubercle suggests *infrapatellar* or, if more medial, *anserine bursitis.*

Palpation. Ask the patient to sit on the edge of the examining table with the knees in flexion. In this position, bony landmarks are more visible, and the muscles, tendons, and ligaments are more relaxed, making them easier to palpate. Pay special attention to any areas of tenderness. Pain is a common complaint in knee problems, and localizing the structure causing pain is important for accurate evaluation.

The Tibiofemoral Joint. Palpate the *tibiofemoral joint.* Facing the knee, place your thumbs in the soft tissue depressions on either side of the *patellar tendon.* Identify the groove of the tibiofemoral joint. Note that the inferior pole of the patella lies at the tibiofemoral joint line. As you press your thumbs downward, you can feel the edge of the tibial plateau. Follow it medially, then laterally, until you are stopped by the converging femur and tibia. By moving your thumbs upward toward the midline to the top of the patella, you can follow the articulating surface of the femur and identify the margins of the joint.

Note any irregular bony ridges along the joint margins.

Bony enlargement at the joint margins, genu varum deformity, and stiffness lasting ≤30 minutes are typical findings in *OA* (LRs 11.8, 3.4, and 3.0, respectively).[57] Crepitus is also common.

■ *Medial and lateral menisci.* Palpate the *medial meniscus.* Press on the medial soft tissue depression along the upper edge of the tibial plateau with the tibia slightly internally rotated. Place the knee in slight flexion and palpate the *lateral meniscus* along the lateral joint line.

A medial meniscus tear with joint line point tenderness is common after trauma and requires prompt further evaluation.[79]

■ *Medial and lateral joint compartments: MCL and LCL.* Palpate *the medial and lateral joint compartments* of the tibiofemoral joint with the knee flexed on the examining table to approximately 90°. Pay special attention to any areas of pain or tenderness.

■ *Medial compartment* (Fig. 16-77). Medially, move your thumbs upward to palpate the *medial femoral condyle.* The *adductor tubercle* is posterior to the medial femoral condyle. Move your thumbs downward to palpate the *medial tibial plateau.*

Also medially, palpate along the joint line and identify the *MCL,* which connects the medial epicondyle of the femur to the medial condyle and superior medial surface of the tibia. Palpate along this broad, flat ligament from its origin to insertion.

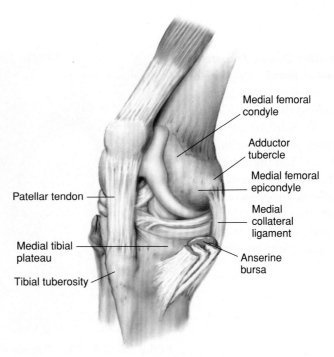

FIGURE 16-77. **Medial compartment of the knee.**

■ *Lateral compartment.* Lateral to the patellar tendon, move your thumbs upward to palpate the *lateral femoral condyle* and downward to palpate the *lateral tibial plateau.* When the knee is flexed, the femoral epicondyles are lateral to the femoral condyles.

■ Also on the lateral surface, ask the patient to cross one leg so that the ankle rests on the opposite knee and find the *LCL,* a firm cord that runs from the lateral femoral epicondyle to the head of the fibula.

■ *Patellofemoral compartment: patellar tendon.* Palpate the *patellofemoral compartment.* Locate the *patella* and trace the *patellar tendon* distally until you palpate the *tibial tuberosity.* Ask the patient to extend the knee to make sure the patellar tendon is intact.

With the patient supine and the knee extended, compress the patella against the underlying femur, and gently move it medially and laterally, assessing for crepitus and pain. Ask the patient to tighten the quadriceps as the patella moves distally in the trochlear groove. Check for a smooth sliding motion (the *patellofemoral grinding test*).

The Suprapatellar Pouch, Prepatellar Bursa, and Anserine Bursa. Palpate for any thickening or swelling in the *suprapatellar pouch* and along the margins of the patella (Fig. 16-78). Start 10 cm above the superior border of the patella, well above the pouch, and feel the soft tissues between your thumb and fingers. Move your hand distally in progressive steps, trying to identify the pouch. Continue your palpation along the sides of the patella. Note any tenderness or increased warmth.

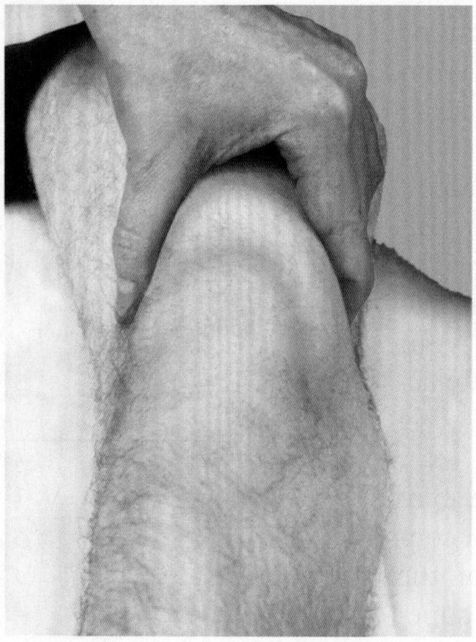

FIGURE 16-78. Palpate the suprapatellar pouch.

MCL tenderness after injury is suspicious for an MCL tear; LCL injuries are less frequent.

Tenderness over the tendon or inability to extend the knee suggests a partial or complete tear of the patellar tendon.

Pain and crepitus arise from the roughened undersurface of the patella as it articulates with the femur. Similar pain may occur when using the stairs, or getting up from a chair.

Pain with compression and patellar movement during quadriceps contraction occurs in *chondromalacia.* Two of three findings are most diagnostic of the *patellofemoral pain syndrome:* pain with quadriceps contraction; pain with squatting; and pain with palpation of the posteromedial/or lateral patellar border.[80,81]

Swelling around the patella points to synovial thickening or effusion of the knee joint (Fig. 16-79).

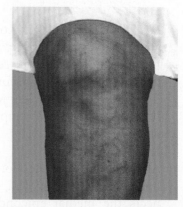

FIGURE 16-79. **Effusion of the knee joint.**

Thickening, bogginess, or warmth occurs with synovitis and nontender effusions from *OA.*

Check three other bursae for bogginess or swelling. Palpate the *prepatellar bursa*. Palpate over the *anserine bursa* on the posteromedial side of the knee between the MCL and the tendons inserting on the medial tibial and plateau. On the posterior surface, with the leg extended, check the medial aspect of the popliteal fossa.

Prepatellar bursitis **is triggered by excessive kneeling;** a*nserine bursitis* **from running, valgus knee deformity, or** *OA;* **and a** *popliteal* **or** *"Baker" cyst* **from distention of the gastrocnemius semimembranosus bursa from underlying arthritis or trauma.**

Palpation Tests for Knee Joint Effusions. Learn to apply three tests for detecting fluid in the knee joint: the bulge sign, the balloon sign, and balloting the patella.

■ The *bulge sign (for minor effusions)*. With the knee extended, place the left hand above the knee and apply pressure on the suprapatellar pouch, displacing or "milking" fluid downward (Fig. 16-80). Stroke downward on the medial aspect of the knee and apply pressure to force fluid into the lateral area (Fig. 16-81). Tap the knee just behind the lateral margin of the patella with the right hand (Fig. 16-82).

A fluid wave or bulge on the medial side between the patella and the femur is a *positive test* **for effusion.**

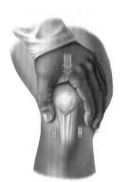

FIGURE 16-80. **Milk downward.**

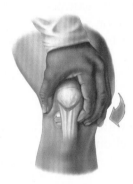

FIGURE 16-81. **Apply medial pressure.**

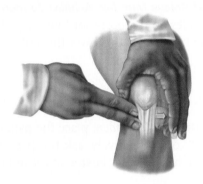

FIGURE 16-82. **Tap and watch for fluid wave.**

■ The *balloon sign (for major effusions)*. Place the thumb and index finger of your right hand on each side of the patella; with the left hand, compress the suprapatellar pouch against the femur (Fig. 16-83). Palpate for fluid ejected or "ballooning" into the spaces next to the patella under your right thumb and index finger.

A palpable fluid wave is a *positive test* **or "balloon sign." A palpable returning fluid wave into the suprapatellar pouch further confirms a major effusion, present in knee fractures (LR 2.5).**[57]

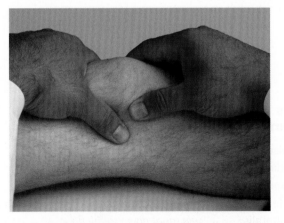

FIGURE 16-83. **Test for the balloon sign.**

■ *Balloting the patella (for major effusions).* To assess large effusions, you can also compress the suprapatellar pouch and "ballotte" or push the patella sharply against the femur (Fig. 16-84). Watch for fluid returning to the suprapatellar pouch.

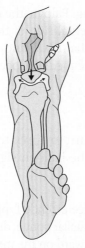

FIGURE 16-84. Ballotte the patella.

A palpable fluid wave returning into the pouch is also a *positive test* for a major effusion.

A palpable patellar click with compression may also occur, but yields more false positives.

Gastrocnemius and Soleus Muscles, Achilles Tendon. Palpate the gastrocnemius and soleus muscles on the posterior lower leg. Their common tendon, the Achilles, is palpable from about the lower third of the calf to its insertion on the calcaneus.

A defect in the muscles, tenderness, and swelling signal a *ruptured Achilles tendon;* tenderness and thickening of the tendon, at times with a protuberant posterolateral bony process of the calcaneus, suggests *Achilles tendinitis.*

To test the integrity of the *Achilles tendon,* place the patient prone with the knee and ankle flexed at 90°, or alternatively, ask the patient to kneel on a chair. Squeeze the calf and watch for plantar flexion at the ankle.

Absent plantar flexion is a *positive test* for Achilles tendon rupture. Sudden severe pain "like a gunshot," an ecchymosis from the calf into the heel, and a flat-footed gait with absent "toe-off" may also be present.

Range of Motion and Maneuvers

Range of Motion. Now assess knee range of motion, referring to the box below for specific muscles responsible for each movement and for instructions to the patient.

Knee Range of Motion

Knee Movement	Primary Muscles Affecting Movement	Patient Instructions
Flexion	Hamstring group: biceps femoris, semitendinosus, and semimembranosus	*"Bend or flex your knee."* OR *"Squat down to the floor."*
Extension	Quadriceps: rectus femoris, vastus medialis, lateralis, and intermedius	*"Straighten your leg."* OR *"After you squat down to the floor, stand up."*
Internal Rotation	Sartorius, gracilis, semitendinosus, semimembranosus	*"While sitting, swing your lower leg toward the midline."*
External Rotation	Biceps femoris	*"While sitting, swing your lower leg away from the midline."*

Crepitus with flexion and extension signals patellofemoral *OA,* a probable precursor of knee *OA.*[82]

Maneuvers. You will often need to test ligamentous stability and integrity of the medial and lateral menisci, the MCL and LCL, the patellar tendon, and the ACL and PCL (not palpable), particularly when there is a history of trauma or knee pain.[57,80,83–85] Always examine both knees and compare findings.

ACL tears are notably more frequent in women, attributed to ligamentous laxity related to estrogen cycling and to differences in anatomy and neuromuscular control. ACL injury prevention programs are now common.

Maneuvers for Examining the Knee

Structure	Maneuver	
Medial Meniscus and Lateral Meniscus 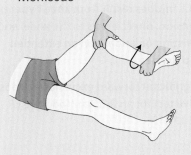	**McMurray Test.** With the patient supine, grasp the heel and flex the knee. Cup your other hand over the knee joint with fingers and thumb along the medial joint line. From the heel, externally rotate the lower leg, then push on the lateral side to apply a valgus stress on the medial side of the joint. At the same time, slowly extend the lower leg in external rotation. The same maneuver with internal rotation of the foot stresses the lateral meniscus. If a click is felt or heard at the joint line during flexion and extension of the knee, or if tenderness is noted along the joint line, further assess the meniscus for a posterior tear.	A palpable click or pop along the medial or lateral joint line is a *positive test* for a tear of the posterior portion of the medial meniscus (positive LR of 4.5).[57] The tear may displace meniscal tissue, causing "locking" on full knee extension.
Medial Collateral Ligament (MCL) 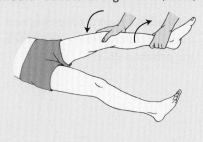	**Abduction (or Valgus) Stress Test.** With the patient supine and the knee slightly flexed, move the thigh about 30° laterally to the side of the table. Place one hand against the lateral knee to stabilize the femur and the other hand around the medial ankle. Push medially against the knee and pull laterally at the ankle to open the knee joint on the medial side (*valgus stress*).	Pain or a gap in the medial joint line is a *positive test* for an MCL injury (sensitivity 79–89%; specificity 49–99%).[57]
Lateral Collateral Ligament (LCL) 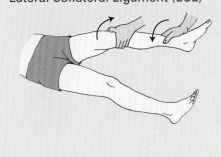	**Adduction (or Varus) Stress Test.** With the thigh and knee in the same position, change your position so that you can place one hand against the medial surface of the knee and the other around the lateral ankle. Push laterally against the knee and pull medially at the ankle to open the knee joint on the lateral side (*varus stress*).	Pain or a gap in the lateral joint line points is a *positive test* for LCL injury (less common than MCL injuries).

(*continued*)

Maneuvers for Examining the Knee (*continued*)

Structure	Maneuver	
Anterior Cruciate Ligament (ACL) 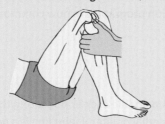	**Anterior Drawer Sign.** With the patient supine, hips flexed and knees flexed to 90° and feet flat on the table, cup your hands around the knee with the thumbs on the medial and lateral joint line and the fingers on the medial and lateral insertions of the hamstrings. Draw the tibia forward and observe if it slides forward (like a drawer) from under the femur. Compare the degree of forward movement with that of the opposite knee.	A few degrees of forward movement are normal if equally present on the opposite side. A forward jerk showing the contours of the upper tibia is a *positive test,* or *anterior drawer sign,* with a positive LR of 11.5 for an ACL tear.[57] ACL injuries result from knee hyperextension, direct blows to the knee, and twisting or landing on an extended hip or knee.
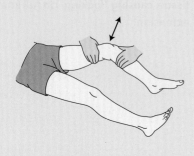	**Lachman Test.** Place the knee in 15° of flexion and external rotation. Grasp the distal femur on the lateral side with one hand and the proximal tibia on the medial side with the other. With the thumb of the tibial hand on the joint line, simultaneously pull the tibia forward and the femur back. Estimate the degree of forward excursion.	Significant forward excursion is a positive test for an *ACL tear* (positive LR of 17.0).[57]
Posterior Cruciate Ligament (PCL) 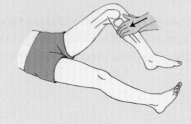	**Posterior Drawer Sign.** Position the patient and place your hands in the positions described for the anterior drawer test. Push the tibia posteriorly and observe the degree of backward movement in the femur.	If the proximal tibia falls back, this is a *positive test* for PCL injury (positive LR of 97.8).[57] Isolated PCL tears are less common, usually resulting from a direct blow to the proximal tibia.

The Ankle and Foot

Overview.   The total weight of the body is transmitted through the ankle to the foot. The ankle and foot must balance the body and absorb the impact of the heel strike and gait. Despite thick padding along the toes, sole, and heel and stabilizing ligaments at the ankles, the ankle and foot are frequent sites of sprain and bony injury.

Bony Structures and Joints.   The ankle is a hinge joint formed by the *tibia,* the *fibula,* and the *talus.* The tibia and fibula act as a mortise, stabilizing the joint while bracing the talus like an inverted cup.

The principal joints of the ankle are the *tibiotalar joint,* between the tibia and the talus, and the *subtalar (talocalcaneal) joint* (Fig. 16-85).

Note the principal landmarks of the ankle: the *medial malleolus,* the bony prominence at the distal end of the tibia, and the *lateral malleolus,* at the distal end of the fibula. Lodged under the talus and jutting posteriorly is the *calcaneus,* or heel bone.

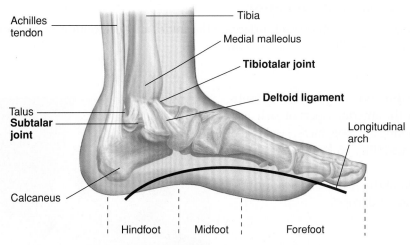

FIGURE 16-85. Ankle, medial view.

An imaginary line, the *longitudinal arch,* spans the foot, extending from the calcaneus of the hind foot along the tarsal bones of the midfoot (see cuneiform, navicular, and cuboid bones in Fig. 16-86) to the forefoot metatarsals and toes. The *heads of the metatarsals* are palpable in the ball of the foot. In the forefoot, identify the *metatarsophalangeal joints,* proximal to the webs of the toes, and the *PIP and DIP joints* of the toes.

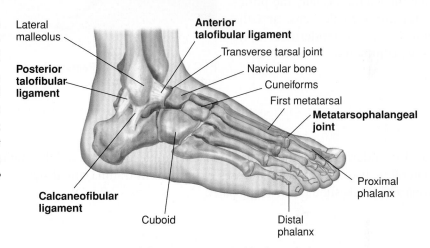

FIGURE 16-86. Ankle, lateral view.

Muscle Groups and Additional Structures. Movement at the ankle (tibiotalar) joint is limited to dorsiflexion and plantar flexion. *Plantar flexion* is powered by the gastrocnemius, the posterior tibial muscle, and the toe flexors. Their tendons run behind the malleoli. The *dorsiflexors* include the anterior tibial muscle and the toe extensors. They lie prominently on the anterior surface, or dorsum, of the ankle, anterior to the malleoli.

Ligaments extend from each malleolus onto the foot.

- Medially, the triangle-shaped *deltoid ligament* fans out from the inferior surface of the medial malleolus to the talus and proximal tarsal bones, protecting against stress from eversion (heel bows outward).

- Laterally, the three ligaments are less substantial, with higher risk for injury: the *anterior talofibular ligament,* most at risk in injury from inversion (heel bows inward) injuries; the *calcaneofibular ligament;* and the *posterior talofibular ligament* (Fig. 16-86). The strong Achilles tendon attaches the gastrocnemius and soleus muscles to the posterior calcaneus. The plantar fascia inserts on the medial tubercle of the calcaneus.

Techniques of Examination

Inspection. Observe all surfaces of the ankles and feet, noting any deformities, nodules, swelling, calluses, or corns.

See Table 16-9, Abnormalities of the Feet (p. 706) and Table 16-10, Abnormalities of the Toes and Soles (p. 707).

Palpation. With your thumbs, palpate the anterior aspect of each *ankle joint*, noting any bogginess, swelling, or tenderness (Fig. 16-87).

Localized tenderness is often present in arthritis, ligamentous injury, or infection.

Feel along the *Achilles tendon* for nodules and tenderness.

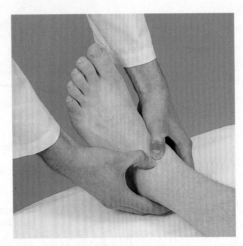

FIGURE 16-87. Palpate the anterior ankle joint.

Check for rheumatoid nodules and tenderness, commonly found in Achilles tendinitis, bursitis, or partial tear from trauma.

Palpate the heel, especially the posterior and inferior calcaneus, and the plantar fascia for tenderness. Bone spurs are common on the calcaneus.

Focal heel tenderness at the attachment site of the plantar fascia is typical of *plantar fasciitis;* risk factors are anatomic (overpronation, flat feet), improper footwear, excessive use, and overtraining with prolonged heel-strike exercise. Presence or absence of a heel spur does not change the diagnosis.[86]

Palpate for tenderness over the medial and lateral ankle ligaments and the medial and lateral malleolus, especially in cases of trauma. In trauma, the distal tip of the tibia and fibula should also be palpated.

Most ankle sprains involve foot inversion and injury to the weaker lateral ligaments (anterior talofibular and calcaneofibular), with overlying tenderness, swelling, and ecchymosis.

After trauma, pain in the malleolar zone plus either bone tenderness over the posterior aspects of either malleolus (or over the navicular or base of the fifth metatarsal) or an inability to bear weight for four steps is suspicious for ankle fracture and warrants radiography (known as the *Ottawa ankle and foot rules*).[87–89]

Palpate the *metatarsophalangeal (MTP) joints* for tenderness (Fig. 16-88). Compress the forefoot between the thumb and fingers. Exert pressure just proximal to the heads of the first and fifth metatarsals.

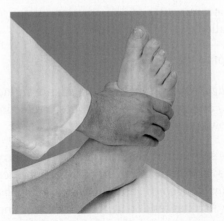

FIGURE 16-88. Palpate the MTP joints.

Tenderness along the posterior medial malleolus is seen in *posterior tibial tendinitis.*

Tenderness on compression is an early sign of *RA.* Acute inflammation of the first MTP joint is common in *gout.*

Palpate the heads of the five metatarsals and the grooves between them with your thumb and index finger (Fig. 16-89). Place your thumb on the dorsum of the foot and your index finger on the plantar surface.

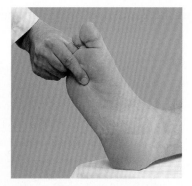

FIGURE 16-89. **Palpate the metatarsal heads.**

Pain and tenderness, called *metatarsalgia,* occurs in trauma, arthritis, and vascular compromise.

Tenderness over the third and fourth metatarsal heads on the plantar surface is suspicious for *Morton neuroma* (see p. 706).

Forefoot abnormalities like hallux valgus, metatarsalgia, and *Morton neuroma* are more common with wear of high-heeled shoes with narrow toe boxes.

Range of Motion and Maneuvers

Range of Motion. Assess flexion and extension at the tibiotalar (ankle) joint. In the foot, assess inversion and eversion at the subtalar and transverse tarsal joints.

Ankle and Foot Range of Motion

Ankle and Foot Movement	Primary Muscles Affecting Movement	Patient Instructions
Ankle Flexion (Plantar Flexion)	Gastrocnemius, soleus, plantaris, tibialis posterior	*"Point your foot toward the floor."*
Ankle Extension (Dorsiflexion)	Tibialis anterior, extensor digitorum longus, and extensor hallucis longus	*"Point your foot toward the ceiling."*
Inversion	Tibialis posterior and anterior	*"Bend your heel inward."*
Eversion	Peroneus longus and brevis	*"Bend your heel outward."*

Maneuvers

- *The ankle (tibiotalar) joint.* Dorsiflex and plantar flex the foot at the ankle.

- *The subtalar (talocalcaneal) joint.* Stabilize the ankle with one hand, grasp the heel with the other, and invert and evert the foot by turning the heel inward then outward (Figs. 16-90 and 16-91).

Pain during movements of the ankle and the foot helps to localize possible arthritis.

An arthritic joint frequently causes pain when moved in any direction, whereas a ligamentous sprain produces pain when the ligament is stretched. For example, often, ankle sprain inversion with plantar flexion of the foot causes pain, whereas eversion with plantar flexion is relatively pain free.

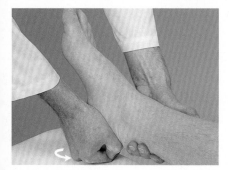

FIGURE 16-90. **Invert the heel.**

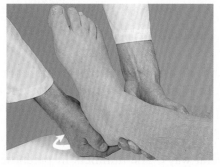

FIGURE 16-91. **Evert the heel.**

■ *The transverse tarsal joint.* Stabilize the heel and invert and evert the forefoot (Figs. 16-92 and 16-93).

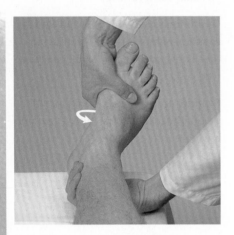

FIGURE 16-92. **Invert the forefoot.**

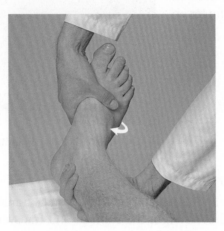

FIGURE 16-93. **Evert the forefoot.**

■ *The metatarsophalangeal joints.* Move the proximal phalanx of each toe up and down.

Pain suggests acute synovitis. Instability occurs in chronic synovitis and claw-toe deformity.

Special Techniques

Measuring the Length of Legs.   To measure leg length, the patient should be relaxed in the supine position and symmetrically aligned with legs extended. With a tape, measure the distance between the anterior superior iliac spine and the medial malleolus (Fig. 16-94). The tape should cross the knee on its medial side.

Measured leg length is the same in scoliosis.

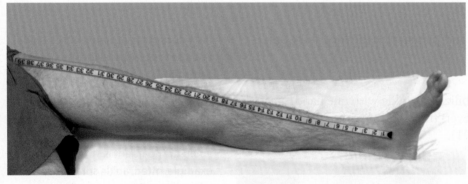

FIGURE 16-94. **Measure leg length.**

Describing Limited Motion of a Joint.   Use a goniometer to measure range of motion in degrees. In Figures 16-95 and 16-96, the red lines show the range of the patient's range of motion, and the black lines show the normal range.

Observations may be described in several ways. The numbers in parentheses show abbreviated descriptions.

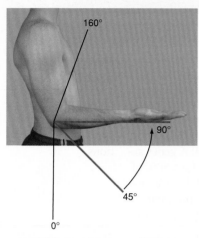

FIGURE 16-95. **Degrees of elbow flexion.**

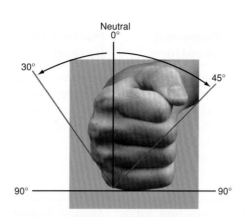

FIGURE 16-96. **Degrees of elbow supination and pronation.**

A. The elbow flexes from 45° to 90° (45° → 90°),

-or-

The elbow has a flexion deformity of 45° and can be flexed farther to 90° (45° → 90°).

B. Supination at elbow = 30° (0° → 30°)
Pronation at elbow = 45° (0° → 45°)

Recording Your Findings

Use anatomical terms specific to the structure and function of individual joint problems to make your write-up of musculoskeletal findings more meaningful and informative.

Recording the Examination—The Musculoskeletal System

"Full range of motion in all joints of the upper and lower extremities. No evidence of swelling or deformity."
OR
"Full range of motion in all joints. Hand with Heberden nodes at the DIP joints, Bouchard nodes at PIP joints. Mild pain with flexion, extension, and rotation of both hips. Full range of motion in the knees, with moderate crepitus; no effusion but bony enlargement along the tibiofemoral joint line bilaterally. Both feet with hallux valgus at the first MTP joints."
OR
"Right knee with moderate effusion and tenderness over medial meniscus along the joint line. Moderate laxity of ACL on Lachman test; PCL, MCL, and LCL intact—no posterior drawer sign or tenderness with varus or valgus stress. Patellar tendon intact—patient able to extend lower extremity. All other joints with good range of motion; no other deformity or swelling."

These findings suggest *OA.*

These findings suggest *partial tear of medial meniscus and ACL,* possibly from sports injury or trauma and require prompt evaluation.

Table 16-1 Patterns of Pain in and Around the Joints

Problem	Process	Common Locations	Pattern of Spread	Onset	Progression and Duration
Rheumatoid Arthritis[8-10]	Chronic inflammation of *synovial membranes* with secondary erosion of adjacent cartilage and bone, and damage to ligaments and tendons	Hands—initially small joints (PIP and MCP joints), feet (MTP joints), wrists, knees, elbows, ankles	Symmetrically additive: progresses to other joints while persisting in initial joints	Usually insidious; human leukocyte antigen (HLA) and non-HLA genes account for >50% of risk of disease; involves proinflammatory cytokines	Often chronic (in >50%), with remissions and exacerbations
Osteoarthritis *(Degenerative Joint Disease)*[12]	Degeneration and progressive loss of joint *cartilage* from mechanical stress, with damage to underlying bone, and formation of new bone at the cartilage margins	Knees, hips, hands (distal, sometimes PIP joints), cervical and lumbar spine, and wrists (first carpometacarpal joint); also joints previously injured or diseased	Additive; however, may involve only one joint.	Usually insidious; genetics may account for >50% of risk of disease; repetitive injury and obesity increase risk	Slowly progressive, with temporary exacerbations after periods of overuse
Gouty Arthritis[7,91]					
Acute Gout	An inflammatory reaction to microcrystals of monosodium urate	Base of the big toe (the first MTP joint), the instep or dorsa of feet, the ankles, knees, and elbows	Early attacks usually confined to one joint	Sudden; often at night; often after injury, surgery, fasting, or excessive food or alcohol intake	Occasional isolated attacks lasting days up to 2 wks; they may get more frequent and severe, with persisting symptoms
Chronic Tophaceous Gout	Multiple local accumulations of sodium urate in the joints and other tissues (*tophi*), with or without inflammation	Feet, ankles, wrists, fingers, and elbows	Additive, not so symmetric as RA	Gradual development of chronicity with repeated attacks	Chronic symptoms with acute exacerbations
Polymyalgia Rheumatica[11]	A disease of unclear etiology in people older than age 50 yrs, especially women; overlaps with giant cell arteritis	Muscles of the hip, shoulder girdle, and neck; symmetric		Insidious or abrupt, even appearing overnight	Chronic but ultimately self-limiting
Fibromyalgia Syndrome[90]	Widespread musculoskeletal pain and tender points. Central pain sensitivity syndrome that may involve aberrant pain signaling and amplification	Multiple specific and symmetric "tender points," often unrecognized until examined; especially in the neck, shoulders, hands, low back, and knees	Shifts unpredictably or worsens in response to immobility, excessive use, or exposure to cold	Variable	Chronic, with "ups and downs"

Swelling	Redness, Warmth, and Tenderness	Stiffness	Limitation of Motion	Generalized Symptoms
Frequent swelling of synovial tissue in joints or tendon sheaths; also subcutaneous nodules	Tender, often warm, but seldom red	Prominent, often for an hour or more in the mornings, also after inactivity	Often develops; affected by associated joint contractures and subluxation, bursitis, and tendinopathy	Weakness, fatigue, weight loss, and low fever are common
Small joint effusions may be present, especially in the knees; also bony enlargement	Possibly tender, seldom warm, and rarely red. Inflammation may accompany disease flares and progression	Frequent but brief (usually 5–10 min), in the morning and after inactivity	Often develops	Usually absent
Present, within and around the involved joint, usually in men (have higher serum urate levels); often polyarticular later in course	Exquisitely tender, hot, and red	Not evident	Motion is limited primarily by pain	Fever may be present; also consider also septic arthritis
Present as tophi in joints, bursae, and subcutaneous tissues; check ears and extensor surfaces for tophi	Tenderness, warmth, and redness may be present during exacerbations	Present	Present	Possibly fever; patients may also develop renal failure and renal stones
Swelling and edema may be present over dorsum of hands, wrists, feet	Muscles often tender, but not warm or red	Prominent, especially in the morning	Pain restricts movement, especially in shoulders	Malaise, depression, anorexia, weight loss, and fever, but no true weakness
None	Multiple specific and symmetric tender "trigger points," often not recognized until the examination	Present, especially in the morning—often confused with inflammatory conditions	Absent, though stiffness is greater at the extremes of movement	Sleep disturbance, usually with fatigue on awakening; overlaps with depression and other pain syndromes

Table 16-2 Pains in the Neck

Patterns	Possible Causes	Physical Signs
Mechanical Neck Pain Aching pain in the cervical paraspinal muscles and ligaments with associated muscle spasm and stiffness and tightness in the upper back and shoulder, lasting up to 6 wks. No associated radiation, paresthesias, or weakness. Headache may be present.	Mechanism poorly understood, possibly sustained muscle contraction. Associated with poor posture, stress, poor sleep, poor head position during activities such as computer use, watching television, and driving.	Local muscle tenderness, pain on movement. No neurologic deficits. Possible trigger points in *fibromyalgia*. *Torticollis* if prolonged abnormal neck posture and muscle spasm.
Mechanical Neck Pain— Whiplash[18,19] Mechanical neck pain with aching paracervical pain and stiffness, often beginning the day after injury. Occipital headache, dizziness, malaise, and fatigue may be present. Chronic whiplash syndrome if symptoms last more than 6 mo; occurs in 20%–40% of injuries.	Musculoligamentous sprain or strain from forced hyperflexion—hyperextension injury to the neck, as in rear-end collisions.	Localized paracervical tenderness, decreased neck range of motion, perceived weakness of the upper extremities. Causes of cervical cord compression such as fracture, herniation, head injury, or altered consciousness are excluded.
Cervical Radiculopathy—from Nerve Root Compression[18,19] Sharp burning or tingling pain in the neck and one arm, with associated paresthesias and weakness. Sensory symptoms often in myotomal pattern, deep in muscle, rather than dermatomal pattern.	Dysfunction of cervical spinal nerve, nerve roots, or both from foraminal encroachment of the spinal nerve (~75%), herniated cervical disc (~25%). Rarely from tumor, syrinx, or multiple sclerosis. Mechanisms may involve hypoxia of the nerve root and dorsal ganglion and release of inflammatory mediators.	C7 nerve root affected most often (45–60%), with weakness in triceps and finger flexors and extensors. C6 nerve root involvement also common, with weakness in biceps, brachioradialis, wrist extensors.
Cervical Myelopathy—from Cervical Cord Compression[18,19] Neck pain with bilateral weakness and paresthesias in both upper and lower extremities, often with urinary frequency. Hand clumsiness, palmar paresthesias, and gait changes may be subtle. Neck flexion often exacerbates symptoms.	Usually from cervical *spondylosis,* defined as cervical degenerative disc disease from spurs, protrusion of ligamentum flavum, and/or disc herniation (~80%); also from cervical stenosis from osteophytes, ossification of ligamentum flavum, and *RA.* Large central or paracentral disc herniation may also compress cord.	Hyperreflexia; clonus at the wrist, knee, or ankle; extensor plantar reflexes (positive Babinski signs); and gait disturbances. May also see *Lhermitte sign:* neck flexion with resulting sensation of electrical shock radiating down the spine. Confirmation of cervical myelopathy warrants neck immobilization and neurosurgical evaluation.

Table 16-3 Low Back Pain

Patterns	Possible Causes	Physical Signs
Mechanical Low Back Pain[4,20,21,24,28] Aching pain in the lumbosacral area; may radiate into lower leg, especially in L5 (lateral leg) or S1 (posterior leg) dermatomes. Signifies anatomic or functional abnormality in absence of neoplastic, infectious, or inflammatory disease. Usually acute (<3 mo), idiopathic, benign, and self-limiting; represents 97% of symptomatic low back pain. Commonly work related and occurring in patients 30–50 yrs. Risk factors include heavy lifting, poor conditioning, obesity.	Often arises from muscle and ligament injuries (~70%) or age-related intervertebral disc or facet disease (~4%). Causes also include herniated disc (~4%), spinal stenosis (~3%), compression fractures (~4%), and spondylolisthesis (2%).	Paraspinal muscle or facet tenderness, pain with back movement, loss of normal lumbar lordosis; motor, sensory, and reflex findings are normal. In *osteoporosis,* check for thoracic kyphosis, percussion tenderness over a spinous process, or fractures in the thoracic spine or hip.[90]
Sciatica (Radicular Low Back Pain)[4,21,57] Shooting pain below the knee, commonly into the lateral leg (L5) or posterior calf (S1); typically accompanies low back pain, often with associated paresthesias and weakness. Bending, sneezing, coughing, straining during bowel movements can worsen the pain.	Sciatic pain is sensitive, ~95%, and specific, ~88%, for disc herniation. Usually from herniated intervertebral disc with compression or traction of nerve root(s) in people ages 50 yrs or older. L5 and S1 roots are involved in ~95% of disc herniations; root or spinal cord compression from neoplastic conditions in fewer than 1% of cases. Tumor or midline disc herniation may cause bowel or bladder dysfunction, leg weakness from *cauda equina syndrome* (S2–S4).	Disc herniation most likely if calf wasting, weak ankle dorsiflexion, absent ankle jerk, positive crossed straight-leg raise (pain in affected leg when healthy leg tested); negative straight-leg raise makes diagnosis highly unlikely. Ipsilateral straight-leg raise sensitive, about 65–98%, but not specific, about 10–60%.
Lumbar Spinal Stenosis[92,93] Neurogenic claudication with gluteal and/or lower extremity pain and/or fatigue that may occur with or without back pain. Pain is provoked by lumbar extension (as in walking uphill) due to reduced space in the lumbar spine from degenerative changes in the spinal canal. Positive LR is >6.0 if pain is absent when seated, improved with bending forward, or present in both buttocks and legs. Positive LR is <4.0 if gait is wide-based and Romberg test is abnormal.	Arises from hypertrophic degenerative disease of one or more vertebral facets and thickening of the ligamentum flavum, causing narrowing of the spinal canal centrally or in lateral recesses. More common after age 60 yrs.	Posture may be flexed forward to reduce symptoms, with lower extremity weakness and hyporeflexia. Thigh pain typically occurs after 30 s of lumbar extension. Straight-leg raise is usually negative.
Chronic Back Stiffness[70,94]	*Ankylosing spondylitis,* an inflammatory polyarthritis, most common in men younger than 40 yrs. *Diffuse idiopathic hyperostosis (DISH)* affects men more than women, usually age ≥50 yrs.	
Nocturnal Back Pain, Unrelieved by Rest[4]	Consider *metastatic malignancy* to the spine from cancer of the prostate, breast, lung, thyroid, and kidney, and multiple myeloma.	Loss of the normal lumbar lordosis, muscle spasm, limited anterior and lateral flexion. Lateral immobility of the spine, especially in thoracic area improves with exercise.
Pain Referred from the Abdomen or Pelvis Usually a deep, aching pain; the level varies with the source. Accounts for ~2% of low back pain.	Peptic ulcer, pancreatitis, pancreatic cancer, chronic prostatitis, endometriosis, dissecting aortic aneurysm, retroperitoneal tumor, and other causes.	Variable with the source. Local vertebral tenderness may be present. Spinal movements are not painful and range of motion is not affected. Look for signs of the primary disorder.

Table 16-4 Painful Shoulders

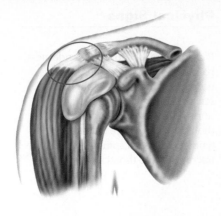

Shoulder-shrugging effort

Limited abduction   Normal abduction

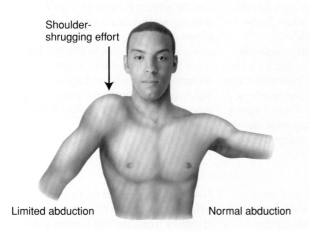

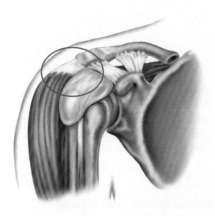

Rotator Cuff Tendinitis (Impingement Syndrome)

Repeated shoulder motion, for example, from throwing or swimming, can cause edema and hemorrhage followed by inflammation, most commonly involving the supraspinatus tendon. Acute, recurrent, or chronic pain may result, often aggravated by activity. Patients report sharp catches of pain, grating, and weakness when lifting the arm overhead. When the supraspinatus tendon is involved, *tenderness is maximal just below the tip of the acromion.* In older adults, bone spurs on the undersurface of the acromion may contribute to symptoms.

Rotator Cuff Tears

The rotator cuff muscles and tendons compress the humeral head into the concave glenoid fossa and strengthen arm movement—the subscapularis in internal rotation, the supraspinatus in elevation, and the infraspinatus and teres minor in external rotation. Injury from a fall, trauma, or repeated impingement against the acromion and the coracoacromial ligament may cause a partial- or full-thickness tear of the rotator cuff, the most common clinical problem of the shoulder, especially in older patients. Patients complain of chronic shoulder pain, night pain, or catching and grating when raising the arm overhead. Weakness or tears of the tendons usually start in the supraspinatus tendon and progress posteriorly and anteriorly. Look for atrophy of the deltoid, supraspinatus, or infraspinatus muscles. Palpate anteriorly over the anterior greater tuberosity of the humerus to check for a defect in muscle attachment and below the acromion for crepitus during arm rotation. In a complete tear, active abduction and forward flexion at the glenohumeral joint are severely impaired, producing a characteristic shrug of the shoulder and a *positive "drop arm" test* (see p. 655).

Calcific Tendinitis

Calcific tendinitis is a degenerative process in the tendon associated with the deposition of calcium salts that usually involves the supraspinatus tendon. Acute disabling attacks of shoulder pain may occur, usually in patients ages ≥30 yrs, especially in women. The arm is held close to the side, and all motions are severely limited by pain. *Tenderness is maximal below the tip of the acromion.* The subacromial bursa, which overlies the supraspinatus tendon, may be inflamed. Chronic less severe pain may also occur.

Bicipital Tendinitis

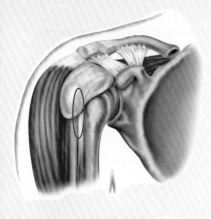

Inflammation of the long head of the biceps tendon and tendon sheath causes anterior shoulder pain resembling and often coexisting with rotator cuff tendinitis. Both conditions may involve impingement injury. *Tenderness is maximal in the bicipital groove.* Externally rotate and abduct the arm to separate this area from the subacromial tenderness of supraspinatus tendinitis. With the patient's arm at the side, elbow flexed to 90°, ask the patient to supinate the forearm against your resistance. Increased pain in the bicipital groove confirms this condition. Pain during resisted forward flexion of the shoulder with the elbow extended is also characteristic.

Adhesive Capsulitis (Frozen Shoulder)

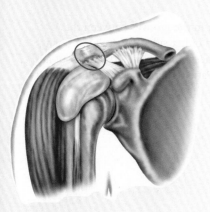

Adhesive capsulitis refers to fibrosis of the glenohumeral joint capsule, manifested by diffuse, dull, aching pain in the shoulder and *progressive restriction of active and passive range of motion,* especially in external rotation, with localized tenderness. The condition is usually unilateral and occurs in people ages 40–60 yrs. There is often an antecedent disorder of the shoulder or another condition (such as myocardial infarction) that has decreased shoulder movements. The disorder may take 6 mo to 2 yrs to resolve. Stretching exercises may help.

Acromioclavicular Arthritis

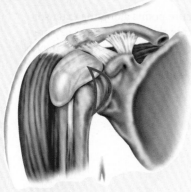

Acromioclavicular arthritis is relatively common, usually arising from prior direct injury to the shoulder girdle with resulting degenerative changes. *Tenderness is localized over the acromioclavicular joint.* Patients report pain with movements of the scapula and arm abduction.

Anterior Dislocation of the Humerus

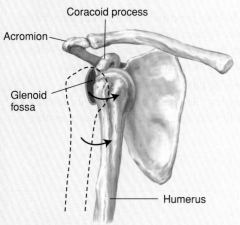

Coracoid process

Acromion

Glenoid fossa

Humerus

Shoulder instability from anterior subluxation or dislocation of the humerus usually results from a fall or forceful throwing motion, then can become common unless treated or the precipitating motion is avoided. The shoulder seems to "slip out of the joint" when the arm is abducted and externally rotated, causing a *positive apprehension sign* for anterior instability when the examiner places the arm in this position. Any shoulder movement may cause pain, and patients hold the arm in a neutral position. The rounded lateral aspect of the shoulder appears flattened. Dislocations may also be inferior, posterior (relatively rare), and multidirectional.

Table 16-5 Swollen or Tender Elbows

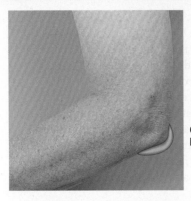

Olecranon
bursitis

Olecranon Bursitis

Swelling and inflammation of the olecranon bursa may result from trauma, gout, or rheumatoid arthritis (RA). The swelling is superficial to the olecranon process and may reach 6 cm in diameter. Consider aspiration for both diagnosis and symptomatic relief.

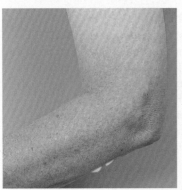

Rheumatoid
nodules

Rheumatoid Nodules

Subcutaneous nodules may develop at pressure points along the extensor surface of the ulna in patients with RA or acute rheumatic fever. They are firm and nontender. They are not attached to the overlying skin but may be attached to the underlying periosteum. They can develop in the area of the olecranon bursa, but often occur more distally.

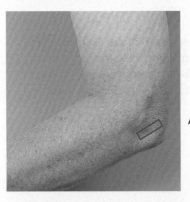

Arthritis

Arthritis of the Elbow

Synovial inflammation or fluid is felt best in the grooves between the olecranon process and the epicondyles on either side. Palpate for a boggy, soft, or fluctuant swelling and for tenderness. Causes include RA, gout and pseudogout, osteoarthritis, and trauma. Patients report pain, stiffness, and restricted motion.

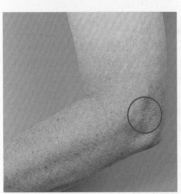

Epicondylitis

Epicondylitis

Lateral epicondylitis (tennis elbow) follows repetitive extension of the wrist or pronation–supination of the forearm. *Pain and tenderness develop 1 cm distal to the lateral epicondyle* and possibly in the extensor muscles close to it. When the patient tries to extend the wrist against resistance, pain increases.

Medial epicondylitis (pitcher's, golfer's, or Little League elbow) follows repetitive wrist flexion such as throwing. *Tenderness is maximal just lateral and distal to the medial epicondyle.* Wrist flexion against resistance increases the pain.

Table 16-6 Arthritis in the Hands

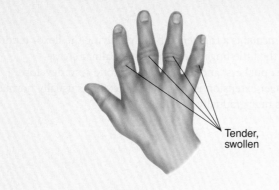

Acute Rheumatoid Arthritis

Tender, painful, stiff joints in *RA,* usually with *symmetric* involvement on both sides of the body. The distal interphalangeal (DIP), metacarpophalangeal (MCP), and wrist joints are the most frequently affected. Note the fusiform or spindle-shaped swelling of the PIP joints in acute disease.

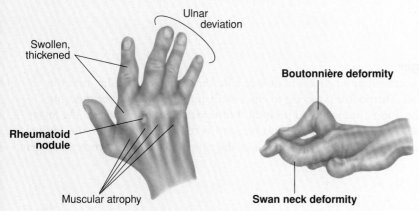

Chronic Rheumatoid Arthritis

In chronic disease, note the swelling and thickening of the MCP and PIP joints. Range of motion becomes limited, and fingers may deviate toward the ulnar side. The interosseous muscles atrophy. The fingers may show *"swan neck" deformities* (hyperextension of the PIP joints with fixed flexion of the distal interphalangeal [DIP] joints). Less common is a *boutonnière deformity* (persistent flexion of the PIP joint with hyperextension of the DIP joint). Rheumatoid nodules are seen in the acute or the chronic stage.

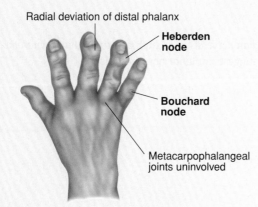

Osteoarthritis (Degenerative Joint Disease)

Heberden nodes on the dorsolateral aspects of the DIP joints from bony overgrowth of OA. Usually hard and painless, they affect middle-ages or older adults; they are often associated with arthritic changes in other joints. Flexion and deviation deformities may develop. *Bouchard nodes* on the PIP joints are less common. The MCP joints are spared.

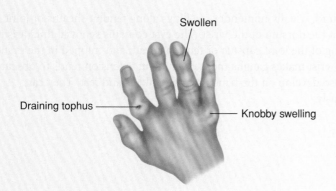

Chronic Tophaceous Gout[8]

Urate crystal deposits, often with surrounding inflammation, cause deformities in subcutaneous tissues, bursae, cartilage, and subchondral bone that mimic RA and OA. Joint involvement is usually less symmetric than in RA. Acute inflammation may be present. Knobby swellings around the joints ulcerate and discharge white chalk-like urates.

Table 16-7 Swellings and Deformities of the Hands

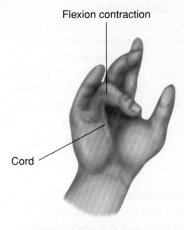

Flexion contraction

Cord

Dupuytren Contracture

The first sign of a *Dupuytren contracture* is a thickened band overlying the flexor tendon of the fourth finger and possibly the little finger near the distal palmar crease. Subsequently, the skin in this area puckers, and a thickened fibrotic cord develops between the palm and finger. Finger extension is limited, but flexion is usually normal. Flexion contracture of the fingers may gradually develop.

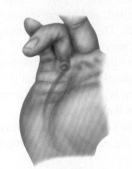

Trigger Finger

Trigger finger is caused by a painless nodule in a flexor tendon in the palm, near the metacarpal head. The nodule is too big to enter easily into the tendon sheath during extension of the fingers from a flexed position. With extra effort or assistance, the finger extends and flexes with a palpable and audible snap as the nodule pops into the tendon sheath. Watch, listen, and palpate the nodule as the patient flexes and extends the fingers.

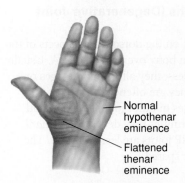

Normal hypothenar eminence

Flattened thenar eminence

Thenar Atrophy

Thenar atrophy suggests a *median nerve disorder* such as *carpal tunnel syndrome* (see p. 664). Hypothenar atrophy suggests an *ulnar nerve disorder*.

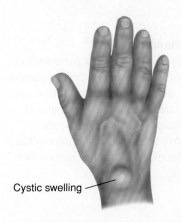

Cystic swelling

Ganglion

Ganglia are cystic, round, usually nontender swellings along tendon sheaths or joint capsules, frequently at the dorsum of the wrist. The cyst contains synovial fluid arising from erosion or tearing of the joint capsule or tendon sheath and trapped in the cystic cavity. Flexion of the wrist makes ganglia more prominent; extension tends to obscure them. Ganglia may also develop on the hands, wrists, ankles, and feet. They can disappear spontaneously.

Table 16-8 Tendon Sheath, Palmar Space, and Finger Infections

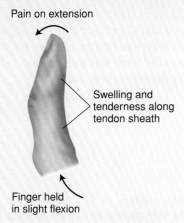

Pain on extension

Swelling and tenderness along tendon sheath

Finger held in slight flexion

Acute Tenosynovitis

Inflammation of the flexor tendon sheaths, *acute tenosynovitis,* may follow local injury, overuse, or infection. Unlike arthritis, tenderness and swelling develop not in the joint but along the course of the tendon sheath, from the distal phalanx to the level of the metacarpophalangeal joint. The finger is held in slight flexion; finger extension is very painful. Causative infectious agents include *Staphylococcus* and *Streptococcus species,* disseminated gonorrhea, and *Candida albicans.*

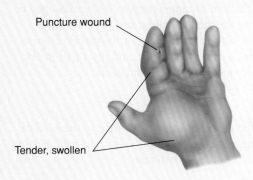

Puncture wound

Tender, swollen

Acute Tenosynovitis and Thenar Space Involvement

If the infection progresses, it may extend from the tendon sheath into the adjacent fascial spaces within the palm. Infections of the index finger and thenar space are illustrated. Early diagnosis and treatment are important.

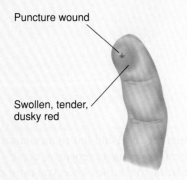

Puncture wound

Swollen, tender, dusky red

Felon

Injury to the fingertip may result in infection of the enclosed fascial spaces of the distal pulp or phalanx pad of the fingertip, usually from *Staphylococcus aureus.* Severe pain, localized tenderness, swelling, and dusky redness are characteristics. Early diagnosis and treatment, usually incision and drainage, are important for preventing abscess formation. If vesicles are present, consider *herpetic whitlow* instead, usually seen in health care workers exposed to *herpes simplex virus* in human saliva.

Table 16-9 Abnormalities of the Feet

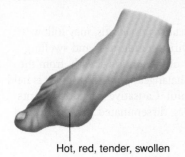

Acute Gouty Arthritis

The metatarsophalangeal joint of the great toe is the initial site of attack in 50% of the episodes of *acute gouty arthritis.* It is characterized by a very painful and tender, hot, dusky red swelling that extends beyond the margin of the joint. It is easily mistaken for a cellulitis. The ankle, tarsal joints, and knee are also commonly involved.

Hot, red, tender, swollen

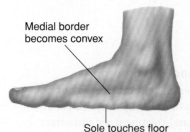

Medial border becomes convex

Flat Feet

Signs of *flat feet* may be apparent only when the patient stands, or they may become permanent. The longitudinal arch flattens so that the sole approaches or touches the floor. The normal concavity on the medial side of the foot becomes convex. Tenderness may be present from the medial malleolus down along the medial plantar surface of the foot. Swelling may develop anterior to the malleoli. Flat feet may be a normal variant or arise from posterior tibial tendon dysfunction, seen in obesity, diabetes, and prior foot injury. Inspect the shoes for excess wear on the inner sides of the soles and heels.

Sole touches floor

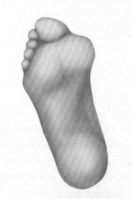

Hallux Valgus

In *hallux valgus,* there is lateral deviation of the great toe and enlargement of the head of the first metatarsal on its medial side, forming a bursa or bunion. This bursa may become inflamed. Women are 10 times more likely to be affected than men.

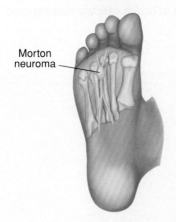

Morton neuroma

Morton Neuroma

Look for tenderness over the plantar surface between the third and fourth metatarsal heads, from perineural fibrosis of the common digital nerve due to repetitive nerve irritation (not a true neuroma). Check for pain radiating to the toes when you press on the plantar interspace and squeeze the metatarsals with your other hand. Symptoms include hyperesthesia, numbness, aching, and burning from the metatarsal heads into the third and fourth toes.

Table 16-10 Abnormalities of the Toes and Soles

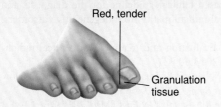

Red, tender

Granulation tissue

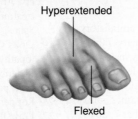

Hyperextended

Flexed

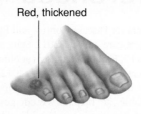

Red, thickened

Ingrown Toenail

The sharp edge of a toenail may dig into and injure the lateral nail fold, resulting in inflammation and infection. A tender, reddened, overhanging nail fold, sometimes with granulation tissue and purulent discharge, results. The great toe is most often affected.

Hammer Toe

Usually involving the second toe, a hammer toe is characterized by hyperextension at the metatarsophalangeal joint with flexion at the proximal interphalangeal (PIP) joint. A corn frequently develops at the pressure point over the PIP joint.

Corn

A corn is a painful conical thickening of skin that results from recurrent pressure on normally thin skin. The apex of the cone points inward and causes pain. Corns characteristically occur over bony prominences such as the fifth toe. When located in moist areas such as pressure points between the fourth and fifth toes, they are called *soft corns*.

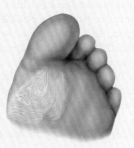

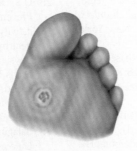

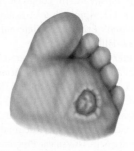

Callus

Like a corn, a callus is an area of greatly thickened skin that develops in a region of recurrent pressure. Unlike a corn, a callus involves skin that is normally thick, such as the sole, and is usually painless. If a callus is painful, suspect an underlying plantar wart.

Plantar Wart

A plantar wart is a hyperkeratotic lesion caused by *human papillomavirus,* located on the sole of the foot. It may look like a callus. Look for the characteristic small dark spots that give a stippled appearance to a wart. Normal skin lines stop at the wart's edge. It is tender if pinched side to side, whereas a callus is tender to direct pressure.

Neuropathic Ulcer

When pain sensation is diminished or absent, as in diabetic neuropathy, neuropathic ulcers may develop at pressure points on the feet. Although often deep, infected, and indolent, they are painless. Underlying osteomyelitis and amputation may ensue. Early detection of loss of sensation using a nylon filament is the standard of care in diabetes.

References

1. Centers for Disease Control and Prevention. National ambulatory medical care survey: 2012 State and National Summary Tables: Table 15, Primary diagnosis at office visits, classified by major disease category: United States, 2012; Table 16, Twenty leading primary diagnosis groups for office visits: United States, 2012. Available at http://www.cdc.gov/nchs/data/ahcd/namcs_summary/2012_namcs_web_tables.pdf. Accessed September 7, 2015.

2. Centers for Disease Control and Prevention. Arthritis-related statistics. Updated March 17, 2014. Available at http://www.cdc.gov/arthritis/data_statistics/arthritis_related_stats.htm#1. Accessed September 8, 2015.

3. Centers for Disease Control and Prevention. Summary Health Statistics for U.S. Adults: National Health Interview Survey, 2010. Table 9. Frequencies of migraines and pain in neck, lower back, face, or jaw among persons aged 18 and over... p. 40. http://www.cdc.gov/nchs/data/series/sr_10/sr10_252.pdf. Accessed September 8, 2015.

4. Chou R. In the clinic. Low back pain. *Ann Intern Med.* 2014; 160:ITC6–1.

5. Cush JJ, Lipsky PE. In: Longo DL, Fauci AS, Kasper DL, et al. (eds). *Chapter 331, Approach to Articular and Musculoskeletal Disorders, in Harrison's Principles of Internal Medicine.* 18th ed. New York: McGraw-Hill; 2012.

6. Carpenter CR, Schuur JD, Everett WW, et al. Evidence-based diagnostics: adult septic arthritis. *Acad Emerg Med.* 2011;18:781.

7. Mead T, Arabindoo K, Smith B. Managing gout: there's more we can do. *J Fam Pract.* 2014;63:707.

8. American College of Physicians. Approach to the Patient with Rheumatic Disease, in Rheumatology. Collier V (ed), *Medical Knowledge Self-Assessment Program (MKSAP) 16.* Philadelphia, PA: American College of Physicians; 2012.

9. Anderson J, Caplan L, Yazdany J, et al. Rheumatoid arthritis disease activity measures: American College of Rheumatology recommendations for use in clinical practice. *Arthritis Care Res (Hoboken).* 2012;64:640.

10. Davis JM 3rd, Matteson EL; American College of Rheumatology; European League Against Rheumatism. My treatment approach to rheumatoid arthritis. *Mayo Clin Proc.* 2012;87:659.

11. Dejaco C, Singh YP, Perel P, et al. 2015 Recommendations for the management of polymyalgia rheumatica: a European League Against Rheumatism/American College of Rheumatology collaborative initiative. *Arthritis Rheumatol.* 2015;67:2569.

12. Gelber AC. In the clinic. Osteoarthritis. *Ann Intern Med.* 2014; 161:ITC1–1.

13. Davatchi F. Behçet's disease. *Int J Rheum Dis.* 2014;17:355.

14. Hatemi G, Yaziel Y, Yazici H. Behçet's syndrome. *Rheum Dis N Am.* 2013;39:245.

15. Michaleff ZA, Maher CG, Verhagen AP, et al. Accuracy of the Canadian C-spine rule and NEXUS to screen for clinically important cervical spine injury in patients following blunt trauma: a systematic review. *CMAJ.* 2012;184:E867.

16. Hoffman JR, Mower WR, Wolfson AB, et al. Validity of a set of clinical criteria to rule out injury to the cervical spine in patients with blunt trauma. *N Engl J Med.* 2000;343:94.

17. Stiell IG, Wells GA, Vandemheen KL, et al. The Canadian C-spine rule for radiography in alert and stable trauma patients. *JAMA.* 2001;286:1841.

18. Bono CM, Ghiselli G, Gilbert TJ, et al; North American Spine Society. An evidence-based clinical guideline for the diagnosis and treatment of cervical radiculopathy from degenerative disorders. *Spine J.* 2011;11:64.

19. Onks CA, Billy G. Evaluation and treatment of cervical radiculopathy. *Prim Care.* 2013;40:837.

20. Rozenberg S, Foltz V, Fautrel B. Treatment strategy for chronic low back pain. *Joint Bone Spine.* 2012;79:555.

21. Ropper AH, Zafonte RD. Sciatica. *N Engl J Med.* 2015;372:1240.

22. Lurie JD, Gerber PD, Sox HC. Clinical problem-solving. A pain in the back. *N Engl J Med.* 2000;343:723.

23. Deyo RA. Biopsychosocial care for chronic back pain. Supporting evidence looks promising but far from complete. *BMJ.* 2015;350: h538.

24. Chou R, Shekelle P. Will this patient develop persistent disabling low back pain? *JAMA.* 2010;303:1295.

25. U.S. Department of Health and Human Services. Office of Disease Prevention and Health Promotion. *Healthy People 2020. Arthritis, osteoporosis, and chronic back conditions.* Washington, D.C. Available at: http://www.healthypeople.gov/202020202020/topics objectives/topic/Arthritis-Osteoporosis-and-Chronic-Back-Conditions. Accessed June 19, 2015.

26. U.S. Department of Health and Human Services. Office of Disease Prevention and Health Promotion. *Healthy People 2020. Physical activity objectives.* Washington, DC. Available at: http://www.healthypeople.gov/2020202020202020/topics-objectives/topic/physical-activity/objectives. Accessed June 19, 2015.

27. Davis MA, Onega T, Weeks WB, et al. Where the United States spends its spine dollars: expenditures on different ambulatory services for the management of back and neck conditions. *Spine.* 2012;37:1693.

28. Balague F, Mannion AF, Pellise F, et al. Non-specific low back pain. *Lancet.* 2012;379:482.

29. National Ambulatory Medical Care Survey. Factsheet. Outpatient Department. Centers for Disease Control and Prevention. National Center for Health Statistics. 2011. Available at: http://www.cdc.gov/nchs/data/ahcd/NHAMCS_2011_opd_factsheet.pdf. Accessed June 19, 2015.

30. Dagenais S, Tricco AC, Haldeman S. Synthesis of recommendations for the assessment and management of low back pain from recent clinical practice guidelines. *Spine J.* 2010;10:514.

31. Waddell G, McCulloch JA, Kummel E, et al. Nonorganic physical signs in low-back pain. *Spine.* 1980;5:117.

32. Chou R. Pharmacological management of low back pain. *Drugs.* 2010;70:387.

33. Looker AC, Borrud LG, Dawson-Hughes B, et al. Osteoporosis or low bone mass at the femur neck or lumbar spine in older adults: United States, 2005 2008. *NCHS Data Brief.* 2012;93:1.

34. U.S. Preventive Services Task Force. Screening for osteoporosis: U.S. preventive services task force recommendation statement. *Ann Intern Med.* 2011;154:356.

35. Brauer CA, Coca-Perraillon M, Cutler DM, et al. Incidence and mortality of hip fractures in the United States. *JAMA.* 2009;302: 1573.

36. Looker AC, Melton LJ 3rd, Harris TB, et al. Prevalence and trends in low femur bone density among older US adults: NHANES 2005–2006 compared with NHANES III. *J Bone Miner Res.* 2010;25:64.

37. Qaseem A, Snow V, Shekelle P, et al. Screening for osteoporosis in men: a clinical practice guideline from the American College of Physicians. *Ann Intern Med.* 2008;148:680.

REFERENCES

38. National Institutes of Health. Office of Dietary Supplements. Calcium. Dietary Supplement Fact Sheet. 2013. Available at: http://ods.od.nih.gov/factsheets/Calcium HealthProfessional./ Accessed June 19, 2015.

39. Ross AC, Manson JE, Abrams SA, et al. The 2011 report on dietary reference intakes for calcium and vitamin D from the Institute of Medicine: what clinicians need to know. *J Clin Endocrinol Metab.* 2011;96:53.

40. LeFevre ML, U.S. Preventive Services Task Force. Screening for vitamin D deficiency in adults: U.S. Preventive Services Task Force recommendation statement. *Ann Intern Med.* 2015;162:133.

41. Moyer VA, U.S. Preventive Services Task Force. Vitamin D and calcium supplementation to prevent fractures in adults: U.S. Preventive Services Task Force recommendation statement. *Ann Intern Med.* 2013;158:691.

42. Reid IR, Bristow SM, Bolland MJ. Cardiovascular complications of calcium supplements. *J Cell Biochem.* 2015;116:494.

43. Heaney RP, Kopecky S, Maki KC, et al. A review of calcium supplements and cardiovascular disease risk. *Adv Nutr.* 2012;3:763.

44. Islam MR, Ahmed MU, Mitu SA, et al. Comparative analysis of serum zinc, copper, manganese, iron, calcium, and magnesium level and complexity of interelement relations in generalized anxiety disorder patients. *Biol Trace Elem Res.* 2013;154:21.

45. Tripkovic L, Lambert H, Hart K, et al. Comparison of vitamin D2 and vitamin D3 supplementation in raising serum 25-hydroxyvitamin D status: a systematic review and meta analysis. *Am J Clin Nutr.* 2012;95:1357.

46. Nelson HD, Haney EM, Dana T, et al. Screening for osteoporosis: an update for the U.S. Preventive Services Task Force. *Ann Intern Med.* 2010;153:99.

47. North American Menopause Society. Management of osteoporosis in postmenopausal women: 2010 position statement of Menopause Society. *Menopause.* 2010;17:25.

48. Hodsman A, Papaioannou A, Ann C. Clinical practice guidelines for the use of parathyroid hormone in the treatment of osteoporosis. *CMAJ.* 2006;175:48.

49. Michael YL, Lin JS, Whitlock EP, et al. *Interventions to prevent falls in older adults: An updated systematic review.* Rockville, MD; 2010. Available at: http://www.ncbi.nlm.nih.gov/pubmed/21595101. 21595101.21595101.21595101. Accessed June 19, 2015.

50. Centers for Disease Control and Prevention. *Hip Fractures Among Older Adults.* Atlanta, GA; 2015. Available at: http://www.cdc.gov/HomeandRecreationalSafety/Falls/adulthipfx.html. Accessed June 19, 2015.

51. Moyer VA. U.S. Preventive Services Task Force. Prevention of falls in community dwelling older adults: U.S. Preventive Services Task Force recommendation statement. *Ann Intern Med.* 2012;157:197.

52. Singh JA, Furst DE, Bharat A, et al. 2012 update of the 2008 American College of Rheumatology recommendations for the use of disease-modifying antirheumatic drugs and biologic agents in the treatment of rheumatoid arthritis. *Arthritis Care Res (Hoboken).* 2012;64:625.

53. Aletaha D, Neogi T, Silman AJ, et al. 2010 Rheumatoid arthritis classification criteria: an American College of Rheumatology/European League Against Rheumatism collaborative initiative. *Arthritis Rheum.* 2010;62:2569.

54. Nagy G, van Vollenhoven RF. Sustained biologic-free and drug-free remission in rheumatoid arthritis, where are we now? *Arthritis Res Ther.* 2015;17:181.

55. Durham J, Newton-John TR, Zakrzewska JM. Temporomandibular disorders. *BMJ.* 2015;350:h1154.

56. Schiffman E, Ohrbach R, Truelove E, et al. Diagnostic Criteria for Temporomandibular Disorders (DC/TMD) for clinical and research applications: recommendations of the International RDC/TMD Consortium Network and Orofacial Pain Special Interest Group. *J Oral Facial Pain Headache.* 2014;28:6.

57. McGee S. Chapter 55, Examination of the musculoskeletal system—the shoulder. In: *Evidence-based Physical Diagnosis.* 3rd ed. St. Louis, MO: Saunders; 2012.

58. Whittle S, Buchbinder R. In the clinic. Rotator cuff disease. *Ann Intern Med.* 2015;162:ITC1–1.

59. Hermans J, Luime JJ, Meuffels DE, et al. Does this patient with shoulder pain have rotator cuff disease?: The Rational Clinical Examination systematic review. *JAMA.* 2013;310:837.

60. Hanchard NC, Lenza M, Handoll HH, et al. Physical tests for shoulder impingements and local lesions of bursa, tendon or labrum that may accompany impingement. *Cochrane Database Syst Rev.* 2013;4:CD007427.

61. Murrell GA, Walton. Diagnosis of rotator cuff tears. *Lancet.* 2001; 357:769.

62. Appleboam A, Reuben AD, Benger JR, et al. Elbow extension test to rule out elbow fracture: multicentre prospective validation and observational study of diagnostic accuracy in adults and children. *BMJ.* 2008;337:2428.

63. Darracq MA, Vinson DR, Panacek EA. Preservation of active range of motion after acute elbow trauma predicts absence of elbow fracture. *Am J Emerg Med.* 2008;26:779.

64. Arundel D, Williams P, Townend W. Deriving the East Riding Elbow Rule (ER2): a maximally sensitive decision tool for elbow injury. *Emerg Med J.* 2014;31:380.

65. Kleopa KA. In the clinic. Carpal tunnel syndrome. *Ann Intern Med.* 2015;163:ITC1–1.

66. Kenney RJ, Hammert WC. Physical examination of the hand. *J Hand Surg Am.* 2014;39:2324.

67. Sauvé PS, Rhee PC, Shin AY, et al. Examination of the wrist: radial-sided wrist pain. *J Hand Surg Am.* 2014;39:2089.

68. McGee S. Chapter 62, Disorders of the nerve roots, plexuses. In: *Evidence-based Physical Diagnosis.* 3rd ed. St. Louis, MO: Saunders; 2012.

69. D'Arcy CA, McGee S. Does this patient have carpal tunnel syndrome? The rational clinical examination. *JAMA.* 2000;283:3110.

70. Raychaudhuri SP, Deodhar A. The classification and diagnostic criteria of ankylosing spondylitis. *J Autoimmun.* 2014;48:128.

71. Al Nezari NH, Schneiders AG, Hendrick PA. Neurological examination of the peripheral nervous system to diagnose lumbar spinal disc herniation with suspected radiculopathy: a systematic review and meta-analysis. *Spine J.* 2013;13:657.

72. Scaia V, Baxter D, Cook C. The pain provocation-based straight leg raise test for diagnosis of lumbar disc herniation, lumbar radiculopathy, and/or sciatica: a systematic review of clinical utility. *J Back Musculoskelet Rehabil.* 2012;25:215.

73. Iversen T, Solberg TK, Romner B, et al. Accuracy of physical examination for chronic lumbar radiculopathy. *BMC Musculoskelet Disord.* 2013;14:206.

74. Frank RM, Slabaugh MA, Grumet RC, et al. Hip pain in active patients: what you may be missing. *J Fam Pract.* 2012;61:736.

75. Suarez JC, Ely EE, Mutnal AB, et al. Comprehensive approach to the evaluation of groin pain. *J Am Acad Orthop Surg.* 2013;21:558.

76. Karrasch C, Lynch S. Practical approach to hip pain. *Med Clin N Am.* 2014;98:737.

REFERENCES

77. Reiman MP, Goode AP, Hegedus EJ, et al. Diagnostic accuracy of clinical tests of the hip: A systematic review with meta-analysis. *Br J Sports Med.* 2012;47:893.

78. Prather H, Harris-Hayes M, Hunt DM, et al. Reliability and agreement of hip range of motion and provocative physical examination tests in asymptomatic volunteers. *PM R.* 2010;2:888.

79. Smith BE, Thacker D, Crewesmith A, et al. Special tests for assessing meniscal tears within the knee: a systematic review and meta-analysis. *Evid Based Med.* 2015;20:88.

80. Lester JD, Watson JN, Hutchinson MR. Physical examination of the patellofemoral joint. *Clin Sports Med.* 2014;33:403.

81. Morelli V, Braxton TM Jr. Meniscal, plica, patellar, and patellofemoral injuries of the knee: updates, controversies and advancements. *Prim Care.* 2013;40:357.

82. Schiphof D, van Middelkoop M, de Klerk BM, et al. Crepitus is a first indication of patellofemoral osteoarthritis (and not of tibiofemoral osteoarthritis). *Osteoarthritis Cartilage.* 2014;22:631.

83. Knutson T, Bothwell J, Durbin R. Evaluation and management of traumatic knee injuries in the emergency department. *Emerg Clin North Am.* 2015;33:345.

84. Karrasch C, Gallo RA. The acutely injured knee. *Med Clin North Am.* 2014;98:719.

85. Young C. In the clinic. Plantar fasciitis. *Ann Intern Med.* 2012; 156:ITC1–1.

86. Papaliodis DN, Vanushkina MA, Richardson NG, et al. The foot and ankle examination. *Med Clin North Am.* 2014;98:181.

87. Czajka CM, Tran E, Cai AN. Ankle sprains and instability. *Med Clin North Am.* 2014;98:313.

88. Tiemstra JD. Update on acute ankle sprains. *Am Fam Phys.* 2012; 85:1170.

89. Clauw DJ. Fibromyalgia: a clinical review. *JAMA.* 2014;311:1547.

90. Golub AL, Laya MB. Osteoporosis: screening, prevention, and management. *Med Clin N Am.* 2015;99:587.

91. Neogi T. Gout. *New Engl J Med.* 2011;364:443.

92. Kreiner DS, Shaffer WO, Baisden JL, et al. An evidence-based clinical guideline for the diagnosis and treatment of degenerative lumbar spinal stenosis (update). *Spine J.* 2013;13:734.

93. Suri P, Rainville J, Kalichman L, et al. Does this older adult with lower extremity pain have the clinical syndrome of lumbar spinal stenosis? *JAMA.* 2010;304:2628.

94. Assassi S, Weisman MH, Lee M, et al. New population-based reference values for spinal mobility measures based on the 2009–2010 National Health and Nutrition Examination Survey. *Arthritis Rheumatol.* 2014;66:2628.

The Nervous System

The Bates' suite offers these additional resources to enhance learning and facilitate understanding of this chapter:

- Bates' *Pocket Guide to Physical Examination and History Taking,* 8th edition
- Bates' *Visual Guide to Physical Examination* (Vols. 17 and 18: Nervous System)
- thePoint online resources, for students and instructors: http://thepoint.lww.com

The focus of this chapter is the evaluation of the cranial nerves (CNs), the motor system with all its components, the sensory system, and the reflexes. The complex anatomy and physiology of the nervous system make examination and assessment especially challenging, but attainable with practice and dedication. For many of the body systems, the history provides the essential clues to diagnosis. While this is true for the nervous system, the neurologic examination allows you to assess all levels of nervous system function to a degree that is unique.

Because the nervous system affects all body systems, knowledge of neural function plays a role in the evaluation of any illness. Begin by reviewing the key structures of the brain illustrated in Figure 17-1.

The history and neurologic examination seek to answer four guiding questions.[1] These questions are not answered separately, but iteratively as you learn about the patient from the patient's spontaneous responses during the interview and from

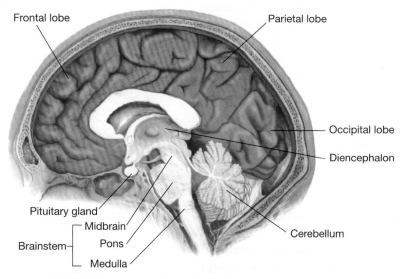

FIGURE 17-1. **Right half of the brain, medial view.**

your neurologic findings. As you acquire the skills of nervous system examination, it is important to test your findings against those of your teachers and neurologists to refine your clinical expertise.

Guiding Questions for Examination of the Nervous System

- Does the patient have neurologic disease?
- If so, what is the localization of the lesion or lesions? Are your findings symmetric?
- What is the pathophysiology of abnormal findings?
- What is the preliminary differential diagnosis?

Assessment of the nervous system begins with the first moments of the patient encounter and continues throughout the interview. If you suspect that the patient's mental status is abnormal, proceed directly to formal mental status testing, described in Chapter 5. If there is significant impairment, for example, disorientation to person or place, the history may be unreliable, so you will need other observers to obtain critical information.

See Chapter 5, Behavior and Mental Status, pp. 147–171, techniques to conduct the formal mental status examination.

The Challenges of Neurologic Diagnosis

Neurologic diagnosis is considered difficult by many. Lesions at different levels of the nervous system can cause the same physical finding. For example, weakness of foot dorsiflexion can be caused by disease of the brain, brainstem, spinal cord, spinal nerve root, peripheral nerve, and muscles. In addition, neurologic pathophysiology can have positive or negative effects, or both. Loss of sensory or motor function may be transient or permanent. Alternatively, some nervous system structures have inhibitory effects. When destroyed, there may be increased function such as heightened muscle tone or pathologic hyperreflexia from upper corticospinal tract lesions. There may be irritative phenomena such as the pins-and-needles sensation of paresthesias, myoclonus, or focal seizures with jerking of a limb on one side of the body. In addition, some parts of the nervous system are relatively silent—extensive lesions can even be present without causing symptoms or abnormal findings.

In many neurologic conditions the neurologic examination may be normal, as when a patient recovers from attacks of epilepsy or a transient ischemic attack (TIA). In some neurologic diseases such as migraine, normal findings are expected—abnormal findings would trigger alarm and further evaluation. In some instances, symptoms in the absence of findings would raise concern, as with a TIA.

When you conduct the neurologic examination, it is wise to adopt a fixed routine or examination sequence to minimize omission of one of its important components. Pursue more detailed testing of areas targeted by symptoms and abnormal function. Follow-up examination over time is important for determining whether the patient's condition is getting worse, improving spontaneously, or responding to treatment. The goal of your assessment is not just diagnosis, but treating and restoring the patient to health and the full range of activities of daily living.[2]

Anatomy and Physiology

Central Nervous System

The Brain.   The brain has four regions: the cerebrum, the diencephalon, the brainstem, and the cerebellum. Each cerebral hemisphere is subdivided into frontal, parietal, temporal, and occipital lobes.

The *central nervous system* (CNS) of the brain is a vast network of interconnecting nerve cells, or *neurons,* consisting of cell bodies and their *axons*—single long fibers that conduct impulses to other parts of the nervous system.

Brain tissue may be gray or white. *Gray matter* consists of aggregations of neuronal cell bodies. It rims the surfaces of the cerebral hemispheres, forming the cerebral cortex. *White matter* consists of neuronal axons that are coated with myelin. The myelin sheaths, which create the white color, allow nerve impulses to travel more rapidly.

Deep in the brain lie additional clusters of gray matter (Fig. 17-2). These include the *basal ganglia,* which affect movement, and the thalamus and the hypothalamus structures in the diencephalon. The *thalamus* processes sensory impulses and relays them to the cerebral cortex. The *hypothalamus* maintains homeostasis

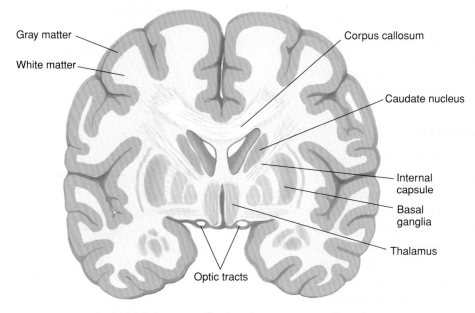

FIGURE 17-2.   Brain anatomy—coronal section.

and regulates temperature, heart rate, and blood pressure. The hypothalamus affects the endocrine system and governs emotional behaviors such as anger and sexual drive. Hormones secreted in the hypothalamus act directly on the pituitary gland.

The *internal capsule* is a white-matter structure where myelinated fibers converge from all parts of the cerebral cortex and descend into the brainstem. The *brainstem,* which connects the upper part of the brain with the spinal cord, has three sections: the midbrain, the pons, and the medulla.

Consciousness relies on the interaction between intact cerebral hemispheres and a structure in the diencephalon and upper brainstem, the *reticular activating (arousal) system.*

The *cerebellum,* which lies at the base of the brain, coordinates all movement and helps maintain the body upright in space.

The Spinal Cord.   Below the medulla, the CNS extends into the elongated *spinal cord,* encased within the bony vertebral column and terminating at the first or second lumbar vertebra. The cord provides a series of segmental relays with the periphery, serving as a conduit for information flow to and from the brain. The motor and sensory nerve pathways relay neural signals that enter and exit the cord through posterior and anterior nerve roots and the spinal and peripheral nerves.

The spinal cord is divided into segments: cervical, from C1 to C8; thoracic, from T1 to T12; lumbar, from L1 to L5; sacral, from S1 to S5; and coccygeal (Fig. 17-3). The spinal cord is thickest in the cervical segment, which contains nerve tracts to and from both the upper and lower extremities.

Note that the spinal cord is not as long as the vertebral canal. The lumbar and sacral roots travel the longest intraspinal distance and fan out like a horse's tail at L1–L2, giving rise to the term *cauda equina.* To avoid injury to the spinal cord, most lumbar punctures are performed at the L3–L4 or L4–L5 vertebral interspaces.[3,4]

Peripheral Nervous System

The *peripheral nervous system* (PNS) consists of both CNs and peripheral nerves that project to the heart, visceral organs, skin, and limbs. It controls the *somatic nervous system,* which regulates muscle movements and response to the sensations of touch and pain, and the *autonomic nervous system* that connects to internal organs and generates autonomic reflex responses. The autonomic nervous system consists of the *sympathetic nervous system,* which "mobilizes organs and their functions during times of stress and arousal, and the *parasympathetic nervous system,* which conserves energy and resources during times of rest and relaxation."[5]

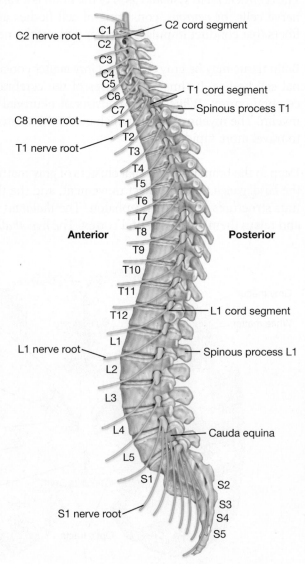

FIGURE 17-3.   Spinal cord, lateral view.

The Cranial Nerves. Twelve pairs of special nerves called *cranial nerves* (CNs) emerge from the cranial vault through skull foramina and canals to structures in the head and neck. They are numbered sequentially with Roman numerals in rostral to caudal order as they arise from the brain. CNs III through XII arise from the diencephalon and the brainstem, as illustrated in Figure 17-4. CNs I and II are actually fiber tracts emerging from the brain. Some CNs are limited to general motor and/or sensory functions, whereas others are specialized, serving smell, vision, or hearing (I, II, VIII).

Functions of the CNs most relevant to the physical examination are summarized on the next page.

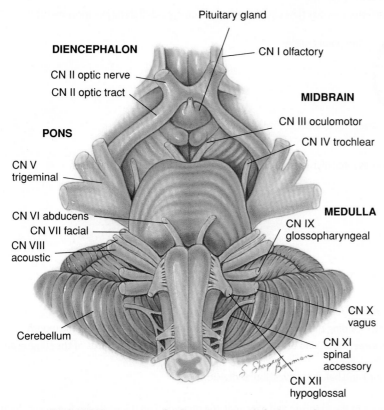

FIGURE 17-4. **Brain anatomy—inferior surface.**

The Peripheral Nerves. The PNS includes spinal and peripheral nerves that carry impulses to and from the cord. A total of 31 pairs of spinal nerves attach to the spinal cord: 8 cervical, 12 thoracic, 5 lumbar, 5 sacral, and 1 coccygeal. Each nerve has an anterior (ventral) root containing motor fibers, and a posterior (dorsal) root containing sensory fibers. The anterior and posterior roots merge to form a short *spinal nerve,* <5 mm long. Spinal nerve fibers commingle with similar fibers from other levels in plexuses outside the cord, from which *peripheral nerves* emerge. Most peripheral nerves contain both *sensory* (afferent) and *motor* (efferent) fibers.

Cranial Nerves

No.	Name	Function
I	Olfactory	Sense of smell
II	Optic	Vision

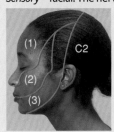

III	Oculomotor	Pupillary constriction, opening the eye (lid elevation), and most extraocular movements
IV	Trochlear	Downward, internal rotation of the eye
V	Trigeminal	*Motor*—temporal and masseter muscles (jaw clenching), lateral pterygoids (lateral jaw movement)

Temporal muscle

Masseter muscle

Sensory—facial. The nerve has three divisions: (1) ophthalmic, (2) maxillary, and (3) mandibular.

(1) C2
(2)
(3)

VI	Abducens	Lateral deviation of the eye
VII	Facial	*Motor*—facial movements, including those of facial expression, closing the eye, and closing the mouth
		Sensory—taste for salty, sweet, sour, and bitter substances on the anterior two thirds of the tongue and sensation from the ear
VIII	Acoustic	Hearing (cochlear division) and balance—(vestibular division)
IX	Glossopha-ryngeal	*Motor*—pharynx
		Sensory—posterior portions of the eardrum and ear canal, the pharynx, and the posterior tongue, including taste (salty, sweet, sour, bitter)
X	Vagus	*Motor*—palate, pharynx, and larynx
		Sensory—pharynx and larynx
XI	Spinal acces-sory	*Motor*—the sternocleidomastoid and upper portion of the trapezius

Sternocleidomastoid muscle
Trapezius muscle

XII	Hypoglossal	*Motor*—tongue

Like the brain, the spinal cord contains both gray matter and white matter (Fig. 17-5). The gray matter consists of aggregations of nerve cell nuclei and dendrites that are surrounded by white tracts of nerve fibers connecting the brain to the PNS. Note the butterfly appearance of the gray matter nuclei and their anterior and posterior horns.

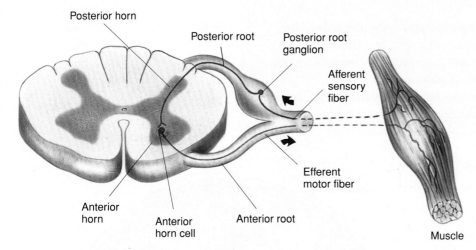

FIGURE 17-5. **Spinal cord, cross section.**

Motor Pathways

Motor pathways are complex avenues that extend from *upper motor neurons* through long white matter tracts to synapses with *lower motor neurons,* and continue to the periphery through peripheral nerve structures. Upper motor neurons, or nerve cell bodies, lie in the motor strip of the cerebral cortex and in several brainstem nuclei; their axons synapse with motor nuclei in the brainstem (for CNs) and in the spinal cord (for peripheral nerves). Lower motor neurons have cell bodies in the spinal cord, termed anterior horn cells; their axons transmit impulses through the anterior roots and spinal nerves into peripheral nerves, terminating at the neuromuscular junction.

Three kinds of motor pathways impinge on the anterior horn cells: the corticospinal tract, the basal ganglia system, and the cerebellar system. Additional pathways originating in the brainstem mediate flexor and extensor tone in limb movement and posture, most notably in coma (see Table 17-14, p. 793).

The Principal Motor Pathways

- The *corticospinal (pyramidal) tract.* The corticospinal tracts mediate voluntary movement and integrate skilled, complicated, or delicate movements by stimulating selected muscular actions and inhibiting others. They also carry impulses that inhibit *muscle tone,* the slight tension maintained by normal muscle even when it is relaxed. The corticospinal tracts originate in the motor cortex of the brain (Fig. 17-6). Motor fibers travel down into the lower medulla, where they form an anatomical structure resembling a pyramid.

(continued)

The Principal Motor Pathways (*continued*)

There, most of these fibers cross to the opposite or *contralateral* side of the medulla, continue downward, and synapse with anterior horn cells or with intermediate neurons. Tracts synapsing in the brainstem with motor nuclei of the CNs are termed *corticobulbar*.

- The *basal ganglia system*. This exceedingly complex system includes motor pathways between the cerebral cortex, basal ganglia, brainstem, and spinal cord. It helps to maintain muscle tone and to control body movements, especially gross automatic movements such as walking.
- The *cerebellar system*. The cerebellum receives both sensory and motor input and coordinates motor activity, maintains equilibrium, and helps to control posture.

All of these higher motor pathways affect movement only through the lower motor neuron systems, sometimes called the "final common pathway." Any movement, whether initiated voluntarily in the cortex, "automatically" in the basal ganglia, or reflexly via the sensory receptors, must ultimately be translated into action by the anterior horn cells. A lesion in any of these areas will affect movement or reflex activity.

When the corticospinal tract is damaged or destroyed, its functions are reduced or lost below the level of injury. When upper motor neuron systems are damaged above their crossover in the medulla, motor impairment develops on the opposite or contralateral side. In damage below the crossover, motor impairment occurs on the same or ipsilateral side of the body. The affected limb becomes weak or paralyzed, and skilled, complicated, or delicate movements are performed poorly when compared with gross movements.

In upper motor neuron lesions, muscle tone is increased and deep tendon reflexes are exaggerated. Damage to the lower motor neuron systems causes ipsilateral weakness and paralysis, but in this case, muscle tone and reflexes are decreased or absent.

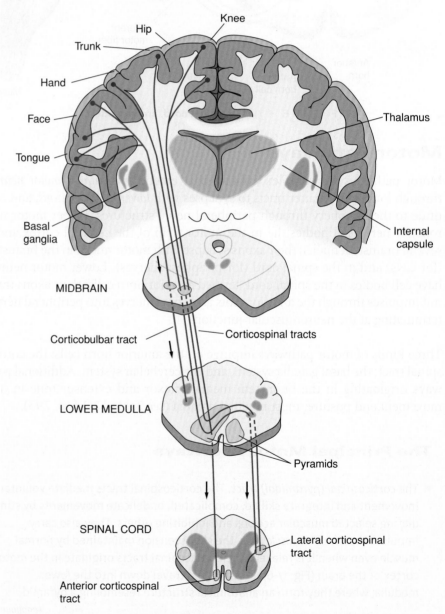

FIGURE 17-6. Motor pathways: corticospinal and corticobulbar tracts.

Disease of the basal ganglia system or cerebellar system does not cause paralysis, but can be disabling. Damage to the basal ganglia system produces changes in muscle tone (most often an increase), disturbances in posture and gait, a slowness or lack of spontaneous and automatic movements termed *bradykinesia,* and various involuntary movements. Cerebellar damage impairs coordination, gait, and equilibrium, and decreases muscle tone.

Sensory Pathways

Sensory impulses participate not only in reflex activity, as previously described, but also give rise to conscious sensation, locate body position in space, and help regulate internal autonomic functions such as blood pressure, heart rate, and respiration.

A complex system of sensory receptors relays impulses from skin, mucous membranes, muscles, tendons, and viscera that travel through peripheral projections into the posterior root ganglia, where a second projection of the ganglia directs impulses centrally into the spinal cord (Fig. 17-7). Sensory impulses then travel to the sensory cortex of the brain via one of two pathways: the *spinothalamic tract,* consisting of smaller sensory neurons with unmyelinated or thinly myelinated axons, and the *posterior columns,* which have larger neurons with heavily myelinated axons.[6]

The peripheral component of the small-fiber *spinothalamic tract* arises in free nerve endings in the skin that register *pain, temperature,* and *crude touch.* Within one or two spinal segments from their entry into the cord, these fibers pass into the posterior horn and synapse with secondary neurons. The secondary neurons then cross to the opposite side and pass upward into the thalamus.

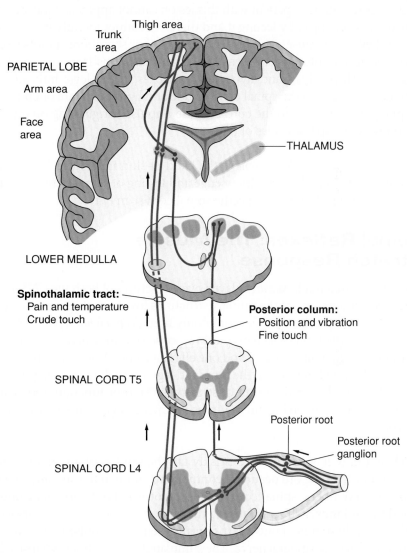

FIGURE 17-7. **Sensory pathways: spinothalamic tract and posterior columns.**

In the *posterior column* system, the peripheral large-fiber projections of the dorsal root ganglia transmit the sensations of *vibration, proprioception, kinesthesia, pressure,* and *fine touch* from skin and joint position receptors to the dorsal root ganglia, where they travel through central projections in the posterior columns to second-order sensory neurons in the medulla. Fibers projecting from the secondary neurons cross to the opposite side at the medullary level and continue on to the thalamus.

Diabetic patients with small-fiber neuropathy report sharp, burning, or shooting foot pain, whereas those with large-fiber neuropathy experience numbness and tingling or even no sensation at all.[7,8]

At the *thalamic level,* the general quality of sensation is perceived (e.g., pain, cold, pleasant, unpleasant), but not fine distinctions. For full perception, a third group of sensory neurons sends impulses from the thalamus to the *sensory cortex* of the brain. Here, stimuli are localized and higher-order discriminations are made.

Lesions at different points in the sensory pathways produce different kinds of sensory loss. Patterns of sensory loss, together with their associated motor findings, help you locate the causative lesions. A lesion in the sensory cortex may not impair the perception of pain, touch, and position, for example, but does impair finer discrimination. A patient with this lesion cannot appreciate the size, shape, or texture of an object by feeling it and therefore cannot identify it. Loss of position and vibration sense, with preservation of other sensations, points to disease of the posterior columns, whereas loss of all sensations from the waist down, together with paralysis and hyperactive reflexes in the legs, indicates severe transverse damage to the spinal cord. Crude and light touch are often preserved despite partial damage to the cord because impulses originating on one side of the body travel up both sides of the cord.

See Table 17-1, Disorders of the Central and Peripheral Nervous Systems, pp. 774–775.

Dermatomes.   A *dermatome* is the band of skin innervated by the sensory root of a single spinal nerve. Knowledge and testing of dermatomes are valuable when localizing a lesion to a specific spinal cord segment.

See the dermatome "maps" on pp. 756 and 757.

Spinal Reflexes: The Muscle Stretch Response

The muscle stretch reflexes are relayed over structures of both the CNS and PNS. Since the tendons are not the primary structures involved, the term *muscle stretch reflexes* is more precise than the commonly used *deep tendon reflexes.* Recall that a *reflex* is an involuntary stereotypical response that may involve as few as two neurons, one afferent (sensory) and one efferent (motor), across a single synapse. The muscle stretch reflexes in the arms and legs are such monosynaptic reflexes. They illustrate the simplest unit of sensory and motor function. Other reflexes are polysynaptic, involving interneurons interposed between sensory and motor neurons.

To elicit a muscle stretch reflex, briskly tap the tendon of a partially stretched muscle. For the reflex to occur, all components of the reflex arc must be intact: sensory nerve fibers, spinal cord synapse, motor nerve fibers, neuromuscular junction, and muscle fibers. Tapping the tendon activates special sensory fibers in the partially stretched muscle, triggering a sensory impulse that travels to the spinal cord via a peripheral nerve. The stimulated sensory fiber synapses directly with the anterior horn cell innervating the same muscle. When the impulse crosses the neuromuscular junction, the muscle suddenly contracts, completing the reflex arc.

Because each muscle stretch reflex involves specific spinal segments, together with their sensory and motor fibers, an abnormal reflex helps you locate a pathologic lesion. Learn the segmental levels of the muscle stretch reflexes. You can remember them easily by their numerical sequence in ascending order from ankle to triceps: S1, L2–L4, C5–C6, C6–C7.

Muscle Stretch Reflexes

Ankle reflex	Sacral 1 primarily
Knee reflex	Lumbar 2, 3, 4
Supinator (brachioradialis) reflex	Cervical 5, 6
Biceps reflex	Cervical 5, 6
Triceps reflex	Cervical 6, 7

Reflexes may be initiated by stimulating skin as well as muscle. Stroking the skin of the abdomen, for example, produces a localized muscular twitch. Superficial (cutaneous) reflexes and their corresponding spinal segments include the following:

Cutaneous Stimulation Reflexes

Abdominal reflexes—upper	Thoracic 8, 9, 10
—lower	Thoracic 10, 11, 12
Cremasteric reflex	Lumbar 1, 2
Plantar responses	Lumbar 5, sacral 1
Anal reflex	Sacral 2, 3, 4

The Health History

Common or Concerning Symptoms

- Headache
- Dizziness or vertigo
- Weakness (generalized, proximal, or distal)
- Numbness, abnormal or absent sensation
- Fainting and blacking out (near-syncope and syncope)
- Seizures
- Tremors or involuntary movements

Two of the most common symptoms in neurologic disorders are *headache* and *dizziness*. Review the discussions of these symptoms in Chapter 7, Head and Neck, pp. 215–302.

Headache. Headaches have many causes, ranging from benign to life threatening, and always warrant thorough assessment. Neurologic causes such as subarachnoid hemorrhage, meningitis, or mass lesions are especially ominous. The careful clinician pays close attention to the history and a detailed neurologic examination.

See Table 7-1, Primary Headaches, p. 267, and Table 7-2, Secondary Headaches, pp. 268–269.

Primary headaches include migraine, tension, cluster, and trigeminal autonomic cephalagias; *secondary headaches* arise from underlying structural, systemic, or infectious causes and may be life threatening.[9]

Always assess the severity of the headache and its location, duration, and any associated symptoms such as double vision, visual changes, weakness, or loss of sensation. Does the headache get worse with coughing, sneezing, or sudden head movements, which can alter intracranial pressure dynamics? Is there fever, stiff neck, or a parameningeal focus like ear, sinus, or throat infection that may signal meningitis?[10]

Subarachnoid hemorrhage classically presents as "the worst headache of my life" with instantaneous onset.[11–13] Severe headache and stiff neck accompany *meningitis*.[14–16] Dull headache increased by coughing and sneezing, especially when recurring in the same location, occurs in mass lesions from *brain tumors* or *abscess*.[17,18]

An atypical presentation of the patient's usual migraine may be suspicious for stroke, especially in women using hormonal contraceptives.[19–22]

Migraine headache is often preceded by an aura or prodrome, and is highly likely if three of the five "POUND" features are present: **P**ulsatile or throbbing; **O**ne-day duration, or lasts 4 to 72 hours if untreated; **U**nilateral; **N**ausea or vomiting; **D**isabling or intensity causing interruption of daily activity.[22,23]

Always look for unusual headache warning signs, such as sudden onset "like a thunderclap," onset after age 50 years, and associated symptoms such as fever and stiff neck. Examine for papilledema and focal neurologic signs.[10]

See box "Headache Warning Signs" on p. 216 in Chapter 7.

Dizziness or Vertigo. As you learned in Chapter 7, Head and Neck, *dizziness* and *light-headedness* are common, somewhat vague, complaints that prompt a more specific history and neurologic examination, with emphasis on detection of nystagmus and focal neurologic signs. Especially in older patients, ask about medications.

Feeling light-headed, weak in the legs, or about to faint points to *presyncope* from vasovagal stimulation, orthostatic hypotension, arrhythmia, or side effects from blood pressure and other medications. See Table 17-3, Syncope and Similar Disorders, pp. 778–779.

Does the patient feel faint or about to fall or pass out (*presyncope*)? Or unsteady and off balance (*disequilibrium* or *ataxia*)? Or is there *true vertigo*, a spinning sensation within the patient or of the surroundings? If there is true vertigo, establish the time course of symptoms, which helps distinguish among the different types of peripheral vestibular disorders.

Vertigo often reflects vestibular disease, usually from peripheral causes in the inner ear such as *benign positional vertigo, labyrinthitis,* or *Ménière disease*.[24]

See Table 7-4, Dizziness and Vertigo, p. 271, for distinguishing symptoms and time course.

If there are localizing symptoms or signs like double vision (*diplopia*), difficulty forming words (*dysarthria*), or problems with gait or balance (*ataxia*), investigate the central causes of vertigo.

Ataxia, diplopia, and dysarthria are suspicious for vertebrobasilar *TIA* or *stroke*.[25–30] Also consider *posterior fossa tumor* and *migraine with brainstem aura*.

See Table 17-2, Types of Stroke, pp. 776–777.

Weakness.   Weakness is another common symptom with many causes which bears careful investigation. It is important to clarify what the patient means—fatigue, apathy, drowsiness, or actual loss of strength. True motor weakness can arise from the CNS, a peripheral nerve, the neuromuscular junction, or a muscle. Time course and location are especially relevant. Is the onset sudden, gradual or subacute, or chronic, over a long period of time?

Abrupt onset of motor and sensory deficits occurs in *TIA* and *stroke*.[25–30] Progressive subacute onset of lower extremity weakness suggests *Guillain–Barré syndrome*.[31] Chronic, more gradual, onset of lower extremity weakness occurs in primary and metastatic spinal cord tumors.

What areas of the body are involved? Is the weakness generalized, or focal to the face or a limb? Does it involve one side of the body or both sides? What movements are affected? As you listen to the patient's story, identify the patterns below:

Focal or asymmetric weakness has both central (ischemic, thrombotic, or mass lesions) and peripheral causes ranging from nerve injury to the neuromuscular junction disorders to *myopathies*.

- *Proximal*—in the shoulder and/or hip girdle, for example

- *Distal*—in the hands and/or feet

- *Symmetric*—in the same areas on both sides of the body

- *Asymmetric*—types of weakness include focal, in a portion of the face or extremity; monoparesis, in an extremity; paraparesis, in both lower extremities; and hemiparesis, in one side of the body

Proximal limb weakness, when symmetric with intact sensation, occurs in myopathies from alcohol, drugs like glucocorticoids, and inflammatory muscle disorders like *polymyositis* and *dermatomyositis*. In the neuromuscular junction disorder *myasthenia gravis*, there is proximal typically asymmetric weakness that gets worse with effort (fatigability), often with associated *bulbar symptoms* such as diplopia, ptosis, dysarthria, and dysphagia.[32,33]

To identify *proximal weakness*, ask about difficulty with movements such as combing hair, reaching up to a shelf, getting up out of a chair, or climbing stairs. Does the weakness get worse with repetition and improve after rest (suggesting *myasthenia gravis*)? Are there associated sensory or other symptoms?

To identify *distal weakness*, ask about hand strength when opening a jar or using scissors or a screwdriver, or problems tripping when walking.

Bilateral predominantly distal weakness, often with sensory loss, suggests a *polyneuropathy*, as in diabetes.

Numbness, Abnormal or Absent Sensation.   In a patient who reports numbness, ask the patient to be more precise. Is there tingling like "pins and needles," which are altered sensations called *paresthesias*, distorted sensations (*dysesthesias*), or is sensation reduced or completely absent?

Sensory changes can arise at several levels: local nerve compression or "entrapment," seen in hand numbness in distributions specific to the median, ulnar, or radial nerve; nerve root compression with dermatomal sensory loss from vertebral bone spurs or herniated discs; or central lesions from *stroke* or *multiple sclerosis*.

In dysesthesias, light touch or pinprick, for example, may cause a burning or irritating sensation.

Establish the pattern of sensory loss. Is there a stocking-glove distribution? Are sensory deficits patchy, nondermatomal, and occurring in more than one limb?

A pattern of stocking, then glove, sensory loss occurs in *polyneuropathies,* especially from diabetes; multiple patchy areas of sensory loss in different limbs suggest *mononeuritis multiplex,* seen in diabetes and rheumatoid arthritis.

Fainting and Blacking Out (Near-Syncope and Syncope). Patient reports of fainting or "passing out" are common and warrant a meticulous history to guide management and possible hospital admission.[36] Begin by finding out whether the patient has actually lost consciousness. Did the patient hear external noise or voices throughout the episode, feel light-headed or weak, but fail to actually lose consciousness, consistent with *near syncope* or *presyncope*? Or did the patient actually experience complete loss of consciousness, a more serious symptom representing *true syncope,* defined as a sudden but temporary loss of consciousness and postural tone from transient global hypoperfusion of the brain?

See Table 17-3, Syncope and Similar Disorders, pp. 778–779.

Causes include seizures, "neurocardiogenic" conditions such as *vasovagal syncope, postural tachycardia syndrome, carotid sinus syncope,* and *orthostatic hypotension,* and cardiac disease causing arrhythmias, especially ventricular tachycardia and bradyarrhythmias.[37] Stroke or subarachnoid hemorrhage are unlikely causes of syncope unless both hemispheres are affected.

Elicit a complete description of the event. What was the patient doing when the episode occurred? Was the patient standing, sitting, or lying down? Were there any triggers or warning symptoms? How long did the episode last? Could voices still be heard? Importantly, were onset and offset slow or fast? Were there any palpitations? Is there a history of heart disease, which has a sensitivity for a cardiac cause of more than 95% (with a specificity of ~45%)?[36]

In *vasovagal syncope,* the most common cause of syncope, look for the prodrome of nausea, diaphoresis, and pallor triggered by a fearful or unpleasant event, then vagally mediated hypotension, often with slow onset and offset. In syncope from arrhythmias, onset and offset are often sudden, reflecting loss and recovery of cerebral perfusion.

Try to interview any witnesses. Consider the possibility of a seizure based on the features described in the following section, especially if the onset was abrupt and without warning.

Seizures. Patients may report "spells" or fainting that raises suspicion of *seizure,* a sudden excessive electrical discharge from cortical neurons. Seizures may be symptomatic, with an identifiable cause, or idiopathic. A careful history is important to rule out other causes of loss of consciousness and acute symptomatic seizures that have discernible explanations.

See Table 17-4, Seizure Disorders, pp. 780–781.

If there is more than one seizure, consider *epilepsy*, defined as two or more seizures that are not provoked by other illnesses or circumstances.[38,39] The incidence of epilepsy in the United States is 3%; in more than 60% to 70% of affected patients, no cause is identified.

Epilepsy does not always involve loss of consciousness, depending on the type. It is usually classified as generalized or partial, based on the location in the cortex of the initial seizure focus. If available, ask a witness how the patient looked before, during, and after the episode. Was there any seizure-like movement of the arms or legs? Any incontinence of the bladder or bowel? What about any drowsiness or impaired memory after the event suggestive of a postictal state?

Ask about age at onset, frequency, change in frequency or symptom pattern, and use of medications, alcohol, or illicit drugs. Check for any history of head injury.

Tremors or Invountary Movements.

Tremor, "a rhythmic oscillatory movement of a body part resulting from the contraction of opposing muscle groups," is the most common movement disorder.[41,42] It may be an isolated finding or part of a neurologic disorder. Ask about any tremor, shaking, or body movements that the patient seems unable to control. Does the tremor occur at rest? Does it get worse with voluntary intentional movement or with sustained postures?

Distinct from these symptoms is *restless legs syndrome,* present in 6% to 12% of the U.S. population, described as an unpleasant sensation in the legs, especially at night, that gets worse with rest and improves with movement of the symptomatic limb(s).[45,46]

Common causes of *acute symptomatic seizures* include: head trauma; alcohol, cocaine, and other drugs; withdrawal from alcohol, benzodiazepines, and barbiturates; metabolic insults from low or high glucose or low calcium or sodium; acute stroke; and meningitis or encephalitis.[40]

Tonic–clonic motor activity, bladder or bowel incontinence, and *postictal state* characterize generalized seizures. Unlike syncope, tongue biting or bruising of limbs may occur.

***Epilepsy* is more common in infants and older adults. The baseline neurologic examination is frequently normal.**

Generalized epilepsy syndromes usually begin in childhood or adolescence; adult-onset seizures are usually partial.

See Table 17-5, Tremors and Involuntary Movements, pp. 782–783.

Low-frequency unilateral resting tremor, rigidity, and bradykinesia typify *Parkinson disease*.[43,44] *Essential tremors* are high-frequency, bilateral, upper extremity tremors that occur with both limb movement and sustained posture and subside when the limb is relaxed; head, voice, and leg tremor may also be present.[42]

Reversible causes of restless legs syndrome include pregnancy, renal disease, and iron deficiency.

Health Promotion and Counseling: Evidence and Recommendations

Important Topics for Health Promotion and Counseling

- Preventing stroke and transient ischemic attack
- Carotid artery screening
- Reducing risk of peripheral neuropathy
- Herpes zoster vaccination
- Detecting the "three D's": delirium, dementia, and depression

Preventing Stroke and Transient Ischemic Attack. *Stroke* is a sudden neurologic deficit caused by cerebrovascular ischemia (87%) or hemorrhage (13%). *Hemorrhagic strokes* may be intracerebral (10% of all strokes) or subarachnoid (3% of all strokes). Stroke is the fourth leading cause of death in the United States and a leading cause of long-term disability.[47]

See Table 17-2, Types of Stroke, pp. 776–777.

The American Heart Association (AHA) and the American Stroke Association (ASA) have established tissue-based definitions for ischemic stroke and transient ischemic attack (TIA) that have important implications for assessing and preventing strokes.[48] These definitions encourage early neurodiagnostic imaging following a TIA and risk stratification for subsequent stroke.

- *Ischemic stroke* is "an infarction of CNS tissue" that may be symptomatic or silent. "Symptomatic ischemic strokes are manifest by clinical signs of focal or global cerebral, spinal, or retinal dysfunction caused by CNS infarction. A silent stroke is a documented CNS infarction that was asymptomatic."

- *TIA* is now defined as "a transient episode of neurological dysfunction caused by focal brain, spinal cord, or retinal ischemia, without acute infarction." The AHA/ASA guidelines recommend neurodiagnostic imaging within 24 hours of symptom onset and routine noninvasive imaging of the carotid and intracranial vessels.

The AHA/ASA report cites the well-validated *ABCD2 scoring system* for predicting ischemic stroke within 2, 7, and 90 days after TIA: **A**ge ≥60 years, initial **B**lood pressure ≥140/90 mm Hg, **C**linical features of focal weakness or impaired speech without focal weakness, **D**uration 10 to 59 minutes or ≥60 minutes, and **D**iabetes.[48]

TIAs are a major risk factor for stroke, which occurs in 3% to 10% of patients within 2 days and in 9% to 17% within 90 days.[47] Short-term stroke risk is highest in those with age 60 years and older, diabetes, focal symptoms of weakness or impaired speech, and a TIA lasting more than 10 minutes. One population-based study found a combined risk for recurrent TIA/stroke/and death of 25% within the 3 months following a TIA.[50]

Stroke at a Glance

Key Facts for Prevention and Patient Education

- Stroke affects nearly 800,000 Americans each year, including more than 600,000 suffering a first stroke, and accounts for about 1 in every 20 deaths.
- The total annual costs associated with stroke are estimated to be about $34 billion.
- Stroke prevalence and mortality are disproportionately higher in *African Americans* compared to whites:
  - Prevalence, black versus white men: 4.2% versus 2.2%; black versus white women: 4.7% versus 2.5%
  - Mortality per 100,000, black versus white men: 55 versus 36; black versus white women: 47 versus 36

- Although younger and middle-aged women have lower age-specific stroke incidence rates than men, rates increase with age so that women, who on average live longer than men, have an overall higher lifetime risk for stroke. Risk factors for women include autoimmune collagen vascular disease and history of preeclampsia, gestational diabetes, and pregnancy-induced hypertension.
- The prevalence of silent stroke, estimated to range from 6% to 28%, increases with age.
- Individuals with TIA have a 1-year mortality of ~12%; 10-year risks for stroke and death from cardiovascular disease are 19% and 43%, respectively.
- Only 51% of the United States population is aware of the five stroke warning signs (see below) and would call 911 if they thought someone was having a stroke.
- Stroke outcomes improve significantly when thrombolytic therapy is given within 3 to 4.5 hours of symptom onset; however, only a minority of those suffering a stroke reaches an emergency room within this time window.

Sources: Mozaffarian D, Benjamin EJ, Go AS, et al. Heart disease and stroke statistics—2015 update: a report from the American Heart Association. *Circulation.* 2015;131:e29; Bushnell C, McCullough LD, Awad IA, et al. Guidelines for the prevention of stroke in women: a statement for healthcare professionals from the American Heart Association/American Stroke Association. *Stroke.* 2014;45:1545; Jauch EC, Saver JL, Adams HP, Jr., et al. Guidelines for the early management of patients with acute ischemic stroke: a guideline for healthcare professionals from the American Heart Association/American Stroke Association. *Stroke.* 2013;44:870.

Cardiovascular causes of death, including stroke, are the greatest contributors to the 5-year disparity in life expectancy for African American men compared to white men and the 4-year racial disparity for women.[49] However, the racial gap in life expectancy has recently been declining.

See Chapter 9, Cardiovascular System, for discussion of the AHA 2011 guidelines for preventing cardiovascular disease in women that address the increased risk of mid-life stroke and death from coronary heart disease, pp. 362–363.[52]

Symptoms and signs of stroke depend on the vascular territory affected in the brain. The most common cause of ischemic symptoms is occlusion of the middle cerebral artery, which causes visual field cuts and contralateral hemiparesis and sensory deficits. Occlusion of the left middle cerebral artery often produces aphasia; and occlusion of the right middle cerebral artery, neglect or inattention to the opposite side of the body.

See Table 17-2, Types of Stroke, pp. 776–777.

See Chapter 5, p. 160, and Table 17-6, Disorders of Speech, p. 784, for discussion of *aphasia*.

Stroke Warning Signs. The AHA and the ASA urge patients to seek immediate care for any of the warning signs below. It is important to teach these to your patients.

AHA/ASA Stroke Warning Signs and Symptoms

F **Face Drooping**—Does one side of the face droop or is it numb?[53] Ask the person to smile. Is the person's smile uneven?

A **Arm Weakness**—Is one arm weak or numb? Ask the person to raise both arms. Does one arm drift downward?

S **Speech Difficulty**—Is speech slurred? Is the person unable to speak or hard to understand? Ask the person to repeat a simple sentence, like "The sky is blue." Is the sentence repeated correctly?

T **Time to call 9-1-1**—If someone shows any of these symptoms, even if the symptoms go away, call 9-1-1 and get the person to the hospital immediately. Check the time so you'll know when the first symptoms appeared

Beyond FAST: Other important symptoms

- Sudden numbness or weakness of the leg, arm, or face
- Sudden confusion or trouble understanding
- Sudden trouble seeing in one or both eyes
- Sudden trouble walking, dizziness, loss of balance or coordination
- Sudden severe headache with no known cause

Stroke Risk Factors—Primary Prevention. Recognizing that stroke and coronary heart disease share common cardiovascular risk factors and threats to health, in 2010, Healthy People 2020 and the AHA presented a new concept of "cardiovascular health" that encompasses seven health behaviors and health factors, and a new set of combined impact goals for the coming decade:

By 2020, to improve the cardiovascular health of all Americans by 20%, while reducing deaths from cardiovascular disease and stroke by 20%.[54]

For primary prevention, target documented modifiable risk factors, detailed in the box below. Learn the indications for using aspirin in healthy and diabetic individuals.[55,56]

Optimal blood pressure control is essential for preventing *hemorrhagic stroke.* Additional risk factors for the most common cause of hemorrhagic stroke— ruptured aneurysms in the circle of Willis—include smoking, alcohol use, oral contraceptives, and family history in a first-degree relative.

See Chapter 9, Cardiovascular System, for discussion of the new more aggressive guidelines for cardiovascular screening and the table on cardiovascular health behaviors and health factors, pp. 363–364.

Stroke Risk Factors—Primary Prevention of Ischemic Stroke

Documented and Modifiable Risk Factors

Hypertension	Hypertension is the leading risk factor for both ischemic and hemorrhagic stroke. Pharmacologic reduction of blood pressure significantly reduces stroke risk, particularly among African Americans and older adults.
Smoking	Smoking is associated with doubling the risk of ischemic stroke and a 2- to 4-fold increased risk of subarachnoid hemorrhage. Smoking cessation rapidly reduces the risk of stroke, but never to the level of never-smokers.
Dyslipidemia	Statin treatment reduces the risk of all strokes by about 20% for patients with or at risk for atherosclerotic cardiovascular disease.
Diabetes	Stroke risk is doubled with diabetes and 20% of diabetic patients will die of stroke. Good blood pressure control and statin therapy reduce stroke risk in diabetic patients.
Weight	Obesity increases the risk of ischemic stroke by 64%.
Diet and nutrition	Dietary factors affect stroke risk primarily by elevating blood pressure. Decreasing salt and saturated fat intake and diets emphasizing fruits, vegetables, nuts, and low-fat dairy products may reduce stroke risk.
Physical inactivity	Moderate exercise, like brisk walking for 150 minutes a week or 30 minutes on most days, improves cardiovascular health.
Alcohol use	Alcohol use has a direct dose-dependent effect on the risk of hemorrhagic stroke. Heavy alcohol use increases the risk for all types of stroke due to effects on hypertension, hypercoagulable states, cardiac arrhythmias, and reduced cerebral blood flow.

Disease-Specific Risk Factors

Atrial fibrillation	Valvular (rheumatic) and nonvalvular atrial fibrillation increases risk of stroke between 2- to 7-fold and 17-fold, respectively, compared to the general population.
	Antiplatelet agents and anticoagulants can reduce the risk for ischemic stroke. When considering antithrombotic therapy, experts recommend individual risk stratification into high-, moderate-, and low-risk groups to balance risk of stroke against risk of bleeding. $CHADS_2$ is a commonly used scoring system based on **C**ongestive heart failure, **H**ypertension, **A**ge ≥75 years, **D**iabetes, and prior **S**troke/TIA. The CHA_2DS_2-VASc, which adds an age category of 65 to 74 years, female sex, and vascular disease to the scoring system, improves risk stratification for individuals estimated as low or moderate risk with $CHADS_2$.

(continued)

Stroke Risk Factors—Primary Prevention of Ischemic Stroke (*continued*)

Carotid artery disease	The estimated prevalence of clinically important carotid artery stenosis in the United States population over age 65 years is 1%. Medical therapy, including statins, antiplatelet agents, treatment of diabetes and hypertension, and smoking cessation, has reduced the risk of stroke in individuals with asymptomatic carotid artery stenosis to less than 2% annually. Experts recommend carotid endarterectomy for selected asymptomatic patients with carotid artery stenosis >60%—provided that the surgeon and center have very low perioperative risks for stroke and mortality.
Obstructive sleep apnea	Sleep apnea is an independent risk factor for stroke, particularly in men. Stroke risk increases with increasing sleep apnea severity as measured by the number of respiratory events (cessation or air flow reduction) per hour. Sleep apnea is usually treated with continuous positive airway pressure (CPAP), though its effectiveness for reducing stroke risk is unknown.

Sources: Meschia JF, Bushnell C, Boden-Albala B, et al. Guidelines for the primary prevention of stroke: a statement for healthcare professionals from the American Heart Association/American Stroke Association. *Stroke*. 2014;45:3754; Mozaffarian D, Benjamin EJ, Go AS, et al. Heart disease and stroke statistics—2015 update: a report from the American Heart Association. *Circulation*. 2015;131:e29; Bushnell C, McCullough LD, Awad IA, et al. Guidelines for the prevention of stroke in women: a statement for healthcare professionals from the American Heart Association/American Stroke Association. *Stroke*. 2014;45:1545; Fuster V, Ryden LE, Cannom DS, et al. 2011 ACCF/AHA/HRS focused updates incorporated into the ACC/AHA/ESC 2006 Guidelines for the management of patients with atrial fibrillation: a report of the American College of Cardiology Foundation/American Heart Association Task Force on Practice Guidelines developed in partnership with the European Society of Cardiology and in collaboration with the European Heart Rhythm Association and the Heart Rhythm Society. *J Am Coll Cardiol*. 2011;57:e101.

Screening for Asymptomatic Carotid Artery Stenosis. Carotid duplex ultrasound accurately and safely detects significant carotid artery stenosis and is widely used for evaluating symptomatic patients. Although asymptomatic carotid artery stenosis is a stroke risk, it accounts for only a small proportion of ischemic strokes. Based on a systematic review, the U.S. Preventive Services Task Force (USPSTF) recommended against screening for asymptomatic carotid artery stenosis in the general adult population (grade D).[57] The USPSTF found no evidence that ultrasound screening reduced the risk for ipsilateral stroke.[58] Given that the population prevalence of asymptomatic carotid artery stenosis is only 1%, screening would lead to many false-positive results. Furthermore, treating asymptomatic patients incurs risks for strokes, death, and other harms.

TIA and Stroke—Secondary Prevention. For the patient who has already suffered TIA or stroke, focus on: identifying the underlying cause including noncardiac emboli, cardiac emboli, and carotid artery stenosis; reducing cardiovascular risk factors, including inactivity, hyperlipidemia, poorly controlled diabetes or hypertension, smoking, and heavy alcohol consumption; and identifying the most appropriate interventions for secondary prevention,

History and careful neurologic examination to assess level of consciousness and focal findings are essential for diagnosing stroke, followed by neuroimaging to distinguish ischemic from hemorrhagic stroke.

including antiplatelet agents, anticoagulants, and carotid revascularization.[59] Strokes in young adults often have a different set of causes—patent foramen ovale and less commonly, carotid or vertebral/basilar artery dissection, hypercoagulable states, or cocaine and illicit drug use.[60]

Reducing Risk of Diabetic Peripheral Neuropathy. Diabetes causes several types of peripheral neuropathy.[62] Maintaining optimal glycemic control can prevent or delay the onset of neuropathy, particularly from type I diabetes.

- *Distal symmetric sensorimotor polyneuropathy.* This is the most common type of diabetic neuropathy. It is slowly progressive, often asymptomatic, and a risk factor for ulcerations, arthropathy, and amputation. Symptomatic patients report burning electrical pain in the lower extremities, usually at night.

- *Autonomic dysfunction, mononeuropathies,* and *polyradiculopathies,* including *diabetic amyotrophy,* which initially causes unilateral thigh pain and proximal lower extremity weakness.

Diabetic patients should have their feet examined regularly for neuropathy, including testing pinprick sensation, ankle reflexes, vibration perception (with a 128-Hz tuning fork) and plantar light touch sensation (with a Semmes-Weinstein monofilament), as well as checking for skin breakdown, poor circulation, and musculoskeletal abnormalities.[63] The monofilament test involves pressing the perpendicular monofilament against the skin at the great toe and metatarsals until it bends (Fig. 17-8), or against the dorsal arch if without calluses; the test is positive if the patient cannot feel the monofilament.

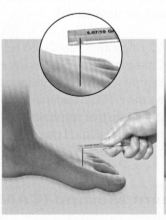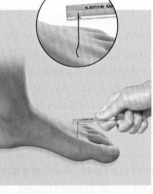

FIGURE 17-8. Monofilament test.

Herpes Zoster Vaccination. Herpes zoster, which results from reactivation of latent varicella (chicken pox) virus infection within the sensory ganglia, usually causes painful unilateral vesicular rashes in a dermatomal distribution.[64] The lifetime risk of herpes zoster infection is about one in three, and is higher for women than for men. Up to one in four adults experience complications following infection, including postherpetic neuralgia (persistent pain in the area of the rash), bacterial skin infections, ophthalmic complications, cranial and peripheral neuropathies, encephalitis, pneumonitis, and hepatitis.[65] Herpes zoster risk is increased in immunocompromised conditions including cancer, HIV, bone marrow or organ transplantation, and immunosuppressive therapies. Increasing age is also strongly associated with developing both herpes zoster infection and postherpetic neuralgia.

The herpes zoster vaccine effectively reduces the short-term risks for zoster and postherpetic neuralgia in adults ≥50 years.[66] The Advisory Committee on

Immunization Practices (ACIP) currently recommends routinely offering one-time vaccination for adults ≥60 years; the Federal Drug Administration has approved the vaccine for adults ≥50 years. Because the long-term efficacy of the herpes zoster vaccine is uncertain, the ACIP is re-evaluating the best age to administer the vaccine and the need for revaccination.

Detecting the "Three Ds": Delirium, Dementia, and Depression. Delirium and dementia are increasingly common conditions in clinical practice and can present with subtle findings. Keep them in mind as you assess cognition and mental status. Differentiating depression, cognitive impairment, and altered consciousness can be challenging. Review the discussion of these disorders in Chapter 20 and Chapter 5.

See Chapter 20, The Older Adult, pp. 955–1008, and Table 20-2, Delirium and Dementia, p. 1001.

See also Chapter 5, Behavior and Mental Status, pp. 147–171.

Delirium. Delirium, a multifactorial syndrome, is an acute confusional state marked by sudden onset, fluctuating course, inattention, and at times changing levels of consciousness. Risk for developing delirium depends on both predisposing conditions which increase susceptibility and the immediate pre-cipitating factors. About one third of older adults experience delirium during hospitalizations on medical services; rates are even higher following major elective surgeries. Intensive care unit admissions are associated with a high incidence of delirium regardless of age. Even though delirium is associated with poor patient outcomes, more than 50% of cases are undetected.

The Confusional Assessment Method (CAM) algorithm, displayed below, is recommended for screening at-risk patients. The CAM instrument can quickly and accurately detect delirium at the bedside[67]; a CAM severity (CAM-S) measure can be used to predict risks for death and nursing home placement.[68] The National Institutes of Health (NIH) have issued guidelines for preventing delirium that emphasize multicomponent interventions by interdisciplinary teams targeting key clinical precipitants.[69]

The Confusion Assessment Method (CAM) Diagnostic Algorithm

1. Acute change in mental status and fluctuating course
   - Is there evidence of an acute change in cognition from baseline?
   - Does the abnormal behavior fluctuate during the day?
2. Inattention
   - Does the patient have difficulty focusing attention?
3. Disorganized thinking
   - Does the patient have rambling or irrelevant conversations, unclear or illogical flow of ideas, or unpredictable switching from subject to subject?
4. Abnormal level of consciousness
   - Is the patient anything besides alert—hyperalert, lethargic, stuporous, or comatose?

Diagnosing delirium requires features 1 and 2 and either 3 or 4.

Dementia. Dementia is characterized by declines in memory and cognitive ability that interfere with activities of daily living.[70,71] The most common types are *Alzheimer disease* (affecting 5 million Americans over age 65 years), *vascular dementia, Lewy body dementia,* and *frontotemporal dementia.*[70,72] Diagnosing dementia requires exclusion of delirium and depression. Teasing out age-related changes in cognition from *mild cognitive impairment* is also challenging. Less than 2% of patients with dementia have potentially reversible causes, such as hypothyroidism, medication side effects, normal pressure hydrocephalus, or major depression.

A meta-analysis identified potentially modifiable risk factors for developing Alzheimer disease, including physical inactivity, depression, smoking, midlife hypertension, midlife obesity, cognitive inactivity or low educational attainment, and diabetes.[73] However, a 2011 NIH review concluded "currently, no evidence of even moderate scientific quality exists to support the association of any modifiable factors…with reduced risk for Alzheimer disease."[74] The USPSTF did not find convincing evidence that pharmacologic or nonpharmacologic interventions could benefit patients with mild to moderate cognitive impairment.[75] Consequently, the USPSTF issued an I statement (insufficient evidence) regarding screening for cognitive impairment.

Depression. Depression is more common in individuals with significant medical conditions, including several neurologic disorders—dementia, epilepsy, multiple sclerosis, and Parkinson disease—and is also underdiagnosed. Two screening questions, with an area under the receiver operating curve (ROC) of 0.93, can accurately identify major depressive disorders: "Have you been feeling down, depressed, or hopeless (depressed mood)?" and, "Have you felt little interest or pleasure in doing things (anhedonia)?"[76] Be sure to assess suicidality and the possibility of bipolar disorder in depressed patients.

The Mini-Mental State Examination, which takes 7 to 10 minutes to administer, is the best studied, and at a score cutpoint of 23 to 24, has a median likelihood ratio (LR) of 6.3 for a positive test and 0.19 for a negative test.[77]

See also discussion of the Mini-Cog on p. 984 and the Mini-Cog screening tool in Table 20-5, Screening for Dementia: The Mini-Cog, on p. 1002.

Techniques of Examination

Important Areas of Examination

- Mental status—see Chapter 5, Behavior and Mental Status
- CNs I through XII
- Motor system: muscle bulk, tone, and strength; coordination, gait, and stance
- Sensory system: pain and temperature, position and vibration, light touch, discriminative sensation
- Deep tendon, abdominal, and plantar reflexes

Return to the four important questions that govern your neurologic evaluation:

- Does the patient have neurologic disease?

- If so, what is the localization of the lesion(s)? Are your findings symmetric?

- What is the pathophysiology of the process?

- What is the preliminary differential diagnosis?

This section presents the techniques you will need for a practical and reasonably comprehensive examination of the nervous system aligned with recommendations of the American Academy of Neurology.[78–80] At first, learning the numerous techniques for a thorough examination may seem difficult. Be an active learner; seek feedback from your teachers and consulting neurologists to make sure you are using skilled and proper techniques. Take advantage of the Bates Visual Guide videos on the nervous system and teaching videos posted by the American Academy of Neurology and Wright State University.[81–83] With supervision and practice your skills for assessing important neurologic disorders will deepen.

The amount of detail in an appropriate neurologic examination varies widely. In healthy patients your examination will be relatively brief, as outlined in the Screening Neurologic Examination recommended by the American Academy of Neurology provided below. If you detect abnormal findings, your examination should be more comprehensive. Be aware that neurologists use many additional techniques in specific situations. Whether you conduct a comprehensive or screening examination, organize your thinking into five categories: (1) mental status, speech, and language; (2) CNs; (3) the motor system; (4) the sensory system; and (5) reflexes. If your findings are abnormal, begin to group them into patterns of central or peripheral disorders.

For efficiency, you should integrate neurologic assessment with other parts of your examination. Survey the patient's mental status and speech during the interview even if you do more detailed testing later during the neurologic examination. Assess the CNs as you examine the head and neck, and any neurologic abnormalities in the arms and legs as you evaluate the peripheral vascular and musculoskeletal systems. Chapter 1 provides an outline for this kind of integrated approach. Think about, describe, and record your findings, however, in terms of the nervous system as a whole.

See Chapter 1, Overview Examination and History Taking table on "The Physical Examination: Suggested Sequence," p. 20.

American Academy of Neurology: Guidelines for a Screening Neurologic Examination

Perform a screening neurologic examination in all patients, even those without neurologic complaints, that is sufficient for detection of significant neurologic disease.[78] Although the screening examination sequence may vary, it should cover the major components of the full examination—mental status, CNs, motor system (strength, gait, and coordination), sensation, and reflexes. One example of a screening examination is given here.

(continued)

American Academy of Neurology: Guidelines for a Screening Neurologic Examination (continued)

Mental Status—level of alertness, appropriateness of responses, orientation to date and place

Cranial Nerves

- Vision—visual fields, funduscopic examination
- Pupillary light reflex
- Eye movements
- Hearing
- Facial strength—smile, eye closure

Motor System

- Strength—shoulder abduction, elbow extension, wrist extension, finger abduction, hip flexion, knee flexion, ankle dorsiflexion
- Gait—casual, heel walk, toe walk, tandem walk
- Coordination—fine finger movements, finger-to-nose, heel-knee-shin

Sensory System—one modality at toes—can be light touch, pain/temperature, or proprioception

Reflexes

- Deep tendon reflexes—biceps, patellar, Achilles
- Plantar responses

Note: If there is reason to suspect neurologic disease based on the patient's history or the results of any components of the screening examination, a more complete neurologic examination is necessary.

Source: Adapted from the American Academy of Neurology. Available at https://www.aan.com/uploadedFiles/4CME_and_Training/2Training/3Fellowship_Resources/5Core_Curricula/skilz.pdf. Accessed July 23, 2015.

The Cranial Nerves

Overview. The examination of the CNs can be summarized as follows.

Summary: Cranial Nerves I–XII

I	Smell
II	Visual acuity, visual fields, and ocular fundi
II, III	Pupillary reactions
III, IV, VI	Extraocular movements
V	Corneal reflexes, facial sensation, and jaw movements
VII	Facial movements
VIII	Hearing
IX, X	Swallowing and rise of the palate, gag reflex
V, VII, X, XII	Voice and speech
XI	Shoulder and neck movements
XII	Tongue symmetry, position, and movement

Cranial Nerve I—Olfactory. Test the *sense of smell* by presenting the patient with familiar nonirritating odors. First, make sure that each nasal passage is patent by compressing one side of the nose and asking the patient to sniff through the other. Then ask the patient to close both eyes. Occlude one nostril and test smell in the other with substances like cloves, coffee, soap, or vanilla. Avoid noxious odors like ammonia that might stimulate CN V. Ask the patient to identify each odor. Test smell on the other side. Normally the patient perceives odors on each side and identifies them correctly.

Loss of smell occurs in sinus conditions, head trauma, smoking, aging, use of cocaine, and *Parkinson disease.*

Cranial Nerve II—Optic. Test visual acuity.

See Chapter 7, Head and Neck, for more detailed discussion of the techniques for examining Visual Acuity and Visual Fields, pp. 231–233, Pupils, pp. 235–236, and the optic fundi using an ophthalmoscope, pp. 238–242.

Inspect the optic fundi with your ophthalmoscope, paying special attention to the optic discs.

Inspect each disc carefully for bulging and blurred margins (*papilledema*); pallor (*optic atrophy*); and cup enlargement (*glaucoma*).

Test the visual fields by confrontation. Test each eye separately, and both eyes together. Occasionally, in stroke patients, for example, patients will complain of partial loss of vision, and testing of both eyes reveals a *visual field defect,* an abnormality in peripheral vision such as *homonymous hemianopsia.* Testing only one eye would miss this finding.

See Table 7-6, Visual Field Defects, p. 273. Look for prechiasmal, or anterior, defects seen in *glaucoma, retinal emboli, optic neuritis* (visual acuity poor); bitemporal hemianopsias from defects at the optic chiasm, usually from *pituitary tumor;* and homonymous hemianopsias or quadrantanopsias in postchiasmal lesions, usually in the *occipital or parietal lobe,* with associated findings of stroke (visual acuity normal).[84]

Cranial Nerves II and III—Optic and Oculomotor. Inspect the size and shape of the pupils, and compare one side with the other. *Anisocoria,* or a difference of >0.4 mm in the diameter of one pupil compared to the other, is seen in up to 38% of healthy individuals. Test the *pupillary reactions to light.*

See Table 7-10, Pupillary Abnormalities, p. 277. If the large pupil reacts poorly to light or anisocoria worsens in light, the large pupil has abnormal pupillary constriction, seen in *CN III palsy.* If ptosis and ophthalmoplegia are also present, consider *intracranial aneurysm* if the patient is awake, and *transtentorial herniation* if the patient is comatose.

Also check the *near response* (p. 230), which tests pupillary constriction (pupillary constrictor muscle), convergence (medial rectus muscles), and accommodation of the lens (ciliary muscle).

If both pupils react to light and anisocoria worsens in darkness, the small pupil has abnormal pupillary dilation, seen in *Horner syndrome* and *simple anisocoria.*[85]

Cranial Nerves III, IV, and VI—Oculomotor, Trochlear, and Abducens. Test the *extraocular movements* in the six cardinal directions of gaze, and look for loss of conjugate movements in any of the six directions, which causes *diplopia*. Ask the patient which direction makes the diplopia worse and inspect the eye closely for asymmetric deviation of movement. Determine if the diplopia is *monocular* or *binocular* by asking the patient to cover one eye, then the other.

Check convergence of the eyes.

Identify any *nystagmus*, an involuntary jerking movement of the eyes with quick and slow components. Note the direction of gaze in which it appears, the plane of the nystagmus (horizontal, vertical, rotary, or mixed), and the direction of the quick and slow components. Nystagmus is named for the direction of the quick component. Ask the patient to fix his or her vision on a distant object and observe if the nystagmus increases or decreases.

Look for *ptosis* (drooping of the upper eyelids). A slight difference in the width of the palpebral fissures is a normal variant in approximately one third of patients.

Cranial Nerve V—Trigeminal

Motor. While palpating the temporal and masseter muscles in turn, ask the patient to firmly clench the teeth (Figs. 17-9 and 17-10). Note the strength of muscle contraction. Ask the patient to open and move the jaw from side to side.

See Chapter 7, Head and Neck (pp. 237–238) for a more detailed discussion of testing extraocular movements.

See Table 7-11, Dysconjugate Gaze, p. 278. Monocular diplopia is seen in local problems with glasses or contact lenses, cataracts, astigmatism, or ptosis. Binocular diplopia occurs in *CN III, IV, and VI neuropathy* (40% of patients), and eye muscle disorders from *myasthenia gravis, trauma, thyroid ophthalmopathy,* and *internuclear ophthalmoplegia.*[86]

See Table 17-7, Nystagmus, pp. 785–786. Nystagmus is seen in *cerebellar disease,* especially with gait ataxia and dysarthria (increases with retinal fixation), and *vestibular disorders* (decreases with retinal fixation); and in *internuclear ophthalmoplegia.*

Ptosis is seen in *3rd nerve palsy* (CN III), *Horner syndrome* (ptosis, miosis, forehead anhidrosis), or *myasthenia gravis.*

Difficulty clenching the jaw or moving it to the opposite side suggests masseter and lateral pterygoid weakness, respectively. Jaw deviation during opening points to weakness on the deviating side.

Look for unilateral weakness in CN V pontine lesions; bilateral weakness in bilateral hemispheric disease.

CNS patterns from stroke include ipsilateral facial and body sensory loss from contralateral cortical or thalamic lesions; ipsilateral face, but contralateral body sensory loss in brainstem lesions.

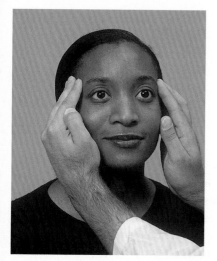

FIGURE 17-9. Palpate the temporal muscles.

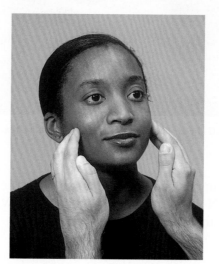

FIGURE 17-10. Palpate the masseter muscles.

Sensory. After explaining what you plan to do, test the forehead, cheeks, and chin on each side for *pain sensation* in the circled areas in Figure 17-11. The patient's eyes should be closed. Use a suitable sharp object such as a pin or cotton swab. You can create a sharp wood splinter by breaking or twisting a cotton swab. To avoid transmitting infection, use a new object for each patient. While testing, occasionally substitute the blunt end for the point as a contrasting stimulus. Ask the patient to report whether each stimulus is "sharp" or "dull" and to compare sides.

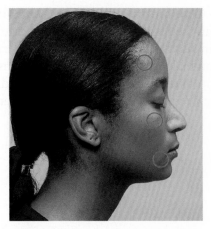

FIGURE 17-11. **Test for facial sensory loss.**

Isolated sensory loss occurs in peripheral nerve disorders, including lesions of the trigeminal nerve (CN V).

If you detect sensory loss, confirm it by testing *temperature sensation.* Two test tubes, filled with hot and ice-cold water, are the traditional stimuli. You can also use a tuning fork, which usually feels cool, and make it warm or cool with running water. Dry it, then touch the skin and ask the patient to identify "hot" or "cold."

Then test for *light touch,* using a fine wisp of cotton. Ask the patient to respond whenever you touch the skin.

Corneal Reflex. Test the *corneal reflex.* Ask the patient to look up and away from you and approach from the opposite side, out of the patient's line of vision. Avoiding the eyelashes, lightly touch the cornea (not just the conjunctiva) with a fine wisp of cotton (Fig. 17-12). If the patient is apprehensive touching the conjunctiva first may be helpful.

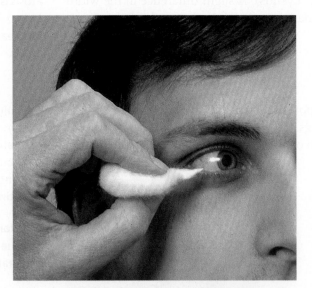

FIGURE 17-12. **Test the corneal reflex.**

Inspect for blinking of both eyes, the normal reaction to this stimulus. The sensory limb of this reflex is carried in CN V, and the motor response in CN VII on both sides. Contact lenses interfere with this testing.

Blinking is absent in both eyes in CN V lesions and on the side of weakness in lesions of CN VII. Absent blinking and sensorineural hearing loss occur in *acoustic neuroma.*

Cranial Nerve VII—Facial. Inspect the face both at rest and during conversation with the patient. Note any asymmetry, often visible in the nasolabial folds, and observe any tics or other abnormal movements.

Ask the patient to:

1. Raise both eyebrows.

2. Frown.

3. Close both eyes tightly so that you cannot open them. Test muscular strength by trying to open them, as illustrated in Figure 17-13.

4. Show both upper and lower teeth.

5. Smile.

6. Puff out both cheeks.

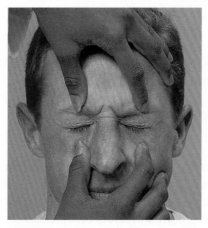

FIGURE 17-13. **Test the eye muscles.**

Cranial Nerve VIII—Acoustic and Vestibular. Assess hearing with the whispered voice test. Ask the patient to repeat numbers whispered into one ear while blocking or rubbing your fingers next to the contralateral ear.

If hearing loss is present, determine if the loss is *conductive,* from impaired "air through ear" transmission, or *sensorineural,* from damage to the cochlear branch of CN VIII. Test for *air and bone conduction,* using the Rinne test, and *lateralization,* using the Weber test.

Specific tests of the vestibular function of CN VIII are rarely included in the typical neurologic examination. Consult textbooks of neurology or otolaryngology as the need arises.

Cranial Nerves IX and X—Glossopharyngeal and Vagus. Listen to the patient's *voice.* Is it hoarse, or does it have a nasal quality?

Is there difficulty in swallowing?

Flattening of the nasolabial fold and drooping of the lower eyelid suggest facial weakness.

A peripheral injury to CN VII, as seen in *Bell palsy,* affects both the upper and lower face; a central lesion affects mainly the lower face. Loss of taste, hyperacusis, and increased or decreased tearing also occur in *Bell palsy.*[87] See Table 17-8, Types of Facial Paralysis, p. 787.

In unilateral facial paralysis, the mouth droops on the paralyzed side when the patient smiles or grimaces.

The whispered voice test is both sensitive (>90%) and specific (>80%) when assessing presence or absence of hearing loss.[88]

See techniques for Weber and Rinne tests on pp. 247–248 and Table 7-21, Patterns of Hearing Loss, p. 289.

Excess cerumen, otosclerosis, and *otitis media* cause conductive hearing loss; *presbyacusis* from aging is usually from sensorineural hearing loss.

Vertigo with hearing loss and nystagmus typifies *Ménière disease.* See Table 7-4, Dizziness and Vertigo, p. 271, and Table 17-7, Nystagmus, pp. 785–786. For caloric stimulation testing of comatose patients, see p. 270.

Hoarseness occurs in vocal cord paralysis; nasal voice in paralysis of the palate.

Difficulty swallowing suggests pharyngeal or palatal weakness.

Ask the patient to say "ah" or to yawn as you watch the *movements of the soft palate and the pharynx*. The soft palate normally rises symmetrically, the uvula remains in the midline, and each side of the posterior pharynx moves medially, like a curtain. The slightly curved uvula seen occasionally as a normal variation should not be mistaken for a uvula deviated by a lesion of CN IX or X.

Warn the patient that you are going to test the *gag reflex*, which some patients may refuse. This reflex consists of elevation of the tongue and soft palate and constriction of the pharyngeal muscles. Stimulate the back of the throat lightly on each side in turn and observe the gag reflex. This reflex is diminished in many normally healthy people.

The palate fails to rise with a bilateral lesion of CN X. In unilateral paralysis, one side of the palate fails to rise and, together with the uvula, is pulled toward the normal side (see Chapter 7, p. 257).

Unilateral absence of this reflex suggests a lesion of CN IX, and perhaps CN X.

Cranial Nerve XI—Spinal Accessory. Standing behind the patient, look for atrophy or fasciculations in the trapezius muscles, and compare one side with the other. *Fasciculations* are fine flickering irregular movements in small groups of muscle fibers. Ask the patient to shrug both shoulders upward against your hands (Fig. 17-14). Note the strength and contraction of the trapezii.

Trapezius weakness with atrophy and fasciculations points to a peripheral nerve disorder. In trapezius muscle paralysis, the shoulder droops, and the scapula is displaced downward and laterally.

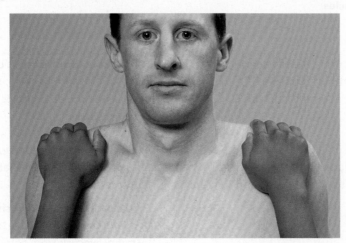

FIGURE 17-14. **Test trapezius strength.**

Ask the patient to turn his or her head to each side against your hand (Fig. 17-15). Observe the contraction of the opposite sternocleidomastoid (SCM) muscle and note the force of the movement against your hand.

A supine patient with bilateral weakness of the SCM muscles has difficulty raising the head off the pillow.

Cranial Nerve XII—Hypoglossal. Listen to the articulation of the patient's words. This depends on CNs V, VII, IX, and X, as well as XII. Inspect the patient's tongue as it lies on the floor of the mouth. Look for any atrophy or fasciculations. Some coarser restless movements are normal. Then, with the patient's tongue protruded, look for asymmetry, atrophy, or deviation from the midline. Ask the patient to move

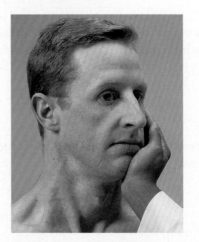

FIGURE 17-15. **Test sternocleidomastoid strength.**

For poor articulation, or *dysarthria*, see Table 17-6, Disorders of Speech, p. 784. Tongue atrophy and fasciculations are present in *amyotrophic lateral sclerosis* and past *polio*.

In a unilateral cortical lesion, the protruded tongue deviates away from the side of the cortical lesion. In CN XII lesions, the tongue deviates to the weak side.

the tongue from side to side, and note the symmetry of the movement. In ambiguous cases, ask the patient to push the tongue against the inside of each cheek in turn as you palpate externally for strength.

The Motor System

As you assess the motor system, focus on body position, involuntary movements, characteristics of the muscles (bulk, tone, and strength), and coordination. You can use this sequence for assessing overall motor function, or check each component in the arms, legs, and trunk in turn. If you detect an abnormality, identify the muscle(s) involved and if it is central or peripheral in origin. Learn which nerves innervate the major muscle groups.

Body Position.   Observe the patient's body position during movement and at rest.

Abnormal positions alert you to conditions such as mono- or hemiparesis from stroke.

Involuntary Movements.   Watch for involuntary movements such as tremors, tics, chorea, or fasciculations. Note their location, quality, rate, rhythm, and amplitude, and their relation to posture, activity, fatigue, emotion, and other factors.

See Table 17-5, Tremors and Involuntary Movements, pp. 782–783.

Muscle Bulk.   Inspect the size and contours of muscles. Do the muscles look flat or concave, suggesting loss of muscle bulk from *atrophy* or wasting? If so, is the process unilateral or bilateral? . . . proximal or distal?

When inspecting for atrophy, pay particular attention to the hands, shoulders, thighs, and legs. The spaces between the metacarpals, where the dorsal interosseous muscles lie, should be full or only slightly depressed (Fig. 17-16). The thenar

Atrophy results from PNS disorders such as diabetic neuropathy and diseases of the muscles themselves. *Hypertrophy* is an increase in bulk with normal or increased strength; increased bulk with diminished strength is called *pseudohypertrophy*, seen in the *Duchenne form of muscular dystrophy*. Corticospinal tract injury can cause mild atrophy due to decreased muscle use.

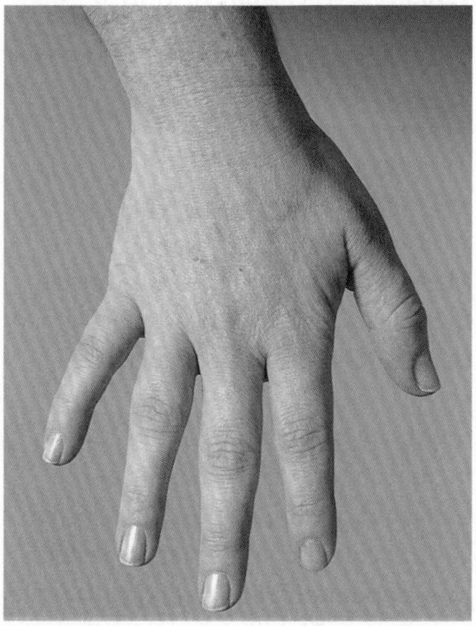

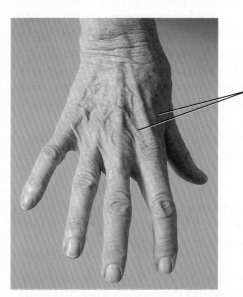

Interosseous atrophy

Furrowing between the metacarpals, and flattening of the thenar and hypothenar eminences (also seen in median and ulnar nerve damage respectively), suggest atrophy.

FIGURE 17-16.   **No atrophy— 44-year-old woman.**

FIGURE 17-17.   **Atrophy—84-year-old woman.**

and hypothenar eminences of the hands should be full and convex (Fig. 17-17). Atrophy of the hand muscles occurs in normal aging (Figs. 17-18 and 17-19).

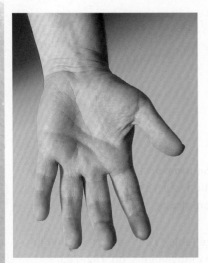 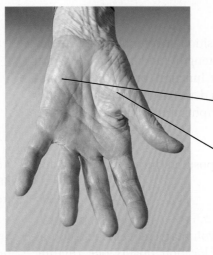

Hypothenar atrophy

Thenar flattening from atrophy

FIGURE 17-18. **No atrophy—44-year-old woman.**

FIGURE 17-19. **Atrophy—84-year-old woman.**

Other causes of muscular atrophy include motor neuron diseases, diseases affecting the peripheral motor system projecting from the spinal cord, and protein–calorie malnutrition.

Inspect for fasciculations in atrophic muscles. If absent, tap on the muscles with a reflex hammer, which stimulates them.

Fasciculations with atrophy and muscle weakness suggest peripheral motor neuron disease.

Muscle Tone. When a normal muscle with an intact nerve supply is relaxed voluntarily, it maintains a slight residual tension known as *muscle tone*. This is best assessed by feeling the muscle's resistance to passive stretch. Persuade the patient to relax. Hold one hand with yours and, while supporting the elbow, flex and extend the patient's fingers, wrist, and elbow, and put the shoulder through a moderate range of motion. With practice, you can combine these actions into a single smooth movement. On each side, note muscle tone—the resistance offered to your movements. Tense patients may show increased resistance. With repeated practice, you will learn the feel of normal resistance.

Decreased resistance suggests disease of the PNS or cerebellum, or the acute stages of spinal cord injury. See Table 17-9, Disorders of Muscle Tone, p. 788.

If you suspect decreased resistance, hold the forearm and shake the hand loosely back and forth. Normally the hand moves back and forth freely but is not completely floppy.

Marked floppiness indicates muscle *hypotonia* or *flaccidity,* usually from a peripheral motor system disorder.

If resistance is increased, determine if it varies as you move the limb or persists throughout the range of movement and in both directions, for example, during both flexion and extension. Feel for any jerkiness in the resistance.

To assess muscle tone in the legs, support the patient's thigh with one hand, grasp the foot with the other, and flex and extend the patient's knee and ankle on each side. Note the resistance to moving the limb.

Spasticity is velocity-dependent increased tone that worsens at the extremes of range. Spasticity, seen in central corticospinal tract diseases, is rate-dependent, increasing with rapid movement. *Rigidity* is increased resistance throughout the range of movement and in both directions; it is not rate-dependent.

Muscle Strength. Normal strength varies widely, so your standard of normal should allow for factors like age, sex, and muscular training. The patient's dominant side is usually slightly stronger than the nondominant side, though differences can be hard to detect. Keep this difference in mind as you compare sides.

Test muscle strength by asking the patient to actively resist your movement. Remember that a muscle is strongest when shortest, and weakest when longest. Give the *patient* the advantage as you try to overcome the resistance and judge true the muscle's true strength. Some patients give way during tests of muscle strength due to pain, misunderstanding of the test, an effort to help the examiner, conversion disorder, or malingering.

If the muscles are too weak to overcome resistance, test them against gravity alone or with gravity eliminated. When the forearm rests in a pronated position, for example, dorsiflexion at the wrist can be tested against gravity alone. When the forearm is midway between pronation and supination, extension at the wrist can be tested with gravity eliminated. Finally, if the patient fails to move the body part, observe or palpate for weak muscular contraction.

Impaired strength or weakness is called *paresis*. Absent strength is *paralysis*, or *plegia*. *Hemiparesis* refers to weakness of one half of the body; *hemiplegia* refers to paralysis of one half of the body. *Paraplegia* means paralysis of the legs; *quadriplegia* means paralysis of all four limbs.

See Table 17-1, Disorders of the Central and Peripheral Nervous Systems, pp. 774–775.

Scale for Grading Muscle Strength

Muscle strength is graded on a 0 to 5 scale:

0—No muscular contraction detected
1—A barely detectable flicker or trace of contraction
2—Active movement of the body part with gravity eliminated
3—Active movement against gravity
4—Active movement against gravity and some resistance
5—Active movement against full resistance without evident fatigue. This is normal muscle strength.

Source: Medical Research Council. Aids to the examination of the peripheral nervous system. London: Bailliere Tindall, 1986.

Many clinicians make further distinctions by adding plus or minus signs toward the stronger end of this scale. Thus, 4+ indicates good but not full strength, while 5– means a trace of weakness.

Methods for testing individual major muscle groups are described in the text that follows. The spinal root innervations and the muscles affected are shown in parentheses. To localize lesions in the spinal cord or the PNS more precisely, consult texts of neurology for specialized additional testing.

Test flexion (C5, C6—biceps and brachioradialis) *and extension* (C6, C7, C8—triceps) *at the elbow* by having the patient pull and push against your hand (Figs. 17-20 and 17-21).

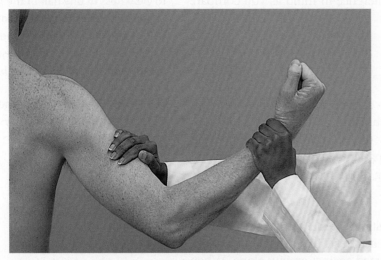

FIGURE 17-20. **Test elbow flexion.**

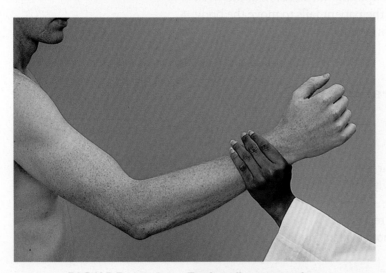

FIGURE 17-21. **Testing elbow extension.**

Test extension at the wrist (C6, C7, C8, radial nerve—extensor carpi radialis longus and brevis) by asking the patient to make a fist and resist as you press down (Fig. 17-22). Or ask the patient to extend the forearms with fingers straight and palms up, then press the palms downward.

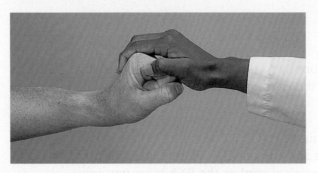

FIGURE 17-22. **Test wrist extension.**

Extensor weakness is seen in peripheral radial nerve damage, and in the hemiplegia of CNS disease seen in *stroke* or *multiple sclerosis*.

Test the grip (C7, C8, T1). Ask the patient to squeeze two of your fingers as hard as possible and not let them go (Fig. 17-23). To avoid getting hurt by strong grips, place your own middle finger on top of your index finger. Normally it should be difficult for you to pull your fingers from the patient's grip. Test both grips simultaneously with the patient's arms extended or in the lap to help compare the right handgrip with the left.

A weak grip is seen in cervical radiculopathy, median or ulnar peripheral nerve disease, and pain from *de Quervain tenosynovitis, carpal tunnel syndrome,* arthritis, and epicondylitis.

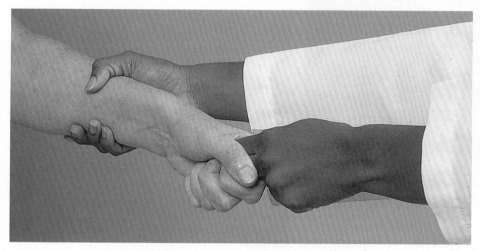

FIGURE 17-23. **Test grip strength.**

Test finger abduction (C8, T1, ulnar nerve). Position the patient's hand with palm down and fingers spread. Instruct the patient to prevent you from moving any fingers as you try to force them together (Fig. 17-24).

Weak finger abduction occurs in ulnar nerve disorders.

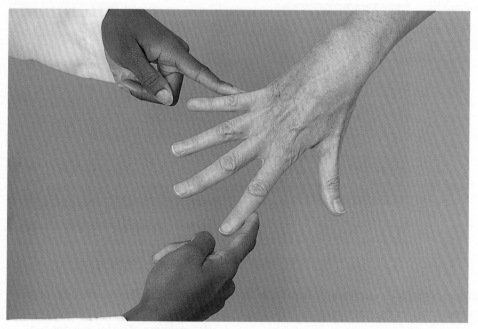

FIGURE 17-24. **Test finger abduction.**

Test opposition of the thumb (C8, T1, median nerve). Ask the patient to touch the tip of the little finger with the thumb, against your resistance (Fig. 17-25).

Inspect for weak opposition of the thumb in median nerve disorders such as *carpal tunnel syndrome* (see Chapter 16, p. 664).

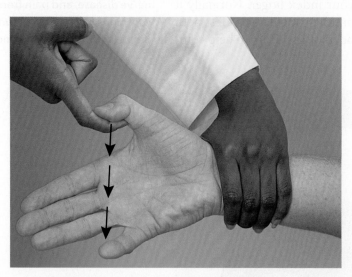

FIGURE 17-25. **Test opposition of the thumb.**

You may already have assessed *muscle strength of the trunk* during other segments of the examination, namely:

- Flexion, extension, and lateral bending of the spine

- Thoracic expansion and diaphragmatic excursion during respiration.

Test flexion at the hip (L2, L3, L4—iliopsoas) by placing your hand on the patient's mid-thigh and asking the patient to raise the leg against your hand (Fig. 17-26).

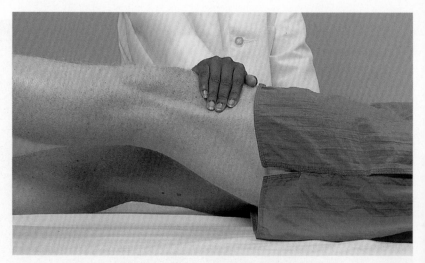

FIGURE 17-26. **Test hip flexion.**

Test adduction at the hips (L2, L3, L4—adductors). Place your hands firmly on the bed between the patient's knees. Ask the patient to bring both legs together.

Test abduction at the hips (L4, L5, S1—gluteus medius and minimus). Place your hands firmly outside the patient's knees. Ask the patient to spread both legs against your hands.

Symmetric weakness of the proximal muscles suggests *myopathy;* symmetric weakness of distal muscles suggests *polyneuropathy,* or disorders of peripheral nerves.

Test extension at the hips (S1—gluteus maximus). Have the patient push the mid posterior thigh down against your hand.

Test extension at the knee (L2, L3, L4—quadriceps). Support the knee in flexion and ask the patient to straighten the leg against your hand (Fig. 17-27). The quadriceps is the strongest muscle in the body, so expect a forceful response.

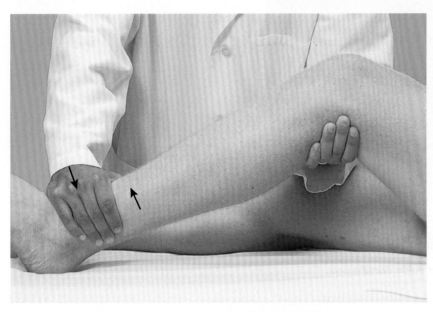

FIGURE 17-27. **Test knee extension.**

Test flexion at the knee (L4, L5, S1, S2—hamstrings) as shown below. Position the patient's leg so that the knee is flexed with the foot resting on the bed. Tell the patient to keep the foot down as you try to straighten the leg (Fig. 17-28).

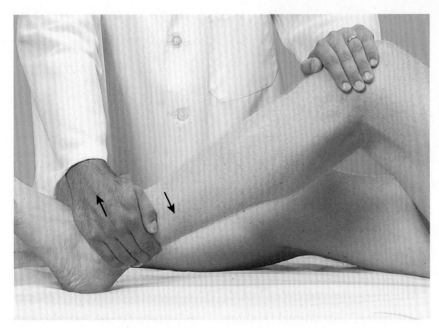

FIGURE 17-28. **Test knee flexion.**

Test foot dorsiflexion (mainly L4, L5—tibialis anterior) and *plantar flexion* (mainly S1—gastrocnemius, soleus) at the ankle by asking the patient to pull up and push down against your hand (Figs. 17-29 and 17-30). Heel and toe walk also assess foot dorsiflexion and plantar flexion, respectively.

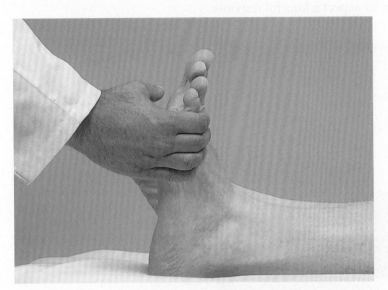

FIGURE 17-29. **Test ankle dorsiflexion.**

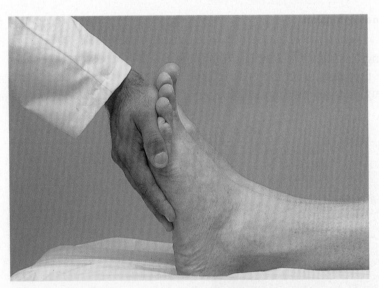

FIGURE 17-30. **Testing plantar flexion.**

Coordination. Coordination of muscle movement requires four areas of the nervous system to function in an integrated way:

■ The motor system, for muscle strength

■ The cerebellar system (also part of the motor system), for normal rhythmic movement and steady posture

In cerebellar disease, look for nystagmus, dysarthria, hypotonia, and ataxia.

- The vestibular system, for balance and for coordinating eye, head, and body movements

- The sensory system, for position sense

To assess coordination, observe the patient performing:

- Rapid alternating movements

- Point-to-point movements

- Gait and other related body movements

- Standing in specified ways

Rapid Alternating Movements

Arms. Show the patient how to strike one hand on the thigh, raise the hand, turn it over, and then strike the back of the hand down on the same place. Urge the patient to repeat these alternating movements as rapidly as possible (Fig. 17-31).

Observe the speed, rhythm, and smoothness of the movements. Repeat with the other hand. The nondominant hand may perform less well.

In cerebellar disease, instead of alternating quickly, these movements are slow, irregular, and clumsy, an abnormality called *dysdiadochokinesis*. Upper motor neuron weakness and basal ganglia disease can also impair these movements, but not in the same manner.

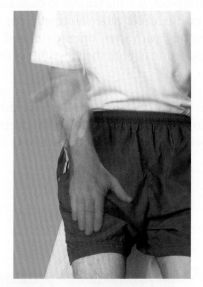

FIGURE 17-31. **Test rapid alternating arm movement.**

Show the patient how to tap the distal joint of the thumb with the tip of the index finger, again as rapidly as possible (Fig. 17-32). Again, observe the speed, rhythm, and smoothness of the movements. The nondominant side often performs less well.

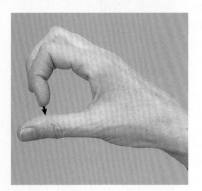

FIGURE 17-32. **Test rapid finger tapping.**

Legs. Ask the patient to tap the ball of each foot in turn as quickly as possible on your hand or the floor. Note any slowness or awkwardness. Normally the feet do not perform as well as the hands.

Dysdiadochokinesis points to cerebellar disease.

Point-to-Point Movements

Arms—Finger-to-Nose Test. Ask the patient to touch your index finger and then his or her nose alternately several times. Move your finger so that the patient has to change directions and extend the arm fully to reach your finger. Observe the accuracy and smoothness of movement, and watch for any tremor.

In cerebellar disease, movements are clumsy, unsteady, and inappropriately variable in their speed, force, and direction. In *dysmetria* the patient's finger may initially overshoot the mark, but then reach it fairly well. An *intention tremor* may appear toward the end of the movement. See Table 17-5, Tremors and Involuntary Movements, p. 782.

Now hold your finger in one place so that the patient can touch it with one arm and finger outstretched. Ask the patient to raise the arm overhead and lower it again to touch your finger. After several repeats, ask the patient to close both eyes and try several more times. Repeat on the other side. Normally the patient touches the examiner's finger successfully with eyes open or closed. These maneuvers test position sense and the function of both the labyrinth of the inner ear and the cerebellum.

In cerebellar disease, incoordination modestly worsens with eyes closed, indicating loss of position sense. Consistent deviation to one side which worsens with the eyes closed, referred to as *past pointing,* suggests cerebellar or vestibular disease.

Legs—Heel-to-Shin Test. Ask the patient to place one heel on the opposite knee, then run it down the shin to the big toe. Observe this movement for smoothness and accuracy. Repetition with the patient's eyes closed tests for position sense. Repeat on the other side.

In cerebellar disease, the heel may overshoot the knee, then oscillate from side to side down the shin. If position sense is absent, the heel lifts too high and the patient tries to look. With eyes closed, performance is poor.

Gait. Ask the patient to:

Gait abnormalities increase risk of falls.

- *Walk across the room* or down the hall, then turn and come back. Observe posture, balance, swinging of the arms, and movements of the legs. Normally balance is intact, the arms swing symmetrically at the sides, and turns are smooth.

A uncoordinated gait with reeling and instability is *ataxic.* Ataxia is seen in cerebellar disease, loss of position sense, and intoxication. See Table 17-10, Abnormalities of Gait and Posture, p. 789.

- *Walk heel-to-toe* in a straight line—called *tandem walking* (Fig. 17-33).

Tandem walking may reveal ataxia that is not otherwise obvious.

- *Walk on the toes, then on the heels*—this tests plantar flexion and dorsiflexion of the ankles as well as balance.

Walking on toes and heels may reveal distal leg weakness. Inability to heel-walk is a sensitive test for corticospinal tract damage.

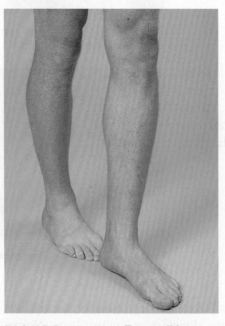

FIGURE 17-33. **Test walking heel-to-toe.**

■ *Hop in place* on each foot in turn (if the patient is not too ill)—this tests proximal and distal muscle strength in the legs and requires both normal position sense and cerebellar function.

Difficulty hopping points to weakness, lack of position sense, or cerebellar dysfunction.

■ *Do a shallow knee bend,* first on one leg, then on the other (Fig. 17-34). Steady the patient if you think the patient might fall.

■ *Or* alternatively, *rise from a sitting position* without arm support and *step up on a sturdy stool*—if the patient is unsteady, neurologically impaired, or frail these tests are more suitable than hopping or knee bends.

Difficulty doing shallow knee bends suggests proximal weakness (extensors of the hip), weakness of the quadriceps (extensor of the knee), or both.

Proximal muscle weakness in the pelvic girdle and legs causes difficulty with both of these activities. See Chapter 20, "Get up and go test," p. 996.

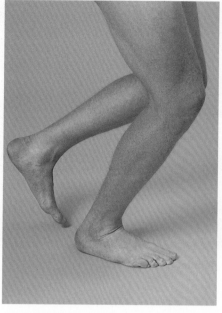

FIGURE 17-34. **Test shallow knee bends.**

Stance. The following two tests can often be performed concurrently. They differ only in the patient's arm position and in what you are assessing. In each case, stand close enough to the patient to prevent a fall.

The Romberg Test. This is mainly a test of *position sense.* The patient should first stand with feet together and eyes open and then close both eyes for 30 to 60 seconds without support. Note the patient's ability to maintain an upright posture. Normally any swaying is minimal.

In ataxia from dorsal column disease and loss of position sense, vision compensates for the sensory loss. The patient stands fairly well with eyes open but loses balance when they are closed, a *positive Romberg sign.* In *cerebellar ataxia,* the patient has difficulty standing with feet together whether the eyes are open or closed.

Test for Pronator Drift. The patient should stand for 20 to 30 seconds with eyes closed and both arms held straight forward with palms up (Fig. 17-35). Normally patients hold this arm position well. If necessary, patients can be tested in the sitting position.

Pronator drift occurs when one forearm and palm turn inward and down (Fig. 17-36) and is both sensitive and specific for a corticospinal tract lesion in the contralateral hemisphere. Downward drift of the arm with flexion of fingers and elbow is also seen.[89–92]

Next, instruct the patient to keep the arms out and eyes shut and *tap the arms briskly downward.* The arms normally return smoothly to the horizontal position. This response requires muscular strength, coordination, and good position sense.

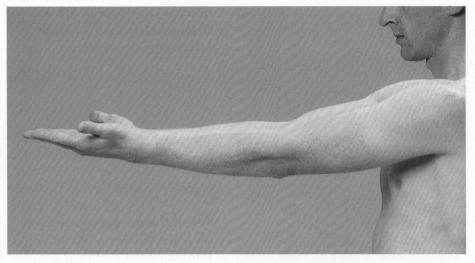

FIGURE 17-35. **Test for pronator drift.**

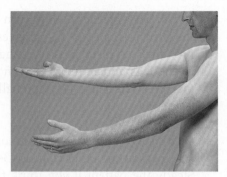

FIGURE 17-36. **Positive test for pronator drift.**

In *loss of position sense* the arms drift sideward or upward, sometimes with writhing movements of the hands; the patient may not recognize the displacement and when asked, corrects it poorly. In *cerebellar incoordination,* the arm returns to its original position but overshoots and bounces.

The Sensory System

To evaluate the sensory system, you will test several kinds of sensation:

- Pain and temperature (spinothalamic tracts)

- Position and vibration (posterior columns)

- Light touch (both of these pathways)

- Discriminative sensations, which depend on some of the above sensations but also involve the cortex

Assess the patient carefully as you consider the following questions: Is the underlying lesion central or peripheral? Is the sensory loss bilateral or unilateral? Does the pattern of sensory loss suggest a dermatomal distribution, a polyneuropathy, or a spinal cord syndrome with a loss of pain and temperature sensation but intact touch and vibration below a given spinal level?

See Table 17-1, Disorders of the Central and Peripheral Nervous Systems, pp. 774–775.

Learn to perform tests for different kinds of sensation when indicated. Correlate any abnormal findings with motor and reflex activity to establish the location of the causative lesion. To improve your physical diagnosis of the many conditions with impaired sensation, it is important to work closely with specialists and refine your skills of examination.

Refer to specialty textbooks for discussion of *spinal cord syndromes* with crossed sensory findings, both ipsilateral and contralateral to the spinal cord injury.

Patterns of Testing. Because sensory testing is tiring for many patients and can produce unreliable results, conduct the examination as efficiently as possible. Focus on areas that have numbness or pain, motor or reflex abnormalities suggesting a lesion of the spinal cord or PNS, and trophic changes such as absent or excessive sweating, atrophic skin, or cutaneous ulceration. You will often need to retest at another time to confirm abnormalities.

The following patterns of testing help you to identify sensory deficits accurately and efficiently.

Meticulous sensory mapping helps establish the level of a spinal cord lesion and whether a more peripheral lesion is in a nerve root, a major peripheral nerve, or one of its branches.

Tips for Detecting Sensory Deficits

- *Compare symmetric areas* on the two sides of the body, including the arms, legs, and trunk.

A hemisensory loss pattern suggests a lesion in the contralateral cerebral hemisphere; a *sensory level* (when one or more sensory modalities are reduced below a dermatome on one or both sides) suggests a *spinal cord lesion.*

- For pain, temperature, and touch sensation, *compare distal to proximal areas* of the extremities. Scatter the stimuli to sample most of the dermatomes and major peripheral nerves (see pp. 756–757). One suggested pattern is to include:
  - both shoulders (C4)
  - the inner and outer aspects of the forearms (C6 and T1)
  - the thumbs and little fingers (C6 and C8)
  - the fronts of both thighs (L2)
  - the medial and lateral aspects of both legs (L4 and L5)
  - the little toes (S1)
  - the medial aspect of each buttock (S3)
- For vibration and position sensation, test the fingers and toes first. If these are normal, you may safely assume that more proximal areas are also be normal.
- *Vary the pace of your testing* so that the patient does not merely respond to your repetitive rhythm.
- When you detect an area of sensory loss or hypersensitivity, *map out its boundaries* in detail. Stimulate first at a point of reduced sensation, then in progressive steps until the patient reports a change to normal sensation. An example is shown here.

Symmetric distal sensory loss suggests a *diabetic polyneuropathy.* You may miss this finding unless you compare distal and proximal sensation.

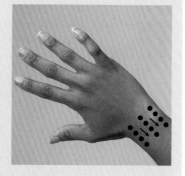

Here, all sensation in the hand is lost. Repetitive testing in a proximal direction reveals a gradual return to normal sensation at the wrist. This pattern does not fit either peripheral nerve damage or dermatomal loss (see pp. 756–757). If bilateral, it suggests the "glove" of the "stocking-glove" sensory loss of *polyneuropathy,* often seen in *alcoholism* and *diabetes.*

Before each of the following tests, show the patient what you plan to do and explain how you would like the patient to respond. The patient's eyes should be closed during actual testing.

Pain. Use a sharp safety pin, the stick portion of a broken cotton swab, or other suitable tool. Occasionally, substitute the blunt end for the point. Ask the patient, "Is this sharp or dull?" or, when making comparisons, "Does this feel the same as this?" Apply the lightest pressure needed for the stimulus to feel sharp; avoid heavy pricks that draw blood.

To prevent transmitting a bloodborne infection, discard the pin or other device safely. Do not reuse it on another person.

Temperature. Testing skin temperature is often omitted if pain sensation is normal. If there are sensory deficits, use two test tubes filled with hot and cold water, or a tuning fork heated or cooled by running water. Touch the skin and ask the patient to identify "hot" or "cold."

Light Touch. With a fine wisp of cotton, touch the skin lightly, avoiding pressure. Ask the patient to respond whenever a touch is felt, and to compare one area with another. Avoid testing calloused skin, which is normally relatively insensitive.

Vibration. Use a relatively low-pitched tuning fork of 128 Hz. Tap it on the heel of your hand and place it firmly over a distal interphalangeal joint of the patient's finger, then over the interphalangeal joint of the big toe (Fig. 17-37). Ask what the patient feels. If you are not sure whether the patient is feeling pressure or vibration, ask the patient to tell you when the vibration stops. Then touch the tuning fork to stop it from vibrating and confirm this change with the patient. If vibration sense is impaired, proceed to more proximal bony prominences (e.g., wrist, elbow; medial malleolus, shin, patella, anterior superior iliac spine, spinous processes, and clavicles).

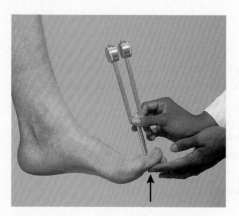

FIGURE 17-37. Test vibration sense.

Proprioception (Joint Position Sense). Grasp the patient's big toe, *holding it by its sides* between your thumb and index finger, then pull it away from the other toes (Fig. 17-38). This prevents extraneous tactile stimuli from affecting testing. Demonstrate "up" and "down" as you move the patient's toe clearly upward and downward. Then, with the patient's eyes closed, ask the patient to say "up" or "down" when moving the large toe in a small arc.

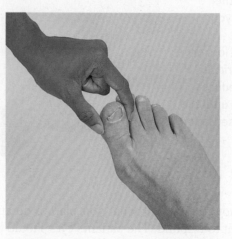

FIGURE 17-38. Test proprioception.

Analgesia refers to absence of pain sensation, *hypalgesia* refers to decreased sensitivity to pain, and *hyperalgesia* refers to increased pain sensitivity.

Anesthesia is absence of touch sensation, *hypesthesia* is decreased sensitivity to touch, and *hyperesthesia* is increased sensitivity.

Vibration sense is often the first sensation lost in a peripheral neuropathy and increases the likelihood of peripheral neuropathy 16-fold.[8] Causes include *diabetes, alcoholism,* and posterior column disease, seen in *tertiary syphilis* or *vitamin B$_{12}$ deficiency.*[93]

Testing vibration sense in the trunk is useful when identifying the level of a cord lesion.

Loss of position sense, like loss of vibration sense, is seen in *tabes dorsalis, multiple sclerosis,* or *B$_{12}$ deficiency* from posterior column disease, and in diabetic neuropathy.

Repeat the test several times on each side. If position sense is impaired, move proximally to test the ankle joint. In a similar fashion, test position in the fingers, moving proximally, if indicated, to the metacarpophalangeal joints, wrist, and elbow.

Discriminative Sensations. Several additional techniques test the ability of the sensory cortex to correlate, analyze, and interpret sensations. Because discriminative sensations depend on touch and position sense, they are useful only when these sensations are either intact or only slightly impaired.

Screen a patient with *stereognosis,* and proceed to other methods, if indicated. The patient's eyes should be closed during all these tests.

If touch and position sense are normal, decreased or absent discriminative sensation indicates a lesion in the sensory cortex. Stereognosis, number identification, and two-point discrimination are also impaired in posterior column disease.

- *Stereognosis.* Stereognosis refers to the ability to identify an object by feeling it. Place a familiar object such as a coin, paper clip, key, pencil, or cotton ball, in the patient's hand and ask the patient to tell you what it is. Normally a patient will manipulate it skillfully and identify it correctly within 5 seconds. Asking the patient to distinguish "heads" from "tails" on a coin is a sensitive test of stereognosis.

Astereognosis refers to the inability to recognize objects placed in the hand.

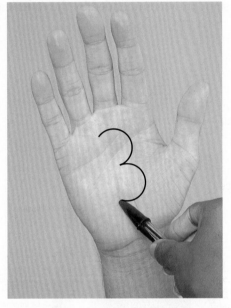

FIGURE 17-39. **Test stereognosis.**

- *Number identification (graphesthesia).* If arthritis or other conditions prevent the patient from manipulating an object well enough to identify it, test the ability to identify numbers. With the blunt end of a pen or pencil, draw a large number in the patient's palm (Fig. 17-39). A normally abled person can identify most such numbers.

The inability to recognize numbers, or *graphanesthesia,* indicates a lesion in the sensory cortex.

- *Two-point discrimination.* Using the two ends of an opened paper clip, or two pins, touch a finger pad in two places simultaneously (Fig. 17-40). Alternate the double stimulus irregularly with a one-point touch. Be careful not to cause pain.

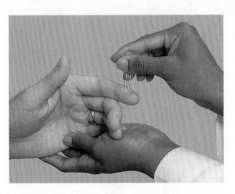

FIGURE 17-40. **Test two-point discrimination.**

Find the minimal distance at which the patient can discriminate one from two points (normally <5 mm on the finger pads). This test may be used on other parts of the body, but normal distances vary widely from one body region to another.

Lesions of the sensory cortex increase the distance between two recognizable points.

■ *Point localization.* Briefly touch a point on the patient's skin. Then ask the patient to open both eyes and point to the place touched. Normally a person can do so accurately.

Lesions of the sensory cortex impair the ability to localize points accurately.

■ *Extinction.* Stimulate one side or simultaneously stimulate corresponding areas on both sides of the body. Ask where the patient feels your touch. Normally both stimuli are felt.

With lesions of the sensory cortex, only one stimulus may be recognized. The stimulus to the side opposite the damaged cortex is extinguished.

Dermatomes. Knowledge of dermatomes helps you localize neurologic lesions to a specific level of the spinal cord, particularly in spinal cord injury. *A dermatome is the band of skin innervated by the sensory root of a single spinal nerve.* Dermatome and peripheral nerve patterns are illustrated in Figures 17-41 to 17-44, which reflect the international standard recommended by the American

In spinal cord injury, the sensory level may be several segments *lower* than the spinal lesion, for reasons that are not well understood. Percussing for the level of vertebral pain may be helpful.

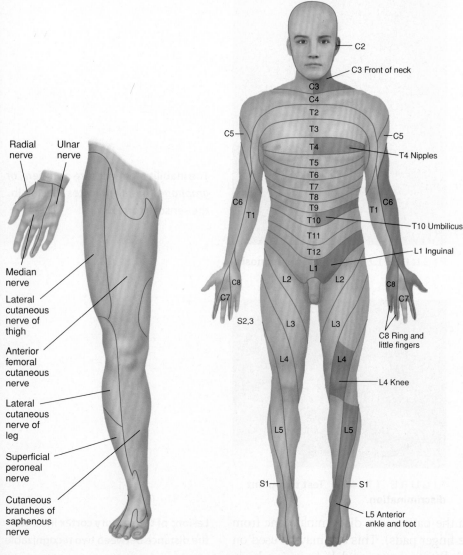

FIGURE 17-41. **Areas innervated by peripheral nerves.**

FIGURE 17-42. **Dermatomes innervated by posterior roots.**

Spinal Injury Association.[94] Dermatome levels are more variable than these diagrams suggest. They overlap at their upper and lower margins and also slightly across the midline.

Do not try to memorize all the dermatomes. Instead, focus on learning the dermatomes shaded in green.

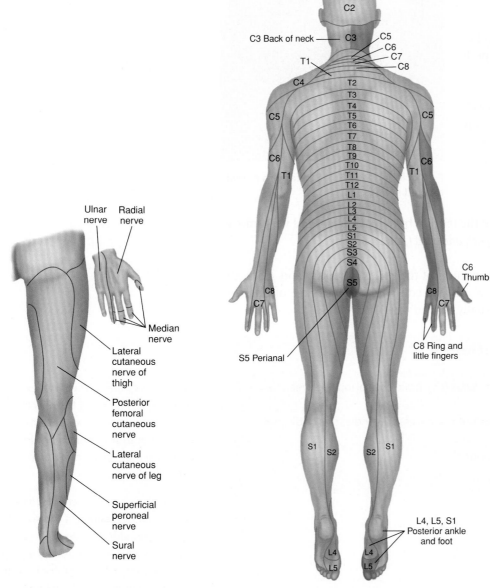

FIGURE 17-43. **Areas innervated by peripheral nerves.**

FIGURE 17-44. **Dermatomes innervated by posterior roots.**

Muscle Stretch Reflexes

Eliciting the *muscle stretch reflexes* requires special handling of the reflex hammer. Select a properly weighted reflex hammer, and learn the different uses of the pointed end and the flat end. For example, the pointed end is useful for striking small areas, such as your finger as it overlies the biceps tendon. Test the reflexes as follows:

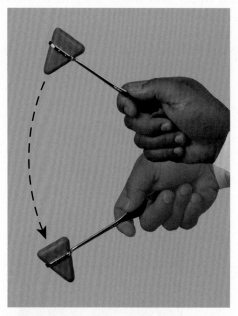

FIGURE 17-45. **Strike with a brisk relaxed swing.**

■ Encourage the patient to relax, then position the limbs properly and symmetrically.

Hold the reflex hammer loosely between your thumb and index finger so that it swings freely in an arc within the limits set by your palm and other fingers (Fig. 17-45).

■ With your wrist relaxed, strike the tendon briskly using a rapid wrist movement. Your strike should be *quick and direct,* not glancing.

Note the speed, force, and amplitude of the reflex response and grade the response using the scale below. Always compare the response of one side with the other. Reflexes are usually graded on a 0 to 4 scale.[95]

Scale for Grading Reflexes

4	Very brisk, hyperactive, with *clonus* (rhythmic oscillations between flexion and extension)
3	Brisker than average; possibly but not necessarily indicative of disease
2	Average; normal
1	Somewhat diminished; low normal
0	Reflex absent

Hyperactive reflexes (hyperreflexia) are seen in CNS lesions of the descending corticospinal tract. Look for associated upper motor neuron findings of weakness, spasticity, or a positive Babinski sign.

Hypoactive or *absent reflexes (hyporeflexia)* occur in lesions of the spinal nerve roots, spinal nerves, plexuses, or peripheral nerves. Look for associated findings of lower motor unit disease, namely weakness, atrophy, and fasciculations.

Reflex response depends partly on the force of your strike on the tendon. Use only enough force to provoke a definite response. Differences between sides are usually easier to detect than symmetric changes on both sides. Symmetrically increased, diminished, or even absent reflexes can be normal.

Reinforcement.   If the patient's reflexes are symmetrically diminished or absent, use reinforcement, a technique involving isometric contraction of other muscles for up to 10 seconds that may increase reflex activity. To reinforce the arm reflexes, for example, ask the patient to clench his or her teeth or to squeeze both knees together. If leg reflexes are diminished or absent, ask the patient to lock fingers and pull one hand against the other. Tell the patient to pull just before you strike the patellar or Achilles tendon (Fig. 17-46).

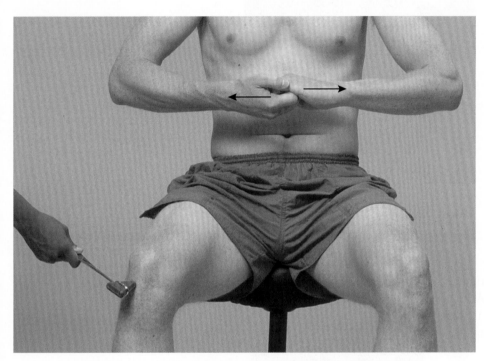

FIGURE 17-46. **Reinforce the quadriceps (patellar) reflex.**

The Biceps Reflex (C5, C6).   The patient's elbow should be partially flexed and the forearm pronated with palm down. Place your thumb or finger firmly on the biceps tendon. Aim the strike with the reflex hammer directly through your digit toward the biceps tendon (Figs. 17-47 and 17-48).

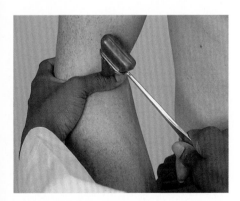

FIGURE 17-47. **Biceps reflex—patient sitting.**

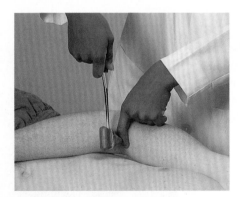

FIGURE 17-48. **Biceps reflex—patient lying down.**

Observe flexion at the elbow, and watch for and feel the contraction of the biceps muscle.

The Triceps Reflex (C6, C7). The patient may be sitting or supine. Flex the patient's arm at the elbow, with palm toward the body, and pull it slightly across the chest. Strike the triceps tendon with a direct blow directly behind and just above the elbow (Figs. 17-49 and 17-50). Watch for contraction of the triceps muscle and extension at the elbow.

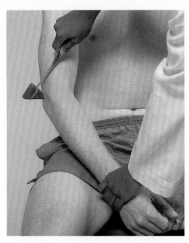

FIGURE 17-49. Triceps reflex—patient sitting.

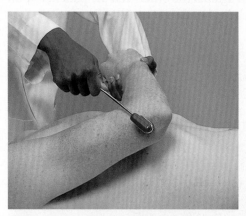

FIGURE 17-50. Triceps reflex—patient supine.

If you have difficulty getting the patient to relax, try supporting the upper arm. Ask the patient to let the arm go limp, as if it were "hung up to dry." Then strike the triceps tendon (Fig. 17-51).

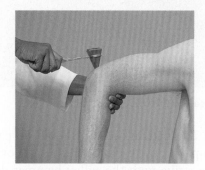

FIGURE 17-51. Triceps reflex—elbow supported.

The Brachioradialis Reflex (C5, C6). The patient's hand should rest on the abdomen or the lap, with the forearm partly pronated. Strike the radius with the point or flat edge of the reflex hammer, about 1 to 2 inches above the wrist (Fig. 17-52). Watch for flexion and supination of the forearm.

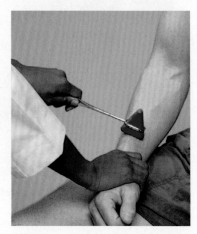

FIGURE 17-52. Brachioradialis reflex.

The Quadriceps (Patellar) Reflex (L2, L3, L4). The patient may be either sitting or lying down as long as the knee is flexed. Briskly tap the patellar tendon just below the patella (Fig. 17-53). Note contraction of the quadriceps with extension at the knee. Placing your hand on the patient's anterior thigh lets you feel this reflex.

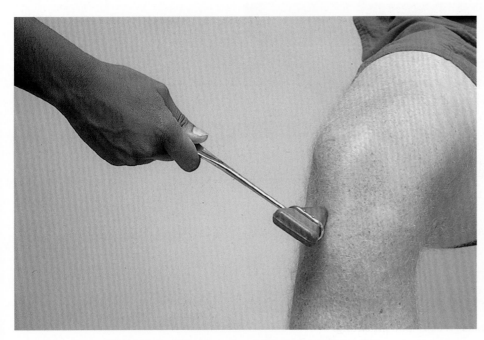

FIGURE 17-53. **Quadricepts (patellar) reflex.**

There are two options for examining the supine patient. Supporting both knees at once allows you to assess small differences between quadriceps reflexes by repeatedly testing one reflex and then the other (Fig. 17-54). If supporting both legs is uncomfortable for you or the patient, you can place your supporting arm under the patient's leg (Fig. 17-55). Some patients find it easier to relax with this method.

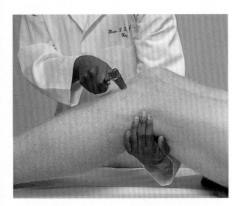

FIGURE 17-54. **Quadriceps reflex—both legs supported.**

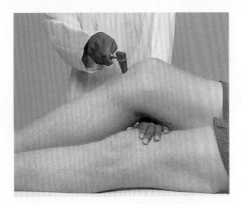

FIGURE 17-55. **Quadriceps reflex—one leg supported.**

The Achilles (Ankle) Reflex (Primarily S1).   If the patient is sitting, partially dorsiflex the foot at the ankle. Persuade the patient to relax. Strike the Achilles tendon, and watch and feel for plantar flexion at the ankle (Fig. 17-56). Also note the speed of relaxation after muscular contraction.

The slowed relaxation phase of reflexes in *hypothyroidism* is often best detected during the ankle reflex.

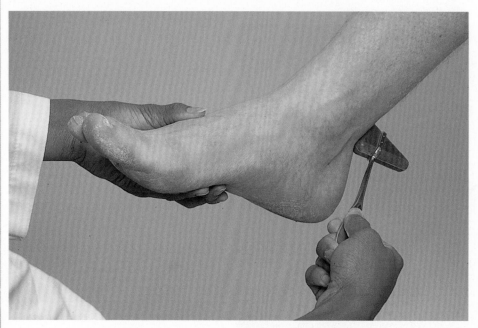

FIGURE 17-56.   Achilles reflex—patient sitting.

When the patient is lying down, flex one leg at both hip and knee and rotate it externally so that the lower leg rests across the opposite shin. Then dorsiflex the foot at the ankle and strike the Achilles tendon (Fig. 17-57).

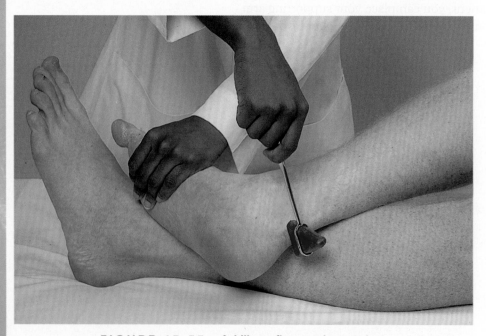

FIGURE 17-57.   Achilles reflex—patient supine.

Clonus.   If the reflexes seem hyperactive, test for *ankle clonus*. Support the knee in a partly flexed position. With your other hand, dorsiflex and plantar flex the foot a few times while encouraging the patient to relax, then sharply dorsiflex the foot and maintain it in dorsiflexion (Fig. 17-58). Look and feel for rhythmic oscillations between dorsiflexion and plantar flexion. Normally the ankle does not react to this stimulus. There may be a few clonic beats if the patient is tense or has exercised.

Sustained clonus points to CNS disease. The ankle plantar flexes and dorsiflexes repetitively and rhythmically. Clonus must be present for a reflex to be graded 4 (see p. 758).

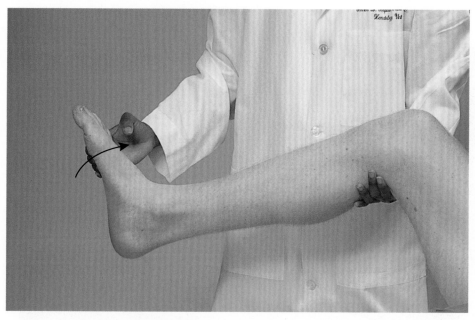

FIGURE 17-58.   **Test for ankle clonus.**

Other joints may display clonus. A sharp downward displacement of the patella, for example, may elicit patellar clonus in the extended knee.

Cutaneous or Superficial Stimulation Reflexes

The Abdominal Reflexes.   Test the abdominal reflexes by lightly but briskly stroking each side of the abdomen, above (T8, T9, T10) and below (T10, T11, T12) the umbilicus in the directions illustrated (Fig. 17-59). Use a key, the wooden end of a cotton-tipped applicator, or a tongue blade twisted and split longitudinally. Note the contraction of the abdominal muscles and movement of the umbilicus toward the stimulus. If obesity or previous abdominal surgery masks the abdominal reflexes, retract the patient's umbilicus away from the side being tested with your finger and feel for the muscular contraction.

Abdominal reflexes may be absent in both central and peripheral nerve disorders.

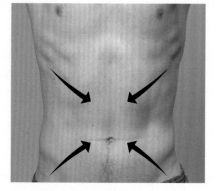

FIGURE 17-59.   **Test the abdominal reflexes.**

The Plantar Response (L5, S1). With a key or the wooden end of an applicator stick, stroke the lateral aspect of the sole from the heel to the ball of the foot, curving medially across the ball (Fig. 17-60). Use the lightest stimulus needed to provoke a response, but increase firmness if necessary. Closely observe movement of the big toe, normally plantar flexion.

Dorsiflexion of the big toe is a *positive Babinski response* (Fig. 17-61), arising from a CNS lesion affecting the corticospinal tract (sensitivity ~50%; specificity 99%).[96] The Babinski response can be transiently positive in unconscious states from drug or alcohol intoxication and during the postictal period following a seizure.

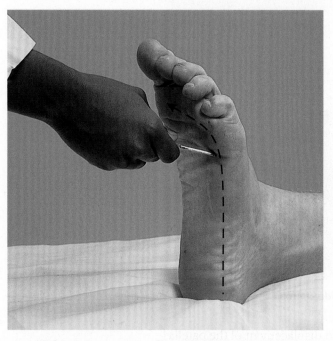

FIGURE 17-60. **Test the plantar response.**

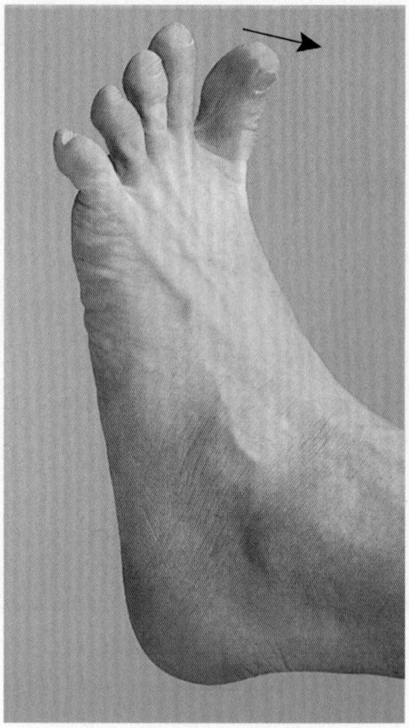

FIGURE 17-61. **Babinski response (abnormal).**

Some patients withdraw from this stimulus by flexing the hip and the knee. Hold the ankle, if necessary, to complete your observation. At times it is difficult to distinguish withdrawal from a Babinski response.

A marked Babinski response is occasionally accompanied by reflex flexion at hip and knee.

The Anal Reflex. Using a broken applicator stick or pinprick, lightly scratch the anus on both sides. Watch for reflex contraction of the external anal sphincter. Detection of the reflex contraction is facilitated by placing a gloved finger in the anus during testing.

Loss of the anal reflex suggests a lesion in the S2–3–4 reflex arc, seen in cauda equina lesions.

Special Techniques

Meningeal Signs. Test for these important signs whenever you suspect meningeal inflammation from meningitis or subarachnoid hemorrhage.

Neck Mobility/Nuchal Rigidity. First, make sure there is no injury or fracture to the cervical vertebrae or cervical cord. In trauma settings, this often requires radiologic evaluation. Then, with the patient supine, place your hands behind the patient's head and flex the neck forward, if possible until the chin

Inflammation in the subarachnoid space causes resistance to movement that stretches the spinal nerves (neck flexion), the femoral nerve (Brudzinski sign), and the sciatic nerve (Kernig sign).

touches the chest. Normally the neck is supple, and the patient can easily bend the head and neck forward.

Neck stiffness with resistance to flexion is found in ~84% of patients with *acute bacterial meningitis* and 21% to 86% of patients with *subarachnoid hemorrhage.*[97] It is most reliably present in severe meningeal inflammation but its overall diagnostic accuracy is low.[98]

Brudzinski Sign.   As you flex the neck, watch the hips and knees in reaction to your maneuver. Normally they should remain relaxed and motionless.

Flexion of both the hips and knees is a *positive Brudzinski sign.*

Kernig Sign.   Flex the patient's leg at both the hip and the knee, and then slowly extend the leg and straighten the knee (Fig. 17-62). Discomfort behind the knee during full extension is normal but should not produce pain.

Pain and increased resistance to knee extension are a *positive Kernig sign.*

The mechanism of this sign is similar to the positive straight leg raise test. Irritation or compression of a lumbar or sacral nerve root or the sciatic nerve causes radicular or sciatic pain radiating into the leg when the nerve is stretched by extending the leg.

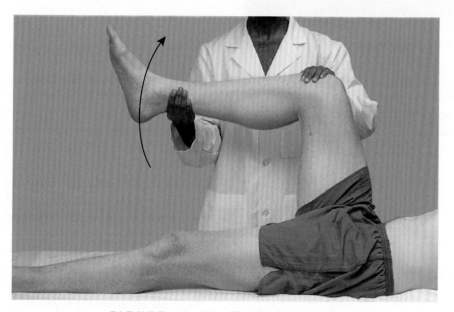

The frequency of Brudzinski and Kernig signs in patients with meningitis has a reported range of 5% to 60%.[97] Sensitivity and specificity for Brudzinski and Kernig signs are reported as ~5% and 95% in limited study sets but are used in emerging scoring systems and merit more systematic investigation.[98,99]

FIGURE 17-62. **Test for Kernig sign.**

Lumbosacral Radiculopathy: Straight-Leg Raise.   If the patient has low back pain that radiates down the thigh and leg, commonly called *sciatica* if in the sciatic nerve distribution, test straight-leg raising on each side in turn. Place the patient in the supine position. Raise the patient's relaxed and straightened leg, flexing the thigh at the hip (Fig. 17-63). Some examiners first raise the patient's leg with the knee flexed, then extend the leg.

See Table 16-3, Low Back Pain, p. 699.

Compression of the spinal nerve root as it passes through the vertebral foramen causes a painful *radiculopathy* with associated muscle weakness and dermatomal sensory loss, usually from a herniated disc. More than 95% of disc herniations occur at L4–L5 or L5–S1, where the spine angles sharply posterior. Look for confirming ipsilateral leg wasting or weak ankle dorsiflexion, which make the diagnosis of sciatica five times more likely.[100]

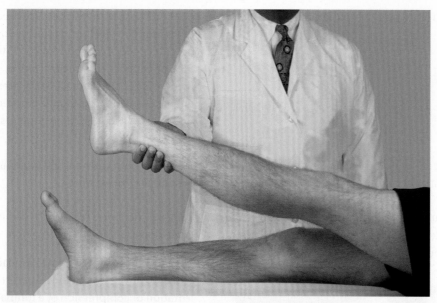

FIGURE 17-63. **Test the straight-leg raise.**

Assess the degree of elevation at which pain occurs, the quality and distribution of the pain, and the effects of foot dorsiflexion. Tightness or discomfort in the buttocks or hamstrings is common during these maneuvers and should not be interpreted as "radiating pain" or a positive test.

Pain radiating into the ipsilateral leg is a *positive straight leg test* for *lumbosacral radiculopathy.* Foot dorsiflexion can further increase leg pain in *lumbosacral radiculopathy, sciatic neuropathy,* or both. Increased pain when the contralateral healthy leg is raised is a *positive crossed straight-leg raise sign.* These maneuvers stretch the affected nerve roots and sciatic nerve.

In addition, be sure to examine motor and sensory function and reflexes at the lumbosacral levels.

Sensitivity and specificity of positive ipsilateral straight leg raise for lumbosacral radiculopathy in patients with sciatica are relatively low, with an LR of only 1.5. For the crossed straight-leg raise the LR is higher, 3.4.[100]

Asterixis.   Asterixis suggests metabolic encephalopathy in patients whose mental functions are impaired. Asterixis is caused by abnormal function of the diencephalic motor centers that regulate agonist and antagonist muscle tone and maintain posture.[101]

Sudden, brief, nonrhythmic flexion of the hands and fingers followed by recovery indicates asterixis, seen in liver disease, uremia, and hypercapnia.

Ask the patient to "stop traffic" by extending both arms, with hands cocked up and fingers spread (Fig. 17-64). Watch for 1 to 2 minutes, coaxing the patient as necessary to maintain this position.

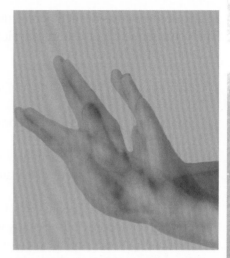

FIGURE 17-64. **Test for asterixis.**

Winging of the Scapula.

When the shoulder muscles seem weak or atrophic, inspect for scapular winging. Ask the patient to extend both arms and push against your hand or against a wall (Fig. 17-65). Observe the scapulae. Normally they lie close to the thorax.

In winging, the medial border of the scapula juts backward (Fig. 17-66), suspicious for weakness of the trapezius or serratus anterior muscle (seen in *muscular* dystrophy), or injury to the long thoracic nerve.

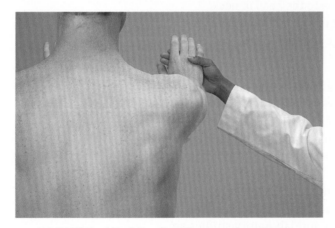

FIGURE 17-65. **Test for scapular winging.**

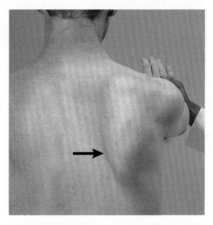

FIGURE 17-66. **Positive scapular winging.**

In very thin but normal people, the scapulae may appear "winged" even when the musculature is intact.

The Stuporous or Comatose Patient.

Coma, a state of impaired arousal and awareness, signals a potentially life-threatening event affecting the two hemispheres, the brainstem, or both. Accurate assessment is critical.[102–107] Although the arousal and awareness functions are interrelated, "a change in one is not always associated with a similar change in the other."[102] Arousal occurs in the ascending reticular activating system of the brainstem which projects through the thalamus to several areas of the cortex, which "processes, integrates, and gives context to the information provided to it thus generating awareness. Injury

Determining prognosis after coma is complex and is complicated by use of therapeutic hypothermia. Research targets include clinical examination, EEG patterns, serum biomarkers, and imaging. Careful neurologic examination remains a mainstay of prognosis, especially after 72 hours.[109,110]

to any of these areas or their connections can result in impaired consciousness." The usual sequence of history, physical examination, and laboratory evaluation does not apply. Instead, you must:

■ First assess and stabilize the ABCs (airway, breathing, and circulation)

■ Establish the patient's level of consciousness

■ Perform the neurologic examination. Identify any focal or asymmetric findings and determine if the cause of impaired consciousness is structural or metabolic.

■ Interview relatives, friends, or witnesses to establish the speed of onset and duration of unconsciousness, any warning symptoms, precipitating factors, or previous episodes, and the premorbid appearance and behavior of the patient. Any history of past medical and psychiatric illnesses is also important.

Be familiar with the Glasgow Coma Scale.[108] See Table 17-12, Glasgow Coma Scale, p. 791.

During your examination, remember two cardinal DON'Ts:

"Don'ts" When Assessing the Comatose Patient

- *Don't* dilate the pupils, the single most important clue to the underlying cause of coma (structural vs. metabolic).
- *Don't* flex the neck if there is any question of trauma to the head or neck. Immobilize the cervical spine and get an x-ray first to rule out fractures of the cervical vertebrae that could compress and damage the spinal cord.

See Table 17-11, Metabolic and Structural Coma, p. 790.

Airway, Breathing, and Circulation. Quickly check the patient's color and pattern of breathing. Inspect the posterior pharynx and listen over the trachea for stridor to make sure the airway is clear. If respirations are slowed or shallow, or if the airway is obstructed by secretions, consider intubating the patient as soon as possible while stabilizing the cervical spine.

Assess the remaining vital signs: pulse, blood pressure, and *rectal* temperature. If hypotension or hemorrhage is present, establish intravenous access and begin intravenous fluids. (Further emergency management and laboratory studies are beyond the scope of this text.)

Level of Consciousness. Level of consciousness primarily reflects the patient's capacity for arousal, or wakefulness. Testing targets the level of activity that the patient can be aroused to perform in response to escalating stimulation by the examiner.

Five clinical levels of consciousness are listed in the table below, with related techniques for examination. Increase your stimuli in a stepwise manner, depending on the patient's response. When you examine patients with an altered level of consciousness, describe and record exactly what you see and hear. Imprecise use of terms such as lethargy, obtundation, stupor, or coma may mislead other examiners.

Level of Consciousness (Arousal): Techniques and Patient Response

Level	Technique	Patient Response
Alertness	Speak to the patient in a normal tone of voice.	The alert patient opens the eyes, looks at you, and responds fully and appropriately to stimuli (arousal intact).
Lethargy	Speak to the patient in a loud voice. For example, call the patient's name or ask "How are you?"	The patient appears drowsy but opens the eyes and looks at you, responds to questions, and then falls asleep.
Obtundation	Shake the patient gently as if awakening a sleeper.	The obtunded patient opens the eyes and looks at you but responds slowly and is somewhat confused. Alertness and interest in the environment are decreased.
Stupor	Apply a painful stimulus. For example, pinch a tendon, rub the sternum, or roll a pencil across a nail bed. (No stronger stimuli needed!)	The stuporous patient arouses from sleep only after painful stimuli. Verbal responses are slow or even absent. The patient lapses into an unresponsive state when the stimulus ceases. There is minimal awareness of self or the environment.
Coma	Apply repeated painful stimuli.	A comatose patient remains unarousable with eyes closed. There is no evident response to inner need or external stimuli.

Neurologic Evaluation

Respirations.   Observe the rate, rhythm, and pattern of respiration. Because neural structures that govern breathing in the cortex and brainstem overlap with those that govern consciousness, abnormalities of respiration often occur in coma.

See Table 17-11, Metabolic and Structural Coma, p. 790, and Table 8-4 Abnormalities in Rate and Rhythm of Breathing, p. 335.

Pupils.   Observe the size and equality of the pupils and test their reaction to light. The presence or absence of the light reaction is one of the most important signs distinguishing structural from metabolic causes of coma. The light reaction often remains intact in metabolic coma.

See Table 17-13, Pupils in Comatose Patients, p. 792.

Structural lesions from stroke, abscess, or tumor mass may lead to asymmetrical pupils and loss of the light reaction.

Ocular Movement.   Observe the position of the eyes and eyelids at rest. Check for horizontal deviation of the eyes to one side (*gaze preference*). When the oculomotor pathways are intact, the eyes look straight ahead.

In structural hemispheric lesions, the eyes "look at the lesion" in the affected hemisphere.

In irritative lesions from epilepsy or a unilateral pontine lesion, the eyes "look away" from the affected hemisphere.

Oculocephalic Reflex (Doll's Eye Movements). This reflex helps assess brainstem function in the comatose patient. Holding the upper eyelids open so that you can see the eyes, turn the head quickly, first to one side and then to the other (Fig. 17-67). Make sure the patient has no neck injury before performing this test.

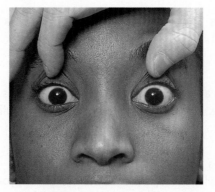

FIGURE 17-67. **Test the oculocephalic reflex.**

In a comatose patient with an intact brainstem, as the head is turned in one direction, the eyes move toward the opposite side (the *doll's eye movements*). In Figure 17-68, for example, the patient's head has been turned to the right; her eyes have moved to the left. Her eyes still seem to gaze at the camera. The doll's eye movements are intact.

In a comatose patient with absent doll's eye movements, the ability to move both eyes to one side is lost, suspicious for a lesion of the midbrain or pons (Fig. 17-69).

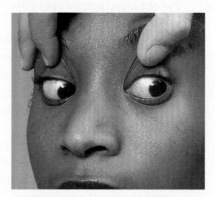

FIGURE 17-68. **Oculocephalic reflex intact.**

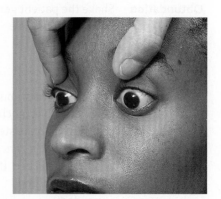

FIGURE 17-69. **Oculocephalic reflex absent.**

Oculovestibular Reflex (with Caloric Stimulation). If the oculocephalic reflex is absent and you seek further testing of brainstem function, test the oculovestibular reflex. Note that this test is usually not performed in an awake patient.

Make sure the eardrums are intact and the ear canals clear. Elevate the patient's head to 30° to perform the test accurately. Place a kidney basin under the ear to catch any water that spills over. With a large syringe, inject ice water through a small catheter that is lying in (but not plugging) the ear canal. Watch for deviation of the eyes in the horizontal plane. You may need to use up to 120 mL of ice water to elicit a response. In the comatose patient with an *intact brainstem,* the eyes drift *toward* the irrigated ear. Repeat on the opposite side, waiting 3 to 5 minutes if necessary for the first response to disappear.

No response to stimulation indicates brainstem injury.

Posture and Muscle Tone. Observe the patient's posture. If there is no spontaneous movement, you may need to apply a painful stimulus (see p. 769). Classify the resulting pattern of movement as:

See Table 17-14, Abnormal Postures in Comatose Patients, p. 793. Two stereotypic responses predominate: *decorticate rigidity* and *decerebrate rigidity*.

■ *Normal–avoidant*—the patient purposefully pushes the stimulus away or withdraws.

■ *Stereotypic*—the stimulus evokes abnormal postural responses of the trunk and extremities.

No response on one side suggests a corticospinal tract lesion.

■ *Flaccid paralysis or no response*

Test muscle tone by grasping each forearm near the wrist and raising it to a vertical position. Note the position of the hand, which is usually only slightly flexed at the wrist (Fig. 17-70).

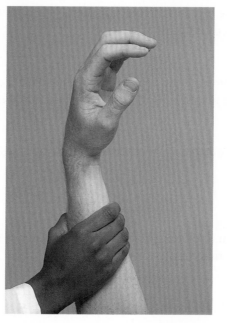

FIGURE 17-70. **Test muscle tone in the arm.**

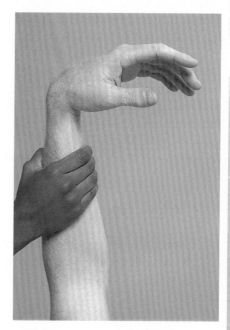

FIGURE 17-71. **Arm tone flaccid.**

The hemiplegia of acute cerebral infarction is usually flaccid at first. The limp hand drops to form a right angle with the wrist (Fig. 17-71).

Then lower the arm to about 12 or 18 inches off the bed and drop it. Watch how it falls. A normal arm drops somewhat slowly.

A flaccid arm drops rapidly, like a rock.

Support the patient's flexed knees. Then extend one leg at a time at the knee and let the leg fall (Fig. 17-72). Compare the speed with which each leg falls.

In *acute hemiplegia,* the flaccid leg falls more rapidly.

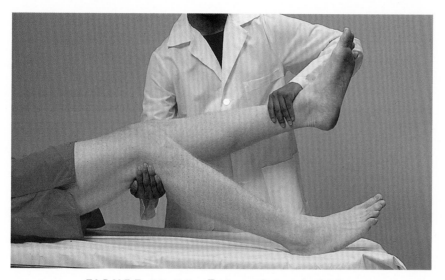

FIGURE 17-72. **Test muscle tone in the leg.**

Flex both legs so that the heels rest on the bed and then release them. The normal leg returns slowly to its original extended position.

In acute hemiplegia, the weak leg falls rapidly into extension, with external rotation at the hip.

Further Examination. As you complete the *neurologic examination,* check for facial asymmetry and asymmetries in motor, sensory, and reflex function. Test for meningeal signs if indicated.

Meningeal signs are suspicious for *meningitis or subarachnoid hemorrhage.*[11,12]

As you proceed to the *general physical examination,* include the following assessments.

- Check for unusual odors.

Consider alcohol, liver failure, or uremia.

- Inspect for abnormalities of the skin, including color, moisture, evidence of bleeding disorders, needle marks, and other lesions.

Note any jaundice, cyanosis, or the cherry red color of carbon monoxide poisoning.

- Inspect and palpate the scalp and skull for signs of trauma.

Look for bruises, lacerations, or swelling.

- Examine the fundi carefully.

Examine closely for *hypertensive retinopathy* and *papilledema,* an important sign of elevated intracranial pressure.

- Test the corneal reflexes to make sure they are intact. Remember that contact lenses may abolish these reflexes.

Corneal reflex loss occurs in coma and lesions affecting CN V or CN VII.

- Inspect the ears and nose, and examine the mouth and throat.

Blood or cerebrospinal fluid in the nose or the ears suggests a skull fracture; otitis media suggests a possible brain abscess. Tongue injury suggests a seizure.

- Be sure to evaluate the heart, lungs, and abdomen.

Recording Your Findings

Note that initially you may use sentences to describe your findings; later you will use phrases. The style below contains phrases appropriate for most write-ups. Note the five components of the examination and write-up of the nervous system.

Recording the Examination—The Nervous System

"*Mental Status:* Alert, relaxed, and cooperative. Thought process coherent. Oriented to person, place, and time. Detailed cognitive testing deferred. *Cranial Nerves:* I—not tested; II through XII intact. *Motor:* Good muscle bulk and tone. Strength 5/5 throughout. Cerebellar—Rapid alternating movements (RAMs), finger-to-nose (F→N), heel-to-shin (H→S) intact. Gait with normal base. Romberg—maintains balance with eyes closed. No pronator drift. *Sensory:* Pinprick, light touch, position, and vibration intact. *Reflexes:* 2 and symmetric with plantar reflexes downgoing."

OR

"*Mental Status:* The patient is alert and tries to answer questions but has difficulty finding words. *Cranial Nerves:* I—not tested; II—visual acuity intact; visual fields full; III, IV, VI—extraocular movements intact; V motor—temporal and masseter strength intact, corneal reflexes present; VII motor—prominent right facial droop and flattening of right nasolabial fold, left facial movements intact, sensory—taste not tested; VIII—hearing intact bilaterally to whispered voice; IX, X—gag intact; XI—strength of sternocleidomastoid and trapezius muscles 5/5; XII—tongue midline. *Motor:* strength in right biceps, triceps, iliopsoas, gluteals, quadriceps, hamstring, and ankle flexor and extensor muscles 3/5 with good bulk but increased tone and spasticity; strength in comparable muscle groups on the left 5/5 with good bulk and tone. Gait—unable to test. Cerebellar—unable to test on right due to right arm and leg weakness; RAMs, F→N, H→S intact on left. Romberg—unable to test due to right leg weakness. Right pronator drift present. *Sensory:* decreased sensation to pinprick over right face, arm, and leg; intact on the left. Stereognosis and two-point discrimination not tested. *Reflexes* (can record in two ways):

	Biceps	Triceps	Brach	Knee	Ankle	Plantar
RT	++++	++++	++++	++++	++++	↑
LT	++	++	++	++	+	↓

OR

These findings are suspicious for left hemispheric cerebral infarction in the distribution of the left middle cerebral artery, with right-sided hemiparesis.

Table 17-1 Disorders of the Central and Peripheral Nervous Systems

Central Nervous System Disorders

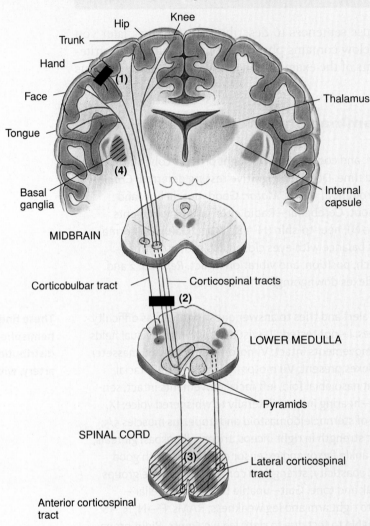

Typical Findings

Location of Lesion	Motor	Sensory	Deep Tendon Reflexes	Examples of Cause
Cerebral Cortex (1)	Chronic contralateral corticospinal-type weakness and spasticity; flexion is stronger than extension in the arm, plantar flexion is stronger than dorsiflexion in the foot, and the leg is externally rotated at the hip	Contralateral sensory loss in the face, limbs, and trunk on the same side as the motor deficits	↑	Cortical stroke
Brainstem (2)	Weakness and spasticity as above, plus CN deficits such as diplopia (from weakness of the extraocular muscles) and dysarthria	Variable; no typical sensory findings	↑	Brainstem stroke, acoustic neuroma

Typical Findings

Location of Lesion	Motor	Sensory	Deep Tendon Reflexes	Examples of Cause
Spinal Cord (3)	Weakness and spasticity as above, but often affecting both sides (when cord damage is bilateral), causing paraparesis or quadriparesis depending on the level of injury	Dermatomal sensory deficit on the trunk on one or both sides at the level of the lesion, and sensory loss from tract damage below the level of the lesion	↑	Trauma, spinal cord tumor
Subcortical Gray Matter: Basal Ganglia (4)	Slowness of movement (bradykinesia), rigidity, and tremor	Sensation not affected	Normal or ↓	Parkinsonism
Cerebellar (not illustrated)	Hypotonia, ataxia, nystagmus, dysdiadochokinesis, and dysmetria	Sensation not affected	Normal or ↓	Cerebellar stroke, brain tumor

Peripheral Nervous System Disorders

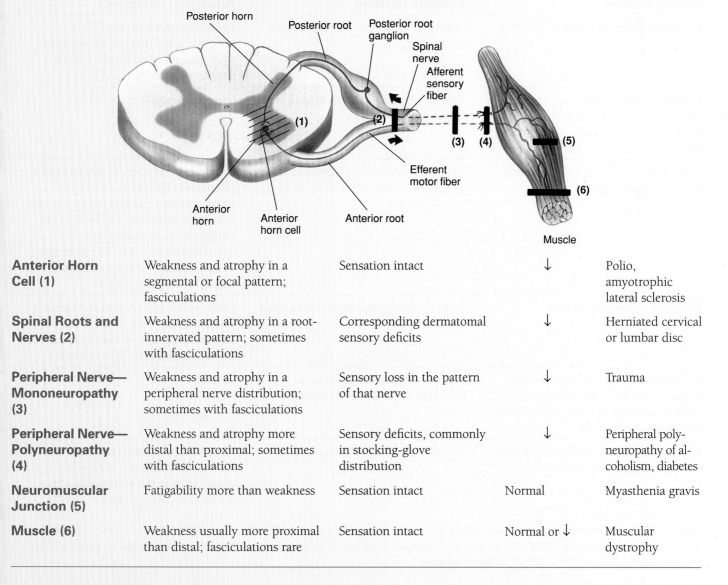

	Motor	Sensory	Deep Tendon Reflexes	Examples of Cause
Anterior Horn Cell (1)	Weakness and atrophy in a segmental or focal pattern; fasciculations	Sensation intact	↓	Polio, amyotrophic lateral sclerosis
Spinal Roots and Nerves (2)	Weakness and atrophy in a root-innervated pattern; sometimes with fasciculations	Corresponding dermatomal sensory deficits	↓	Herniated cervical or lumbar disc
Peripheral Nerve—Mononeuropathy (3)	Weakness and atrophy in a peripheral nerve distribution; sometimes with fasciculations	Sensory loss in the pattern of that nerve	↓	Trauma
Peripheral Nerve—Polyneuropathy (4)	Weakness and atrophy more distal than proximal; sometimes with fasciculations	Sensory deficits, commonly in stocking-glove distribution	↓	Peripheral poly-neuropathy of alcoholism, diabetes
Neuromuscular Junction (5)	Fatigability more than weakness	Sensation intact	Normal	Myasthenia gravis
Muscle (6)	Weakness usually more proximal than distal; fasciculations rare	Sensation intact	Normal or ↓	Muscular dystrophy

Table 17-2 Types of Stroke

Assessment of stroke requires careful history taking and a detailed physical examination, and should focus on three fundamental questions: What brain area and related vascular territory explain the patient's findings? Is the stroke ischemic or hemorrhagic? If ischemic, is the mechanism thrombosis or embolus? Stroke is a medical emergency, and timing is of the essence. Answers to these questions are critical to patient outcomes and use of antithrombotic therapies.

In *acute ischemic stroke,* ischemic brain injury begins with a central core of very low perfusion and often irreversible cell death. This core is surrounded by an *ischemic penumbra* of metabolically disturbed cells that are still potentially viable, depending on the restoration of blood flow and duration of ischemia. Because most irreversible damage occurs in the first 3–6 hrs after onset of symptoms, therapies targeted to the 3-hr window achieve the best outcomes, with recovery in up to 50% of patients in some studies.

Clinician performance in diagnosing stroke improves with training and experience. Understanding the pathophysiology of stroke takes dedication, expert supervision to improve techniques of neurologic examination, and perseverance. *This brief overview is intended to prompt further study and practice.* Accuracy in clinical examination is achievable, and more important than ever in determining patient therapy.[25,27,28,59] Turn to pp. 728–731 and review the discussion of *stroke risk factors—primary and secondary prevention.*

Clinical Features and Vascular Territories of Stroke

Clinical Finding	Vascular Territory	Additional Comments
Contralateral leg weakness	*Anterior circulation*—anterior cerebral artery (ACA)	Includes stem of circle of Willis connecting internal carotid artery to ACA, and the segment distal to ACA and its anterior choroidal branch
Contralateral face, arm > leg weakness, sensory loss, visual field loss, apraxia, aphasia (left MCA), or neglect (right MCA)	*Anterior circulation*—middle cerebral artery (MCA)	Largest vascular bed for stroke
Contralateral motor or sensory deficit without cortical signs	*Subcortical circulation*[a]—lenticulostriate deep penetrating branches of MCA	Small vessel subcortical *lacunar infarcts* in internal capsule, thalamus, or brainstem; five classical syndromes are seen: pure motor stroke (hemiplegia/hemiparesis), pure sensory stroke (hemianesthesia), ataxic hemiparesis, clumsy-hand/dysarthria syndrome, and mixed sensorimotor stroke
Contralateral visual field loss	*Posterior circulation*—posterior cerebral artery (PCA)	Includes paired vertebral and basilar artery, paired PCAs. Bilateral PCA infarction causes cortical blindness but preserved pupillary light reaction.
Dysphagia, dysarthria, tongue/palate deviation, and/or ataxia with crossed sensory/motor deficits (= ipsilateral face with contralateral body)	*Posterior circulation*—brainstem, vertebral, or basilar artery branches	
Oculomotor deficits and/or ataxia with crossed sensory/motor deficits	*Posterior circulation*—basilar artery	Complete basilar artery occlusion—"locked-in syndrome" with intact consciousness but with inability to speak and quadriplegia

[a]Learn to differentiate cortical from subcortical involvement. *Subcortical or lacunar syndromes* do not affect higher cognitive function, language, or visual fields.

Source: Adapted with permission from Medical Knowledge Self-Assessment Program, 14th edition (MKSAP 14), Neurology. Philadelphia, PA: American College of Physicians; 2006. Copyright 2006, American College of Physicians.

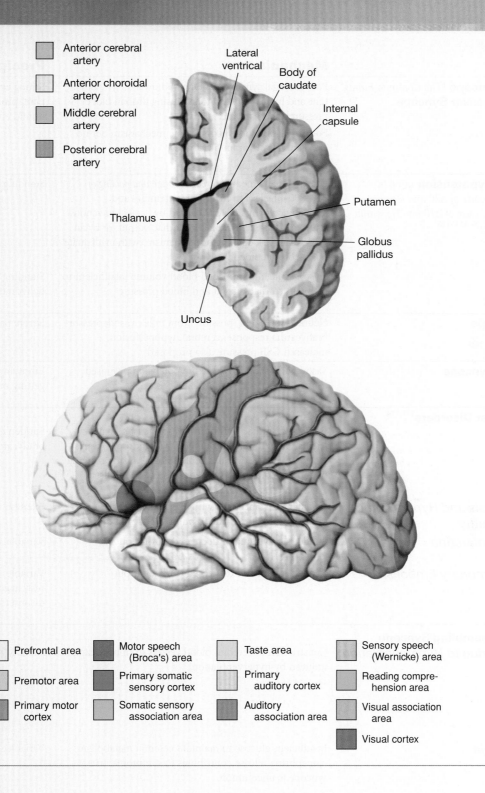

Anterior cerebral artery

Anterior choroidal artery

Middle cerebral artery

Posterior cerebral artery

Lateral ventrical

Body of caudate

Internal capsule

Putamen

Globus pallidus

Thalamus

Uncus

Prefrontal area

Premotor area

Primary motor cortex

Motor speech (Broca's) area

Primary somatic sensory cortex

Somatic sensory association area

Taste area

Primary auditory cortex

Auditory association area

Sensory speech (Wernicke) area

Reading comprehension area

Visual association area

Visual cortex

Table 17-3 Syncope and Similar Disorders Problem

	Mechanism	Precipitating Factors
Vasovagal Syncope (*The Common Faint*) **and Vasodepressor Syncope**	For vasovagal syncope: reflex withdrawal of sympathetic tone and increased vagal tone causing drop in blood pressure and heart rate For vasodepressor syncope: same mechanism but no vagal surge or drop in heart rate Baroreflexes normal	Strong emotion such as fear or pain, prolonged standing, hot humid environment
Orthostatic Hypotension (*drop in systolic blood pressure of ≥20 mm Hg or in diastolic blood pressure of ≥10 mm Hg within 3 min of standing*)[37,111–113]	Gravitationally mediated *redistribution and pooling of 300–800 mL blood* in the lower extremities and splanchnic venous system, caused by decreased venous return and an excessive fall in cardiac output, or by an inadequate vasoconstrictor mechanism (with inadequate release of norepinephrine) *Hypovolemia,* a diminished blood volume insufficient to maintain cardiac output and blood pressure	Standing up Standing up after hemorrhage or dehydration
Cough Syncope	Neurally mediated, possibly from reflex vasodepressor-bradycardia response; cerebral hypoperfusion, increased CSF pressure also proposed	Severe paroxysm of coughing
Micturition Syncope	Vasovagal response, sudden hypotension proposed	Emptying the bladder after getting out of bed to void
Cardiovascular Disorders[111,114] *Arrhythmias*	Decreased cardiac output from cardiac ischemia, ventricular arrhythmias, prolonged QT syndrome, persistent bradycardia, infrafascicular block causing cerebral hypoperfusion; often sudden onset, sudden offset	Sudden change in rhythm to bradycardia or tachyarrhythmia
Aortic Stenosis and Hypertrophic Cardiomyopathy	Vascular resistance falls with exercise, but cardiac output does not rise due to outflow obstruction.	Exercise
Myocardial Infarction	Sudden arrhythmia or decreased cardiac output	Variable, often exertion
Massive Pulmonary Embolism	Sudden hypoxia or decreased cardiac output	Variable, including prolonged bed rest, major surgery, clotting disorders, pregnancy
Disorders Resembling Syncope *Hypocapnia due to Hyperventilation*	Constriction of cerebral blood vessels from hypocapnia induced by hyperventilation	Anxiety, panic disorder
Hypoglycemia	Insufficient glucose to maintain cerebral metabolism; epinephrine release contributes to symptoms; true syncope is uncommon	Variable, including fasting
Fainting from Conversion Disorder (*Termed "Functional Neurologic Symptom Disorder" in DSM-5*)	The symbolic expression of an unacceptable idea through behavior; skin color, vital signs may be normal; sometimes with bizarre purposeful movements; usually occurs when other people present	Stress or trauma, psychological or physical

Predisposing Factors	Prodromal Manifestations	Postural Associations	Recovery
Fatigue, hunger, preload reduction from dehydration, diuretics, vasodilators	Usually >10 s. Palpitations, nausea, blurred vision, warmth, pallor, diaphoresis, light-headedness	Usually occurs when standing, at times when sitting	Prompt return of consciousness after lying down, but pallor, weakness, nausea, and slight confusion may persist for a time Most common type of syncope
Aging; central and peripheral neuropathies: Parkinson disease, multiple system atrophy; Lewy body disease diabetes, amyloidosis; antihypertensive vasodilator drugs; prolonged bed rest	Lightheadedness, dizziness, cognitive slowing, fatigue Often none	Occurs soon after standing Supine hypertension is common	Prompt return to normal when lying down
Bleeding from the GI tract or trauma, potent diuretics, vomiting, diarrhea, polyuria	Light-headedness and palpitations (tachycardia) on standing up	Occurs soon after standing up	Improves with volume repletion
COPD, asthma, pulmonary hypertension. Typically occurs in overweight middle-aged patients.	Often none except for cough; blurred vision, light-headedness may occur	May occur in any position	Prompt return to normal after a few seconds
Nocturia, usually in elderly or adult men	Often none	Commonly just after (or during) voiding after standing up	Prompt return to normal
Ischemic or valvular heart disease; conduction abnormalities; pericardial disease; cardiomyopathy Aging decreases tolerance of abnormal rhythms.	Palpitations, usually lasting <5 s. Often none	May occur in any position	Prompt return to normal when arrhythmia resolves. Most common cause of cardiac syncope. Cardiogenic syncope has a 6-mo mortality >10%
Cardiac disorders	Chest pain, often none; onset is sudden	Occurs with or after exercise	Usually a prompt return to normal
Coronary artery disease, coronary ischemia or vasospasm	Ischemic chest pain; may be silent	May occur in any position	Variable; related to time to diagnosis and treatment
Deep vein thrombosis, bed rest, hypercoagulable states (systemic lupus erythematosus, cancer), protein S or C deficiency antithrombin III deficiency. Estrogen therapy	Tachypnea, chest or pleuritic pain, dyspnea, anxiety, cough	May occur in any position	Related to time to diagnosis and treatment
Anxiety	Dyspnea, palpitations, chest discomfort, numbness, and tingling in hands and around the mouth lasting several minutes; consciousness is often maintained	May occur in any position	Slow improvement as hyperventilation ceases
Insulin therapy and a variety of metabolic disorders	Sweating, tremors, palpitations, hunger, headache, confusion, abnormal behavior, coma	May occur in any position	Variable, depending on severity and treatment
History of multiple somatic symptoms Often dissociative symptoms such as depersonalization, derealization, dissociative amnesia, or maladaptive personality traits Associated with past child abuse or neglect	Variable	A slump to the floor, often from a standing position, without injury	Variable; may be prolonged, often with fluctuating responsiveness and inconsistent neurologic findings

Table 17-4 Seizure Disorders

Seizures were reclassified in 2010 as focal or generalized to better reflect current medical science. Underlying causes should be identified as genetic, structural/metabolic, or unknown. The complexities of the reclassification scheme are best explored by turning to the report of the International League Against Epilepsy (ILAE) Commission on Classification and Terminology, 2005–2009 and to more detailed references. This table presents only basic concepts from the ILAE report.

Focal Seizures

Focal seizures "are conceptualized as originating within networks limited to *one hemisphere*.

- They may be discretely localized or more widely distributed.
- Focal seizures may originate in subcortical structures.
- For each seizure type, ictal onset is *consistent* from one seizure to another, with preferential propagation patterns that can involve the contralateral hemisphere. In some cases, however, there is more than one network, and more than one seizure type, but each individual seizure type has a consistent site of onset.
- Focal seizures do not fall into any recognized set of natural causes."

The distinction between simple partial and partial complex is eliminated, but clinicians are urged to recognize and describe "impairment of consciousness/awareness or other dyscognitive features, localization, and progression of ictal events."

Type	Clinical Manifestations	Postictal State
Focal Seizures without Impairment of Consciousness With observable motor and autonomic symptoms		
■ Jacksonian	Tonic then clonic movements that start unilaterally in the hand, foot, or face and spread to other body parts on the same side	Normal consciousness
■ Other motor	Turning of the head and eyes to one side, or tonic and clonic movements of an arm or leg without the Jacksonian spread	Normal consciousness
■ With autonomic symptoms	A "funny feeling" in the epigastrium, nausea, pallor, flushing, lightheadedness	Normal consciousness
With subjective sensory or psychic phenomena	Numbness, tingling; simple visual, auditory, or olfactory hallucinations such as flashing lights, buzzing, or odors	Normal consciousness
	Anxiety or fear; feelings of familiarity (déjà vu) or unreality; dreamy states; fear or rage; flashback experiences; more complex hallucinations	Normal consciousness
Focal Seizures with Impairment of Consciousness	The seizure may or may not start with the autonomic or psychic symptoms outlined above; consciousness is impaired, and the person appears confused Automatisms include automatic motor behaviors such as chewing, smacking the lips, walking about, and unbuttoning clothes; also more complicated and skilled behaviors such as driving a car	The patient may remember initial autonomic or psychic symptoms (which are then termed an *aura*), but is amnesic for the rest of the seizure. Temporary confusion and headache may occur
Focal Seizures That Become Generalized	Partial seizures that become generalized resemble tonic–clonic seizures (see next page); the patient may not recall the focal onset	As in a tonic–clonic seizure, described on the next page; two attributes indicate a partial seizure that has become generalized: (1) the recollection of an *aura*, and (2) a *unilateral* neurologic deficit during the postictal period

Generalized Seizures and Pseudoseizures

Generalized seizures "are conceptualized as originating at some point within, and rapidly engaging, bilaterally distributed networks . . . that include cortical and subcortical structures, but do not necessarily include the entire cortex . . ."

- The location and lateralization are *not consistent* from one seizure to another.
- Generalized seizures can be asymmetric.
- They may begin with body movements, impaired consciousness, or both.
- If onset of tonic–clonic seizures begins after age 30 yrs, suspect either a partial seizure that has become generalized or a generalized seizure caused by a toxic or metabolic disorder.

Toxic and metabolic causes include withdrawal from alcohol or other sedative drugs, uremia, hypoglycemia, hyperglycemia, hyponatremia, drug toxicity, and bacterial meningitis.

Problem	Clinical Manifestations	Postictal (*Postseizure*) State
Generalized Seizures		
Tonic–Clonic (Grand Mal)[a]	The patient loses consciousness suddenly, sometimes with a cry, and the body stiffens into tonic extensor rigidity. Breathing stops, and the patient becomes cyanotic. A clonic phase of rhythmic muscular contraction follows. Breathing resumes and is often noisy, with excessive salivation. Injury, tongue biting, and urinary incontinence may occur.	Confusion, drowsiness, fatigue, headache, muscular aching, and sometimes the temporary persistence of bilateral neurologic deficits such as hyperactive reflexes and Babinski responses. The patient is amnestic about the seizure and aura.
Absence	A sudden brief lapse of consciousness, with momentary blinking, staring, or movements of the lips and hands but no falling. Two subtypes are: *typical absence*—lasts <10 s and stops abruptly; *atypical absence*—may last >10 s.	No aura recalled. In typical absence, a prompt return to normal; in atypical absence, some postictal confusion
Myoclonic	Sudden, brief, rapid jerks, involving the trunk or limbs. Associated with a variety of disorders.	Variable.
Myoclonic Atonic (Drop Attack)	Sudden loss of consciousness with falling but no movements. Injury may occur.	Either a prompt return to normal or a brief period of confusion.
Pseudoseizures		
May mimic seizures but are due to a conversion disorder (termed "Functional Neurologic Symptom Disorder" in *DSM-5*).	The movements may have personally symbolic significance and often do not follow a neuroanatomic pattern. Injury is uncommon.	Variable.

[a]*Febrile convulsions* that resemble brief tonic–clonic seizures occur in infants and young children. They are usually benign but may also be the first manifestation of a seizure disorder.

Source: Commission on Classification and Terminology of the International League Against Epilepsy (Berg AT, Berkovic SF, Brodie MJ, et al.). A proposed diagnostic scheme for people with epileptic seizures and with epilepsy: report of the ILAE Task Force on Classification and Terminology, 2005–2009. *Epilepsia*. 2010;51:676. Available at http://onlinelibrary.wiley.com/doi/10.1111/j.1528-1167.2010.02522.x/full. Accessed July 31, 2015.

Table 17-5 Tremors and Involuntary Movements

Tremors

Tremors are rhythmic oscillatory movements, which may be roughly subdivided into three groups: resting (or static) tremors, postural tremors, and intention tremors.

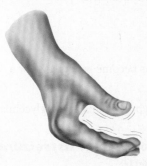

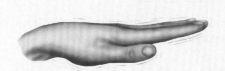

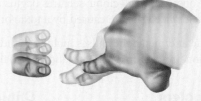

Resting (Static) Tremors

These tremors are most prominent at rest and may decrease or disappear with voluntary movement. Illustrated is the common relatively slow, fine pill-rolling tremor of parkinsonism, about 5 per second.

Postural Tremors

These tremors appear when the affected part is actively maintaining a posture. Examples include the fine rapid tremor of hyperthyroidism, the tremors of anxiety and fatigue, and benign essential (and often familial) tremor.

Intention Tremors

Intention tremors, absent at rest, appear with movement and often get worse as the target gets closer. Causes include cerebellar disorders such as multiple sclerosis.

Involuntary Movements

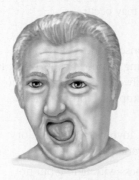 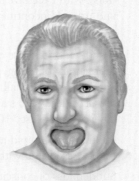 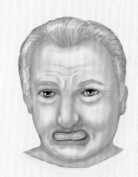

Oral–Facial Dyskinesias

Oral–facial dyskinesias are arrhythmic, repetitive, bizarre movements that chiefly involve the face, mouth, jaw, and tongue: grimacing, pursing of the lips, protrusions of the tongue, opening and closing of the mouth, and deviations of the jaw. The limbs and trunk are involved less often. These movements may be a late complication of psychotropic drugs such as phenothiazines, termed *tardive* (late) dyskinesias. They also occur in long-standing psychoses, in some elderly individuals, and in some edentulous persons.

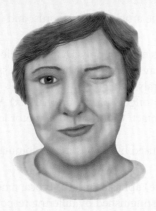

Tics

Tics are brief, repetitive, stereotyped, coordinated movements occurring at irregular intervals. Examples include repetitive winking, grimacing, and shoulder shrugging. Causes include Tourette syndrome and late effects of drugs such as phenothiazines.

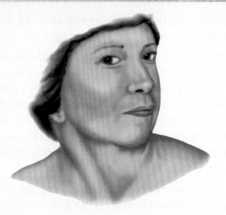

Dystonia

Dystonic movements are similar to athetoid movements, but often involve larger parts of the body, including the trunk. Grotesque, twisted postures may result. Causes include drugs such as phenothiazines, primary torsion dystonia, and as illustrated, spasmodic torticollis.

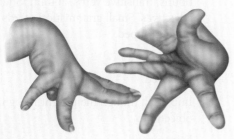

Athetosis

Athetoid movements are slower and more twisting and writhing than choreiform movements, and have a larger amplitude. They most commonly involve the face and the distal extremities. Athetosis is often associated with spasticity. Causes include cerebral palsy.

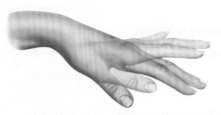

Chorea

Choreiform movements are brief, rapid, jerky, irregular, and unpredictable. They occur at rest or interrupt normal coordinated movements. Unlike tics, they seldom repeat themselves. The face, head, lower arms, and hands are often involved. Causes include Sydenham chorea (with rheumatic fever) and Huntington disease.

Table 17-6 Disorders of Speech

Disorders of speech fall into three groups affecting: (1) phonation of the voice, (2) the articulation of words, and (3) the production and comprehension of language.

- *Aphonia* refers to a loss of voice that accompanies disease affecting the larynx or its nerve supply. *Dysphonia* refers to less severe impairment in the volume, quality, or pitch of the voice. For example, a person may be hoarse or only able to speak in a whisper. Causes include laryngitis, laryngeal tumors, and unilateral vocal cord paralysis (CN X).
- *Dysarthria* refers to a defect in the muscular control of the speech apparatus (lips, tongue, palate, or pharynx). Words may be nasal, slurred, or indistinct, but the central symbolic aspect of language remains intact. Causes include motor lesions of the CNS or PNS, parkinsonism, and cerebellar disease.
- *Aphasia* refers to a disorder in producing or understanding language. It is often caused by lesions in the dominant cerebral hemisphere, usually the left.

Compared below are two common types of aphasia: (1) Wernicke, a fluent (receptive) aphasia, and (2) Broca, a nonfluent (or expressive) aphasia. There are other less common kinds of aphasia, which are distinguished by differing responses on the specific tests listed. Neurologic consultation is usually indicated.

	Wernicke Aphasia	Broca Aphasia
Qualities of Spontaneous Speech	Fluent; often rapid, voluble, and effortless. Inflection and articulation are good, but sentences lack meaning and words are malformed (paraphasias) or invented (neologisms). Speech may be totally incomprehensible.	Nonfluent; slow, with few words and laborious effort. Inflection and articulation are impaired but words are meaningful, with nouns, transitive verbs, and important adjectives. Small grammatical words are often dropped.
Word Comprehension	Impaired	Fair to good
Repetition	Impaired	Impaired
Naming	Impaired	Impaired, though the patient recognizes objects
Reading Comprehension	Impaired	Fair to good
Writing	Impaired	Impaired
Location of Lesion	Posterior superior temporal lobe	Posterior inferior frontal lobe

Although it is important to recognize aphasia early in your encounter with a patient, integrate this information with your neurologic examination as you generate your differential diagnosis.

Table 17-7 Nystagmus

Nystagmus is a rhythmic oscillation of the eyes, analogous to a tremor in other parts of the body. It has multiple causes, including impairment of vision in early life, disorders of the labyrinth and the cerebellar system, and drug toxicity. Nystagmus occurs normally when a person watches a rapidly moving object (e.g., a passing train). Study the three characteristics of nystagmus described in this table so that you can correctly identify the type of nystagmus. Then refer to textbooks of neurology for differential diagnoses.

Direction of Gaze in Which Nystagmus Appears
Example: Nystagmus on Right Lateral Gaze

Nystagmus Present (Right Lateral Gaze)

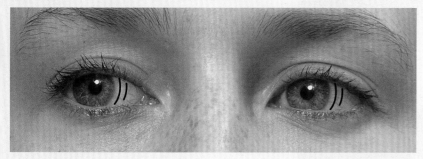

Although nystagmus may be present in all directions of gaze, it may appear or become accentuated only on deviation of the eyes (e.g., to the side or upward). On extreme lateral gaze, the normal person may show a few beats resembling nystagmus. Avoid making assessments in such extreme positions, and *observe for nystagmus only within the field of full binocular vision.*

Nystagmus Not Present (Left Lateral Gaze)

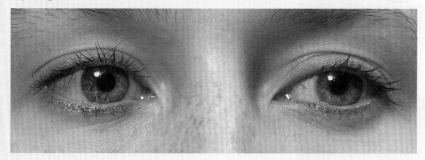

Direction of the Quick and Slow Phases
Example: Left-Beating Nystagmus—a Quick Jerk to the Left in Each Eye, then a Slow Drift to the Right

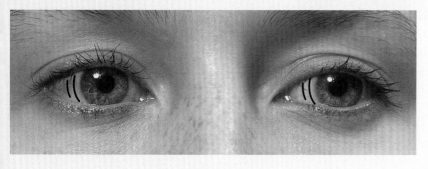

Nystagmus usually has both slow and fast movements, but *is defined by its fast phase.* For example, if the eyes jerk quickly to the patient's left and drift back slowly to the right, the patient is said to have *left-beating nystagmus.* Occasionally, nystagmus consists only of coarse oscillations without quick and slow components, described as *pendular.*

(*continued*)

Table 17-7 Nystagmus (*Continued*)

Plane of the Movements
Horizontal Nystagmus

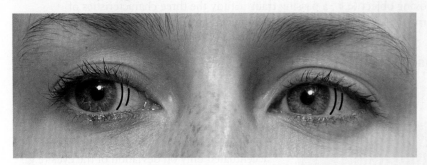

The movement of nystagmus may occur in one or more planes, namely horizontal, vertical, or rotary. It is the plane of the movements, not the direction of the gaze, that defines this variable.

Vertical Nystagmus

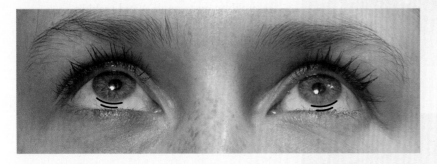

Rotary Nystagmus

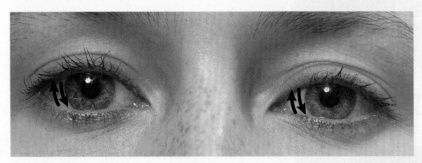

Table 17-8 Types of Facial Paralysis

Facial weakness or paralysis may result from either (1) a peripheral lesion of CN VII, the facial nerve, anywhere from its origin in the pons to its periphery in the face, or (2) a central lesion involving the upper motor neuron system between the cortex and the pons. A peripheral lesion of CN VII, exemplified here by a Bell palsy, is compared with a central lesion, exemplified by a left hemispheric cerebral infarction. These can be distinguished by their different effects on the upper portion of the face. The lower portion of the face is normally controlled by upper motor neurons located on only one side of the cortex—the opposite side. *Left hemispheric damage to these pathways, as in stroke, weakens the right lower face.* The upper face, however, is controlled by pathways from both sides of the cortex. Even though the upper motor neurons on the left are destroyed, others on the right remain, and the right upper face continues to function fairly well.

CN VII—Peripheral Lesion

Peripheral nerve damage to CN VII paralyzes the entire right side of the face, including the forehead.

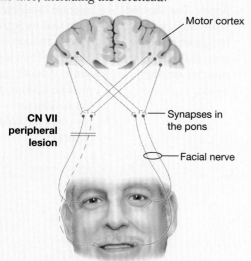

Motor cortex

CN VII peripheral lesion

Synapses in the pons

Facial nerve

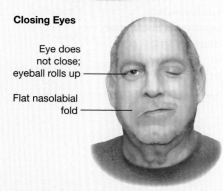

Closing Eyes

Eye does not close; eyeball rolls up

Flat nasolabial fold

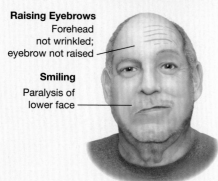

Raising Eyebrows
Forehead not wrinkled; eyebrow not raised

Smiling
Paralysis of lower face

CN VII—Central Lesion

Central nerve damage to CN VII paralyzes the lower face but cortical innervation to the forehead is preserved.

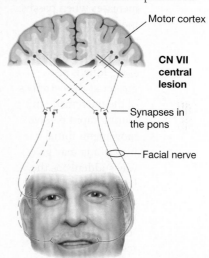

Motor cortex

CN VII central lesion

Synapses in the pons

Facial nerve

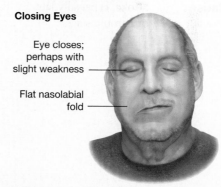

Closing Eyes

Eye closes; perhaps with slight weakness

Flat nasolabial fold

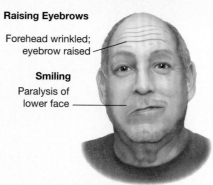

Raising Eyebrows
Forehead wrinkled; eyebrow raised

Smiling
Paralysis of lower face

Table 17-9 Disorders of Muscle Tone

	Spasticity	Rigidity	Flaccidity (*or Hypotonia*)	Paratonia
Location of Lesion	Upper motor neuron or corticospinal tract systems.	Basal ganglia system.	Lower motor neuron system at any point from the anterior horn cell to the peripheral nerves, and in cerebellar disease.	Both hemispheres, usually in the frontal lobes.
Description	Increased muscle tone (*hypertonia*) is rate dependent. Tone increases when passive movement is rapid, and decreases when passive movement is slow. Tone is also greater at the extremes of the movement arc. During rapid passive movement, initial hypertonia may give way suddenly as the limb relaxes. This spastic "catch" and relaxation is known as "clasp-knife" resistance.	Increased resistance that persists throughout the movement arc, independent of rate of movement, is called *lead-pipe rigidity.* During flexion and extension of the wrist or forearm, a superimposed ratchet-like jerkiness is called *cogwheel rigidity,* and can be due to underlying tremor.	Loss of muscle tone (*hypotonia*) causes the limb to be loose or floppy. The affected limbs may be hyperextensible or even flail-like. Flaccid muscles are often weak.	Sudden changes in tone accompany passive range of motion. Sudden loss of tone that increases the ease of motion is called *mitgehen* (moving with). Sudden increase in tone making motion more difficult is called *gegenhalten* (holding against).
Common Cause	Stroke, especially late or chronic stage.	Parkinsonism.	Guillain–Barré syndrome; also initial phase of spinal cord injury (spinal shock) or stroke.	Dementia.

Table 17-10 Abnormalities of Gait and Posture

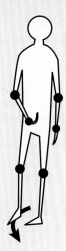

Spastic Hemiparesis

Seen in corticospinal tract lesions that cause poor control of flexor muscles during swing phase (for example, from stroke).

- Affected arm is flexed, immobile, and held close to the side, with elbow, wrists, and interphalangeal joints flexed.
- Affected leg extensors are spastic; ankles are plantar-flexed and inverted.
- Patients may drag toe, circle leg stiffly outward and forward (*circumduction*), or lean trunk to contralateral side to clear affected leg during walking.

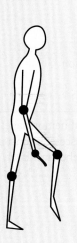

Steppage Gait

Seen in foot drop, usually secondary to peripheral motor unit disease.

- Patients either drag the feet or lift them high, with knees flexed, and bring them down with a slap onto the floor, appearing to be walking up stairs.
- Patients cannot walk on their heels.
- Gait may involve one or both legs.
- Tibialis anterior and toe extensors are weak.

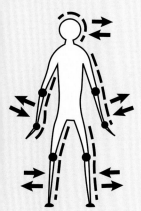

Cerebellar Ataxia

Seen in disease of the cerebellum or associated tracts.

- Gait is staggering and unsteady, with feet wide apart and exaggerated difficulty on turns.
- Patients cannot stand steadily with feet together, whether eyes are open or closed.
- Other cerebellar signs are present such as dysmetria, nystagmus, and intention tremor.

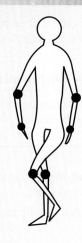

Scissors Gait

Seen in spinal cord disease, causing bilateral lower extremity spasticity, including adductor spasm.

- Gait is stiff. Patients advance each leg slowly, and the thighs tend to cross forward on each other at each step.
- Steps are short.
- Patients appear to be walking through water, and there may be compensating sway of the trunk away from the side of the advancing leg.
- Scissoring is seen in all spasticity disorders, most commonly cerebral palsy.

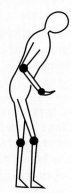

Parkinsonian Gait

Seen in the basal ganglia defects of Parkinson disease.

- Posture is stooped, with flexion of head, arms, hips, and knees.
- Patients are slow getting started.
- Steps are short and shuffling, with involuntary hastening (*festination*).
- Arm swings are decreased, and patients turn around stiffly—"all in one piece."
- Postural control is poor (*anteropulsion* or *retropulsion*).

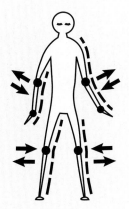

Sensory Ataxia

Seen in loss of position sense in the legs from polyneuropathy or posterior column damage.

- Gait is unsteady and wide based (with feet wide apart).
- Patients throw their feet forward and outward and bring them down, first on the heels and then on the toes, with a double tapping sound.
- Patients watch the ground for guidance when walking.
- With eyes closed, patients cannot stand steadily with feet together (positive Romberg sign), and the staggering gait worsens.

Table 17-11 Metabolic and Structural Coma

Although there are many causes of coma, most can be classified as either *structural* or *metabolic*. Findings vary widely in individual patients; the features listed are general guidelines rather than strict diagnostic criteria. Remember that psychiatric disorders may mimic coma.

	Toxic—Metabolic	Structural
Pathophysiology	Arousal centers poisoned or critical substrates depleted	Lesion destroys or compresses brainstem arousal areas, either directly or secondary to more distant expanding mass lesions
Clinical Features		
■ Respiratory pattern	If regular, may be normal or hyperventilation	Irregular, especially Cheyne–Stokes or ataxic breathing
	If irregular, usually Cheyne–Stokes	Also with selected stereotypical patterns like "apneustic" respiration (peak inspiratory arrest) or central hyperventilation
■ Pupillary size and reaction	Equal, reactive to light. If *pinpoint* from opiates or cholinergics, you may need a magnifying glass to see the reaction	Unequal or unreactive to light (fixed) *Midposition, fixed—suggests midbrain compression*
	May be unreactive if *fixed and dilated* from anticholinergics or hypothermia	*Dilated, fixed—suggests compression* of CN III from herniation
■ Level of consciousness	Changes *after* pupils change	Changes *before* pupils change
Examples of Cause	Uremia, hyperglycemia alcohol, drugs, liver failure hypothyroidism, hypoglycemia, anoxia, ischemia meningitis, encephalitis hyperthermia, hypothermia	Epidural, subdural, or intracerebral hemorrhage; large cerebral infarction; tumor, abscess; brainstem infarct, tumor, or hemorrhage; cerebellar infarct, hemorrhage, tumor, or abscess

Table 17-12 Glasgow Coma Scale

Activity		Score
Eye Opening		
None	1 = Even to supraorbital pressure	
To pain	2 = Pain from sternum/limb/supraorbital pressure	
To speech	3 = Nonspecific response, not necessarily to command	
Spontaneous	4 = Eyes open, not necessarily aware	_____
Motor Response		
None	1 = To any pain; limbs remain flaccid	
Extension	2 = Shoulder adducted and shoulder and forearm internally rotated	
Flexor response	3 = Withdrawal response or assumption of hemiplegic posture	
Withdrawal	4 = Arm withdraws to pain, shoulder abducts	
Localizes pain	5 = Arm attempts to remove supraorbital/chest pressure	
Obeys commands	6 = Follows simple commands	_____
Verbal Response		
None	1 = No verbalization of any type	
Incomprehensible	2 = Moans/groans, no speech	
Inappropriate	3 = Intelligible, no sustained sentences	
Confused	4 = Converses but confused, disoriented	
Oriented	5 = Converses and is oriented	_____
		TOTAL (3–15)[a]

_____

[a]**Interpretation:** Patients with scores of 3–8 usually are considered to be in a coma.

Source: Teasdale G, Jennett B. Assessment of coma and impaired consciousness. A practical scale. *Lancet.* 1974;304(7872):81.

Table 17-13 Pupils in Comatose Patients

Pupillary size, equality, and light reactions are important signs in assessing the cause of coma the region of the brain that is impaired. Keep in mind that unrelated pupillary abnormalities may precede coma, for example from use of miotic drops for glaucoma or mydriatic drops for viewing the ocular fundi (not recommended).

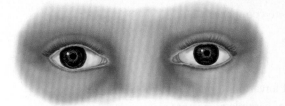

Small or Pinpoint Pupils

Bilaterally small pupils (1–2.5 mm) suggest damage to the sympathetic pathways in the hypothalamus, or metabolic encephalopathy, a diffuse failure of cerebral function that has many causes, including drugs. Light reactions are usually normal.

Pinpoint pupils (<1 mm) suggest a hemorrhage in the pons, or the effects of morphine, heroin, or other narcotics. The light reactions may be seen with a magnifying glass.

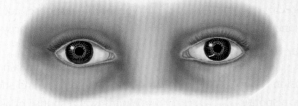

Midposition Fixed Pupils

Pupils that are in the *midposition or slightly dilated* (4–6 mm) and are *fixed to light* suggest structural damage in the midbrain.

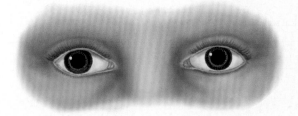

Large Pupils

Bilaterally fixed and dilated pupils may be due to severe anoxia and its sympathomimetic effects, as seen after cardiac arrest. They may also result from atropine-like agents, phenothiazines, or tricyclic antidepressants.

Bilaterally large reactive pupils may be due to cocaine, amphetamine, LSD, or other sympathetic nervous system agonists.

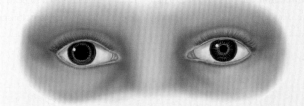

One Large Pupil

A pupil that is *fixed and dilated* warns of herniation of the temporal lobe, causing compression of the oculomotor nerve and midbrain. A single large pupil is commonly seen in diabetic patients with infarction of CN III.

Table 17-14 Abnormal Postures in Comatose Patients

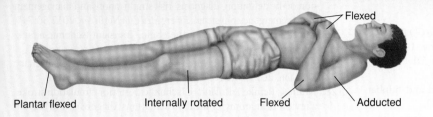

Flexed

Plantar flexed   Internally rotated   Flexed   Adducted

Decorticate Rigidity (Abnormal Flexor Response)

In *decorticate rigidity,* the upper arms are flexed tight to the sides with elbows, wrists, and fingers flexed. The legs are extended and internally rotated. The feet are plantar flexed. This posture implies a destructive lesion of the corticospinal tracts within or very near the cerebral hemispheres. When unilateral, this is the posture of chronic spastic hemiplegia.

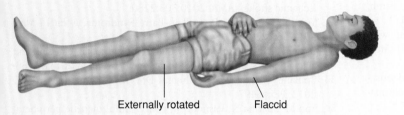

Externally rotated   Flaccid

Hemiplegia (Early)

Sudden unilateral brain damage involving the corticospinal tract may produce a *hemiplegia* (one-sided paralysis), which is flaccid early in its course. Spasticity will develop later. The paralyzed arm and leg are slack. They fall loosely and without tone when raised and dropped to the bed. Spontaneous movements or responses to noxious stimuli are limited to the opposite side. The leg may lie externally rotated. One side of the lower face may be paralyzed, and that cheek puffs out on expiration. Both eyes may be turned away from the paralyzed side.

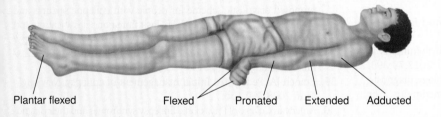

Plantar flexed   Flexed   Pronated   Extended   Adducted

Decerebrate Rigidity (Abnormal Extensor Response)

In *decerebrate rigidity,* the jaws are clenched and the neck is extended. The arms are adducted and stiffly extended at the elbows, with forearms pronated, wrists and fingers flexed. The legs are stiffly *extended at the knees,* with the feet plantar flexed. This posture may occur spontaneously or only in response to external stimuli such as light, noise, or pain. It is caused by a lesion in the diencephalon, midbrain, or pons, although may also arise from severe metabolic disorders such as hypoxia or hypoglycemia.

References

1. Wiebers DO, Dale AJD, Kokmen E, et al. (eds). *Mayo Clinic Examinations in Neurology*. 7th ed. Philadelphia, PA: Mosby; 1998.

2. Campbell WW. *DeJong's The Neurologic Examination*. 7th ed. Philadelphia, PA: Lippincott Williams & Wilkins; 2013.

3. Wright BL, Lai JT, Sinclair AJ. Cerebrospinal fluid and lumbar puncture: a practical review. *Neurol*. 2012;259:1530.

4. Straus SE, Thorpe KE, Holroyd-Leduc J. How do I perform a lumbar puncture and analyze the results to diagnose bacterial meningitis? *JAMA*. 2006;296:2012.

5. National Institute of Neurologic Disorders and Stroke, National Institutes of Health. Spinal cord injury: hope through research. Updated February 23, 2015. Available at http://www.ninds.nih.gov/disorders/sci/detail_sci.htm. Accessed April 23, 2015.

6. Chad DA, Stone JH, Gupta R. Case 14-2011: A woman with asymmetric sensory loss and paresthesias. *N Engl J Med*. 2011;364:1856.

7. Dyck PJ, Herrmann DN, Staff NP, et al. Assessing decreased sensation and increased sensory phenomena in diabetic polyneuropathies. *Diabetes*. 2013;62:3677.

8. Kanji JN, Anglin RE, Hunt DL, et al. Does this patient with diabetes have large-fiber peripheral neuropathy? *JAMA*. 2010;303:1526.

9. International Headache Society. The International Classification of Headache Disorders. 3rd ed. (beta version). *Cephalalgia*. 2013;33:629.

10. De Luca GC, Bartleson JD. When and how to investigate the patient with headache. *Semin Neurol*. 2010;30:131.

11. D'Souza S. Aneurysmal subarachnoid hemorrhage. *J Neurosurg Anesthesiol*. 2015;27:222.

12. Mortimer AM, Bradley MD, Stoodley NG, et al. Thunderclap headache: diagnostic considerations and neuroimaging features. *Clin Radiol*. 2013;68:e101.

13. Dill E. Thunderclap headache. *Curr Neurol Neurosci Rep*. 2014;14:437.

14. Bhimraj A. Acute community-acquired bacterial meningitis in adults: an evidence-based review. *Cleve Clin J Med*. 2012;79:393.

15. Brouwer MC, Tunkel AR, van de Beek D. Epidemiology, diagnosis, and antimicrobial treatment of acute bacterial meningitis. *Clin Microbiol Rev*. 2010;23:467.

16. Logan SA, MacMahon E. Viral meningitis. *BMJ*. 2008;336(7634):36.

17. Omuro A, DeAngelis LM. Glioblastoma and other malignant gliomas. *JAMA*. 2013; 310:1842.

18. Brouwer MC, Tunkel AR, McKhann GM, et al. Brain abscess. *N Engl J Med*. 2014;371:447.

19. Bushnell C, McCullough L. Stroke prevention in women: synopsis of the 2014 American Heart Association/American Stroke Association guideline. *Ann Intern Med*. 2012;160:853.

20. Sacco S, Ornello R, Ripa P, et al. Migraine and hemorrhagic stroke: a meta-analysis. *Stroke*. 2012;44:3032.

21. Sacco S, Ricci S, Degan D, et al. Migraine in women: the role of hormones and their impact on vascular diseases. *J Headache Pain*. 2012;13:177.

22. McGregor EA. In the clinic: migraine. *Ann Intern Med*. 2013;159:ITC5-1.

23. Detsky ME, McDonald DR, Baerlocher MO, et al. Does this patient with headache have a migraine or need neuroimaging? *JAMA*. 2006;296:1274.

24. Wipperman J. Dizziness and vertigo. *Prim Care*. 2014;41:115.

25. Siket MS, Edlow JA. Transient ischemic attack: reviewing the evolution of the definition, diagnosis, risk stratification, and management for the emergency physician. *Emerg Med Clin North Am*. 2012;30:745.

26. Cucchiara B, Kasner SE. In the clinic. Transient ischemic attack. *Ann Intern Med*. 2011;154:ITC-1.

27. Karras C, Aitchison R, Aitchison P, et al. Adult stroke summary. *Dis Mon*. 2013;59:210.

28. Nouh A, Remke J, Ruland S. Ischemic posterior circulation stroke: a review of anatomy, clinical presentations, diagnosis, and current management. *Front Neurol*. 2014;5:30.

29. Ishiyama G, Ishiyama A. Vertebrobasilar infarcts and ischemia. *Otolaryngol Clin North Am*. 2011;44:415.

30. Runchey S, McGee S. Does this patient have a hemorrhagic stroke? Clinical findings distinguishing hemorrhagic stroke from ischemic stroke. *JAMA*. 2010;303:2280.

31. Yuki N, Hartung H-P. Guillain-Barré Syndrome. *N Engl J Med*. 2012;366:2294.

32. Baggi F, Andreetta F, Maggi L, et al. Complete stable remission and autoantibody specificity in myasthenia gravis. *Neurology*. 2013;80:188.

33. Spillane J, Higham E, Kullmann DM. Myasthenia gravis. *BMJ*. 2012;345:e8497.

34. Yoo M, Sharma N, Pasnoor M, et al. Painful diabetic peripheral neuropathy: presentations, mechanisms, and exercise therapy. *J Diabetes Metab*. 2013;Suppl 10:005.

35. Gilron I, Baron R, Jensen T. Neuropathic pain: principles of diagnosis and treatment. *Mayo Clin Proc*. 2015;90:532.

36. Benditt DG, Adkisson WO. Approach to the patient with syncope: venues, presentations, diagnoses. *Cardiol Clin*. 2013;31:9.

37. Low PA, Tomalia VA. Orthostatic hypotension: mechanisms, causes, management. *J Clin Neurol*. 2015;11:220.

38. Commission on Classification and Terminology of the International League Against Epilepsy (Berg AT, Berkovic SF, Brodie MJ, et al). A proposed diagnostic scheme for people with epileptic seizures and with epilepsy: report of the ILAE Task Force on Classification and Terminology, 2005–2009. *Epilepsia*. 2010;51:676. Available at http://onlinelibrary.wiley.com/doi/10.1111/j.1528-1167.2010.02522.x/full. Accessed July 31, 2015.

39. French JA, Pedley TA. Initial management of epilepsy. *New Engl J Med*. 2008;359:166.

40. American College of Physicians. Epilepsy syndromes and their diagnosis. In: *Neurology, Medical Knowledge Self-Assessment Program (MKSAP) 15*. Philadelphia, PA: American College of Physicians; 2006:74.

41. Elias WJ, Shah BB. Tremor. *JAMA*. 2014;311:948.

42. Benito-Leon J. Essential tremor: a neurodegenerative disease? *Tremor Other Hyperkinet Mov (NY)*. 2014;4:252.

43. Connolly BS, Lang AE. Pharmocological treatment of Parkinson disease, a review. *JAMA*. 2014; 311:1670.

44. Jankovic J. Parkinson's disease: clinical features and diagnosis. *J Neurol Neurosurg Psychiatry*. 2008;79:368.

45. Wijemanne S, Jankovic J. Restless legs syndrome: clinical presentation diagnosis and treatment. *Sleep Med*. 2015;16:678.

46. Silber MH, Becker PM, Earley C, et al. Willis-Ekbom Disease Foundation revised consensus statement on the management of restless legs syndrome. *Mayo Clin Proc*. 2013;88:977.

47. Mozaffarian D, Benjamin EJ, Go AS, et al. Heart disease and stroke statistics—2015 update: a report from the American Heart Association. *Circulation*. 2015;131:e29.

48. Easton JD, Saver JL, Albers GW, et al. Definition and evaluation of transient ischemic attack: a scientific statement for healthcare professionals from the American Heart Association/American

REFERENCES

Stroke Association Stroke Council; Council on Cardiovascular Surgery and Anesthesia; Council on Cardiovascular Surgery and Anesthesia; Council on Cardiovascular Radiology and Intervention; Council on Cardiovascular Nursing; and the Interdisciplinary Council on Peripheral Vascular Disease. The American Academy of Neurology affirms the value of this statement as an educational tool for neurologists. *Stroke.* 2009;40(6):2276.

49. Kleindorfer DO, Lindsell C, Broderick JP, et al. Impact of socioeconomic status on stroke incidence: A population-based study. *Ann Neurol.* 2006;60:480.

50. Kleindorfer D, Panagos P, Pancioli A, et al. Incidence and short-term prognosis of transient ischemic attack in a population-based study. *Stroke.* 2005;36:720.

51. Harper S, Rushani D, Kaufman JS. Trends in the black-white life expectancy gap, 2003–2008. *JAMA.* 2012;307:2257.

52. Mosca L, Benjamin EJ, Berra K, et al. Effectiveness-based guidelines for the prevention of cardiovascular disease in women—2011 update: a guideline from the American Heart Association. *Circulation.* 2011;123:1243.

53. American Heart Association, American Stroke Association. Stroke warning signs and symptoms. Available at http://www.strokeassociation.org/STROKEORG/WarningSigns/Stroke-Warning-Signs-and-Symptoms_UCM_308528_SubHomePage.jsp. Accessed July 22, 2015.

54. U.S. Department of Health and Human Services, Office of Disease Prevention and Health Promotion. Healthy People 2020—Heart disease and stroke, objectives. Available at http://www.healthypeople.gov/2020/topics-objectives/topic/heart-disease-and-stroke/objectives. Accessed July 22, 2015.

55. Wolff T, Miller T, Ko S. Aspirin for the primary prevention of cardiovascular events: an update of the evidence for the U.S. Preventive Services Task Force. *Ann Intern Med.* 2009;150:405.

56. Pignone M, Alberts MJ, Colwell JA, et al. Aspirin for primary prevention of cardiovascular events in people with diabetes: a position statement of the American Diabetes Association, a scientific statement of the American Heart Association, and an expert consensus document of the American College of Cardiology Foundation. *Diabetes Care.* 2010;33:1395.

57. U.S. Preventive Services Task Force. *Final Recommendation Statement. Carotid artery stenosis: screening, July 2014.* U.S. Department of Health and Human Services; 2014. Available at http://www.uspreventiveservicestaskforce.org/Page/Document/UpdateSummaryFinal/carotid-artery-stenosis-screening?ds=1&s=carotid artery. Accessed August 3, 2015.

58. Jonas DE, Feltner C, Amick HR, et al. Screening for asymptomatic carotid artery stenosis: a systematic review and meta-analysis for the U.S. Preventive Services Task Force. *Ann Intern Med.* 2014;161:336.

59. Kernan WN, Ovbiagele B, Black HR, et al. Guidelines for the prevention of stroke in patients with stroke and transient ischemic attack: a guideline for healthcare professionals from the American Heart Association/American Stroke Association. *Stroke.* 2014;45:2160.

60. Ji R, Schwamm LH, Pervez MA, et al. Ischemic stroke and transient ischemic attack in young adults: risk factors, diagnostic yield, neuroimaging, and thrombolysis. *JAMA Neurol.* 2013;70:51.

61. American College of Physicians. *Stroke, in Neurology. Medical Knowledge Self-Assessment Program (MKSAP) 16.* Philadelphia, PA: American College of Physicians; 2012:24.

62. Tesfaye S, Boulton AJ, Dyck PJ, et al. Diabetic neuropathies: update on definitions, diagnostic criteria, estimation of severity, and treatments. *Diabetes Care.* 2010;33:2285.

63. American Diabetes Association. Microvascular complications and foot care. *Diabetes Care.* 2015;38(Suppl):S58.

64. Centers for Disease Control and Prevention. Prevalence of stroke—United States, 2006–2010. *MMWR Morb Mortal Wkly Rep.* 2012;61:379.

65. Yawn BP, Saddier P, Wollan PC, et al. A population-based study of the incidence and complication rates of herpes zoster before zoster vaccine introduction. *Mayo Clin Proc.* 2007;82:1341.

66. Hales CM, Harpaz R, Ortega-Sanchez I, et al.; Centers for Disease Control and Prevention. Update on recommendations for use of herpes zoster vaccine. *MMWR Morb Mortal Wkly Rep.* 2014;63:729.

67. Wong CL, Holroyd-Leduc J, Simel DL, et al. Does this patient have delirium?: value of bedside instruments. *JAMA.* 2010;304:779.

68. Inouye SK, Kosar CM, Tommet D, et al. The CAM-S: development and validation of a new scoring system for delirium severity in 2 cohorts. *Ann Intern Med.* 2014;160:526.

69. O'Mahony R, Murthy L, Akunne A, et al.; Guideline Development Group. Synopsis of the National Institute for Health and Clinical Excellence guideline for prevention of delirium. *Ann Intern Med.* 2011;154:746.

70. Rabins PV, Blass DM. In the clinic. Dementia. *Ann Intern Med.* 2014;161:ITC1; quiz ITC16.

71. American Psychiatric Association. *Diagnostic and Statistical Manual of Mental Disorders.* 5th ed. (DSM-5). Washington, DC: America Psychiatric Association; 2013.

72. Centers for Disease Control and Prevention. Dementia/Alzheimer's disease. Updated October 4, 2013. Available at http://www.cdc.gov/mentalhealth/basics/mental-illness/dementia.htm. Accessed July 22, 2015.

73. Barnes DE, Yaffe K. The projected effect of risk factor reduction on Alzheimer's disease prevalence. *Lancet Neurol.* 2011;10:819.

74. Daviglus ML, Bell CC, Berrettini W, et al. National Institutes of Health State-of-the-Science Conference statement: preventing Alzheimer disease and cognitive decline. *Ann Intern Med.* 2010;153:176.

75. Moyer VA. Screening for cognitive impairment in older adults: U.S. Preventive Services Task Force recommendation statement. *Ann Intern Med.* 2014;160:791.

76. Kroenke K, Spitzer RL, Williams JB. The Patient Health Questionnaire-2: validity of a two-item depression screener. *Med Care.* 2003;41:1284.

77. Holsinger T, Deveau J, Boustani M, et al. Does this patient have dementia? *JAMA.* 2007;297:2391.

78. American Academy of Neurology. Neurology clerkship core curriculum guidelines. See also Appendix 2: Guidelines for a Screening Neurologic Examination, p. 7. Available at https://www.aan.com/uploadedFiles/4CME_and_Training/2Training/3Fellowship_Resources/5Core_Curricula/skilz.pdf. Accessed July 23, 2015.

79. Gelb D, Gunderson C, Henry K, Kirshner H, Józefowicz R, for the Consortium of Neurology Clerkship Directors and the Undergraduate Education Subcommittee of the American Academy of Neurology. The neurology clerkship core curriculum. *Neurology.* 2002;58(6):849–852.

80. Moore FG, Chalk C. The essential neurologic examination. *Neurology.* 2009;72:2020.

81. Bates' Visual Guide to Physical Examination. Videos 17, 18—The Nervous System. Available at https://batesvisualguide.com/. Accessed July 23, 2015.

82. American Academy of Neurology. Educational resources. Available at https://www.aan.com/residents-and-fellows/clerkship-and-course-director-resources/educational-resources/ and http://www.aan.com/go/education/curricula/internal/toc. Accessed July 23, 2015.

83. Wright State University (Pearson JC, Nieder GL, Mathews T, et al.). Neurological teaching videos—a database-driven website for distribution of quicktime streaming videos to neuroscience educators. Available at http://corescholar.libraries.wright.edu/ncbp/383/. Accessed July 23, 2015.

84. McGee S. *Ch 56, Visual field testing, in Evidence-Based Physical Diagnosis.* 3rd ed. Philadelphia, PA: Saunders; 2012:513–520.

85. McGee S. *Ch 20, The pupils, in Evidence-Based Physical Diagnosis.* 3rd ed. Philadelphia, PA: Saunders; 2012:176–178.

86. McGee S. *Ch 57, Nerves of the eye muscles, in Evidence-Based Physical Diagnosis.* 3rd ed. Philadelphia, PA: Saunders; 2012:521–531.

87. Zandian A, Osiro S, Hudson R, et al. The neurologist's dilemma: a comprehensive clinical review of Bell's palsy, with emphasis on current management trends. *Med Sci Monit.* 2014;20:83.

88. McGee S. *Ch 22, Hearing, in Evidence-Based Physical Diagnosis.* 3rd ed. Philadelphia, PA: Elsevier Saunders; 2012:190.

89. Darcy P, Moughty AM. Pronator drift. *N Engl J Med.* 2013;369:320.

90. Daum C, Aybek S. Validity of the "drift without pronation" sign in conversion disorder. *BMC Neurol.* 2013;13:31.

91. Stone J, Carson A, Duncan R, et al. Which neurological diseases are most likely to be associated with "symptoms unexplained by organic disease." *J Neurol.* 2012;259:33.

92. Stone J, Carson A, Sharpe M. Functional symptoms and signs in neurology: assessment and diagnosis. *J Neurol Neurosurg Psychiatry.* 2005;76(Suppl 1):i2.

93. Stabler SP. Clinical practice. Vitamin B_{12} deficiency. *N Engl J Med.* 2013; 368:149.

94. Kirshblum SC, Burns SP, Biering-Sorensen F, et al. International Standards for Neurological Classification of Spinal Cord Injury (Revised 2011). *J Spinal Cord Med.* 2011;34:535.

95. Hallett M. NINDS myotatic reflex scale. *Neurology.* 1993;43:2723.

96. Isaza Jaramillo SP, Uribe Uribe CS, García Jimenez FA, et al. Accuracy of the Babinski sign in the identification of pyramidal tract dysfunction. *J Neurol Sci.* 2014;343:66.

97. McGee S. *Ch 24, Meninges, in Evidence-Based Physical Diagnosis.* 3rd ed. Philadelphia, PA: Elsevier Saunders; 2012:210–214.

98. Thomas KE, Hasbun R, Jekel J, et al. The diagnostic accuracy of Kernig's sign, Brudzinski's sign, and nuchal rigidity in adults with suspected meningitis. *Clin Infect Dis.* 2002;35:46.

99. Ward MA, Greenwood TM, Kumar DR, et al. Josef Brudzinski and Vladimir Mikhailovich Kernig: signs for diagnosing meningitis. *Clin Med Res.* 2010;8:13.

100. McGee S. *Ch 62, Disorders of nerve roots, plexuses, in Evidence-Based Physical Diagnosis.* 3rd ed. Philadelphia, PA: Elsevier Saunders; 2012:607–609.

101. Mendizabal M, Silva MO. Asterixis. *N Engl J Med.* 2010;363:e14.

102. Edlow JA, Rabinstein A, Traub SJ, et al. Diagnosis of reversible causes of coma. *Lancet.* 2014;384(9959):2064.

103. Moore SA, Wijdicks EF. The acutely comatose patient: clinical approach and diagnosis. *Semin Neurol.* 2013;33:110.

104. Wijdicks EF. *The Comatose Patient.* 2nd ed. New York, NY: Oxford University Press; 2014.

105. Henry TR, Ezzeddine MA. Approach to the patient with transient alteration of consciousness. *Neurol Clin Pract.* 2012;2:179.

106. Pope JV, Edlow JA. Avoiding misdiagnosis in patients with neurological emergencies. *Emerg Med Int.* 2012;2012:949275.

107. Brown EN, Lydic R, Schiff ND. General anesthesia, sleep, and coma. *N Engl J Med.* 2010;363:2638.

108. Teasdale G, Jennett B. Assessment of coma and impaired consciousness. A practical scale. *Lancet.* 1974;304(7872):81.

109. Sandroni C, Geocadin RG. Neurological prognostication after cardiac arrest. *Curr Opin Crit Care.* 2015;21:209.

110. Sandroni C, Cariou A, Cavallaro F, et al. Prognostication in comatose survivors of cardiac arrest: an advisory statement from the European Resuscitation Council and the European Society of Intensive Care Medicine. *Resuscitation.* 2014;85:1779.

111. American College of Physicians. Syncope. In: *General Internal Medicine, Medical Knowledge Self-Assessment Program (MKSAP) 16.* Philadelphia, PA: American College of Physicians; 2012:45.

112. Freeman R, Wieling W, Axelrod FB, et al. Consensus statement on the definition of orthostatic hypotension, neutrally mediated syncope and the postural tachycardia syndrome. *Clin Auton Res.* 2011;21:69.

113. Vijayan J, Sharma VK. Neurogenic orthostatic hypotension—management update and role of droxidopa. *Ther Clin Risk Manag.* 2015;8:915.

114. Chen LY, Benditt DG, Shen WK. Management of syncope in adults: an update. *Mayo Clin Proc.* 2008;83:1280.

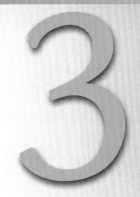

Special Populations

Assessing Children: Infancy through Adolescence

Peter G. Szilagyi, MD, MPH

The Bates' suite offers these additional resources to enhance learning and facilitate understanding of this chapter:

- Bates' *Pocket Guide to Physical Examination and History Taking*, 8th edition
- Bates' *Visual Guide to Physical Examination* (Vol. 2: Head-to-Toe Assessment: Infant; Vol. 3: Head-to-Toe Assessment: Child)
- thePoint online resources, for students and instructors: http://thepoint.lww.com

This chapter highlights clinical assessment for each pediatric age group, beginning with general principles of development and key components of health promotion. Newborns, infants, young and school-aged children, and adolescents are covered in separate sections, with relevant discussions of development, history taking, health promotion and counseling, and techniques of examination for each (Figs. 18-1 to 18-3).

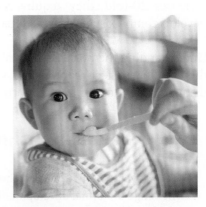

FIGURE 18-1. Infants have surprising abilities.

Guide to Chapter Organization

General Principles of Child Development
Health Promotion and Counseling: Key Components
Assessing the Newborn
Assessing the Infant
Assessing Young and School-Aged Children
Assessing Adolescents
Recording Your Findings

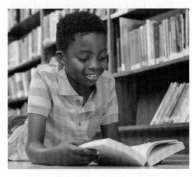

FIGURE 18-2. A drive for independence appears in school-aged children.

Inexperienced examiners are often intimidated when approaching a tiny baby or an upset child, especially under the critical eyes of anxious parents. Although it is initially challenging, you will come to enjoy almost all pediatric encounters.

Review Chapter 1, Overview: Physical Examination and History Taking, for the methods and sequence of examining adults. When examining infants and children, the sequence should vary according to the child's age and comfort level. *Perform less invasive maneuvers early and potentially distressing maneuvers near the end of the examination.* For example, palpate the head and neck and auscultate the heart and lungs early, and examine the ears and mouth and palpate the abdomen near the end. *If the child reports pain in one area examine that area last.*

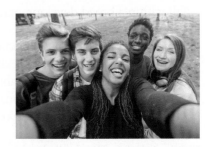

FIGURE 18-3. Social interactions become important in adolescence.

The format of the clinical record is the same for both children and adults. Although the sequence of the physical examination may vary, convert your clinical findings into the traditional written or electronic format.

General Principles of Child Development

Childhood is a period of remarkable physical, cognitive, and social growth—by far the greatest in a person's lifetime. Within a few short years, children's size increases 20-fold, they acquire sophisticated language and reasoning, they develop complex social interactions, and they progress toward mature adults.

Understanding the normal physical, cognitive, and social development of children facilitates effective interviews and physical examinations and is the basis for distinguishing normal from abnormal findings.

Four Principles of Child Development

1. Child development proceeds along a predictable pathway.
2. The range of normal development is wide.
3. Various physical, social, and environmental factors, as well as diseases, can affect child development and health.
4. The child's developmental level affects how you conduct the history and physical examination.[1,2]

- Principle #1: *Child development proceeds along a predictable pathway* governed by the maturing brain. You can measure age-specific milestones and use them to characterize development as normal or abnormal. Because your health care visit and physical examination take place at one point in time, you need to determine where the child fits along a developmental trajectory. Milestones are achieved in an order than can be anticipated. *Loss of milestones is always concerning.*

- Principle #2: *The range of normal development is wide.* Children mature at different rates. Each child's physical, cognitive, and social development should fall within a broad developmental range.

- Principle #3: *Various physical, social, and environmental factors, as well as diseases, can affect child development and health.* For example, chronic illnesses, child abuse, and poverty can all cause detectable physical abnormalities and alter the rate and course of development. Additionally, *children with physical or cognitive disabilities may not follow the expected age-specific developmental trajectory* (Fig. 18-4).

- Principle #4: *The child's developmental level affects how you conduct the clinical history and physical examination.* For example, interviewing a 5-year-old is

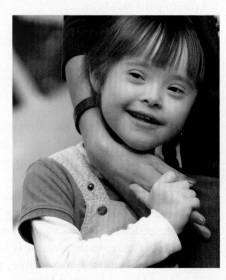

FIGURE 18-4. Child development is affected by many factors.

fundamentally different than interviewing an adolescent. Both order and style differ from the adult examination. Before performing a physical examination, attempt to ascertain the child's approximate developmental level and adapt your physical examination to that level. An understanding of normal child development helps you achieve these tasks.

Health Promotion and Counseling: Key Components

Benjamin Franklin noted that "an ounce of prevention is worth a pound of cure." This adage is particularly true for children and adolescents because prevention and health promotion at a young age can result in improved health outcomes for decades. Pediatric clinicians dedicate substantial time to health supervision visits and health promotion activities.

Several national and international organizations have developed guidelines for health promotion in children.[3–5] Current concepts of health promotion include the detection and prevention of disease as well as active promotion of the well-being of children and their families spanning physical, cognitive, emotional, and social health.

Every interaction with a child and family is an opportunity for health promotion. From the interview to the physical examination, think of your interactions as an opportunity for two important tasks: the detection of clinical problems and the promotion of health. Capitalize on the examination to offer age-appropriate guidance about the child's development. Provide suggestions about reading, conversing, playing music, and optimizing opportunities for gross and fine motor development. Advise parents about upcoming developmental stages and strategies to encourage their child's development. *Parents are the major agents of health promotion for children and your advice is implemented through them.*

The American Academy of Pediatrics (AAP) publishes guidelines for *health supervision visits* and the key age-appropriate components of these visits (see www.healthychildren.org). Remember that children and adolescents who have a chronic illness or high-risk family or environmental circumstances will probably require more frequent visits and more intensive health promotion. Key health promotion issues and strategies, tailored for specific age groups, are found throughout this chapter.

Integrate explanations of your physical findings with health promotion. Provide advice about expected maturational changes or how health behaviors can affect physical findings (e.g., exercise may reduce blood pressure and prevent obesity). Be sure to demonstrate the relationship between healthy lifestyles and physical health. For example, give parents a copy of their child's body mass index (BMI) result along with a "prescription" for healthy living.

Childhood immunizations are a mainstay for health promotion and have been heralded as the most significant clinical achievement in public health worldwide.

The childhood immunization schedule changes yearly. Updates are published widely and disseminated on websites of the Centers for Disease Control and Prevention (CDC) (see www.cdc.gov) and the AAP.[6,7]

Age-specific screening procedures are performed at specific ages. These include growth parameters and developmental screening at all ages, blood pressure screening after age 3 years, BMI screening after age 2 years, vision and hearing screening at key ages, and behavioral and mental health screening. Increasingly, standardized screening instruments are being used to assist clinicians in identifying abnormalities. In addition, screening procedures recommended for all children at certain ages or for specific high-risk patients (depending on the test) include tests for lead poisoning, anemia, tuberculosis exposure, dyslipidemia, urinary tract infections, and sexually transmitted infections. There is variation worldwide in recommendations for screening tests; the AAP recommendations are provided at www.aap.org.

Anticipatory guidance is a major component of the pediatric visit.[4] Key areas cover a broad range of topics, from clinical to developmental, social, and emotional health.

Key Components of Pediatric Health Promotion

1. Age-appropriate developmental achievement of the child
   - Physical (maturation, growth, puberty)
   - Motor (gross and fine motor skills)
   - Cognitive (developmental milestones, language, school performance)
   - Emotional (self-regulation, mood, temperament, self-efficacy, self-esteem, independence)
   - Social (social competence, self-responsibility, integration with family and community, peer interactions)
2. Health supervision visits
   - Periodic assessment of clinical and oral health
   - More frequent health supervision visits for children with special health care needs
3. Integration of physical examination findings with health promotion
4. Immunizations
5. Screening procedures
6. Anticipatory guidance[4,8]
   - Healthy habits
   - Nutrition and healthy eating
   - Safety and prevention of injury
   - Physical activity
   - Sexual development and sexuality
   - Self-responsibility, efficacy, and healthy self-esteem
   - Family relationships (interactions, strengths, supports)
   - Positive parenting strategies

(continued)

Key Components of Pediatric Health Promotion (*continued*)

- Emotional and mental health
- Oral health
- Recognition of illness
- Sleep
- Screen time
- Prevention of risky behaviors (e.g., tobacco, alcohol and drug use, unprotected sex)
- School and vocation
- Peer relationships
- Community interactions
7. Partnership among health care provider, child/adolescent, and family

ASSESSING THE NEWBORN

The first year of life, or infancy, is divided into the neonatal period (the first 28 days) and the postneonatal period (29 days to 1 year).

Tips for Examining Newborns

- Examine the newborn in the presence of the parents.
- Swaddle and then undress the newborn as the examination proceeds.
- Dim the lights and rock the newborn to encourage the eyes to open.
- Observe feeding, if possible, particularly breast-feeding.
- Demonstrate calming maneuvers to parents (e.g., swaddling).
- Observe and teach parents about transitions as the newborn arouses.
- A typical sequence for the examination of the newborn:
  - Careful observation before (and during) the examination
  - Heart
  - Lungs
  - Head, neck, and clavicles
  - Ears and mouth
  - Hips
  - Abdomen and genitourinary system
  - Lower extremities, back
  - Eyes, whenever they are spontaneously open or at end of examination
  - Skin, as you go along
  - Neurologic system

The first pediatric examination is performed immediately after delivery by obstetrical or pediatric clinicians. A comprehensive pediatric examination is then generally performed within 24 hours of birth (Fig. 18-5). Subsequent physical examinations occur at regular intervals or when the infant is ill. Assessment techniques for these examinations are described in detail in the following sections.

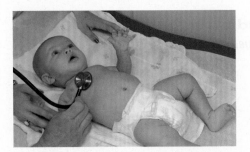

FIGURE 18-5. **Physical examination starts soon after birth.**

If possible, do the physical examination in front of the parents so that they can interact with you and ask questions. Parents may question their baby's physical appearance, so stating normal findings as you go can be reassuring. Observe parent interaction with their newborn and reinforce positive parenting behaviors. If a mother has concerns about breast-feeding technique, you can watch how well the breast-feeding baby latches on and sucks. Breast-feeding is physiologically and psychologically optimal, but many mothers will need help and support at first. Early detection of difficulties and anticipatory guidance can promote and sustain breast-feeding. This is an excellent opportunity to educate parents about their baby and what their baby can do.

Newborns are most responsive 1 to 2 hours after a feeding, when they are neither too satiated (and less responsive) nor too hungry (and more agitated). Start with the newborn swaddled and comfortable. Then, for gradual stimulation and arousal, undress the newborn as the examination proceeds. If the newborn becomes agitated, use a pacifier or a bottle of formula (if not breast-feeding) or allow the baby to suck on your gloved finger. Reswaddle the baby long enough to complete the parts of the examination that require a quiet baby.

Immediate Assessment at Birth

Examining newborns immediately after birth is important for determining general condition, developmental status, abnormalities in gestational development, and any congenital abnormalities. This examination may reveal diseases of cardiac, respiratory, or neurologic origin. Listen to the anterior thorax with your stethoscope, palpate the abdomen, and inspect the head, face, oral cavity, extremities, genitalia, and perineum. *Refer to the section "Assessing the Infant" for a complete physical examination.*

Apgar Score. The Apgar score is an assessment of the newborn immediately after birth. Its five components classify the newborn's neurologic recovery from the stress of birth and immediate adaptation to extrauterine life. Score each newborn at 1 and 5 minutes after birth according to the following table. Scoring is based on a 3-point scale (0, 1, or 2) for each component. Total scores range from 0 to 10. Scoring may continue at 5-minute intervals until the score is >7. If the 5-minute Apgar score is 8 or more, proceed to a more complete examination.[9]

The Apgar Scoring System

Clinical Sign	Assigned Score		
	0	1	2
Heart rate	Absent	<100	>100
Respiratory effort	Absent	Slow and irregular	Good; strong
Muscle tone	Flaccid	Some flexion of the arms and legs	Active movement
Reflex irritability[a]	No responses	Grimace	Vigorous cry, sneeze, or cough
Color	Blue, pale	Pink body, blue extremities	Pink all over

1-Min Apgar Score		5-Min Apgar Score	
8–10	Normal	8—10	Normal
5–7	Some nervous system depression	0—7	High risk for subsequent central nervous system and other organ system dysfunction
0–4	Severe depression, requiring immediate resuscitation		

[a]Reaction to suction of nares with bulb syringe.

Example of Apgar score calculation for a newborn with hypoxia:

> Heart rate = 110 [2]
>
> Respiratory effort = slow, irregular [1]
>
> Muscle tone = some flexion of arms/legs [1]
>
> Reflex irritability = grimace [1]
>
> Color = blue, pale [0]
>
> Apgar score = 5

Gestational Age and Birth Weight.   Classify newborns according to their gestational age of maturity and birth weight. These classifications help predict clinical problems and morbidity. Some clinical practice guidelines address the potential challenges of infants born before a certain gestational age or below a specific birth weight.

Gestational age is based on specific neuromuscular signs and physical characteristics that change with gestational maturity. The *Ballard Scoring System*[10] estimates gestational age to within 2 weeks, even in extremely premature infants. A complete Ballard Scoring System, with instructions for assessing neuromuscular and physical maturity, is included in Figure 18-6.

Classification by Gestational Age and Birth Weight

Gestational Age Classification	Gestational Age
• Preterm	• <34 wks
• Late preterm	• 34–36 wks
• Term	• 37–42 wks
• Postterm	• >42 wks

Birth Weight Classification	Weight
• Extremely low birth weight	• <1,000 g
• Very low birth weight	• <1,500 g
• Low birth weight	• <2,500 g
• Normal birth weight	• ≥2,500 g

Preterm infants are at risk for both short-term complications (mainly respiratory and cardiovascular) as well as long-term sequelae (e.g., neurodevelopmental).

Late preterm infants are at considerable risk for prematurity-related complications.

Postterm infants are at increased risk of perinatal mortality or morbidity such as asphyxia and meconium aspiration.

The New Ballard Score for Determining Gestational Age in Weeks

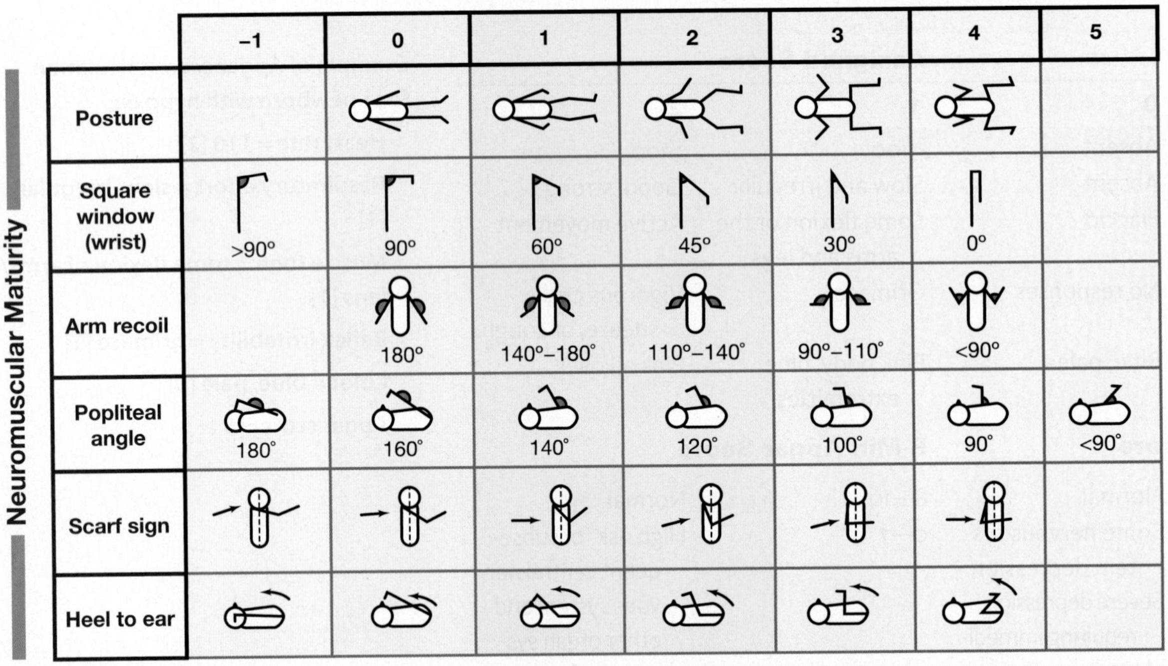

		−1	0	1	2	3	4	5
Neuromuscular Maturity	Posture							
	Square window (wrist)	>90°	90°	60°	45°	30°	0°	
	Arm recoil		180°	140°–180°	110°–140°	90°–110°	<90°	
	Popliteal angle	180°	160°	140°	120°	100°	90°	<90°
	Scarf sign							
	Heel to ear							
Physical Maturity	Skin	Sticky friable transparent	Gelatinous red, translucent	Smooth pink, visible veins	Superficial peeling and/or rash, few veins	Cracking pale areas rare veins	Parchment deep cracking no vessels	Leathery cracked wrinkled
	Lanugo	None	Sparse	Abundant	Thinning	Bald areas	Mostly bald	
	Plantar surface	heel — toe 40–50 mm: −1 <40 mm: −2	>50 mm no crease	Faint red marks	Anterior transverse crease only	Creases anterior 2/3	Creases over entire sole	
	Breast	Imperceptible	barely preceptible	flat areola no bud	Stippled areola 1–2-mm bud	Raised areola 3–4-mm bud	Full areola 5–10-mm bud	
	Eye/ear	Lids fused loosely: −1 Tightly: −2	Lids open, pinna flat stays folded	Slightly curved pinna; soft, slow recoil	Well-curved pinna; soft, but ready recoil	Formed and firm instant recoil	Thick cartilage, ear stiff	
	Genitals male	Scrotum flat, smooth	Scrotum empty, faint rugae	Testes in upper canal, rare rugae	Testes descending, few rugae	Testes down, good rugae	Testes pendulous, deep rugae	
	Genitals female	Clitoris prominent, labia flat	Prominent clitoris, small labia minora	Prominent clitoris, enlarging minora	Majora and minora equally prominent	Majora large, minora small	Majora cover clitoris and minora	

Maturity Rating

Score	Weeks
−10	20
−5	22
0	24
5	26
10	28
15	30
20	32
25	34
30	36
35	38
40	40
45	42
50	44

FIGURE 18-6. **The sum of the scores for all of the neuromuscular and physical maturity items provides an estimate of gestational age in weeks, using the maturity rating scale at the lower right potion of the figure.** (Redrawn from Ballard JL, Khoury JC, Wedig K, et al. New Ballard Score, expanded to include extremely premature infants. *J Pediatr.* 1991;119:417.)

A useful classification, shown below, is derived from the gestational age and birth weight on the intrauterine growth curve.

Newborn Classifications

Category	Abbreviation	Percentile
Small for gestational age	SGA	<10th
Appropriate for gestational age	AGA	10–90th
Large for gestational age	LGA	>90th

Figure 18-7 displays the intrauterine growth curves for the 10th and 90th percentiles and depicts the categories of maturity for newborns based on gestational age and birth weight.

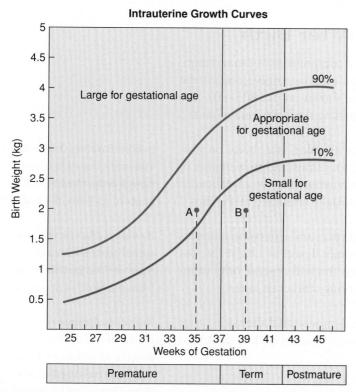

Intrauterine Growth Curves

LGA infants may experience difficulties during birth. Infants of mothers with diabetes are often LGA and may have metabolic abnormalities shortly after birth, as well as congenital anomalies.

A common complication among LGA newborns is *hypoglycemia*, which can result in jitteriness, irritability, cyanosis, or other health issues.

While no etiology is noted for many SGA infants, known causes include fetal, placental, and maternal factors. Maternal smoking is associated with SGA newborns.

FIGURE 18-7. Level of intrauterine growth based on gestational age and birth weight of liveborn, single, white infants. Point A represents a premature infant; point B indicates an infant of similar birth weight who is mature but SGA. (Adapted from Sweet YA. Classification of the low-birth-weight infant. In: Klaus MH, Fanaroff AA. Care of the High-Risk Neonate, 3rd ed. Philadelphia, PA: WB Saunders; 1986. Reproduced with permission.)

The three babies shown in Figure 18-8 were all born at 32 weeks gestational age and weighed 600 g (SGA), 1,400 g (AGA), and 2,750 g (LGA). Each of these categories has a different mortality rate, highest for preterm SGA and LGA infants, and lowest for term AGA infants.

Preterm AGA infants are more prone to respiratory distress syndrome, apnea, patent ductus arteriosus (PDA) with left-to-right shunt, and infection. *Preterm SGA infants* are more likely to experience asphyxia, hypoglycemia, and hypocalcemia.

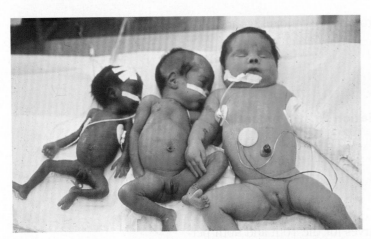

FIGURE 18-8. Infants who are small, average, and large for their gestational age.
(Reprinted with permission from Korones SB: High-Risk Newborn Infants: The Basis for Intensive Nursing Care, 4th ed. St. Louis: CV Mosby; 1986.)

Assessment Several Hours After Birth

During the first day of life, newborns should have a comprehensive examination. Wait until 1 or 2 hours after a feeding, when the baby is most responsive, and ask the parents to remain in the room. Follow the sequence shown on pp. 803–807. See *Techniques of Examination* (p. 813) for details on examining newborns and infants.

Observe the undressed newborn. Note the newborn's color, size, body proportions, nutritional status, and posture, as well as respirations and movements of the head and extremities. Most normal, full-term newborns lie in a symmetric position, with the limbs semiflexed and the legs partially abducted at the hip.

In *breech babies* (buttock first), the knees are flexed in utero; in a *frank breech baby*, the knees are extended in utero. In both, the hips are flexed.

Note the baby's spontaneous motor activity with flexion and extension alternating between the arms and legs. The fingers are usually flexed in a tight fist, but may extend in slow athetoid posturing movements. You will observe brief tremors of the body and extremities during vigorous crying, and even at rest.

By 4 days after birth, tremors at rest signal central nervous system disease from various possible causes, ranging from *asphyxia* to *drug withdrawal*.

Studies by Dr. T. Berry Brazelton and others have demonstrated the wide range of abilities in newborns which are described below.[11] Parents will be delighted by these abilities.

Asymmetric movements of the arms or legs at any time suggest *central* or *peripheral neurologic deficits, birth injury* (such as a fractured clavicle or brachial plexus injury), or *congenital anomalies*.

What a Newborn Can Do

Core Elements[11]

- Newborns use all five senses. For example, they will look at human faces and turn to a parent's voice.
- Newborns are unique individuals. Marked differences exist in temperaments, personality, behavior, and learning.
- Newborns interact dynamically with caregivers—a two-way street!

Newborns who do not demonstrate these behaviors may have a neurologic condition, drug withdrawal, or a serious illness such as infection.

(continued)

What a Newborn Can Do (continued)

Examples of Complex Newborn Behavior

Habituation	Ability to selectively and progressively shut out negative stimuli (e.g., a repetitive sound)
Attachment	A reciprocal, dynamic process of interacting and bonding with the caregiver
State regulation	Ability to modulate the level of arousal in response to different degrees of stimulation (e.g., self-consoling)
Perception	Ability to regard faces, turn to voices, quiet in presence of singing, track colorful objects, respond to touch, and recognize familiar scents

ASSESSING THE INFANT

Development

Physical Development.   Physical growth during infancy is faster than at any other age.[12] By 1 year, the infant's birth weight should have tripled and height increased by 50% from weight and height at birth.

Newborns have surprising abilities, such as fixing upon and following human faces. Neurologic development progresses centrally to peripherally. Thus, newborns learn head control before trunk control and use of arms and legs before use of hands and fingers (Fig. 18-9).

Activity, exploration, and environmental manipulation contribute to learning. By 3 months, normal infants lift the head and clasp the hands. By 6 months, they roll over, reach for objects, turn to voices, and possibly sit with support. With increasing peripheral coordination, infants reach for objects, transfer them from hand to hand, crawl, stand by holding on, and play with objects by banging and grabbing. At 1 year a child may be standing and putting objects in the mouth (Fig. 18-10).[13]

Cognitive and Language Development.   Exploration fosters increased understanding of self and environment. Infants learn cause and effect (e.g., shaking a rattle produces sound), object permanence, and use of tools. By 9 months, they may recognize the examiner as a stranger deserving wary cooperation, seek comfort from parents during examinations, and actively manipulate reachable objects (e.g., your stethoscope). Language development proceeds from cooing at 2 months, to babbling at 6 months, to saying one to three words by 1 year.[14]

Social and Emotional Development.   Understanding of self and family also matures. Social tasks include bonding, attachment to caregivers, and trust that caregivers will meet their needs (Fig. 18-11). Temperaments vary. Some infants are predictable, adaptable, and respond positively to new stimuli; others are less so and respond intensely or negatively. Because environment affects social development, observe the infant's interactions with caregivers.

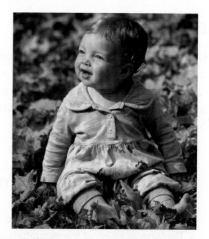

FIGURE 18-9.   **Sitting up is a developmental milestone among infants.**

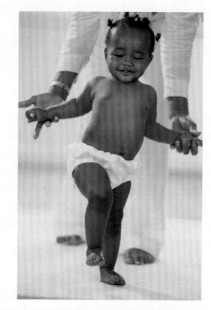

FIGURE 18-10.   **Children often take their first steps after one year.**

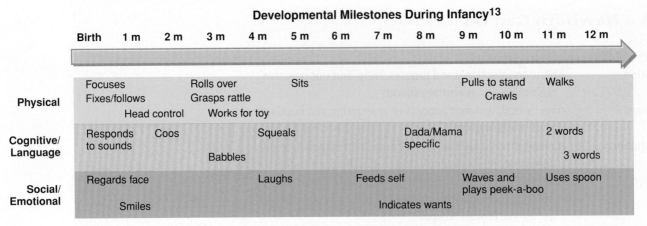

Developmental Milestones During Infancy[13]

	Birth	1 m	2 m	3 m	4 m	5 m	6 m	7 m	8 m	9 m	10 m	11 m	12 m
Physical	Focuses Fixes/follows			Rolls over Grasps rattle		Sits					Pulls to stand Crawls		Walks
		Head control			Works for toy								
Cognitive/ Language	Responds to sounds		Coos			Squeals			Dada/Mama specific			2 words	
				Babbles								3 words	
Social/ Emotional	Regards face					Laughs			Feeds self	Waves and plays peek-a-boo		Uses spoon	
		Smiles								Indicates wants			

FIGURE 18-11. Developmental milestones during infancy.

General Guidelines

Use developmentally appropriate methods such as *distraction* and *play* to examine the infant. Because infants pay attention to one thing at a time, it is relatively easy to distract the infant from the examination as it is performed. You can use a moving object, a flashing light, a game of peek-a-boo (for older infants), tickling, or any sort of noise.

If you cannot distract the infant or engage the awake infant with an object, your face, or a sound, consider a possible *visual* or *hearing deficit*.

Tips for Examining Infants

- Approach the infant gradually, using a toy or object for distraction.
- Perform as much of the examination as possible with the infant in the parent's lap.
- Speak softly to the infant or mimic the infant's sounds to attract attention.
- If the infant is cranky, make sure he or she is well fed before proceeding.
- Ask a parent about the infant's strengths to elicit useful developmental and parenting information.
- Don't expect to do a head-to-toe examination in a specific order. Work with what the infant gives you and save the mouth and ear examination for last.

Start with the infant sitting or lying in the parent's lap (Fig. 18-12). If the infant is tired, hungry, or ill, ask the parent to hold the baby against the parent's chest. Make sure appropriate toys, a blanket, or other familiar objects are nearby. A hungry infant may need to be fed before you initiate the examination.

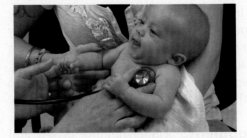

FIGURE 18-12. Start the exam while the child is still on the parent's lap.

Many neurologic conditions can be diagnosed during this general part of the examination. For example, you can detect *hypotonia*, conditions associated with *irritability* or signs of *cerebral palsy* (see neurologic examination below).

Close observation of an awake infant sitting on the parent's lap can reveal potential abnormalities such as *hypotonia* or *hypertonia*, conditions with abnormal skin color, jaundice or cyanosis, jitteriness, or respiratory problems.

Observe parent–infant interactions. Watch the parent's affect when talking about the infant. Note the parent's manner of holding, moving, dressing, and comforting the infant. Assess and comment on positive interactions, such as the obvious pride in the mother's face in Figure 18-13.

Infants do not object to having their clothing removed. To keep yourself and your surroundings dry, it is wise to leave the diaper in place throughout the examination; remove it only to examine the genitals, rectum, and hips.

Testing for Developmental Milestones. Because you want to measure the infant's best performance, check milestones at the end of the interview, just before the examination. This "fun and games" interlude also enhances cooperation during the examination. Experienced clinicians can weave the developmental examination into the other parts of the examination. The table on p. 810 shows some key

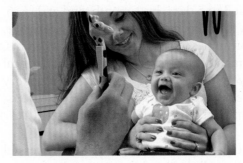

FIGURE 18-13. **Children can have fun during the developmental exam.**

physical or motor, cognitive or language, and social–emotional milestones during the first year. As an example, the infant in Figure 18-13 can squeal and laugh and interact with the examiner.

The AAP recommends that health care providers use a standardized developmental screening instrument for infants as young as several months of age.[15] Several developmental screening instruments have been tested widely and validated in many nations. In general, these instruments assess five *critical domains of infant/child development: gross motor, fine motor, cognitive (or problem-solving), communication, and personal/social domains of development.* Pediatric health care providers are recommended to use these standardized instruments periodically during preventive health visits because they perform better than a clinician's physical examination in identifying developmental delays, which can often be subtle and challenging to determine because of the wide spectrum of normal development in children. These screening instruments are practical to use in clinical settings and have reasonable sensitivity and specificity for identifying developmental delays. Some useful developmental screening instruments include the Ages and Stages Questionnaire (ASQ), the Early Language Milestone Scale (ELM Scale-2), the Modified Checklist for Autism in Toddlers (MCHAT), and the Parents' Evaluation of Developmental Status (PEDS). Combined with your findings on interview and physical examination, results from these screening tests can help determine an appropriate management strategy.

Use these screening instruments as adjuncts to a comprehensive developmental examination. Suspected delays warrant further examination. *For babies born prematurely, adjust expected developmental milestones for the gestational age up to 24 months.*

Observation of the infant's communication with the parent can reveal abnormalities such as *developmental delay, language delay, hearing deficits,* or *inadequate parental attachment.* Likewise, such observations may identify maladaptive nurturing patterns that may stem from *maternal depression* or *inadequate social support.*

Many disorders cause delays in more than one milestone. For most children with developmental delay, the causes are unknown. Some known causes include *abnormality in embryonic development* (e.g., prenatal insult); *hereditary and genetic disorders* (e.g., inborn errors, genetic abnormalities); *environmental and social problems* (e.g., insufficient stimulation); *pregnancy or perinatal problems* (e.g., placental insufficiency, prematurity); and *childhood diseases* (e.g., infection, trauma, chronic illness).

If a cooperative infant fails items on a standardized screening instrument, developmental delay is possible, necessitating more precise testing and evaluation.

An infant or toddler who has developmental skills that plateau or are out of sequence may have *autism* or *cerebral palsy.*

As an example, an infant who was born 8 weeks prematurely at 32-week gestation will have abnormal findings on developmental screening if expected milestones are not adjusted for prematurity. At a visit at 12 months of age, the infant should be expected to have attained milestones appropriate for a 10-month old.

Health Promotion and Counseling: Evidence and Recommendations

The AAP and the group Bright Futures[4] recommend health supervision visits for infants at the following ages: at birth, at 3 to 5 days, by 1 month, and at 2, 4, 6, 9, and 12 months (Fig. 18-14). This is called the *Infant Periodicity Schedule*. Health supervision visits provide opportunities to answer questions for parents, assess the infant's growth and development, perform a comprehensive physical examination, and provide anticipatory guidance. Age-appropriate anticipatory guidance includes healthy habits and behaviors, social competence of caregivers, parenting techniques, family relationships, and community interactions.

Regular visits provide an opportunity to plot a course for healthy and successful development. That infants generally are well during these visits enhances the quality of the experience. Parents are usually receptive to suggestions about health promotion which can have major, long-term influences on the child and family. Strong interviewing skills are necessary as you discuss strategies to optimize the health and well-being of their infants. Adjust the content to the appropriate developmental level of the infant. As an exercise, review the critical components of a health supervision visit for a 6-month-old.

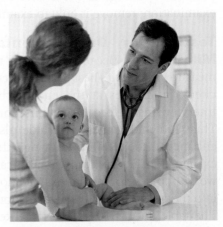

FIGURE 18-14. **Regular health supervision serves many purposes.**

Components of a Health Supervision Visit for a 6-Month-Old

Discussions with Parents

- Address parents' concerns/questions
- Provide advice
- Obtain social history
- Assess development, nutrition, sleep, elimination, safety, oral health, family relationships, stressors, parenting beliefs, community factors

Developmental Assessment

- Use a standardized developmental instrument to measure milestones
- Assess milestones by history
- Assess milestones by examination

Physical Examination

- Perform a careful examination, including growth parameters with percentiles for age

Screening Tests

- Vision and hearing (by examination), possibly hematocrit and lead (if high risk), screen for social risk factors

Immunizations

- See schedule (AAP or CDC website)

Anticipatory Guidance

Healthy Habits and Behaviors

- Injury and illness prevention
  Use infant seat, watch for rolling, caution on walkers, poisons, tobacco exposure
- Nutrition
  Breastfeeding or bottle, solids, no juice, prevent choking, overfeeding
- Oral health
  No bottle in bed, fluoride, brushing teeth

Parent–Infant Interaction

- Promoting development (play, reading, music, talking)

Family Relationships

- Time for self; babysitters

Community Interaction

- Child care, resources

Techniques of Examination

General Survey and Vital Signs

Measure the infant's body size and vital signs. Tables on the World Health Organization website (www.who.int) show norms for blood pressure, height, weight, BMI (starting age 2 years), and head circumference. Compare vital signs or body proportions with age-specific norms because *they change dramatically as children grow.* Pediatric practitioners also assess pain regularly, using standardized pain scales.

Variations beyond two standard deviations for age or above the 95th percentile or below the 5th percentile are indications for more detailed evaluation. These deviations may be the first and only indicators of disease (see examples on the website tables).

Somatic Growth. Measurement of growth is one of the most important indicators of infant health. Deviations may provide an early indication of an underlying problem. Compare growth parameters with respect to normal values for age and sex, as well as prior readings on the same child, to assess trends. Confirm abnormalities in somatic growth by repeat measurement to account for potential measurement error.

Measure growth parameters carefully using consistent technique and, optimally, the same scales to measure height and weight.

The most important tools for assessing somatic growth are the growth charts which are published by the National Center for Health Statistics (www.cdc.gov/nchsv)[16] and also the World Health Organization (www.who.int).[17] All charts include height, weight, and head circumference for children up to 36 months and height and weight for children 2 to 18 years. Charts plotting weight by length as well as BMI are also available. These growth charts have percentile lines indicating the percentage of normal children above and below the child's measurement by chronologic age. Special growth charts are available for use in infants born prematurely to correct for this result.

Although many healthy infants cross percentiles on growth charts, a sudden or significant change in growth may indicate systemic disease due to various possible organ systems or inappropriate excess weight gain usually due to overfeeding.

Abnormalities that can cause deviation from normal growth patterns include chronic disease or *prematurity*. Growth charts are also available for children with specific conditions such as *Down syndrome* or *Turner syndrome*.

The AAP, NIH, and CDC now recommend that clinicians use the 2006 WHO International growth charts for children 0 to 23 months of age. CDC growth charts should be used in the United States to assess growth in children 2 to 19 years of age.

Length. For children younger than age 2 years, measure body length by placing the child supine on a measuring board or in a measuring tray, as shown in Figure 18-15. Direct measurement of the infant using a tape measure is inaccurate unless an assistant holds the child still with hips and knees extended. Velocity growth curves are helpful for older children, especially those who are suspected of having endocrine disorders.

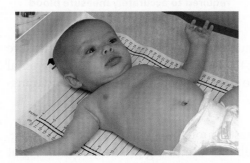

FIGURE 18-15. Accurate length measurement requires careful assistance.

Reduced growth velocity, shown by a drop in height percentile on a growth curve, may signify a chronic condition. Comparison with normal standards is essential because growth velocity is normally less during the second year than during the first year.

Chronic conditions causing reduced length or height include *neurologic, renal, cardiac, gastrointestinal,* and *endocrine disorders as well as cystic fibrosis.*

Weight. Weigh infants directly with an infant scale. Infants should be weighed naked or be clothed only in a diaper.

Head Circumference. The head circumference should always be measured during the first 2 years of life, but measurement can be useful at any age to assess growth of the head (Fig. 18-16). The head circumference in infants reflects the rate of growth of the cranium and the brain.

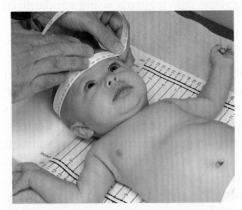

FIGURE 18-16. **Head circumference is a vital metric during early childhood.**

Vital Signs

Blood Pressure. Although obtaining accurate blood pressure readings in infants is challenging (Fig. 18-17), this measurement is nevertheless important for some high-risk infants and should be routinely performed after age 3 years. You will need your skills in distraction or play.

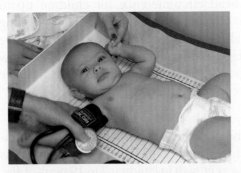

FIGURE 18-17. **Practice is required to accurately measure blood pressure in early childhood.**

An alternative to using the blood pressure cuff, and the most easily used measure of systolic blood pressure in infants, is the *Doppler method* which detects arterial blood flow vibrations, converts them to systolic blood pressure levels, and transmits them to a digital read-out device.

Systolic blood pressure gradually increases throughout childhood. For example, normal systolic pressure in males is about 70 mm Hg at birth, 85 mm Hg at 1 month, and 90 mm Hg at 6 months (see WHO or CDC website).

Failure to thrive is inadequate weight gain for age. Common indicators are: (a) growth <5th percentile for age; (b) drop >2 quartiles in 6 months; or (c) weight for length <5th percentile. Causes include environmental or psychosocial factors and a variety of gastrointestinal, neurologic, cardiac, endocrine, renal, and other diseases.

A small head size may result from premature closure of the sutures or microcephaly, which may be familial or due to *chromosomal abnormalities*, *congenital infections*, *maternal metabolic disorders*, and *neurologic insults*.

An abnormally large head size (>95th percentile or 2 standard deviations above the mean) is *macrocephaly*, which may result from *hydrocephalus*, *subdural hematoma*, or rare causes like *brain tumor* or *inherited syndromes*. *Familial megaloencephaly* (large head) is a benign familial condition.

Causes of sustained hypertension in newborns include *renal artery disease* (stenosis, thrombosis), *congenital renal malformations*, and *coarctation of the aorta*.

Pulse. The heart rate of infants is more sensitive to the effects of illness, exercise, and emotion than that of adults.

Heart Rates from Birth to 1 Year

Age	Average Heart Rate	Range
Birth–1 mo	140	90–190
1–6 mo	130	80–180
6–12 mo	115	75–155

While *sinus tachycardia* may be extremely rapid, a pulse rate that is too rapid to count (usually >180/min) may indicate *paroxysmal supraventricular tachycardia (PSVT)*.

Bradycardia may be from *drug ingestion, hypoxia, intracranial* or *neurologic conditions*, or, rarely, *cardiac dysrhythmia* such as *heart blockage*.

You may have trouble obtaining an accurate pulse rate in a squirming infant. Palpate the femoral arteries in the inguinal area or the brachial arteries in the antecubital fossa, or auscultate the heart.

Respiratory Rate. As with heart rate, the respiratory rate in infants has a greater range and is more responsive to illness, exercise, and emotion than that of adults or older children. The rate of respirations per minute ranges between 30 and 60 in the newborn.

Extremely rapid and shallow respiratory rates are seen in newborns with *cyanotic cardiac disease* and *right-to-left shunting,* and *metabolic acidosis*.

The respiratory rate may vary considerably from moment to moment in the newborn, with alternating periods of rapid and slow breathing (called "periodic breathing"). The sleeping respiratory rate is most reliable. Respiratory rates during active sleep compared with quiet sleep may be up to 10 breaths per minute faster. The respiratory pattern should be observed for at least 60 seconds to asses both the rate and the pattern. In infancy and early childhood, diaphragmatic breathing is predominant; thoracic excursion is minimal.

Fever can raise respiratory rates in infants by up to 10 respirations per minute for each degree centigrade of fever.

Commonly accepted cutoffs for defining *tachypnea* are >60/min from birth to 2 months, and >50/min from 2 to 12 months.

Tachypnea and increased respiratory effort in an infant are signs of lower respiratory disease such as *bronchiolitis* or *pneumonia*.

Temperature. Because fever is so common in infants and children, obtain an accurate body temperature when you suspect infection. Axillary and thermal-tape skin temperature recordings in infants and children are inaccurate. Auditory canal temperatures are accurate.

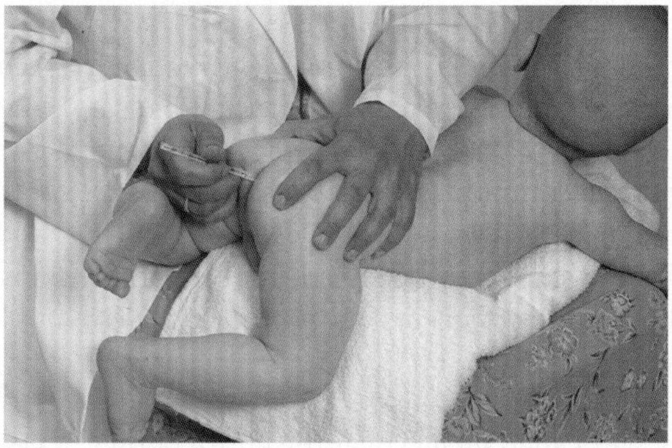

Fever (>38°C or >100.4°F) in infants younger than age 2 to 3 months may be a sign of *serious infection* or disease. These infants should be evaluated promptly and thoroughly.

Rectal temperatures are the most accurate for infants. The technique for obtaining a rectal temperature is relatively simple. One method is illustrated in Figure 18-18. Place the infant prone, separate the buttocks with the thumb and forefinger on one

FIGURE 18-18. **Rectal thermometers are the most accurate tool for infants.**

Potentially sick febrile infants under 3 months of age may have *serious bacterial infection* and should have temperatures assessed using a rectal thermometer.

hand and with the other hand gently insert a well-lubricated rectal thermometer to a depth of 2 to 3 cm. Keep the thermometer in place for at least 2 minutes.

Body temperature in infants and children is less constant than in adults. The average rectal temperature is higher in infancy and early childhood, usually above 99°F (37.2°C) until after age 3 years. Body temperature may fluctuate as much as 3°F during a single day, approaching 101°F (38.3°C) in normal children, particularly in late afternoon and after vigorous activity.

Anxiety may elevate the body temperature of children. *Excessive bundling* of infants may elevate skin temperature but not core temperature.

Temperature instability in a newborn may result from *sepsis, metabolic abnormality,* or other serious conditions. Older infants rarely manifest temperature instability.

The Skin

Inspection. Examine the skin of the newborn or infant carefully to identify both normal markings and potentially abnormal ones. The photos on pp. 818–820 demonstrate normal markings. The newborn's skin has a unique characteristic *texture and appearance.* The texture is soft and smooth because it is thinner than the skin of older children. Within the first 10 minutes after birth a normal newborn progresses from generalized cyanosis to pinkness. In lighter-skinned infants, an erythematous flush, giving the skin the appearance of a "boiled lobster," is common during the first 8 to 24 hours after which the normal pale pink coloring predominates.

Some newborns with *polycythemia* have a "ruddy" complexion. This is a reddish purple color.

Vasomotor changes in the dermis and subcutaneous tissue—a response to cooling or chronic exposure to radiant heat—can produce a lattice-like, bluish mottled appearance (*cutis marmorata*), particularly on the trunk, arms, and legs. This response to cold may last for months in normal infants. *Acrocyanosis,* a blue cast to the hands and feet when exposed to cold (see p. 818), is very common in newborns for the first few days and may recur throughout early infancy. Occasionally in newborns, a remarkable color change (*harlequin dyschromia*) appears with transient cyanosis of one half of the body or one extremity, presumably from temporary vascular instability.

Cutis marmorata is prominent in *premature infants* and in infants with *congenital hypothyroidism* and *Down syndrome.* If acrocyanosis does not disappear within 8 hours or with warming, *cyanotic congenital heart disease* should be considered.

The amount of melanin in the skin of newborns varies, affecting *pigmentation.* Black newborns may have a lighter skin color initially, except in the nail beds, genitalia, and ear folds which are dark at birth. A dark or bluish pigmentation over the buttocks and lower lumbar regions is common in newborns of African, Asian, and Mediterranean descent. These areas, called *slate blue patches,* result from pigmented cells in the deep layers of the skin; they become less noticeable with age and usually disappear during childhood. *Document these pigmented areas to avoid later concern about bruising.*

Central cyanosis in a baby or child of any age should raise suspicion of *congenital heart disease.* The best area to look for central cyanosis is the tongue and oral mucosa, not the nail beds, lips, or the extremities.

At birth, there is a fine, downy growth of hair called *lanugo* over the entire body, especially the shoulders and back. This hair is shed within the first few weeks. Lanugo is prominent in premature infants. Hair thickness on the head varies considerably among newborns and is not predictive of later hair growth. All of

Pigmented light-brown lesions (<1 to 2 cm at birth) are *café-au-lait spots.* Isolated lesions have no significance, but multiple lesions with sharp borders may suggest *neurofibromatosis* (see

the original hair is shed within months and is replaced with a new crop, sometimes of a different color.

Inspect the newborn closely for a series of common skin conditions. At birth, a cheesy white material called *vernix caseosa*, composed of sebum and desquamated epithelial cells, covers the body. Some newborns have *edema* over their hands, feet, lower legs, pubis, and sacrum; this disappears within a few days. Superficial desquamation of the skin is often noticeable 24 to 36 hours after birth, particularly in postterm babies (>40 weeks gestation), and it can last for 7 to 10 days.

You should be able to identify four common dermatologic conditions in newborns—*miliaria rubra, erythema toxicum, pustular melanosis,* and *milia*—which are shown on p. 819. None of these is clinically significant.

Note any signs of trauma from the birth process and the use of forceps or suction; these signs disappear but should prompt a careful neurologic examination.

Jaundice. Carefully examine and touch the newborn's skin to assess the level of jaundice. Normal "physiologic" jaundice, which occurs in half of all newborns, appears on the second or third day, peaks at about the fifth day, and usually disappears within a week (although it may persist longer in breast-fed infants). Jaundice is best seen in natural daylight rather than artificial light. Newborn jaundice appears to progress from head to toe, with more intense jaundice on the upper body and less intense yellow color in the lower extremities.

To detect jaundice, apply pressure to the skin (Fig. 18-19) to press out the normal pink or brown color. A yellowish "blanching" indicates jaundice.

Table 18-2, Common Skin Rashes and Skin Findings in Newborns and Infants, p. 911).

Skin desquamation is normal in full-term newborns but may rarely be a sign of *placental circulatory insufficiency* or *congenital ichthyosis*.

Both erythema toxicum and pustular melanosis may appear similar to the pathologic vesiculopustular rash of *herpes simplex* or *Staphylococcus aureus skin infection*.

Midline hair tufts over the lumbosacral spine region suggest a possible *spinal cord defect*.

Jaundice within the first 24 hours of birth may be from *hemolytic disease of the newborn*.

Late-appearing jaundice or jaundice that persists beyond 2 to 3 weeks should raise suspicions of *biliary obstruction* or *liver disease*.

A common source of jaundice during the first couple of weeks is breast-feeding jaundice, which resolves around 10 to 14 days of life. Persistent jaundice requires evaluation.

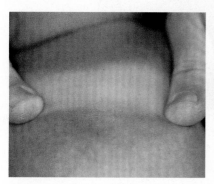 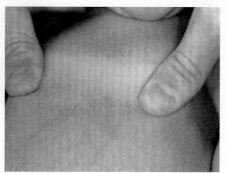

FIGURE 18-19. **Pressing the red color from the skin allows better recognition of the yellow of normal skin (left) or jaundice (right).** (From Fletcher M. *Physical Diagnosis in Neonatology.* Philadelphia, PA: Lippincott-Raven; 1998.)

Vascular Markings. A common *vascular marking* is the "salmon patch" (also known as *nevus simplex,* "flame nevi," telangiectatic nevus, or capillary hemangioma). These flat, irregular, light pink patches (see p. 819) are most often seen on the nape of the neck ("stork bite"), upper eyelids, forehead, or upper lip ("angel kisses"). They are not true nevi, but result from distended capillaries. They often disappear by 1 year of age and are covered by the hairline.

A unilateral dark, purplish lesion, or "port wine stain" over the distribution of the ophthalmic branch of the trigeminal nerve may be a sign of *Sturge–Weber syndrome,* which is associated with seizures, hemiparesis, glaucoma, and mental retardation.

Palpation. Palpate the newborn or infant's skin to assess the degree of hydration, or turgor. Roll a fold of loosely adherent skin on the abdominal wall between your thumb and forefinger to determine its consistency. The skin in well-hydrated infants returns to its normal position immediately upon release. Delay in return is a phenomenon called "tenting" and usually occurs in children with significant dehydration.

Significant edema of the hands and feet of a newborn girl may be suggestive of *Turner syndrome.* Other features such as a webbed neck would reinforce this diagnosis.

Dehydration is a common problem in infants. Usual causes are insufficient intake or excess loss of fluids from diarrhea.

Newborn Skin Findings

Finding/Description	Finding/Description
Common Nonpathologic Conditions Acrocyanosis This bluish discoloration usually appears in the palms and soles. *Cyanotic congenital heart disease can present with severe acrocyanosis.*	Jaundice Physiologic jaundice occurs during days 2 to 5 of life and progresses from head to toe as it peaks. *Extreme jaundice may signify a hemolytic process or biliary or liver disease.*

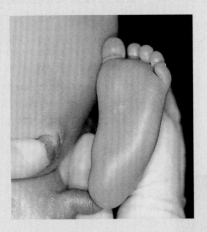

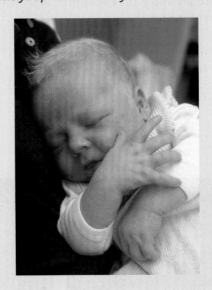

(continued)

Newborn Skin Findings (*continued*)

Finding/Description

Common Benign Rashes

Miliaria Rubra

Scattered vesicles on an erythematous base, usually on the face and trunk, result from obstruction of the sweat gland ducts; this condition disappears spontaneously within weeks.

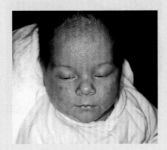

Pustular Melanosis

Seen more commonly in black infants, the rash presents at birth as small vesiculopustules over a brown macular base; these can last for several months.

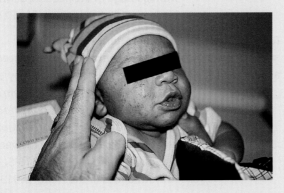

Benign Birthmarks

Eyelid Patch

This birthmark fades, usually within the first year of life.

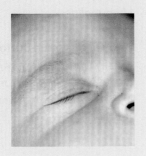

Finding/Description

Erythema Toxicum

Usually appearing on days 2 to 3 of life, this rash consists of erythematous macules with central pinpoint vesicles scattered diffusely over the entire body. They appear similar to flea bites. These lesions are of unknown etiology but disappear within 1 week of birth.

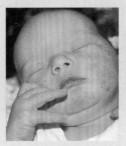

Milia

Pinhead-sized smooth white raised areas without surrounding erythema on the nose (seen here), chin, and forehead result from retention of sebum in the openings of the sebaceous glands. Although occasionally present at birth, milia usually appear within the first few weeks and disappears over several weeks.

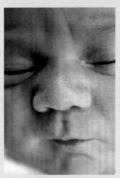

Salmon Patch

Also called the "stork bite," or "angel kiss," this splotchy pink mark fades with age.

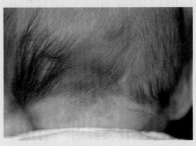

(*continued*)

Newborn Skin Findings (continued)

Finding/Description

Café-au-lait Spots

These light-brown pigmented lesions usually have borders and are uniform. They are noted in more than 10% of black infants. *If more than five café-au-lait spots exist, consider the diagnosis of neurofibromatosis (see Table 18-2, Common Skin Rashes and Skin Findings in Newborns and Infants, p. 911).*

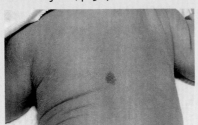

Finding/Description

Slate Blue Patches

These are more common among dark-skinned babies. It is important to note them so that they are not mistaken for bruises.

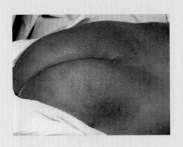

The Head

At birth, a baby's head may seem large relative to the body. A newborn's head accounts for one fourth of the body length and one third of the body weight; these proportions change, so that by adulthood the head accounts for one eighth of the body length and about one tenth of the body weight.

Sutures and Fontanelles.   Membranous tissue spaces called *sutures* separate the bones of the skull from one another. The areas where the major sutures intersect in the anterior and posterior portions of the skull are known as *fontanelles*. Examine the *sutures* and *fontanelles* carefully (Fig. 18-20).

On palpation, the sutures feel like ridges and the fontanelles like soft concavities. The *anterior fontanelle* at birth measures 4 to 6 cm in diameter and usually closes between 2 and 26 months of age (90% between 7 and 19 months). The *posterior fontanelle* measures 1 to 2 cm at birth and usually closes by 2 months.

An enlarged posterior fontanelle may be present in *congenital hypothyroidism.*

Overlap of the cranial bones at the sutures at birth, called *molding,* results from passage of the head through the birth canal; it disappears within 2 days.

A bulging, tense fontanelle is observed in infants with *increased intracranial pressure,* which may be caused by *central nervous system infections, neoplastic disease,* or *hydrocephalus* (obstruction of the circulation of cerebrospinal fluid within the ventricles of the brain) (see Table 18-5, Abnormalities of the Head, p. 913).

Early closure of the fontanelles can be due to developing *microcephaly* or to *craniosynostosis* or some *metabolic abnormalities.*

Delayed closure of the fontanelles is usually a normal variant, but can be due to *hypothyroidism, megalocephaly, increased intracranial pressure,* or *rickets.*

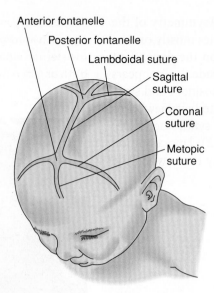

FIGURE 18-20. **Sutures and fontanelles.**

Carefully examine the fontanelle, because its fullness reflects *intracranial pressure*. Palpate the fontanelle while the baby is sitting quietly or being held upright. Clinicians often palpate the fontanelles at the beginning of the examination. In normal infants, the anterior fontanelle is soft and flat. A full anterior fontanelle with increased intracranial pressure is seen when a baby cries or vomits. Pulsations of the fontanelle reflect the peripheral pulse and are normal (and parents often inquire about them). Learn to palpate the fontanelle because a bulging fontanelle is concerning for increased intracranial pressure and a depressed fontanelle may suggest dehydration.

A depressed anterior fontanelle may be a sign of *dehydration.*

Inspect the scalp veins carefully to assess for dilatation.

Dilated scalp veins are indicative of long-standing *increased intracranial pressure.*

Skull Symmetry and Head Circumference.

Carefully assess *skull symmetry* (Fig. 18-21). Various conditions can cause asymmetry; some are benign, while others reflect underlying pathology.

Look for asymmetric head swelling. A newborn's scalp may be swollen over the occipitoparietal region. This is called *caput succedaneum* and results from capillary distention and extravasation of blood and fluid resulting from the vacuum effect of rupture of the amniotic sac. This swelling *typically crosses suture lines* and resolves in 1 to 2 days.

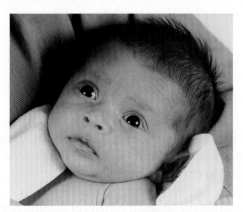

FIGURE 18-21. **Skull shape and symmetry should be assessed.**

A common type of localized swelling of the scalp is a *cephalohematoma,* caused by subperiosteal hemorrhage from the trauma of birth. This swelling does not cross over suture lines and resolves within 3 weeks. As the hemorrhage resolves and calcifies, there may be a palpable bony rim with a soft center (see Table 18-5, Abnormalities of the Head, p. 913).

The premature infant's head at birth is relatively long in the occipitofrontal diameter and narrow in the bitemporal diameter (*dolichocephaly*). Usually, the skull shape normalizes within 1 to 2 years.

Pick up the infant and examine the skull shape from behind. Asymmetry of the cranial vault (*positional plagiocephaly*) occurs when an infant lies mostly on one side, resulting in a flattening of the parieto-occipital region on the dependent side and a prominence of the frontal region on the ipsilateral side. It disappears as the baby becomes more active and spends less time in one position, and symmetry is almost always restored. Interestingly, the current trend to have newborns sleep on their backs to reduce the risk for sudden infant death syndrome (SIDS) has resulted in more cases of positional plagiocephaly (Fig. 18-22). This condition can be prevented by frequent repositioning (providing "tummy time" when the infant is awake).

Plagiocephaly may also reflect pathology such as *torticollis* from injury to the sternocleidomastoid muscle at birth or *lack of stimulation* of the infant.

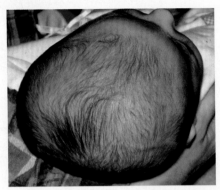

FIGURE 18-22. Careful assessment may reveal plagiocephaly.

Measure the head circumference (p. 814) to detect abnormally large head size (*macrocephaly*) or small head size (*microcephaly*), both of which may signify an underlying disorder affecting the brain.

Premature closure of cranial sutures causes *craniosynostosis* (p. 913) and an abnormally shaped skull. *Sagittal suture* synostosis causes a narrow head from lack of growth of the parietal bones.

Palpate along the suture lines. A raised, bony ridge at a suture line suggests craniosynostosis.

Palpate the infant's skull with care. The cranial bones generally appear "soft" or pliable; they will normally become firmer with increasing gestational age.

In *craniotabes,* the cranial bones feel springy. Craniotabes can result from increased intracranial pressure, as with *hydrocephaly,* metabolic disturbances such as *rickets,* and infection such as *congenital syphilis.*

Facial Symmetry. Check the *face* of infants for symmetry. In utero positioning may result in transient facial asymmetries. If the head is flexed on the sternum, a shortened chin (*micrognathia*) may result. Pressure of the shoulder on the jaw may create a temporary lateral displacement of the mandible.

Micrognathia may also be part of a syndrome, such as the *Pierre Robin syndrome.*

Examine the face for an overall impression of the *facies*; it is helpful to compare with the face of the parents. A systematic assessment of a child with abnormal-appearing facies can identify specific syndromes.[18] The box on the next page describes steps for evaluating facies.

Evaluating a Newborn or Child with Possible Abnormal Facies

Carefully review the history, especially:
- Family history
- Pregnancy
- Perinatal history

Note abnormalities on other parts of the physical examination, especially:
- Growth
- Development
- Other dysmorphic somatic features

Perform measurements (and plot percentiles), especially:
- Head circumference
- Height
- Weight

Consider the three mechanisms of facial dysmorphogenesis:
- Deformations from intrauterine constraint
- Disruptions from amniotic bands or fetal tissue
- Malformations from intrinsic abnormality in face/head or brain

Examine the parents and siblings:
- Similarity to a parent may be reassuring (e.g., large head) but may also be an indication of a familial disorder

Try to determine whether the facial features fit a recognizable syndrome, comparing with:
- References (including measurements) and pictures of syndromes
- Tables/databases of combinations of features

Most developmental and genetic syndromes with abnormal facies also have other abnormalities.

An infant with *congenital hyperthyroidism* may have coarse facial features and other abnormal facial features (Table 18-6, Diagnostic Facies in Infancy and Childhood, pp. 914–915).

A child with abnormal shape or length of palpebral fissures (see Table 18-6, Diagnostic Facies in Infancy and Childhood, pp. 914–915):
   Upslanting (*Down syndrome*)
   Downslanting (*Noonan syndrome*)
   Short (*fetal alcohol effects*)

Chvostek Sign. Percuss the cheek to check for *Chvostek sign,* which is present in some metabolic disturbances and occasionally in normal infants. Percuss at the top of the cheek just below the zygomatic bone in front of the ear, using the tip of your index or middle finger.

A positive Chvostek sign produces facial grimacing caused by repeated contractions of the facial muscles. A Chvostek's sign is noted in cases of *hypocalcemic tetany, tetanus, and tetany due to hyperventilation.*

The Eyes

Inspection. Newborns keep their eyes closed except during brief awake periods. If you attempt to separate their eyelids, they will tighten them even more. Bright light causes infants to blink, so use subdued lighting. Awaken the baby gently and support the baby in a sitting position; often the eyes open.

A newborn who truly cannot open an eye (even when awake and alert) may have *congenital ptosis.* Causes include birth trauma and third cranial nerve palsy.

To examine the eyes of infants and young children, use some tricks to encourage cooperation. Small colorful toys are useful as fixation devices in examining the eyes.

Subconjunctival hemorrhages are common in neonates born via vaginal delivery.

Newborns may look at your face and follow a bright light if you catch them during an alert period. Some newborns can follow your face and turn their heads 90° to each side. Examine infants for *eye movements*. Hold the baby upright, supporting the head. Rotate yourself with the baby slowly in one direction. This usually causes the baby's eyes to open, allowing you to examine the sclerae, pupils, irises, and extraocular movements (Fig. 18-23). The baby's eyes gaze in the direction you are turning. When the rotation stops, the eyes look in the opposite direction, after a few nystagmoid movements.

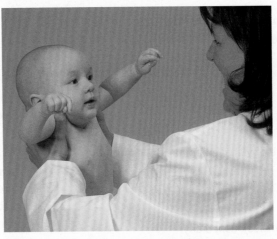

FIGURE 18-23. **Carefully assess gaze and eye movements.**

Nystagmus (wandering or shaking eye movements) persisting after a few days or persisting after the maneuver described on the left may indicate *poor vision* or *central nervous system disease.*

If a newborn fails to gaze at you and follow your face during alert periods, pay particular attention to the rest of the ocular examination. The newborn may have *visual impairment* from congenital cataracts or other disorders.

During the first 10 days of life, the eyes may stare in one direction if just the head is turned without moving the body (*doll's eye reflex*).

During the first few months of life, some infants have intermittent crossed eyes (*intermittent alternating convergent strabismus,* or *esotropia*) or laterally deviated eyes (*intermittent alternating divergent strabismus,* or *exotropia*).

Alternating convergent or divergent *strabismus* persisting beyond 3 months, or persistent strabismus of any type, may indicate *ocular motor weakness* or another abnormality in the visual system.

Look for abnormalities or congenital problems in the *sclera* and *pupils*. Subconjunctival hemorrhages are common in newborns and resolve within a couple of weeks. The eyes of many newborns are edematous from the birth process.

Colobomas may be seen with the naked eye and represent defects in the iris.

Observe pupillary reactions by response to light or by covering each eye with your hand and then uncovering it. Although there may be initial asymmetry in the size of the pupils, over time they should be equal in size and reaction to light.

Inspect the irises carefully for abnormalities.

Brushfield spots (seen with an ophthalmoscope) are a ring of white specks in the iris (see Table 18-7, Abnormalities of the Eyes, Ears, and Mouth, p. 916). Although sometimes present in normal children, these strongly suggest *Down syndrome.*

Examine the *conjunctiva* for swelling or redness. Most newborn nurseries use an antibiotic eye ointment to help prevent gonococcal eye infection.

You will not be able to measure the *visual acuity* of newborns or infants. You can use visual reflexes to indirectly assess vision: direct and consensual pupillary constriction in response to light, blinking in response to bright light (*optic blink reflex*), and blinking in response to quick movement of an object toward the eyes. During the first year of life, visual acuity sharpens as the ability to focus improves. Infants achieve the following visual milestones:

Persistent ocular discharge and tearing beginning at birth may be from *dacryocystitis* or *nasolacrimal duct obstruction*.

Visual Milestones of Infancy

Birth[19]	Blinks, may regard face
1 month	Fixes on objects
1½–2 months	Coordinated eye movements
3 months	Eyes converge, baby reaches toward a visual stimulus
12 months	Acuity around 20/60–20/80

Failure to progress along these visual developmental milestones may indicate *delayed visual maturation*.

Ophthalmoscopic Examination. For the *ophthalmoscopic examination*, with the newborn awake and eyes open, examine the red retinal (fundus) reflex by setting the ophthalmoscope at 0 diopters and viewing the pupil from about 10 inches. Normally, a red or orange color is reflected from the fundus through the pupil.

Congenital glaucoma may cause cloudiness of the cornea. A dark light reflex can result from *cataracts, retinopathy of prematurity,* or other disorders. A white retinal reflex (*leukokoria*) is abnormal, and *cataract, retinal detachment, chorioretinitis,* or *retinoblastoma* should be suspected.

A thorough ophthalmoscopic examination is difficult in young infants but may be needed if ocular or neurologic abnormalities are noted. The cornea can ordinarily be seen at +20 diopters, the lens at +15 diopters, and the fundus at 0 diopters.

Occlusion of the lens may represent a *cataract*.

Examine the optic disc area as you would for an adult. In infants, the optic disc is difficult to visualize but is lighter in color, with less macular pigmentation. The foveal light reflection may not be visible. Papilledema is rare in infants because the fontanelles and open sutures accommodate any increased intracranial pressure, sparing the optic discs.

Small retinal hemorrhages may occur in normal newborns. Extensive hemorrhages may suggest severe *anoxia, subdural hematoma, subarachnoid hemorrhage,* or *trauma*.

The Ears

The physical examination of the ears of infants is important because many abnormalities can be detected, including structural problems, otitis media, and hearing loss.

The goals are to determine the *position, shape,* and *features of the ear* and to detect abnormalities. Note ear position in relation to the eyes. An imaginary line drawn across the inner and outer canthi of the eyes should cross the pinna or auricle; if the pinna is below this line the infant has low-set ears. Draw this imaginary line across the face of the baby on p. 821; note that it crosses the pinna.

Small, deformed, or low-set auricles may indicate associated *congenital defects,* especially renal disease.

Otoscopic examination of the newborn's ear can detect only patency of the *ear canal* because accumulated vernix caseosa obscures the tympanic membrane for the first few days of life.

A small skin tab, cleft, or pit found just forward of the tragus represents a remnant of the *first branchial cleft* and usually has no significance. However, occasionally it may also be associated with renal disease and acquired hearing loss if there is a family history of hearing loss.

The infant's ear canal is directed downward from the outside; therefore, pull the auricle gently downward, not upward, for the best view of the eardrum. Once the tympanic membrane is visible, note that the light reflex is diffuse; it does not become cone-shaped for several months.

Otitis media (see pp. 869–870) can occur in infants.

The *acoustic blink reflex* is a blinking of the infant's eyes in response to a sudden sharp sound. You can produce it by snapping your fingers or using a bell, beeper, or other noisemaking device approximately 1 foot from the infant's ear. Be sure you are not producing an airstream that may cause the infant to blink. This reflex may be difficult to elicit during the first 2 to 3 days of life. After it is elicited several times within a brief period, the reflex disappears, a phenomenon known as *habituation*. This crude test of hearing certainly is not diagnostic. Most newborns in the United States undergo hearing screenings, which are mandatory in the majority of states.

Perinatal problems raising the risk for *hearing defects* include birth weight <1,500 g, anoxia, treatment with potentially ototoxic medications, congenital infections, severe hyperbilirubinemia, and meningitis.

Signs That an Infant Can Hear

Age	Sign
0–2 mo	Startle response and blink to a sudden noise
	Calming down with soothing voice or music
2–3 mo	Change in body movements in response to sound
	Change in facial expression to familiar sounds
	Turning eyes and head to sound
3–4 mo	Turning to listen to voices and conversation
6–7 mo	Appropriate language development

In the absence of universal hearing screening, many children with *hearing deficits* are not diagnosed until 2 years. Clues to hearing deficits include parental concern about hearing, delayed speech, and lack of developmental indicators of hearing.

The Nose and Sinuses

The most important component of the examination of the infant nose is to *test for patency of the nasal passages*. You can do this by gently occluding each nostril alternately while holding the infant's mouth closed. This usually will not cause stress because most infants are nasal breathers. Some infants are *obligate nasal breathers* and have difficulty breathing through their mouths. Do not occlude both nares simultaneously, as this will cause considerable distress.

Inspect the nose to ensure that the nasal septum is midline.

At birth, the maxillary and the ethmoid sinuses are present. Palpation of the sinuses of newborns is not helpful.

The nasal passages in newborns may be obstructed in *choanal atresia*. In severe cases, nasal obstruction can be assessed by attempting to pass a no. 8 feeding tube through each nostril into the posterior pharynx. This is usually done in the delivery room to assess for choanal atresia.

The Mouth and Pharynx

Use both inspection with a tongue depressor and flashlight and palpation to inspect the mouth and pharynx (Fig. 18-24). One method employs the parent to hold the infant's head and arms. The newborn's mouth is edentulous and the alveolar mucosa is smooth with finely serrated borders. Occasionally, pearl-like retention cysts are seen along the alveolar ridges and are easily mistaken for teeth; these disappear within 1 or 2 months. Petechiae are commonly found on the soft palate after birth.

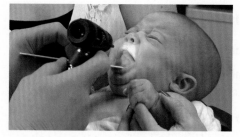

FIGURE 18-24. **Parental assistance helps with oral assessment.**

Palpate the upper hard palate to make sure it is intact. *Epstein pearls*, tiny white or yellow, rounded mucous retention cysts, are located along the posterior midline of the hard palate. They disappear within months.

Cysts may be noted on the tongue or mouth. Thyroglossal duct cysts may open under the tongue.

Infants produce little saliva during the first 3 months. Older infants produce a lot of saliva and drool frequently.

Inspect the tongue. The frenulum varies in tightness; sometimes it extends almost to the tip and other times it is short, limiting protrusion of the tongue (*ankyloglossia* or *tongue tie*).

You will often see a whitish covering on the tongue. If this coating is from milk, it can be easily removed by scraping or wiping it away. Use a tongue depressor or your gloved finger to wipe away the coating.

While there is a predictable *pattern of tooth eruption,* there is wide variation in the age at which teeth appear. A rule of thumb is that a child will have 1 tooth for each month of age between 6 and 26 months, up to a maximum of 20 primary teeth.

The pharynx of the infant is best seen while the baby is crying. You will likely have difficulty using a tongue depressor because it produces a strong gag reflex. Infants do not have prominent lymphoid tissue so you will probably not visualize the tonsils which increase in size as children grow.

Listen to the quality of the *infant's cry*. Normal infants have a lusty, strong cry. The following box lists some unusual types of infant cries.

Rarely, *supernumerary teeth* are noted. These are usually dysmorphic and are shed within days but are removed to prevent aspiration.

Although unusual, a prominent, protruding tongue may signal *congenital hypothyroidism* or *Down syndrome.*

Oral candidiasis (thrush) is common in infants. The white plaques are difficult to wipe away and have an erythematous raw base (see Table 18-7, Abnormalities of the Eyes, Ears, and Mouth, p. 916). They are found on the buccal mucosa, palate, and tongue.

Natal teeth are teeth that are present at birth. They are usually simply early eruptions of normal teeth, but they can be part of syndromes.

Macroglossia is associated with several systemic conditions. If associated with hypoglycemia and omphalocele, the diagnosis is likely *Beckwith–Wiedemann syndrome.*

Abnormal Infant Cries (If Persistent)

Type	Possible Abnormality
Shrill or high-pitched	Increased intracranial pressure. Also in newborns born to narcotic-addicted mothers.
Hoarse	Hypocalcemic tetany or congenital hypothyroidism
Continuous inspiratory and expiratory stridor	Upper airway obstruction from various lesions (e.g., a polyp or hemangioma), a relatively small larynx (*infantile laryngeal stridor*), or a delay in the development of the cartilage in the tracheal rings (*tracheomalacia*)
Absence of cry	Severe illness, vocal cord paralysis, or profound brain damage

A congenital fissure of the median line of the palate is a *cleft palate.*

Inspiratory stridor beginning at birth suggests a congenital abnormality as described in this table. Stridor that appears following birth can be due to infections such as *croup, a foreign body, or gastroesophageal reflux.*

The Neck

Palpate the *lymph nodes of the neck* and assess for any additional masses such as *congenital cysts* (Fig. 18-25). Because the necks of infants are short, it is best to palpate the neck while infants are lying supine, whereas older children are best examined while sitting. Check the position of the thyroid cartilage and trachea.

Branchial cleft cysts appear as small dimples or openings anterior to the midportion of the sternocleidomastoid muscle. They may be associated with a sinus tract.

Preauricular cysts and sinuses are common, pinhole-size pits, usually located anterior to the helix of the ear. They are often bilateral and may be associated with *hearing deficits* and renal disorders.

Thyroglossal duct cysts are located at the midline of the neck, just above the thyroid cartilage. These small, firm, mobile masses move upward with tongue protrusion or with swallowing. They are usually detected after 2 years.

Congenital torticollis, or a "wry neck," is from bleeding into the sternocleidomastoid muscle during the stretching process during delivery. A firm fibrous mass is felt within the muscle 2 to 3 weeks after birth and generally disappears over months.

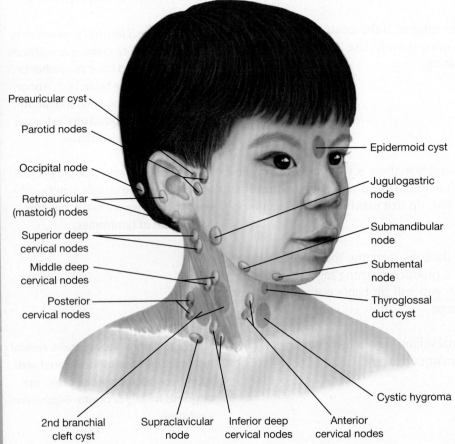

Preauricular cyst
Parotid nodes
Occipital node
Retroauricular (mastoid) nodes
Superior deep cervical nodes
Middle deep cervical nodes
Posterior cervical nodes
2nd branchial cleft cyst
Supraclavicular node
Inferior deep cervical nodes
Anterior cervical nodes
Cystic hygroma
Thyroglossal duct cyst
Submental node
Submandibular node
Jugulogastric node
Epidermoid cyst

FIGURE 18-25. **Nodes and cysts of the head and neck.**

In newborns, palpate the *clavicles* and look for evidence of a fracture. If present, you may feel a break in the contour of the bone, tenderness, crepitus at the fracture site, and may notice limited movement of the arm on the affected side.

A *fracture of the clavicle* may occur during birth, particularly during delivery of a difficult arm or shoulder extraction.

The Thorax and Lungs

The infant's *thorax* is more rounded than that of adults. The thin chest wall has little musculature; thus, lung and heart sounds are transmitted quite clearly. The bony and cartilaginous rib cage is soft and pliant. The tip of the xiphoid process often protrudes anteriorly, immediately beneath the skin.

Two types of chest wall abnormalities noted in childhood include *pectus excavatum*, or "funnel chest," and *pectus carinatum*, or "chicken breast deformity."

Inspection. Carefully *assess respirations* and *breathing patterns*. Newborns, especially those born prematurely, show periods of normal rate (30 to 40 per minute) alternating respirations that may even cease for 5 to 10 seconds. This alternating pattern of rapid and slow breathing is called "periodic respiration" or "periodic breathing."

Apnea is cessation of breathing for more than 20 seconds. It is often accompanied by bradycardia and may indicate *respiratory disease, central nervous system disease,* or, rarely, a *cardiopulmonary condition.* Apnea may be a high-risk factor for *SIDS.*

Do not rush to the stethoscope. Instead, observe the infant carefully as demonstrated in Figure 18-26, which demonstrates locations for retractions among infants. Inspection is easiest when infants are not crying; thus, work with the parents to settle the child. Observe for 30 to 60 seconds, note general appearance, respiratory rate, color, nasal component of breathing, audible breath sounds, and work of breathing, as described below.

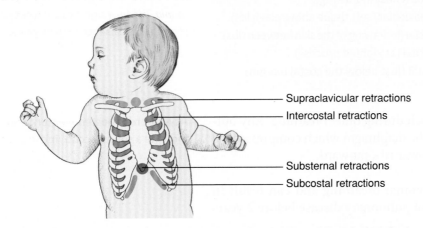

Supraclavicular retractions
Intercostal retractions

Substernal retractions
Subcostal retractions

FIGURE 18-26. **Anatomic locations of retractions (chest indrawing).**

Because infants are obligate nasal breathers, observe their nose as they breathe. Look for *nasal flaring.* Observe breathing with the infant's mouth closed or during nursing or sucking on a bottle to assess for nasal patency. Listen to the sounds of breathing; note any *grunting, audible wheezing,* or *lack of breath sounds (obstruction).* *Nasal flaring, grunting, retractions, and wheezing are all signs of respiratory distress.*

In newborns and young infants, nasal flaring may be the result of *upper respiratory infections,* with subsequent obstruction of their small nares, but it may also be caused by *pneumonia* or other serious respiratory infections.

Observe two aspects of the infant's breathing: *audible breath sounds* and *work of breathing.* These are particularly relevant in assessing both upper and lower respiratory illness. Studies in countries with poor access to chest radiographs have

Lower respiratory infections, defined as infections below the vocal cords, are common in infants and include *bronchiolitis* and *pneumonia.*

found these signs at least as useful as auscultation. Any of the abnormalities listed below should raise concern about underlying respiratory pathology.

Observing Respiration— Before You Touch the Child

Type of Assessment	Specific Observable Pathology
General appearance	Inability to feed or smile Lack of consolability
Respiratory rate	Tachypnea (see p. 815), apnea
Color	Pallor or cyanosis
Nasal component of breathing	Nasal flaring (enlargement of both nasal openings during inspiration)
Audible breath sounds	Grunting (repetitive, short expiratory sound) Wheezing (musical expiratory sound) Stridor (high-pitched, inspiratory noise) Obstruction (lack of breath sounds)

Work of breathing	Nasal flaring (excessive movement of nares)
	Grunting (expiratory noises)
	Retractions (chest indrawing):
	    Supraclavicular (soft tissue above clavicles)
	    Intercostal (indrawing of the skin between ribs)
	    Substernal (at xiphoid process)
	    Subcostal (just below the costal margin)

Acute stridor is a potentially serious condition; causes include *laryngotracheobronchitis (croup), epiglottitis, bacterial tracheitis, foreign body, hemangioma,* or *a vascular ring.*

In infants, abnormal work of breathing plus abnormal findings on auscultation are the best findings for ruling in *pneumonia*. The best sign for ruling *out* pneumonia is the absence of tachypnea.

In healthy infants, the ribs do not move much during quiet breathing. Any outward movement is produced by descent of the diaphragm which compresses the abdominal contents and in turn shifts the lower ribs outward.

Asymmetric chest movement may indicate a space-occupying lesion.

Pulmonary disease causes increased abdominal breathing and can result in *retractions (chest indrawing),* an indicator of pulmonary disease before 2 years of age.

Chest indrawing is inward movement of the skin between the ribs during inspiration. Movement of the diaphragm primarily affects breathing with little assistance from the thoracic muscles. As mentioned in the preceding table, four types of retractions can be noted in infants: suprasternal, intercostal, substernal, and subcostal.

Airway obstruction or lower respiratory tract disease in infants can result in the *Hoover sign,* or paradoxical (seesaw) breathing in which the abdomen moves outward while the chest moves inward during inspiration.

Thoracoabdominal paradox, inward movement of the chest and outward movement of the abdomen during inspiration (abdominal breathing), is a *normal finding in newborns (but not older infants)*. It persists during active, or rapid eye movement (REM), sleep even when it is no longer seen during wakefulness or quiet sleep because of the decreased muscle tone of active sleep. As muscle strength increases and chest wall compliance decreases with age, abdominal breathing should no longer be noted. If observed, it may signify respiratory disease.

Children with *muscle weakness* may be noted to have thoracoabdominal paradox at several years of age.

Palpation. Assess tactile fremitus by *palpation*. Place your hand on the chest when the infant cries or makes noise. Place your hand or fingertips over each side of the chest and feel for symmetry in the transmitted vibrations. Percussion is not helpful in infants except in extreme instances. The infant's chest is hyperresonant throughout, and it is difficult to detect abnormalities on percussion.

Because of the excellent transmission of sounds throughout the chest, any abnormalities of tactile fremitus or on percussion suggest severe pathology, such as a large *pneumonic consolidation*.

Auscultation. After performing these maneuvers, you are ready for *auscultation*. Infant breath sounds are louder and harsher than those of adults because the stethoscope is closer to the origin of the sounds. It is often difficult to distinguish transmitted upper airway sounds from sounds originating in the chest. Upper airway sounds tend to be loud, transmitted symmetrically throughout the chest, and loudest as you move your stethoscope toward the neck. They are usually coarse inspiratory sounds. Lower airway sounds are loudest over the site of pathology, are often asymmetric, and often occur during expiration.

Biphasic sounds imply severe obstruction from intrathoracic airway narrowing or severe obstruction from extrathoracic airway narrowing.

Distinguishing Upper Airway from Lower Airway Sounds in Infants

Technique	Upper Airway	Lower Airway
Compare sounds from nose/stethoscope	Same sounds	Often different sounds
Listen to harshness of sounds	Harsh and loud	Variable
Note symmetry (left/right)	Symmetric	Often asymmetric
Compare sounds at different locations (higher or lower)	Sounds are louder as stethoscope is moved up chest	Often sounds are louder lower in chest toward abdomen
Inspiratory vs. expiratory	Almost always inspiratory	Often has expiratory phase

Diminished breath sounds in one side of the chest of a newborn suggest unilateral lesions (e.g., *congenital diaphragmatic hernia or pneumothorax*).

Expiratory sounds usually arise from an intrathoracic source, whereas inspiratory sounds can arise from an extrathoracic airway such as the trachea or from an intrathoracic source. During expiration, the diameter of the intrathoracic airways decreases because radial forces from the surrounding lung do not "tether" the airways open as occurs during inspiration. Higher flow rates during inspiration produce turbulent flow, resulting in appreciable sounds.

Upper respiratory infections are not serious in infants but can produce loud inspiratory sounds that are often transmitted to the chest.

The characteristics of the *breath sounds,* such as vesicular and bronchovesicular, and of the adventitious lung sounds, such as crackles, wheezes, and rhonchi, are the same as those for adults, except that they may be more difficult to distinguish in infants and often occur together. Wheezes and rhonchi are common in infants. *Wheezes,* often audible without the stethoscope, occur more frequently because of the smaller size of the tracheobronchial tree. *Rhonchi* reflect obstruction of larger airways, or bronchi. *Crackles* (rales) are discontinuous sounds (see p. 325), near the end of inspiration; they are usually caused by lung disorders and are far less likely to represent cardiac failure in infants than in adults. They tend to be harsher than in adults.

Wheezes in infants occur commonly from *asthma* or *bronchiolitis*.

Rhonchi in infants occur with *upper respiratory infections*.

Crackles (rales) can be heard with *pneumonia* and *bronchiolitis*.

The Heart

Inspection. Before examining the heart itself, observe the infant carefully for any cyanosis. Acrocyanosis in the newborn is discussed on pages 816 and 918. It is important to detect central cyanosis because it is always abnormal and because many congenital cardiac abnormalities, as well as respiratory diseases, present with cyanosis.[20]

Central cyanosis without acute respiratory symptoms suggests *cardiac disease*. See Table 18-9, Cyanosis in Children, p. 918, and Table 18-10, Congenital Heart Murmurs, pp. 919–920.

Recognizing minimal degrees of cyanosis requires care. Look inside the body (i.e., the inside of the mouth, the tongue, or the conjunctivae) in addition to assessing skin color. A true strawberry pink is normal, whereas any hint of raspberry red suggests desaturation and requires urgent evaluation.

The distribution of the cyanosis should be evaluated. An oximetry reading will confirm desaturation.

In general, cardiac causes of central cyanosis involve right-to-left shunting and can be caused by a variety of congenital cardiac lesions.

Cardiac Causes of Central Cyanosis in Infants and Children

Age of Onset	Potential Cardiac Cause
Immediately at birth	Transposition of the great arteries
	Pulmonary valve atresia
	Severe pulmonary valve stenosis
	Possibly Ebstein malformation
Within a few days after birth	All of the above plus:
	Total anomalous pulmonary venous return
	Hypoplastic left heart syndrome
	Truncus arteriosus (sometimes)
	Single ventricle variants
Weeks, months, or years of life	All of the above plus:
	Pulmonary vascular disease with atrial,
	ventricular, or great vessel shunting
	(right-to-left shunting)

Observe the infant for *general signs of health.* The infant's nutritional status, responsiveness, irritability, and fatigue are all clues that may be useful in evaluating cardiac disease. Note that noncardiac findings (see box on the next page) are often present in infants with cardiac disease.

The combination of tachypnea, tachycardia, and hepatomegaly in infants suggests *heart failure*.

Noncardiac Findings Commonly Present in Infants with Cardiac Disease

Poor feeding	Tachypnea	Poor overall appearance
Failure to thrive	Hepatomegaly	Weakness
Irritability	Clubbing	Fatigue

Observe the respiratory rate and pattern to help distinguish the degree of illness and cardiac versus pulmonary diseases. An increase in respiratory effort is expected from pulmonary diseases, whereas in cardiac disease there may be tachypnea without increased work of breathing (called "peaceful tachypnea") until heart failure becomes significant.

Palpation. *Palpation* of the chest wall will allow you to assess volume changes within the heart. For example, a hyperdynamic precordium reflects a big volume change.

The *point of maximal cardiac impulse,* or *PMI*, is not always palpable in infants and is affected by respiratory patterns, a full stomach, and the infant's positioning. It is usually an interspace higher than in adults during the first few years of life because the heart lies more horizontally within the chest.

Thrills are palpable when turbulence within the heart or great vessels is transmitted to the surface. Knowledge of the structures of the precordium helps pinpoint the origin of the thrill. Thrills are easiest to feel with your palm or the base of your fingers rather than your fingertips. Thrills have a somewhat rough, vibrating quality. Figure 18-27 shows locations of thrills that occur in infants and children from various cardiac abnormalities.

A diffuse bulge outward of the left side of the chest suggests long-standing *cardiomegaly.*

A *"rolling" heave* at the left sternal border suggests an *increase in right ventricular work,* whereas the same kind of motion closer to the apex suggests the same thing for the left ventricle.

PDA is associated with hyperdynamic precordium and bounding distal pulses.

Visible and palpable chest pulsations suggest a hyperdynamic state from either increased metabolic rate or inefficient pumping as a result of an underlying *cardiac defect.*

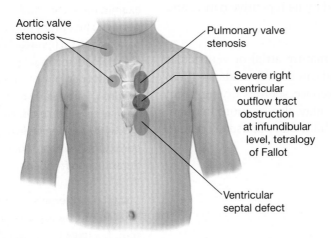

Aortic valve stenosis

Pulmonary valve stenosis

Severe right ventricular outflow tract obstruction at infundibular level, tetralogy of Fallot

Ventricular septal defect

FIGURE 18-27. Location of thrills in infants and children.

Pulses. The major branches of the aorta can be assessed by evaluation of the *peripheral pulses*. All neonates should have an evaluation of all pulses at the time of their newborn examination. In neonates and infants, *the brachial artery pulse in the antecubital fossa is easier to feel than the radial artery pulse at the wrist.* Both temporal arteries should be felt just in front of the ear.

Palpate the femoral pulses. They lie in the midline just below the inguinal crease, between the iliac crest and the symphysis pubis. Take your time to search for femoral pulses; they are difficult to detect in chubby, squirming infants. If you first flex the infant's thighs on the abdomen, this may overcome the reflex flexion that occurs when you then extend the legs.

Palpate the pulses in the lower extremities using your index or middle finger. The dorsalis pedis and posterior tibial pulses (Fig. 18-28) may be difficult to feel unless there is an abnormality involving aortic run-off. Normal pulses should have a sharp rise and should be firm and well localized.

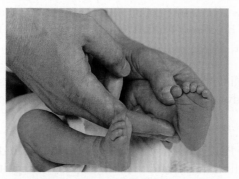

FIGURE 18-28. Palpating pulses in lower extremity.

As discussed on p. 814, carefully measure the *blood pressure* of infants and children (using an appropriate-sized infant blood pressure cuff) as part of the cardiac examination.

Auscultation. You can evaluate the *heart rhythm* more easily in infants by listening to the heart than by feeling the peripheral pulses; in older children assess the rhythm either way.

Infants and children commonly have a normal sinus dysrhythmia, with the heart rate increasing on inspiration and decreasing on expiration, sometimes quite abruptly. This normal finding can be identified by its repetitive nature and its correlation with respiration.

Many neonates and some older children have premature atrial or ventricular beats that are often described as "skipped" beats. You can usually eradicate them by increasing their intrinsic sinus rate through exercise such as crying in an infant or jumping in an older child, although they may also be more frequent in the postexercise period. In a completely healthy child, they are usually benign and rarely persist.

The absence or diminution of femoral pulses is indicative of *coarctation of the aorta.* If you cannot detect femoral pulses, measure blood pressures of one of the lower and both upper extremities. Normally, the blood pressure in the lower extremity is slightly higher than in the upper extremities. If they are equal or lower in the leg, coarctation is likely to be present.

A weak or thready, difficult-to-feel pulse may reflect *myocardial dysfunction* and *heart failure,* particularly if associated with an unusual degree of tachycardia.

Although the pulses in the feet of neonates and infants are often faint, several conditions can cause full pulses, such as *PDA* or *truncus arteriosus.*

The most common abnormal dysrhythmia in infants is *paroxysmal atrial tachycardia (PAT).* It can occur at any age, including in utero. It is remarkably well tolerated by some infants and children and is found on examination. The child may look perfectly healthy or may be mildly pale or with tachypnea. The heart rate is sustained and regular at around 240 beats per minute or more. Some children, particularly neonates, may appear very ill. In older children, this dysrhythmia is more likely to be truly paroxysmal, with episodes of varying duration and frequency.

Distant heart tones suggest *pericardial effusion;* mushy, less distinct heart sounds suggest *myocardial dysfunction.*

Heart Sounds. Heart sounds are very challenging to assess in infants because they are rapid and often obscured by respiratory or other sounds. Nevertheless, evaluate the S_1 and S_2 heart sounds carefully and systematically. They are normally crisp. You can usually hear the second sounds (S_2) at the base separately, but they should fuse into a single sound in deep expiration. In the neonate, you should be able to detect a split S_2 if you examine the infant when the infant is completely quiet or asleep. Detecting this split eliminates many, but not all, of the more serious congenital cardiac defects.

Pathologic arrhythmias in children can be from structural cardiac lesions but also from other causes such as drug ingestion, metabolic abnormalities, endocrine disorders, serious infections, and postinfectious states, or conduction disturbances without structural heart disease.

Characteristics of Normal Variants of Heart Rhythms in Children

Characteristics	Atrial Premature Contractions (APCs) or Ventricular Premature Contractions (VPCs)	Normal Sinus Dysrhythmias
Most common age	Neonates (may occur at any time)	After infancy Throughout childhood
Correlation with respiration	No	Yes: Increases on inspiration, decreases on expiration
Effect of exercise on tachycardia	Eradicated by exercise May be more frequent postexercise	Disappears
Characteristic of rhythm	Skipped or missed beat Irregularly occurring	Gradually faster with inspiration Often suddenly slower on expiration
Number of beats	Usually single abnormal beats	Several beats, usually in repetitive cycles
Severity	Usually benign	Benign (by definition)

Although ventricular premature contractions generally occur in otherwise healthy infants, they can occur with underlying cardiac disease, particularly *cardiomyopathies* and *congenital heart disorders*. Electrolyte or metabolic disturbances are also causes.

In addition to trying to detect splitting of the S_2, listen for the intensity of A_2 and P_2. The aortic, or first component of the second sound at the base, is normally louder than the pulmonic, or second component (Fig. 18-29).

A louder-than-normal pulmonic component, particularly when louder than the aortic sound, suggests *pulmonary hypertension*.

Persistent splitting of S_2 may indicate a right ventricular volume load such as *atrial septal defect, anomalies of pulmonary venous return,* or *chronic anemia.*

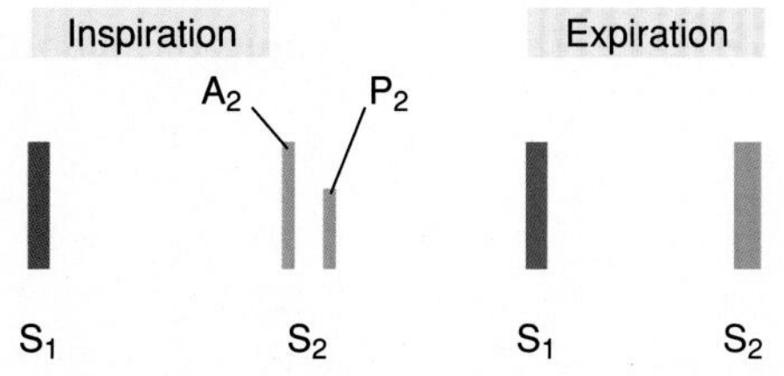

FIGURE 18-29. **Healthy heart sounds in infants.**

You may detect *third heart sounds* which are low-pitched, early diastolic sounds best heard at the lower left sternal border, or apex; they reflect rapid ventricular filling. These are frequently heard in children and are normal.

Fourth heart sounds represent decreased ventricular compliance, suggesting *heart failure*.

You may also detect an *apparent gallop* (widely split S_2 that varies), in the presence of a normal heart rate and rhythm. This is frequently found in normal children and does not represent pathology.

Heart Murmurs.

One of the most challenging aspects of the cardiac examination in children is the evaluation of *heart murmurs*. In addition to listening to a squirming, perhaps uncooperative child, a major challenge is distinguishing common benign murmurs from unusual or pathologic ones. Characterize heart murmurs in infants and children by noting their specific location (e.g., left upper sternal border, not just left sternal border), timing, intensity, and quality. If each murmur is delineated completely, the diagnosis is usually made clinically, and laboratory tools such as ECG, chest x-ray, and echocardiography are needed for confirmation and better characterization.

An important rule of thumb is that, by definition, *benign murmurs in children have no associated abnormal findings*. Many (but not all) children with serious cardiac malformations have signs and symptoms other than a heart murmur obtainable on careful history or examination. Many have noncardiac signs and symptoms, including evidence of genetic defects that may offer helpful diagnostic clues.

Most children, if not all, will have one or more *functional, or benign, heart murmurs* before reaching adulthood.[21–23] It is important to identify functional murmurs by their specific qualities rather than by their intensity. You will learn to recognize the common functional murmurs of infancy and childhood, which under most circumstances do not require evaluation.

The box on the next page characterizes two *benign* heart murmurs in infants according to their locations and key characteristics.

The third heart sound (S_3) should be differentiated from the higher-intensity third heart sound gallop, which is a sign of underlying pathology.

Fourth heart sounds (S_4), not often heard in children, are low-frequency, late diastolic sounds, occurring just before the first heart sound.

A true *gallop rhythm* (in contrast to a widely split S_2 which gives an apparent gallop)—tachycardia plus a loud S_3, S_4, or both—is pathologic and indicates *heart failure (poor ventricular function)*.

Any of the *noncardiac findings* that frequently accompany cardiac disease in children markedly raises the possibility that a murmur is pathologic.

Some *pathologic murmurs of congenital heart disease* are present at birth. Others are not apparent until later, depending on their severity, drop in pulmonary vascular resistance following birth, or changes associated with growth of the child. Table 18-10, Congenital Heart Murmurs, on pp. 919–920, shows examples of pathologic murmurs of childhood.

Two Common Benign Murmurs in Infants

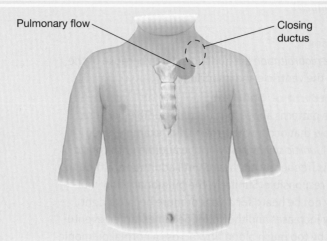

Typical Age	Name	Characteristics	Description and Location
Newborn	*Closing ductus*		Transient, soft, ejection, systolic Upper left sternal border
Newborn to 1 yr	*Peripheral pulmonary flow murmur*	S_1 S_2	Soft, slightly ejectile, systolic Upper left sternal border, radiating to lung fields and axillae

In some infants, you will detect a soft, somewhat ejectile murmur, not over the precordium but over the lung fields, particularly in the axillae. This represents peripheral pulmonary artery flow and is partly the result of inadequate pulmonary artery growth in utero (when there is little pulmonary blood flow) and the sharp angle at which the pulmonary artery curves backward. In the absence of any physical findings to suggest additional underlying diseases, this *peripheral pulmonary flow murmur* (which is common) can be considered benign and usually disappears by 1 year.

A pulmonary flow murmur in the newborn with other signs of disease is more likely to be pathologic. Diseases may include *Williams syndrome, congenital rubella syndrome,* and *Alagille syndrome.*

Physiologic Basis for Some Pathologic Heart Murmurs

Change in Pulmonary Vascular Resistance
Heart murmurs that are dependent on a postnatal drop in pulmonary vascular resistance, allowing turbulent flow from the high-pressure systemic circuit to the lower-pressure pulmonary circuit, are not audible until such a drop has occurred. Except in premature infants, murmurs of a *ventricular septal defect* or *PDA* are not heard in the first few days of life and usually become audible after a week to 10 days.

Obstructive Lesions
Obstructive lesions, such as *pulmonic and aortic stenosis,* are caused by normal blood flow through two small valves. They are not dependent on a drop in pulmonary vascular resistance. They are audible at birth.

Characteristics of specific pathologic heart murmurs in children are described in Table 18-10, Congenital Heart Murmurs, pp. 919–920.

(continued)

Physiologic Basis for Some Pathologic Heart Murmurs (*continued*)

Pressure Gradient Differences

Murmurs of *atrioventricular valve regurgitation* are audible at birth because of the high-pressure gradient between the ventricle and its atrium.

Changes Associated with Growth of Children

Some murmurs do not follow the patterns above, but become audible because of alterations in normal blood flow that occur with growth. For example, even though it is an obstructive defect, *aortic stenosis* may not be audible until considerable growth has occurred and is frequently not heard until adulthood, although a congenitally abnormal valve is responsible. Similarly, the pulmonary flow murmur of an *atrial septal defect* may not be heard for a year or more because right ventricular compliance gradually increases and the shunt becomes larger, eventually producing a murmur caused by too much blood flow across a normal pulmonic valve.

When you detect a murmur in a child, note all of the qualities as described in Chapter 9, The Cardiovascular System, to help you distinguish *pathologic murmurs* from benign murmurs. Heart murmurs that reflect underlying structural heart disease are easier to evaluate if you have a good knowledge of intrathoracic anatomy and the functional cardiac changes following birth and if you understand the physiologic basis for heart murmurs. Understanding these physiologic changes can help you distinguish pathologic murmurs from benign heart murmurs in children.

A newborn with a heart murmur and central cyanosis is likely to have congenital heart disease and requires urgent cardiac evaluation.

The Breasts

The breasts of the newborn in both males and females are often enlarged from maternal estrogen effect; this may last several months. The breasts may also be engorged with a white liquid, sometimes colloquially called "witch's milk," which may last 1 or 2 weeks.

In *premature thelarche*, breast development occurs, most often between 6 months and 2 years. Other signs of puberty or hormonal abnormalities are not present.

The Abdomen

Inspection. Inspect the abdomen with the infant lying supine (and, optimally, asleep). The infant's abdomen is protuberant as a result of poorly developed abdominal musculature. You will easily notice abdominal wall blood vessels and intestinal peristalsis.

Inspect the newborn's *umbilical cord* to detect abnormalities. Normally, there are two thick-walled umbilical arteries and one larger but thin-walled umbilical vein which is usually located at the 12 o'clock position.

A *single umbilical artery* may be associated with congenital anomalies or be an isolated anomaly.

The umbilicus in the newborn may have a long cutaneous portion (*umbilicus cutis*) which is covered with skin, and an amniotic portion (*umbilicus amnioticus*) which is covered by a firm gelatinous substance. The amniotic portion dries up and falls off within 2 weeks, whereas the cutaneous portion retracts to be flush with the abdominal wall.

An *umbilical granuloma* at the base of the navel is the development of pink granulation tissue formed during the healing process.

Inspect the area around the umbilicus for redness or swelling.

Infection of the umbilical stump (*omphalitis*) can be a serious condition and is characterized by periumbilical edema and erythema.

Umbilical hernias are detectable by a few weeks of age. Most disappear by 1 year, nearly all by 5 years.

Umbilical hernias in infants are caused by a defect in the abdominal wall and can be quite protuberant with increased intra-abdominal pressure (i.e., during crying).

In some normal infants, you will notice a *diastasis recti*. This involves separation of the two rectus abdominis muscles, causing a midline ridge most apparent when the infant contracts the abdominal muscles. A benign condition in most cases, it resolves during early childhood.

Auscultation. *Auscultation* of a quiet infant's abdomen is easy. You may hear an orchestra of musical tinkling bowel sounds upon placement of your stethoscope on the infant's abdomen.

An increase in pitch or frequency of bowel sounds is heard with *gastroenteritis* or, rarely, with *intestinal obstruction*.

Percussion and Palpation. You can *percuss* an infant's abdomen as you would an adult's, but may note greater tympanitic sounds because of the infant's propensity to swallow air. Percussion is useful for determining the size of organs and abdominal masses.

A silent, tympanic, distended, and tender abdomen suggests *peritonitis*.

It is easy to *palpate* an infant's abdomen because infants like being touched. A useful technique to relax the infant is to hold the legs flexed at the knees and hips with one hand and palpate the abdomen with the other. A pacifier may quiet the infant in this position.

When palpating the liver, start gently low in the abdomen, moving upward with your fingers. This technique helps to identify an extremely enlarged liver that extends down into the pelvis. With a careful examination, you can feel the liver edge in most infants, 1 to 3 cm below the right costal margin.

An enlarged, tender liver may be due to *heart failure* or due to *storage diseases*. Among newborns, causes of hepatomegaly include *hepatitis*, *storage diseases*, *vascular congestion*, and *biliary obstruction*.

One technique for assessing liver size in infants is simultaneous percussion and auscultation.[24] Percuss and simultaneously auscultate, noting a change in sound as you percuss over the liver or beyond it. Of note, a scratch test (described on page 880 for older children) can be attempted in infants.

Liver Size in Healthy Term Newborns

By palpation and percussion[25]	Mean, 5.9 ± 0.7 cm
Projection below right costal margin	Mean, 2.5 ± 1.0 cm

The *spleen*, like the liver, is felt easily in most infants. It is soft with a sharp edge and it projects downward like a tongue from under the left costal margin. The spleen is moveable and rarely extends more than 1 to 2 cm below the left costal margin.

Several diseases can cause spleno-megaly, including *infections, hemolytic anemias, infiltrative disorders, inflammatory* or *autoimmune diseases,* and *portal hypertension.*

Palpate the *other abdominal structures.* You will commonly note pulsations in the epigastrium caused by the aorta. This is felt on deep palpation to the left of the midline.

Abnormal abdominal masses in infants can be associated with the kidney (e.g., *hydronephrosis*), bladder (e.g., *urethral obstruction*), bowel (e.g., *Hirschsprung disease,* or *intussusception*), and tumors.

You may be able to palpate the kidneys of infants by carefully placing the fingers of one hand in front of and those of the other behind each kidney. The descending colon is a sausage-like mass in the left lower quadrant.

Once you have identified the normal structures in the infant's abdomen, use palpation to identify abnormal masses.

In *pyloric stenosis,* deep palpation in the right upper quadrant or midline can reveal an "olive," or a 2-cm firm pyloric mass. While feeding, some infants with this condition will have visible peristaltic waves pass across their abdomen, followed by projectile vomiting. Infants present at about 4 to 6 weeks of age.

Male Genitalia

Inspect the male genitalia with the infant supine noting the appearance of the penis, testes, and scrotum. The *foreskin completely covers the glans penis.* It is nonretractable at birth though you may be able to retract it enough to visualize the external urethral meatus. The foreskin gradually loosens over months to years and becomes retractable. The rate of circumcision had declined over several decades in North America and varies worldwide, depending on cultural practices, but is now recommended by the AAP and by experts in many parts of the world due to reduced rates of HIV and other infections among circumcised males.

Hypospadias refers to an abnormal location of the urethral orifice to some point along the ventral surface of the glans or shaft of the penis (see Table 18-12, The Male Genitourinary System, p. 922). The foreskin is incompletely formed ventrally.

Inspect the *shaft of the penis,* noting any abnormalities on the ventral surface. Make sure the penis appears straight.

A fixed, downward bowing of the penis is a *chordee;* this may accompany a hypospadias.

Inspect the *scrotum* noting rugae which should be present by 40 weeks gestation. Scrotal edema may be present for several days following birth because of the effect of maternal estrogen.

Palpate the testes in the scrotal sacs, proceeding downward from the external inguinal ring to the scrotum. If you feel a testis up in the inguinal canal, gently milk it downward into the scrotum. The newborn's testes should be about 10 mm in width and 15 mm in length and should lie in the scrotal sacs most of the time.

In newborns with an *undescended testicle* (*cryptorchidism*), the scrotum often appears underdeveloped and tight, and palpation reveals an absence of scrotal contents (see Table 18-12, The Male Genitourinary System, p. 922).

In about 3% of neonates, one or both *testes* cannot be felt in the scrotum or inguinal canal. This raises concern of *cryptorchidism*. In two thirds of these cases, both testes are descended by 1 year of age.

Examine the testes for swelling within the scrotal sac and over the inguinal ring. If you detect swelling in the scrotal sac try to differentiate it from the testis. Note whether the size changes when the infant increases abdominal pressure by crying. See if your fingers can get above the mass, trapping it in the scrotal sac. Apply gentle pressure to try to reduce the size of the mass and note any tenderness. Note whether it transilluminates (Fig. 18-30).

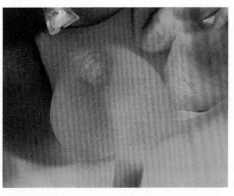

FIGURE 18-30. **Transillumination of a hydrocele.** From Fletcher M. *Physical Diagnosis in Neonatology.* Philadelphia, PA: Lippincott-Raven; 1998.

Two common scrotal masses in newborns are *hydroceles* and *inguinal hernias;* frequently both coexist, and both are more common on the right side. Hydroceles overlie the testes and the spermatic cord, are not reducible, and can be transilluminated (Fig. 18-30). Most resolve by 18 months. Hernias are separate from the testes, are usually reducible, and often do not transilluminate. They do not resolve. Sometimes a thickened spermatic cord (called the *silk sign*) is noted.

Female Genitalia

Become familiar with the anatomy of an infant's female genitalia. Examine the female genitalia with the infant supine.

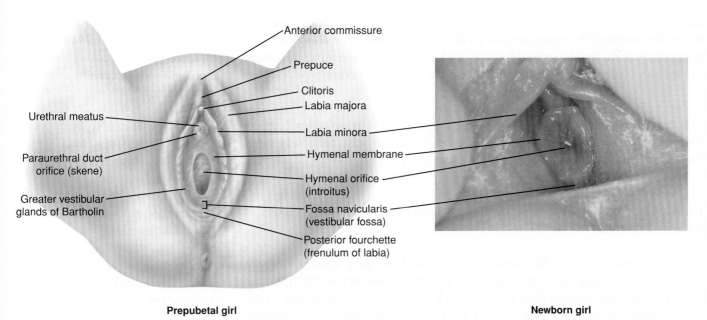

Prepubetal girl

Newborn girl

FIGURE 18-31. **Highly estrogenized hymen of a newborn with thickening and hypertrophy of hymenal tissue.**

In the newborn female, the genitalia will be prominent due to the effects of maternal estrogen. The labia majora and minora have a dull pink color in light-skinned infants and may be hyperpigmented in dark-skinned infants. During the first few weeks of life there is often a milky white vaginal discharge that may be blood tinged and is not a cause for concern. This estrogenized appearance of the genitalia decreases during the first year of life.

Ambiguous genitalia, involving masculinization of the female external genitalia, is a rare condition caused by endocrine disorders such as *congenital adrenal hyperplasia.*

Examine the different structures systematically, including the size of the clitoris, the color and size of the labia majora, and any rashes, bruises, or external lesions (Fig. 18-31). Next, separate the labia majora at their midpoint with the thumb of each hand, or as shown in Figs. 18-83 and 18-84 below.

Labial adhesions occur frequently, tend to be paper thin, and often disappear without treatment. The paper-thin adhesions attach the labial minora to each other at the midline.

Inspect the urethral orifice and the labia minora. Assess the hymen, which in newborns and infants is a thickened, avascular structure with a central orifice, covering the vaginal opening. You should note a vaginal opening, although the hymen will be thickened and redundant. Note any discharge.

An imperforate hymen may be noted at birth.

Rectal Examination

The rectal examination generally is not performed for infants or children unless there is question of patency of the anus or an abdominal mass. In such cases, flex the infant's hips and fold the legs to the head. Use your lubricated and gloved pinky to perform the examination.

A common cause of blood in the stool of infants is an *anal fissure* which is a superficial break in the surface of the anus and observable with the naked eye.

The Musculoskeletal System

Enormous changes in the musculoskeletal system occur during infancy. Much of the examination of the infant focuses on detection of congenital abnormalities, particularly in the hands, spine, hips, legs, and feet. Combine the musculoskeletal examination with the neurologic and developmental examination.

Careful inspection can reveal gross deformities such as *dwarfism, congenital abnormalities* of the *extremities* or *digits,* and *annular bands* that *constrict* an *extremity.*

The *newborn's hands* are clenched. Because of the palmar grasp reflex (see the discussion on the nervous system, p. 849) you will need to help the infant extend the fingers. Inspect the fingers carefully, noting any defects.

Skin tags, remnants of digits, polydactyly (extra fingers), or *syndactyly* (webbed fingers) are congenital defects noted at birth.

Palpate along the *clavicle* noting any lumps, tenderness, or crepitus; these may indicate a fracture.

A *fracture of the clavicle* can occur during a difficult birth.

Inspect the *spine* carefully. Although major defects of the spine such as *meningomyelocele* are obvious and often detected by ultrasound before birth, subtle abnormalities may include pigmented spots, hairy patches, or deep pits. These abnormalities, if present within 1 cm or so of the midline, may overlie external openings of sinus tracts that extend to the spinal canal. Do not probe sinus tracts because of the potential risk for introducing infection. Palpate the spine in the lumbosacral region, noting any deformities of the vertebrae.

Spina bifida occulta (a defect of the vertebral bodies) may be associated with defects of the spinal cord, which can cause severe neurologic dysfunction.

Examine the newborn and infant's *hips* carefully at each examination for signs of dislocation.[26,27] Figures 18-32 to 18-36 and discussion cover the two major techniques, one to test for the presence of a posteriorly dislocated hip (*Ortolani test*) (Fig. 18-32), and another to test for the ability to sublux or dislocate an intact but unstable hip (*Barlow test*) (Fig. 18-33).

Developmental dysplasia of the hip is important to detect as early treatment has excellent outcomes.

A soft audible "click" heard with these maneuvers does not prove a *dislocated hip*, but should prompt a careful examination.

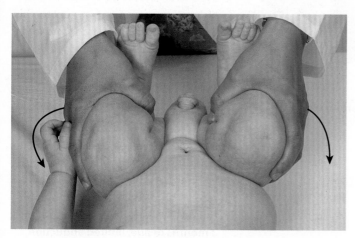

FIGURE 18-32. **Ortolani test, overhead view.**

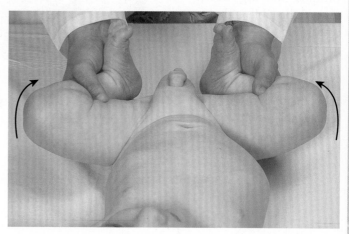

FIGURE 18-33. **Barlow test, overhead view.**

Make sure the baby is relaxed for these techniques. For the *Ortolani test*, place the baby supine with the legs pointing toward you. Flex the legs to form right angles at the hips and knees, placing your index fingers over the greater trochanter of each femur and your thumbs over the lesser trochanters (Fig. 18-34). Abduct both hips simultaneously until the lateral aspect of each knee touches the examining table (Fig. 18-35).

With a *developmental dysplasia of the hip,* you feel a "clunk" as the femoral head, which lies posterior to the acetabulum, enters the acetabulum. A palpable movement of the femoral head back into place constitutes a *positive Ortolani sign.*

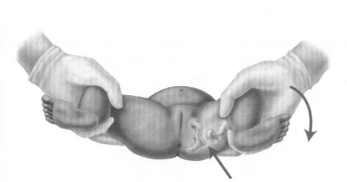

FIGURE 18-34. **Ortolani test, starting position.**

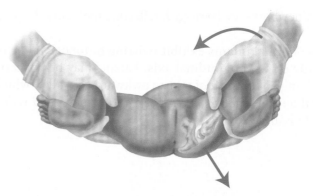

FIGURE 18-35. **Ortolani test, ending position.**

For the *Barlow test,* place your hands in the same position as for the Ortolani test. Pull the leg forward and adduct with posterior force; that is, press in the opposite direction with your thumbs moving down toward the table and outward (Fig. 18-36). Feel for any movement of the head of the femur laterally. Normally, there is no movement and the hip feels "stable."

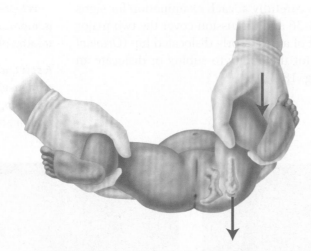

FIGURE 18-36. **Barlow test.**

A positive Barlow sign is not diagnostic of a *dysplastic hip,* but indicates laxity and a potentially dislocatable hip. If a Barlow sign is present, the baby needs to be followed very closely. If you feel the head of the femur slipping out onto the posterior lip of the acetabulum, this constitutes a *positive Barlow sign.* If you feel this dislocation movement, abduct the hip by pressing with your index and middle fingers back inward and feel for the movement of the femoral head as it returns to the hip socket.

Children older than age 3 months may have a negative Ortolani or Barlow sign and still have a *dislocated hip* due to tightening of the hip muscles and ligaments. Of note, all babies should receive serial hip examinations until they are walking. In infants beyond 3 months of age, limited abduction is concerning for developmental dysplasia of the hip.

Test for femoral shortening using the *Galeazzi* or *Allis sign.* Place the feet (with knee flexed and sacrum flat on the table) together and note any difference in knee heights.

Examine a newborn or infant's *legs and feet* to detect developmental abnormalities. Assess symmetry, bowing, and torsion of the legs. There should be no discrepancy in leg length. It is common for normal infants to have asymmetric thigh skin folds, but if you do detect asymmetry, make sure you perform the instability tests because dislocated hips are commonly associated with this finding.

Severe bowing of the knees can be normal, but it can also be due to *rickets* or *Blount disease.* The most common cause of bowing is tibial torsion.

Most newborns are *bowlegged,* reflecting their curled-up intrauterine position.

Some normal infants exhibit twisting or *torsion of the tibia* inwardly or outwardly on its longitudinal axis. Parents may be concerned about a toeing in or toeing out of the foot and an awkward gait, all of which are usually normal. *Tibial torsion usually corrects itself during the second year of life after months of weight bearing.*

Pathologic tibial torsion occurs only in association with *deformities of the feet or hips.*

Examine the feet of new-borns and infants. *At birth, the feet may appear deformed from retaining their intra-uterine positioning,* often turned inward (Fig. 18-37). You should be able to cor-rect the feet to the neutral and even to an overcor-rected position (Fig. 18-38). Scratch or stroke along the outer edge to see if the foot assumes a normal position.

True *deformities of the feet* do not return to the neutral position even with manipulation.

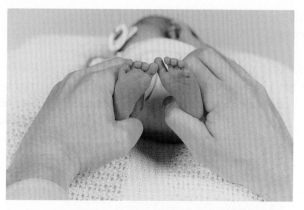

FIGURE 18-37. **Assess alignment of the feet.**

The normal newborn's foot has several benign features that may initially cause con-cern. The newborn's foot appears flat because of a plantar fat pad. There is often inversion of the foot, elevating the outer margin (see p. 922). Other babies will have adduction of the forefoot without inversion, called *metatarsus adductus* which requires close follow-up. Still others will have adduc-tion of the entire foot. Finally, most toddlers have some pronation during early stages of weight-bearing with eversion of the foot. In all of these normal variants the abnormal position can be easily overcorrected past midline. They all tend to resolve within 1 or 2 years.

The most common severe congenital foot deformity is talipes equinovarus or *clubfoot.*

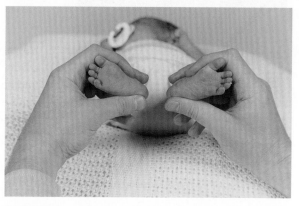

FIGURE 18-38. **Assess alignment by turning to an overcorrected position.**

See Table 18-13, Common Musculo-skeletal Findings in Young Children, p. 922.

The Nervous System

The examination of the nervous system in infants includes techniques that are highly specific to this particular age. Unlike many neurologic abnormalities in adults that produce asymmetric localized findings, neurologic abnormalities in infants often present as developmental abnormalities such as failure to do age-appropriate tasks. Therefore, the neurologic and developmental examinations need to proceed together. *A developmental abnormality should prompt you to pay particular attention to the neurologic examination.*

Signs of severe neurologic disease in infants include extreme irritability, persistent asymmetry of posture, per-sistent extension of extremities, con-stant turning of the head to one side, marked extension of the head, neck, and extremities (opisthotonus), severe flaccidity, and limited response to pain, and sometimes seizures.

The neurologic screening examination of all newborns should include assess-ment of mental status, gross and fine motor function, tone, cry, deep tendon reflexes, and primitive reflexes. More detailed examination of cranial nerve func-tion and sensory function are indicated if you suspect any abnormalities from the history or screening.[28]

Subtle neonatal behaviors such as fine tremors, irritability, and poor self-regulation may indicate *withdrawal from nicotine* if the mother smoked during pregnancy.

The neurologic examination can reveal extensive disease but will not pinpoint specific functional deficits or minute lesions.

Mental Status.   Assess the *mental status* of newborns by observing the newborn activities discussed on p. 808 ("What a Newborn Can Do"). Make sure you test the newborn during alert periods. A detailed description of the assessment of development follows.

Persistent irritability in the newborn may be a sign of *neurologic insult* or may reflect a variety of *metabolic, infectious,* or other *constitutional abnormalities,* or environmental conditions such as *drug withdrawal.*

Motor Function and Tone.   Assess the *motor tone* of newborns and infants, first by carefully observing their position at rest and testing their resistance to passive movement.

Further, assess *tone* as you move each major joint through its range of motion, noting any spasticity or flaccidity. Hold the baby in your hands to determine whether the tone is normal, increased, or decreased (Fig. 18-39). *Either increased or decreased tone may indicate intracranial disease* although such disease is usually accompanied by a number of other signs.

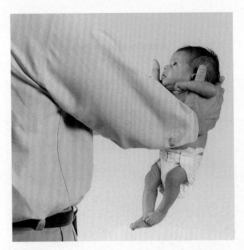

FIGURE 18-39.   **Assessing motor tone.**

Newborns with *hypotonia* often lie in a frog-leg position, with arms flexed and hands near the ears. Hypotonia can be caused by a variety of *central nervous system abnormalities* and *disorders of the motor unit.*

Sensory Function.   You can test for *sensory function* of the newborn in only a limited way. Test for pain sensation by flicking the infant's palm or sole with your finger. Observe for withdrawal, arousal, and change in facial expression. Do not use a pin to test for pain.

If changes in facial expression or cry follow a painful stimulus but no withdrawal occurs, weakness or *paralysis* may be present.

Cranial Nerves.   The *cranial nerves* of the newborn or infant can be tested. The following table provides useful strategies.

Abnormalities in the cranial nerves suggest an intracranial lesion such as *hemorrhage* or a *congenital malformation.*

Strategies to Assess Cranial Nerves in Newborns and Infants

Cranial Nerve		Strategy
I	Olfactory	Very difficult to test
II	Visual acuity	Have infant regard your face and look for facial response and tracking.
II, III	Response to light	Darken room, raise infant to sitting position to open eyes.
		Use light and test for *optic blink reflex* (blink in response to light).
		Use the otoscope's light (without speculum) to assess pupillary responses.

(continued)

Strategies to Assess Cranial Nerves in Newborns and Infants (*continued*)

Cranial Nerve		Strategy
III, IV, VI	Extraocular movements	Observe how well the infant tracks your smiling face (or a bright light) and whether the eyes move together.
V	Motor	Test rooting reflex. Test sucking reflex (watch infant suck breast, bottle, or pacifier) and strength of suck.
VII	Facial	Observe infant crying and smiling; note symmetry of face.
VIII	Acoustic	Test acoustic blink reflex (blinking of both eyes in response to a loud noise). Observe tracking in response to sound.
IX, X	Swallow	Observe coordination during swallowing.
	Gag	Test for gag reflex.
XI	Spinal accessory	Observe symmetry of shoulders.
XII	Hypoglossal	Observe coordination of sucking, swallowing, and tongue thrusting. Pinch nostrils; observe reflex opening of mouth with tip of tongue to midline.

Congenital facial nerve palsy can result from birth trauma or developmental defects.

Dysphagia, or difficulty in swallowing, can occasionally be due to injury to cranial nerve IX, X, and XII.

Deep Tendon Reflexes. The *deep tendon reflexes* are present in newborns but may be difficult to elicit and may vary in their intensity because the corticospinal pathways are immature. Their exaggerated presence or their absence has little diagnostic significance, unless this response is different from results of previous testing or extreme responses are observed or they are very asymmetric.

Use the same techniques to elicit deep tendon reflexes as you would for an adult. You can substitute your index or middle finger for the reflex hammer as shown in Figure 18-40.

A progressive increase in deep tendon reflexes during the first year of life may indicate central nervous system disease such as *cerebral palsy,* especially if it is coupled with increased tone. Another common pattern of presentation is central hypotonia followed by progressively increased tone.

As in adults, asymmetric reflexes suggest a lesion of the peripheral nerves or spinal segment.

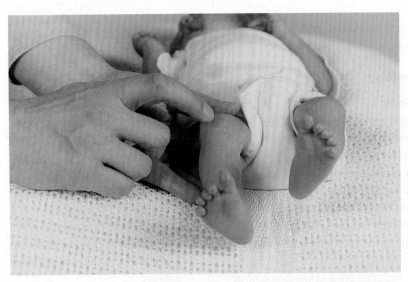

FIGURE 18-40. **Assessing deep tendon reflexes with finger.**

The triceps, brachioradialis, and abdominal reflexes are difficult to elicit before 6 months of age. The *anal reflex* is present at birth and important to elicit if a spinal cord lesion is suspected.

An absent anal reflex suggests loss of innervation of the external sphincter muscle caused by a spinal cord abnormality such as a congenital anomaly (e.g., *spina bifida*), *tumor*, or *injury*.

In newborns, a *positive Babinski response* to plantar stimulation (dorsiflexion of big toe and fanning of other toes) can be elicited and may persist for several months.

In order to best elicit the ankle reflex of an infant, grasp the infant's malleolus with one hand and abruptly dorsiflex the ankle (Fig. 18-41). You may note rapid, rhythmic plantar flexion of the newborn's foot (*ankle clonus*) in response to this maneuver. Up to 10 beats are normal in newborns and young infants; this is *unsustained ankle clonus*.

When the contractions are continuous (*sustained ankle clonus*), *central nervous system disease* should be suspected.

A newborn who is irritable, jittery and has tremors, hypertonicity, and hyperactive reflexes may have *drug withdrawal* from maternal substance use during pregnancy.

***Neonatal abstinence syndrome* results from the use of opioids by the mother while pregnant. In addition to the signs listed above, the newborn may also have autonomic signs, as well as poor feeding and seizures.**

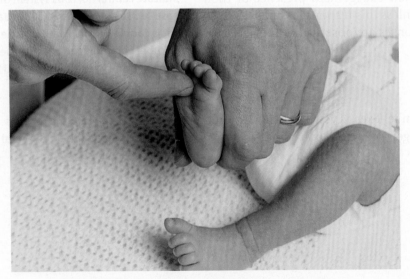

FIGURE 18-41. **Assessing ankle reflexes.**

Primitive Reflexes. Evaluate the newborn's and infant's developing central nervous system by assessing *infantile automatisms*, called *primitive reflexes*. These develop during gestation, are generally demonstrable at birth, and disappear at defined ages. Abnormalities in these primitive reflexes suggest neurologic disease and merit more intensive investigation.[29]

A *neurologic* or *developmental abnormality* is suspected if primitive reflexes are:

- Absent at appropriate age
- Present longer than normal
- Asymmetric
- Associated with posturing or twitching

The most important primitive reflexes are illustrated below.

Development. Refer to the developmental milestones on p. 810 and to the items on a standardized developmental screening instrument to learn which age-specific developmental tasks to evaluate. By observation and play with the infant, you can do both a developmental screening examination and an assessment for gross and fine motor achievement. Specifically, look for *weakness* by observing sitting, standing, and transitions. Note *station*, or the posture of sitting or standing. Assess fine motor development in a similar way, combining the neurologic and developmental examination. Key milestones include the development of the pincer grasp, ability to manipulate objects with the hands, and more precise tasks, such as building a tower of cubes or scribbling. Fine and gross motor development progresses in a proximal to distal direction.

Many causes of developmental delay exist but often no cause is identified. Etiologies include *prenatal* (genetic, central nervous system, congenital hypothyroidism), *perinatal* (preterm, asphyxia, infection, trauma), and *postnatal* (trauma, infection, toxin, abuse).

Assess the infant's cognitive and social–emotional development as you proceed with the comprehensive neurologic and developmental examination. Some neurologic abnormalities produce deficits or slowing in cognitive and social development. Infants who have developmental delay may have abnormalities on the neurologic examination because much of the examination is based on age-specific norms.

Developmental delay across more than one domain (e.g., motor plus cognitive) suggests more severe disease.

Primitive Reflex

Primitive Reflex		Maneuver	Ages	
Palmar Grasp Reflex		Place your fingers into the infant's hands and press against the palmar surfaces. The infant will flex all fingers to grasp your fingers.	Birth to 3–4 mo	Persistence of palmar grasp reflex beyond 4 months suggests pyramidal tract dysfunction. Persistence of clenched hand beyond 2 months suggests central nervous system damage, especially if fingers overlap the thumb.
Plantar Grasp Reflex		Touch the sole at the base of the toes. The toes will curl.	Birth to 6–8 mo	Persistence of plantar grasp reflex beyond 8 months suggests pyramidal tract dysfunction.

(*continued*)

Primitive Reflex (continued)

Primitive Reflex		Maneuver	Ages	
Rooting Reflex	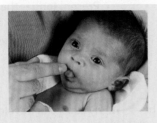	Stroke the perioral skin at the corners of the mouth. The mouth will open and the infant will turn the head toward the stimulated side and suck.	Birth to 3–4 mo	Absence of rooting indicates severe generalized or central nervous system disease.
Moro Reflex (Startle Reflex)	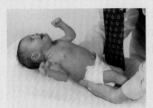	Hold the infant supine, supporting the head, back, and legs. Abruptly lower the entire body about 2 feet. The arms will abduct and extend, hands will open, and legs will flex. The infant may cry.	Birth to 4 mo	Persistence beyond 4 months suggests neurologic disease (e.g., cerebral palsy); persistence beyond 6 months strongly suggests it. Asymmetric response suggests fracture of clavicle or humerus or brachial plexus injury.
Asymmetric Tonic Neck Reflex	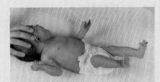	With the infant supine, turn head to one side, holding jaw over shoulder. The arms/legs on side to which head is turned will extend while the opposite arm/leg will flex. Repeat on other side.	Birth to 2 mo	Persistence beyond 2 months suggests asymmetric central nervous system development and sometimes predicts the development of cerebral palsy.
Trunk Incurvation (Galant) Reflex	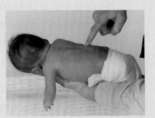	Support the infant prone with one hand and stroke one side of the back 1 cm from midline, from shoulder to buttocks. The spine will curve toward the stimulated side.	Birth to 2 mo	Absence suggests a transverse spinal cord lesion or injury. Persistence may indicate delayed development.

(continued)

Primitive Reflex (continued)

Primitive Reflex		Maneuver	Ages	
Landau Reflex	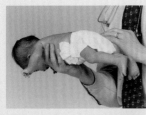	Suspend the infant prone with one hand. The head will lift up, and the spine will straighten.	Birth to 6 mo	Persistence may indicate delayed development.
Parachute Reflex	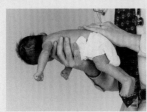	Suspend the infant prone and slowly lower the head toward a surface. The arms and legs will extend in a protective fashion.	8 mo and does not disappear	Delay in appearance may predict future delays in voluntary motor development.
Positive Support Reflex	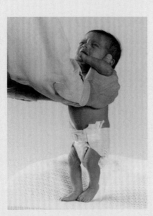	Hold the infant around the trunk and lower until the feet touch a flat surface. The hips, knees, and ankles will extend, the infant will stand up, partially bearing weight, sagging after 20–30 seconds.	Birth or 2 mo until 6 mo	Lack of reflex suggests hypotonia or flaccidity. Fixed extension and adduction of legs (scissoring) suggests spasticity from neurologic disease, such as cerebral palsy.
Placing and Stepping Reflexes	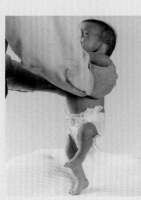	Hold the infant upright as in positive support reflex. Have one sole touch the tabletop. The hip and knee of that foot will flex and the other foot will step forward. Alternate stepping will occur.	Birth (best after 4 days; variable age to disappear)	Absence of placing may indicate paralysis. Newborns born by breech delivery may not have a placing reflex.

A normative measure of development is the developmental quotient,[30] shown here:

$$\text{Development quotient} = \frac{\text{Development age}}{\text{Chronologic age}} \times 100$$

Assess the development of an infant or child using standard scales for each type of development. Assign to each child a gross motor developmental quotient, a fine motor developmental quotient, a cognitive developmental quotient, and so forth. Importantly, these estimates are never a perfect assessment of a child's development or potential because both can change over time.[31]

Developmental Quotients

>85	Normal
70–85	Possibly delayed; follow-up needed
<70	Delayed

Case Examples of Gross and Fine Motor Development

Gross Motor Development

A 12-mo-old child who is just pulling to stand (gross motor developmental age of 9 mo), cruising (10 mo), and walking when both hands are held (10 mo) has a gross motor developmental age of 10 mo. This child's gross motor developmental quotient is:

$$\left(\tfrac{10}{12} \times 100\right) = 83$$

This child is in the gray zone, is likely to do well without intervention, but requires close follow-up.

Fine Motor Development

A 12-mo-old child can transfer objects from hand to hand (a fine motor developmental age of 6 mo), rake objects into his palm (7 mo), and pull things (7 mo). He cannot hold blocks in each hand and does not have thumb and finger grasp (8–9 mo).

He has normal primitive reflexes (most absent), increased tone, scissoring of legs when held, spasticity, and delays on the gross motor part of a standardized developmental screening instrument.

This child's fine motor developmental quotient is:

$$\left(\tfrac{7}{12} \times 100\right) = 58$$

This child is delayed in fine motor development and has signs of *cerebral palsy*.

ASSESSING YOUNG AND SCHOOL-AGED CHILDREN

Development

Early Childhood: 1 to 4 Years

Physical Development. After infancy, the rate of physical growth slows by approximately half. *After 2 years, toddlers gain about 2 to 3 kg and grow 5 cm per year.* Physical changes are impressive. Chubby, clumsy toddlers transform into leaner, more muscular preschoolers.

Gross motor skills also develop quickly. Almost all children walk by 15 months, run well by 2 years, and pedal a tricycle and jump by 4 years. Fine motor skills develop through neurologic maturation and environmental manipulation (Fig. 18-42). The 18-month-old who scribbles becomes a 2-year-old who draws lines and then a 4-year-old who makes circles.

Cognitive and Language Development. Toddlers move from sensorimotor learning (through touching and looking) to symbolic thinking, solving simple problems, remembering songs, and engaging in imitative play. Language develops with extraordinary speed. An 18-month-old with 10 to 20 words becomes a 2-year-old with three-word sentences, and a 3-year-old who converses well. By 4 years, preschoolers form complex sentences. They remain preoperational, however, without sustained logical thought processes.

Social and Emotional Development. New intellectual pursuits are surpassed only by an emerging drive for independence (Fig. 18-43). Because toddlers are impulsive and have poor self-regulation, temper tantrums are common. Self-regulation is an important developmental task with a wide range of normal (Fig. 18-44).

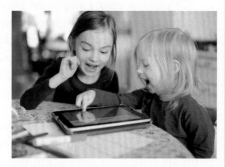

FIGURE 18-42. **Fine motor skills develop along with cognition.**

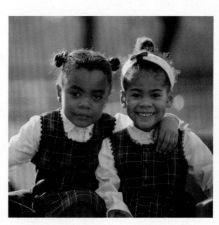

FIGURE 18-43. **Individual personalities emerge as the intellect grows.**

Developmental Milestones During Early Childhood

	1 yr	2 yr	3 yr	4 yr	5 yr
Physical/ Motor	Walks	Throws a ball overhand	Pedals tricyle	Cuts with scissors	Copies
	Runs		Jumps in place	Hops	Skips
			Feeds self with utensils	Balances on 1 foot	Balances well on 1 foot
					Walks on tiptoes
Cognitive/ Language	2–3 single words	2-3 word phrases	Knows colors	100% of speech understandable	Says ABCs
		Draws circle	Sentences	Talks in paragraphs	Copies figures
			Asks "why?"		Defines words
Social/ Emotional	Plays peek-a-boo	Imitates activities	Sings songs	Imaginative	Dresses self, buttons, zips
	Separation anxiety	Prefers to do tasks by self at times	Knows self in mirror	Sings	Plays games
			Knows gender	Imaginary play	Knows whole name and telephone number
				Takes turns	
				Puts on clothes	

FIGURE 18-44. **Developmental milestones during early childhood.**

Middle Childhood: 5 to 10 Years. Middle childhood is an active period of growth and development. *Goal-directed exploration, increased physical and cognitive abilities, and achievements by trial and error mark this stage.* The physical examination is more straightforward during this age period, but always consider the developmental stages and tasks that school-aged children are facing.

Physical Development. Children grow steadily but more slowly. Strength and coordination improve dramatically with more participation in activities (Fig. 18-45). This is also when children with physical disabilities or chronic illnesses become more aware of their limitations.

Cognitive and Language Development. Children become "concrete operational"—capable of limited logic and more complex learning. They remain rooted in the present with little ability to understand consequences or abstractions. School, family, and environment greatly influence learning (Fig. 18-46). A major developmental task is self-efficacy, or the ability to thrive in different situations. Language becomes increasingly complex.

Social and Emotional Development. Children become progressively more independent, initiating activities and enjoying accomplishments. Achievements are critical for self-esteem and developing a "fit" within major social structures—family, school, and peer activity groups. Guilt and poor self-esteem also may emerge. Family and environment contribute enormously to the child's self-image. Moral development remains simple and concrete with a clear sense of "right and wrong."

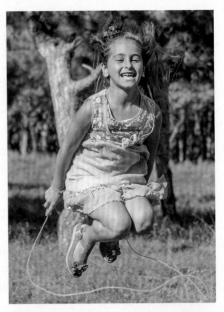

FIGURE 18-45. Physical abilities rapidly progress in early childhood.

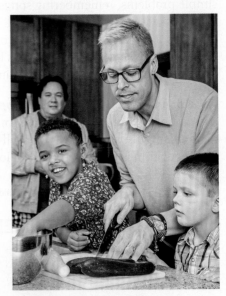

FIGURE 18-46. A child's cognitive development is shaped by family relationships.

Developmental Tasks during Middle Childhood

Task	Characteristic	Health Care Needs
Physical	Enhanced strength and coordination	Screening for strengths, assessing problems
	Competence in various tasks and activities	Involving parents
		Support for disabilities
		Anticipatory guidance: safety, exercise, nutrition, sleep
Cognitive	"Concrete operational:" focus on the present	Emphasis on short-term consequences
	Achievement of knowledge and skills, self-efficacy	Support; screening for skills and school performance
Social	Achieving good "fit" with family, friends, school	Assessment, support, advice about interactions including peer relationships
	Sustained self-esteem	Support, emphasis on strengths
	Evolving self-identity	Understanding, advice, support

The Health History

An important aspect of examining children is that parents are usually watching and taking part in the interaction, providing you the opportunity to observe the parent–child interaction. Note whether the child displays age-appropriate behaviors. Assess the "goodness of fit" between parents and child. Although some abnormal interactions may result from the unnatural setting of the examination room, others may be a consequence of interactional problems. Careful observation of the child's interactions with parents and the child's unstructured play in the examination room can reveal *abnormalities in physical, cognitive, and social development or issues with parent–child relationship.*

Normal toddlers are occasionally terrified or angry at the examiner. Often, they are completely uncooperative. Most eventually warm up to you. If this behavior continues or is not developmentally appropriate, there may be an *underlying behavioral or developmental abnormality.* Older, school-aged children have more self-control and prior experience with clinicians and are generally cooperative with the examination.

Abnormalities Detected While Observing Play

Behavioral[a]
Poor parent–child interactions
Sibling rivalry
Inappropriate parental discipline
"Difficult temperament"

Developmental
Gross motor delay
Fine motor delay
Language delay (expressive or receptive)
Delay in social or emotional tasks

Social or Environmental
Parental stress, depression
Risk for abuse or neglect

Neurologic
Weakness
Abnormal posture
Spasticity
Clumsiness
Attentional problems, hyperactivity
Autistic features
Musculoskeletal abnormalities

[a]Note: The child's behavior during the visit may not represent typical behavior but your observations may serve as a springboard for discussion with parents.

Assessing Younger Children

One challenge in examining children in this age group is avoiding a physical struggle, a crying child, or a distraught parent. Accomplishing this successfully is one aspect of the "art of medicine" in the practice of pediatrics.

Gain the child's confidence and allay the child's fears from the start of the encounter. Your approach will vary with the circumstances of the visit. A health supervision visit allows greater rapport than a visit when the child is ill.

The child should remain dressed during the interview to minimize the child's apprehension. It also allows you to interact more naturally and observe the child playing, interacting with the parents, and undressing and dressing.

Toddlers who are of 9 to 15 months may have *stranger anxiety,* a fear of strangers that is developmentally normal. It signals the toddler's growing awareness that the stranger is new. You should not approach these toddlers quickly. Play can help the child warm up to you. Make sure they remain solidly in their parent's lap throughout much of the examination and that the parent remains close when the child is on the examination table.

Some Tips for Examining Young Children (1- to 4-Year-Olds)

Useful Strategies for Examination

Examine a child sitting on parent's lap. Try to be at the child's eye level.

First examine the child's toy or teddy bear, then the child.

Let the child do some of the examination (e.g., move the stethoscope). Then go back and "get the places we missed."

Ask the toddler who keeps pushing you away to "hold your hand." Then have the toddler "help you" with the examination.

Some toddlers believe that if they can't see you, then you aren't there. Perform the examination while the child stands on the parent's lap, facing the parent.

If 2-yr-olds are holding something in each hand (such as tongue depressors), it is more difficult for them to fight or resist.

Hand the child an age-appropriate book and engage the child in reading.

Useful Toys and Aids

"Blow out" the otoscope light.

"Beep" the stethoscope on your nose.

Make tongue-depressor puppets.

Use the child's own toys for play.

Jingle your keys to test for hearing.

Shine the otoscope through the tip of your finger (or the child's finger) to show it doesn't hurt, "lighting it up," and then examine the child's ears with it.

Use age-appropriate toys and books.

Engage children in age-appropriate conversation. Ask simple questions about their illness or toys. Compliment their appearance or behavior, tell a story, or play a simple game (Fig. 18-47). If a child is shy, turn your attention to the parent to allow the child to warm up gradually. Also, sometimes the parent is anxious. Helping the parent relax or asking them to help by reading to the child or playing with the child can help relax everyone in the examination room.

With certain exceptions, physical examination does not require use of the examining table; it can be done on the floor or with the child in a parent's lap. The key is to engage the child's cooperation. For young children who resist undressing, expose only the body part being examined. When examining siblings, begin with the oldest child who is more likely to cooperate and set a good example. Approach the child pleasantly. Explain each step as you perform it. Continue conversing with the family to provide distraction.

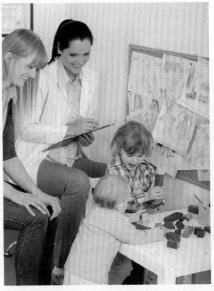

FIGURE 18-47. Engaging children in play is sometimes part of the assessment.

Plan the examination to start with the least distressing procedures and end with the most distressing ones, usually involving the throat and ears. Begin with parts that can be done with the child sitting such as examining the eyes or palpating the neck. Lying down may make a child feel vulnerable, so change positions with care. Once a child is supine, begin with the abdomen, saving throat and ears or genitalia for last. You may need a parent's help to restrain the child for examination of

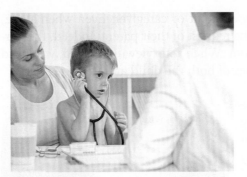

FIGURE 18-48. **Familiarizing the child with the equipment and procedures can reduces anxiety in children.**

the ears or throat; however, use of formal restraints is inappropriate. *Patience, distraction, play, flexibility in the order of the examination, and a caring but firm and gentle approach, are all key to successfully examining the young child* (Fig. 18-48).

More Tips for Examining the Young Child

Use a reassuring voice throughout the examination.

Let the child see and touch the examination tools you will be using.

Avoid asking permission to examine a body part because you will do the examination anyway. Instead, ask the child which ear or which part of the body he or she would like you to examine first.

Examine the child in the parent's lap. Let the parent undress the child.

If unable to console the child, give the child a short break.

Make a game out of the examination! For example, "Let's see how big your tongue is!" or "Is Elmo in your ear? Let's see!"

Reassure parents that resistance to examination is developmentally appropriate. Some embarrassed parents scold the child, compounding the problem. Involve parents in the examination. Learn which techniques and approaches work best and are most comfortable for you.

Assessing Older Children

Examining children after they reach school age usually poses few difficulties. Although some have unpleasant memories of previous clinical encounters, most children respond well when the examiner is attuned to their developmental level.

Many children at this age are modest (Fig. 18-49). Providing gowns and leaving underwear in place as long as possible are wise approaches. Suggest that children disrobe behind a curtain. Consider leaving the room while they change with their parents' help. Some children may prefer opposite-sex siblings to leave, but most prefer a parent of either sex to remain in the room. *Parents of children younger than 11 years should stay with them.*

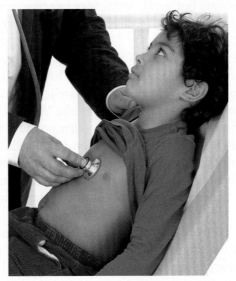

FIGURE 18-49. **Clinicians need to be aware of older children's developing modesty.**

Children are usually accompanied by a parent or caregiver. Even when alone, they are often seeking health care at the request of their parent; indeed, the parent is usually sitting in the waiting room. When interviewing a child, you need to consider the needs and perspectives of both the child and the caregivers.

Establishing Rapport. Begin the interview by greeting and establishing rapport with each person present (Fig. 18-50). Refer to the child by name rather than by "him" or "her." Clarify the role or relationship of all of the adults and children. "Now, are you Jimmy's grandmother?" "Please help me by telling me Jimmy's relationship to everyone here." Address the parents as "Mr. Smith" and "Ms. Smith" rather than by their first names or "Mom" or "Dad." When the family structure is not immediately clear, you may avoid

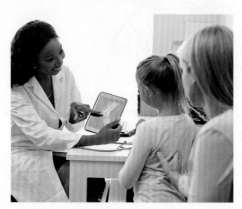

FIGURE 18-50. Establishing rapport enables more effective evaluation.

embarrassment by asking directly about other members. "Who else lives in the home?" "Who is Jimmy's father?" "Do you live together?" Do not assume that just because parents are separated, only one parent is actively involved in the child's life. Families come in many varieties—these include traditional families, single parents, separated/divorced parents, blended, same-sex parents, kinship families, foster families, and adoptive families.

Use your personal experiences with children to guide how you interact in a health care setting. To establish rapport, meet children on their own level. Eye contact on their level, participating in playful engagement, and talking about what interests them are always good strategies. Ask children about their clothes, one of their toys, what book or TV show they like, or their adult companion in an enthusiastic but gentle style. *Spending time at the beginning of the interview to calm and connect with an anxious child can put both the child and the caregiver at ease.*

Working with Families. One challenge when several people are present is deciding to whom to direct your questions. While eventually you need to get information from both the child and the parent, it is useful to start with the child. Asking simple open-ended questions like "Are you sick? . . . Tell me about it," followed by more specific questions, often provides much of the clinical data. The parents can then verify the information, add details that give you the larger context, and identify other issues you need to address. Sometimes children are embarrassed to begin, but once the parent has started the conversation, direct questions back to the child. Characterize symptom attributes the same way you do with adults.

> Your mom tells me that you get stomachaches. Tell me about them.
> Show me where you get the pain. What does it feel like?
> Is it sharp like a pinprick, or does it ache?
> Does it stay in the same spot, or does it move around?
> What helps make it go away? What makes it worse?
> What do you think causes it?

The presence of family members allows you to observe how they interact with the child. A child may be able to sit still or may get restless and start fidgeting. Watch how the parents set, or fail to set, limits when needed.

Multiple Agendas.   Each individual in the room, including the clinician, may have a different idea about the nature of the problem and what needs to be done about it. Discover as many of these perspectives and agendas as possible. Family members who are not present (e.g., the absent parent or grandparent) may also have concerns. Ask about those concerns, too. "If Suzie's father were here today, what questions or concerns would he have?" "Have you, Mrs. Jones, discussed this with your mother or anyone else?" "What does she think?"

For example, Mrs. Jones brings Suzie in for abdominal pain because she is worried that Suzie may have an ulcer and is also worried about Suzie's eating habits. Suzie is not worried about the belly pain, but is uneasy about the changes in her body and about getting fat. Mr. Jones thinks that Suzie's schoolwork is not getting enough attention. You, as the clinician, need to balance these concerns with what you see as a healthy 12-year-old girl in early puberty with some mild functional abdominal pain and appropriate concern for possible emerging obesity. Your goals need to include uncovering the concerns of each person and helping the family to be realistic about the range of "normal."

The Family as a Resource.   In general, family members provide most of the care and are your natural allies in promoting the child's health. Being open to a wide range of parenting behaviors helps to make this alliance. Raising a child reflects cultural, socioeconomic, and family practices. It is important to respect the tremendous variation in these practices. A good strategy is to *view the parents as experts in the care of their child and yourself as their consultant.* This demonstrates respect for the parents' care and minimizes their likelihood of discounting or ignoring your advice. Parents face many challenges raising children, so practitioners need to be supportive, not judgmental. Comments like, "Why didn't you bring him in sooner?" or "What did you do that for?" do not improve your rapport with the parent. Statements acknowledging the hard work of parenting and praising successes are always appreciated. "Mr. Smith, you are doing such a wonderful job with Bobby. Being a parent takes so much work and Bobby's behavior here today clearly shows your efforts. We might have some suggestions for you at the end of the visit." Or to the child, "Bobby you are so lucky to have such a wonderful dad."

Hidden Agendas.   As with adults, the chief complaint may not relate to the real reason the parent has brought the child to see you (Fig. 18-51). The complaint may be a bridge to concerns that may not seem like a legitimate reason to go to the clinician. Create a trusting atmosphere that allows parents to be open about all their concerns by asking facilitating questions such as:

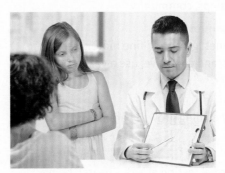

> Do you have any other concerns about Randy?
> Was there anything else that you wanted to tell/ask me today?

FIGURE 18-51. Talking with parents about their children can reveal hidden agendas.

Health Promotion and Counseling: Evidence and Recommendations

Children 1 to 4 Years

The AAP and Bright Futures periodicity schedules for children include health supervision visits at 12, 15, 18, and 24 months followed by annual visits when the child is 3 and 4 years old.[8] An additional visit at 30 months is also recommended to assess the child's development.

During these health supervision visits clinicians address concerns and questions from parents, evaluate the child's growth and development, perform a comprehensive physical examination, and provide anticipatory guidance about healthy habits and behaviors, social competence of caregivers, family relationships, and community interactions.

This is a critical age for preventing childhood obesity as *many children begin their trajectory toward obesity between ages 3 and 4 years.* It is also important to assess the child's development. Standardized developmental screening instruments are recommended to measure the different dimensions of a child's development (see p. 853). Similarly, it is important to differentiate normal (but potentially challenging) childhood behavior from abnormal behavioral or mental health problems.[32]

The following box demonstrates the major components of a health supervision visit for a 3-year-old, stressing health promotion. You do not have to wait for a health supervision visit to address many of these health promotion issues; they can be addressed during other types of visits, even when the child is mildly ill.

Components of a Health Supervision Visit for a 3-Year-Old

Discussions with Parents
- Parental concerns[8]
- Providing advice
- Child care, school, social
- Major topic areas: development, nutrition, safety, oral health, family relationships, community

Developmental Assessment
- Assessment of milestones: gross and fine motor, personal–social, language, and cognitive; use a validated developmental screener.

Physical Examination
- Careful examination, including growth parameters with percentiles for age.

Screening Tests
- Vision and hearing (formal testing at age 4 years), hematocrit and lead (if high risk or at ages 1 to 3 years), screen for social risk factors

Immunizations
- See updated AAP schedule

Anticipatory Guidance

Healthy Habits and Behaviors
- Injury and illness prevention
  Car seats, poisons, tobacco exposure, supervision
- Nutrition and exercise
  Obesity assessment; healthy meals and snacks
- Oral health
  Brushing teeth; dentist

Parent–Child Interaction
- Reading and fun times, child-directed play, limiting screen time

Family Relationships
- Activities, babysitters

Community Interaction
- Child care, resources

Children 5 to 10 Years

The AAP and Bright Futures periodicity schedules for children recommend annual health supervision visits during this period.[8] As for earlier ages, these visits present opportunities to assess the child's physical, mental, and developmental health and the parent–child relationship and the child's relationships with peers and school performance (Fig. 18-52). Once again, health promotion should be incorporated into all interactions with children and families.

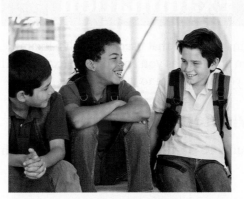

FIGURE 18-52. As children develop, mental health and peer relationships become increasingly important.

Older children enjoy talking directly with the examiner. In addition to discussing health, safety, development, and anticipatory guidance with parents, include the child in these conversations using age-appropriate language and concepts. Discuss the child's experience and perceptions of school, interactions with peers, and other cognitive and social activities. Focus on healthy habits such as good nutrition, exercise, reading, stimulating activities, health sleep hygiene, screen time, and safety.

About 12% to 20% of children have some type of chronic physical, developmental, or mental condition.[33] These children should be seen more frequently for monitoring, disease management, and preventive care (Fig. 18-53). Some behaviors that become established at this age can lead to or exacerbate chronic conditions such as obesity or eating disorders. Health promotion is critical to optimize healthy habits and minimize unhealthy ones. Helping families and children with chronic diseases deal most effectively with these disorders is a key part of health promotion.

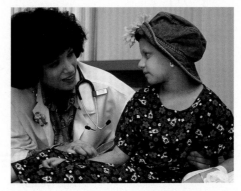

FIGURE 18-53. Connecting with children with chronic conditions can positively affect health outcomes.

For all children, health promotion involves assessing and promoting the family's overall health.

The specific components of the health supervision visit for older children are the same as the components for younger children. Emphasize school performance and experiences as well as appropriate and safe sports and activities and healthy peer relationships.

Techniques of Examination

The order of the examination now begins to follow that used for adults. Examine painful areas last and forewarn children about areas you are going to examine. If a child resists part of the examination you can return to it at the end.

General Survey and Vital Signs

Somatic Growth. Figures 18-54 and 18-55 demonstrate somatic growth patterns in children.

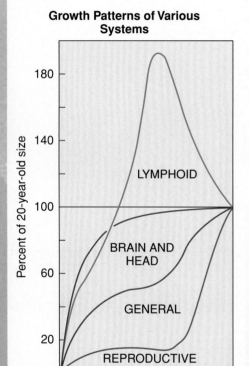

Growth Patterns of Various Systems

FIGURE 18-54. **Growth patterns of various systems.**

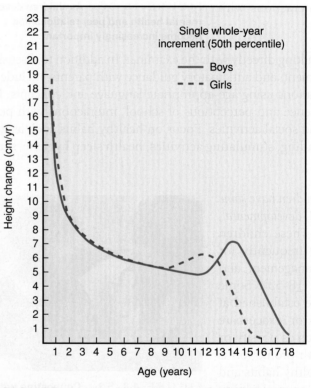

FIGURE 18-55. **Velocity curves for length and height for boys and girls based on intervals of 1 year.**
(From Lowrey GH. Growth and Development of Children, 8th ed. Chicago: Mosby, 1986.)

Height. For children older than 2 years measure standing height, optimally using wall-mounted stadiometers. Have the child stand with heels, back, and head against a wall or the back of the stadiometer. If using a wall with a marked ruler, make sure to place a flat board or surface against the top of the child's head and at right angles to the ruler. Stand-up weight scales with a height attachment are not very accurate.

Short stature, defined as height <5th percentile, can be a normal variant or caused by endocrine or other diseases. Normal variants include *familial short stature* and *constitutional delay*. Chronic diseases include *growth hormone deficiency*, other endocrine diseases, *gastrointestinal disease, renal* or *metabolic disease*, and *genetic syndromes*.

After age 2 years children should grow at least 5 cm per year. During puberty, growth velocity increases.

Young children can have inadequate weight and height gain if caloric intake is insufficient. Etiologies include *psychosocial, interactional, gastrointestinal, and endocrine disorders.*

Weight. Children who can stand should be weighed in a gown (or in clothing without shoes) on a stand-up scale. Use the same scales across successive visits to optimize comparability.

Head Circumference. In general, head circumference is measured until the child reaches 24 months. Afterward, head circumference measurement may be helpful if you suspect a genetic or a central nervous system disorder.

Body Mass Index for Age. Age- and sex-specific charts are now available to assess BMI in children. BMI in children is associated with body fat, related to subsequent health risks for obesity. BMI measurements are helpful for early detection of obesity in children older than 2 years. BMI growth charts for children take into account differences by sex and age. Obesity is now a major childhood epidemic and it often begins before age 6 to 8 years. Consequences of childhood obesity include *hypertension, diabetes, metabolic syndrome, and poor self-esteem.* Childhood obesity *often leads to adult obesity and shortened lifespan.* It is helpful to give parents their child's BMI results together with information about the impact of healthy eating and physical activity.

Most children with exogenous obesity are also tall for their age. Children with endocrine causes of obesity tend to be short.

Childhood obesity is a major epidemic: 32% of U.S. children have a BMI greater than the 85th percentile, and 17% have a BMI in the 95th percentile or greater.[34] Long-term morbidity from childhood obesity spans many organ systems, including cardiovascular, endocrine, renal, musculoskeletal, gastrointestinal, and psychological. Prevention, early detection, and aggressive management are needed.

Interpreting BMI in Children

Group	BMI-for-Age
Underweight	<5th percentile
Healthy weight	5th–85th percentile
Overweight	85th–95th percentile
Obese	≥95th percentile

Vital Signs

Blood Pressure. Hypertension during childhood is more common than previously thought and it is important to recognize, confirm, and appropriately manage it.

Children have elevated blood pressure during exercise, crying, and anxiety. The procedure for measuring blood pressure was explained and demonstrated beforehand. Most children are cooperative with blood pressure measurement. If the blood pressure is initially elevated you can perform blood pressure readings again at the end of the examination. Leave the cuff on the arm (deflated) and repeat the reading later. Elevated readings must always be confirmed by subsequent measurements.

A very common cause of apparent hypertension is anxiety or "white-coat hypertension." The most frequent "cause" of an elevated blood pressure in children is probably an *improperly performed examination,* often due to an incorrect cuff size.

A proper cuff size is essential for accurate determinations of blood pressure in children. Select the blood pressure cuff as you would for adults; it should be wide enough to cover two thirds of the upper arm or leg (Fig. 18-56). *A narrower cuff falsely elevates the blood pressure reading,* whereas *a wider cuff lowers it* and may interfere with proper placement of the stethoscope diaphragm over the artery.

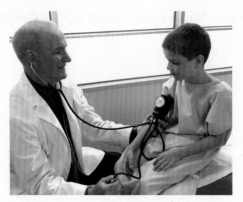

FIGURE 18-56. Blood pressure monitoring in childhood can be challenging.

With children, as with adults, the first Korotkoff sound indicates systolic pressure and the point at which the Korotkoff sounds disappear constitutes the diastolic pressure. At times, especially among chubby young children, the Korotkoff sounds are not easily heard. In such instances, you can use palpation to determine the systolic blood pressure, remembering that the systolic pressure obtained is approximately 10 mm Hg lower by palpation than by auscultation.

A relatively inaccurate method is "inspection." If unable to obtain the blood pressure by auscultation/palpation, watch for the needle to bounce by about 10 mm Hg. The systolic blood pressure obtained by "inspection" is about 1 mm Hg higher than that obtained by auscultation.

In 2004, the National Heart, Lung, and Blood Institute's National High Blood Pressure Working Group on Hypertension Control in Children and Adolescents defined normal, high-normal, and high blood pressure as follows, with measurements on at least three separate occasions.[36]

In children, as in adults, blood pressure readings from the thigh are approximately 10 mm Hg higher than those from the upper arm. If they are the same or lower, *coarctation of the aorta* should be suspected.

Transient hypertension in children can be caused by some *common childhood medications*, including those to treat asthma (e.g., prednisone) and ADHD (e.g., Ritalin).

Causes of *sustained hypertension*[35] in childhood include primary hypertension (with no underlying etiology) and secondary hypertension (which has an underlying etiology). Causes of secondary hypertension include: renal, endocrine, and neurologic disease, vascular causes, drugs or medications and psychological causes. Obesity is highly associated with hypertension in childhood.

The epidemic of childhood obesity has also resulted in a rising prevalence of childhood hypertension.[37,38]

Blood Pressure in Children and Adolescents

Blood Pressure Category	Average Systolic and/or Diastolic Blood Pressure for Age, Sex, and Height
Normal	<90th percentile
Prehypertensive	90th–95th percentile
Hypertensive	≥95th percentile
• stage 1	95th percentile to 5 mm Hg above 99th percentile
• stage 2	≥99th percentile plus 5 mm Hg[a]

[a]Refer to standard blood pressure tables based on age.

Children who have hypertension should be evaluated extensively to determine the cause. For infants and young children, a specific cause can often be found. An increasing proportion of older children and adolescents, however, have essential or primary hypertension. In all cases it is important to repeat measurements to reduce the possibility that the elevation reflects anxiety. Sometimes, repeating measurements in school is a way to obtain readings in a more relaxed environment. *Hypertension and obesity often coexist in children.*

It is important not to *falsely label* a child or adolescent as having hypertension because of the stigma of labeling, potential limitations to activities, and possible side effects of treatment.

Pulse. Average heart rates and normal ranges are shown in the table below. Measure the heart rate over a 60-second interval.

Average Heart Rate of Children at Rest

Age	Average Rate	Range (Two Standard Deviations)
1–2 yrs	110	70–150
2–6 yrs	103	68–138
6–10 yrs	95	65–125

Sinus bradycardia is a heart rate <100 beats per minute in infants and toddlers and <60 beats per minute in children 3 to 9 years.

Respiratory Rate. The rate of respirations per minute ranges from 20 to 40 during early childhood and 15 to 25 during late childhood, reaching adult levels at around 15 years of age.[39]

For young children, observe the movements of the chest wall for two 30-second intervals or over 1 minute, preferably before stimulating them. Direct auscultation of the chest or placing the stethoscope in front of the mouth is also useful for counting respirations, but the measurement may be falsely elevated if the child becomes agitated. For older children use the same technique as that used for adults.

Children with respiratory diseases such as *bronchiolitis* or *pneumonia* have rapid respirations (up to 80 to 90/min) and increased work of breathing such as grunting, nasal flaring, or use of accessory muscles.

The commonly accepted standard for tachypnea in children older than age 1 year is a respiratory rate >40 breaths per minute. The best single physical finding for ruling out *pneumonia* is an absence of tachypnea.

Temperature. In children, auditory canal temperature recordings are preferable because they can be obtained quickly with essentially no discomfort.

Children younger than 3 years, who appear very ill with a fever, should be evaluated for *sepsis, urinary tract infection, pneumonia,* or other *serious infection.*

The Skin

After a child's first year of life, the techniques of examination are the same as those for the adult (see Chapter 6, The Skin, Hair, and Nails).

The Head

In examining the head and neck, tailor your examination to the child's stage of growth and development.

Even before touching the child, carefully observe the shape of the head, its symmetry, and the presence of abnormal facies. Abnormal facies may not be apparent until later in childhood; therefore, carefully examine the face as well as the head of all children.

There are diagnostic facies in childhood (Table 18-6, Diagnostic Facies in Infancy and Childhood, pp. 914–915, shows several) that reflect chromosomal abnormalities, endocrine defects, chronic illness, and other disorders.

Fetal alcohol syndrome can cause abnormal facies (p. 914), microcephaly, and developmental delay.

The Eyes

The two most important components of the eye examination for young children are to determine whether the gaze is conjugate or symmetric and to test visual acuity in each eye.

Strabismus (see Table 18-7, Abnormalities of the Eyes, Ears, and Mouth, p. 916) in children requires treatment by an ophthalmologist.

Conjugate Gaze. Use the methods described in Chapter 7 for adults to assess conjugate gaze, or the position and alignment of the eyes, and the function of the extraocular muscles. The corneal light reflex test and the cover–uncover test are particularly useful in young children (Figs. 18-57 and 18-58).

Both *ocular strabismus* and *anisometropia* (eyes with significantly different refractive errors) can result in *amblyopia,* or reduced vision in an otherwise normal eye. *Amblyopia* can lead to a "lazy eye," with permanently reduced visual acuity if not corrected early.

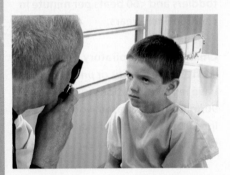

FIGURE 18-57. **Corneal light reflex test.**

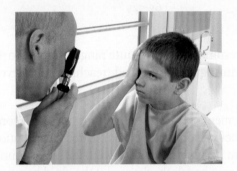

FIGURE 18-58. **Cover–uncover test.**

Perform the cover–uncover test as a game by having the young child watch your nose or tell you if you are smiling or not while you cover one of the child's eyes. When you uncover the eye, watch for any deviation of that eye. Repeat for the other eye. Latent strabismus is indicated by movement of either eye when uncovered.

The common forms of strabismus in children involve horizontal deviation: nasal ("eso") or temporal ("exo"). A *latent strabismus* ("phoria") occurs when you disrupt fixation, whereas *manifest strabismus* ("tropia") is present without interruption.

Visual Acuity. It may not be possible to measure the *visual acuity* of children younger than 3 years who cannot identify pictures on an eye chart. For these children, the simplest examination is to assess for fixation preference by alternately covering one eye; the child with normal vision will not object, but a child with poor vision in one eye will object to having the good eye covered. Importantly, if you or the parent have any doubts about visual acuity, it is wise to refer to an optometrist or ophthalmologist because this aspect of the physical examination is insensitive. In all tests of visual acuity it is important that both eyes show the same result because of the risk for amblyopia.

Reduced visual acuity is more likely among children who were born prematurely and among those with other neurologic or developmental disorders.

Visual Acuity

Age	Acuity
3 mo	Eyes converge, baby reaches
12 mo	~20/200
Younger than 4 yrs	20/40
4 yrs and older	20/30

Any difference in visual acuity between the eyes (e.g., 20/20 on the left and 20/30 on the right) is abnormal by age 5 years (Figs. 18-59 and 18-60).

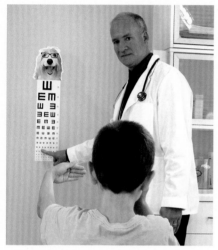

FIGURE 18-59. **Testing visual acuity with a simple chart.**

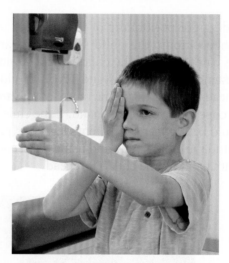

FIGURE 18-60. **Test each eye and note the difference in acuity.**

Visual acuity in children 4 years and older can usually be formally tested using an eye chart with one of a variety of optotypes (characters or symbols).[40] A child who does not know letters or numbers reliably can be tested using pictures, symbols, or the "E" chart. Using the "E" chart, most children will cooperate by telling you in which direction the "E" is pointing.

The most common visual disorder of childhood is *myopia,* which can be easily detected using this examination technique.

Some children develop *abnormalities in near vision,* which can lead to reading difficulties, headaches, and school problems, as well as double vision.

Visual Fields. While it is often challenging, the *visual fields* can be examined in infants and young children with the child sitting on the parent's lap. One eye should be tested at a time with the other eye covered. Hold the child's head in the midline while bringing an object such as a toy into the field of vision from behind the child. The overall method is the same as that for adults, except that you will have to make this into a game for your patient.

The Ears

Examining the *ear canal and drum* can be difficult in young children who are sensitive and fearful because they cannot observe the procedure. With a little practice though, you can master this technique. Unfortunately, *many young children need to be briefly restrained during this examination, which is why you may want to leave it for the end.*

If the child is not too fearful, you may examine the ears with the child sitting on a parent's lap. Make a game out of the otoscopic examination, such as finding an imaginary object in the child's ear or talking playfully to allay fears. It may help to place the otoscopic speculum gently into the external auditory canal of one ear and then withdraw it so that the child gets used to the procedure before the actual examination. It is also helpful to show the child that the speculum does not hurt by letting the child touch it and shine a light through your finger.

Ask the parent for a preference regarding the positioning of the child for the examination. There are two common positions: the child lying down and restrained, and the child sitting in the parent's lap. If the child is held supine, have the parent hold the arms either extended (Figs. 18-61 and 18-62) or close to the sides to limit motion. Hold the head and pull the pinna (auricle) upwards with one hand while you hold the otoscope with your other hand. If the child is on the parent's lap, the child's legs should be between the parent's legs. The parent could help by placing one arm around the child's body and using the second arm to steady the head (with the parent's hand on the child's forehead).

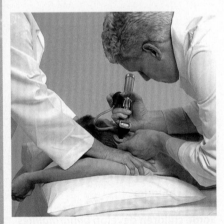

FIGURE 18-61. **Gently holding the child's arms reduces reactions to the otoscope.**

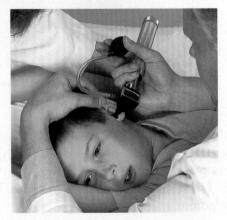

FIGURE 18-62. **Hand positions for standard otoscope approach.**

Gently move and pull on the *pinna* before or during your otoscopic examination. Carefully inspect the area behind the pinna, over the mastoid bone. Many offices now use a tympanometer, which measures the compliance of the tympanic membrane and helps to diagnose a middle ear effusion.

Tympanic Membranes. Many students have difficulty visualizing a child's tympanic membrane. In young children, the external auditory canal is directed upward and backward from the outside, and *the auricle must be pulled upward, outward, and backward to afford the best view.* Press the child's head with one hand, and with that same hand pull up on the auricle. Position the otoscope with your other hand.

With acute *mastoiditis,* the auricle may protrude forward and outward, and the area over the mastoid bone is red, swollen, and tender.

Tips for Conducting the Otoscopic Examination

- Use the best angle of the otoscope.
- Use the largest possible speculum.
  - A larger speculum allows you to better visualize the tympanic membrane and is less painful since it is not inserted as far as a smaller speculum.
  - A small speculum may not provide a seal for pneumatic otoscopy.
- Don't apply too much pressure which will cause the child to cry and may cause false-positive results on pneumatic otoscopy.
- Insert the speculum ¼ to ½ inch into the canal.
- First find the landmarks.
  - Careful—sometimes the ear canal resembles the tympanic membrane.
- Note whether the tympanic membrane is abnormal.
- Remove cerumen if it is blocking your view, using one of the following:
  - Special plastic curettes
  - A moistened microtipped cotton swab
  - Flushing of ears for older children
  - Special instruments that can also be purchased.

There are two ways to hold the otoscope, as illustrated by the following figures:

- The first is the method generally used in adults, with the otoscope handle pointing upward or laterally while you pull up on the auricle. Hold the lateral aspect of your hand that has the otoscope against the child's head to provide a buffer against sudden movements by the patient (Figs. 18-61 and 18-62).

- The second position, with the handle of the otoscope pointing down toward the child's feet, is preferred by many pediatricians because of the angle of the auditory canal in children. While holding the otoscope with the handle pointing down, pull up on the auricle. Steady your hand against the child's head and pull up on the auricle with that hand, while you hold the otoscope with the other hand (Figs. 18-63 and 18-64).

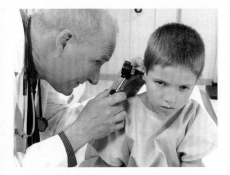

FIGURE 18-63. Gently pulling up on the auricle gives a better otoscope view with many children.

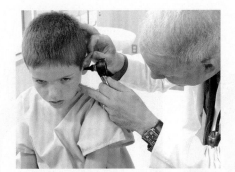

FIGURE 18-64. Auricle pulled up, handle pointed down, assessing left ear.

Acute otitis media is a common condition of childhood. A symptomatic child typically has a red, bulging tympanic membrane with a dull or absent light reflex and diminished movement on pneumatic otoscopy. Purulent material may also be seen behind the tympanic membrane. See Table 18-7, Abnormalities of the Eyes, Ears, and Mouth, p. 916. The most useful symptom in making the diagnosis is ear pain, if combined with the above signs.[41–43]

You can use a *pneumatic otoscope* to improve the accuracy of diagnosis of otitis media in children (Fig. 18-65). This allows you to assess the mobility of the tympanic membrane as you increase and decrease the pressure in the external auditory canal by squeezing the rubber bulb of the pneumatic otoscope.

First, check the pneumatic otoscope for leaks by placing your finger over the tip of the speculum and squeezing the bulb. Note the pressure on the bulb. Then insert the speculum, obtaining a proper seal; this is critical because failure to obtain a seal can produce a false-positive finding (lack of movement of the tympanic membrane). Of note, this process requires a cooperative patient.

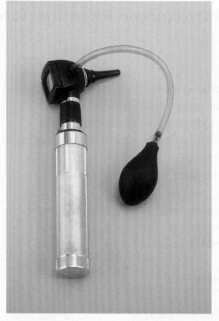

FIGURE 18-65. **Pneumatic otoscope.**

Sometimes when you are examining acute otitis media leads to a *ruptured tympanic membrane*, leading to pus in the auditory canal. In these cases, you will generally not visualize the tympanic membrane.

With *otitis externa* (but not otitis media), movement of the pinna elicits pain.

When air is introduced into the normal ear canal, the tympanic membrane and its light reflex move inward. When air is removed, the tympanic membrane moves outward. This rapid, subtle to-and-fro movement of the tympanic membrane has been likened to the luffing of a sail. If the tympanic membrane fails to move perceptibly as you introduce positive or negative pressure, the child is likely to have a middle ear effusion (or the technique was poor). A child with acute otitis media may flinch because of pain due to the air pressure.

Hearing Testing. Formal hearing testing is necessary for accurate detection of hearing deficits in young children. Once the child is old enough to cooperate, use a formal hearing test method. You can grossly test for hearing in very young children by using the whispered voice test. Stand behind the child (so that the child cannot read your lips), cover one of the child's ear canals, and rub the

Movement of the tympanic membrane is absent in middle ear effusion (*otitis media with effusion*).

Significantly, *temporary hearing loss* for several months can accompany otitis media with effusion.

Younger children who fail these screening maneuvers or who have speech delay should have audiometric testing. These children may have *hearing deficits* or central auditory processing disorders.

Up to 15% of school-aged children have at least *mild hearing loss*, emphasizing the importance of screening for hearing prior to school age.[41]

The two types of hearing loss seen in children are *conductive* and *sensorineural* hearing loss.

Causes of *conductive hearing loss* include congenital abnormalities, trauma, recurrent otitis media, and tympanic membrane perforation.

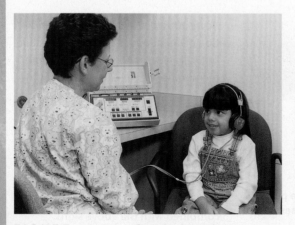

FIGURE 18-66. **Standardized testing equipment provides more precise metrics.**

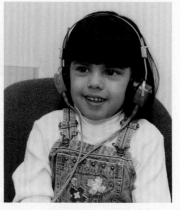

FIGURE 18-67. **Children often enjoy a full-scale acoustic screening test.**

tragus, using a circular motion. Whisper letters, numbers, or a word and have the child repeat it, and then test the other ear. This technique has relatively high sensitivity and specificity compared to formal testing.[44]

The AAP recommends that *all children older than 4 years have a full-scale acoustic screening test using standardized equipment* (Figs. 18-66 and 18-67).[4] Even though a normal hearing screen at birth is reassuring, some hearing loss is acquired as children age and hearing loss can dramatically affect a child's language and development. If you do use an acoustic screening test, be sure to test the entire acoustic range, including the speaking range (500 to 6,000 Hz). The table below shows one classification of hearing ranges.

Hearing Ranges on Formal Acoustic Screening Tests	
Normal hearing	0–20 dB
Mild hearing loss	21–40 dB
Moderate hearing loss	41–60 dB
Severe hearing loss	61–90 dB
Profound hearing loss	>90 dB

Causes of *sensorineural hearing loss* include hereditary congenital infections, ototopic drugs, trauma, and some infections such as meningitis.

The Nose and Sinuses

Inspect the anterior portion of the nose by using a large speculum on your otoscope. Inspect the nasal mucous membranes, noting their color and condition. Look for nasal septal deviation and the presence of polyps (Fig. 18-68).

Maxillary sinuses are noted on x-rays by age 4 years, sphenoid sinuses by age 6 years, and frontal sinuses by age 6 to 7 years. The sinuses of older children can be palpated as in adults, looking for tenderness.[45] Transillumination of the paranasal sinuses of younger children has poor sensitivity and specificity for diagnosing sinusitis or fluid in the sinuses.

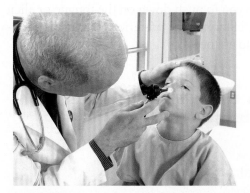

FIGURE 18-68. **Nasal inspection of children often has different results than adults.**

Pale, boggy nasal mucous membranes are found in children with *allergic rhinitis.*

Purulent rhinitis is common in viral infections but may be part of the constellation of symptoms of *sinusitis.*

Foul-smelling, purulent, unilateral discharge from the nose may be due to a *foreign body.* This most often occurs among *young preschool children* who tend to stick objects into body orifices.

Nasal polyps are flesh-colored growths inside the nares. They are generally isolated findings, but can be part of a syndrome.

Children with purulent rhinorrhea (generally unilateral) for more than 10 days, and also headache, sore throat, fever, and tenderness over the sinuses may have *sinusitis.*

The Mouth and Pharynx

For anxious or young children, it is wise to leave the examination of the mouth and pharynx until the end because it may require parental restraint. The young, cooperative child may be more comfortable sitting in the parent's lap.

Healthy children are more likely to cooperate with this examination than sick children, especially if the sick child sees the tongue depressor or has had previous experience with throat cultures.

Figure 18-69 demonstrates how to get children to open their mouths. The child who can say "ahhh" will usually offer a sufficient (albeit brief) view of the posterior pharynx so that a tongue depressor is unnecessary.

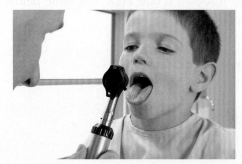

FIGURE 18-69. Children generally imitate well enough to allow you to inspect the back of their mouths.

If you need to use a tongue depressor, push down and pull slightly forward toward yourself while the child says "ahhh," being careful not to place the depressor too far posteriorly, eliciting a gag reflex. Sometimes, young and anxious children will need to be restrained and will clamp their teeth and purse their lips. In these cases, carefully slip the tongue depressor between the teeth and onto the tongue. This will either allow you to push down on the tongue or elicit a gag reflex, which should permit a brief look at the posterior pharynx and tonsils. Careful planning and parental help are needed.

How to Get Children to Open Their Mouths (a.k.a., "Would You Please Say 'Ahhh'?")

- Turn it into a game.
  - "Now let's see what's in your mouth."
  - "Can you stick out your *whole tongue*?"
  - "I bet you can't open your mouth *really wide*!"
  - "Let me see the inside of your teeth."
  - "Can you pant like a dog on a hot day?"
- Don't show a tongue depressor unless really necessary.
- Demonstrate first on an older sibling (or even the parent).
- Offer enthusiastic praise for opening their mouths a little and encourage them to open even wider.

Dental caries are the *most common health problem in children.* They are particularly prevalent in impoverished populations and can cause both short-term and long-term problems.[46] Caries are highly treatable but require a dental visit.

Examine the *teeth* for the timing and sequence of eruption, number, character, condition, and position. Abnormalities of the enamel may reflect local or general disease.

Carefully inspect the upper teeth as shown in Figure 18-70. This is a common location for *nursing-bottle caries*. The technique shown in the photo, called "lift the lip," can help visualize dental caries.

Visualize the inside of the upper teeth by having the child look up at the ceiling with the mouth wide open.

The box below displays the common pattern of tooth eruption. In general, lower teeth erupt a bit earlier than upper teeth.

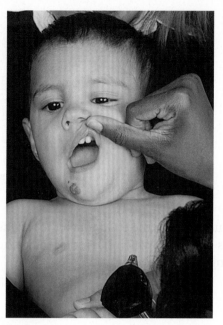

FIGURE 18-70. Lift the lip to check for dental caries.

Dental caries are caused by bacterial activity. Caries are more likely among young children who have prolonged bottle-feeding ("nursing-bottle caries"). See Table 18-8, Abnormalities of the Teeth, Pharynx, and Neck, p. 917, for different stages of caries.

Staining of the teeth may be intrinsic or extrinsic. Intrinsic stains may be from tetracycline use before 8 years (yellow, gray, or brown stain). Iron preparation (black stain) and fluoride (white stain) are examples of extrinsic stains. Extrinsic stains can be polished off; intrinsic stains cannot (see Table 18-8, Abnormalities of the Teeth, Pharynx, and Neck, p. 917).

Tooth Types and Age of Eruption

Tooth Type	Approximate Age of Eruption[47]	
	Primary (mo)	Permanent (yrs)
Central incisor	5–8	6–8
Lateral incisor	5–11	7–9
Cuspids	24–30	11–12
First bicuspids	—	10–12
Second bicuspids	—	10–12
First molars	16–20	6–7
Second molars	24–30	11–13
Third molars	—	17–22

Look for abnormalities of the position of the teeth. These include malocclusion, maxillary protrusion (*overbite*), and mandibular protrusion (*underbite*). You can demonstrate the latter two by asking the child to bite down hard while either you or the child parts the lips. Normally, the lower teeth are contained within the arch formed by the upper teeth.

Malocclusion and misalignment of teeth can be from thumb sucking, a hereditary condition, or premature loss of primary teeth.

Carefully inspect the *tongue,* including the underside (Fig. 18-71). Most children will happily stick their tongue out at you, move it from side to side, and demonstrate its color.

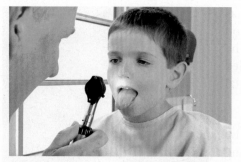

FIGURE 18-71. **Inspect all parts of the tongue.**

Some young children have a tight frenulum. Have the child touch the tongue to the roof of the mouth to diagnose this condition which often does not require treatment unless it interferes with eating or speech.

Note the size, position, symmetry, and appearance of the *tonsils.* The peak growth of tonsillar tissue is between 8 and 16 years (Fig. 18-54). The size of the tonsils varies considerably in children and is often categorized on a scale of 1+ to 4+, with 1+ being easy visibility of the gap between the tonsils, and 4+ being tonsils that touch in the midline with the mouth wide open. The tonsils in children often appear more obstructive than they really are.

Tonsils in children usually have deep crypts on their surfaces, which often have white concretions or food particles protruding from their depths. This does not indicate disease.

Look for clues of a submucosal cleft palate such as notching of the posterior margin of the hard palate or a bifid *uvula.* Because the mucosa is intact, the underlying defect is easily missed, but needs referral to otolaryngology.

Extremely rarely, you may encounter a child who has a sore throat and has difficulty swallowing saliva and who is sitting up stiffly in a "tripod" position because of throat obstruction. Do not open this child's mouth because he may have acute epiglottitis, or obstruction from another cause, and examination of the throat may induce gagging and laryngeal obstruction.

Note the quality of the child's voice. Certain abnormalities can change the pitch and quality of the voice.

Common abnormalities include *coated tongue* in viral infections, and *strawberry tongue,* from scarlet fever.

Children who are severely "tongue-tied" might have a speech impediment.

A *geographic tongue* is a benign but chronic condition in which a portion of the tongue has a rough, unusual appearance.

Streptococcal pharyngitis typically produces a strawberry tongue, white or yellow exudates on the tonsils or posterior pharynx, a beefy-red uvula, and palatal petechiae; see Table 18-8, p. 917.[48]

A *peritonsillar abscess* is suggested by erythema and asymmetric enlargement of one tonsil, pain, and lateral displacement of the uvula.

Acute epiglottitis is now rare in the United States because of immunization against *Haemophilus influenzae* type B.

Bacterial tracheitis can cause airway obstruction.

Tonsillitis can be caused by bacteria, such as *Streptococcus,* or viruses. The "rocks in the mouth" voice is accompanied by enlarged tonsils with exudates.

Voice Changes— Clues to Underlying Abnormalities

Voice Change	Possible Abnormality
Hypernasal speech	Submucosal cleft palate
Nasal voice plus snoring	Adenoidal hypertrophy
Hoarse voice plus cough	Viral infection (croup)
"Rocks in mouth"	Tonsillitis

The epidemic of childhood obesity has resulted in many children who snore and have sleep apnea.

You may note an abnormal breath odor which may help lead to a specific diagnosis.

Halitosis in a child can be caused by upper respiratory, pharyngeal, or mouth infection, foreign body in the nose, sinusitis, dental disease, and gastroesophageal reflux.

The Neck

Beyond infancy, the techniques for examining the neck are the same as for adults. Lymphadenopathy is unusual during infancy but very common during childhood. The child's lymphatic system reaches its zenith of growth at 12 years, and cervical or tonsillar lymph nodes reach their peak size between 8 and 16 years (Fig. 18-54).

Lymphadenopathy is usually from viral or bacterial infections (see Table 18-8, Abnormalities of the Teeth, Pharynx, and Neck, p. 917).

The vast majority of enlarged lymph nodes in children are due to infections (mostly viral, but sometimes bacterial) and not due to malignant disease, even though the latter is a concern for many parents. It is important to differentiate normal lymph nodes from abnormal ones or from congenital cysts of the neck.

Malignancy is more likely if the node is *>2 cm, is hard, or is fixed to the skin or underlying tissues* (i.e., not mobile) and is *accompanied by serious systemic signs* such as weight loss.

Figure 18-25 on p. 828 demonstrates the typical anatomical locations of lymph nodes and congenital cysts of the neck.

Check for *neck mobility*. It is important to ensure that the neck of all children is supple and easily mobile in all directions. This is particularly important when the patient is holding the head in an asymmetric manner and when central nervous system disease such as meningitis is suspected.

In young children with small necks, it may be difficult to differentiate low posterior cervical lymph nodes from *supraclavicular lymph nodes* (which are always abnormal and raise suspicion for malignancy).

In children, the presence of *nuchal rigidity* is a more reliable indicator of meningeal irritation than *Brudzinski sign* or *Kernig sign*. To detect nuchal rigidity in older children, ask the child to sit with legs extended on the examining table. Normally, children should be able to sit upright and touch their chins to their chests. Younger children can be persuaded to flex their necks by having them follow a small toy or light beam. You also can test for nuchal rigidity with the child lying on the examining table, as shown in Figure 18-72. Nearly all children with nuchal rigidity will be extremely sick, irritable, and difficult to examine. In many countries the incidence of bacterial meningitis has plummeted because of vaccinations.

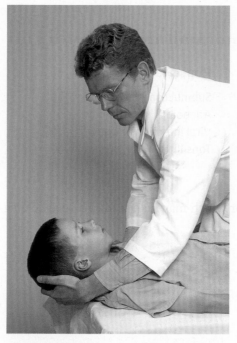

FIGURE 18-72. Inspect the neck for nuchal rigidity.

Nuchal rigidity is marked resistance to movement of the head in any direction. It suggests meningeal irritation due to *meningitis, bleeding, tumor,* or *other causes.* These children are extremely irritable and difficult to console and may have "paradoxical irritability"—increased irritability when being held.

When meningeal irritation is present, the child may assume the *tripod position* and is unable to assume a full upright position to perform the chin-to-chest maneuver.

The Thorax and Lungs

As children age, the lung examination becomes similar to that for adults. Cooperation is critical. Auscultation is usually easiest when a child barely notices (as when in a parent's lap). Let a toddler who seems fearful of the stethoscope play with it before it touches the child's chest.

Assess the relative proportion of time spent on inspiration versus expiration. *The normal ratio is about 1:1.* Prolonged inspirations or expirations are a clue to disease location. Degree of prolongation and effort or "work of breathing" are related to disease severity.

With upper airway obstruction such as croup, inspiration is prolonged and accompanied by other signs such as stridor, cough, or rhonchi.

With lower airway obstruction such as asthma, expiration is prolonged and often accompanied by wheezing.

Young children asked to "take deep breaths" often hold their breath, further complicating auscultation. It is easier to let preschoolers breathe normally. Demonstrate to older children how to take nice, quiet, deep breaths. Make it a game. To accomplish a forced expiratory maneuver, ask the child to blow out candles on an imaginary birthday cake or use pinwheels (Fig. 18-73).

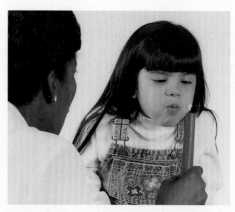

FIGURE 18-73. Getting a child to perform a forced expiration.

Pneumonia in young children is generally manifested by fever, tachypnea, dyspnea, and increased work of breathing.

Although *upper respiratory infections* due to viruses can cause young infants to appear quite ill, in children they present with the same signs as in adults and children generally appear well without lower respiratory signs.

Childhood asthma is an extremely common condition throughout the world. Children with acute asthma present with varying severity and often have increased work of breathing. Expiratory wheezing and a prolonged expiratory

Older children will be cooperative for the respiratory examination and can even go through the maneuvers of assessing fremitus or listening to "E to A" changes (see pp. 326–327). As children grow, the evaluation by observation discussed on the previous page, such as assessing the work of breathing, nasal flaring, and grunting, becomes less helpful in assessing for respiratory pathology. Palpation, percussion, and auscultation achieve greater importance in a careful examination of the thorax and lungs.

Children in respiratory distress may assume a "*tripod position*" in which they lean forward to optimize airway patency (Fig. 18-74). This same position can also be caused by pharyngeal obstruction (see p. 874).

phase, caused by reversible broncho-spasm, may be heard without the stethoscope and are apparent on auscultation. Wheezes are often accompanied by inspiratory rhonchi caused by upper respiratory congestion.[49] Asthma flares often occur with viral infections.

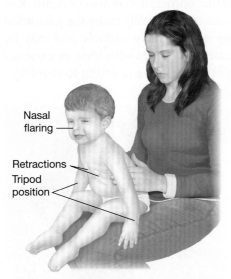

Nasal flaring

Retractions
Tripod position

FIGURE 18-74. **A child in respiratory distress**

The Heart

The examination of the heart and vascular systems in infants and children is similar to that in adults. However, a child's fearfulness or inability to cooperate may make the examination difficult while the desire to play will make the examination easier and more productive. Use your knowledge of the developmental stage of each child. A 2-year-old may be the easiest to examine while standing or sitting on the mother's lap, facing her shoulder, or being held (Fig. 18-75). Give young children something to hold in each hand. They cannot figure out how to drop one object and, therefore, have no hand free to push you away. Endless chatter to small children will hold their attention and they may forget you are examining them. Let older children move the stethoscope themselves, going back to listen properly.

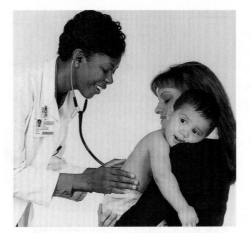

FIGURE 18-75. **Young children are easiest to examine when held by a parent.**

General abnormalities may suggest increased likelihood of congenital cardiac disease as exemplified by Down syndrome or Turner syndrome.

Blood Pressure. Measure the blood pressure in both arms and one leg at one time around age 3 to 4 years to check for possible *coarctation of the aorta*. Thereafter, only the right arm blood pressure needs to be measured.

Benign Murmurs. Preschool and school-aged children often have benign murmurs (see figure on p. 879). The most common (*Still's murmur*) is a grade I–II/VI, musical, vibratory, early and midsystolic murmur with multiple overtones located over the mid or lower left sternal border; it may also be heard over the carotid arteries. Carotid artery compression will usually cause the precordial murmur to disappear. This murmur may be extremely variable and may be accentuated when cardiac output is increased, as occurs with fever or exercise. The murmur will diminish as the child goes from supine to sitting to standing.

In preschool or school-aged children, you may detect a *venous hum*. This is a soft, hollow, continuous sound, louder in diastole, heard just below the right clavicle (Fig. 18-76). It can be completely eliminated by maneuvers that affect venous return, such as lying supine, changing head position, or jugular venous compression. It has the same quality as breath sounds and is therefore frequently overlooked.

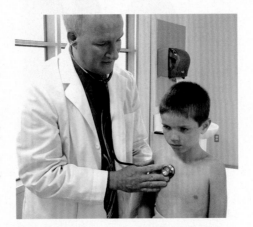

FIGURE 18-76. **Listening for venous hum.**

Among young children, murmurs without the recognizable features of the common benign murmurs may signify underlying heart disease and should be evaluated thoroughly by a pediatric cardiologist.

Pathologic murmurs that signify cardiac disease can first appear after infancy and during childhood. Examples include aortic stenosis and mitral valve disease.

The murmur heard in the carotid area or just above the clavicles is known as a *carotid bruit*. It is early and midsystolic with a slightly harsh quality. It is usually louder on the left and may be heard alone or in combination with the Still's murmur. It may be completely eradicated by carotid artery compression (Fig. 18-77).

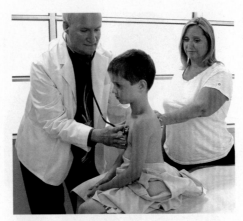

FIGURE 18-77. **Carotid artery compression while listening to murmur.**

Location and Characteristics of Benign Heart Murmurs in Children[a]

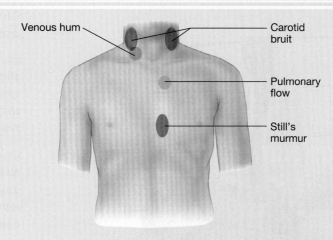

Typical Age	Name	Characteristics	Description and Location
Preschool or early school age	*Still's murmur*		Grade I–II/VI, musical, vibratory Multiple overtones Early and midsystolic Mid/lower left sternal border Frequently also a carotid bruit
Preschool or early school age	*Venous hum*		Soft, hollow, continuous Louder in diastole Under clavicle Can be eliminated by maneuvers
Preschool and later	*Carotid bruit*		Early and midsystolic Usually louder on left Eliminated by carotid compression
Preschool and school age	*Pulmonary flow murmur*	S_1 S_2	Grade 2–3 systolic ejection Loudest at pulmonary auscultation area Harsh, nonvibratory Intensity increases when in the supine position

[a]See the table on p. 896 for location and characteristics of benign heart murmurs in older children and adolescents.

The Abdomen

Toddlers and young children commonly have protuberant abdomens, most apparent when they are upright. The examination can follow the same order as for adults except that you may need to distract the child during the examination.

Most children are ticklish when you first place your hand on their abdomens for *palpation*. This reaction tends to disappear, particularly if you distract the child with conversation and place your whole hand flush on the abdominal surface for a few moments without probing. For children who are particularly sensitive and who tighten their abdominal muscles you can start by placing the child's hand under yours. Eventually, you will be able to remove the child's hand and palpate the abdomen freely.

An exaggerated "pot-belly appearance" may indicate malabsorption from *celiac disease, cystic fibrosis,* or *constipation* or *aerophagia.*

A common condition of childhood that can occasionally cause a protuberant abdomen is *constipation.* The abdomen is often tympanitic on percussion, and stool is sometimes felt on palpation.

Try flexing the knees and hips to relax the child's abdominal wall, as shown in Figure 18-78. Palpate lightly in all areas, then deeply, leaving the site of potential pathology to the end.

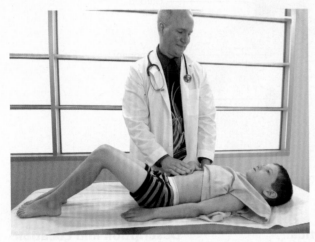

FIGURE 18-78. Position child as shown to palpate abdomen.

Expected Liver Span of Children by Percussion

Age in Yrs	Mean Estimated Liver Span (cm)	
	Males	Females
2	3.5	3.6
3	4.0	4.0
4	4.4	4.3
5	4.8	4.5
6	5.1	4.8
8	5.6	5.1
10	6.1	5.4

One method to determine the lower border of the liver involves the *scratch test,* shown in Figures 18-79 and 18-80. Place the diaphragm of your stethoscope just above the right costal margin at the midclavicular line. With your fingernail, lightly scratch the skin of the abdomen along the midclavicular line, moving from below the umbilicus toward the costal margin. When your scratching finger reaches the liver's edge you will hear a change in the scratching sound as it passes through the liver to your stethoscope. The accuracy of the scratch test has not been well studied.[50]

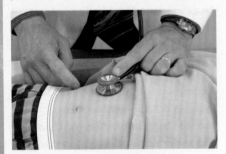

FIGURE 18-79. Palpate the lower border of the liver starting low.

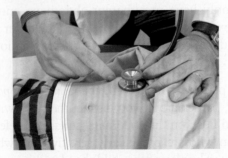

FIGURE 18-80. Move your finger cephalad to the rib.

Chronic or recurrent abdominal pain is relatively common in children. Causes include both *functional disorders* and *organic disorders.*

Functional disorders causing abdominal pain include *irritable bowel syndrome, functional dyspepsia,* and *childhood functional abdominal pain syndrome.*

Organic causes of chronic or recurrent abdominal pain in children include *gastritis* or *ulcer, gastroesophageal reflux, constipation,* and *inflammatory bowel disease.*

Many children present with abdominal pain from *acute gastroenteritis.* Despite pain, their physical examination is relatively normal except for increased bowel sounds on auscultation and mild tenderness on palpation.

The childhood obesity epidemic has resulted in many children who have extremely obese abdomens. While it is difficult to accurately examine these children, the steps to the examination are the same as for normal children.

Hepatomegaly in young children is unusual. It can be caused by *cystic fibrosis, protein malabsorption,* parasites, *fatty liver,* and *tumors.*

If hepatomegaly is accompanied by splenomegaly, *portal hypertension, storage diseases, chronic infections,* and *malignancy* should be considered.

Various diseases can cause splenomegaly, including infections, hematologic disorders such as hemolytic anemias, infiltrative disorders, and inflammatory or autoimmune diseases, as well as congestion from portal hypertension.

The *spleen,* like the liver, is felt easily in most children. It too is soft with a sharp edge, and it projects downward like a tongue from under the left costal margin. The spleen is moveable and rarely extends more than 1 to 2 cm below the costal margin.

Palpate the *other abdominal structures.* You will commonly note pulsations in the epigastrium caused by the aorta. This is felt most easily to the left of the midline, on deep palpation.

An abdominal mass felt on palpation may represent stool from constipation, or a serious condition such as a tumor.

Palpating for abdominal tenderness in an older child is the same as for the adult; however, the causes of abdominal pain are often different, encompassing a wide spectrum of acute and chronic diseases. Localization of tenderness may help you pinpoint the abdominal structures most likely to be causing the abdominal pain.

In a child with an acute abdomen, as in *acute appendicitis,* check for involuntary rigidity, rebound tenderness, a Rovsing sign, or a positive psoas or obturator sign (see pp. 485–486).[51] *Gastroenteritis, constipation,* and *gastrointestinal obstruction* are other possible etiologies of acute abdominal pain.

Male Genitalia

Inspect the penis. The size in prepubertal children has little significance unless it is abnormally large. In obese boys, the fat pad over the symphysis pubis may obscure the penis.

In *precocious puberty,* the penis and testes are enlarged with signs of pubertal changes. Other pubertal changes also occur.

Precocious puberty is due to excess androgens and can be caused by multiple conditions including *adrenal or pituitary tumors.*

There is an art to *palpation* of the young boy's scrotum and testes because many have an extremely active cremasteric reflex that may cause the testis to retract upward into the inguinal canal and thereby appear to be undescended. Examine the child when he is relaxed because anxiety stimulates the cremasteric reflex. With warm hands, *palpate the lower abdomen, working your way downward toward the scrotum along the inguinal canal. This will minimize retraction of the testes* into the canal.

A useful technique is to have the boy sit cross-legged on the examining table, as shown in Figure 18-81. You can also give him a balloon to inflate or an object to lift to increase intra-abdominal pressure. If you can detect the testis in the scrotum it is descended, even if it spends much time in the inguinal canal. A painful testicle requires rapid treatment.

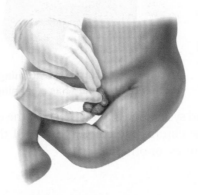

FIGURE 18-81. Position of child to palpate scrotum.

Cryptorchidism **may be noted at this age. It requires surgical correction. It should be differentiated from a retractile testis.**

Possible causes of a painful testicle include infection such as *epididymitis* or *orchitis, torsion of the testicle,* or *torsion of the appendix testis.*

A painless scrotal mass in a young boy is usually due to a hydrocele or a nonincarcerated inguinal hernia. Other rare causes include a varicocele or tumor.

The cremasteric reflex can be tested by scratching the medial aspect of the thigh. The testis on the side being scratched will move upward.

Examine the inguinal canal as you would for adults noting any swelling that may reflect an *inguinal hernia*. Have the boy increase abdominal pressure as described above and note whether a bulge in the inguinal canal increases with Valsalva.

Inguinal hernias in older boys present as they do in adult men with swelling in the inguinal canal, particularly following a Valsalva maneuver.

Female Genitalia

The genital examination can be anxiety provoking for the older child and adolescent (especially if you are of the opposite sex) and for parents. Nevertheless, not performed, a significant finding may be missed. Depending on the child's developmental stage, explain what parts of the body you will check and that this is part of the routine examination.

The appearance of pubic hair before age 7 years should be considered *precocious puberty* and requires evaluation to determine the cause.

After infancy, the labia majora and minora flatten out and the hymenal membrane becomes thin, translucent, and vascular, with the edges easily identified.

Rashes on the external genitals can be from physical irritation, sweating, and candidal or bacterial infections including streptococcal infection.

The genital examination is the same for all ages of children, from late infancy until adolescence. Use a calm, gentle approach including a developmentally appropriate explanation as you do the examination. A bright light source is essential. Most children can be examined in the supine, frog-leg position.

Vulvovaginal pruritis and *erythema* can be caused by external irritants, bubble baths, masturbatory activity, pinworms, or other infections such as *Candida* or *sexually transmitted infections.*

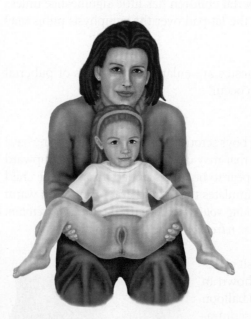

If the child seems reluctant, it may be helpful to have the parent sit on the examination table with the child; alternatively, the examination may be performed while the child sits in the parent's lap. Do not use stirrups as these may frighten the child. Figure 18-82 demonstrates a 5-year-old girl sitting on her parent's lap with the parent holding her knees outstretched.

FIGURE 18-82. Positioning mother behind child has a calming effect.

Examine the genitalia in an efficient and systematic manner. Inspect the external genitalia for pubic hair, the size of the clitoris, the color and size of the labia majora, and the presence of rashes, bruises, or other lesions.

Next, visualize the structures by separating the labia with your fingers, as shown in Figure 18-83. You can also apply gentle traction by grasping the labia between your thumb and index finger of each hand, separating the labia majora laterally and posteriorly to examine the inner structures as shown in Figure 18-84. *Labial adhesions,* or fusion of the labia minora, may be noted in prepubertal children and can obscure the vaginal and urethral orifices. They may be a normal variant. Vaginal bleeding is always cause for concern.

A *vaginal discharge* in early childhood can be from *perineal irritation* (e.g., bubble baths or soaps), *foreign body, nonspecific vulvovaginitis, Candida, pinworms,* or a *sexually transmitted infection* from sexual abuse.

Precocious puberty can induce menses in a young girl.

Purulent, profuse, malodorous, and blood-tinged discharge should be evaluated for the presence of *infiltration, foreign body,* or *trauma.*

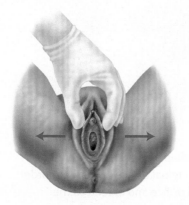

FIGURE 18-83. **Separate labia to assess genital structures.**

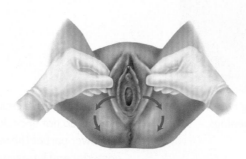

FIGURE 18-84. **Using thumb and forefinger to examine inner structures.**

Note the condition of the labia minora, urethra, hymen, and proximal vagina. If you are unable to visualize the edges of the hymen, ask the child to take a deep breath to relax the abdominal muscles. Another useful technique (to be performed by an experienced pediatric examiner) is to position her in the knee–chest position, as shown in Figures 18-85 and 18-86. These maneuvers will often open the hymen. Experienced examiners can also use saline drops to make the edges of the hymen less sticky.

Sexual abuse is unfortunately far too common throughout the world. Up to 25% of women report some history of sexual abuse; while many of these do not involve severe physical trauma, some do.[52–54]

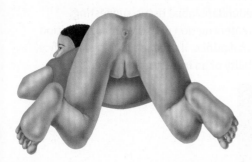

FIGURE 18-85. **Position for more advanced technique to visualize hymen.**

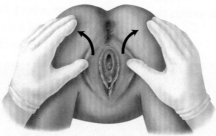

FIGURE 18-86. **Using thumbs to separate labia to open the hymen.**

Avoid touching the hymenal edges because the hymen is exquisitely tender without the protective effects of hormones. Examine for discharge, labial adhesions, lesions, estrogenization (indicating onset of puberty), hymenal variations (such as imperforate or septate hymen, which are rare), and hygiene. A thin, white discharge (leukorrhea) is often present. *A speculum examination of the vagina and cervix is contraindicated in a prepubertal child unless there is suspicion of severe trauma or foreign body.*

Abrasions or signs of trauma of the external genitalia can be from benign causes such as masturbation, irritants, or accidental trauma, but should also raise the possibility of *sexual abuse.* See Table 18-11, Physical Signs of Sexual Abuse, p. 932.

The normal hymen in infants and young girls can have various configurations, as shown below.

Normal Configurations of the Hymen in Prepubertal and Adolescent Females

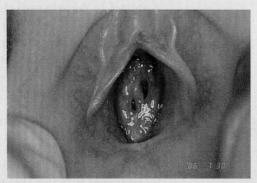

6-yr-old girl with a septate hymen causing two orifices. Traction is needed to visualize the two openings.

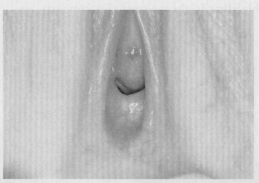

7-yr-old girl with a crescent-shaped hymen. Crescentic hymens do not encircle the vaginal orifice but rather border the lower part of the vaginal orifice and extend to the posterior and lateral margins of the hymenal ring.

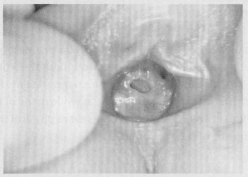

2-yr-old girl with an annular hymen, visible with labial traction. Annular means that the hymen surrounds the orifice circumferentially.

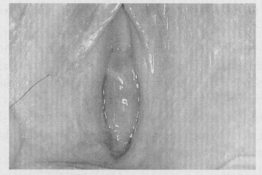

9-yr-old girl with redundant labial tissue suggesting estrogen effect. Greater traction or a knee–chest position would reveal a normal orifice. If unable to locate an orifice, consider the possibility of an imperforate hymen.

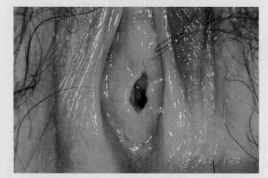

12-yr-old girl with annular hymen and hormonal influence of puberty, causing thickened, pink tissue.

Source of photos: Reece R, Ludwig S (eds). Child Abuse: Medical Diagnosis and Management, 2nd ed. Philadelphia: Lippincott Williams & Wilkins, 2001.

The physical examination may reveal signs that suggest *sexual abuse,* and the examination is particularly important if there are suspicious clues in the history. Even with known abuse, the majority of examinations will be unremarkable; a normal genital examination does not rule out sexual abuse. Mounds, notches, and tags on the hymen may all be normal variants. The size of the orifice can vary with age and the examination technique. *If the hymenal edges are smooth and without interruption in the inferior half, the hymen is probably normal* (but does not rule out abuse since the hymen, like most other tissues, can heal over 7 to 10 days). Certain physical findings, however, suggest the possibility of sexual abuse and require more complete evaluation by an expert in the field. See Table 18-11, Physical Signs of Sexual Abuse, p. 921.

As demonstrated in Table 18-11, Physical Signs of Sexual Abuse, p. 921, physical signs strongly suggestive of *sexual abuse* include lacerations, ecchymoses and newly healed scars of the hymen, lack of hymenal tissue from 3 to 9 o'clock, and healed hymenal transections. Other signs such as purulent discharge and herpetic lesions are concerning as well.

The Rectal Examination

The rectal examination is not routine but should be done whenever intra-abdominal, pelvic, or perirectal disease is suspected.

The rectal examination of the young child can be performed with the child in either the side-lying or lithotomy position. For many young children, the lithotomy position is less threatening and easier to perform. Have the child lie on the back with the knees and hips flexed and the legs abducted. Drape the child from the waist down. Provide frequent reassurance during the examination, and ask the child to breathe in and out through the mouth to relax. Spread the buttocks and observe the anus. You can use your lubricated gloved index finger, even in small children. Palpate the abdomen with your other hand, both to distract the child and to note the abdominal structures between your hands. The prostate gland is not palpable in young boys.

Anal skin tags are present in *inflammatory bowel disease* but are more often an incidental finding when located in the midline.

Tenderness noted on rectal examination of a child usually indicates an infectious or inflammatory cause, such as an *abscess* or *appendicitis.*

The Musculoskeletal System

In older children, abnormalities of the upper extremities are rare in the absence of injury.

The normal young child has increased lumbar concavity and decreased thoracic convexity compared with the adult, and often has a protuberant abdomen.

Observe the child standing and walking barefoot. Ask the child to touch the toes, rise from sitting, run a short distance, and pick up objects. You will detect most abnormalities by watching carefully from both front and behind. To indirectly assess the child's gait pattern, note the soles of the shoes to see whether one side of the soles is worn down.

Toddlers may acquire *nursemaid's elbow* or subluxation of the radial head from a tugging injury. They will hold their arms slightly flexed at the elbows.

The cause of *acute limp* in childhood is usually trauma or injury, although infection of the bone, joint, or muscle should be considered. In an obese child, consider *slipped capital femoral epiphysis.*

During early infancy, there is a common and normal progression from bowleggedness (Fig. 18-87) that begins to disappear at about 18 months of age, often followed by transition toward knock-knees. The *knock-knee pattern* (Fig. 18-88) is usually maximal by age 3 to 4 years and gradually corrects by age 9 or 10 years.

Severe bowing of the legs (genu varum) may still be physiologic bowing that will spontaneously resolve. Extreme bowing or unilateral bowing may be from pathologic causes such as *rickets* or *tibia vara (Blount disease)*.

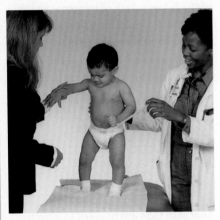

FIGURE 18-87. **Bowleggedness is normal in early childhood.**

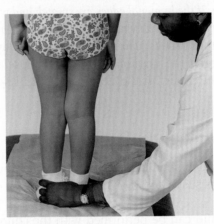

FIGURE 18-88. **Knock-knee is not unusual in childhood.**

The presence of tibial torsion can be assessed in several ways[55]; one method is shown in Figure 18-89. Have the toddler lie prone on the examination table, with the knees flexed to 90°. Note the thigh–foot axis. Usually there is ±10° of internal or external rotation noted by a foot pointing off in a direction. Check the position of the malleoli—they should be symmetric.

Children may *toe in* when they begin to walk. This may increase up to 4 years of age and then gradually disappear by about 10 years of age.

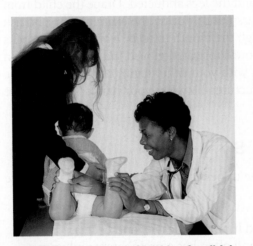

FIGURE 18-89. **Checking for tibial torsion.**

The most common lower-extremity pathology in childhood is injury from accidents. Joint injuries, fractures, sprains, strains, and serious ligament injuries such as anterior cruciate ligament tears of the knee are all too common in children.

A *chronic limp* in childhood could be caused by Blount disease, hip disorders such as *avascular necrosis of the hip,* leg length discrepancy, spinal disorder, and serious systemic disease such as leukemia.

Inspect any child who can stand for *scoliosis* using techniques described under "Adolescents."

Determine any *leg shortening* that may accompany hip disease by comparing the distance from the anterior superior spine of the ilium to the medial malleolus on each side. Straighten the child by pulling gently on the legs, and then compare the levels of the medial malleoli with each other. Put a small ink dot over the prominent malleoli and touch them together for a direct measure.

Have the child stand straight and place your hands horizontally over the iliac crests from behind. Small discrepancies can be noted. If such a discrepancy is noted and you suspect leg length discrepancy, with one iliac crest higher than the other, place a book under the shorter leg; this should eliminate the discrepancy.

Test for severe hip disease with its associated weakness of the gluteus medius muscle. Observe from behind as the child shifts weight from one leg to the other (Figs. 18-90 and 18-91). A pelvis that remains level when weight is shifted from one foot to the other is a *negative Trendelenburg sign.*[56] With an abnormal positive sign in *severe hip disease,* the *pelvis tilts toward the unaffected hip* during weight-bearing on the affected side (positive Trendelenburg sign).

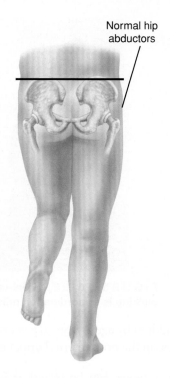

FIGURE 18-90. Negative Trendelenberg sign.

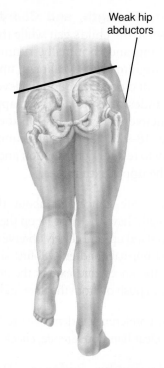

FIGURE 18-91. Positive Trendelenberg sign.

The Nervous System

Beyond infancy, the neurologic examination includes the components evaluated in adults. Combine the neurologic and developmental assessment; turn this into a game with the child to assess optimal development and neurologic performance.

Use a validated developmental screen for preschool children. Children usually enjoy this component, and you can too. Many neurologic conditions in children are accompanied by developmental abnormalities.

Sensation. The sensory examination can be performed by using a cotton ball or tickling the child. This is best performed with the child's eyes closed. Do not use pin pricks.

Children with *spastic diplegias* will often have hypotonia as infants and then excessive tone with spasticity, scissoring, and perhaps clenched fists as toddlers and young children.

Problems with social interaction, verbal and nonverbal communication, restricted interests, and repetitive behaviors could be signs of *autism.*

Gait, Strength, and Coordination.
Observe the child's gait while the child is walking and, optimally, running. Note any asymmetries, weakness, undue tripping, or clumsiness. Follow developmental milestones to test for appropriate maneuvers such as heel-to-toe walking (Fig. 18-92), hopping, and jumping. Use a toy to test for coordination and strength of the upper extremities.

If you are concerned about the child's strength, have the child lie on the floor and then stand up, and closely observe the stages. Most normal children will first sit up, then flex the knees, and extend the arms to the side to push off from the floor and stand up.

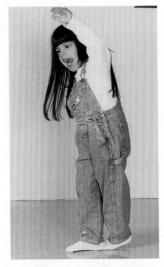

FIGURE 18-92. **Heel-to-toe walking is a coordination milestone.**

In children with uncoordinated gait, be sure to distinguish *orthopedic causes* such as positional deformities of the hip, knee, or foot from *neurologic abnormalities* such as *cerebral palsy, ataxia,* or *neuromuscular conditions.*

In certain forms of *muscular dystrophy* with weakness of the pelvic girdle muscles, children will rise to standing by rolling over prone and pushing off the floor with the arms while the legs remain extended (*Gower sign*).

Hand preference is demonstrated in most children by age 2 years. If a younger child has clear hand preference, check for weakness in the nonpreferred upper extremity.

Deep Tendon Reflexes. Deep tendon reflexes can be tested as in adults. First, demonstrate the use of the reflex hammer on the child's hand, assuring the child that it will not hurt. Children love to feel their legs bounce when you test their patellar reflexes. Have the child keep the eyes closed during some of this examination because tensing will disrupt the results.

Children with mild cerebral palsy may have both slightly increased tone and hyperreflexia.

Cognitive Development. You can ask children older than 3 years to draw a picture or copy objects and then discuss their pictures to test simultaneously for fine motor coordination, cognition, and language.

Among school-aged children, the best test for development is their school performance. You can obtain school records or psychological testing results, obviating the need for the clinician to formally test an older child's development.

Distinguish between isolated delays in one aspect of development (e.g., coordination or language) and more generalized delays that occur in several components. The latter is more likely to reflect global neurologic disorders such as *cognitive disability* that can have many etiologies.

Cerebellar Function. The cerebellar examination can be tested using finger-to-nose and rapid alternating movements of the hands or fingers (Figs. 18-93 and 18-94). Children older than 5 years should be able to tell right from left so you can assign them right–left discrimination tasks as is done in the adult patient.

Some children with *attention deficit disorder with hyperactivity (ADHD)* will have great difficulty in cooperating with your neurologic and developmental examination because of problems focusing. These children often have high energy levels, cannot stay still for extended periods, and have a history of difficulty in school or structured situations. However, other conditions may have similar symptoms, so a complete history and physical examination is warranted.

Delayed or disordered development in early childhood can lead to early school failure as well as social, behavioral, and emotional problems.

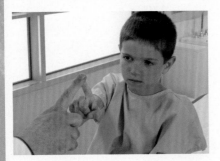

FIGURE 18-93. **Finger-to-nose test—first have child touch your finger.**

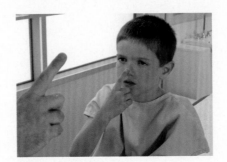

FIGURE 18-94. **Then have child touch her/his nose.**

Cranial Nerves. The cranial nerves can be assessed quite well using developmentally appropriate strategies, as shown in the following table:

Strategies to Assess Cranial Nerves in Young Children

Cranial Nerve		Strategy
I	Olfactory	Testable in older children.
II	Visual acuity	Use Snellen chart after age 3 yrs. Test visual fields as for an adult. A parent may need to hold the child's head.
III, IV, VI	Extraocular movements	Have the child track a light or an object (a toy is preferable). A parent may need to hold the child's head.
V	Motor	Play a game with a soft cotton ball to test sensation. Have the child clench the teeth and chew or swallow some food.
VII	Facial	Have the child "make faces" or imitate you as you make faces (including moving your eyebrows) and observe symmetry and facial movements.
VII	Acoustic	Perform auditory testing after age 4 yrs. Whisper a word or command behind the child's back and have the child repeat it.
IX, X	Swallow and gag	Have the child stick the "whole tongue out" or "say 'ah'." Observe movement of the uvula and soft palate. Test the gag reflex.
XI	Spinal accessory	Have the child push your hand away with his head. Have the child shrug his shoulders while you push down with your hands to "see how strong you are."
XII	Hypoglossal	Ask the child to "stick out your tongue all the way."

Localizing neurologic signs are rare in children but can be caused by *trauma*, *brain tumor*, *intracranial bleed*, or *infection*. Children with *increased intracranial pressure* can develop cranial nerve abnormalities as well as papilledema and altered mental status.

Children with meningitis, encephalitis, or cerebral abscess can have abnormalities of cranial nerves, although they also have altered consciousness and other signs.

Although *facial nerve palsy* can be congenital, it is often caused by infection or trauma.

ASSESSING ADOLESCENTS

Development: 11 to 20 Years

Adolescence can be divided into three stages: early, middle, and late. Interview and examination techniques vary widely depending on the adolescent's physical, cognitive, and social–emotional levels of development.

Physical Development. Adolescence is the period of transition from childhood to adulthood. The physical transformation generally occurs over a period of years, beginning at an average age of 10 years in girls and 11 years in boys. On average, girls end pubertal development with a growth spurt by age 14 years and boys by age 16 years. The age of onset and duration of puberty vary widely, although the stages follow the same sequence in all adolescents. *Early adolescents are preoccupied with these physical changes.*

Cognitive Development. Although less obvious, cognitive changes during adolescence are as dramatic as changes in physique. Most adolescents progress from concrete to formal operational thinking, acquiring an ability to reason logically and abstractly and to consider future implications of current actions (Fig. 18-95). Although the interview and examination resemble those of adults, keep in mind the wide variability in cognitive development of adolescents and their often erratic and still limited ability to see beyond simple solutions. Moral thinking becomes sophisticated with lots of time spent debating issues. Recent evidence shows that brain development (especially in the right prefrontal cortex) probably continues well into the twenties.

Social and Emotional Development. Adolescence is a tumultuous time, marked by the transition from family-dominated influences to increasing autonomy and peer influence (Fig. 18-96). The struggle for identity, independence, and eventually intimacy leads to stress, health-related problems, and often, high-risk behaviors. This struggle also provides an important opportunity for health promotion.

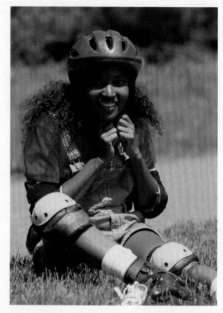

FIGURE 18-95. **Cognitive development is often overshadowed by continuing physical changes in adolescents.**

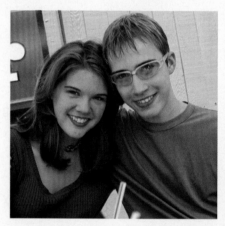

FIGURE 18-96. **In adolescence, peers often become more influential than family.**

Developmental Tasks of Adolescence

Task	Characteristic	Health Care Approaches
Early Adolescence (10- to 14-yr-olds)		
Physical	Puberty (F: 10–14; M: 11–16)	Confidentiality; privacy
Cognitive	Concrete operational	Emphasis on short-term
Social identity	Am I normal? Peers increasingly important	Reassurance and positive attitude
Independence	Ambivalence (family, self, peers)	Support for growing autonomy

(*continued*)

Developmental Tasks of Adolescence (*continued*)

Task	Characteristic	Health Care Approaches
Middle Adolescence (15- to 16-yr-olds)		
Physical	Females more comfortable, males awkward	Support if patient varies from normal
Cognitive	Transition; many ideas, often highly emotional thinker	Problem solving; decision making, increased responsibility
Social identity	Who am I? Much introspection; global issues	Nonjudgmental acceptance
Independence	Limit testing; experimental behaviors; dating	Consistency; limit setting
Late Adolescence (17- to 20-yr-olds)		
Physical	Adult appearance	Minimal unless chronic illness
Cognitive	Formal operational (for many but not all)	Approach as an adult
Social identity	Role with respect to others; sexuality; future	Encouragement of identity to allow growth; safety and healthy decision-making
Independence	Separation from family; toward real independence	Support, anticipatory guidance

The Health History

The key to successfully examining adolescents is a *comfortable, confidential environment.* This makes the examination more relaxed and informative. Consider the teen's cognitive and social development when deciding issues of privacy, parental involvement, and confidentiality (Fig. 18-97).

Adolescents usually respond positively to anyone demonstrating a genuine interest in them. Show such interest early and then sustain the connection for effective communication.

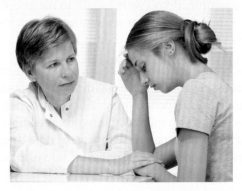

FIGURE 18-97. **Trust-building is vital with the adolescent patient.**

Adolescents are more likely to open up when the *interview focuses on them rather than on their problems.* In contrast to most other interviews, *start with specific questions* to build trust and rapport and get the conversation going. You may have to do more talking than usual at the beginning. Chat informally about friends, school, hobbies, and family. Using silence in an attempt to get adolescents to talk or asking about feelings directly is usually not a good idea.

It is particularly important to use summarization and transitional statements and to explain what you are going to do during the physical examination. The physical examination can also be an opportunity to engage young persons. *Once you have established rapport, return to more open-ended questions.* At that point, make sure to ask what concerns or questions the adolescent may have. Because adolescents are often reluctant to ask their most important questions (which are sometimes about sensitive topics), ask if the adolescent has anything else to discuss. A useful phrase to use is "tell me what other questions you have." Another trick is to use the phrase: "other kids your age often have questions about ..."

Adolescents' behavior is related to their developmental stage and not necessarily to chronologic age or physical maturation. Their appearance may fool you into assuming that they are functioning on a more future-oriented and realistic level. This is particularly true regarding "early bloomers," who look older than their age. The reverse can also be true, especially in teens with delayed puberty or chronic illness.

Issues of *confidentiality* are important in adolescence. Explain to both parents and adolescents that the best health care allows adolescents some degree of independence and confidentiality. It helps if the clinician starts asking the parent to leave the room for part of the interview when the child is aged 11 years. This prepares both parents and teens for future visits when the patient spends time alone with the clinician.

Before the parent leaves, obtain relevant clinical history from him or her, such as certain elements of past history, and clarify the parent's agenda for the visit. Adolescents need to know that you will hold in confidence what they discuss with you. However, never make confidentiality unlimited. Always state explicitly that you may need to act on information that makes you concerned about safety: "I will not tell your parents what we talk about unless you give me permission or I am concerned about your safety. For example, if you were to talk to me about hurting yourself or someone else and I thought that you really were at risk to follow through, I would need to discuss it with others in order to help you."

An important goal is to help adolescents bring their concerns or questions to their parents. Encourage adolescents to discuss sensitive issues with their parents and offer to be present or help. Although young people may believe that their parents would "disown them if they only knew," you may be able to promote more open dialogue. Occasionally, you will encounter a parent who is very rigid and punitive. It is important to carefully assess the parents' perspective prior to further discussion, and to obtain the explicit consent of the young person.

As in middle childhood, modesty is important. The patient should remain dressed until the examination begins (Fig. 18-98). Leave the room while the patient puts on a gown. Not all adolescents are willing to don a gown, so partially uncovering as the examination proceeds to preserve the patient's modesty is important. Most adolescents older than 13 years prefer to be examined without a parent in the room, but

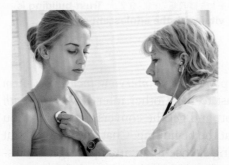

FIGURE 18-98. **Some adolescents will request to remain in their clothes.**

this depends on the patient's developmental level, familiarity with the examiner, relationship with the parent, and culture. Ask younger adolescents and their parent their preferences. It is advisable for clinicians to have a chaperone in the room when examining an adolescent of a different gender, for example, a male clinician examining a female patient's breasts or genitalia. However, miscommunication and embarrassing situations can occur with concordant gender between clinicians and patients, and it is best to discuss the issue of chaperones with patients/parents and record the shared decision in the clinical chart.[57]

The sequence and content of the physical examination of the adolescent are similar to those in the adult. Keep in mind, however, issues unique to adolescents such as puberty, growth, development, family and peer relationships, sexuality, healthy decision making, and high-risk behaviors.

Health Promotion and Counseling: Evidence and Recommendations

The AAP recommends annual health supervision visits for adolescents.[8] Be sure to include health promotion during all health encounters with youth. Adolescents with chronic problems or high-risk behaviors may require additional visits for health promotion and anticipatory guidance.

Most chronic diseases of adults have their antecedents in childhood or adolescence. For example, obesity, cardiovascular disease, addiction (to drugs, tobacco, or alcohol), and depression are all influenced by childhood and teen experiences and by behaviors established during adolescence. For example, most obese adults were obese as adolescents or had abnormal indicators such as elevated BMI scores. As a second example, *almost all adults who are addicted to tobacco began their tobacco habits before 18 years.* Therefore, a major component of health promotion for adolescents includes discussions about health behaviors or habits (Fig. 18-99). Effective health promotion can help patients develop healthy habits and lifestyles and avoid several chronic health problems.

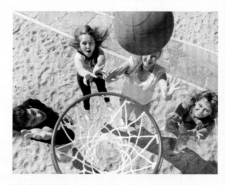

FIGURE 18-99. **Inquire about and encourage adolescents to participate in healthy activities.**

Because some health promotion topics involve confidential issues such as mental health, addiction, sexual behavior, and eating disorders, speak to adolescents (particularly older youth) privately during part of a visit that involves health supervision.

Self-completed screening questionnaires can be completed before the visit to facilitate comprehensive assessment of youth risk behaviors. This approach saves time so that you can better address the specific risk behaviors the adolescent endorses during the visit. An excellent instrument is the Guidelines for Adolescent Preventive Services (GAPS).[58,59]

Components of a Health Supervision Visit for Adolescents Aged 11 to 18 Years

Discussions with Parents

- Address parent concerns
- Provide advice about supervision, encouraging progressively responsible decision-making
- Ask about school, activities, social interactions
- Assess youth's behaviors and habits, mental health

Discussions with Adolescent

- *Social and Emotional:* mental health, friends, family
- *Physical Development:* puberty, self-concept
- *Behaviors and Habits:* nutrition, exercise, TV or computer screen time, drug/alcohol, sleep
- *Relationships and Sexuality:* dating, sexual activity, sexual orientation, forced sex
- *Family Functioning:* relations with parents and siblings
- *School Performance:* activities, strengths, goals

Physical Examination

- Perform a careful examination; note growth parameters, sexual maturity ratings

Screening Tests

- Vision and hearing, blood pressure; consider hematocrit (especially in females); assess emotional health and risk factors (using a validated instrument)

Immunizations

- See schedule from the AAP

Anticipatory Guidance—Teen

- *Promote Healthy Habits and Behaviors:*
  - Injury and illness prevention
    - Seat belts, drunk driving, helmets, sun, weapons
  - Nutrition
    - Healthy meals/snacks, obesity prevention
  - Oral health: dentist, brushing
    - Physical activity and screen time
- *Sexuality:*
  - Confidentiality, sexual behaviors, safer sex, contraception if needed
- *High-risk Behaviors:*
  - Prevention strategies
  - Parent–teen interaction, peer interactions
  - Communication, rules
- *Social Achievement:*
  - Activities, school, future
  - Community interaction
  - Resources, involvement

Anticipatory Guidance—Parent

- Positive interactions, support, safety, limit setting, family values, modeling behaviors, increased responsibility

Techniques of Examination

General Survey and Vital Signs

Somatic Growth. Adolescents should wear gowns to be weighed or have them remove their shoes and heavy clothing. This is particularly important for adolescent girls being evaluated for underweight problems. Ideally, serial weights (and heights) should use the same scale.

Both obesity and eating disorders (anorexia and bulimia) among adolescent girls are major public health problems requiring regular assessments of weight, monitoring for complications, and promoting healthy choices and self-concept.

Vital Signs. Ongoing evaluations of blood pressure are important for adolescents.[33] The average heart rate from age 10 to 14 years is 85 beats per minute, with a range of 55 to 115 beats per minute considered normal. Average heart rate for those 15 years and older is 60 to 100 beats per minute. Percentiles for blood pressure are shown on p. 864.

Causes of sustained hypertension for this age group include primary hypertension, renal parenchymal disease, and drug use.

The Skin

Examine the adolescent's skin carefully. Many adolescents will have concerns about various skin lesions, such as acne, dimples, blemishes, warts, and moles. Pay particular attention to the face and back in examining adolescents for acne. Stretch marks have become more common with the epidemic of obesity.

Adolescent acne, a common skin condition, tends to resolve eventually, but often benefits from proper treatment. It tends to begin during middle to late puberty.

Many adolescents spend considerable time in the sun and at tanning salons. You may detect this during a comprehensive health history or by noticing signs of tanning during the physical examination. This is a good opportunity to counsel adolescents about the dangers of excessive ultraviolet exposure, the need for sunscreen, and the risks of tanning salons.

Moles or benign nevi may appear during adolescence. Their characteristics differentiate them from atypical nevi, described on p. 912.

Counsel older adolescents to begin performing a regular self-examination of the skin, as shown on pp. 187–188.

Head, Ears, Eyes, Throat, and Neck

The examination of these body parts is generally the same as for adults.

The methods used to examine the eye, including testing for visual acuity, are the same as those for adults. Refractive errors become common, and it is important to test visual acuity monocularly at regular intervals, such as during the annual health supervision visit.

The ease and techniques of examining the ears and testing the hearing approach the methods used for adults. There are no ear, mouth, throat, or neck abnormalities or variations of normal unique to this age group.

An adolescent with persistent fever, tonsillar pharyngitis, and cervical lymphadenopathy may have infectious mononucleosis.

The Heart

The technique and sequence of examination are the same as those for adults. Murmurs are a continued cardiovascular issue for evaluation.

The benign *pulmonary flow murmur* is a grade I–II/VI soft, nonharsh murmur with the timing characteristics of an ejection murmur, beginning after the first sound and ending before the second sound, but without the marked crescendo–decrescendo quality of an organic ejection murmur. If you hear this murmur, evaluate whether the

A pulmonary flow murmur accompanied by a fixed split second heart sound suggests right-heart volume load such as an atrial septal defect.

Location and Characteristics of Benign Heart Murmurs in Adolescents

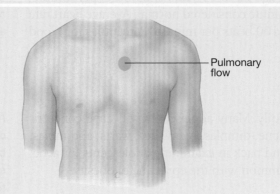

Typical Age	Name	Characteristics	Description and Location
Older child, adolescence and later	*Pulmonary flow murmur*	S_1 S_2	Grade I–II/VI soft, nonharsh Ejection in timing Upper left sternal border Normal P_2

pulmonary closure sound is of normal intensity and whether splitting of the second heart sound is eliminated during expiration. *An adolescent with a benign pulmonary ejection murmur will have normal intensity and normally split second heart sounds.*

The pulmonary flow murmur may also be heard in the presence of volume overload from any cause such as chronic anemia, and following exercise. It may persist into adulthood.

The Breasts

Physical changes in a girl's breasts are one of the first signs of puberty. As in most developmental changes, there is a systematic progression. Generally, over a 4-year period, the breasts progress through five stages, called Tanner stages or *Tanner sex maturity rating* stages, as shown in the box on the next page. Breast buds in the preadolescent stage enlarge, changing the contour of the breasts and areola. The areola also darkens in color. These stages are accompanied by the development of pubic hair and other secondary sexual characteristics, as shown on p. 901. Menarche usually occurs when a girl is in breast stage 3 or 4. By then, she has passed her peak growth spurt (see the figure on p. 897).

For years, the normal range for onset of breast development and pubic hair was 8 to 13 years (average, 11 years), with earlier onset considered abnormal.[60–62] Some studies suggest that the *lower age cutoff should be as low as age 7 years for white girls and 6 years for African American and Hispanic girls.* Breast development varies by age, race, and ethnicity.[61,62] Breasts develop at different rates in approximately 10% of girls, with resultant asymmetry of size or Tanner stage. Reassurance that this generally resolves is helpful to the patient.

Breast buds (pea-size firm masses inferior to the nipple) are common among both girls and boys entering puberty or during early puberty.

Breast asymmetry is common in adolescents, particularly when adolescents are between Tanner stages 2 and 4. This is nearly always a benign condition.

Guidelines for the usefulness of clinical breast examinations by a clinician are changing, and the American Cancer Society no longer recommends clinical breast examinations for women of any age to screen for breast cancer.[63] However, professional organizations consistently recommend providing female patients with instructions for self-examination (see p. 442). It is useful to begin this process with adolescent females. In the event of a clinical breast examination, a chaperone (parent or nurse) should assist male clinicians.

Breasts in boys consist of a small nipple and areola. During puberty, about one third of boys develop a breast bud 2 cm or more in diameter, usually in one breast. Obese boys may develop substantial breast tissue.

Many adolescent boys develop *gynecomastia* (enlarged breasts) on one or both sides. Although usually slight, it can be embarrassing. It generally resolves in a few years.

Sexual Maturity Ratings in Girls: Breasts

Stage 1
Preadolescent: elevation of nipple only

Masses or nodules in the breasts of adolescent girls should be examined carefully. They are usually *benign fibroadenomas* or *cysts;* less likely, etiologies include *abscesses* or *lipomas*. Breast carcinoma is extremely rare in adolescence and nearly always occurs in families with a strong history of the disease.[64]

Stage 2

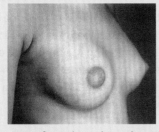

Breast bud stage: elevation of breast and nipple as a small mound; enlargement of areolar diameter

Stage 3

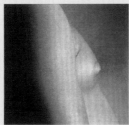

Further enlargement of elevation of breast and areola, with no separation of their contours

Stage 4

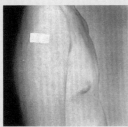

Projection of areola and nipple to form a secondary mound above the level of breast

Stage 5

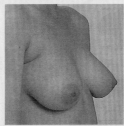

Mature stage: projection of nipple only; areola has receded to general contour of the breast (although in some normal individuals the areola continues to form a secondary mound)

Photos used with permission of the American Academy of Pediatrics, *Assessment of Sexual Maturity Stages in Girls,* 1995.

The Abdomen

Techniques of abdominal examination are the same as for adults. The size of the liver approaches the adult size as the teen progresses through puberty, and is related to the adolescent's overall height. Although data are lacking about the usefulness of different techniques to assess liver size, it is likely that evidence from adult studies apply, particularly for older adolescents. Palpate the liver. If it is nonpalpable, hepatomegaly is highly unlikely. If you can palpate the lower edge, use light percussion to assess liver span.

Hepatomegaly in teens may be from *infections* such as hepatitis or infectious mononucleosis, inflammatory bowel disease, or tumors.

Male Genitalia

The genital examination of the adolescent boy proceeds like the examination of the adult male. Be aware of the embarrassment many boys experience during this aspect of the examination.

Important anatomical changes in the male genitalia accompany puberty and help to define its progress. The first reliable sign of puberty (Fig. 18-100), starting between ages 9 and 13.5 years is an increase in the size of the testes. Next, pubic hair appears, along with progressive enlargement of the penis. The complete change from preadolescent to adult anatomy requires about 3 years, with a range of 1.8 to 5 years.

Delayed puberty is suspected in boys who have no signs of pubertal development by 14 years of age.

An axiom of development is that pubertal changes follow a well-established sequence. The age range for start and completion is wide, but the sequence for each boy is the same (Fig. 18-100). This progression is helpful when counseling anxious adolescents about current and future maturation and the wide range of normal for puberty.

When examining the adolescent male, assign a sexual maturity rating. The five stages of sexual development, first described by Tanner, are outlined and illustrated

The most common cause of delayed puberty in males is *constitutional delay*, frequently a familial condition involving delayed bone and physical maturation, but normal hormonal levels.

Although nocturnal or daytime ejaculation tends to begin around Sexual Maturity Rating 3, a finding on either history or physical examination of penile discharge may indicate a *sexually transmitted infection*.

In addition to constitutional delay, less common causes of *delayed puberty* in boys include primary or secondary hypogonadism as well as congenital GnRH deficiency.[65]

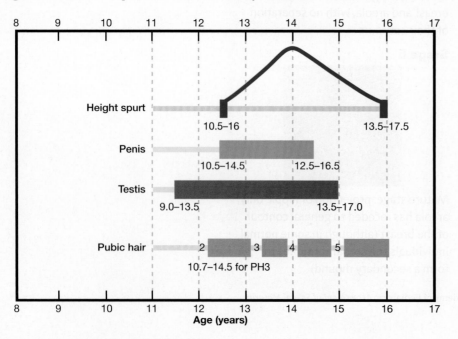

Numbers below the bars indicate the ranges in age within which the changes occur.

FIGURE 18-100. Male adolescents.

in the box below. These involve changes in the penis, testes, and scrotum. In about 80% of men, pubic hair spreads farther up the abdomen in a triangular pattern pointing toward the umbilicus; this phase is not completed until the 20s.

Observe the penis for sores and discharge as you would in an adult male.

In uncircumcised males, the foreskin should be easily retractable by adolescence. This is also an opportunity to discuss normal hygiene. Discuss testicular examination in older boys by age 18 years.

Sexual Maturity Rating in Boys

In assigning sexual maturity rating in boys, observe each of the three characteristics separately because they may develop at different rates. Record two separate ratings: pubic hair and genital. If the penis and testes differ in their stages, average the two into a single figure for the genital rating. These photos demonstrate pubertal development in an uncircumcised male.

		Pubic Hair	Penis	Testes and Scrotum
Stage 1		Preadolescent—no pubic hair except for the fine body hair (vellus hair) similar to that on the abdomen	Preadolescent—same size and proportions as in childhood	Preadolescent—same size and proportions as in childhood
Stage 2		Sparse growth of long, slightly pigmented, downy hair, straight or only slightly curled, chiefly at the base of the penis	Slight or no enlargement	Testes larger; scrotum larger, somewhat reddened, and altered in texture
Stage 3		Darker, coarser, curlier hair spreading sparsely over the pubic symphysis	Larger, especially in length	Further enlarged
Stage 4		Coarse and curly hair, as in the adult; area covered greater than in stage 3, but not as great as in the adult and not yet including the thighs	Further enlarged in length and breadth, with development of the glans	Further enlarged; scrotal skin darkened
Stage 5		Hair adult in quantity and quality, spreads to the medial surfaces of the thighs but not up over the abdomen	Adult in size and shape	Adult in size and shape

Photos reprinted from Wales JKH, Wit JM. Pediatric Endocrinology and Growth, 2nd ed. Philadelphia, W. B. Saunders, 2003.

Female Genitalia

The external examination of adolescent female genitalia proceeds in the same manner as for school-aged children. If clinically necessary to perform a pelvic examination, the technique is the same as for an adult female. Of note, indications for performing pelvic examinations in adolescents have become much more stringent. When performing a pelvic examination, a full explanation of the steps of the examination, demonstration of the instruments, and a gentle, reassuring approach are necessary because the adolescent is usually quite anxious. A chaperone (parent or nurse) must be present. An adolescent's first pelvic examination should be performed by an experienced health care provider.

A girl's initial signs of puberty are hymenal thickening and redundancy secondary to estrogen, widening of the hips, and beginning of a height spurt, although these changes are difficult to detect. The first easily detectable sign of puberty is usually the appearance of breast buds although pubic hair sometimes appears earlier. The average age of the appearance of pubic hair has decreased in recent years, and current consensus is that the appearance of pubic hair as early as 7 years can be normal, particularly in dark-skinned girls who develop secondary sexual characteristics at an earlier age.

Assign a sexual maturity rating to every female, irrespective of chronologic age. The assessment of sexual maturity in girls is based on both growth of pubic hair and the development of breasts.[59] The sexual maturity rating of pubic hair growth is shown in the box on page 901. See p. 897 for breast development assessment. Counsel girls about this sequence and their current stage.

Although there is a wide variation in the age of onset and completion of puberty in girls, the stages occur in a predictable sequence, as shown in Figure 18-101.

Vaginal discharge in a young adolescent should be treated as in the adult. Causes include physiologic leukorrhea, sexually transmitted infections from consensual sexual activity or sexual abuse, bacterial vaginosis, foreign body, and external irritants.

Pubertal development prior to the normal age range may signify precocious puberty which has a variety of endocrine and central nervous system causes. Premature adrenarche is usually benign, but may occasionally be associated with polycystic ovary syndrome, insulin resistance, and metabolic syndrome.

Delayed puberty (no breasts or pubic hair development by age 12 years) is usually caused by inadequate gonadotropin secretion from the anterior pituitary due to defective hypothalamic GnRH production. A common cause is anorexia nervosa.

Delayed puberty in an adolescent female below the third percentile in height may be from Turner syndrome or chronic disease. The two most common causes of delayed sexual development in an extremely thin adolescent girl are anorexia nervosa and chronic disease.

Obesity in females can be associated with early onset of puberty.

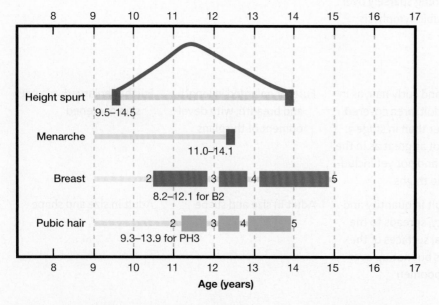

Numbers below the bars indicate the ranges in age within which the changes occur.

FIGURE 18-101. Female adolescents.

Sexual Maturity Ratings in Girls: Pubic Hair

Stage 1
Preadolescent—no pubic hair except for the fine body hair (vellus hair) similar to that on the abdomen

Stage 2

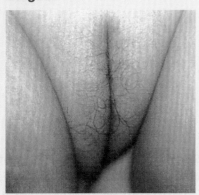

Sparse growth of long, slightly pigmented, downy hair, straight or only slightly curled, chiefly along the labia

Stage 3

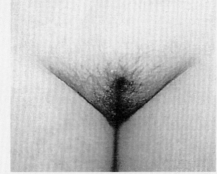

Darker, coarser, curlier hair, spreading sparsely over the pubic symphysis

Stage 4

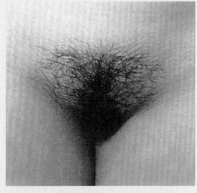

Coarse and curly hair as in adults; area covered greater than in stage 3 but not as great as in the adult and not yet including the thighs

Stage 5

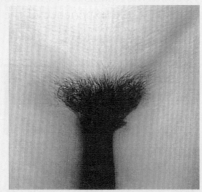

Hair adult in quantity and quality, spreads on the medial surfaces of the thighs but not up over the abdomen

Photos used with permission of the American Academy of Pediatrics, *Assessment of Sexual Maturity Stages in Girls*, 1995.

Amenorrhea in adolescence can be primary (no menarche by age 16 years) or secondary (cessation of menses in an adolescent who had previously menstruated). While primary amenorrhea is usually due to anatomic or genetic causes, secondary amenorrhea can be due to a variety of etiologies such as *stress, excessive exercise, and eating disorders.*

The Musculoskeletal System

Evaluations for scoliosis and screening for participation in sports (pp. 902–905) remain common components of examination in adolescents. Other segments of the musculoskeletal examination are the same as for adults.

Assessing for Scoliosis. First, examine the patient standing assessing symmetry of shoulders, scapula, and hips. Then have the child bend forward with the knees straight and head hanging straight down between extended arms (Adams forward bend test). Next, evaluate any asymmetry in positioning. Scoliosis in a young child is unusual and abnormal; mild scoliosis in an older child is not uncommon. Scoliosis appears as an asymmetrical rise in the thoracic region (as shown in Fig. 18-102) or lumbar region, or both.

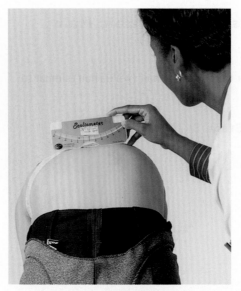

FIGURE 18-102. **Measure and record scoliosis with a scoliometer.**

If you detect scoliosis use a *scoliometer* to test for the degree of scoliosis. Have the teen bend forward again as described above. Place the scoliometer over the spine at a point of maximum prominence making sure that the spine is parallel to the floor at that point, as shown in Figure 18-102. If needed, move the scoliometer up and down the spine to find the point of maximal prominence. An angle greater than 7° on the scoliometer is a reason for concern and often used as a threshold for referral to a specialist. Of note, the sensitivity and specificity of both the Adams forward bend test and scoliometer vary greatly according to the skill and experience of the examiner.

You can also use a *plumb line,* a string with a weight attached, to assess symmetry of the back (Fig. 18-103). Place the top of the plumb line at C7 and have the child stand straight. The plumb line should extend to the gluteal crease (not shown here).

Scoliosis is more common among children and adolescents with neurologic or musculoskeletal abnormalities.

The remainder of the musculoskeletal examination is similar to that for adults, except for the sports preparticipation screening examination described below.

Apparent scoliosis, including an abnormal plumb line test, can be caused by a *leg-length discrepancy* (see p. 886).

Several types of *scoliosis* may present during childhood. Idiopathic scoliosis (75% of cases), seen mostly in girls, is usually detected in early adolescence. As seen in the girl in Figure 18-102, the right hemithorax is generally prominent. Other causes include neuromuscular and congenital.

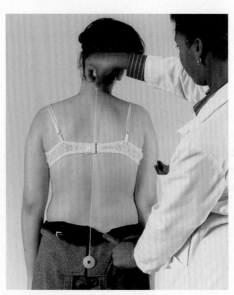

FIGURE 18-103. **Measuring scoliosis with a plumb line.**

The Sports Preparticipation Physical Evaluation.   More than 25 million children and adolescents in the United States and several other countries participate in organized sports and often require "medical clearance." Start the evaluation with a thorough medical history focusing on cardiovascular risk factors, prior surgeries, prior injuries, other medical problems, and a family history. In fact, a complete history is the most sensitive and specific part of the evaluation for detection of risk factors or abnormalities that would preclude participation in sports. The preparticipation physical evaluation is often one of the few times a healthy adolescent will see a clinical professional, so it is important to include some screening questions and anticipatory guidance (see the discussion in Health Promotion and Counseling). Finally, perform a general physical examination, with special attention to the heart and lungs and a vision and hearing screening. Include a *focused, thorough musculoskeletal examination, looking for weakness, limited range of motion, and evidence of previous injury.*

A 2-minute preparticipation screening musculoskeletal examination shown below has been recommended.[67,68]

Important risk factors for sudden cardiovascular death during sports include episodes of *dizziness or palpitations, prior syncope* (particularly if associated with exercise), or family history of *sudden death* or cardiomyopathy in young or middle-aged relatives.

During the preparticipation sports physical examination, assess carefully for *cardiac murmurs* and *wheezing* in the lungs. Also, if the adolescent has had head injuries or a *concussion,*[66] perform a careful, focused neurologic examination.[67,68]

Screening Musculoskeletal Examination for Sports

Position and Instruction to Patient

Step 1: Stand straight, facing forward.   **Step 2:** Move neck in all directions.

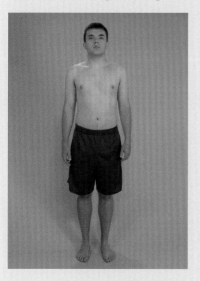

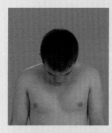
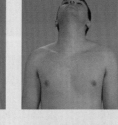
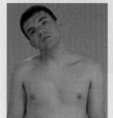
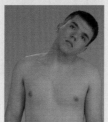

(*continued*)

Common Abnormalities from Prior Injury

Step 1: Asymmetry, swelling of joints
Step 2: Loss of range of motion

Screening Musculoskeletal Examination for Sports (*continued*)

Position and Instruction to Patient

Common Abnormalities from Prior Injury

Step 3: Shrug shoulders against resistance.

Step 4: Hold arms out to the side against resistance.

Step 3: Weakness of shoulder, neck, or trapezius muscles

Step 4: Loss of strength of deltoid muscle

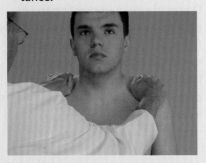

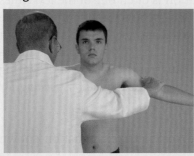

Step 5: Hold arms out to side with elbows bent 90°; raise and lower arms.

Step 6: Hold arms out, completely bend, and straighten elbows.

Step 5: Loss of external rotation and injury of glenohumeral joint

Step 6: Reduced range of motion of elbow

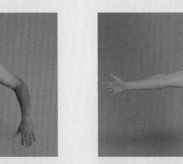

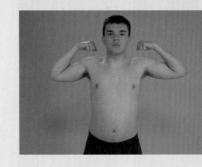

(*continued*)

Screening Musculoskeletal Examination for Sports (continued)

Position and Instruction to Patient

Step 7: Hold arms down, bend elbows 90°, and pronate and supinate forearms.

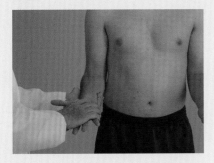

Step 8: Make a fist, clench, and then spread fingers.

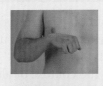
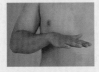

Step 9: Squat and duck-walk for four steps forward.

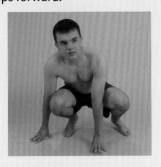

Step 10: Stand straight with arms at sides, facing back.

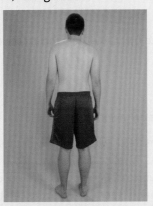

Step 11: Bend forward with knees straight and touch toes.

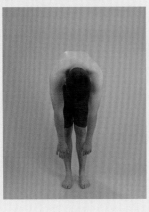

Step 12: Stand on heels and rise to the toes.

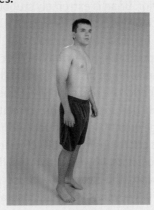

Common Abnormalities from Prior Injury

Step 7: Reduced range of motion from injury to forearm, elbow, or wrist

Step 8: Protruding knuckle, reduced range of motion of fingers from prior sprain or fracture

Step 9: Inability to fully flex knees and difficulty standing up from prior knee or ankle injury

Step 10: Asymmetry from scoliosis, leg-length discrepancy, or weakness from injury

Step 11: Asymmetry from scoliosis and twisting of back from low back pain

Step 12: Wasting of calf muscles from ankle or Achilles tendon injury

The Nervous System

The neurologic examination of the adolescent and the adult is the same. Assess the adolescent's developmental achievement according to age-specific milestones, as described on pp. 890–891.

Recording Your Findings

Initially, you may use sentences to describe your findings; later you will use phrases. The style here contains phrases appropriate for most write-ups. As you read through this write-up, you will note some atypical findings. Try to test yourself. See if you can interpret these findings in the context of all you have learned about the examination of children. You will also note the modifications necessary to accommodate reports from the small child's parent, rather than from the child. If you are using electronic clinical records, make sure your write-up includes sufficient detail and text to adequately summarize your findings.

Recording the Examination: The Pediatric Patient

3/4/2016

Brian is an active, 26-month-old boy accompanied by his mother who is concerned about his development and behavior.

Referral. None

Source and Reliability. Mother (Mom), reliable.

Chief Complaint: Slow development and difficult behavior.

Present Illness: Brian appears to be developing more slowly than his older sister did. He uses only single words and simple phrases, rarely combines words, and appears frustrated with not being able to communicate. People understand less than one quarter of his speech. Physical development seems normal: he can throw a ball, kick, scribble, and dress himself well. He has had no head trauma, chronic illnesses, seizures, or regression in his milestones.

Brian's mom is also concerned about his behavior. Brian is extremely stubborn, frequently has tantrums, gets angry easily (especially with his older sister), throws objects, bites, and physically strikes others when he doesn't get his way. His behavior seems worse around his mother who reports that he is "fine" at his child care center. He moves from one activity to another with an inability to sit still to read or play a game. Of note, he is sometimes affectionate and cuddly. He does make eye contact and plays normally with toys. He has no unusual movements.

Brian is an extremely picky eater who eats a large quantity of junk food and little else. He will not eat fruits or vegetables and drinks enormous quantities of juice and soda. His mother has tried everything to get him to eat healthy food, to no avail.

The family has been under substantial stress during the past year because Brian's father has been unemployed. Although Brian now has Medicaid insurance, the parents are uninsured.

Brian's sleep is considered normal.

Medications. One multivitamin daily.

(continued)

Recording the Examination:
The Pediatric Patient (*continued*)

Past History

Pregnancy. Uneventful. Mom reduced tobacco intake to a half-pack a day and drank alcohol at times. She denies use of other drugs or any infections.

Newborn Period. Born vaginally at 40 weeks; left the hospital in 2 days. Birth weight 2.5 kg (5 lb, 8 oz). Mom does not know why Brian was small at birth.

Illnesses. Only minor illnesses; no hospitalizations.

Accidents. Required sutures last year for a facial laceration secondary to a fall on the road. He did not lose consciousness and had no sequelae.

Preventive Care. Brian has had regular preventive check-ups. At the last appointment 6 months ago, his regular physician said that Brian was a bit behind on some developmental milestones and suggested a child care center that he knew was excellent, as well as increased parental attention to reading, speaking, playing, and stimulation. Immunizations are up to date. His lead level was elevated mildly last year and Mom reports that he had "low blood." His physician recommended iron supplements and foods high in iron, but Brian really won't eat these foods.

Family History

Strong family history of diabetes (two grandparents, none with diabetes as children) and hypertension. No family history of childhood developmental, psychiatric, or chronic illnesses.

Developmental History: Sat up at 6 months, crawled at 9 months, and walked at 13 months. First words ("mama" and "car") said at approximately 1 year.

Personal and Social History: Parents are married and live with the two children in a rented apartment. Dad has not had a steady job for 1 year, but has worked intermittently in construction. Mom works as a waitress part-time while Brian is in child care.

Mom had depression during Brian's first year and attended some counseling sessions but stopped because she could not pay for them or medications. She gets support from her mother who lives 30 minutes away, and many friends, some of whom babysit occasionally.

Despite substantial family stress, Mom describes a loving and intact family. They try to eat dinner together daily, limit television, read to both children (although Brian won't sit still), and go to the nearby park regularly to play.

Environmental Exposures. Both parents smoke, although generally outside the house.

Safety. Mom reports this as a major concern: she can barely leave Brian out of her sight without him getting into something. She fears he will run under a car; the family is thinking of fencing in their small yard. Brian sits in his car seat most of the time; smoke detectors work in the home. Dad's guns are locked; medications are in a cabinet in the parents' bedroom.

Review of Systems

General. No major illnesses.

Skin. Dry and itchy. Last year he was prescribed hydrocortisone for it.

Head, Eyes, Ears, Nose, and Throat (HEENT). *Head:* No trauma. *Eyes:* Vision fine. *Ears:* Multiple infections in the past year. Frequently ignores parents' requests;

(*continued*)

Recording the Examination:
The Pediatric Patient (*continued*)

they can't tell if this is purposeful or if he can't hear well. *Nose:* Often runny; Mom wonders about allergies. *Mouth:* No dentist visit yet. Brushes teeth sometimes (a frequent source of dispute).

Neck. No lumps. Glands in neck seem large.

Respiratory. Frequent cough and whistle in chest. Mom cannot identify trigger; it tends to go away. He can run around all day without seeming to get tired.

Cardiovascular. No known heart disease. He had a murmur when younger, but it went away.

Gastrointestinal. Appetite and eating habits described above. Regular bowel movements. He is in the process of toilet training and wears pull-ups at night, but not at child care.

Urinary. Good stream. No prior urinary tract infections.

Genital. Normal.

Musculoskeletal. He is "all boy" and never gets tired. Minor bumps and bruises occasionally.

Neurologic. Walks and runs well; seems coordinated for age. No stiffness, seizures, or fainting. Mom says his memory seems great, but his attention span is poor.

Psychiatric. Generally seems happy. Cries easily; bounces back and forth from trying to be independent to needing cuddling and comforting.

Physical Examination

Brian is an active and energetic toddler. He plays with the reflex hammer, pretending it is a truck. He appears closely bonded with his mother, looking at her occasionally for comfort. She seems concerned that Brian will break something. His clothes are clean.

Vital Signs. Ht 90 cm (90th percentile). Wt 16 kg (>95th percentile). BMI 19.8 (>95th percentile). Head circumference 50 cm (75th percentile). BP 108/58. Heart rate 90 beats per minute and regular. Respiratory rate 30/minute; varies with activity. Temperature (ear) 37.5°C. Obviously no pain.

Skin. Normal except for bruises on the anterior aspects of his legs, and patchy, dry skin over external surface of elbows.

HEENT. *Head:* Normocephalic; no lesions. *Eyes:* Difficult to examine because he won't sit still. Symmetric with normal extraocular movements. Pupils 4 to 5 mm, and symmetrically reactive to light. Discs difficult to visualize; no hemorrhages noted. *Ears:* Normal pinna; no external abnormalities. Normal external canals and tympanic membranes (TMs). *Nose:* Normal nares; septum midline. *Mouth:* Several darkened teeth (inside surface of upper incisors). One clear cavity on upper right incisor. Tongue normal. Cobblestoning of posterior pharynx; no exudates. Tonsils large but adequate gap (1.5 cm) between them. No allergic shiners.

Neck. Supple, midline trachea, no thyroid palpable.

Lymph Nodes. Easily palpable (1.5 to 2 cm), firm, mobile anterior cervical lymph nodes bilaterally. Small (0.5 cm) nodes in inguinal canal bilaterally. All lymph nodes mobile and nontender.

(*continued*)

Recording the Examination:
The Pediatric Patient (*continued*)

Lungs. Good expansion. No tachypnea or dyspnea. Congestion audible, but seems to be upper airway (louder near mouth, symmetric). No rhonchi, rales, or wheezes. Clear to auscultation.

Cardiovascular. PMI in 4th or 5th interspace and midsternal line. Normal S_1 and S_2. No murmurs or abnormal heart sounds. Normal femoral pulses; dorsalis pedis pulses palpable bilaterally.

Breasts. Normal, with some fat under both.

Abdomen. Protuberant but soft; no masses or tenderness. Liver span 2 cm below right costal margin (RCM) and not tender. Spleen and kidneys not palpable.

Genitalia. Tanner I circumcised penis; no pubic hair, lesions, or discharge. Testes descended, difficult to palpate because of active cremasteric reflex. Normal scrotum both sides.

Musculoskeletal. Normal range of motion of upper and lower extremities and all joints. Spine straight. Gait normal.

Neurologic. *Mental Status:* Happy, cooperative, active child. *Developmental:* Gross motor—Jumps and throws objects. Fine motor—Imitates vertical line. Language—Does not combine words; single words only, three to four noted during examination. Personal–social—Washes face, brushes teeth, and puts on shirt. Overall—Normal, except for language, which appears delayed. *Cranial Nerves:* Intact, although several difficult to elicit. *Cerebellar:* Normal gait; good balance. *Deep tendon reflexes (DTRs):* Normal and symmetric throughout with downgoing toes. *Sensory:* Deferred.

Table 18-1 Abnormalities in Heart Rhythm and Blood Pressure

Supraventricular Tachycardia

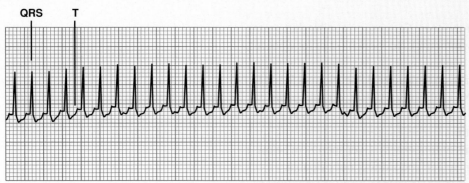

Paroxysmal supraventricular tachycardia (PSVT) is the most common dysrhythmia in children. Some infants with SVT look well or may be somewhat pale with tachypnea but have a heart rate of ≥240 beats per minute. Others are ill and in cardiovascular collapse. P waves have different morphology or are not seen.

SVT in infants is usually sustained, requiring clinical therapy for conversion to a normal rate and rhythm. In older children, it is more likely to be truly paroxysmal, with episodes of varying duration and frequency.

Hypertension in Childhood—A Typical Example

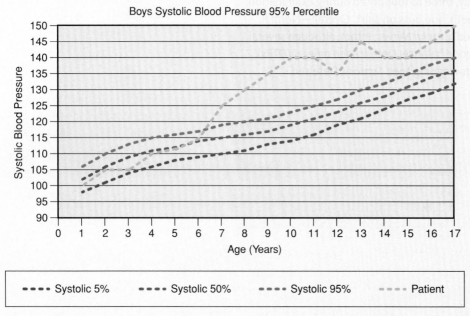

Hypertension can start in childhood.[35,36] Although elevated blood pressure in young children is more likely to have a renal, cardiac, or endocrine cause, older children and adolescents with hypertension are most likely to have primary or essential hypertension.

This child developed hypertension, and it "tracked" into adulthood. Children tend to remain in the same percentile for blood pressure as they grow. This tracking of blood pressure continues into adulthood, supporting the concept that adult essential hypertension often begins during childhood.

The consequences of untreated hypertension can be severe and include cardiac, renal, and visual sequelae.

Table 18-2 Common Skin Rashes and Skin Findings in Newborns and Infants

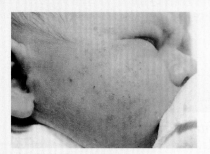

Erythema Toxicum
These common yellow or white pustules are surrounded by a red base.

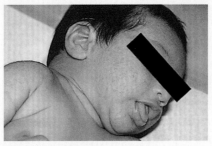

Neonatal Acne
Red pustules and papules are most prominent over the cheeks and nose of some normal newborns.

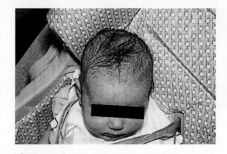

Seborrhea
The salmon red, scaly eruption often involves the face, neck, axilla, diaper area, and behind the ears.

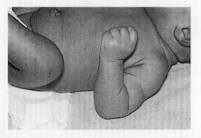

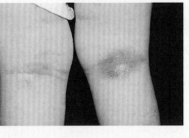

Atopic Dermatitis (Eczema)
Erythema, scaling, dry skin, and intense itching characterize this condition.

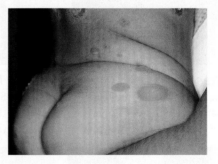

Neurofibromatosis
Characteristic features include more than 5 café-au-lait spots and axillary freckling. Later findings include neurofibromas and Lisch nodules (not shown).

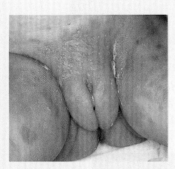

Candidal Diaper Dermatitis
This bright red rash involves the intertriginous folds, with small "satellite lesions" along the edges.

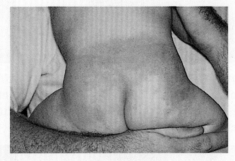

Contact Diaper Dermatitis
This irritant rash is secondary to diarrhea or irritation and is noted along contact areas (here, the area touching the diaper).

Impetigo
This infection is due to bacteria and can appear bullous or crusty and yellowed with some pus.

Table 18-3 Warts, Lesions That Resemble Warts, and Other Raised Lesions

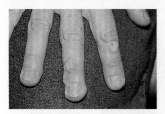

Verruca Vulgaris
Dry, rough warts on hands

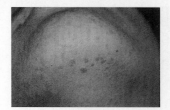

Verruca Plana
Small, flat warts

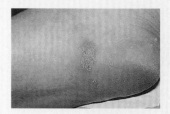

Plantar Warts
Tender warts on feet

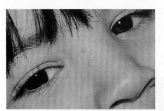

Molluscum Contagiosum
Dome-shaped, fleshy lesions

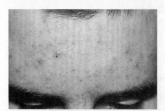

Adolescent Acne
Acne in adolescents involves open comedones (blackheads) and closed comedones (whiteheads) shown at the left, and inflamed pustules (right).

Table 18-4 Common Skin Lesions During Childhood

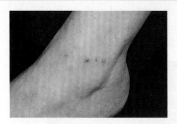

Bites
Intensely pruritic, red, distinct papules characterize these lesions.

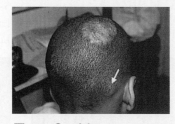

Tinea Capitis
Scaling, crusting, and hair loss are seen in the scalp, along with a painful plaque (kerion) and occipital lymph node (*arrow*).

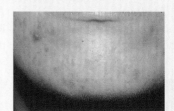

Urticaria (Hives)
This pruritic, allergic sensitivity reaction changes shape quickly.

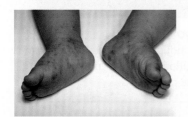

Scabies
Intensely itchy papules and vesicles, sometimes burrows, most often on extremities

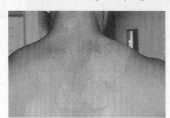

Tinea Corporis
This annular lesion has central clearing and papules along the border.

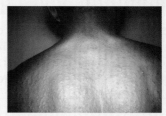

Pityriasis Rosea
Oval lesions on trunk, in older children, often in a Christmas tree pattern, sometimes a herald patch (a large patch that appears first)

Source of *Bites, Tinea Capitis,* and *Tinea Corporis* photos—Goodheart HA. *Photoguide of Common Skin Disorders.* Baltimore: Williams & Wilkins; 1999.

Table 18-5 Abnormalities of the Head

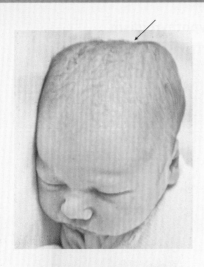

Cephalohematoma

Although not present at birth, cephalohematomas appear within the first 24 hours from subperiosteal hemorrhage involving the outer table of one of the cranial bones. The swelling, shown at the *arrow*, does not extend across a suture though it is occasionally bilateral following a difficult birth. The swelling is initially soft, then develops a raised bony margin within a few days from calcium deposits at the edge of the periosteum. It tends to resolve within several weeks.

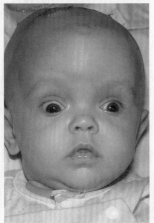

Hydrocephalus

In hydrocephaly, the anterior fontanelle is bulging and the eyes may be deviated downward revealing the upper scleras and creating the *setting sun* sign, as shown on the left. The setting sun sign is also seen briefly in some normal newborns. (From Zitelli BJ, Davis HW. Atlas of Pediatric Physical Diagnosis, 3rd ed. St. Louis: Mosby–Year Book, 1997. Courtesy of Dr. Albert Briglan, Children's Hospital of Pittsburgh.)

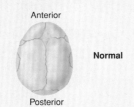

Anterior

Normal

Posterior

Craniosynostosis

Craniosynostosis is a condition of premature closure of one or more sutures of the skull. This results in an abnormal growth and shape of the skull because growth will occur across sutures that are not affected but not across sutures that are affected.

The figures demonstrate different skull shapes associated with the various types of craniosynostosis. The prematurely closed suture line is noted by the absence of a suture line in each figure. Scaphocephaly and frontal plagiocephaly are the most common forms of craniosynostosis. The *blue shading* shows areas of maximal flattening. The *red arrows* show the direction of continued growth across the sutures, which is normal.

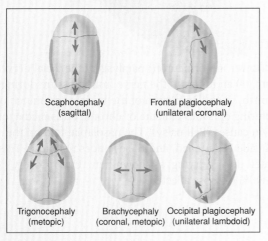

Scaphocephaly (sagittal)

Frontal plagiocephaly (unilateral coronal)

Trigonocephaly (metopic)

Brachycephaly (coronal, metopic)

Occipital plagiocephaly (unilateral lambdoid)

Table 18-6 Diagnostic Facies in Infancy and Childhood

Fetal Alcohol Syndrome

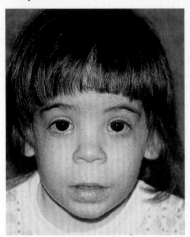

Babies born to women with chronic alcoholism are at increased risk for growth deficiency, microcephaly, and intellectual disability. Facial characteristics include short palpebral fissures, a wide and flattened philtrum (the vertical groove in the midline of the upper lip), and thin lips.

Congenital Syphilis

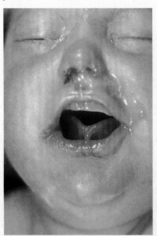

In utero infection by *Treponema pallidum* usually occurs after the 16th week of gestation and affects virtually all fetal organs. If it is not treated, 25% of infected babies die before birth and another 30% shortly thereafter. Signs of illness appear in survivors within the first month of life. Facial stigmata often include bulging of the frontal bones and nasal bridge depression (*saddle nose*), both from periostitis; rhinitis from weeping nasal mucosal lesions (*snuffles*); and a circumoral rash. Mucocutaneous inflammation and fissuring of the mouth and lips (*rhagades*), not shown here, may also occur as stigmata of congenital syphilis, as may craniotabes tibial periostitis (*saber shins*) and dental dysplasia (*Hutchinson teeth*—see p. 296).

Congenital Hypothyroidism

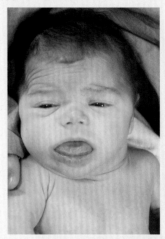

The child with congenital hypothyroidism (*cretinism*) has coarse facial features, a low-set hair line, sparse eyebrows, and an enlarged tongue. Associated features include a hoarse cry, umbilical hernia, dry and cold extremities, myxedema, mottled skin, and intellectual disability. Most infants with congenital hypothyroidism have no physical stigmata; this has led to screening of all newborns in the United States and most other developed countries for congenital hypothyroidism.

Facial Nerve Palsy

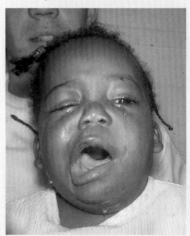

Peripheral (lower motor neuron) paralysis of the facial nerve may be from (1) an injury to the nerve from pressure during labor and birth, (2) inflammation of the middle ear branch of the nerve during episodes of acute or chronic otitis media, or (3) unknown causes (Bell palsy). The nasolabial fold on the affected left side is flattened, and the eye does not close. This is accentuated during crying, as shown here. Full recovery occurs in ≥90% of those affected.

Down Syndrome

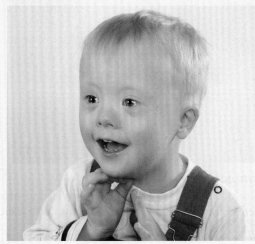

The child with Down syndrome (trisomy 21) usually has a small, rounded head, a flattened nasal bridge, oblique palpebral fissures, prominent epicanthal folds, small, low-set, shell-like ears, and a relatively large tongue. Associated features include generalized hypotonia, transverse palmar creases (*simian lines*), shortening and incurving of the fifth fingers (*clinodactyly*), Brushfield spots (see p. 916), and mild to moderate cognitive impairment.

Battered Child Syndrome

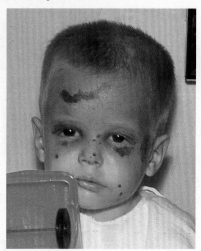

The child who has been physically abused (battered) may have *old and fresh bruises* on the head and face. Other stigmata include bruises in areas (axilla and groin) not usually subject to injury rather than the bony prominences; x-ray evidence of fractures of the skull, ribs, and long bones in various stages of healing; and skin lesions that are morphologically similar to implements used to inflict trauma (hand, belt buckle, strap, rope, coat hanger, or lighted cigarette). Of note, while many normal children have bruises on bony prominences, abused children are more likely to have bruises on protected areas.

Perennial Allergic Rhinitis

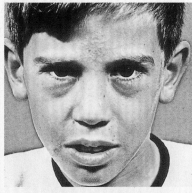

The child suffering from perennial allergic rhinitis has an open mouth (cannot breathe through the nose) and edema and discoloration of the lower orbitopalpebral grooves ("allergic shiners"). Such a child is often seen to push the nose upward and backward with a hand ("allergic salute") and to grimace (wrinkle the nose and mouth) to relieve nasal itching and obstruction.

Hyperthyroidism

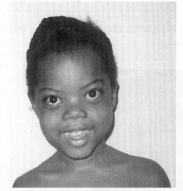 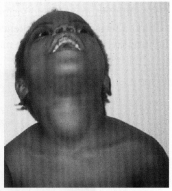

Thyrotoxicosis (*Graves disease*) occurs in approximately 2 per 1,000 children younger than 10 years. Affected children exhibit tachycardia, hypermetabolism, and accelerated linear growth. Facial characteristics shown in this 6-year-old girl are "staring" eyes (not true exophthalmos, which is rare in children) and an enlarged thyroid gland (*goiter*).

Table 18-7 Abnormalities of the Eyes, Ears, and Mouth

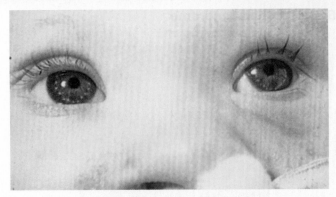

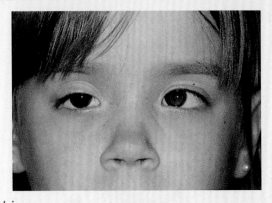

Brushfield Spots

These abnormal speckling spots on the iris suggest Down syndrome.

Strabismus

Strabismus, or misalignment of the eyes, can lead to visual impairment. Esotropia, shown here, is an inward deviation.

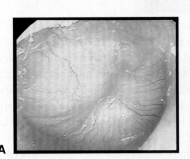 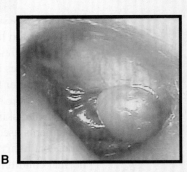 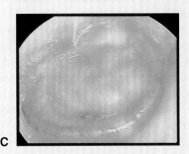

A   B   C

Otitis Media

Otitis media is one of the most common conditions in young children. The spectrum of otitis media is shown here. **A:** Typical acute otitis media with a red, distorted, bulging tympanic membrane in a highly symptomatic child. **B:** Acute otitis media with bullae formation and fluid visible behind the tympanic membrane. **C:** Otitis media with effusion, showing a yellowish fluid behind a retracted and thickened tympanic membrane. Often you can no longer visualize the normal landmarks such as the light reflex and handle of the malleus.

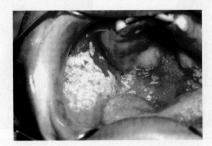

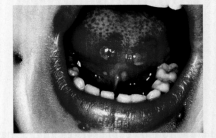

Oral Candidiasis ("Thrush")

This infection is common in infants. The white plaques do not rub off.

Herpetic Stomatitis

Tender ulcerations on the oral mucosa are surrounded by erythema.

Source of photos: *Otitis Media*—Courtesy of Alejandro Hoberman, Children's Hospital of Pittsburgh, University of Pittsburgh.

Table 18-8 Abnormalities of the Teeth, Pharynx, and Neck

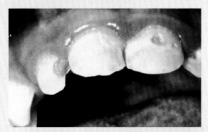

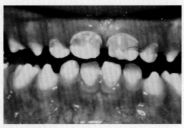

Nursing-Bottle Caries   Erosion of Teeth

Dental Caries

Dental caries is a major global health and pediatric problem. White spots on the teeth often reflect early caries. The photographs to the left show different characteristics of caries.

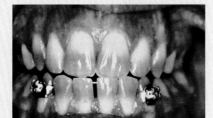

Staining of the Teeth

Various causes can lead to staining of the teeth of children, including intrinsic stains such as tetracycline (*left*) or extrinsic stains such as poor oral hygiene (not shown). Extrinsic stains can be removed.

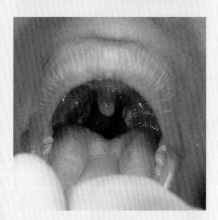

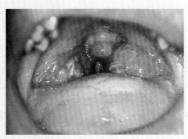

Streptococcal Pharyngitis ("Strep Throat")

This common childhood infection has a classic presentation of erythema of the posterior pharynx and palatal petechiae. A foul-smelling exudate is also commonly noted.

Lymphadenopathy

Enlarged and tender cervical lymph nodes are common in children. The most likely causes are viral and bacterial infections. Lymph node enlargement can be bilateral, as shown in the figure to the left.

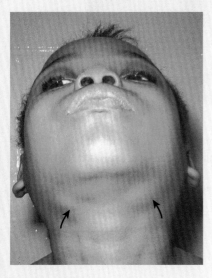

Sources of photos: *Dental Caries* and *Staining of the Teeth*—Courtesy of American Academy of Pediatrics.

Table 18-9 Cyanosis in Children

It is important to recognize cyanosis. The best location to examine is the mucous membranes. Cyanosis is a "raspberry" color, whereas normal mucous membranes should have a "strawberry" color. Try to identify the cyanosis in these photographs before reading the captions.

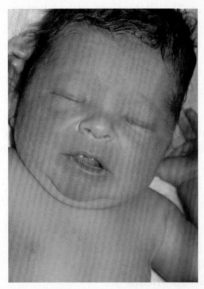

Generalized Cyanosis

This baby has total anomalous pulmonary venous return and an oxygen saturation level of 80%.

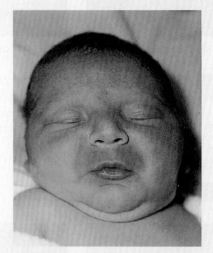

Perioral Cyanosis

This baby has mild cyanosis above the lips, but the mucous membranes remain pink.

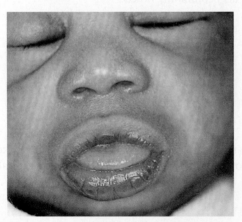

Bluish Lips, Giving Appearance of Cyanosis

Normal pigment deposition in the vermilion border of the lips gives them a bluish hue, but the mucous membranes are pink.

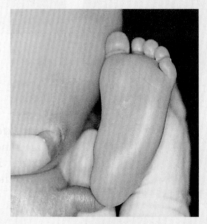

Acrocyanosis

This commonly appears on the feet and hands of babies shortly after birth. This infant is a 32-week-old newborn.

Source of photos (except *Generalized Cyanosis*): Fletcher M. *Physical Diagnosis in Neonatology*. Philadelphia: Lippincott-Raven; 1998.

Table 18-10 Congenital Heart Murmurs

Some heart murmurs reflect underlying heart disease. If you understand their physiologic causes, you will more readily be able to identify and distinguish them from innocent heart murmurs. Obstructive lesions result when blood flows through under-sized valves. Because this problem does not depend on the drop in pulmonary vascular resistance following birth, these murmurs are audible at birth. Defects with left-to-right shunts, on the other hand, depend on the drop in pulmonary vascular resistance that occurs shortly after birth. High-pressured shunts such as ventricular septal defect, patent ductus arteriosus, and persistent truncus arteriosus are not heard until 1 wk or more after birth. Low-pressured left-to-right shunts, such as atrial septal defects, may not be heard until age 1 yr or more. Many children with congenital cardiac defects have combinations of defects or variations of abnormalities, so findings on cardiac examination may not follow these classic patterns. This table shows a limited selection of the more common murmurs, starting with murmurs that appear in the newborn period.

Congenital Defect and Mechanism	Characteristics of the Murmur	Associated Findings
Pulmonary Valve Stenosis Usually a normal valve annulus with fusion of some or most of the valve leaflets, restricting flow across the valve *Mild* 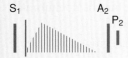 *Severe* 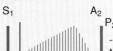	*Location.* Upper left sternal border *Radiation.* In mild degrees of stenosis, the murmur may be heard over the course of the pulmonary arteries in the lung fields. *Intensity.* Increases in intensity and duration as the degree of obstruction increases *Quality.* Ejection, peaking later in systole as the obstruction increases	Usually a prominent ejection click in early systole Pulmonary component of the second sound at the base (P_2) becomes delayed and softer, disappearing as obstruction increases. Inspiration may increase murmur; expiration may increase click. Growth is usually normal. Newborns with severe stenosis may be cyanotic from right-to-left atrial shunting and rapidly develop heart failure as the ductus arteriosus closes.
Aortic Valve Stenosis Usually a bicuspid valve with progressive obstruction, but may occur as a result of a dysplastic valve or damage from rheumatic fever or degenerative disease 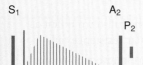	*Location.* Midsternum, upper right sternal border *Radiation.* To the carotid arteries and suprasternal notch; may also be a thrill *Intensity.* Varies, louder with increasingly severe obstruction *Quality.* An ejection, often harsh, systolic murmur	May be an associated ejection click The aortic closure sound may be increased in intensity. There may be a diastolic murmur of aortic valve regurgitation (not shown in the diagram). Newborns with severe stenosis may have weak or absent pulses and severe heart failure. May not be audible until adulthood even though the valve is congenitally abnormal
Tetralogy of Fallot Complex defect with ventricular septal defect, infundibular and usually valvular right ventricular outflow obstruction, malrotation of the aorta, and right-to-left shunting at ventricular septal level *With Pulmonic Stenosis* 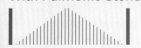 *With Pulmonic Atresia* 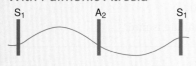	*General.* Variable cyanosis, increasing with activity *Location.* Mid-to-upper left sternal border. If pulmonary atresia, the continuous murmur of ductus arteriosus flow at upper left sternal border or in the back. *Radiation.* Little, to upper left sternal border, occasionally to lung fields *Intensity.* Usually grade III–IV *Quality.* Systolic ejection murmur	Normal pulses The pulmonary closure sound is usually not heard. May have abrupt hypercyanotic spells with sudden increase in cyanosis, air hunger, altered level of awareness Failure to gain weight with persistent and increasingly severe cyanosis Long-term persistence of cyanosis accompanied by clubbing of fingers and toes Persistent hypoxemia leads to polycythemia, which will accentuate the cyanosis.

(continued)

Table 18-10 Congenital Heart Murmurs (*Continued*)

Transposition of the Great Arteries

A severe defect with failure of rotation of the great vessels, leaving the aorta to arise from the right ventricle and the pulmonary artery from the left ventricle

General. Intense generalized cyanosis

Location. No characteristic murmur. If present, it may reflect an associated defect such as ventricular septal defect (VSD).

Radiation and Quality. Depends on associated abnormalities

Single loud second sound of the anterior aortic valve

Frequent rapid development of heart failure

Frequent associated defects as described at the left

Ventricular Septal Defect

Blood going from a high-pressure left ventricle through a defect in the septum to the lower-pressure right ventricle creates turbulence, usually throughout systole.

Small to Moderate

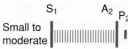

Location. Lower left sternal border

Radiation. Little

Intensity. Variable, only partially determined by the size of the shunt. Small shunts with a high-pressure gradient may have very loud murmurs. Large defects with elevated pulmonary vascular resistance may have no murmur. Grade II–IV/VI with a thrill if grade IV/VI or higher.

Quality. Pansystolic, usually harsh, may obscure S_1 and S_2 if loud enough

With large shunts, there may be a low-pitched middiastolic murmur of relative mitral stenosis at the apex.

As pulmonary artery pressure increases, the pulmonic component of the second sounds at the base increases in intensity. When pulmonary artery pressure equals aortic pressure there may be no murmur and P_2 will be very loud.

In low-volume shunts, growth is normal.

In larger shunts, heart failure may occur by 6–8 wks; poor weight gain, poor feeding.

Associated defects are frequent.

Patent Ductus Arteriosus

Continuous flow from aorta to pulmonary artery throughout the cardiac cycle when ductus arteriosus does not close after birth

Small to Moderate

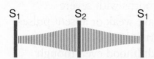

Location. Upper left sternal border and to left

Radiation. Sometimes to the back

Intensity. Varies depending on size of the shunt, usually grade II–III/VI.

Quality. A rather hollow, sometimes machinery-like murmur that is continuous throughout the cardiac cycle, although occasionally almost inaudible in late diastole, uninterrupted by the heart sounds, louder in systole

Full to bounding pulses

Noticed at birth in the premature infant who may have bounding pulses, a hyperdynamic precordium, and an atypical murmur

Noticed later in the full-term infant as pulmonary vascular resistance falls

May develop heart failure at 4–6 wks if large shunt

Poor weight gain related to size of shunt

Pulmonary hypertension affects murmur as above.

Atrial Septal Defect

Left-to-right shunt through an opening in the atrial septum, possible at various levels

Location. Upper left sternal border

Radiation. To the back

Intensity. Variable, usually grade II–III/VI

Quality. Ejection but without the harsh quality

Widely split second sounds throughout all phases of respiration, normal intensity

Usually not heard until after age of 1 yr

Gradual decrease in weight gain as shunt increases

Decreased exercise tolerance, subtle, not dramatic

Heart failure is rare.

Table 18-11 Physical Signs of Sexual Abuse

Possible Indications

1. Marked and immediate dilatation of the anus in knee–chest position, with no constipation, stool in the vault, or neurologic disorders
2. Hymenal notch or cleft that extends >50% of the inferior hymenal rim (confirmed in knee–chest position)
3. Condyloma acuminata in a child older than 3 yrs
4. Bruising, abrasions, lacerations, or bite marks of labia or perihymenal tissue
5. Herpes of the anogenital area beyond the neonatal period
6. Purulent or malodorous vaginal discharge in a young girl (culture and view all discharges under a microscope for evidence of a sexually transmitted infection)

Strong Indications

1. Lacerations, ecchymoses, and newly healed scars of the hymen or the posterior fourchette
2. No hymenal tissue from 3 o'clock to 9 o'clock (confirmed in various positions)
3. Healed hymenal transections especially between 3 and 9 o'clock (complete cleft)
4. Perianal lacerations extending to external sphincter

A child with concerning physical signs must be evaluated by a sexual abuse expert for a complete history and sexual abuse examination.

Any physical sign must be evaluated in light of the entire history, other parts of the physical examination, and laboratory data.

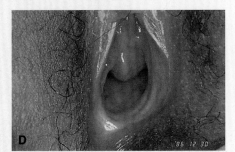

A

Acute hemorrhage and ecchymoses of tissues (10-mo-old)

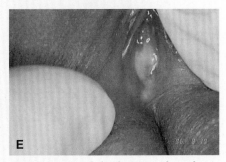

B

Erythema and superficial abrasions to the labia minora (5-yr-old)

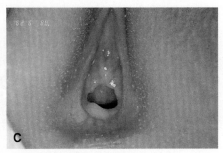

C

Healed interruption of hymenal membrane at 9 o'clock (4-yr-old)

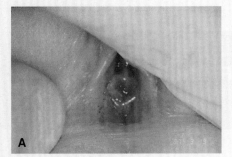

D

Narrowed posterior ring continuous with floor of vagina (12-yr-old)

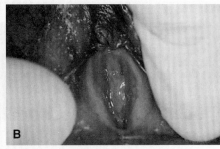

E

Copious vaginal discharge and erythema (9-yr-old)

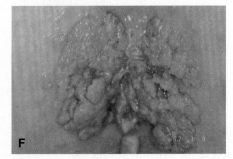

F

Extensive condylomata around the anus (2-yr-old)

Source: Reece R, Ludwig S, eds. *Child Abuse Medical Diagnosis and Management*, 2nd ed. Philadelphia: Lippincott Williams & Wilkins; 2001.

Table 18-12 The Male Genitourinary System

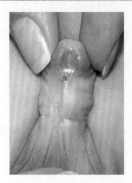

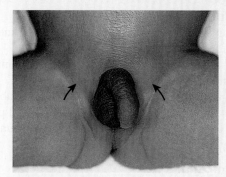

Hypospadias

Hypospadias is the most common congenital penile abnormality. The urethral meatus opens abnormally on the ventral surface of the penis. One form is shown above; more severe forms involve openings on the lower shaft or scrotum.

Undescended Testicle

You should distinguish between undescended testes, shown above, (with testes in the inguinal canals—see *arrows*), from highly retractile testes from an active cremasteric reflex.

Sources of photos: *Hypospadias*—Courtesy of Warren Snodgrass, MD, UT–Southwestern Medical Center at Dallas; *Undescended Testicle*—Fletcher M. *Physical Diagnosis in Neonatology*. Philadelphia: Lippincott-Raven; 1998.

Table 18-13 Common Musculoskeletal Findings in Young Children

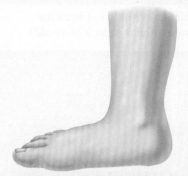

Flat feet or *pes planus* from laxity of the soft tissue structures of the foot

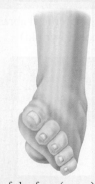

Inversion of the foot (*varus*)

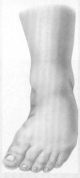

Metatarsus adductus in a child. The forefoot is adducted and not inverted.

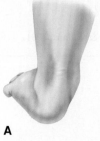

A

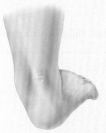

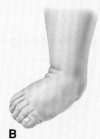

B

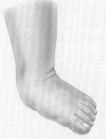

Pronation in a toddler. **A:** When viewed from behind, the hindfoot is everted. **B:** When viewed from the front, the forefoot is everted and abducted.

Table 18-14 The Power of Prevention: Vaccine-Preventable Diseases

This table shows photographs of children with vaccine-preventable diseases. Childhood vaccines have been named the single most important clinical intervention in the world in terms of influence on public health. Because of vaccinations, we hope you will never see many of these conditions, but you should be able to identify them. Try to identify the diseases before reading the captions.

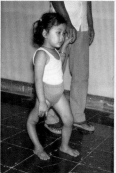

Polio
The deformed leg of this child is from polio

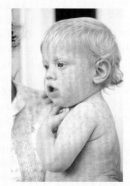

Measles
Characteristic rash of measles, in the presence of a child who also has coryza, conjunctivitis, fever, and this diffuse rash

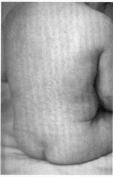

Rubella
Rubella rash on a child's back

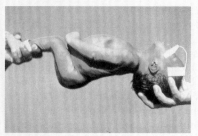

Tetanus
Rigid newborn with neonatal tetanus

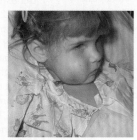

Haemophilus Influenzae Type b
Buccal cellulitis from this invasive bacterial disease

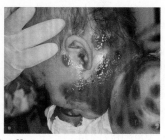

Varicella
An infant with a severe form of varicella

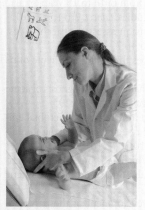

Meningitis
Nuchal rigidity

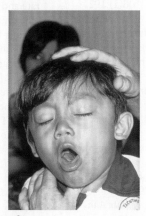

Pertussis
Paroxysmal cough with a "whoop" at the end

Cervical Cancer
Largely prevented through vaccination with human papillomavirus vaccine

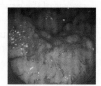

Sequelae of Human Papillomavirus

Sources of photos: *Polio*—Courtesy of World Health Organization; *Haemophilus influenzae*—Courtesy of American Academy of Pediatrics; *Varicella*—Courtesy of Barbara Watson, MD, Albert Einstein Medical Center and Division of Disease Control, Philadelphia Department of Health; *Tetanus*—Courtesy of Centers for Disease Control and Prevention. *Pertussis*—Courtesy of the Immunization Action Coalition.

References

1. Carey WB. *Developmental-Behavioral Pediatrics.* 4th ed. Philadelphia, PA: Saunders/Elsevier; 2009.

2. Levine MD, Carey WB, Crocker AC. *Developmental-Behavioral Pediatrics.* 3rd ed. Philadelphia, PA: Saunders; 1999.

3. Clark EM. *Well-Child Care: A Bright Futures Pocket Guide For Pediatric Providers.* 1st ed. Washington, DC: Georgetown University, 2008.

4. American Academy of Pediatrics. Bright Futures. Available at https://brightfutures.aap.org/Pages/default.aspx. Accessed June 2, 2015.

5. United States Department of Health and Human Services. U.S. Preventive Services Task Force (USPSTF). Available at http://www.ahrq.gov/professionals/clinicians-providers/guidelines-recommendations/guide/. Accessed June 2, 2015.

6. Centers for Disease Control and Prevention. Immunization Schedules. Available at http://www.cdc.gov/vaccines/schedules/index.html. Accessed June 2, 2015.

7. American Academy of Pediatrics. Immunization. Available at http://www2.aap.org/immunization/izschedule.html. Accessed June 2, 2015.

8. Hagan JF, Shaw JS, Duncan PM. *Bright Futures: Guidelines For Health Supervision Of Infants, Children, And Adolescents.* 3rd ed. Elk Grove Village, IL: American Academy of Pediatrics; 2008.

9. Casey BM, McIntire DD, Leveno KJ. The continuing value of the Apgar score for the assessment of newborn infants. *N Engl J Med.* 2001;344(7):467.

10. Ballard JL, Khoury JC, Wedig K. Ballard scoring system for determining gestational age in weeks. *J Pediatr.* 1991;119:417.

11. Brazelton TB. Working with families: opportunities for early intervention. *Pediatr Clin North Am.* 1995;42(1):1.

12. Johnson CP, Blasco PA. Infant growth and development. *Pediatr Rev.* 1997;18(7):224.

13. Colson ER, Dworkin PH. Toddler development. *Pediatr Rev.* 1997; 18(8):255.

14. Copelan J. Normal speech and development. *Pediatr Rev.* 1995;18:91.

15. American Academy of Pediatrics. Developmental surveillance and screening of infants and young children. *Pediatrics.* 2001;108(1):192.

16. Grummer-Strawn LM, Reinold C, Krebs NF, et al. Use of World Health Organization and CDC growth charts for children aged 0–59 months in the United States. *MMWR Recomm Rep.* 2010;59:1.

17. Wright CM, Williams AF, Elliman D, et al. Using the new UK-WHO growth charts. *BMJ.* 2010;340:c1140.

18. Fong CT. Clinical diagnosis of genetic diseases. *Pediatr Ann.* 1993; 22(5):277.

19. Hyvarinen L. Assessment of visually impaired infants. *Ophthalmol Clin North Am.* 1994;7:219.

20. Lees MH. Cyanosis of the newborn infant: recognition and clinical evaluation. *J Pediatr.* 1970;77:484.

21. Frank JE, Jacobe KM. Evaluation and management of heart murmurs in children. *American Fam Physician.* 2011;84:793.

22. Gessner IH. What makes a heart murmur innocent? *Pediatr Ann.* 1997;26(2):82.

23. Wierwille L. Pediatric heart murmurs: evaluation and management in primary care. *J Nurse Pract.* 2011;36:22–8;quiz 8.

24. Callahan CW Jr, Alpert B. Simultaneous percussion auscultation technique for the determination of liver span. *Arch Pediatr Adolesc Med.* 1994;148(8):873.

25. Reiff MI, Osborn LM. Clinical estimation of liver size in newborn infants. *Pediatrics.* 1983;71:46.

26. Burger BJ, Burger JD, Bos CF, et al. Neonatal screening and staggered early treatment for congenital dislocation or dysplasia of the hip. *Lancet.* 1990;336(8730):1549.

27. American Academy of Pediatrics. Clinical practice guideline: early detection of developmental dysplasia of the hip. Committee on Quality Improvement, Subcommittee on Developmental Dysplasia of the Hip. *Pediatrics.* 2000;105:896.

28. Zafeiriou DI. Primitive reflexes and postural reactions in the neurodevelopmental examination. *Pediatr Neurol.* 2004;31(1):1.

29. Schott JM, Rossor MN. The grasp and other primitive reflexes. *J Neurol Neurosurg Psychiatry.* 2003;74(5):558.

30. Luiz DM, Foxcroft CD, Stewart R. The construct validity of the Griffiths Scales of Mental Development. *Child Care Health Dev.* 2001;27:73.

31. Aylward GP. Developmental screening and assessment: what are we thinking? *J Dev Behav Pediatr.* 2009;30:169.

32. Sheldrick RC, Merchant S, Perrin EC. Identification of developmental-behavioral problems in primary care: a systematic review. *Pediatrics.* 2011;128:356.

33. Newacheck PW, Strickland B, Shonkoff JP, et al. An epidemiologic profile of children with special health care needs. *Pediatrics.* 1998; 102:117.

34. Ogden CL, Carroll MD, Kit BK, et al. Prevalence of obesity and trends in body mass index among US children and adolescents, 1999–2010. *JAMA.* 2012;307:483.

35. Ingelfinger JR. The child or adolescent with elevated blood pressure. *N Engl J Med.* 2014;370:2316.

36. National High Blood Pressure Education Program Working Group on High Blood Pressure in Children and Adolescents. The Fourth Report on the Diagnosis, Evaluation, and Treatment of High Blood Pressure in Children and Adolescents. *Pediatrics.* 2004;114:555.

37. Lurbe, Empar, et al. "Management of high blood pressure in children and adolescents: recommendations of the European Society of Hypertension." *Journal of Hypertension* 2009;27.9:1719–1742.

38. Falkner, Bonita, Empar Lurbe, and Franz Schaefer. "High blood pressure in children: clinical and health policy implications." *The Journal of Clinical Hypertension* 2010;12.4:261–276.

39. Fleming S, Thompson M, Stevens R, et al. Normal ranges of heart rate and respiratory rate in children from birth to 18 years of age: a systematic review of observational studies. *Lancet.* 2011;377:1011.

40. Shamis DI. Collecting the "facts": vision assessment techniques: perils and pitfalls. *Am Orthop J.* 1996;46:7.

41. Rothman R, Owens T, Simel DL. Does this child have acute otitis media? *JAMA.* 2003;290:1633.

42. Blomgren K, Pitkaranta A. Current challenges in diagnosis of acute otitis media. *Intl J Ped Otorhinolaryngol.* 2005;69(3):295.

43. Coker TR, Chan LS, Newberry SJ, et al. Diagnosis, microbial epidemiology, and antibiotic treatment of acute otitis media in children: a systematic review. *JAMA.* 2010;304:2161.

44. Pirozzo S, Papinczak T, Glasziou P. Whispered voice test for screening for hearing impairment in adults and children: systematic review. *BMJ.* 2003;327(7421):967.

45. Wolf G, Anderhuber W, Kuhn F. Development of the paranasal sinuses in children: implications for paranasal sinus surgery. *Ann Otol Rhinol Laryngol.* 1993;102(9):705.

46. Tinanoff N, Reisine S. Update on early childhood caries since the Surgeon General's Report. *Acad Pediatr.* 2009;9:396.

47. Lunt RC, Law DB. A review of the chronology of eruption of deciduous teeth. *J Am Dent Assoc.* 1974;89:872.

48. Ebell MH, Smith MA, Barry HC, et al. Does this patient have strep throat? *JAMA.* 2000;284:2912.

REFERENCES

49. Moorman JE, Zahran H, Truman BI, et al. Current asthma prevalence—United States, 2006–2008. *MMWR Surveill Summ.* 2011; 60(Suppl):84.

50. Naylor C. Physical Examination of the Liver. *JAMA.* 1994;271(23): 1859–1865. doi:10.1001/jama.1994.03510470063036.

51. Ashcraft KW. Consultation with the specialist: acute abdominal pain. *Pediatr Rev.* 2000;21:363.

52. Hymel KP, Jenny C. Child sexual abuse. *Pediatr Rev.* 1996; 17(7):236–249; quiz, 249.

53. Maniglio R. The impact of child sexual abuse on the course of bipolar disorder: a systematic review. *Bipolar Disord.* 2013;15:341.

54. Stoltenborgh M, van Ijzendoorn MH, Euser EM, et al. A global perspective on child sexual abuse: meta-analysis of prevalence around the world. *Child Maltreat.* 2011;16:79.

55. Scherl S. Common lower extremity problems in children. *Pediatr Rev.* 2004;25:43.

56. Bruce RW. Torsional and angular deformities. *Pediatr Clin North Am.* 1996;43:867.

57. Committee on Practice and Ambulatory Medicine. Use of chaperones during the physical examination of the pediatric patient. *Pediatrics.* 2011;127:991.

58. American Medical Association. Guidelines for Adolescent Preventive Services (GAPS). Available at http://www.ama-assn.org/ama/upload/mm/39/gapsmono.pdf. Accessed February 19, 2008.

59. Elster AB, Kuznets MJ. *AMA Guidelines for Adolescent Preventive Services (GAPS): Recommendations and Rationale.* Baltimore, MD: Williams & Wilkins; 1993.

60. Herman-Giddens ME, Slora EJ, Wasserman RC, et al. Secondary sexual characteristics and menses in young girls seen in office practice: a study from the Pediatric Research in Office Settings Network. *Pediatrics.* 1997;99(4):505.

61. Biro FM, Galvez MP, Greenspan LC, et al. Pubertal assessment method and baseline characteristics in a mixed longitudinal study of girls. *Pediatrics.* 2010;126(3):e583–e590.

62. Biro FM, Greenspan LC, Galvez MP, et al. Onset of breast development in a longitudinal cohort. *Pediatrics.* 2013;132:1019.

63. Oeffinger KC, Fontham EH, Etzioni R, et al. Breast Cancer Screening for Women at Average Risk: 2015 Guideline Update From the American Cancer Society. *JAMA.* 2015;314(15):1599–1614.

64. ACOG Committee on Adolescent Health Care. ACOG Committee. Opinion no. 350, November 2006: Breast concerns in the adolescent. *Obstet Gynecol.* 2006;108(5):1329.

65. Herman-Giddens ME, Steffes J, Harris D, et al. Secondary sexual characteristics in boys: data from the Pediatric Research in Office Settings Network. *Pediatrics.* 2012;130:e1058.

66. McCrory P, Meeuwisse WH, Aubry M, et al. Consensus statement on concussion in sport: the 4th International Conference on Concussion in Sport held in Zurich, November 2012. *Brit J Sports Med.* 2013; 47:250.

67. Metzl JD. Preparticipation examination of the adolescent athlete: part 1. *Pediatr Rev.* 2001;22(6):119.

68. Metzl JD. Preparticipation examination of the adolescent athlete: part 2. *Pediatr Rev.* 2001;22(7):227.

The Pregnant Woman

The Bates' suite offers these additional resources to enhance learning and facilitate understanding of this chapter:
■ Bates' *Pocket Guide to Physical Examination and History Taking*, 8th edition
■ thePoint online resources, for students and instructors: http://thepoint.lww.com

This chapter presents the history and physical examination of the healthy pregnant woman. Many of the techniques of examination are similar to those of the nonpregnant woman; however, the clinician must distinguish the changes of pregnancy from abnormal findings. This chapter reviews common anatomic and physiologic changes as they evolve throughout pregnancy, elements of the health history specific to the pregnant woman, recommendations for prenatal health promotion and counseling, and physical examination techniques specific to pregnancy (Figs. 19-1 to 19-3).

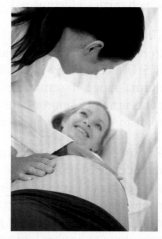

FIGURE 19-1. Support a healthy pregnancy.

Anatomy and Physiology

Physiologic Hormonal Changes

The hormonal changes of pregnancy alter many of the body systems. Because these normal but complex variations result in visible changes in anatomy, in this chapter, the physiologic changes of pregnancy precede the discussion of anatomy and are briefly summarized here.

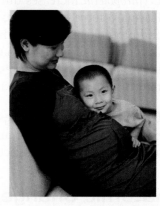

FIGURE 19-2. Sharing and discovering.

■ *Estrogen* promotes endometrial growth that supports the early embryo. It appears to stimulate marked enlargement of the pituitary gland (by up to 135%) and increased prolactin output from its anterior lobe, which readies breast tissue for lactation.[1] Estrogen also contributes to the hypercoagulable state that puts pregnant women at four to five times higher risk for thromboembolic events, primarily in the venous system.[2]

■ *Progesterone* levels increase throughout pregnancy, leading to increased tidal volume and alveolar minute ventilation, though respiratory rate remains constant; respiratory alkalosis and subjective shortness of breath result from these changes.[3] Lower esophageal sphincter tone resulting from rising levels of estradiol and progesterone contributes to gastroesophageal reflux. Progesterone relaxes tone in the ureters and bladder, causing hydronephrosis (in the right ureter more than the left) and an increased risk of bacteriuria.[1]

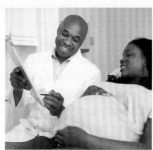

FIGURE 19-3. Support a healthy delivery.

■ *Human chorionic gonadotropin (HCG)* has five variant subtypes. Two are produced by the placenta and support progesterone synthesis in the corpus luteum, stabilizing the endometrium and effectively preventing loss of the early embryo to menstruation. Serum and urine pregnancy assays test primarily for the two pregnancy-related HCG variants; three isoforms are produced by different cancers and the pituitary gland.[4]

■ *Placental growth hormone* influences fetal growth and the development of preeclampsia.[1] Placental growth hormone and other hormones have been implicated in insulin resistance after midpregnancy and in gestational diabetes, which carries a lifetime risk of progressing to type 2 diabetes of up to 60%.[5,6]

■ *Thyroid function* changes include an increase in thyroid-binding globulin due to rising levels of estrogen and stimulation of thyroid-stimulating hormone (TSH) receptors by HCG. This results in a slight increase, usually in the normal range, in serum concentrations of free T3 and T4, while serum TSH concentrations appropriately decrease. This transient apparent "hyperthyroidism" should be considered physiologic.[7]

■ *Relaxin* is secreted by the corpus luteum and placenta and is involved in the remodeling of reproductive tract connective tissue to facilitate delivery, increased renal hemodynamics, and increased serum osmolality. Despite its name, relaxin does not affect peripheral joint laxity during pregnancy. Weight gain, especially around the gravid uterus, and shifts in the center of gravity contribute to lumbar lordosis and other musculoskeletal strain.

■ *Erythropoietin* increases during pregnancy, which raises erythrocyte mass. Plasma volume increases to a greater extent, causing relative hemodilution and physiologic anemia, which can protect against blood loss during birth. Cardiac output increases but systemic vascular resistance decreases, resulting in a net fall in blood pressure, especially during the second trimester and returning to normal by the third trimester.

■ *Basal metabolic rate* increases 15% to 20% during pregnancy, increasing daily energy demands by an estimated 85, 285, and 475 kcal/d in the first, second, and third trimesters, respectively.[1]

Anatomic Changes

Changes in the breasts, abdomen, and urogenital tract are the most visible signs of pregnancy. Review the anatomy and physiology of these body systems in Chapter 10, Breasts and Axillae; Chapter 11, Abdomen; and Chapter 14, Female Genitalia.

Breasts. The breasts become moderately enlarged due to hormonal stimulation that causes increased vascularity and glandular hyperplasia. By the third month of gestation, the breasts become more nodular. The nipples become larger and more erectile, with darker areolae and more pronounced Montgomery glands. The venous pattern over the breasts becomes visibly more prominent as pregnancy progresses. In the second and third trimesters, some women secrete colostrum, a thick, yellowish, nutrient-rich precursor to milk. Breast tenderness may make them more sensitive during examination.

Uterus. Muscle cell hypertrophy, increases in fibrous and elastic tissue, and development of blood vessels and lymphatics all contribute to growth of the uterus. The uterus increases in weight from ~70 g at conception to almost 1,100 g at delivery, when it accommodates from 5 to 20 L of fluid.[1] In the first trimester, the uterus is confined to the pelvis and shaped like an inverted pear; it may retain its prior anteverted (forward-leaning), retroverted (backward-leaning), or retroflexed (backward-bent) position. By 12 to 14 weeks, the gravid uterus becomes externally palpable as it expands into a globular shape beyond the pelvic brim.

Beginning in the second trimester, the enlarging fetus pushes the uterus into an anteverted position that encroaches into the space usually occupied by the bladder, triggering frequent voiding. The intestines are displaced laterally and superiorly. The uterus stretches its own supporting ligaments, causing "round ligament pain" in the lower quadrants. Often, slight dextrorotation to accommodate the rectosigmoid structures on the left side of the pelvis leads to greater discomfort on the right side as well as increased right-sided hydronephrosis.[1] Growth patterns of the gravid uterus are shown in Figure 19-4. Sagittal depictions of the gravid abdomen during each trimester appear in Figures 19-5 to 19-7.

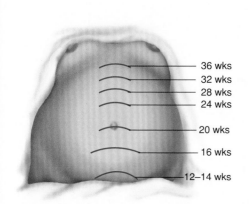

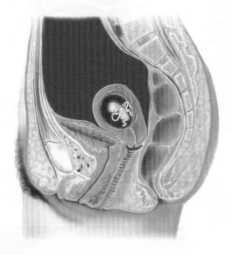

FIGURE 19-4. Growth patterns of the uterine fundus by weeks of pregnancy.

FIGURE 19-5. First trimester.

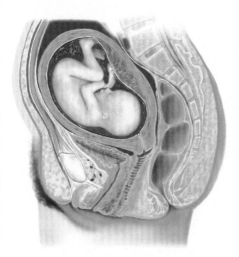

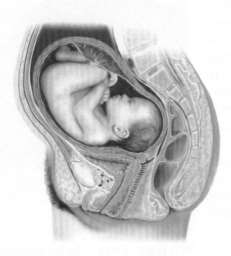

FIGURE 19-6. Second trimester.

FIGURE 19-7. Third trimester.

Vagina. Increased vascularity throughout the pelvis gives the vagina a bluish color, known as *Chadwick sign.* The vaginal walls appear deeply rugated due to thicker mucosa, loosening of connective tissue, and hypertrophy of smooth muscle cells. Normal vaginal secretions may become thick, white, and more profuse, known as *leukorrhea of pregnancy.* Increased glycogen stores in the vaginal epithelium give rise to a proliferation of *Lactobacillus acidophilus,* which lowers the vaginal pH. This acidification protects against some vaginal infections, but at the same time, increased glycogen may contribute to higher rates of vaginal candidiasis.

Cervix. At ~1 month after conception, the cervix softens and also turns bluish or cyanotic in color, reflecting the increased vascularity, edema, and glandular hyperplasia throughout the cervix.[1] *Hegar sign* is the palpable softening of the cervical isthmus, the portion of the uterus that narrows into the cervix, illustrated in Figure 19-8. This cervical remodeling involves rearrangement of the cervical connective tissue that decreases collagen concentration and facilitates dilatation during delivery. Copious cervical secretions fill the cervical canal soon after conception with a tenacious *mucus plug* that protects the uterine environment from outside pathogens and is expelled as *bloody show* at delivery.

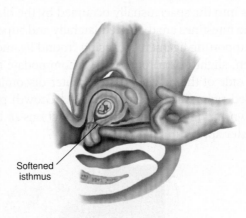

Softened isthmus

FIGURE 19-8. **Hegar sign.**

Adnexae. Early in pregnancy, the corpus luteum, which is the ovarian follicle that has discharged its ovum, may be prominent enough to be felt on the affected ovary as a small nodule; this disappears by midpregnancy.

External Abdomen. As the skin over the abdomen stretches to accommodate the fetus, purplish *striae gravidarum* or "stretch marks" and a *linea nigra,* a brownish black pigmented vertical stripe along the midline skin, may appear (Fig. 19-9). As tension on the abdominal wall increases with advancing pregnancy, the rectus abdominis muscles may separate at the midline, called *diastasis recti.* If diastasis is severe, especially in multiparous women, only a layer of skin, fascia, and peritoneum may cover the anterior uterine wall, and fetal parts may be palpable through this muscular gap.

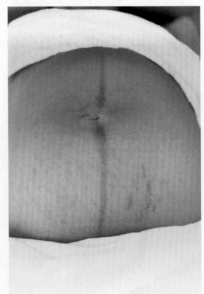

FIGURE 19-9. **Striae and linea nigra.**

Common Concerns During Pregnancy and Their Explanations

Common Concerns	Trimester	Explanation
Missed periods (amenorrhea)	All	High levels of estrogen, progesterone, and HCG build up the endometrium and prevent menses, causing missed periods which are often the first noticeable sign of pregnancy.
Heartburn	All	Progesterone relaxes the lower esophageal sphincter, allowing gastric contents to reflux into the esophagus. The gravid uterus also exerts physical pressure against the stomach, contributing to reflux symptoms.[1]
Urinary frequency	All	Increases in blood volume and filtration rate through the kidneys result in increased urine production, while pressure from the gravid uterus reduces potential space for the bladder. Dysuria or suprapubic pain should be investigated for urinary tract infection.
Vaginal discharge	All	Asymptomatic milky white discharge, *leukorrhea,* results from increased secretions from vaginal and cervical epithelium due to vasocongestion and hormonal changes. Any foul-smelling or pruritic discharge should be investigated.
Constipation	All	Constipation results from slowed gastrointestinal transit due to hormonal changes, dehydration from nausea and vomiting, and the supplemental iron in prenatal vitamins.
Hemorrhoids	All	Hemorrhoids may be caused by constipation, decreased venous return from increasing pressure in the pelvis, compression by fetal parts, and changes in activity level during pregnancy.
Backache	All	Hormonally induced relaxation of the pelvic ligaments contributes to musculoskeletal aches. Lordosis required to balance the gravid uterus contributes to lower back strain. Breast enlargement may contribute to upper backaches.
Nausea and/or vomiting	First	This is poorly understood but appears to reflect hormonal changes, slowed gastrointestinal peristalsis, alterations in smell and taste, and sociocultural factors. *Hyperemesis gravidarum* is vomiting with weight loss of >5% of prepregnancy weight.
Breast tenderness/ tingling	First	Pregnancy hormones stimulate the growth of breast tissue, which causes swelling and possible aching, tenderness, and tingling. Increased blood flow can make delicate veins more visible beneath the skin.
Fatigue	First/Third	Fatigue is related to the rapid change in energy requirements, sedative effects of progesterone, changes in body mechanics due to the gravid uterus, and sleep disturbance. Many women report increased energy and well-being during the second trimester.
Lower abdominal pain	Second	Rapid growth in the second trimester causes tension and stretching of the round ligaments that support the uterus, causing sharp or cramping pain with movement or position change.
Abdominal striae	Second or third	Stretching of the skin and tearing of the collagen in the dermis contribute to thin, usually pink, bands, or *striae gravidarum* (stretch marks). These may persist or fade over time after delivery.
Contractions	Third	Irregular and unpredictable uterine contractions (*Braxton Hicks contractions*) are rarely associated with labor. Contractions that become regular or painful should be evaluated for onset of labor.
Loss of mucus plug	Third	Passage of the mucus plug is common during labor but may occur prior to the onset of contractions. As long as there are no regular contractions, bleeding, or loss of fluid, loss of the mucus plug is unlikely to trigger the onset of labor.
Edema	Third	Decreased venous return, obstruction of lymphatic flow, and reduced plasma colloid oncotic pressure commonly cause lower extremity edema. However, sudden severe edema and hypertension may signal *preeclampsia.*

The Health History

Common Concerns

- Initial prenatal history
  - Confirmation of pregnancy
  - Symptoms of pregnancy
  - Concerns and attitudes toward the pregnancy
  - Current health and past clinical history
  - Past obstetric history
  - Risk factors for maternal and fetal health
  - Family history of patient and father of the newborn
  - Plans for breastfeeding
  - Plans for postpartum contraception
- Determining gestational age and expected date of delivery

Prenatal care focuses on optimizing health and minimizing risk for the mother and fetus. The goals of the initial prenatal visit are to define the health status of the mother and fetus, confirm the pregnancy and estimate gestational age, develop a plan for continuing care, and counsel the mother about her expectations and concerns. During subsequent visits, you should assess any interim changes in the health status of the mother and fetus, review specific physical examination findings related to the pregnancy, and provide counseling and timely preventive screenings.

Initial Prenatal History. Initial prenatal visits are best timed early in pregnancy, but may occur at later in gestation; tailor your history to where it falls during the mother's gestational cycle.

Confirmation of Pregnancy. Ask about *confirmation of pregnancy:* Has the patient had a confirmatory urine pregnancy test, and when? When was her last menstrual period (LMP)? Has she had an ultrasound to establish dates? Explain that serum pregnancy tests are rarely required to confirm pregnancy.

Symptoms of Pregnancy. Has the patient had missed periods, breast tenderness, nausea or vomiting, fatigue, or urinary frequency?

See the table on "Common Concerns During Pregnancy and Their Explanations" for a list of normal as well as concerning symptoms, p. 931.

Concerns and Attitudes Toward Pregnancy. Ask how the patient feels about the pregnancy. Is she excited, concerned, or scared? Was the pregnancy planned and desired? If not, does she plan to complete the pregnancy to term, terminate, or consider adoption? Is a partner, father of the baby, or other family support network involved? As you elicit her viewpoints, use open-ended questions and be flexible and nonjudgmental. Respect diverse family structures, such as extended family support, single motherhood, or pregnancy conceived by sperm donation with or without a partner of either gender. Support the patient's choices when unexpected admissions arise, such as a pregnancy resulting from a coerced sexual act, or the wish to end the pregnancy.

Current Health and Past Clinical History. Explore any past or present clinical conditions (Fig. 19-10). Pay particular attention to conditions that affect pregnancy, such as abdominal surgeries, hypertension, diabetes, cardiac disorders including childhood surgery for congenital heart disease, asthma, hypercoagulability states from lupus anticoagulant or anticardiolipin antibodies, mental health disorders such as postpartum depression, human immunodeficiency virus (HIV), sexually transmitted infections (STIs), abnormal Pap smears, and exposure to diethylstilbestrol (DES) in utero.

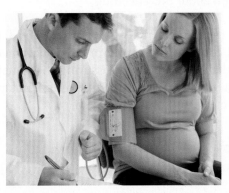

FIGURE 19-10. **Explore the health history.**

Past Obstetric History. How many prior pregnancies has the patient had? How many were term deliveries, preterm deliveries, spontaneous and terminated pregnancies, and how many were live births? Were there any complications from diabetes, hypertension, preeclampsia, intrauterine growth restriction, or preterm labor? Were there any complications during labor and delivery such as large babies (*fetal macrosomia*), fetal distress, or emergency interventions? Were deliveries by vaginal delivery, assisted delivery (vacuum or forceps), or cesarean section?

Risk Factors for Maternal and Fetal Health. Does she use tobacco, alcohol, or illicit drugs? What about medications, over-the-counter drugs, or herbal preparations? Does she have any toxic exposures at work, at home, or in other settings? Is her nutritional intake adequate, or is she at risk from obesity? Does she have an adequate social support network and source of income? Are there unusual sources of stress at home or work? Is there any history of physical abuse or domestic violence?

Family History. Ask about the genetic and family history of the patient and her partner and/or father. What are the ethnic backgrounds of the patient and father? Is there any family history of genetic diseases such as sickle cell anemia, cystic fibrosis, or muscular dystrophy, among others? Have babies in the family had any congenital problems?

Plans for Breastfeeding. Breastfeeding protects the baby against a variety of infectious and noninfectious conditions, and exerts a protective effect on the mother against breast cancer and other conditions.[8-10] Education during pregnancy and clinician encouragement increase the subsequent rate and duration of maternal breastfeeding.

Plans for Postpartum Contraception. Initiate this discussion early, as postpartum contraception reduces the risk of unintended pregnancy and shortened interpregnancy intervals, which are linked to increases in adverse pregnancy outcomes.[11,12] Plans for contraception will depend on the patient's preferences, clinical history, and decision about breastfeeding.

Determining Gestational Age and Expected Date of Delivery. Accurate dating is best done early and contributes to appropriate management of the pregnancy. Dating establishes the timeframe for reassuring the patient about normal progress, establishing paternity, timing screening tests, tracking fetal growth, and effectively triaging preterm and postdated labor.

Determining Gestational Age and the Expected Date of Delivery

- *Gestational age.* To establish gestational age, count the number of weeks and days from the first day of the LMP. Counting this *menstrual age* from the LMP, although biologically distinct from date of conception, is the standard means of calculating fetal age, yielding an average pregnancy length of 40 weeks. If the actual date of conception is known (as with in vitro fertilization), a *conception age* which is 2 weeks less than the menstrual age can be used to calculate menstrual age (i.e., a corrected or adjusted LMP dating) to establish dating.

- *Expected date of delivery (EDD).* The EDD is 40 weeks from the first date of the LMP. Using the *Naegele rule,* the EDD can be estimated by taking the LMP, adding 7 days, subtracting 3 months, and adding 1 year.

- *Tools for calculations.* Pregnancy wheels and online calculators are commonly used to calculate the EDD. However, pregnancy wheels vary widely in quality and accuracy, and are often produced as commercial marketing tools. Online calculators may be more reliable, but should be checked for accuracy before routine use.

- *Limitations on pregnancy dating.* Patient recall of the LMP is highly variable. Even when this date is accurate, the LMP can be affected by hormonal contraceptives, menstrual irregularities, or variations in ovulation that result in atypical cycle lengths. LMP dating should be checked against physical examination markers such as fundal height, and any wide discrepancies should be clarified by ultrasound evaluation. In clinical practice, dating by ultrasound is widespread, regardless of the certainty of the LMP, even though this approach is not currently endorsed by national guidelines.

Concluding the Initial Visit. As you conclude the visit, reaffirm your commitment to the woman's health and her concerns during pregnancy. Review your findings, discuss any tests or screenings that are needed, and ask if she has further questions. Reinforce the need for regular prenatal care and review the timing of future visits. Record your findings in the prenatal record.

Subsequent Prenatal Visits. Though the optimal number of prenatal appointments has not been well established, obstetric visits traditionally follow a set schedule: monthly until 28 gestational weeks, then biweekly until

36 weeks, then weekly until delivery.[13] Update and document the history at every visit, especially fetal movement felt by the patient, contractions, leakage of fluid, and vaginal bleeding. The physical examination findings at every visit should include vital signs (especially blood pressure and weight), fundal height, verification of fetal heart rate (FHR), and determination of fetal position and activity, as described in Techniques of Examination to follow. At each visit, the urine should be tested for infection and protein.

Health Promotion and Counseling: Evidence and Recommendations

Important Topics for Health Promotion and Counseling

- Nutrition
- Weight gain
- Immunizations
- Exercise
- Substance abuse
- Intimate partner violence
- Prenatal laboratory screening

Nutrition.   Evaluate the nutritional status of the pregnant patient during the first prenatal visit. Assess inadequate nutrition as well as obesity.

- *Take a diet history.* What does the patient typically eat for each meal? How often does she eat? Does she have nausea that limits her eating? Does she have any history of conditions that affect food intake like diabetes, eating disorders, or past bariatric surgery?

- *Review the body mass index (BMI) and laboratory findings.* Measure the height and weight, then calculate the BMI; note that later in pregnancy, the BMI reflects the gravid uterus. The hematocrit is a screen for anemia, which may reflect nutritional deficiency, underlying clinical issues, or the expected hemodilution later in pregnancy.

- *Recommend a prenatal multivitamin.* Daily prenatal supplements should include 400 μg of folic acid, 600 International Units of vitamin D, 27 mg of iron, and at least 1,000 mg of calcium.[14] If not present in the prenatal vitamins, recommend 150 to 290 μg of daily iodine in pregnant and breast-feeding women as iodine deficiency is widespread.[15] Patients should be advised that excess amounts of fat-soluble vitamins like vitamins A, D, E, and K can cause toxicity.

■ *Caution the patient about foods to avoid.* Pregnant women are especially vulnerable to *listeriosis.* To help prevent listeriosis, the American College of Obstetricians and Gynecologists (ACOG)[14] encourages pregnant patients to avoid:

   ■ Unpasteurized milk and foods made with unpasteurized milk

   ■ Raw and undercooked seafood, eggs, and meat

   ■ Refrigerated paté, meat spreads, and smoked salmon

   ■ Hot dogs, luncheon meats, and cold cuts unless served steaming hot

■ Regarding *fish and shellfish,* some nutrients like omega-3 fatty acids and dehydroepiandrostenedione (DHEA) may enhance fetal brain development. For pregnant and breastfeeding women, ACOG recommends two servings a week of selected fish and shellfish. Intake should include 8 to 12 ounces a week of fish lower in mercury such as salmon, shrimp, pollock, tuna (light canned), tilapia, catfish, and cod. White tuna consumption should be limited to 6 ounces a week. Pregnant women should avoid fish higher in mercury like tilefish, shark, swordfish, and king mackerel.[16,17]

■ *Make a nutritional plan.* Review goals for weight gain that are tailored to the patient's BMI, as shown below. Weight gain recommendations are incorporated into the Pregnancy Weight Gain Calculator and Super Tracker at the user-friendly ChooseMyPlate.gov website (http://www.choosemyplate. gov/pregnancy-weight-gain-calculator). This calculator displays the daily recommended intake of each of the five food groups for each trimester.[18] Calculations of these amounts are based on the woman's height, prepregnancy weight, due date, and levels of weekly exercise. Small frequent meals may help with mild nausea. Consider a team-based approach involving dieticians or behavioral health specialists in complex cases such as gestational diabetes or eating disorders.

Weight Gain.   Weight gain should be closely monitored during pregnancy as poor birth outcomes are associated with both excess and inadequate weight gain. Ideally, patients should begin pregnancy with a BMI as close to the normal range as possible. Women with a normal BMI should gain 25 to 35 pounds during pregnancy. In 2013, ACOG affirmed the revised 2009 weight gain recommendations by the National Institute of Medicine, shown below.[19,20]

Weigh the patient at each visit and plot the results on a graph so that they are easy for you and the patient to review and discuss.

Recommendations for Total and Rate of Weight Gain During Pregnancy, by Prepregnancy BMI, 2009

Prepregnancy BMI[a]	Total Weight Gain (Range in lbs)	Rates of Weight Gain[b] 2nd and 3rd Trimesters	
		lbs/wk	Mean Range
Underweight, or <18.5	28–40	1	1.0–1.3
Normal weight, or 18.5–24.9	25–35	1	0.8–1.0
Overweight, or 25.0–29.9	15–25	0.6	0.5–0.7
Obese, or ≥30.0	11–20	0.5	0.4–0.6

[a]To calculate BMI, go to Calculate Your Body Mass Index, National Heart, Lung, and Blood Institute at http://www.nhlbi.nih.gov/health/educational/lose_wt/BMI/bmicalc.htm.

[b]Calculations assume a 1.1–4.4 lbs weight gain in the first trimester.

Reprinted with permission from Rasmussen KM, Yaktine AL (eds.) and Institute of Medicine. *Committee to Re-examine IOM Pregnancy Weight Guidelines. Weight Gain During Pregnancy: Re-examining the Guidelines.* Washington, DC: National Academies Press, 2009. Available at http://www.ncbi.nlm.nih.gov/books/NBK32799/table/summary.t1/?report = objectonly. Accessed September 4, 2015.

Immunizations. Given the persistent increase in pertussis infection in the United States, the Centers for Disease Control and Prevention (CDC) Advisory Committee on Immunization Practices and ACOG recommend that *Tdap* be administered during each pregnancy, ideally at 27 to 36 weeks of gestation, regardless of the prior immunization history.[21] Caretakers in direct contact with the infant should also receive Tdap. *Inactivated influenza vaccination* is indicated in any trimester during the influenza season.[22]

The following vaccines are safe during pregnancy: pneumococcal, meningococcal, and hepatitis B. Hepatitis A and B, meningococcal polysaccharide and conjugate, and pneumococcal polysaccharide vaccines can be given, if indicated.[23] The following vaccines are *not* safe during pregnancy: measles/mumps/rubella, polio, and varicella. All women should have rubella titers drawn during pregnancy and be immunized after birth if found to be nonimmune.

Check Rh(D) and antibody typing at the first prenatal visit, at 28 weeks, and at delivery. Anti-D immunoglobulin should be given to all Rh-negative women at 28 weeks' gestation and again within 3 days of delivery to prevent sensitization if the infant is Rh-D positive.[24,25]

Exercise. Physical activity during pregnancy has a number of psychological benefits and reduces risk of excessive gestational weight gain, gestational diabetes, preeclampsia, preterm birth, varicose veins, and deep vein thrombosis (DVT).[26] It may reduce the length of labor and complications during delivery. In contrast, excess activity is associated with low birth weight, so educating your patients about recommended guidelines is important, especially because evidence suggests that physical activity levels in pregnant U.S. women are relatively low.[27]

ACOG recommends that pregnant women should engage in ≥30 minutes of moderate exercise on most days of the week unless there are contraindications.[28] Women initiating exercise during pregnancy should be cautious and consider programs developed specifically for pregnant women. Water-based exercises can temporarily help alleviate musculoskeletal aches, but immersion in hot water should be avoided. After the first trimester, women should avoid exercise in the supine position, which compresses the inferior vena cava and can cause dizziness and decreased placental blood flow. Because the center of gravity shifts in the third trimester, advise against exercises that cause loss of balance. Contact sports or activities that risk abdominal trauma are contraindicated throughout pregnancy. Pregnant women also should avoid overheating, dehydration, and any exertion that causes notable fatigue or discomfort.

Substance Abuse. Abstinence from substances of abuse is a top priority goal during pregnancy. Provide universal screening, which can uncover subtle issues and help you address these topics in a neutral and constructive manner. Incarceration, confrontation, and criminalization of substance abuse have all been shown to worsen outcomes of pregnancy for women and their children.

- *Tobacco.* Tobacco use is implicated in 13% to 19% of all low–birth weight babies and many other poor pregnancy outcomes, including a twofold risk of placenta previa, placental abruption, and preterm labor.[29,30] Risk of spontaneous abortion, fetal death, and fetal digit anomalies is also increased. Cessation is the goal, but any decrease in use is favorable.

- *Alcohol.* Fetal alcohol syndrome, the neurodevelopmental sequela of alcohol exposure during fetal development, is the leading cause of preventable mental retardation in the United States. No safe dose of alcohol has been established. ACOG strongly recommends that women abstain throughout pregnancy.[31] To promote abstinence, make use of the numerous ACOG and CDC resources, professional counseling, inpatient treatment, and Alcoholics Anonymous.

- *Illicit drugs.* Illegal drugs have significant detrimental effects on fetal development; pregnant women with addiction should be referred for treatment immediately and screened for HIV and hepatitis C infection.

- *Abuse of prescription drugs.* Ask about the unusual use of narcotics, stimulants, benzodiazepines, and other commonly abused prescription drugs.

- *Herbal and unregulated supplements.* Herbal supplements during pregnancy have been poorly studied and can harm the developing fetus. Unregulated supplements or vitamins, especially if formulated outside the United States, may contain lead and other toxins. Review and discuss any intake of supplements and consider pregnancy toxicology, for example, through MothertoBaby .org, to determine specific risks related to the timing of ingestion and the extent of fetal exposure.

Intimate Partner Violence. Pregnancy is a time of increased risk from intimate partner violence. Pre-existing patterns of abuse may intensify from verbal to physical abuse or from mild to severe physical abuse. Up to one in five women experiences some form of abuse during pregnancy, which has been associated with delayed prenatal care, low infant birth weight, or even murder of the mother and fetus.[32]

ACOG recommends universal screening of all women for domestic violence without regard to socioeconomic status, including pregnant women at the first prenatal visit and at least once each trimester.[32] For a direct nonjudgmental approach, ACOG recommends the statement and simple questions listed below.

ACOG Screening Approach for Intimate Partner Violence

Initial Statement: "Because violence is so common in many women's lives and because there is help available for women being abused, I now ask every patient about domestic violence."

Screening Questions:

1. "Within the past year—or since you have been pregnant—have you been hit, slapped, kicked, or otherwise physically hurt by someone?"
2. "Are you in a relationship with a person who threatens or physically hurts you?"
3. "Has anyone forced you to have sexual activities that made you feel uncomfortable?"

Source: American Congress of Obstetricians and Gynecologists. Screening tools–domestic violence. Available at http://www.acog.org/About-ACOG/ACOG-Departments/Violence-Against-Women/Screening-Tools–Domestic-Violence. Accessed September 2, 2015.

Watch for nonverbal clues of abuse such as frequent last-minute appointment changes, unusual behavior during visits, partners who refuse to leave the patient alone during the visit, and bruises or other injuries. It may take several visits for the patient to admit to abuse due to fear about safety and reprisal.

Once the patient acknowledges abuse, ask about the best way for you to help her. She may set limits on sharing information. Accept her decisions about how to handle her situation safely, with the caveat that if children are involved, you may be required to report harmful behaviors to the authorities. Maintain an updated list of shelters, counseling centers, hotline numbers, and other trusted local referrals. Plan future appointments at more frequent intervals. Finally, complete as thorough a physical examination as the patient permits, and document all injuries on a body diagram.

National Domestic Violence Hotline

- Website: www.thehotline.org
- 1–800–799-SAFE (7233)
- TTY for hearing impaired: 1–800–787–3224

Prenatal Laboratory Screenings. The standard prenatal screening panel includes blood type and Rh, antibody screen, complete blood count— especially hematocrit and platelet count, rubella titer, syphilis test, hepatitis B surface antigen, HIV test, STI screen for gonorrhea and chlamydia, and urinalysis with culture. Scheduled screenings include an oral glucose tolerance test for gestational diabetes around 24 to 28 weeks and a rectovaginal swab for group B *streptococcus* between 35 and 37 weeks.

Because obesity is associated with insulin resistance, the obese pregnant patient is at increased risk of both gestational diabetes and type 2 diabetes mellitus. Both ACOG and the American Diabetes Association recommend testing for glucose tolerance in the first trimester for obese pregnant patients.[33]

If indicated, pursue additional tests related to the mother's risk factors, such as screening for aneuploidy, Tay–Sachs disease, or other genetic diseases, and amniocentesis.

Techniques of Examination

As you begin the examination, be responsive to the patient's comfort and privacy, as well as her individual and cultural sensitivities. During the initial visit, take the history while she is clothed. If partners or children are present, ask if she wants them to stay during the physical examination. If she has never had a pelvic examination, take the time to explain what is involved and seek her cooperation with each step. Concerns about modesty should be balanced against the need for a complete examination. Patients who have experienced sexual assault may resist the pelvic examination. This reluctance can also stem from personal or cultural boundaries which should be explored and understood. To ease examination of the breasts and abdomen, ask the patient to gown with the opening in front. Make sure that the equipment and examining tables accommodate pregnant patients who are obese.

Positioning

In early pregnancy, the patient can be examined in the supine position. In later trimesters, the patient should adopt the semisitting position with the knees bent (Fig. 19-11). This position is more comfortable and reduces the weight of the gravid uterus on the descending aorta and inferior vena cava. The pregnant

Compression interferes with venous return from the lower extremities and pelvic vessels, causing the patient to feel dizzy and faint, the *supine hypotensive syndrome.*

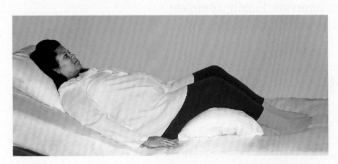

FIGURE 19-11. **Adopt the semisitting position.**

woman should avoid lying supine for long periods. Most portions of the examination (except the pelvic examination) should be done in the sitting or left-side-lying position.

During the examination, encourage the patient to sit upright if she feels light-headed; make sure she takes her time if she needs to stand up. She may need to empty her bladder, especially before the pelvic examination. Complete your examination relatively quickly.

Examining Equipment

Make your touch and hand motions comforting as you examine the pregnant woman. Warm your hands and use firm yet gentle palpation rather than abrupt pressure or kneading. When possible, keep your fingers flattened together in smooth continuous contact with the skin on the abdominal surface. The palmar surfaces of your fingertips are the most sensitive.

Before beginning the examination, gather the equipment listed below.

Equipment for Examining the Pregnant Woman

- *Gynecologic speculum and lubrication:* Due to vaginal wall relaxation during pregnancy, a larger-than-usual speculum may be needed in multiparous patients.
- *Sampling materials:* Because of the increased vascularity of vaginal and cervical structures, the cervical brush may cause bleeding that interferes with Pap smear samples, so the "broom" sampling device is preferred during pregnancy. Use additional swabs as needed to screen for STIs, group B strep, and wet mount preparations.
- *Tape measure:* A plastic or paper tape measure is used to assess the size of the uterus after 20 gestational weeks.
- *Doppler FHR monitor and gel:* A "Doppler" or "Doptone" is a handheld device used to assess FHR after 10 weeks of gestation when applied externally to the gravid belly.

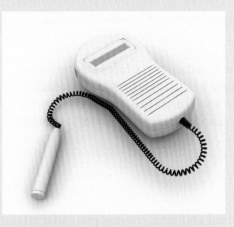

Handheld Doppler monitor.

General Inspection

Assess the general health, emotional state, nutritional status, and neuromuscular coordination of the patient as she walks into the room and moves onto the examining table.

Height, Weight, and Vital Signs

Measure the height and weight. Calculate the BMI with standard tables, using 19 to 25 as normal for the prepregnant state.

Weight loss due to nausea and vomiting that exceeds 5% of prepregnancy weight is considered excessive, representing *hyperemesis gravidarum,* and can lead to adverse pregnancy outcomes.

Measure the blood pressure at every visit. Blood pressure parameters in pregnancy follow the recommendations of the Eighth Joint National Committee (JNC8) (see p. 130).[34] Baseline prepregnancy readings are important for determining the patient's usual range. In the second trimester, blood pressure normally drops below the nonpregnant state.

Hypertensive disorders affect 5% to 10% of all pregnancies, so all elevations in blood pressure must be closely monitored. Hypertension can be both an independent diagnosis and a marker of *preeclampsia syndrome.* This syndrome is "a pregnancy-specific syndrome that can affect virtually every organ system."[35] ACOG issued new recommendations on hypertension in pregnancy in 2013 that no longer depend on proteinuria, recognizing that preeclampsia cannot only be lethal for the mother and fetus, but doubles the risk of later-life cardiovascular disease. Preeclampsia increases cardiovascular disease risk eight- to ninefold in women with preeclampsia giving birth before 34 weeks' gestation.[34]

Gestational hypertension is systolic blood pressure (SBP) >140 mm Hg or diastolic blood pressure (DBP) >90 mm Hg first documented after 20 weeks, without proteinuria or preeclampsia, that resolves by 12 weeks postpartum.

Chronic hypertension is SBP >140 or DBP >90 that predates pregnancy. Chronic hypertension affects almost 2% of U.S. births.[35]

Definition of Preeclampsia

Preeclampsia is SBP ≥140 or DBP ≥90 after 20 weeks on two occasions at least 4 hours apart in a woman with previously normal BP or BP ≥160/110 confirmed within minutes *and* proteinuria ≥300 mg/24 hours, protein:creatinine ≥0.3, or dipstick 1+;

OR

new onset hypertension without proteinuria and any of the following: thrombocytopenia (platelets <100,000/μL), impaired liver function (liver transaminase levels more than twice normal), new renal insufficiency (creatinine >1.1 mg/dL or doubles in the absence of renal disease), pulmonary edema, or new onset cerebral or visual symptoms.[34]

Head and Neck

Face the seated patient and inspect the head and neck, paying particular attention to the following features:

- *Face.* Irregular brownish patches around the forehead, cheeks, nose, and jaw are known as *chloasma* or *melasma,* the "mask of pregnancy," a normal skin finding during pregnancy.

Facial edema after 20 gestational weeks is suspicious for *preeclampsia* and should be investigated.

- *Hair.* Hair may become dry, oily, or sparse during pregnancy; mild hirsutism on the face, abdomen, and extremities is also common.

Localized patches of hair loss should not be attributed to pregnancy (though postpartum hair loss is common).

■ *Eyes.* Assess the conjunctivae and sclera for signs of pallor and jaundice.

Anemia may cause conjunctival pallor.

■ *Nose.* Inspect the mucus membranes and septum. Nasal congestion and nose bleeds are more common during pregnancy.

Erosions and perforations of the nasal septum may represent use of intranasal cocaine.

■ *Mouth.* Examine the teeth and gums. Gingival enlargement with bleeding is common during pregnancy.

Dental problems are associated with poor pregnancy outcomes, so initiate prompt dental referrals for tooth and gum pain or infections.

■ *Thyroid gland.* Modest symmetric enlargement caused by glandular hyperplasia and increased vascularity is normal on inspection and palpation.[1]

Thyroid enlargement, goiters, and nodules are abnormal and require investigation.

Thorax and Lungs

Count the respiratory rate, which should remain normal throughout pregnancy.

Dyspnea accompanied by increased respiratory rate, cough, rales, or respiratory distress point to possible infection, asthma, pulmonary embolus, or peripartum cardiomyopathy.

Inspect the thorax for contours and breathing patterns.

Percuss to observe diaphragmatic elevation that may be seen as early as the first trimester.

Auscultate for clear breath sounds without wheezes, rales, or rhonchi.

Heart

Palpate the apical impulse, which may be rotated upward and to the left toward the fourth intercostal space by the enlarging uterus.

See also Chapter 9, Cardiovascular System, pp. 343–417.

Auscultate the heart. Listen for a *venous hum* or a continuous *mammary souffle* (pronounced *soo-fl*) often found during pregnancy due to increased blood flow through normal vessels. The mammary souffle is commonly heard during late pregnancy or lactation, is strongest in the second or third intercostal space at the sternal border, and is typically both systolic and diastolic, though only the systolic component may be audible.

Assess dyspnea and signs of heart failure for possible *peripartum cardiomyopathy,* particularly in the late stages of pregnancy.

Auscultate for murmurs.

Murmurs may signal anemia. Investigate any diastolic murmur.

Breasts

The breast examination is similar to that of a nonpregnant woman but with some notable differences.

See also Chapter 10, Breasts and Axillae, pp. 419–447.

Inspect the breasts and nipples for symmetry and color. Normal changes include a marked venous pattern, darkened nipples and areolae, and prominent Montgomery glands.

Inverted nipples need attention at the time of birth if breastfeeding is planned.

Palpate for masses and axillary lymph nodes. Normal breasts may be tender and nodular during pregnancy.

Pathologic masses may be difficult to isolate, but warrant immediate attention. Severe focal tenderness with erythema in *mastitis* requires immediate treatment.

Compress each nipple between your thumb and index finger; colostrum may express from the nipples during later trimesters. Reassure the patient that this is normal and that she may also experience "let down," a spontaneous mild leakage often accompanied by a cramping sensation in the breast during a hot shower or orgasm in the third trimester.

Bloody or purulent discharge should not be attributed to pregnancy.

Abdomen

For the abdominal examination, help the patient move into a semisitting position with knees flexed, as shown on pp. 947–950.

Inspect the abdomen for striae, scars, size, shape, and contour. Purplish *striae* and a *linea nigra* are normal in pregnancy.

Cesarean scars on the abdomen may not match the orientation of the scar on the uterus, which is important when evaluating whether vaginal delivery is appropriate after cesarean section.

Palpate the abdomen for:

- *Organs and masses.* The mass of the gravid uterus is expected.

- *Fetal movement.* The examiner can usually feel movements externally after 24 gestational weeks; the mother can usually feel these by 18 to 24 weeks. The maternal sensation of fetal movement is traditionally known as "quickening."

If fetal movement is not felt after 24 weeks, consider a miscalculation of gestational age, fetal death or severe morbidity, or false pregnancy. Confirm fetal health and gestational age with an ultrasound.

- *Uterine contractility.* Irregular uterine contractions occur as early as 12 weeks and may be triggered by external palpation during the third trimester. During contractions, the abdomen feels tense or firm to the examiner, obscuring the palpation of fetal parts; after the contraction, the palpating fingers sense the relaxation of the uterine muscle.

Before 37 weeks, regular uterine contractions with or without pain and bleeding are abnormal, suggesting preterm labor.

- *Measure the fundal height* if gestational age is >20 weeks, when the fundus should reach the umbilicus. With a plastic or paper tape measure, locate the pubic symphysis and place the "zero" end of the tape measure where you can firmly feel that bone (Fig. 19-12). Then extend the tape measure to the very top of uterine fundus and note the number of centimeters measured. Though subject to error between 16 and 36 weeks, measurement in centimeters should roughly equal the number of weeks of gestation. This low-technology, widely used technique may underdetect newborns who are small for gestational age.[36–38]

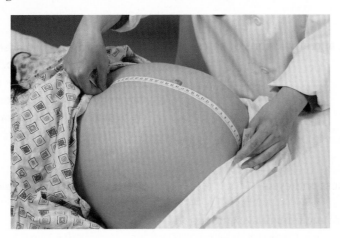

FIGURE 19-12. **Measure fundal height.**

If fundal height is *4 cm greater* than expected, consider multiple gestation, a large fetus, extra amniotic fluid, or uterine leiomyoma. If fundal height is *4 cm smaller* than expected, consider low-level amniotic fluid, missed abortion, intrauterine growth retardation, or fetal anomaly. These conditions should be investigated by ultrasound.

- *Auscultate the fetal heart tones.* The Doppler fetal rate monitor ("Doppler" or "Doptone") is the standard instrument for measuring FHR, which is normally audible as early as 10 to 12 weeks' gestation. Detection of the FHR may be slightly delayed in obese patients.

Inaudible fetal heart tones may indicate fewer weeks of gestation than expected, fetal demise, false pregnancy, or observer error; inability to locate the FHR should always be investigated with formal ultrasound.

- *Location.* From 10 to 18 weeks' gestation, the FHR is located along the midline of the lower abdomen. After that time, the FHR is best heard over the back or chest and depends on fetal position; the Leopold maneuvers can help identify the position. (See pp. 947–948.)

After 24 weeks, auscultation of more than one FHR in different locations with varying rates suggests multiple gestation.

- *Rate.* The FHR ranges between 110 and 160 beats per minute (BPM). A heart rate of 60 to 90 BPM is usually maternal, but an adequate FHR should be confirmed.

Sustained dips in FHR, or "decelerations," have a wide differential diagnosis but always warrant investigation, at least by formal FHR monitoring.

- *Rhythm.* FHR should vary 10 to 15 BPM from second to second, especially later in the pregnancy. After 32 to 34 weeks, the FHR should become more variable and increased with fetal activity. This subtlety can be difficult to assess with a Doppler but can be tracked with an FHR monitor if any questions arise.

Lack of beat-to-beat variability is difficult to discern with a handheld Doppler, so this finding warrants formal FHR monitoring.

Genitalia

For this portion of the examination, the patient will need to be supine with her feet placed in stirrups. Assemble the needed equipment in advance and minimize the time she spends in this position to avert dizziness and hypotension from uterine compression of the major abdominal vessels.

External Genitalia. *Inspect* the external genitalia. Relaxation of the vaginal introitus and enlargement of the labia and clitoris are normal changes of pregnancy. In multiparous women, scars from perineal lacerations or episiotomy incisions may be present.

Inspect for labial varicosities, cystoceles, rectoceles, and any lesions or sores.

Labial varicosities that arise during pregnancy can become tortuous and painful. Cystoceles and rectoceles may be pronounced due to the muscle relaxation of pregnancy. Lesions and sores occur with *herpes simplex* infection.

Palpate the Bartholin and Skene glands for tenderness and cysts.

See also Chapter 14, Female Genitalia, pp. 565–606.

Internal Genitalia. Prepare for both a speculum and bimanual examination.

Speculum Examination. Relaxation of the perineal and vulvar structures during pregnancy may minimize, but not eliminate, discomfort from the speculum examination. The increased vascularity of vaginal and cervical structures promotes friability, so insert and open the speculum gently to prevent tissue trauma and bleeding. During the third trimester, perform this examination only when necessary as descent of the fetal parts into the pelvis can make the examination very uncomfortable.

- *Inspect the cervix for color, shape, and closure.* Typically, the external os in a nulliparous cervix appears as a circular dot, and in a parous cervix more like an arc or "smile." A parous cervix may also look irregular due to healed lacerations from prior deliveries. The inner portion of the cervix everts slightly during pregnancy, called *ectropion,* and appears as a glandular friable darker pink or red area inside the os. *Perform a Pap smear if indicated,* and collect other vaginal specimens such as STI cultures, wet mount samples, or group B strep swabs as appropriate.

A pink cervix suggests a nonpregnant state. Cervical erosion, erythema, discharge, or irritation suggests *cervicitis,* and warrants investigation for STIs.

- *Inspect the vaginal walls* as you withdraw the speculum. Check for color, relaxation, rugae, and discharge. Normal findings include bluish color, deep rugae, and increased milky white discharge, or *leukorrhea.*

Investigate abnormal vaginal discharges for possible *candida* or *bacterial vaginosis,* which can affect pregnancy outcome.

Bimanual Examination. Performing the bimanual examination is often easier during pregnancy due to pelvic floor relaxation. Avoiding sensitive urethral structures, insert two lubricated fingers into the introitus, palmar side down, with slight pressure downward on the perineum. Maintaining downward pressure on the perineum, gently turn the fingers palmar side up.

- *Cervix.* Because of softening during pregnancy, or *Hegar sign,* the cervix may be difficult to identify. If there are nabothian cysts or healed lacerations from prior deliveries, the cervix may feel irregular.

To estimate the cervical length, *palpate the lateral surface of the cervical tip to the lateral fornix.* Prior to 34 to 36 weeks' gestation, the cervix should retain its initial length of 3 cm or greater.

Palpate the cervical os. This may be easier if the patient moves her heels as close to her buttocks as possible, which shortens the vagina, and places her closed fists under her buttocks to tip the pelvis upward, which makes posterior cervices easier to palpate. The *external os* may be open to admit a fingertip in multiparous women. The *internal os,* the narrow passage between the endocervical canal and the uterine cavity, should be closed until late pregnancy, regardless of parity. The internal os may only be palpable by reaching behind or past the fetal parts.

Cervical opening or shortening (effacement) prior to 37 weeks may indicate preterm labor.

As with the speculum examination, in late pregnancy, examine the cervix only when necessary because palpation is very uncomfortable. Warn patients that it may cause cramping and pressure.

■ *Uterus.* With your internal fingers placed at either side of the cervix and the external hand on the patient's abdomen, use the internal fingers to gently lift the uterus upward toward the abdominal hand. Capture the fundal portion of the uterus between your two hands and assess the uterine size, keeping in mind the contours of the gravid uterus at various gestational intervals, depicted in Figure 19-8. *Palpate* for shape, consistency, and position.

An irregularly shaped uterus suggests uterine *leiomyomata,* or fibroids, or a *bicornuate uterus,* one with two distinct cavities separated by a septum.

■ *Adnexa. Palpate the right and left adnexa.* The corpus luteum may be palpable as a small nodule on the affected ovary during the first weeks after conception. After the first trimester, adnexal masses become difficult to feel.

■ *Pelvic floor.* Evaluate pelvic floor strength as you withdraw your examining fingers.

Adnexal tenderness or masses early in gestation require ultrasound evaluation to rule out *ectopic pregnancy.* Acute pelvic inflammatory disease is rare in pregnancy, especially after the first trimester, because the adnexae are sealed by the gravid uterus and mucus plug.

Anus

Inspect for external hemorrhoids. If present, note their size, location, and any evidence of thrombosis.

Hemorrhoids often become engorged late in pregnancy; they may be painful, bleed, or thrombose.

Rectum and Rectovaginal Septum

The rectal examination is not standard in prenatal care unless there are concerning symptoms like rectal bleeding or masses or conditions that compromise the rectovaginal septum. Rectal examination may help you assess the size of a retroverted or retroflexed uterus, but transvaginal ultrasound provides superior information.

Extremities

Ask the woman to resume sitting or to lie on her left side. *Inspect* the legs for varicose veins.

Palpate the extremities for edema in the pretibial, ankle, and pedal distributions, which are rated on a 0 to 4+ scale. Physiologic edema is common in advanced pregnancy, during hot weather, and in women who stand for long periods of time due to decreased venous return from the lower extremities.

Elicit the knee and ankle deep tendon reflexes.

Special Techniques

Leopold Maneuvers.   Leopold maneuvers are used to determine the fetal position in the maternal abdomen beginning in the second trimester; accuracy is greatest after 36 weeks' gestation.[41] Although less accurate for assessing fetal growth,[42] these examination findings help determine readiness for vaginal delivery by assessing:

- The upper and lower fetal pole, namely, the proximal and distal fetal parts

- The maternal side where the fetal back is located

- The descent of the presenting part into the maternal pelvis

- The extent of flexion of the fetal head

- The estimated size and weight of the fetus (an advanced skill that will not be addressed further here)

Varicose veins may begin or worsen during pregnancy.

See Chapter 12, Peripheral Vascular System, for grades of edema, pp. 525–526. Unilateral severe edema with calf tenderness warrants prompt evaluation for *DVT*. Hand or facial edema after 20 gestational weeks is nonspecific for *eclampsia*, but should be investigated.[39,40]

Hyperreflexia may signal cortical irritability from eclampsia, but clinical accuracy is variable.

Common deviations include *breech presentation* (when parts other than the head, such as buttocks or foot, present at the maternal pelvis), and lack of engagement of the presenting part in the maternal pelvis at term. If discovered prior to term, breech presentations may sometimes be corrected by rotational maneuvers.

First Maneuver (Upper Fetal Pole). Stand at the woman's side, facing her head. Palpate the uppermost part of gravid uterus gently, with the fingertips together, to determine what fetal part is located at the fundus, which is the "upper fetal pole" (Fig. 19-13).

The fetal buttocks are usually at the upper fetal pole; they feel firm but irregular, and less globular than the head. The fetal head feels firm, round, and smooth. Occasionally, neither part is easily palpated at the fundus, as when the fetus is in a transverse lie.

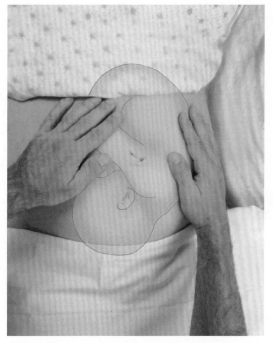

FIGURE 19-13. **Palpate upper fetal pole.**

Second Maneuver (Sides of the Maternal Abdomen). Place one hand on each side of the woman's abdomen, capturing the fetal body between them (Fig. 19-14). Steady the uterus with one hand and palpate the fetus with the other, looking for the back on one side and extremities on the other.

By 32 weeks' gestation, the fetal back has a smooth, firm surface as long or longer than the examiner's hand. The fetal arms and legs feel like irregular bumps. The fetus may kick if awake and active.

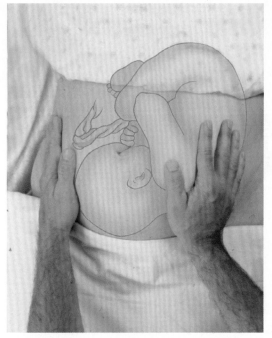

FIGURE 19-14. **Palpate fetal back and extremities.**

Third Maneuver (Lower Fetal Pole and Descent into Pelvis). Face the woman's feet. Place the flat palmar surfaces of the fingertips on the fetal pole just above the pubic symphysis (Fig. 19-15). Palpate the presenting fetal part for texture and firmness to distinguish the head from the buttock. Judge the descent, or engagement, of the presenting part into the maternal pelvis. Alternatively, use the Pawlik grip by grasping the lower fetal pole with the thumb and fingers of one hand to assess the presenting part and descent into pelvis; however, this technique tends to be uncomfortable to the gravid patient.

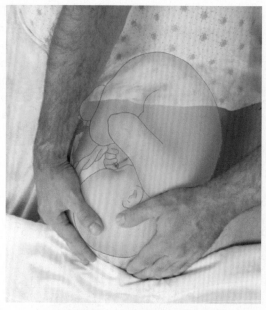

FIGURE 19-15. **Palpate lower fetal pole.**

Again, the fetal head feels very firm and globular; the buttocks feel firm but irregular, and less globular than the head. In a *vertex* or *cephalic* presentation, the fetal head is the presenting part. If the most distal part of the lower fetal pole cannot be palpated, it is usually engaged in the pelvis. If you can depress the tissues over the maternal bladder without touching the fetus, the presenting part is proximal to your fingers.

Fourth Maneuver (Flexion of the Fetal Head). This maneuver assesses the flexion or extension of the fetal head, presuming that the fetal head is the presenting part in the pelvis. Still facing the woman's feet, with your hands positioned on either side of the gravid uterus, identify the fetal front and back sides (Fig. 19-16). Using one hand at a time, slide your fingers down each side of the fetal body until you reach the "cephalic prominence," that is, where the fetal brow or occiput juts out.

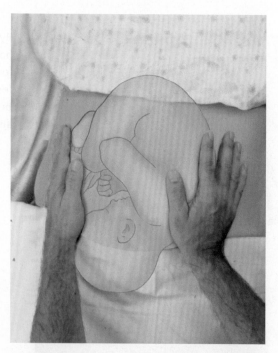

FIGURE 19-16. **Palpate for the cephalic prominence.**

If the cephalic prominence juts out along the line of the fetal back, the head is extended. If the cephalic prominence juts out along the line of the fetal anterior side, the head is flexed.

Recording Your Findings

Like many specialties, obstetrics utilizes a very specific vocabulary, which cannot be fully covered in this textbook.

■ Pregnant women are described in terms of number of pregnancies (gravida) and labors (para) they have experienced. Parity is further broken down into *term deliveries, preterm deliveries, abortions* (spontaneous abortions and terminated pregnancies), and *living children,* which yields the mnemonic "TPAL" when listed in that order.

■ This is expressed in "Gs and Ps"; for example, a woman who has had two prior children and is pregnant with her third pregnancy would be referred to simply as "G3P2." A woman with two spontaneous losses prior to 20 weeks' gestation, three living children who were delivered at term, and a current pregnancy, would be referred to as "G6P3023." This shorthand allows obstetricians to track large amounts of data succinctly.

■ One common error is to assign a multiple pregnancy, for example, twins, as a count of two for either gravity or parity. In practice, each pregnancy receives only one count in any of the categories regardless of the number of fetuses, except for *living children,* when all are counted. So, for a first pregnancy with twins delivered at term, the correct designation is G1P1002.

Typically, the presentation of a pregnant patient follows a standard order: age, Gs and Ps, weeks of gestation, means of determining gestational age (ultrasound vs. LMP), followed by chief complaint, chief pregnancy complications, then important history and examination findings. Two sample presentations are given below.

Recording the Physical Examination—The Pregnant Woman

"32-year-old G3P1102 at 18 weeks' gestation by LMP presents to establish prenatal care. Pregnancy complicated by closely spaced pregnancies, prior preterm birth for preeclampsia, and prior cesarean delivery. Patient reports fetal movement; denies contractions, vaginal bleeding, and leakage of fluids. On external exam, low-transverse cesarean scar is evident; fundus is palpable just below umbilicus. On internal exam, cervix is open to fingertip at the external os but closed at the internal os; cervix is 3 cm long; uterus enlarged to size consistent with 18-week gestation. Speculum exam shows leukorrhea with positive Chadwick sign. FHR by Doppler is between 140 and 145 BPM."

(continued)

These findings describe the examination of a healthy pregnant woman at 18 weeks' gestation.

Recording the Physical Examination—The Pregnant Woman (continued)

OR

"21-year-old G1P0 at 33 weeks' gestation as determined by 19-week ultrasound presents with chief complaint of decreased fetal movement. Pregnancy complicated by poor compliance and homelessness. Patient reports minimal fetal movement over the last 24 hours; denies contractions, vaginal bleeding, and leakage of fluids. On external exam, nontender gravid abdomen with no scars is noted; fundus is measured at 32 cm; fetus is vertex but not engaged in pelvis by Leopold maneuvers. On internal exam, cervix is closed, thick, and high; speculum exam shows thin gray discharge with clue cells on wet mount. FHT by Doppler are between 155 and 160 BPM."

These findings describe the examination of a more complex presentation of a pregnant woman at 33 weeks' gestation.

REFERENCES

References

1. Cunningham FG, Leveno KL, Bloom SL, et al (eds.). *Ch 2, Maternal anatomy, and Chapter 4, Maternal physiology, in Williams Obstetrics.* 24th ed. New York: McGraw Hill, Medical Publishers Division; 2014.

2. James A; Committee on Practice Bulletins—Obstetrics. Practice bulletin no. 123: thromboembolism in pregnancy. *Obstet Gynec.* 2011;118:718.

3. McCormack MC, Wise RA. Respiratory physiology in pregnancy. *Respir Med.* 2009;1:1. Available at http://www.libreriauniverso.it/pdf/9781934115121.pdf. Accessed August 30, 2015.

4. Cole LA. The hCG assay or pregnancy test. *Clin Chem Lab Med.* 2012;50:617.

5. Noctor E, Dunne FP. Type 2 diabetes after gestational diabetes: The influence of changing diagnostic criteria. *World J Diabetes.* 2015; 6:234.

6. Kim C, Newton KM, Knopp RH. Gestational diabetes and the incidence of type II diabetes: a systematic review. *Diabetes Care.* 2002;25:1862.

7. Patton PE, Samuels MH, Trinidad R, et al. Controversies in the management of hypothyroidism during pregnancy. *Obstet Gynecol Surv.* 2014;69:346.

8. Lord SJ, Bernstein L, Johnson KA, et al. Breast cancer risk and hormone receptor status in older women by parity, age of first birth, and breastfeeding: a case-control study. *Cancer Epidemiol Biomarkers Prev.* 2008;17:1723.

9. Ursin G, Bernstein L, Lord SJ, et al. Reproductive factors and subtypes of breast cancer defined by hormone receptor and histology. *Br J Cancer.* 2005;93:364.

10. U.S. Preventive Services Task Force. Final Evidence Summary: Breastfeeding: Counseling. August 2014. Update in progress for 2016. Available at http://www.uspreventiveservicestaskforce.org/Page/Document/final-evidence-summary10/breastfeeding-counseling. Accessed August 31, 2015.

11. DeFranco EA, Ehrlich S, Muglia LJ. Influence of interpregnancy interval on birth timing. *BJOG.* 2014;121;1633.

12. Thiel de Bocanegra H, Chang R, Howell M, et al. Interpregnancy intervals: impact of postpartum contraceptive effectiveness and coverage. *Am J Obstet Gynecol.* 2014;210;311.e1.

13. American College of Obstetricians and Gynecologists, American Academy of Pediatrics. *Guidelines for Perinatal Care.* 7th ed. Available at http://www.acog.org/About-ACOG/ACOG-Departments/Breastfeeding/ACOG-Clinical-Guidelines. Accessed August 31, 2015.

14. American College of Obstetricians and Gynecologists. Frequently asked questions–FAQ001. Nutrition during pregnancy, April 2015. Available at http://www.acog.org/Patients/FAQs/Nutrition-During-Pregnancy. Accessed August 31, 2015.

15. American Academy of Pediatrics. Pregnant and breastfeeding women may be deficient in iodine; AAP recommends supplements. May 26, 2014. https://www.aap.org/en-us/about-the-aap/aap-press-room/Pages/Pregnant-and-Breastfeeding-Women-May-Be-.aspx. Accessed August 29, 2015.

16. American College of Obstetricians and Gynecologists. ACOG Practice Advisory: seafood consumption during pregnancy, June 10, 2014. Available at http://www.acog.org/About-ACOG/News-Room/Practice-Advisories/ACOG-Practice-Advisory-Seafood-Consumption-During-Pregnancy. Accessed August 31, 2015.

17. U.S. Food and Drug Administration. Fish: what pregnant women and parents should know. Draft updated advice by FDA and EPA, June 2014. Updated February 24, 2015. Available at http://sales.acog.org/eBook-Guidelines-for-Perinatal-Care-Seventh-Edition-P729.aspx. Accessed August 31, 2015.

18. U.S. Department of Agriculture. Pregnancy Weight Gain Calculator. ChooseMyPlate.gov. Available at http://www.choosemyplate.gov/pregnancy-weight-gain-calculator. Accessed September 1, 2015.

19. American College of Obstetricians and Gynecologists. ACOG Committee Opinion No. 548. Weight gain during pregnancy. *Obstet Gynecol.* 2013;121:210.

20. Rasmussen KM, Yaktine AL (eds.) and Institute of Medicine. *Committee to Reexamine IOM Pregnancy Weight Guidelines. Weight Gain During Pregnancy: Re-Examining The Guidelines.* Washington, DC: National Academies Press; 2009. Available at http://www.ncbi.nlm.nih.gov/books/NBK32813/. Accessed September 1, 2015.

21. American College of Obstetricians and Gynecologists. Update on immunization and pregnancy: tetanus, diphtheria, and pertussis vaccination. ACOG Committee Opinion, No. 566. *Obstet Gynecol.* 2013;121:1411.

22. American College of Obstetricians and Gynecologists. Influenza vaccination during pregnancy. Committee Opinion No. 608. September 2014. American College of Obstetricians and Gynecologists. *Obstet Gynecol.* 2014;124:648. Available at http://www.acog.org/Resources-And-Publications/Committee-Opinions/Committee-on-Obstetric-Practice/Influenza-Vaccination-During-Pregnancy. Accessed September 1, 2015.

23. Centers for Disease Control and Prevention. Immunization and pregnancy. March 2013. Available at http://www.cdc.gov/vaccines/pubs/downloads/f_preg_chart.pdf. Accessed September 1, 2015.

24. American College of Obstetricians and Gynecologists. ACOG Practice Bulletin No. 75. Management of alloimmunization during pregnancy. *Obstet Gynecol.* 2006;108:457.

25. American College of Obstetrics and Gynecology. ACOG Practice Bulletin No. 4. Prevention of Rh D alloimmunization, May 1999 (replaces educational bulletin Number 147, October 1990). Clinical management guidelines for obstetrician-gynecologists. *Int J Gynaecol Obstet.* 1999;66:63.

26. Evenson KR, Barakat R, Brown WJ, et al. Guidelines for Physical Activity during Pregnancy: Comparisons From Around the World. *Am J Lifestyle Med.* 2014;8:102.

27. Evenson KR, Wen F. National trends in self-reported physical activity and sedentary behaviors among pregnant women: NHANES 1999–2006. *Prev Med.* 2010;50:123.

28. American College of Obstetricians and Gynecologists. Exercise during pregnancy and the postpartum period. ACOG Committee Opinion No. 267. *Obstet Gynecol.* 2002;99:171.

29. Cunningham FG, Leveno KL, Bloom SL, et al (eds.). *Chapter 9, Prenatal care, in Williams Obstetrics.* 24th ed. New York: McGraw Hill, Medical Publishers Division; 2014.

30. American College of Obstetricians and Gynecologists. Smoking cessation during pregnancy. Committee Opinion No. 471, November 2010, Reaffirmed 2013. *Obstet Gynecol.* 2010;116:1241.

31. American College of Obstetricians and Gynecologists. At risk drinking and alcohol dependence: obstetric and gynecologic implications. Committee Opinion No. 496. August 2011, reaffirmed 2013. Available at http://www.acog.org/-/media/Committee-Opinions/Committee-on-Health-Care-for-Underserved-Women/co496.pdf?dmc=1&ts=20150902T1326596732. Accessed September 2, 2015.

32. American College of Obstetricians and Gynecologists. Committee opinion No. 518. Intimate partner violence. *Obstet Gynecol.* 2012;119:412. Available at http://www.acog.org/Resources-

And-Publications/Committee-Opinions/Committee-on-Health-Care-for-Underserved-Women/Intimate-Partner-Violence. Accessed September 4, 2015.

33. Gilmandyar D, Zozzaro-Smith P, Thornburg L. Complications and challenges in management of the obese expectant mother. *Expert Rev Obstet Gynecol.* 2012;7:585.

34. American College of Obstetricians and Gynecologists; Task Force on Hypertension in Pregnancy. Hypertension in pregnancy. Report of the American College of Obstetricians and Gynecologists' Task Force on Hypertension in Pregnancy. *Obstet Gynecol.* 2013;122:1122.

35. Cunningham FG, Leveno KL, Bloom SL, et al (eds.). *Chapter 40, Hypertensive disorders, and Chapter 50, Chronic hypertension, in Williams Obstetrics.* 24th ed. New York: McGraw Hill, Medical Publishers Division; 2014.

36. Pay AS, Wiik J, Backe B, et al. Symphysis-fundus height measurement to predict small-for-gestational-age status at birth: a systematic review. *BMC Pregnancy Childbirth.* 2015;15:22.

37. White LJ, Lee SJ, Stepniewska K, et al. Estimation of gestational age from fundal height: a solution for resource-poor settings. *J R Soc Interface.* 2012;9:503.

38. Neilson JP. Symphysis-fundal height measurement in pregnancy. *Cochrane Database Syst Rev.* 2000;(2):CD000944.

39. Powe CE, Levine RJ, Karumanchi SA. Preeclampsia, a disease of the maternal endothelium: the role of antiangiogenic factors and implications for later cardiovascular disease. *Circulation.* 2011;123:2856.

40. Chen CW, Jaffe IZ, Karumanchi SA. Pre-eclampsia and cardiovascular disease. *Cardiovasc Res.* 2014;101:579.

41. Kirkham C, Harris S, Grzybowski S. Evidence-based prenatal care: part I. General prenatal care and counseling issues. *Am Fam Physician.* 2005;71:1307.

42. Goetzinger KR, Odibo AO, Shanks AL, et al. Clinical accuracy of estimated fetal weight in term pregnancies in a teaching hospital. *J Matern Fetal Neonatal Med.* 2014;27:89.

The Older Adult

The Bates' suite offers these additional resources to enhance learning and facilitate understanding of this chapter:

- Bates' *Pocket Guide to Physical Examination and History Taking,* 8th edition
- Bates' *Visual Guide to Physical Examination* (Vol. 4: Head-to-Toe Assessment: Older Adult)
- thePoint online resources, for students and instructors: http://thepoint.lww.com

Older Americans now number more than 43 million people and are expected to reach 80 million by 2040, over 20% of the population.[1,2] Americans are living longer than previous generations: life span at birth is currently 81 years for women and 76 years for men. The population over age 85 years is projected to more than double from 6 million in 2013 to over 14 million in 2040.[3] Hence, the "*demographic imperative*" to societies worldwide is to maximize not only life span but also "health span," so that older adults maintain full function as long as possible, enjoying rich and active lives in their homes and communities (Fig. 20-1).

Although statistics group aging by decades, aging is hardly chronologic, measured by time in years, but encompasses a wealth of wisdom and lived experience in addition to the complex interplay of health and illness. The aging population is highly heterogeneous—in disposition, social networks, level of physical activity, and biology. Frailty is one of society's common myths about aging; more than 95% of Americans older than 65 years live in the community, and only 5% reside in institutional facilities.[4] For those over age 85 years, only 10% live in institutional facilities.

Self-reported health status and functional status supersede disability as measures of healthy aging. In 2009, 76% rated their health as good to excellent, and there has been a decline in the percentage of older adults reporting functional limitations, from 49% in 1990 to 41% in 2010, even though up to 56% report at least one chronic condition.[5] However, recent trends suggest that obesity may increase future levels of disability, especially in African American and Hispanic adults aged 60 to 69 years. Now, 38% of adults 65 years and above are obese, compared to 22% in the 1988 to 1994 period. Studies show that successful aging is not strictly clinical, but rests on variables such as positive cognition and mental health, physical activity, and social networks.[6] Terminology about aging is in flux. This chapter uses the term "older adult" and at times "senior." Because evidence about these designations is lacking, take the time to find out which term your patients prefer.

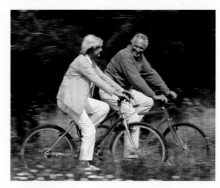

FIGURE 20-1. **Enriching the "health span."**

Promoting healthy aging leads to interactive goals in clinical care—"an informed activated patient interacting with a prepared proactive team, resulting in high-quality satisfying encounters and improved outcomes" and a distinct set of clinical attitudes and skills.[7–9] Experts recommend "goal-oriented patient care" that is patient-centered, defined as "respectful of and responsive to individual patient preferences, needs, and values, and ensuring that patient values guide all clinical decisions."[10] For older adults, this means focusing on the patient's "individual health goals within or across a variety of dimensions (e.g., symptoms; physical functional status, including mobility; and social and role functions) and determin[ing] how these goals are being met."[11] This approach individualizes decision-making and allows patients to express preferences about which "health states are important to them and their relative priority," for example, choosing better symptom control over a longer life span. Goal-oriented care moves beyond "preventive and disease-specific care processes . . . and condition-specific indicators" like targets for HgA1C or blood pressure.

New paradigms also highlight the importance of shifting assessment to *geriatric syndromes* that fall outside traditional disease models but are strongly linked to activities of daily living (ADLs). These syndromes are present in almost 50% of older adults.[12] Managing these conditions—cognitive impairment, falls, incontinence, low body mass index (BMI), dizziness, impaired vision and hearing—presents both opportunities and challenges: the focus on healthy or "successful" aging; the need to understand and mobilize family, social, and community supports; the importance of skills directed to functional assessment, "the sixth vital sign"; and the opportunities for promoting the older adult's long-term health and safety.

The Geriatric Approach for Primary Care

1. Learn to quickly identify frail elderly patients; they are most vulnerable to adverse outcomes and most benefit from a holistic geriatric approach.
2. Look for common geriatric syndromes, including falls, delirium/cognitive impairment, functional dependence, and urinary incontinence in every patient.
3. Learn about efficient assessment tools for geriatrics and geriatric syndromes and teach clinical staff to administer them when possible.
4. Be familiar with community resources, such as fall prevention programs, PACE programs, and senior centers.
5. Take into account a patient's goals, life expectancy, and functional status before considering any test or procedure.
6. Review advanced directives and goals of care periodically.
7. Be knowledgeable about the Beers Criteria (see p. 972) use them to identify potentially inappropriate medications in the elderly and inform periodic comprehensive medication review.
8. Adopt an evidence-based approach to health screening, especially in the frail elderly.

(continued)

The Geriatric Approach for Primary Care (continued)

9. Watch carefully for mood disorders in the frail elderly and consider using geriatric-specific screening tools, such as the five-item Geriatric Depression Scale.
10. Provide caregiver support when possible.

Source: Carlson C, Merel SE, Yukawa M. Geriatric syndromes and geriatric assessment for the generalist. *Med Clin N Am.* 2015:99:263; Adapted from American Geriatrics Society 2012 Beers Criteria Update Expert Panel. American Geriatrics Society updated Beers criteria for potentially inappropriate medication use in older adults. *J Am Geriatr Soc.* 2012;60:616; and Hoyl MT, Alessi CA, Harker JO, et al. Development and testing of a five-item version of the geriatric depression scale. *J Am Geriatr Soc.* 1999;47:873.

Anatomy and Physiology

Primary aging reflects changes in physiologic reserves over time that are independent of changes from disease. Physiologic changes are especially apt to appear during periods of stress, such as exposure to fluctuating temperatures, dehydration, or even shock. In aging, decreased cutaneous vasoconstriction and sweat production can impair responses to heat; declines in thirst may delay recovery from dehydration; and the physiologic drops in maximum cardiac output, left ventricular filling, and maximum heart rate may impair the response to shock.

At the same time, the aging population displays marked heterogeneity. Investigators have identified vast differences in how people age and have distinguished "usual" aging, with its complex of diseases and impairments, from "optimal" aging. Optimal aging occurs in those people who escape debilitating disease entirely and maintain healthy lives late into their 80s and 90s. Studies of centenarians show that genes account for 20% to 30% of their probability of living to age 100 years. Importantly, healthy lifestyles also account for 20% to 30%.[13,14] These findings provide evidence for clinicians to promote modifiable lifestyle choices like optimal nutrition, strength training, and exercise and to promote optimal function for older adults that delay the depletion of physiologic reserves and the onset of frailty.

Vital Signs

Blood Pressure. In Western societies, systolic blood pressure tends to rise with aging (Fig. 20-2). The aorta and large arteries stiffen and become atherosclerotic. As the aorta becomes less distensible, a given stroke volume causes a greater rise in systolic blood pressure; *systolic hypertension* with a *widened pulse pressure (PP)* often ensues. Diastolic blood pressure (DBP) stops rising at approximately the sixth decade. At the other extreme, many older adults develop *orthostatic (postural) hypotension*—a sudden drop in blood pressure when rising to a standing position.

See Table 17-3, Syncope and Similar Disorders, pp. 778–779.

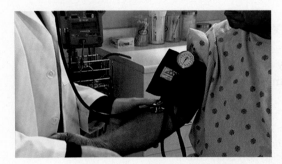

FIGURE 20-2. **Systolic blood pressure increases with age.**

Heart Rate and Rhythm. In older adults, resting heart rate remains unchanged, but there are declines in the pacemaker cells of the sinoatrial node and the maximal heart rate, which affect the response to exercise and physiologic stress.[15] Older adults are more likely to have abnormal heart rhythms such as atrial or ventricular ectopy. Asymptomatic rhythm changes are generally benign. However, some rhythm changes cause *syncope,* which is a temporary loss of consciousness.

Respiratory Rate and Temperature. Respiratory rate and temperature are unchanged, but changes in temperature regulation lead to a susceptibility to *hypothermia.*

Skin, Nails, and Hair. With age, the skin wrinkles, becomes lax, and loses turgor. The dermis is less vascular, causing lighter skin to look paler and more opaque. Skin on the backs of the hands and forearms appears thin, fragile, loose, and transparent. There may be purple patches or macules, termed *actinic purpura,* that fade over time. These spots and patches come from blood that has leaked through poorly supported capillaries and spread within the dermis (Fig. 20-3).

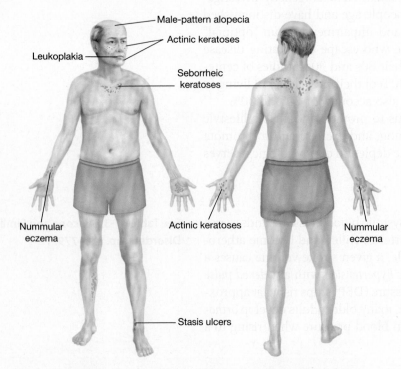

Male-pattern alopecia

Actinic keratoses

Leukoplakia

Seborrheic keratoses

Nummular eczema

Actinic keratoses

Nummular eczema

Stasis ulcers

FIGURE 20-3. **Skin and hair changes in older adults.**

Nails lose luster with age and may yellow and thicken, especially on the toes.

Hair undergoes a series of changes. Scalp hair loses its pigment, changing hair color to gray. Hair loss on the scalp is genetically determined. As early as 20 years, a man's hairline may start to recede at the temples and then at the vertex. In women, hair loss follows a similar but less severe pattern. In both sexes, the number of scalp hairs decreases in a generalized pattern, and the diameter of each hair gets smaller. There is also normal hair loss elsewhere on the body—the trunk, pubic areas, axillae, and limbs. Women over 55 years may develop coarse facial hairs on the chin and upper lip.

Many of these changes are more common in lighter-skinned patients and may not apply to patients with darker skin tones. For example, Native American men have relatively little facial and body hair compared with lighter-skinned men and should be evaluated according to their own norms.

Head and Neck

Eyes and Visual Acuity. The eyes, ears, and mouth show more visible changes of aging. The fat that surrounds and cushions the eyes within the bony orbit may atrophy, making the eyeballs appear to recede. The skin of the eyelids becomes wrinkled and may hang in looser folds. Fat may push the fascia of the eyelids forward, creating soft bulges, especially in the lower lids and the inner third of the upper lids. Because of fewer lacrimal secretions, older patients may complain of dry eyes. The corneas lose some of their luster.

The pupils become smaller, making it more difficult to examine the ocular fundi. The pupils may also become slightly irregular but should continue to respond to light and show the near reaction (see pp. 235–236).

Visual acuity remains fairly constant between ages 20 and 50 years. It diminishes gradually until approximately 70 years and then more rapidly. Nevertheless, most older adults retain good to adequate vision (20/20 to 20/70 as measured by standard charts). Near vision, however, begins to blur noticeably for virtually everyone. From childhood on, the lens gradually loses its elasticity, with progressive loss of accommodation and the ability to focus on nearby objects. Ensuing *presbyopia* usually becomes noticeable during the fifth decade.

Aging increases the risk of developing *cataracts, glaucoma,* and *macular degeneration.* Thickening and yellowing of the lens impairs the passage of light to the retina, requiring more light for reading and doing fine work. Cataracts affect 10% of patients in their 60s and over 30% in their 80s. Because the lens continues to expand with aging, it may push the iris forward, narrowing the angle between iris and cornea and increasing the risk of *narrow-angle glaucoma.*

See Chapter 7, Head and Neck, pp. 215–302.

Hearing. Hearing acuity usually declines with age. Early losses, which start in young adulthood, involve primarily the high-pitched sounds beyond the range of human speech and have relatively little functional significance. Gradually, loss extends to sounds in the middle and lower ranges. When a person fails to hear the higher tones of words but still hears lower tones, words sound distorted and difficult to understand, especially in noisy environments. Hearing loss associated with aging, known as *presbycusis,* becomes increasingly evident, usually after age 50 years.

Mouth, Teeth, and Lymph Nodes. With aging, there are decreased salivary secretions and loss of taste; medications and various diseases can exacerbate these changes. Decreased olfaction and increased sensitivity to bitterness and saltiness also affect taste. Teeth may wear down, become abraded, or fall out due to dental caries or periodontal disease. In patients without teeth, the lower portion of the face looks small and sunken, with accentuated "purse-string" wrinkles radiating from the mouth. Overclosure of the mouth may lead to maceration of the skin at the corners, or *angular cheilitis.* The bony ridges of the jaws that once surrounded the tooth sockets are gradually resorbed, especially in the lower jaw.

See Chapter 7, The Head and Neck, pp. 215–302.

With aging, the cervical lymph nodes become less palpable. In contrast, the submandibular glands become easier to feel.

Thorax and Lungs. As people age, they lose lung capacity during exercise.[16] The chest wall becomes stiffer and harder to move, respiratory muscles may weaken, and the lungs lose some of their elastic recoil. Lung mass and the surface area for gas exchange decline, and residual volume increases as the alveoli enlarge. An increase in closing volumes of small airways predisposes to atelectasis and risk of pneumonia. Diaphragmatic strength declines. The speed of breathing out with maximal effort gradually diminishes, and coughing becomes less effective. There is a decrease in arterial pO_2, but the O_2 saturation normally remains above 90%.

Skeletal changes can accentuate the dorsal curve of the thoracic spine. Osteoporotic vertebral collapse produces *kyphosis,* which increases the anteroposterior diameter of the chest. However, the resulting "barrel chest" has little effect on function.

Cardiovascular System. A number of changes occur in the neck vessels, cardiac output, heart sounds, and murmurs.

Review the effects of aging on blood pressure and heart rate described on p. 355.

Neck Vessels. Lengthening and tortuosity of the aorta and its branches occasionally result in kinking or buckling of the carotid artery low in the neck, especially on the right. The resulting pulsatile mass, occurring chiefly in women with hypertension, may be mistaken for a carotid aneurysm—a true dilatation of the artery. A tortuous aorta occasionally raises the pressure in the jugular veins on the left side of the neck by impairing their drainage within the thorax.

In older adults, systolic bruits heard in the middle or upper portions of the carotid arteries indicate stenosis from atherosclerotic plaque. Cervical bruits in younger people are usually innocent.

See discussion of carotid bruits in Chapter 9, pp. 381–382.

Cardiac Output. Myocardial contraction is less responsive to stimulation from β-adrenergic catecholamines. There is a modest drop in resting heart rate, but a significant drop in the maximum heart rate during exercise. Although heart rate drops, stroke volume increases, so cardiac output is maintained. Diastolic dysfunction arises from decreased early diastolic filling and greater dependence on atrial contraction. There is increased myocardial stiffness, notably in the left ventricle, which also hypertrophies.

Risk of heart failure increases with loss of atrial contraction and onset of atrial fibrillation due to decreased ventricular filling.

Extra Heart Sounds—S₃ and S₄. A physiologic *third heart sound*, commonly heard in children and young adults, may persist as late as age 40 years, especially in women. After age 40 years, however, an S_3 strongly suggests heart failure from volume overload of the left ventricle in conditions like heart failure and valvular heart disease (e.g., mitral regurgitation). In contrast, a *fourth heart sound* is seldom heard in young adults other than well-conditioned athletes. An S_4 can be heard in otherwise healthy older people, but often suggests decreased ventricular compliance and impaired ventricular filling.

See Table 9-8, Extra Heart Sounds in Diastole, p. 407.

Cardiac Murmurs. Middle-aged and older adults commonly have a *systolic aortic murmur*. This murmur is detected in approximately one third of people at age 60 years, and in more than half of those reaching 85 years. With aging, fibrotic changes thicken the bases of the aortic cusps. Calcification follows, resulting in audible vibrations. Turbulence produced by blood flow into a dilated aorta may further augment this murmur. In most older adults, the process of fibrosis and calcification, known as *aortic sclerosis*, does not impede blood flow. In some, the aortic valve leaflets become calcified and immobile, resulting in *aortic stenosis* and outflow obstruction. A brisk carotid upstroke can help distinguish aortic sclerosis from aortic stenosis, which has a delayed carotid upstroke, but clinically distinguishing these conditions is difficult. Both carry increased risk for cardiovascular morbidity and mortality.

Similar changes alter the mitral valve, but usually about one decade later than the aortic valve. Calcification of the mitral valve annulus, or valve ring, impedes normal valve closure during systole, causing the systolic murmur of *mitral regurgitation*. This change in the configuration of the valve may become pathologic as volume overload increases in the left ventricle.

Peripheral Vascular System. The peripheral arteries tend to lengthen, become tortuous, and feel harder and less resilient. There is increased arterial stiffness and decreased endothelial function.[16] The trophic changes of the skin, nails, and hair discussed earlier occur independently, although they may accompany arterial disease. Although arterial and venous disorders, especially atherosclerosis, are more common in older adults, these are not normal changes of aging. Loss of arterial pulsations is not typical and demands careful evaluation. Abdominal or back pain in older adults raises the important concern of possible abdominal aortic aneurysm, especially in male smokers over age 65 years. Rarely, after age 50 years but especially after age 70 years, the temporal arteries may develop *giant cell*, or *temporal, arteritis,* leading to loss of vision in 15% of patients and headache and jaw claudication.

Breasts and Axillae.   The normal adult female breast is soft but may be granular, nodular, or lumpy. This uneven texture represents physiologic nodularity, palpable throughout or only in parts of the breasts. With aging, the female breasts tend to get smaller, more flaccid, and more pendulous as glandular tissue atrophies and is replaced by fat. The ducts surrounding the nipple may become more palpable as firm stringy strands. Axillary hair diminishes. Males may develop gynecomastia or increased breast fullness due to obesity and hormonal changes.

Abdomen.   During the middle and later years, the abdominal muscles tend to weaken, there is decreased activity of lipoprotein lipase, and fat may accumulate in the lower abdomen and near the hips even when the weight is stable. These changes often produce a softer, more protruding, abdomen which patients may interpret as fluid or evidence of disease. The change in abdominal fat distribution increases the risk of cardiovascular disease.

Aging can blunt the manifestations of acute abdominal disease. Pain may be less severe, fever is often less pronounced, and signs of peritoneal inflammation, such as guarding and rebound tenderness, may be diminished or even absent.

See Chapter 11, The Abdomen, pp. 449–507.

Male and Female Genitalia; Prostate.   As men age, sexual interest appears to remain intact, although frequency of intercourse appears to decline after age 75 years. Several physiologic changes accompany decreasing testosterone levels.[16] Erections become more dependent on tactile stimulation and less responsive to erotic cues. The penis decreases in size, and the testicles drop lower in the scrotum. Protracted illnesses, more than aging, lead to decreased testicular size. Pubic hair may decrease and become gray. Erectile dysfunction, or the inability to maintain an erection, affects approximately 50% of older men. Vascular causes are the most common, from both atherosclerotic arterial occlusive disease and corpora cavernosa venous leak. Chronic diseases such as diabetes, hypertension, dyslipidemia, and smoking, as well as medication side effects, all contribute to the prevalence of erectile dysfunction.

In women, ovarian function usually starts to decline during the fifth decade; on average, menstrual periods cease between age 45 and 52 years. As estrogen stimulation falls, many women experience hot flashes, sometimes for up to 5 years. Symptoms range from flushing, sweating, and palpitations to chills and anxiety. Sleep disruption and mood changes are common. Women may report vaginal dryness, urge incontinence, or dyspareunia. Several vulvovaginal changes occur: Pubic hair becomes sparse as well as gray, and the labia and clitoris become smaller. The vagina narrows and shortens, and the vaginal mucosa becomes thin, pale, and dry, with loss of lubrication. The uterus and ovaries diminish in size. Within 10 years after menopause, the ovaries are usually no longer palpable. The suspensory ligaments of the adnexa, uterus, and bladder may also relax. Sexuality and sexual interest are often unchanged, particularly when women are untroubled by partner issues, partner loss, or unusual work or life stress.[17]

The prevalence of *urinary incontinence* increases with age, related to decreased innervation and contractility of the detrusor muscle and loss of bladder capacity, urinary flow rate, and the ability to inhibit voiding. In men, there is androgen-dependent proliferation of prostate epithelial and stromal tissue, termed *benign prostatic hyperplasia (BPH),* that begins in the third decade, continues to the seventh decade, then appears to plateau. Only half of men will have clinically significant enlargement, and of those, only half will report symptoms such as urinary hesitancy, dribbling, and incomplete emptying. These symptoms can often be traced to other causes like coexisting disease, use of medications, and lower urinary tract abnormalities.[18]

Musculoskeletal System. Both men and women lose cortical and trabecular bone mass throughout adulthood; men more slowly, and women more rapidly after menopause, which leads to increased risk of fracture. Calcium resorption from bone, rather than diet, increases with aging as parathyroid hormone levels rise. Subtle losses in height begin soon after maturity; significant shortening is obvious by old age. Most loss of height occurs in the trunk and reflects thinning of the intervertebral discs and shortening or even collapse of the vertebral bodies from osteoporosis, leading to kyphosis and an increase in the anteroposterior diameter of the chest. Added flexion at the knees and hips also contributes to shortened stature. These changes cause the limbs of an elderly person to look long in proportion to the trunk.

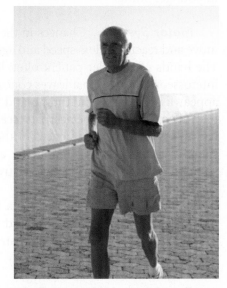

FIGURE 20-4. **Exercise improves strength and bone mass.**

With aging, there is a 30% to 50% decline in muscle mass in relation to body weight in both men and women, and ligaments lose some of their tensile strength. Range of motion diminishes, in part due to osteoarthritis. *Sarcopenia* is the loss of lean body mass and strength with aging.[19] The causes of muscle loss are multifactorial, including inflammatory and endocrine changes as well as sedentary lifestyle. There is substantial evidence that strength training in older adults can slow or reverse this process (Fig. 20-4).

Nervous System. Aging affects all aspects of the nervous system, from mental status to motor and sensory function and reflexes. Brain volume, cortical brain cells, and intrinsic regional connecting networks decrease, and both micro-anatomical and biochemical changes have been identified.[20] Nevertheless, most older adults maintain their self-esteem and adapt well to their changing capacities and circumstances.

Mental Status. Although older adults generally perform well on mental status examinations, they may display selected impairments, especially at advanced ages. Many older people complain about memory problems. This is usually from "benign forgetfulness," which can occur at any age. This term refers to difficulty recalling the names of people or objects or details of specific events.

Identifying this common phenomenon can allay fear of Alzheimer disease. Older adults also retrieve and process data more slowly and take longer to learn new information. Their motor responses may slow and their ability to perform complex tasks may diminish.

Frequently, the clinician must try to distinguish these age-related changes from manifestations of mental disorders that are prevalent in older adults like *depression* and *dementia*. Diagnosis can be difficult because both mood disturbances and cognitive changes can alter the patient's ability to recognize or report symptoms. Older patients are also more susceptible to *delirium*, a temporary state of confusion that may be the first clue to infection, problems with medications, or impending dementia. It is important to recognize these conditions promptly to delay functional decline. Recall that sensory and motor findings in older patients that are physiologic, such as the changes in hearing; vision; extraocular movements; and pupillary size, shape, and reactivity, are abnormal in younger adults.

Review Chapter 5, Behavior and Mental Status, The Mental Status Examination, pp. 147–171, and Table 20-2, Delirium and Dementia, p. 1001.

Motor System.

Changes in the motor system are common. Older adults move and react with less speed and agility and skeletal muscles decrease in bulk. The hands of an older patient often look thin and bony due to atrophy of the interosseous muscles that leaves concavities or grooves. Muscle wasting tends to appear first between the thumb and the hand (first and second metacarpals), then affects the other metacarpals (see pp. 741–742). It may also flatten the thenar and hypothenar eminences of the palms. Arm and leg muscles can show signs of atrophy, exaggerating the apparent size of adjacent joints. Muscle strength, though diminished, is relatively well maintained.

Occasionally, older adults develop a benign essential tremor in the head, jaw, lips, or hands that may be confused with parkinsonism. Unlike parkinsonian tremors, however, benign tremors are slightly faster and disappear at rest, and there is no associated muscle rigidity.

See Chapter 17, The Nervous System, Table 17-5, Tremors and Involuntary Movement, pp. 782–783.

Position and Vibratory Sense; Reflexes.

Aging can also affect vibratory and position sense and reflexes. Older adults frequently lose some or all vibration sense in the feet and ankles (but not in the fingers or over the shins). Less commonly, position sense may diminish or disappear. The gag reflex may be decreased or absent. Abdominal reflexes may diminish or disappear. Ankle reflexes may be symmetrically decreased or absent, even when reinforced. Less commonly, knee reflexes are similarly affected. Partly because of musculoskeletal changes in the feet, the plantar responses become less obvious and more difficult to interpret. If there are associated abnormal neurologic findings, or if atrophy and reflex changes are asymmetric, search for an explanation other than aging.

Older adults experience the death of loved ones and friends, retirement from valued employment, diminution in income, and often growing social isolation in addition to physiologic changes and decreased physical capacity. Including the impact of these significant life events in the assessment of mood and affect and addressing these issues may improve the patient's quality of life.

The Health History

Approach to the Patient

As you interview older adults, you will need to modify your usual approach to obtaining the Health History. As with all patients, your demeanor should convey respect, patience, and cultural awareness. Be sure to address older patients by an appropriate title and their last name.

Approach to the Older Adult Patient

- Adjusting the office environment
- Shaping the content and pace of the visit
- Eliciting symptoms
- Addressing the cultural dimensions of aging

Adjusting the Office Environment. First, take the time to adjust the environment of the office, hospital, or nursing home to put your patient at ease. Recall the physiologic changes in temperature regulation, and make sure that the office is neither too cool nor too warm. Bright lighting helps compensate for changes in lens proteins and allows the older patient to see your facial expressions and gestures more clearly. Face the patient directly, sitting at eye level (Fig. 20-5). Avoid focusing on personal electronic devices or turning away from the patient to search the electronic clinical record.

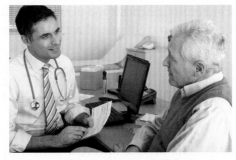

FIGURE 20-5. **Face the patient at eye level.**

More than 50% of older adults have hearing deficits, especially for higher frequency tones, so choose a quiet room that is free of distractions or noise. Turn off the radio or television before you start the conversation. If appropriate, consider using a "pocket talker," a small portable microphone and speaker that amplifies your voice and connects to an earpiece inserted by the patient. Speak in low tones, and make sure the patient is using glasses, hearing aids, and dentures to assist with communication. Patients with quadriceps weakness benefit from chairs with higher seating and a wide stool with a handrail leading up to the examining table.

Shaping the Content and Pace of the Visit. With older adults, rethink the traditional format of the visit. Older patients often measure their lives in terms of years left rather than years lived. They may reminisce about the past and previous experiences. By listening to these life reviews, you gain important insights that help you understand and support them as they work through painful feelings or recapture joys and accomplishments.

At the same time, it is important to weigh the need to assess complex problems against the patient's endurance and possible fatigue. To expand time for listening to the patient but prevent exhaustion, make ample use of brief and well-validated screening tools,[21,22] information from home visits and the clinical record, and reports from family members, caregivers, and allied health disciplines. Consider dividing the initial assessment into two visits. Two or more shorter visits may be more productive to allow more time to respond to questions since explanations may be slow and lengthy.

See the "10-Minute Geriatric Screener," p. 986.

Eliciting Symptoms from the Older Adult.   Eliciting the history calls for an astute clinician: patients may accidentally or intentionally underreport symptoms; the presentation of acute illnesses may differ from younger patients; common symptoms may mask a geriatric syndrome; or patients may have cognitive impairment.

Underreporting.   Older patients tend to give more positive ratings to their overall health than younger adults, even when affected by disease and disability. Some are reluctant to report their symptoms. Some are afraid or embarrassed; others try to avoid clinical expenses or the discomforts of diagnosis and treatment. Still others overlook their symptoms, thinking they are merely part of aging, or they may simply forget about them.

To minimize delayed diagnosis and treatment, ask direct questions, use the well-validated geriatric screening tools, and consult with family members and caregivers.

Atypical Presentations of Illness.   Acute illnesses present differently in older adults. Older patients with infections are less likely to have fever. Older patients having a myocardial infarction are less likely to report chest pain; symptoms of atypical or no chest pain, shortness of breath, palpitations, syncope, and confusion are more common.[23] Older patients with hyperthyroidism and hypothyroidism have fewer symptoms and signs. One third of older adults with hyperthyroidism present with fatigue, weight loss, and tachycardia in lieu of the classic features of heat intolerance, sweating, and hyperreflexia.[24] Up to 35% present with atrial fibrillation. Hyperthyroidism increases the risk of osteoporosis, and, in affected women, the risk of hip and vertebral fractures increases threefold. In older adults, hypothyroidism is most commonly caused by autoimmune thyroiditis (Hashimoto thyroiditis); fatigue, weakness, constipation, dry skin, and cold intolerance are often attributed to other conditions, medication side effects, or aging.

In older adults the prevalence of hyperthyroidism is 0.5%–4% and of hypothyroidism, ~10% in men and 16% in women.[24]

Geriatric Syndromes.   Managing an increasing number of interrelated conditions calls for recognizing the symptom clusters of different *geriatric syndromes*. A geriatric syndrome is "a multifactorial condition that involves the interaction between identifiable situation-specific stressors and underlying age-related risk factors, resulting in damage across multiple organ systems," as shown in

Figure 20-6.[12] These syndromes are strongly linked to functional decline. Examples include dizziness[25–27] as well as functional impairment, frailty, delirium, depression, cognitive impairment, falls, and urinary incontinence.

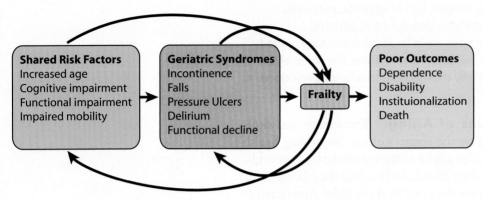

FIGURE 20-6. Geriatric syndromes.

Experts state that "evaluating functional status, frailty, and other geriatric syndromes while simultaneously addressing individual disease processes is at the heart of geriatric approach to primary care." It is especially important to recognize these syndromes because symptoms may cluster in patterns unfamiliar to the patient.[28]

These syndromes have been found in more than half of adults over age 65 years, in contrast to the conventional search in younger patients for a "single unifying diagnosis."[29]

Cognitive Impairment. A number of parameters affects assessment of health status; however, evidence suggests that self-report continues to be reliable in older adults, especially for prevalence of chronic conditions.[30–34] When compared with healthy peers, older adults with mild cognitive impairment provide sufficient history to reveal concurrent disorders. Use simple sentences with prompts to elicit necessary information. For patients with more severe impairments, confirm key symptoms with family members or caregivers in the patient's presence and with his or her consent. To avoid invalid assumptions, explore how older patients view themselves and their situations. Listen for their priorities and coping skills. These insights strengthen your partnerships with both patients and families as you evolve plans for care and treatment.

Tips for Communicating Effectively with Older Adults

- Provide a well-lit, moderately warm setting with minimal background noise, chairs with arms, and access to the examining table.
- Face the patient and speak in low tones; make sure the patient is using glasses, hearing devices, and dentures, if needed.
- Adjust the pace and content of the interview to the stamina of the patient; consider two visits for initial evaluations.
- Allow time for open-ended questions and reminiscing; include family and caregivers when indicated, especially if the patient has cognitive impairment.
- Make use of screening instruments, the clinical record, and reports from allied disciplines.

(continued)

Tips for Communicating Effectively with Older Adults (*continued*)

- Carefully assess symptoms, especially fatigue, loss of appetite, dizziness, weight loss, and pain, for clues to underlying disorders and geriatric syndromes. Make sure written instructions are in large print and easy to read.
- Always give the patient an updated medication that includes the name of the medication, dosage instructions, and why the medication is being prescribed.

Addressing Cultural Dimensions of Aging.   Knowledge and skills about the cultural dimensions of aging are the cornerstone to improving health care for the rapidly growing number of older adults of diverse ethnic backgrounds. In fact, the demographic imperative for older adults can be called the *ethnogeriatric imperative,* "because by mid-century more than one in three older Americans is projected to be from one of the four populations designated as 'minority,'"[35] as shown in Figure 20-7.

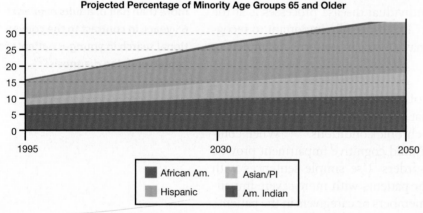

Projected Percentage of Minority Age Groups 65 and Older

Legend: African Am. · Asian/PI · Hispanic · Am. Indian

FIGURE 20-7. **Projected percentage of minority age groups 65 years and older.**
Source: Yeo G. How will the U.S. healthcare system meet the challenge of the ethnogeriatric imperative? *J Am Geriatr Soc.* 2009;57:1278.

Geriatric Diversity—Now and in 2050

- *Hispanic Americans* over age 65 years will increase from 2.7 million in 2010, or 6.9% of older adults, to 17.5 million in 2050, or 19.8% of the older population.[5]
- *African American* older adults will increase from 3.4 million (8.5%) to 10.5 million in 2050 (11.9%).
- *Asian Americans* and other ethnic groups, although smaller in number currently, will increase from 1.4 million to 7.5 million, or from 3.4% to 8.5%.
- *Non-Hispanic whites* will increase from 32.2 million to 58.5 million in 2050, but will drop as a percentage of the older population from 80% to 58.5%.

Source: Federal Interagency Forum on Aging Related Statistics. Older Americans 2012, Key Indicators of Well Being. Indicator 2, Racial and Ethnic Composition, p. 86. Federal Interagency Forum on Aging-Related Statistics. Washington, DC: U.S. Government Printing Office. June 2012. Available at http://agingstats.gov/agingstatsdotnet/Main_Site/Data/2012_Documents/Docs/EntireChartbook.pdf. Accessed August 11, 2015.

The changing demographics of aging only hint at how older adults of different ethnicities experience suffering, illness, and decisions about their health care. Culture and socioeconomic attributes affect the epidemiology of illness and mental health, the process of acculturation in families, individual concerns about aging, choices about healers and when to pursue symptoms, the potential for misdiagnosis, and disparities in health outcomes.[36] Culture shapes beliefs about the entire spectrum of aging: work and retirement, perceptions of health and illness, the utility of medications, use of health care proxies, and preferences about dying, to name just a few.

The CDC Health Disparities and Inequalities Report–United States, 2013 "highlights health disparities and inequalities across a wide range of diseases, behavioral risk factors, environmental exposures, social determinants, and health care access by sex, race and ethnicity, income, education, disability status, and other social characteristics."[37,38] Aging racial/ethnic minority populations have poorer health outcomes in cardiovascular disease, diabetes, cancer, asthma, and human immunodeficiency virus/acquired immunodeficiency syndrome as well as shorter life spans.[39] Despite advances in *ethnogeriatrics,*[40–42] information on racial and ethnic disparities in later life regarding chronic disease, ADLs, and self-rated health status remains "limited and inconsistent," and guidelines for providing individualized culturally appropriate care are sparse.[38]

Improving competence in care for diverse older populations is a critical step in improving health outcomes. The *ETHIC(S)* mnemonic helps clinicians escape the pitfalls of group-labeling by expanding individual history taking to include **Explanation, Treatment, Healers, Negotiate, Intervention, Collaborate,** and **Spirituality.**[43] Nonetheless, this model may miss important information about cultural identity, social supports, and views about health care.[44] Experts recommend letting patients establish their cultural identity by exploring four key areas during the interview: the individual's cultural identity; cultural explanations of the individual's illness; cultural factors related to the psychosocial environment and levels of function; and cultural elements in the clinician–patient relationship. Test your "ethnogeriatric IQ" at the Stanford Geriatrics Education Center website and explore the Stanford curriculum in ethnogeriatrics.[45,46] Learn to convey respect to older adults through culturally specific nonverbal communication. Direct eye contact or handshaking, for example, may not be culturally appropriate. Identify critical life experiences from the country of origin or migration history that affect the patient's outlook and psyche. Ask about family decision making, spiritual advisors, and traditional healers and practices.

See Table 20-1, Interviewing Older Adults: Enhancing Culturally Appropriate Care, p. 1000.

The Office of Minority Health in the Department of Health and Human Services has developed *Think Cultural Health,* a resource center to improve quality of care through cultural and linguistic competencies and continuing education programs.[41]

See Chapter 3, Demonstrating Cultural Humility—A Changing Paradigm, pp. 82–86.

Cultural values particularly affect decisions about the end of life. Elders, family, and even an extended community group may make these decisions with or for the older patient. Such group decision making is quite different from the focus on individual autonomy and informed consent featured in contemporary health care settings. Eliciting the stresses of migration and acculturation, using translators effectively, enlisting "patient navigators" from the family and community, and accessing culturally validated assessment tools like the Geriatric Depression Scale will help you provide empathic care of older adults.

See Chapter 3, Interviewing and the Health History, on working with translators, pp. 90–91.

SPECIAL AREAS OF CONCERN WHEN ASSESSING COMMON SYMPTOMS

Common Concerns

- Activities of Daily Living
- Instrumental activities of daily living
- Medications
- Acute and persistent pain
- Smoking and alcohol
- Nutrition
- Frailty
- Advance directives and palliative care

Symptoms in the older adult can have many meanings and interconnections, as seen with the geriatric syndromes. Explore the full dimensions of these symptoms as you would with all patients, and for older adults, place symptoms in the context of your overall functional assessment of the ADLs. Several topics warrant special attention as you gather the health history. Approach these areas with extra thoroughness and sensitivity, always with the goal of helping your older patients to maintain their optimal level of function and well-being.

See Functional Assessment and the 10-Minute Geriatric Screener, pp. 985 and 986.

Activities of Daily Living.   The daily activities of older adults, especially those with chronic illness, provide an important baseline for future evaluations. First, ask about how well the patient performs the ADLs, which consist of six basic self-care abilities. Then, move on to higher level functions, the instrumental activities of daily living (IADLs). Can the patient perform these activities independently, does he or she need some help, or is the patient entirely dependent on others?

Start with open-ended questions like "Tell me about your typical day" or "Tell me about your day yesterday." Then probe for more detail…"You got up at 8 AM? How is it getting out of bed?… What did you do next?" Ask if activity levels have changed, who is available for help, and what helpers or caregivers actually do. Remember that assessing the patient's safety is a clinical priority.

Activities of Daily Living and Instrumental Activities of Daily Living

Activities of Daily Living (ADLs)	Instrumental Activities of Daily Living (IADLs)
Bathing	Using the telephone
Dressing	Shopping
Toileting	Preparing food
Transferring	Housekeeping
Continence	Laundry
Feeding	Transportation
	Taking medicine
	Managing money

Medications. The magnitude of adverse drug events leading to hospitalization and poor patient outcomes underscores the importance of a thorough medication history. Adults over age 65 years receive approximately 30% of all prescriptions. Approximately 85% of adults over age 65 years have at least one of six chronic conditions—arthritis, current asthma, cancer, cardiovascular disease, chronic obstructive pulmonary disease, or diabetes—and 50% take at least one prescription drug each day.[47,48] Almost 40% take five or more prescription drugs daily. Older adults have more than 50% of all reported adverse drug reactions causing hospital admission, reflecting pharmacodynamic changes in the distribution, metabolism, and elimination of drugs that place them at increased risk.

▪ A thorough *medication history* includes name, dose, frequency, and the *patient's view* of the reason for taking each drug.

▪ Ask the patient to bring in all medication bottles and over-the-counter products to develop an accurate medication list.

▪ Explore all components of polypharmacy—a major cause of morbidity—including suboptimal prescribing, concurrent use of multiple drugs, underuse, inappropriate use, and nonadherence.

▪ Ask specifically about over-the-counter products; vitamin and nutritional supplements; and mood-altering drugs such as narcotics, benzodiazepines, and recreational substances.[49]

▪ Assess medications for drug interactions.

▪ Be particularly careful when treating *insomnia*, estimated to occur in 40% of older adults. A *sleep history* provides information essential for diagnosis; a *sleep diary* may be especially helpful in uncovering the origins of a poor sleep pattern.[50] Increased exercise may be the best remedy. Turn to expert guidelines on types of sleep disorders and recommended management.[51]

Medications are the single most common modifiable risk factor associated with falls. Review strategies for avoiding polypharmacy.[52,53] Keep the number of drugs prescribed to a minimum and "start low, go slow" with respect to dosing. Learn about drug–drug interactions and consult the *Beers criteria,* updated in 2012 by the American Geriatrics Society and widely used by health care providers, educators, and policymakers. These criteria include the list of hazardous drugs for older adults.[54,55] Risk factors for adverse drug reactions in hospitalized older patients are listed below.

Hospitalized Older Adults: Risk Factors for Adverse Drug Reactions

- More than four comorbid conditions
- Heart failure, renal failure, or liver disease
- Age ≥80 years
- Number of drugs, especially if eight or more
- Use of warfarin, insulins, oral antiplatelet agents, or oral hypoglycemic agents
- Previous adverse drug reaction
- Hyperlipidemia
- Raised white cell count
- Use of antidiabetic agents
- Length of stay ≥12 days

Source: Onder G, Petrovic M, Balamurugan T, et al. Less is more. Development and validation of a score to assess risk of adverse drug reactions among the in-hospital patients 65 years or older. *Arch Intern Med.* 2010;170:1142; Tangiisuran B, Scutt G, Stevenson J, et al. Development and validation of a risk model for predicting adverse drug reactions in older people during hospital stay: Brighton Adverse Drug Reactions Risk (BADRI) model. *PLoS One.* 2014;9:e111254; Budnitz DS, Lovegrove MC, Shehab N, et al. Emergency hospitalizations for adverse drug events in older Americans. *N Engl J Med.* 2011;365:2002.

Acute and Persistent Pain. Pain and associated complaints account for 80% of clinician visits. Prevalence of pain may reach 25% to 50% in community-dwelling adults and 40% to 80% in nursing home residents. Pain usually arises from musculoskeletal complaints such as back and joint pain.[56,57] Headache, neuralgias from diabetes and herpes zoster, nighttime leg pain, and cancer pain are also common. Older patients are less likely to report pain, leading to suffering, depression, social isolation, physical disability, and loss of function. The American Geriatrics Society advocates use of the term *persistent pain* to reduce negative stereotypes associated with the term "chronic pain."[56]

Pain is subjective, so some view pain as a spectrum disorder rather than "the fifth vital sign." See discussion, pp. 134–137.

Characteristics of Acute and Persistent Pain

Acute Pain	Persistent Pain
Distinct onset	Lasts more than 3 months
Obvious pathology	Often associated with psychological or functional impairment

(continued)

Characteristics of Acute and Persistent Pain (*continued*)

Acute Pain	Persistent Pain
Short duration	Can fluctuate in character and intensity over time
Common causes: postsurgical, trauma, headache	Common causes: arthritis, cancer, claudication, leg cramps, neuropathy, radiculopathy

Source: Reuben DB, Herr KA, Pacala JT, et al. *Geriatrics at your Fingertips*. 18th ed. New York, NY: American Geriatrics Society; 2016.

Accurate assessment is the basis of effective treatment.[58,59] Inquire about pain each time you meet with an older patient. Assessing pain in older adults is challenging. They may be reluctant to report symptoms due to fear of additional testing, cost of care and medication, denial of disease, cognitive or verbal impairments, or barriers of trust, language, or cultural understanding. Patients may report multiple conditions that complicate assessment. Nonetheless, evidence shows when patients do report pain, even those with even mild to moderate cognitive impairment, self-report is reliable. Ask specifically, "Are you having any pain right now? How about during the past week?" Be alert for signs of untreated pain, such as use of the terms "burning," "discomfort," or "soreness," depressed affect, and nonverbal change in posture or gait. Many pain scales are available that have been validated in multicultural populations. Unidimensional scales such as the Visual Analog Scale, graphic pictures, and the Verbal 0–10 Scale have all been validated and are easy to use.[60,61] Interview caregivers or family members for relevant history in patients with severe cognitive deficits.

It is important to distinguish acute pain from persistent pain, and to thoroughly investigate its cause. In older adults, confusion, restlessness, fatigue, or irritability often accompany conditions causing pain. Assessing pain includes evaluation of these related conditions as well as the effect of pain on quality of life, social interactions, and functional level. Consider multidisciplinary assessment in complex cases where the risks of disability and comorbidity are high. Be familiar with the many modalities of pain relief, ranging from analgesics to numerous nonpharmacologic therapies, especially those that actively engage patients in their treatment plan and build self-reliance. Patient education alone has been shown effective.[56] Relaxation techniques, tai chi, acupuncture, massage, and biofeedback can help reduce escalating doses or the addition of more medications.

See the *10-Minute Geriatric Screener* for functional assessment on p. 986.

Smoking and Alcohol

Smoking. *Smoking* is harmful at all ages. At each visit, advise smokers, approximately 9.5% of older adults, to quit.[62] The commitment to stop smoking may take time, but quitting is crucial for reducing the risk of heart disease, pulmonary disease, malignancy, and loss of daily function.

Alcohol. Recommended drinking limits are lower for adults over age 65 years due to physiologic changes that alter alcohol metabolism, frequent comorbid illness, and risk of drug interactions. Older adults should have no more than three drinks on any one day or seven drinks a week.[63]

More than 40% of adults over age 65 years drink alcohol, about 4.5% are binge-drinkers, and 2% to 4% may have abuse or dependence.[64,65] More than 14% of older adults exceed the recommended limits.[66] When health status is taken into account, more than 53% have harmful or hazardous drinking. From 10% to 15% of older patients in primary care practices and up to 38% of hospitalized older adults are reported to have problem drinking.[67]

Despite the high prevalence of alcohol-related problems, rates of detection and treatment are low. Screening all older adults for harmful alcohol use is especially important due to adverse interactions with most medications and exacerbation of comorbid illnesses, including cirrhosis, gastrointestinal bleeding or reflux disease, gout, hypertension, diabetes, insomnia, gait disorders, and depression in up to 30% of older patients.[65] Watch for clues of excess alcohol consumption, listed below, especially in patients with recent bereavement or losses, pain, disability or depression, or a family history of alcohol disorders.

Clues to Alcohol-Use Disorders in Older Adults

- Memory loss, cognitive impairment
- Depression, anxiety
- Neglect of hygiene, appearance
- Poor appetite, nutritional deficits
- Sleep disruption
- Hypertension refractory to therapy
- Blood sugar control problems
- Seizures refractory to therapy
- Impaired balance and gait, falls
- Recurrent gastritis and esophagitis
- Difficulty managing warfarin dosing
- Use of other addictive substances such as sedatives or narcotic analgesics, illicit drugs, nicotine

Source: American Geriatrics Society. Alcohol use disorders in older adults. AGS clinical practice guidelines screening recommendation. *Ann Long Term Care.* 2006;14(1). Available at http://www.annalsoflongtermcare.com/article/5143. Accessed August 15, 2015.

Use the CAGE questions to uncover problem drinking. Although symptoms and signs are subtler in older adults, making early detection more difficult, the four CAGE questions remain sensitive and specific in this age group, using the conventional cutoff score of 2 or more.

See Chapter 3, Interviewing and the Health History, Alcohol and Illicit Drugs, pp. 96–97.

Nutrition. Taking a dietary history and using nutritional screening tools often reveal nutritional deficits. Prevalence of undernutrition increases with age, affecting up to 10% of nursing home residents and up to 50% of older

See Table 4-3, Nutrition Screening, p. 141.

patients at hospital discharge.[68] Recent data suggest that only 30% to 40% meet recommended guidelines for daily intake of fruit and vegetables.[69] Older adults with chronic diseases are particularly vulnerable, especially those with poor dentition, oral or gastrointestinal disorders, depression or other psychiatric illness, and drug regimens that affect appetite and oral secretions.

Frailty. *Frailty* is a multifactorial geriatric syndrome characterized by an age-related lack of adaptive physiological capacity occurring even in the absence of identifiable illness. Frailty typically signifies loss of muscle mass, decreased energy and exercise intolerance, and decreased physiological reserve, with increasing vulnerability to physiologic stressors. Studies generally use one of two definitions. The narrower definition is based solely on physical conditions such as weight loss, exhaustion, weakness, slowness, and low physical activity; the broader definition also includes mood, cognition, and incontinence. Overall prevalence of frailty in community-dwelling adults is ~10%, but reports of prevalence range from 4% to 59% depending on the definition and measurement indexes used.[70,71]

Screen your patients for the presence of three components identified in the Study for Osteoporotic Fractures and pursue related interventions: weight loss of more than 5% over 3 years, inability to do five chair stands, and self-reported exhaustion.[72]

Advance Directives and Palliative Care. Many older patients are interested in discussing end-of-life decisions and would like providers to initiate these discussions *before* the onset of serious illness.[73] *Advance care planning* involves several tasks: providing information, clarifying the patient's preferences, and identifying the surrogate decision maker. You can begin this discussion by linking these decisions to a current illness or experiences with relatives or friends. Ask the patient about "Do Not Resuscitate" orders specifying life support measures "if the heart or lungs were to stop or give out." Also encourage the patient to designate in writing a health care proxy or durable power of attorney for health care, "someone who can make decisions reflecting your wishes in case of confusion or emergency."

See also Chapter 3, The Patient with Altered Cognition, pp. 87–89, and Death and the Dying Patient, pp. 98–99.

Roughly half of hospitalized older adults require surrogate decision making within 48 hours of admission. Common topics include life-sustaining care, surgeries and procedures, and discharge planning.[74] Conversations about life care choices help patients and their families prepare openly and in advance for a peaceful death. Pursue these discussions during office visits rather than in the stressful environment of the emergency department or intensive care unit.

Experts note that *advance care directives* can be more flexible, depending on the situation. These directives "may range from general statements of values to such specific orders as [Do Not Resuscitate], do not intubate, do not hospitalize, do not provide artificial hydration or nutrition, or do not administer antibiotics. Different situations, including different stages of health and illness, demand different types of advanced care directives, and thus require both different conversations and different training in leading such discussions."[75] Moreover, always consult competent patients about current options because their decisions supercede prior written instructions.

For patients with advanced or terminal illnesses, include the review of advanced directives in an overall plan for *palliative care*. Palliative care encompasses the alleviation of pain and suffering and the promotion of optimal quality of life across all phases of treatment, including curative interventions and rehabilitation. Its goals are "to consider the physical, mental, spiritual, and social well-being of patients and their families in order to maintain hope while ensuring patient dignity and respecting autonomy" both for patients with serious illnesses and for patients considering hospice care at the end of life.[76] To ease patient and family distress, use good communication skills: Make good eye contact; ask open-ended questions; respond to anxiety, depression, or changes in the patient's affect; show empathy; and be sure to consult caregivers.

Health Promotion and Counseling: Evidence and Recommendations

Important Topics for Health Promotion and Counseling in the Older Adult

- When to screen
- Vision and hearing
- Exercise
- Household safety and fall prevention
- Immunizations
- Cancer screening
- Depression
- Dementia, mild cognitive impairment, and cognitive decline
- Elder mistreatment and abuse

When to Screen.   As more adults live into their 80s and beyond, decisions about screening become more complex, and the evidence base for screening decisions becomes more limited.[77,78] The aging population is physiologically heterogeneous, many with numerous chronic diseases and also many with delayed or absent disability. Moreover, level of function in "successful aging" does not always parallel the number of chronic ailments, and there are substantial regional gaps in availability and use of preventive services.[79] Although there is relative consensus about immunization recommendations and falls prevention, screening for specific disease states remains more controversial. In general, individualized screening decisions should be based on each older adult's health and functional status, including presence of comorbidity, rather than age alone.[80,81] This approach is depicted in Figure 20-8. The vertical axis shows the health status distribution of the population age 65 years and older, and the horizontal bars show the variation in importance of specific measures.

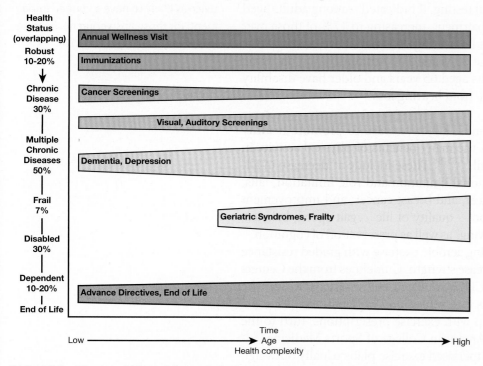

FIGURE 20-8. **Older adults: relative role of screening and preventive services according to functional status.** Source: Nicholas JA, Hall WJ. Screening and preventive services for older adults. *Mt Sinai J Med.* 2011;78:498.

The American Geriatrics Society recommends a five-step approach to screening decisions[82]:

1. Assess patient preferences

2. Interpret the available evidence

3. Estimate prognosis

4. Consider treatment feasibility

5. Optimize therapies and care plans.

If life expectancy is short, give priority to treatment that benefits the patient in the time that remains. Consider deferring screening if it overburdens the older adults who have multiple clinical problems, shortened life expectancy, or dementia. Tests that help with prognosis and planning may still be warranted even if the patient does not want to pursue treatment.

Vision and Hearing. Although the U.S. Preventive Services Task Force (USPSTF) has cited insufficient evidence for screening,[83] geriatricians recommend screening for *vision* and *hearing* insofar as they are vital sensory modalities for daily living. They are key items in the *10-Minute Geriatric Screener.*

See 10-Minute Geriatric Screener, p. 986, and Chapter 7, The Head and Neck, for techniques for assessing hearing, pp. 226–248.

■ Test *vision* objectively using an eye chart.

■ Ask the patient about any *hearing* loss is effective for screening, then proceed to the whisper test and more formal testing, if indicated. Among adults aged 65 to 69 years, 1% have visual impairment, increasing to 17% of those over age 80 years. About a third of adults over age 65 years have hearing loss, increasing to 80% in those over age 80 years. The Administration on Aging reports that a total of 6.5% of adults aged 65 years and older have disability from visual impairment and 17.5% from hearing loss.[2]

Patients reporting hearing loss are twice as likely to have a verified impairment; for those answering no, hearing loss is very unlikely (LR if 0.13).[84]

Exercise.   Exercise is one of the most effective ways to promote healthy aging. Abundant literature documents the many benefits of physical activity in older adults, even in those who are frail.[77,85–88] These include a "decrease in all-cause mortality; reduced risk of functional limitation and role limitation, falls, hypertension, diabetes, colorectal cancer, and breast cancer; and improvement in cognitive function, physical function…quality of life…gait speed, balance, and performance of activities of daily living" as well as preservation of cognition.[77] Recommendations emphasize combining aerobic exercise with graded resistance training in major muscle groups to increase strength. Guidelines from the Centers for Disease Control and Prevention (CDC) are listed below. The CDC website provides information on higher targets for exercise and explanations of aerobic and muscle-strength training. For help with exercise prescriptions, turn to the Exercise in Medicine program of the American College of Sports Medicine.[89,90] The many benefits of individualized supervised exercise plans usually outweigh the risks of joint pain, falls, and cardiac events.

CDC Exercise Recommendations for Older Adults

Adults need at least:

- 2 hours and 30 minutes (150 minutes) of moderate-intensity aerobic activity (i.e., brisk walking) every week **and**
- muscle-strengthening activities on two or more days a week that work all major muscle groups (legs, hips, back, abdomen, chest, shoulders, and arms).

OR

- 1 hour and 15 minutes (75 minutes) of vigorous-intensity aerobic activity (i.e., jogging or running) every week **and**
- muscle-strengthening activities on two or more days a week that work all major muscle groups (legs, hips, back, abdomen, chest, shoulders, and arms).

OR

- An equivalent mix of moderate- and vigorous-intensity aerobic activity **and**
- muscle-strengthening activities on two or more days a week that work all major muscle groups (legs, hips, back, abdomen, chest, shoulders, and arms).

Source: Centers for Disease Control and Prevention. How much physical activity do older adults need?

Physical activity is essential to healthy aging. Updated June 4, 2015. Available at http://www.cdc.gov/physicalactivity/basics/older_adults/index.htm. Accessed August 16, 2015.

Household Safety and Falls Prevention.   In 2013, the CDC reported that 2.5 million nonfatal falls among older adults were treated in emergency departments, and more than 734,000 of these patients were hospitalized at a direct clinical cost of $34 billion.[91] Many have hip fractures and traumatic brain injuries that impact daily function and independence. Emergency room visits and deaths are most likely to involve yard and garden equipment, ladders and stepstools, personal-use items like hair dryers and flammable clothing, and bathroom and sports injuries. Encourage older adults to adopt corrective measures for poor lighting, chairs at awkward heights, slippery or irregular surfaces, and environmental hazards.

See also Further Assessment for Preventing Falls, pp. 987–989.

Home Safety Tips for Older Adults[91]

- Install bright lighting and lightweight curtains or shades.
- Install handrails and lights on all staircases. Pathways and walkways should be well-lit.
- Remove items that cause tripping like papers, books, clothes, and shoes from stairs and walkways.
- Remove or secure small throw rugs and other rugs with double-sided tape.
- Wear shoes both inside and outside the house. Avoid bare feet and wearing slippers.
- Store medications safely.
- Keep commonly used items in cabinets that are easy to reach without using a step stool.
- Install grab bars and nonslip mats or safety strips in baths and showers.
- Repair faulty plugs and electrical cords.
- Install smoke alarms and have a plan for escaping fire.
- Secure all firearms.
- Have a clinical alert device/system for emergency contacts or easy access to 911.

Immunizations.   Recommend vaccination for influenza; pneumonia, both PPSV23 and PCV13; herpes zoster (shingles); and tetanus/diphtheria and pertussis (Tdap and Td). For the most up-to-date recommendations, consult the updated annual guidelines and contraindications provided by the CDC at *http://www.cdc.gov/vaccines*.[92,93] Note that vaccination rates still lag for Hispanics and African Americans.

See also Chapter 8, The Thorax and Lungs, Immunizations, pp. 316–317.

Older Adult Immunizations 2015

Influenza Vaccine[94]
The influenza vaccine protects against up to two strains of influenza A and influenza B in both trivalent and quadrivalent formulations. The following groups should receive the influenza vaccine each year:

- All adults ≥50 years
- Adults with chronic pulmonary and cardiovascular disorders including asthma (but excluding hypertension), and renal, hepatic, neurologic, hematologic, or metabolic disorders including diabetes

(continued)

Older Adult Immunizations 2015 (*continued*)

- Adults who are immunosuppressed from medication or HIV
- Residents of nursing homes and other long-term care facilities; adults with morbid obesity (BMI ≥40)
- Household contacts and caregivers of children under 5 years and adults ≥50 years, especially those with clinical conditions placing them at risk for severe complications from influenza.

Pneumococcal Vaccine[95,96]

PCV13 protects against 13 of the 90 types of pneumococcal bacteria; these types cause infection in about half of the affected adults. PPSV23 protects against 23 types of pneumococcal bacteria.

- *Adults aged ≥65 years:* Older adults who have not previously received PCV13 should receive PCV13 first, followed 6 to 12 months later by PPSV23. Those who have already received one or more doses of PPSV23 should receive PCV13 at least 1 year after the most recent dose of PPSV23. The recommendations for routine PCV13 use among adults aged ≥65 years will be re-evaluated in 2018.
- *Adults aged 19 to 64 years:* This age group should also be vaccinated as above if they have the following conditions: HIV infection, long-term immunosuppressive therapy, chronic renal failure, nephrotic syndrome, functional or anatomic asplenia, cochlear implants, sickle cell disease or other hemoglobinopathies, congenital or acquired immunodeficiencies, generalized malignancy, Hodgkin disease, leukemia, multiple myeloma, solid organ transplant, or cerebrospinal fluid leaks.

Zoster Vaccine[97,98]

The approved herpes zoster vaccine is a live attenuated vaccine. Efficacy against herpes zoster is 70% in people aged 50 to 59 years, falling to 38% in those aged 70 or more years. Efficacy against postherpetic neuralgia after age 60 years is 66%. HZ/su vaccine, a new recombinant subunit vaccine containing varicella-zoster virus glycoprotein E in an $AS01_B$ adjuvant system, is currently being investigated. It has an efficacy of 97% across all age groups, but significant local site injection reactions and myalgias have been reported.[98]

- *All adults aged ≥60 years,* regardless of whether they have already had either chicken pox or shingles, should be vaccinated.
- *Contraindications:* The vaccine should not be given to adults with a history of a primary or acquired immunodeficiency state, including leukemia, lymphoma, or other malignant neoplasm affecting the bone marrow or lymphatic system, or with HIV/AIDS or to those receiving immunosuppressive therapy, including high-dose corticosteroids.

Tetanus/diphtheria (Td) and Tetanus/diphtheria/pertussis (Tdap) Vaccine[99]

- *All adults aged ≥19 years, including those aged ≥65 years:* All adults aged ≥19 years who have not been vaccinated with Tdap should receive a single dose of Tdap regardless of the time interval since last receiving Td. After receiving Tdap, they should receive Td boosters at 10-year intervals. For adults aged ≥65 years, this will reduce the likelihood of transmission to infants aged <12 months.

Cancer Screening. Cancer screening recommendations for older adults remain controversial. In 2015, the American Geriatrics Society stated: "Don't recommend screening for breast, colorectal, prostate or lung cancer without considering life expectancy and the risks of testing, overdiagnosis and overtreatment."[100] Geriatricians advocate *individualized decision making* based on the principles outlined in "When to Screen" discussed earlier, since "guidelines become less robust and evidenced-based as individuals age and/or develop declining health status and disabilities."[78] Recent more complex published frameworks include "weighing quantitative information, such as risk of cancer death and likelihood of beneficial and adverse screening outcomes, as well as qualitative factors, such as individual patients' values and preferences."[101] The American College of Physicians has developed high- and low-value screening strategies that factor in health benefits, frequency of screening, and harms and costs.[102]

The recommendations of the USPSTF as of 2015, which target straightforward age cutoffs, are summarized below.[103]

See "When to Screen," pp. 976–977, and also discussions about screening for breast cancer, pp. 427–433, cervical cancer, pp. 575–578, prostate cancer, pp. 610–615, and colorectal cancer, p. 615.

Screening Recommendations for Older Adults: U.S. Preventive Services Task Force

- **Breast cancer (2016):** Recommends mammography every 2 years for women aged 50 to 74 years and cites insufficient evidence for screening women aged ≥75 years.
- **Cervical cancer (2012):** Recommends against routine screening for women over age 65 years if they have had adequate recent screening with normal Pap smears and are not otherwise at high risk for cervical cancer, based on fair evidence.
- **Colorectal cancer (2008):** Recommends screening with colonoscopy every 10 years, sigmoidoscopy every 5 years with high-sensitivity fecal occult blood tests (FOBTs) every 3 years, or FOBTs every year beginning age 50 years through age 75 years. Recommends against routine screening for adults aged 76 to 85 years, due to moderate certainty that the net benefit is small.
- **Prostate cancer (2012):** Recommends against prostate-specific antigen-based screening for prostate cancer in men of all ages due to evidence that expected harms are greater than expected benefits.
- **Lung cancer (2013):** For adults aged 55 to 80 years with a 30-pack/yr smoking history, and those who currently smoke or have quit within the past 15 years, recommends annual screening with low-dose computed tomography. Screening should be discontinued once a person has not smoked for 15 years or develops a health problem that substantially limits life expectancy or the ability or willingness to have curative lung surgery.
- **Skin cancer (2009; updated in 2015):** States that evidence is insufficient to balance the benefits and harms of whole-body skin examination.

Depression. *Depression* affects 5% to 7% of community-dwelling older adults and approximately 10% of older men and 18% of older women, but is often undiagnosed, untreated, or undertreated.[77,104] Prevalence rises in those with multiple comorbidities and hospitalizations. Screening for the general adult population, with services in place for diagnosis, treatment, and follow-up, is now recommended by the USPSTF (2015)[105] and requires only one or two questions. The single screening question, "Do you often feel sad or depressed?" has a sensitivity of 69% and specificity of 90%. The two screening questions below are 100% sensitive and 77% specific.

See Chapter 5, Behavior and Mental Status, Depression, pp. 156–157.

- "Over the past 2 weeks, have you felt down, depressed, or hopeless?" (screens for depressed mood)

- "Over the past 2 weeks, have you felt little interest or pleasure in doing things?" (screens for anhedonia)

Positive responses should prompt further investigation with scales such as the Geriatric Depression Scale or the 9-item Patient Health Questionnaire (PHQ-9).[104,106,107] Depressed men over age 65 years are at increased risk for suicide and require particularly careful evaluation. Effective treatment for older adults both reduces morbidity and extends life, and includes exercise, supportive and group therapy, and medication.[108]

Dementia, Mild Cognitive Impairment, and Cognitive Decline.
Dementia is "an acquired condition that is characterized by a decline in at least two cognitive domains (e.g., loss of memory, attention, language, or visuospatial or executive functioning) that is severe enough to affect social or occupational functioning." Affected patients may also exhibit behavioral and psychological symptoms. In the *Diagnostic and Statistical Manual of Mental Disorders 5* (*DSM-5*), dementia is classified as a "major neurocognitive disorder."[109] The major dementia syndromes include Alzheimer disease (AD), vascular dementia, frontotemporal dementia, dementia with Lewy bodies, Parkinson disease with dementia, and dementia of mixed etiology. AD, the predominant form, affects 11% of Americans over age 65 years, or roughly 5.1 million people; over two thirds are women.[110] By 2050, prevalence is estimated to increase to 13.8 million cases. Risk factors include advancing age, family history, and the gene mutation apolipoprotein (APOE) ε4. Risk of AD more than doubles in first-degree relatives. Risk doubles in the presence of one APOE ε4 allele and increases fivefold or more in the presence of two alleles, although only 2% of the population carries these genes.[111]

The diagnosis of AD is challenging: the mechanisms of disease are still under intense investigation; the absence of a consistent and uniformly applied definition of disease hampers investigation of risk factors; between 60% and 90% of Alzheimer patients have coexisting ischemic disease; and distinguishing *age-related cognitive decline* from *mild cognitive impairment* and AD can be subtle. Excluding delirium and depression can further complicate diagnosis.[112,113] Some distinguishing clinical features are highlighted on next page.

See Table 20-2, Delirium and Dementia, p. 1001, and Table 20-3, Screening for Dementia: The Mini-Cog, p. 1002.

The Spectrum of Cognitive Decline

Age-related Cognitive Decline

- This diagnosis is suggested by mild forgetfulness, difficulty remembering names, mildly reduced concentration.
- Such symptoms are sporadic and do not affect daily function.

Mild Cognitive Impairment (MCI)

- *Daily function is preserved,* but there is evidence of modest *cognitive decline in one or more cognitive domains* (complex attention, executive function, learning and memory, language, perceptual-motor, or social cognition) based on objective tasks, as reported by the patient, an informant, or the clinician or on clinical testing.[109,114,115]
- *Alertness and attention is preserved* (unlike delirium).
- Other dementias are unlikely (see below).
- AD develops at a higher frequency in MCI patients, progressing to AD at a reported rate of 6% to 15% per year.[116,117]

Alzheimer Disease

- *Probable AD*, based on *DSM-5* criteria, consists of evidence of a causative genetic mutation from family history or genetic testing, or the presence *of cognitive decline in two or more cognitive domains, with all three of the following features:* (1) clear evidence of a decline in memory and learning and at least one other cognitive domain (see above); (2) steady progressive decline in cognition without extended plateaus; and (3) no evidence of mixed etiology from other neurodegenerative, cerebrovascular, mental, or systemic disease.[114]
- *Possible AD* is diagnosed when the patient meets all three criteria by evidence from genetic testing or when family history is absent.
- *Alertness and attention is preserved.*
- Other dementias are unlikely (see below).
- Memory difficulties may take the form of repeating questions, losing objects, or confusion when performing tasks such as shopping. Later stages include impaired judgment and disorientation progressing to aphasia, apraxia, left–right confusion, and ultimately, dependence of IADLs. Psychosis and agitation may also occur.
- "The differentiation of dementia from MCI rests on the determination of whether or not there is significant interference in the ability to function at work or in usual daily activities."[118]

Other Dementias[112,119]

- *Vascular dementia* is suggested by vascular risk factors or cerebrovascular disease causing cognitive impairment. Stepwise decline, especially in executive function, should correlate with the onset of cerebrovascular event, but consider this dementia even if just risk factors are present. At times, there are gait changes and focal findings.
- *Lewy body disease* is suggested by evidence of parkinsonism. Visual hallucinations, delusions, and gait disorder may be early clues. At times, there are extrapyramidal symptoms, fluctuating mental status, and sensitivity to antipsychotic medications.
- *Frontotemporal lobar degeneration* is suggested by prominent behavioral or language disorders, at times with personality changes including impulsivity, aggression, and apathy. At times, there is excessive eating and drinking. There is relative preservation of memory and visual–spatial skills. Onset may occur before age 60 years.

Screening Tests for Dementia. The *Mini Mental State Examination* has the best sensitivity and specificity, over 86%, but is now copyrighted for commercial use, so is less accessible. Recommended screening tests include the *Mini-Cog* and *the Montreal Cognitive Assessment (MoCA)*, both included in Tables 20-3 and 20-4.

See Table 20-3, Screening for Dementia: The Mini-Cog, p. 1003, and Table 20-4, Screening for Dementia: The Montreal Cognitive Assessment (MoCA), p. 1004.

■ The Mini-Cog has a sensitivity and specificity in some studies as high as 91% and 86%, respectively, and is shorter to administer—about 3 minutes.[109,120,121]

■ The MoCA has comparable sensitivity and specificity, 91% and 81% in recent studies, and takes 10 minutes to administer.[119,121–124]

Caring for Patients with Altered Cognition. Once you identify cognitive changes, a number of steps are helpful for planning patient care.

See Chapter 3, The Patient with Altered Cognition, pp. 87–89.

Caring for Patients with Altered Cognition

- **Collateral information:** Obtain collateral information from family members and caretakers.
- **Neuropsychological testing:** Consider formal neuropsychological testing.
- **Contributing factors:** Investigate contributing factors such as medications; metabolic abnormalities; depression; delirium; and other clinical and psychiatric conditions, including vascular risk from diabetes and hypertension.
- **Caregivers:** Counsel families about the challenges for caregivers. The NIH Senior Health website *http://nihseniorhealth.gov/* is especially helpful about "Alzheimer caregiving." Review household safety measures.
- **Drivers with dementia:** Learn the laws about reporting *drivers with dementia* in your state. Consult the American Academy of Neurology evidence-based practice parameters for drivers with dementia, updated in 2010, and guidelines from numerous professional organizations, including the American Medical Association. Note, however, that underlying quantitative evidence linking assessment to road safety is limited.[125] A 2013 Cochrane review details the pitfalls of disqualifying impaired drivers, which can lead to depression and social withdrawal if disqualification is premature.[126,127] The review concludes that for drivers with dementia, there is no good evidence that neuropsychological or on-road assessment will maintain mobility and improve safety. The authors call for more research to develop assessment tools "that can reliably identify unsafe drivers with dementia in an office setting" and determine what changes in function provide a threshold for disqualification, as no single validated test is available.
- **Advance directives:** Encourage patient and family discussion of appointing a health care proxy and arranging for power of attorney, health care power of attorney, and advance directives while the patient can still contribute to active decision making.

Elder Mistreatment and Abuse. Screen vulnerable older adults for possible *elder mistreatment*, which includes abuse, neglect, exploitation, and abandonment. Prevalence ranges from 5% to 10%, depending on the population studied, and is even higher among older adults with depression and dementia.[128–130] Many cases are undetected due to the patient's fear of reprisal, physical or cognitive inability to report, and unwillingness to expose the abuser, of whom 90% are family members. *Self-neglect*, or "the behavior of an elderly person that threatens his/her own health and safety," is also a growing national concern and represents more the 50% of adult protective service referrals.

In a 2013 review, the USPSTF found no valid reliable screening tools to identify abuse of elderly or vulnerable adults in the primary care setting and therefore cited insufficient evidence for recommending screening.[81] Consequently, a careful history and high index of suspicion are important.

Techniques of Examination

Assessment of the older adult has several unique features compared to the customary format of the history and physical examination. It calls for enhanced interviewing techniques, special emphasis on the topics reviewed in the previous sections, and a focus on functional assessment. Because of its importance to older adult health, Techniques of Examination begins with "Assessing Functional Status: the 'Sixth Vital Sign,'" which includes steps for evaluating the patient's risk for falls, one of the primary threats to older adult well-being. Following this section are the components of the traditional "head-to-toe" examination, tailored to the older adult.

Assessing Functional Status: the "Sixth Vital Sign"

All visits are opportunities to promote the patient's independence and optimal level of function. Although the specific goals of care vary from patient to patient, preserving the patient's functional status, the "sixth vital sign," is of primary importance. Functional status is the ability to perform tasks and fulfill social roles associated with daily living across a wide range of complexity.

Establishing *functional status* provides a baseline for making interventions that optimize the patient's level of function and for identifying *geriatric syndromes* that can be treated or delayed, such as cognitive impairment, falls, incontinence, low BMI, dizziness, and impaired vision and hearing. Deficits in function are now recognized as better predictors of patient outcome and mortality after hospitalization than the admitting diagnoses. In 2010, the USPSTF outlined new prevention recommendations for older adults that address the multifactorial nature of geriatric syndromes and combine recommendations on related topics, such as osteoporosis, vitamin D supplementation, and prevention of falls, so that they are "more consistent, interlinked, and comprehensive" and directed at interventions that are effective.[131]

Your assessment of functional status begins as the patient enters the room. The *10-Minute Geriatric Screener* is one of several validated and time-efficient performance-based assessment tools. The *Screener* is brief, has high interrater agreement, and can be easily used by office staff.[132] It covers three important areas:

cognitive, psychosocial, and physical function. It includes vision, hearing, and questions about urinary incontinence, an often hidden source of social isolation and distress. Up to 55% of community-dwelling women aged ≥65 years and 30% of men report bladder leakage, increasing to 70% of long-term nursing home residents.[133]

10-Minute Geriatric Screener

Problem	Screening Measure	Positive Screen
Vision	Two parts: Ask: "Do you have difficulty driving, or watching television, or reading, or doing any of your daily activities because of your eyesight?" If yes, then: Test each eye with Snellen chart while the patient wears corrective lenses (if applicable).	Yes to question and inability to read >20/40 on Snellen chart
Hearing	Use audioscope set at 40 dB Test hearing using 1,000 and 2,000 Hz.	Inability to hear 1,000 or 2,000 Hz in both ears or either of these frequencies in one ear
Leg Mobility–Timed Get Up and Go (TUG) Test	Time the patient after asking: "Rise from the chair. Walk 10 feet briskly, turn, walk back to the chair, and sit down."	Unable to complete task in 10 seconds
Urinary incontinence	Two parts: Ask: "In the last year, have you ever lost your urine and gotten wet?" If yes, then ask: "Have you lost urine on at least 6 separate dates?"	Yes to both questions
Nutrition/weight loss	Two parts: Ask: "Have you lost 10 lbs over the past 6 mo without trying to do so?" Weigh the patient.	Yes to the question or weight <100 lbs
Memory	Three-item recall	Unable to remember all three items after 1 minute
Depression	Ask: "Do you often feel sad or depressed?"	Yes to the question
Physical disability	Six questions: "Are you able to…: "Do strenuous activities like fast walking or bicycling?" "Do heavy work around the house like washing windows, walls, or floors?" "Go shopping for groceries or clothes?" "Get to places out of walking distance?" "Bathe, either a sponge bath, tub bath, or shower?" "Dress, like putting on a shirt, buttoning and zipping, or putting on shoes?"	No to any of the questions

Source: Adapted from Moore AA, Siu AL. Screening for common problems in ambulatory elderly: clinical confirmation of a screening instrument. *Am J Med.* 1996;100:438.

Urinary Incontinence.   For identifying causes of incontinence, two mnemonics may be helpful:

- **DIAPERS: D**elirium, **I**nfection, **A**trophic urethritis/vaginitis, **P**harmaceuticals, **E**xcess urine output from conditions like hyperglycemia or heart failure, **R**estricted mobility, and **S**tool impaction, and

- **DDRRIIPP: D**elirium, **D**rug side effects, **R**etention of feces, **R**estricted mobility, **I**nfection of urine, **I**nflammation, **P**olyuria, and **P**sychogenic.

Further Assessment for Preventing Falls.   Compelling evidence links falls, a multifactorial geriatric syndrome, to fatal and nonfatal injuries, mortality, and burgeoning clinical costs that exceed $34 billion annually.[134] One in three older adults falls each year, but less than half discuss this with their health care provider. Falls are the most common cause of traumatic brain injury in older adults and cause 95% of hip fractures.

In 2010, the American Geriatrics Society and British Geriatrics Society updated an excellent algorithm for individualizing falls prevention in older adults.[135] Recognizing a gap in adoption by clinicians, the CDC's Injury Center has launched the *STEADI (Stopping Elderly Accidents, Deaths, and Injuries) falls prevention toolkit* to help primary care providers to better assess and treat patients at risk and make referrals to community-based falls prevention programs (Fig. 20-9).[136,137] STEADI materials include a risk triage algorithm, a Fall Risk Checklist, videos on how to conduct standard falls assessment tests, and "Stay Independent" brochures for falls prevention for patients and families.

Note the key features of the STEADI algorithm on p. 988 that you should incorporate into your practice. If time, consider functional assessment and environmental/home safety assessment.

STEADI Falls Prevention Algorithm: Key Features for Clinical Practice

- Screen *all* community-dwelling older adults about risk for falls.
- Encourage *all* older patients to pursue gait and balance exercise.
- Do a gait, strength, and balance assessment with the Timed Get Up and Go test in patients who screen positive.
- Stratify patients according to low, moderate, and high risk.
- *Identify high-risk older adults,* namely, those with a gait, strength, or balance problem and at least one fall with an injury.
- In *high-risk older adults,* conduct a multifactorial risk assessment, including:
  - review of the Stay Independent brochure;
  - a falls history and medication review;
  - physical examination including assessment of visual acuity, postural hypotension, a cognitive screen, inspection of the feet and use of footwear, and use of mobility aids;
  - functional assessment; and
  - environmental or home safety assessment.
- Implement individualized interventions, including physical therapy and follow-up in 30 days.

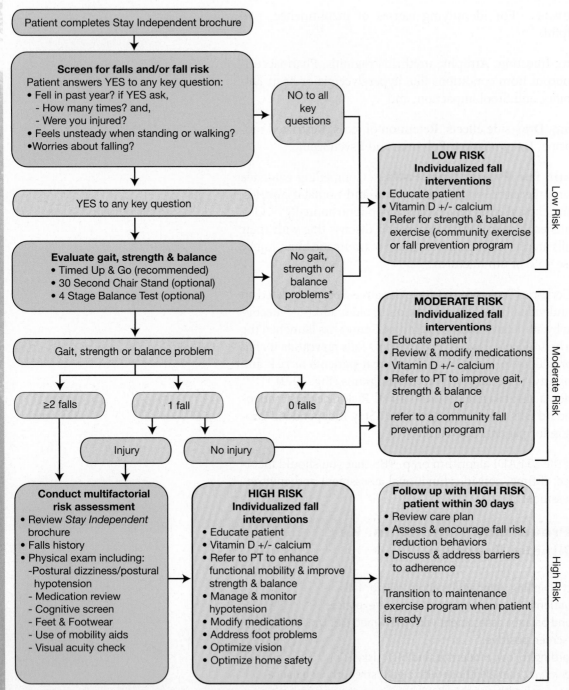

FIGURE 20-9. **STEADI algorithm.** Source: Centers for Disease Control and Prevention. National Center for Injury Prevention and Control. STEADI–Stopping Elderly Accidents, Deaths and Injuries. Available at http://www.cdc.gov/steadi/pdf/algorithm_2015–04-a.pdf. Accessed August 23, 2015.

Although methods for studying individual and multifactorial fall interventions vary greatly, the USPSTF found evidence of falls reduction from the following interventions: gait, balance, and strength training, particularly over an extended period—by 13%; vitamin D supplementation—by 14% to 17%; and minimization or withdrawal of psychoactive and other medications.[138–141] Multifactorial assessment and intervention appear to be more effective than interventions targeting specific risk factors, reducing falls in some studies by up to 25%. Additional prevention strategies that have been evaluated include reducing home hazards, vision correction, and improved management of chronic conditions such as change in postural blood pressure, and numerous types and combinations of exercise.[141]

Physical Examination of the Older Adult

General Survey. As the patient enters the room, how does the patient walk to the chair? Move onto the examining table? Are there changes in posture or involuntary movements? Note the patient's hygiene and dress. Assess the patient's apparent state of health, degree of vitality, and mood and affect. As you talk with the patient, decide if screening for cognitive changes is needed.

Undernutrition, slowed motor performance, loss of muscle mass, or weakness suggests frailty.

Kyphosis or abnormal gait can impair balance and increase risk of falls.

Flat or impoverished affect is seen in *depression, Parkinson disease,* and *Alzheimer disease.*

See Table 20-3, Screening for Dementia: The Mini-Cog, p. 1002, and Table 20-4, Screening for Dementia: The Montreal Cognitive Assessment, p. 1003 for brief and validated screening tools for dementia.[120,121]

Vital Signs. Measure blood pressure using recommended techniques (see pp. 124–132), checking for increased systolic blood pressure (SBP) and widened PP, defined as SBP minus DBP. With aging, SBP and peripheral vascular resistance increase, whereas DBP decreases. For adults aged ≥60 years, the eighth Joint National Committee (JNC8) recommends blood pressure targets of ≤150/90 but notes that if treatment results in SBP <140 and is "well tolerated and without adverse effects to health or quality of live, treatment does not need to be adjusted."[142] However, in the "oldest old," those aged 80 years and older, other experts cite studies showing that blood pressure targets of 140 to <150/70 to 80 appear optimal for notable reductions in stroke, cardiovascular events, and all-cause mortality.[143–146]

Isolated systolic hypertension (SBP ≥ 140) after age 50 years and PP ≥ 60 increase risk of stroke, renal failure, and heart disease.[147]

See JNC8 recommendations on p. 130.

Assess the patient for orthostatic hypotension, defined as a drop in SBP of ≥20 mm Hg or DBP of ≥10 mm Hg within 3 minutes of standing. Measure blood pressure and heart rate in two positions: supine after the patient rests for up to 10 minutes; then within 3 minutes after standing up.

Orthostatic hypotension occurs in 20% of older adults and in up to 50% of frail nursing home residents, especially when they first get up. Symptoms include lightheadedness, weakness, unsteadiness, visual blurring, and, in 20% to 30% of patients, syncope. Causes include medications, autonomic disorders, diabetes, prolonged bed rest, volume depletion, amyloidosis, postprandial state, and cardiovascular disorders.[148–151]

Measure heart rate, respiratory rate, and temperature. The apical heart rate often allows better detection of arrhythmias in older patients than does the radial pulse. Use thermometers accurate for lower temperatures. Obtain oxygen saturation using a pulse oximeter.

Respiratory rate ≥25 breaths per minute points to lower respiratory infection, heart failure, and chronic obstructive pulmonary disease exacerbation.

Hypothermia is more common in older patients.

Weight and height are especially important in the elderly, and are needed for calculation of the BMI. Weight is also a key clinical measure for patients with heart failure and chronic kidney disease. Weight should be measured at every visit, preferably with footwear removed.

Low weight is a key indicator of poor nutrition, seen in depression, alcoholism, cognitive impairment, malignancy, chronic organ failure (cardiac, renal, pulmonary), medication use, social isolation, poor dentition, and poverty. Rapidly increasing daily weights occur in fluid overload.

Skin. Note physiologic changes of aging, such as thinning, loss of elastic tissue and turgor, and wrinkling. Skin may be dry, flaky, rough, and often itchy (*asteatosis*), with a latticework of shallow fissures that creates a mosaic of small polygons, especially on the legs.

Observe any patchy changes in color. Check the extensor surface of the hands and forearms for white depigmented patches, or *pseudoscars,* and for well-demarcated vividly purple macules or patches, *actinic purpura,* that may fade after several weeks (Fig. 20-10).

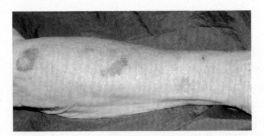

FIGURE 20-10. **Actinic purpura on forearm.**

Look for changes from sun exposure. Areas of skin may appear weather beaten, thickened, yellowed, and deeply furrowed; there may be *actinic lentigines,* or "liver spots," and *actinic keratoses,* superficial flattened papules covered by a dry scale.

Inspect for the benign lesions of aging, namely *comedones,* or blackheads, on the cheeks or around the eyes; *cherry angiomas,* which often appear early in adulthood; and *seborrheic keratoses,* raised yellowish lesions that feel greasy and velvety or warty.

Distinguish such lesions from a *basal cell carcinoma,* a translucent nodule that spreads and leaves a depressed center with a firm elevated border, and *squamous cell carcinoma,* a firm reddish-appearing lesion often emerging in a sun-exposed area. A dark raised asymmetric lesion with irregular borders may be a *melanoma.* See Tables 6-4, 6-5, and 6-6, pp. 197–203, assessment of rough, pink, and brown lesions and related carcinomas.

Watch for any painful vesicular lesions in a dermatomal distribution.

Vesicular lesions occurring in a dermatomal distribution are suspicious for *herpes zoster* from reactivation of latent varicella-zoster virus in the dorsal root ganglia. Risk increases with age and impaired cell-mediated immunity.[98,152]

In older bed-bound patients, especially those emaciated or neurologically impaired, inspect the skin for damage or ulceration on the sacral and perianal areas, the lower back, heels, and elbows where pressure ulcers commonly occur.

Pressure ulcers arise from obliteration of arteriolar and capillary blood flow to the skin or from shear forces during movement across sheets or when lifted upright incorrectly. See Table 6-13, Pressure Ulcers, p. 213.

Head and Neck. Perform a thorough examination of the head and neck.

See Chapter 7, The Head and Neck, pp. 215–302.

Inspect the eyelids, the bony orbit, and the eye. The eye may appear recessed from atrophy of fat in the surrounding tissues. Observe any *senile ptosis* arising from weakening of the levator palpebrae, relaxation of the skin, and increased weight of the upper eyelid. Check the lower lids for ectropion or *entropion*. Note yellowing of the sclera, and *arcus senilis*, a benign whitish ring around the limbus.

See Table 7-7, Variations and Abnormalities of the Eyelids, p. 274, and Table 7-9, Opacities of the Cornea and Lens, p. 276.

Test the best-corrected visual acuity in each eye, using a pocket Snellen chart or wall-mounted chart. Note any *presbyopia*, the loss of near vision arising from decreased elasticity of the lens related to aging.

One in three adults suffers some form of visual loss by age 65 years.[153]

Test pupillary constriction to light, both the direct and consensual response and during the near response. Then swing the light beam several times between the right and left eyes. Test the six directions of gaze. Except for possible impairment in upward gaze, extraocular movements should remain intact.

If the pupil dilates as the light swings over, a relative afferent pupillary defect is present, which is suspicious for optic nerve disease. Refer to an ophthalmologist.

Using your ophthalmoscope, carefully examine the lenses and fundi.

The prevalence of cataracts, glaucoma, and macular degeneration all increases with aging.

Using the ophthalmoscope beam, check at 1 to 2 feet for a red reflex. With the ophthalmoscope lens at +10 diopters, inspect each lens close to the eye for opacities. Do not depend on the flashlight alone because the lens may look clear superficially.

A red reflex is seen with *cataracts* (Figs. 20-11 and 20-12). At +10 diopters, a cataract appears white.[154]

Cataracts are the world's leading cause of blindness. Risk factors include cigarette smoking, exposure to UV-B light, high alcohol intake, diabetes, medications (including steroids), and trauma. See Table 7-9, Opacities of the Cornea and Lens, p. 276.

Retinal microvascular disease is linked to cerebral microvascular changes and cognitive impairment.[155,156]

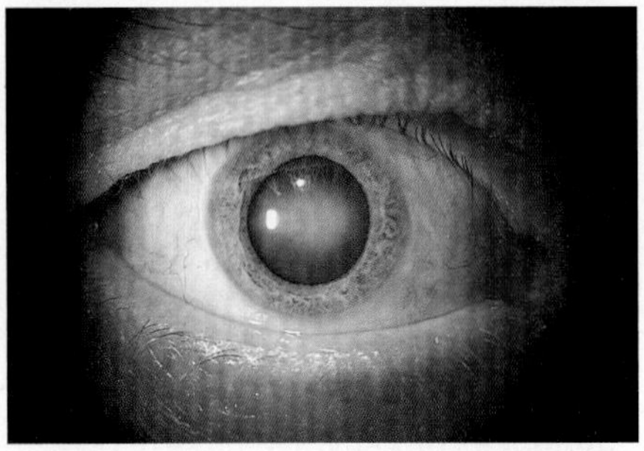

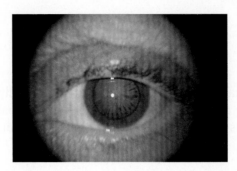

FIGURE 20-11. Nuclear cataract.

FIGURE 20-12. Peripheral cataract.

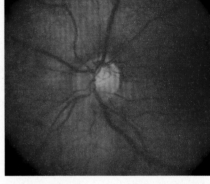

FIGURE 20-13. Glaucoma with disc "cupping."

In older adults, the fundi lose their youthful shine and light reflections, and the arteries look narrowed, paler, straighter, and less brilliant. Assess the cup-to-disc ratio, usually 1:2 or less, for possible glaucoma (Fig. 20-13).

An increased cup-to-disc ratio suggests *primary open angle glaucoma (POAG),* caused by irreversible optic neuropathy and leading to loss of peripheral and central vision and blindness. Prevalence of POAG is four to five times higher in African Americans and Hispanics, though non-Hispanic whites, especially older women, are highest in the number affected.[157,158]

Inspect the fundi for colloid bodies causing alterations in pigmentation, called *drusen.*

Macular degeneration causes poor central vision and blindness (Fig. 20-14).[159] Types include *dry atrophic* (more common but less severe) and *wet exudative,* or neovascular. Drusen may be hard and sharply defined, or soft and confluent with altered pigmentation (see p. 285).

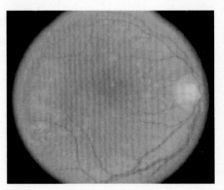

FIGURE 20-14. Age-related macular degeneration and drusen.

Test hearing by occluding one ear and using the whispered voice technique or an audioscope. Be sure to inspect the ear canals for cerumen because removal can quickly improve hearing. Asking if hearing loss is present is an effective screening method. Proceed to audiometry for those saying yes; check acuity to whispered voice for saying no.[84]

See techniques for testing hearing, pp. 242–248.

Examine the oral cavity for odor, appearance of the gingival mucosa, any caries, mobility of the teeth, and quantity of saliva. Inspect closely for lesions on any of the mucosal surfaces. Ask the patient to remove dentures so that you can check the gums for denture sores.

Malodor points to poor oral hygiene, periodontitis, and caries. *Gingivitis* accompanies periodontal disease. Dental plaque and cavitation may cause caries. For increased tooth mobility from abscesses or advanced caries, consider removal to prevent aspiration. Decreased salivation results from medication effects, radiation, Sjögren syndrome, or dehydration. *Oral tumors* can cause lesions, usually on the lateral margins of the tongue and floor of the mouth.[160,161]

Continue with your usual examination of the thyroid gland and lymph nodes.

In older adults, common causes of hyperthyroidism are *Graves disease* and *toxic multinodular goiter*. Causes of hypothyroidism include autoimmune thyroiditis, followed by drugs, neck radiotherapy, thyroidectomy, or radioiodine ablation.[24]

Thorax and Lungs. Complete the usual examination, observing for subtle signs of changes in pulmonary function.

Increased anteroposterior diameter, purse-lipped breathing, and dyspnea with talking or minimal exertion suggest *chronic obstructive pulmonary disease*. There is considerable overlap of asthma and COPD in older adults, heralded by nonspecific symptoms like dyspnea, cough, wheezing, and nocturnal onset. Proceed to objective testing with spirometry, which most tolerate well.[162]

Cardiovascular System. Review your findings from measurement of the blood pressure and heart rate.

Isolated systolic hypertension and a widened PP are cardiac risk factors, prompting a search for *left ventricular hypertrophy (LVH)*.

Begin by inspecting the jugular venous pressure. Palpate the carotid upstrokes and auscultate for carotid bruits.

A *tortuous atherosclerotic aorta* can raise pressure in the left jugular veins by impairing emptying into the right atrium. A tortuous aorta can also cause kinking of the carotid artery low in the neck on the right, chiefly in women with hypertension, which can be mistaken for a *carotid aneurysm*.

Carotid bruits can occur in *aortic stenosis*. The presence of bruits from *carotid stenosis* increases risk of ipsilateral stroke.

Assess the point of maximal impulse (PMI), then auscultate S_1 and S_2. Listen also for the extra sounds of S_3 and S_4.

A *sustained PMI* is present in LVH; a *diffuse PMI* and an S_3 signal left ventricular dilatation from heart failure or cardiomyopathy (see pp. 385–388).[163] An S_4 often accompanies hypertension.

Beginning in the second right interspace, listen for cardiac murmurs in all areas of auscultation (see pp. 393–397). Describe the timing, shape, location of maximal intensity, radiation, intensity, pitch, and quality of each murmur you detect.

A systolic crescendo–decrescendo murmur in the second right interspace suggests *aortic sclerosis* or *aortic stenosis,* seen respectively in up to 40% and 2% to 3% of community-dwelling older adults. Both are associated with an increased risk of cardiovascular disease and death.[164,165]

A harsh holosystolic murmur at the apex radiating to the axilla suggests *mitral regurgitation,* the most common murmur in older adults.

Breasts and Axillae. Palpate the breasts carefully for lumps or masses. Include palpation of the tail of Spence that extends into the axilla. Examine the axillae for lymphadenopathy. Note any scaly, vesicular ulcerated lesions on or near the nipple.

Any lumps or masses in older women, and, more rarely, in older men, mandate further investigation for possible breast cancer.

Paget disease with eczematoid scaling of the nipple is uncommon, but peaks between the ages of 50 and 60 years.[166]

Abdomen. Inspect the abdomen for masses or visible pulsations. Auscultate for bruits over the aorta and the renal and femoral arteries. Palpate to the right and left of the midline for aortic pulsations. Try to assess the width of the aorta by pressing more deeply on each of its lateral margins (see p. 483).

Abdominal bruits are suspicious for atherosclerotic vascular disease.

A widened aorta of ≥3 cm and pulsatile mass occur in *abdominal aortic aneurysm,* especially in older male smokers.

Peripheral Vascular System. Carefully palpate the brachial, radial, femoral, popliteal, and pedal pulses.

Diminished or absent pulses are present in *peripheral arterial disease (PAD)*. Confirm your findings with an office ankle-brachial index (ABI); if <0.9, the ABI has a sensitivity of 70% and specificity of 90%. In patients with PAD, 30% to 60% report no leg symptoms.[167]

See Table 12-3, Using the Ankle-Brachial Index, p. 536.

Female Genitalia and Pelvic Examination. Take the time to explain your plans for the examination and arrange for careful patient positioning.[168] You may need help from an assistant to move the older woman onto the examining table, then into the lithotomy position. Raising the head of the table may make her more comfortable. For the woman with arthritis or spinal deformities who cannot flex her hips or knees, an assistant can gently raise and support the legs, or help the woman into the left lateral position.

Inspect the vulva for changes related to menopause such as thinning of the skin, loss of pubic hair, and decreased distensibility of the introitus. Identify any labial masses. Bluish swellings may be varicosities. Bulging of the anterior vaginal wall below the urethra may be an *urethrocele* or *urethral diverticulum*.

Benign masses include condylomata, fibromas, leiomyomas, and sebaceous cysts. See Table 14-2, Bulges and Swellings of the Vulva, Vagina, and Urethra, p. 597.

Inspect for any vulvar erythema.

Erythema with satellite lesions results from *Candida* infection; erythema with ulceration or a necrotic center is suspicious for *vulvar carcinoma*. Multi-focal reddened lesions with white scaling plaques occur in extramam-mary *Paget disease*, a form of intraepi-thelial adenocarcinoma.

Inspect the urethra for *caruncles,* or prolapse of fleshy erythematous mucosal tissue at the urethral meatus. Note any enlargement of the clitoris.

Clitoral enlargement may accompany *androgen-producing tumors* and use of androgen creams.

Spread the labia, press downward on the introitus to relax the levator muscles, and gently insert the speculum after moistening it with warm water or a water-soluble lubricant. If you find severe vaginal atrophy, a gaping introitus, or an introital stric-ture from estrogen loss, you will need to change the size of the speculum.

The thin patchy atrophic white plaques of *lichen sclerosus* are more common in postmenopausal women and may be precancerous.[169]

Inspect the vaginal walls, which may be atrophic, and the cervix. Note any thin cervical mucus or vaginal or cervical discharge.

Estrogen-stimulated cervical mucus with ferning is seen in use of hormone replacement therapy, *endometrial hyper-plasia,* and *estrogen-producing tumors.*

Discharge may accompany vaginitis or cervicitis. See Table 14-3, Vaginal Discharge, p. 598.

If indicated, use an endocervical brush (or less commonly, a wooden spatula) to obtain endocervical cells for the Pap smear. Consider using a blind swab if the atrophic vagina is too small.

Current USPSTF recommendations are to discontinue screening in low-risk women >age 65 years if adequate prior screening has been negative.[170]

After removing the speculum, ask the patient to bear down to detect uterine prolapse or a cystocele, urethrocele, or rectocele.

See Table 14-7, Positions of the Uterus, p. 601, and Table 14-8, Abnor-malities of the Uterus, p. 602.

Perform the bimanual examination. Check the motion of the cervix and palpate for any uterine or adnexal masses.

Mobility of the cervix is restricted with inflammation, malignancy, or surgical adhesion. Enlarging uterine fibroids, or *leiomyomas,* can be normal or *malig-nant leiomyosarcoma;* ovarian masses or enlargement are seen in *ovarian cancer.*

Perform the rectovaginal examination if indicated. Assess for uterine and adnexal irregularities through the anterior rectal wall, and check for rectal masses. Change gloves after the bimanual examination so that no blood is present on your gloves when you obtain the stool sample.

A uterus that is enlarged, fixed, or irregular may have adhesions or contain a malignancy. Rectal masses are found in *colorectal cancer.*

Male Genitalia and Prostate.   Examine the penis, retracting the foreskin, if present. Examine the scrotum, testes, and epididymis.

Findings include smegma, penile cancer, and scrotal hydroceles.

Proceed with the rectal examination. Assess rectal tone. Palpate for any rectal masses or nodularity or masses of the prostate. The anterior and central lobes of the prostate are inaccessible to palpation, which limits your ability to detect prostate enlargement or malignancy.

A loss of rectal tone can result in fecal incontinence. Rectal masses suggest *colorectal cancer.* Rule out *prostate cancer* if nodules or masses are present. See discussion of prostate cancer screening on pp. 612–615.

Musculoskeletal System.   Your evaluation of this system began with leg mobility testing during the *10-Minute Geriatric Screener,* p. 986, at the outset of the visit. Leg mobility is routinely tested by the *"Timed Get up and Go,"* or *TUG, test* for gait and balance, an excellent screen for risk of falling. Ask the patient to get up from a chair, walk 10 feet, turn, and return to the chair. Older adults should complete this test in 10 seconds.

See Chapter 16, The Musculoskeletal System; see Tables 16-1 to 16-10, pp. 696–707.

If the patient has joint deformities, deficits in mobility, pain with movement, or a delayed "get up and go" perform a more thorough examination of individual joints and a more comprehensive neurologic examination.

Look for degenerative joint changes in *osteoarthritis* and joint inflammation from *rheumatoid* or *gouty arthritis.*

Timed Get Up and Go Test

Performed with patient wearing regular footwear, using usual walking aid if needed, and sitting back in a chair with armrest.

On the word, "Go," the patient is asked to do the following:

1. Stand up from the arm chair
2. Walk 3 m (in a line)
3. Turn
4. Walk back to chair
5. Sit down

Time the second effort.
Observe patient for postural stability, steppage, stride length, and sway.

Scoring:
- **Normal:** completes task in <10 s
- **Abnormal:** completes task in >20 s

Low scores correlate with good functional independence; high scores correlate with poor functional independence and higher risk of falls.

Reproduced from: Get-up and Go Test. In: Mathias S, Nayak USL, Isaacs B. "Balance in elderly patient" The "Get Up and Go" Test. *Arch Phys Med Rehabil.* 1986;67:387; Podsiadlo D, Richardson S. The Timed "Up and Go": A test of basic functional mobility for frail elderly persons. *J Am Geriatr Soc.* 1991;39:142.

Nervous System. As with the musculoskeletal examination, your evaluation began with the *10-Minute Geriatric Screener* (p. 986). Carefully assess memory and affect.

Pay close attention to gait and balance, particularly standing balance; timed 10-foot walk; stride characteristics like width, pace, and length of stride; and careful turning. A recent study of neurologic versus non-neurologic (primarily hip and knee orthopedic) gait disorders showed that neurologic disorders like parkinsonian; sensory ataxic; spastic; higher level gait; and, particularly, multiple neurologic gait disorders tripled the risk for recurrent falls.[171] Investigators are looking at the neurobiology of gait disorders as markers of preclinical dementia and other neurologic conditions that may lead to earlier diagnosis and new preventive strategies.[172]

When gait abnormalities are detected, pursue a more detailed neurologic examination.[173,174] Distinguishing neurologic changes of aging from abnormal findings is challenging, as neurologic abnormalities without identifiable disease are common in the older population and increase with age, occurring in up to 50% of older adults.[175] Examples of age-related abnormalities include unequal pupil size, decreased arm swing and spontaneous movements, increased leg rigidity and abnormal gait, presence of the snout and grasp reflexes, and decreased toe vibratory sense.

Examine for evidence of **T**remor, **R**igidity, **A**kinesia, and **P**ostural instability, or **TRAP**, which are several of the most common features of Parkinson disease.[176] Also look for bradykinesia, the most characteristic clinical sign, and micrographia, shuffling "freezing" gait, and difficulty rising from a chair.

Learn to distinguish delirium from depression and dementia (Table 20-2, p. 1001). Search carefully for underlying causes.[105,106] See Table 20-3, Screening for Dementia: The Mini-Cog, p. 1002 and Table 20-4, The Montreal Cognitive Assessment (MoCA), p. 1003.

Abnormalities of gait and balance, especially widening of base, slowing and lengthening of stride, and difficulty turning, are correlated with risk for falls.[135,138]

These findings are seen in *Parkinson disease*, found in ~60,000 new cases a year and affecting about 1 million people in the United States.[177] Tremor is slow frequency, occurs at rest, has a "pill-rolling" quality, and is aggravated by stress and inhibited during sleep or movement. Prodromal nonmotor symptoms including depression, rapid eye movement behavior disorder, and daytime sleepiness are now being identified.[178,179]

***Essential tremor* is bilateral and symmetric, with a positive family history and commonly diminished by alcohol.**

Recording Your Findings

Note that initially you may use sentences to describe your findings; later you will use phrases. The style below contains phrases appropriate for most write-ups. As you read through this physical examination, you will notice some atypical findings. Try to test yourself. See if you can interpret these findings in the context of all you have learned about the examination of the older adult.

Recording the Physical Examination— The Older Adult

Mr. J is an older adult who appears healthy but overweight, with good muscle bulk and tone. He is alert and interactive, with good recall of his life history. He is accompanied by his son.

Vital Signs: Ht (without shoes) 5′ 10″. Wt (dressed) 195 lbs. BMI 28. BP 145/88 right arm, supine; 154/94 left arm, supine. Heart rate (HR) 98 and regular. Respiratory rate (RR) 18. Temperature (oral) 98.6°F.

10-Minute Geriatric Screener (see p. 986)

Vision: Patient reports difficulty reading. Visual acuity 20/60 on Snellen chart.

Hearing: Cannot hear whispered voice in either ear. Cannot hear 1,000 or 2,000 Hz with audioscope in either ear.

Further evaluation for glasses and possibly a hearing aid is needed.

Leg Mobility: Able to walk 10 feet briskly, turn, walk back to chair, and sit down in 9 seconds.

Urinary Incontinence: Has lost urine and gotten wet on 20 separate days.

Further evaluation for incontinence, including "DIAPERS" assessment (see p. 987), prostate examination, and postvoid residual, which is normally ≤50 mL (requires bladder scan or catheterization) is needed.

Nutrition: Has lost 15 lbs over the past 6 months without trying.

Evaluate and monitor weight loss. Needs nutritional screen, p. 141.

Memory: Can remember three items after 1 minute.

Depression: Does not often feel sad or depressed.

Physical Disability: Can walk fast but cannot ride a bicycle. Can do moderate but not heavy work around the house. Can go shopping for groceries or clothes. Can get to places out of walking distance. Can bathe each day without difficulty. Can dress, including buttoning and zipping, and can put on shoes.

Consider an exercise regimen with strength training.

Physical Examination

Skin. Warm and moist. Nails without clubbing or cyanosis. Hair thinning at crown.

Head, Eyes, Ears, Nose, Throat (HEENT). Scalp without lesions. Skull NC/AT. Conjunctiva pink, sclera muddy. Pupils 2 mm constricting to 1 mm, round, regular,

(continued)

Recording the Physical Examination— The Older Adult (*continued*)

equally reactive to light and accommodation. Extraocular movements intact. Disc margins sharp, without hemorrhages or exudates. Mild arteriolar narrowing. TMs with good cone of light. Weber midline. AC ≥ BC. Nasal mucosa pink. No sinus tenderness. Oral mucosa pink. Dentition fair. Caries present. Tongue midline, slight beefy redness. Pharynx without exudates.

Neck. Supple. Trachea midline. Thyroid lobes slightly enlarged, no nodules.

Lymph Nodes. No cervical, axillary, epitrochlear, or inguinal lymph nodes.

Thorax and Lungs. Thorax symmetric. Kyphosis noted. Lungs resonant with good excursion. Breath sounds vesicular. Diaphragms descend 4 cm bilaterally.

Cardiovascular. JVP 6 cm above the left atrium. Carotid upstrokes brisk, without bruits. PMI tapping, in the 5th ICS, 9 cm lateral to the midsternal line. II/VI harsh holosystolic murmur at the apex, radiating to the axilla. No S_3, S_4, or other murmurs.

Abdomen. Scaphoid, with active bowel sounds. Soft, nontender. No masses or hepatosplenomegaly. Liver span 7 cm in right midclavicular line; edge smooth and palpable at the RCM. No CVAT.

Genitourinary. Circumcised male. No penile lesions. Testes descended bilaterally, smooth without masses or tenderness.

Rectal. Good rectal sphincter tone. Rectal vault without masses. Stool brown, negative for occult blood.

Extremities. Warm and without edema. Calves supple.

Peripheral Vascular. Pulses 2+ and symmetric.

Musculoskeletal. Mild degenerative changes at the knees, with quadriceps wasting. Good range of motion in all joints.

Neurological. Oriented to person, place, and time. Montreal Cognitive Assessment (MoCA): score 29. Cranial nerves II–XII intact. Motor: Decreased quadriceps bulk. Tone intact. Strength 4/5 throughout. RAMs, finger-to-nose intact. Gait with widened base. Sensation intact to pinprick, light touch, position, and vibration. Romberg negative. Reflexes 2+ and symmetric, with plantar response downgoing.

Table 20-1 Interviewing Older Adults: Enhancing Culturally Appropriate Care

Cultural Dimension	Interview
Cultural Identity of the Individual	Where are you and your family from? What is your ancestry? Are there cultural differences between you and your parents or you and your significant other? Do you feel a strong connection to any groups of people? If so, whom? What foods do you eat? What holidays do you celebrate? What languages do you speak? With whom do you speak these languages? What languages would you like to speak with me? What types of activities do you enjoy? What are your sources for news and entertainment? Has this changed over time?
Cultural Explanations of the Individual's Illness	Do you or anyone else have a name for the problem you're having now? Why do you think it's happening to you? What will make it better or worse? When did it start and when do you think you'll get better? Has anyone else you know had this problem? What activities has this problem stopped you from doing that you, your family, or your friends expect? Who else have you seen for help with this problem? Should I talk to anyone else you trust to help you with this problem?
Cultural Factors Related to Psychological Environment and Levels of Functioning	Who lives at home with you? Can they help with this problem? Who else can help you? Is anything going on to make this problem better or worse? How has this problem affected your life? Is it preventing you from working? Moving, grooming, feeding, or sleeping? Do people close to you understand how you feel?
Cultural Elements of the Clinician–Patient Relationship	Do you think your friends or family would be upset if you spoke to me about the problem? What can I do to make you feel more comfortable? How often can you see me? Do you have any wishes for or concerns about treatment? What are your thoughts about medications? Can I share your answers with anyone else you trust?

Source: Aggarwal NK. Reassessing cultural evaluations in geriatrics: insights from cultural psychiatry. *J Am Geriatr Soc.* 2010;58:2191.

Table 20-2 Delirium and Dementia

Delirium and dementia are common and important disorders that affect multiple aspects of mental status. Both have many possible causes. Some clinical features of these two conditions and their effects on mental status are compared below. A delirium may be superimposed on dementia.

	Delirium	Dementia
Clinical Features		
Onset	Acute	Insidious
Course	Fluctuating, with lucid intervals; worse at night	Slowly progressive
Duration	Hours to weeks	Months to years
Sleep/Wake Cycle	Always disrupted	Sleep fragmented
General Clinical Illness or Drug Toxicity	Either or both present	Often absent, especially in Alzheimer disease
Mental Status		
Level of Consciousness	Disturbed. Person less alert to clearly aware of the environment and less able to focus, sustain, or shift attention	Usually normal until late in the course of the illness
Behavior	Activity often abnormally decreased (somnolence) or increased (agitation, hypervigilance)	Normal to slow; may become inappropriate
Speech	May be hesitant, slow or rapid, incoherent	Difficulty in finding words, aphasia
Mood	Fluctuating, labile, from fearful or irritable to normal or depressed	Often flat, depressed
Thought Processes	Disorganized, may be incoherent	Impoverished. Speech gives little information
Thought Content	Delusions common, often transient	Delusions may occur
Perceptions	Illusions, hallucinations, most often visual	Hallucinations may occur
Judgment	Impaired, often to a varying degree	Increasingly impaired over the course of the illness
Orientation	Usually disoriented, especially for time. A known place may seem unfamiliar.	Fairly well maintained, but becomes impaired in the later stages of illness
Attention	Fluctuates, with inattention. Person easily distracted, unable to concentrate on selected tasks	Usually unaffected until late in the illness
Memory	Immediate and recent memory impaired	Recent memory and new learning especially impaired
Examples of Cause	Delirium tremens (due to withdrawal from alcohol)	*Reversible:* Vitamin B_{12} deficiency, thyroid disorders
	Uremia	*Irreversible:* Alzheimer disease, vascular dementia (from multiple infarcts), dementia due to head trauma
	Acute hepatic failure	
	Acute cerebral vasculitis	
	Atropine poisoning	

Table 20-3 Screening for Dementia: The Mini-Cog

Administration

The test is administered as follows:

1. Instruct the patient to listen carefully to and remember three unrelated words and then to repeat the words.

2. Instruct the patient to draw the face of a clock, either on a blank sheet of paper or on a sheet with the clock circle already drawn on the page. After the patient puts the numbers on the clock face, ask him or her to draw the hands of the clock to read a specific time.

3. Ask the patient to repeat the three previously stated words.

Scoring

Give 1 point for each recalled word after the clock drawing test (CDT) distractor.

Patients recalling none of the three words are classified as demented (Score = 0).

Patients recalling all three words are classified as nondemented (Score = 3).

Patients with intermediate word recall of one to two words are classified based on the CDT (Abnormal = demented; Normal = nondemented).

Note: The CDT is considered normal if all numbers are present in the correct sequence and position, and the hands readably display the requested time.

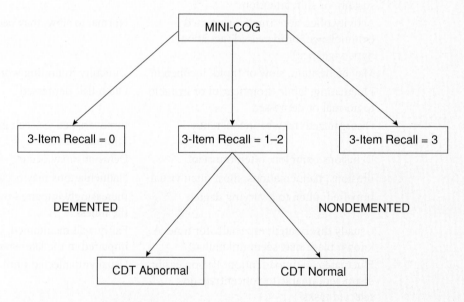

Source: From Borson S, Scanlan J, Brush M, et al. The Mini-Cog: a cognitive 'vital signs' measure for dementia screening in multi-lingual elderly. *Int J Geriatr Psychiatry.* 2000;15:1021. Copyright John Wiley & Sons Limited.

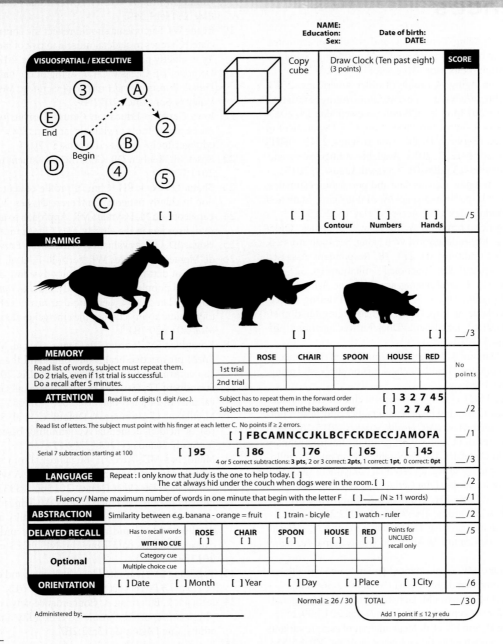

NAME:
Education:
Sex:
Date of birth:
DATE:

VISUOSPATIAL / EXECUTIVE	Copy cube	Draw Clock (Ten past eight) (3 points)	SCORE

[ ]   [ ]   [ ] Contour   [ ] Numbers   [ ] Hands   __/5

NAMING

[ ]   [ ]   [ ]   __/3

MEMORY

Read list of words, subject must repeat them.
Do 2 trials, even if 1st trial is successful.
Do a recall after 5 minutes.

		ROSE	CHAIR	SPOON	HOUSE	RED	No points
	1st trial						
	2nd trial						

ATTENTION   Read list of digits (1 digit /sec.).

Subject has to repeat them in the forward order   [ ] 3 2 7 4 5

Subject has to repeat them in the backward order   [ ] 2 7 4   __/2

Read list of letters. The subject must point with his finger at each letter C. No points if ≥ 2 errors.

[ ] FBCAMNCCJKLBCFCKDECCJAMOFA   __/1

Serial 7 subtraction starting at 100   [ ] 95   [ ] 86   [ ] 76   [ ] 65   [ ] 45   __/3

4 or 5 correct subtractions: **3 pts**, 2 or 3 correct: **2pts**, 1 correct: **1pt**, 0 correct: **0pt**

LANGUAGE   Repeat : I only know that Judy is the one to help today. [ ]

The cat always hid under the couch when dogs were in the room. [ ]   __/2

Fluency / Name maximum number of words in one minute that begin with the letter F   [ ]____ (N ≥ 11 words)   __/1

ABSTRACTION   Similarity between e.g. banana - orange = fruit   [ ] train - bicycle   [ ] watch - ruler   __/2

DELAYED RECALL	Has to recall words WITH NO CUE	ROSE [ ]	CHAIR [ ]	SPOON [ ]	HOUSE [ ]	RED [ ]	Points for UNCUED recall only	__/5
Optional	Category cue							
	Multiple choice cue							

ORIENTATION   [ ] Date   [ ] Month   [ ] Year   [ ] Day   [ ] Place   [ ] City   __/6

Normal ≥ 26 / 30   TOTAL   __/30

Administered by:_____   Add 1 point if ≤ 12 yr edu

References

1. Administration on Aging. Census data and population estimates. 2013. Available at http://www.aoa.gov/AoARoot/Aging_Statistics/Census_Population/Index.aspx. Accessed May 13, 2015.

2. Administration on Aging. A profile of older Americans: 2013. Available at http://www.aoa.gov/AoARoot/Aging_Statistics/Profile/2013/docs/2013profile_508.pdf. Accessed May 13, 2015.

3. Centers for Disease Control and Prevention, U.S. Department of Health and Human Services. Health, United States, 2013. DHHS Publication No. 2014–1232, 2013. Available at http://www.cdc.gov/nchs/data/hus/hus13.pdf#018. Accessed August 5, 2015.

4. Administration on Aging. Census data and population estimates, 2013. Available at http://www.aoa.gov/AoARoot/Aging_Statistics/Census_Population/Index.aspx. Accessed May 13, 2015.

5. Federal Interagency Forum on Aging Related Statistics. Older Americans 2012, Key Indicators of Well Being. See Indicators 16, Chronic Health Conditions (p. 27); 18, Respondent Assessed Health Statistics (p. 29); 20, Functional Limitations (p. 32); and 45, Obesity (p. 41). *Federal Interagency Forum on Aging-Related Statistics.* Washington, DC: U.S. Government Printing Office. June 2012. Available at http://agingstats.gov/agingstatsdotnet/Main_Site/Data/2012_Documents/Docs/EntireChartbook.pdf. Accessed August 5, 2015.

6. Sabia S, Singh-Manoux A, Hagger-Johnson G, et al. Influence of individual and combined healthy behaviours on successful aging. *CMAJ.* 2012;184:1985.

7. Davy C, Bleasel J, Liu H, et al. Effectiveness of chronic care models: opportunities for improving healthcare practice and health outcomes: a systematic review. *BMC Health Serv Res.* 2015;15:194.

8. Partnership for Health in Aging Workgroup on Interdisciplinary Team Training in Geriatrics. Position statement on interdisciplinary team training in geriatrics: an essential component of quality health care for older adults. *J Am Geriatr Soc.* 2014;62:961.

9. Bodenheimer T, Wagner EH, Brumbach K. Improving primary care for patients with chronic illness. *JAMA.* 2002;288:1775.

10. Institute of Medicine. *Crossing The Quality Chasm: A New Health System For The 21st Century.* Washington DC: National Academy Press; 2011.

11. Reuben DB, Tinetti ME. Goal-oriented patient care—an alternative health outcome paradigm. *N Engl J Med.* 2012;366:777.

12. Carlson C, Merel SE, Yukawa M. Geriatric syndromes and geriatric assessment for the generalist. *Med Clin N Am.* 2015;99:263.

13. Sebastiani P, Bae H, Sun FX, et al. Meta-analysis of genetic variants associated with human exceptional longevity. *Aging.* 2014;5:653.

14. Sebastiani P, Sun FX, Andersen SL, et al. Families enriched for exceptional longevity also have increased health-span: findings from the Long Life Family Study. *Front Public Health.* 2013;1:38.

15. Kane EL, Ouslander JG, Abrass IB, et al. *Ch 3, Evaluating the geriatric patient, in Essentials of Clinical Geriatrics.* 7th ed. New York: McGraw Hill Medical; 2013.

16. Morley JE, Tolsen DT. Ch 3, The physiology of aging. In: Vellas BJ, Pathy MS, Sinclair A, et al (eds). *Pathy's Principles and Practice of Geriatric Medicine.* 5th ed. Oxford: John Wiley & Sons, Inc.; 2012:33.

17. Morley JE, Tolsen DT. Ch 9, Sexuality and aging. In: Vellas BJ, Pathy MS, Sinclair A, et al (eds). *Pathy's Principles and Practice of Geriatric Medicine.* 5th ed. Oxford: John Wiley & Sons, Inc.; 2012:93.

18. Hollingsworth JM, Wilt TJ. Lower urinary tract symptoms in men. *BMJ.* 2014;14;349.

19. Evans WJ. Sarcopenia should reflect the contribution of age-associated changes in skeletal muscle to risk of morbidity and mortality in elderly people. *J Am Med Dir Assoc.* 2015;16:5464.

20. Demonet J-F, Celsis P. Ch 5, Aging of the brain. In: Vellas BJ, ed. *Pathy's Principles and Practice of Geriatric Medicine.* 5th ed. John Wiley & Sons, Inc.; 2012:49.

21. Iowa Geriatric Education Center, University of Iowa. Geriatric Assessment Tools. Available at https://www.healthcare.uiowa.edu/igec/tools/. Accessed August 9, 2015.

22. Rosen SL, Reuben DB. Geriatric assessment tools. *Mt Sinai J Med.* 2011;78:489.

23. Bhatia LC, Naik RH. Clinical profile of acute myocardial infarction in elderly patients. *Cardiovasc Dis Res.* 2013;4:107.

24. Papaleontiou M, Haymart MR. Approach to and treatment of thyroid disorders in the elderly. *Med Clin North Am.* 2012;96:297.

25. Hogue JD. Office evaluation of dizziness. *Prim Care.* 2015;42:249.

26. de Moraes SA, Soares WJ, Ferriolli E, et al. Prevalence and correlates of dizziness in community-dwelling older people: a cross sectional population based study. *BMC Geriatr.* 2013;13:4.

27. Lo AX, Harada CN. Geriatric dizziness: evolving diagnostic and therapeutic approaches for the emergency department. *Clin Geriatr Med.* 2013;29:181.

28. Koroukian SM, Warner DF, Owusu C, et al. Multimorbidity redefined: prospective health outcomes and the cumulative effect of co-occurring conditions. *Prev Chronic Dis.* 2015;12:E55.

29. Strandberg TE, Pitkälä KH, Tilvis RS, et al. Geriatric syndromes–vascular disorders? *Ann Med.* 2013;45:265.

30. Montlahuc C, Soumaré A, Dufouil C, et al. Self-rated health and risk of incident dementia: A community-based elderly cohort, the 3C Study. *Neurology.* 2011;77:1457.

31. Mendonça MD, Alves L, Bugalho P. From subjective cognitive complaints to dementia: who is at risk?: A systematic review. *Am J Alzheimers Dis Other Demen.* 2015pii: 1533317515592331.

32. Fernández-Ruiz M, Guerra-Vales JM, Trincado R, et al. The ability of self-rated health to predict mortality among community-dwelling elderly individuals differs according to the specific cause of death: data from the NEDICES cohort. *Gerontology.* 2013;59:368.

33. Vogelsang EM. Self-rated health changes and oldest-old mortality. *J Gerontol B Psychol Sci Soc Sci.* 2014;69:612.

34. Iecovich E, Biderman A. Concordance between self-reported and physician-reported chronic co-morbidity among disabled older adults. *Can J Aging.* 2013;32:287.

35. Yeo G. How will the U.S. healthcare system meet the challenge of the ethnogeriatric imperative? *J Am Geriatr Soc.* 2009;57:1278.

36. Jackson CS, Gracia JN. Addressing health and health-care disparities: the role of a diverse workforce and the social determinants of health. *Pub Health Rep.* 2014;129:57.

37. Centers for Disease Control and Prevention. Health Disparities and Inequalities Report 2013. Available at http://www.cdc.gov/minorityhealth/CHDIReport.html. Accessed August 11, 2015.

38. August KJ, Sorkin DH. Racial and ethnic disparities in indicators of physical health status: do they still exist throughout late life? *J Am Geriatr Soc.* 2010;58:2009.

39. Ng JH, Bierman AS, Elliott MN, et al. Beyond black and white: race/ethnicity and health status among older adults. *Am J Manag Care.* 2014;20:239.

REFERENCES

40. Stanford School of Medicine. Ethnogeriatrics. Available at http://geriatrics.stanford.edu/. Accessed August 11, 2015.

41. Office of Minority Health, Department of Health and Human Services. Think Cultural Health. Available at https://www.thinkculturalhealth.hhs.gov/index.asp. Accessed August 11, 2015.

42. Aggarwal NK, Glass A, Tirado A, et al. The development of the DSM-5 Cultural Formulation Interview-Fidelity Instrument (CFI-FI): a pilot study. *J Health Care Poor Underserved.* 2014;25:1397.

43. Kobylarz FA, Heath JM, Lide RC. The ETHNIC(S) mnemonic: a clinical tool for ethnogeriatric education. *J Am Geriatr Soc.* 2002; 50:1852.

44. Aggarwal NK. Reassessing cultural evaluations in geriatrics: insights from cultural psychiatry. *J Am Geriatr Soc.* 2010;58:2191.

45. Stanford Geriatrics Education Center. "Test your Ethnogeriatric IQ." Available at http://sgec.stanford.edu/resources/training/iq.html. Accessed August 11, 2015.

46. Stanford Geriatric Education Center. Modules—EthnoGeriatrics Overview. Available at https://geriatrics.stanford.edu/culturemed.html. Accessed August 11, 2015.

47. Centers for Disease Control and Prevention, U.S. Department of Health and Human Services. Percent of U.S. adults 55 and over with chronic conditions (2009). Available at http://www.cdc.gov/nchs/health_policy/adult_chronic_conditions.htm. Accessed August 12, 2015.

48. Centers for Disease Control and Prevention, U.S. Department of Health and Human Services. Special feature on prescription drugs, p. 20; see Figure 20, Prescription drug use in the past 30 days, p. 21, in Health, United States, 2013. DHHS Publication No. 2014–1232, 2013. Available at http://www.cdc.gov/nchs/data/hus/hus13.pdf#018. Accessed August 12, 2015.

49. Wang YP, Andrade LH. Epidemiology of alcohol and drug use in the elderly. *Curr Opin Psychiatry.* 2013;26:343.

50. Rodriguez JC, Dzierzewski JM, Alessi CA. Sleep problems in the elderly. *Med Clin North Am.* 2015;99:431.

51. Bloom HG, Ahmed I, Alessi CA, et al. Evidence-based recommendations for the assessment and management of sleep disorders in older persons. *J Am Geriatr Soc.* 2009;57:761.

52. Wooten JM. Rules for improving pharmacotherapy in older adult patients: part 1 (rules 1–5). *South Med J.* 2015;108:97.

53. Wooten JM. Rules for improving pharmacotherapy in older adult patients: part 2 (rules 6–10). *South Med J.* 2015;108:145.

54. American Geriatrics Society 2012 Beers Criteria Update Expert Panel. American Geriatrics Society updated Beers criteria for potentially inappropriate medication use in older adults. *J Am Geriatr Soc.* 2012;60:616.

55. Reuben DB, Herr KA, Pacala JT, et al. *Geriatrics at your Fingertips.* 16th ed., p. 227. New York, NY: American Geriatrics Society; 2014.

56. American Geriatrics Society Panel on the Pharmacologic Management of Persistent Pain in Older Persons. Pharmacologic management of persistent pain in older persons. *J Am Geriatr Soc.* 2009; 57:1331.

57. Budnitz DS, Lovegrove MC, Shehab N, et al. Emergency hospitalizations for adverse drug events in older Americans. *N Engl J Med.* 2011;365:2002.

58. Hadjistavropoulos T, Hadjistavropoulos HD. *Pain Management for Older Adults: A Self-Help Guide.* Washington DC: American Psychological Association; 2015. Available at http://ebooks.iasp-pain.org/pain_management_for_older_adults/. See also International Association for the Study of Pain eBookstore. Available at http://ebooks.iasp-pain.org/. Accessed August 13, 2015.

59. Savage SR. Multidimensional care of chronic pain: reducing reliance on opioids for relief, June 2013. Webinar–American Medical Association. Available at http://eo2.commpartners.com/users/ama/session.php?id=11044. Accessed August 11, 2015.

60. American Academy of Pain Medicine. Pain index. Pain intensity scales. Available at http://www.painmed.org/SOPResources/ClinicalTools/government-websites/. Accessed August 13, 2015.

61. Hjermstad MJ, Fayers PM, Haugen DF, et al. Studies comparing Numerical Rating Scales, Verbal Rating Scales, and Visual Analogue Scales for assessment of pain intensity in adults: a systematic literature review. *J Pain Symptom Manage.* 2011;41:1073.

62. Centers for Disease Control and Prevention. Cigarette Smoking—United States, 2006–2008 and 2009–2010, Table 1. Prevalence of current smoking among persons aged 12–17 years, by selected characteristics—National Survey on Drug Use and Health, United States, 2006–2010, in CDC Health Disparities and Inequalities Report—United States, 2013. *MMWR Suppl.* 62(3):82. Available at http://www.cdc.gov/mmwr/pdf/other/su6203.pdf. Accessed August 13, 2015.

63. National Institute on Aging. Age Page: Alcohol use in older people. Available at http://www.nia.nih.gov/health/publication/alcohol-use-older-people. Accessed August 13, 2015.

64. Centers for Disease Control and Prevention. Binge Drinking, United States, 2011- Table - Prevalence, frequency, and intensity of binge-drinking, by sex, age group, race/ethnicity, education, and disability—Behavioral Risk Factor Surveillance System, United States, 2011. in CDC Health Disparities and Inequalities Report—United States, 2013. *MMWR Suppl.* 62(3):79. Available at http://www.cdc.gov/mmwr/pdf/other/su6203.pdf. Accessed August 13, 2015.

65. American Geriatrics Society. Alcohol use disorders in older adults. AGS clinical practice guidelines screening recommendation. Ann Long Term Care. 2006;14. Available at http://www.annalsoflongtermcare.com/article/5143. Accessed August 15, 2015.

66. Wilson SR, Knowles SB, Huang Q, et al. The prevalence of harmful and hazardous alcohol consumption in older U.S. adults: data from the 2005–2008 National Health and Nutrition Examination Survey (NHANES). *J Gen Intern Med.* 2014;29:312.

67. Bommersbach TJ, Lapid MI, Rummans TA, et al. Geriatric alcohol use disorder: a review for primary care physicians. *Mayo Clin Proc.* 2015;90:659.

68. Morley JE. Undernutrition in older adults. *Fam Pract.* 2012; 29(Suppl 1):i89.

69. National Center for Chronic Disease Prevention and Health Promotion. *Centers for Disease Control and Prevention. Table 1, The national report card on healthy aging. How healthy are older adults in the United States, p. 15.* Atlanta: Centers for Disease Control and Prevention, U.S. Department of Health and Human Services; 2013. Available at http://www.cdc.gov/aging/pdf/state-aging-health-in-america-2013.pdf. Accessed August 14, 2015.

70. Collard RM, Boter H, Schoevers RA, et al. Prevalence of frailty in community-dwelling older persons: a systematic review. *J Am Geriatri Soc.* 2012;60;1487.

71. Song X, Mitnitski A, Rockwood K. Prevalence and 10-year outcomes of frailty in older adults in relation to deficit accumulation. *J Am Geriatr Soc.* 2010;58:681.

72. Clegg A, Rogers L, Young J. Diagnostic test accuracy of simple instruments for identifying frailty in community-dwelling older people: a systematic review. *Age Ageing.* 2015;44:148.

73. O'Sullivan R, Mailo K, Angeles R, et al. Advance directives: survey of primary care patients. *Can Fam Physician.* 2015;61:353.

74. Torke AM, Sachs GA, Helft PR, et al. Scope and outcomes of surrogate decision making among hospitalized older adults. *JAMA Intern Med.* 2014;174:370.

75. Billings JA. The need for safeguards in advance care planning. *J Gen Intern Med.* 2012;27:595.

76. Swetz KM, Kamal AH. In the clinic. Palliative care. *Ann Intern Med.* 2012;156:ITC2–1.

77. Gestuvo MK. Health maintenance in older adults: combining evidence and individual preferences. *Mt Sinai J Med.* 2012;79:560.

78. Nicholas JA, Hall WJ. Screening and preventive services for older adults. *Mt Sinai J Med.* 2011;78:498.

79. Centers for Disease Control and Prevention, Administration on Aging, Agency for Healthcare Research and Quality, Centers for Medicare and Medicaid Services. *Enhancing Use of Clinical Preventive Services Among Older Adults.* Washington, DC: AARP; 2011. Available at http://www.cdc.gov/aging/pdf/Clinical_Preventive_Services_Closing_the_Gap_Report.pdf. Accessed August 15, 2015.

80. Eckstrom K, Feeny DH, Walter LC, et al. Individualizing cancer screening in older adults: a narrative review and framework for future research. *J Gen Intern Med.* 2013;28:292.

81. Leipzig RM, Whitlock EP, Wolff TA, et al. Reconsidering the approach to prevention recommendations for older adults. *Ann Intern Med.* 2010;153:809.

82. American Geriatrics Society Expert Panel on the Care of Older Adults with Multimorbidity. Patient-centered care for older adults with multiple chronic conditions: a stepwise approach from the American Geriatrics Society: American Geriatrics Society Expert Panel on the Care of Older Adults with Multimorbidity. *J Am Geriatr Soc.* 2012;60:1957.

83. U.S. Preventive Services Task Force. Draft Recommendation Statement Impaired Visual Acuity in Older Adults: Screening, 2015. Available at http://www.uspreventiveservicestaskforce.org/Page/Document/draft-recommendation-statement161/impaired-visual-acuity-in-older-adults-screening. Accessed August 15, 2015.

84. Bagai A, Thavendiranathan P, Detsky AS. Does this patient have hearing impairment? *JAMA.* 2006;295:416.

85. Hötting K, Röder B. Beneficial effects of physical exercise on neuroplasticity and cognition. *Neurosci Biobehav Rev.* 2013;37(9 Pt B):2243.

86. Buchman AS, Boyle PA, Yu L, et al. Total daily physical activity and the risk of AD and cognitive decline in older adults. *Neurology.* 2012;78:1323.

87. Lee L, Heckman G, Mohar FJ. Frailty: Identifying elderly patients at high risk of poor outcomes. *Can Fam Physician.* 2015;61:227.

88. Chou CH, Hwang CL, Wu YT. Effect of exercise on physical function, daily living activities, and quality of life in the frail older adults: a meta-analysis. *Arch Phys Med Rehabil.* 2012;93:237.

89. American College of Sports Medicine. Exercise is Medicine–Summary Sheet for Healthcare Providers and Healthcare Providers Action Guide. Available at http://www.exerciseismedicine.org/support_page.php?p = 8. Accessed August 15, 2015.

90. Crookham J. A guide to exercise prescription. *Prim Care.* 2013;40:801.

91. Centers for Disease Control and Prevention. Preventing falls in older adults. Updated September 23 2013. Available at http://www.cdc.gov/Features/OlderAmericans/. Accessed August 17, 2015.

92. Centers for Disease Control and Prevention. Vaccine information statements. Updated August 7, 2015. Available at http://www.cdc.gov/vaccines/hcp/vis/. Accessed August 17, 2015.

93. Kim DK, Bridges CB, Harriman KH. Advisory Committee on Immunization Practices recommended immunization schedule for adults aged 19 years or older: United States, 2015. *Ann Intern Med.* 2015;162:214.

94. Centers for Disease Control and Prevention. Influenza vaccination. A summary for clinicians. Updated August 7, 2015. Available at http://www.cdc.gov/flu/professionals/vaccination/vax-summary.htm. Accessed August 16, 2015.

95. Centers for Disease Control and Prevention. Pneumococcal vaccination. Who needs it? Updated June 19, 2015. Available at http://www.cdc.gov/vaccines/vpd-vac/pneumo/vacc-in-short.htm. Accessed August 16, 2015.

96. Tomczyk S, Bennett NM, Stoecker C, et al. Use of 13-valent pneumococcal conjugate vaccine and 23-valent pneumococcal polysaccharide vaccine among adults aged > 65 years: recommendations of the Advisory Committee on Immunization Practices (ACIP). *MMWR.* 2014;63:822.

97. Hales CM, Harpaz MD, Ortega-Sanchez I, et al. Update on recommendations for use of Herpes Zoster vaccine. *MMWR.* 2014;63:729. Available at http://www.cdc.gov/mmwr/preview/mmwrhtml/mm6333a3.htm. Accessed August 17, 2015.

98. Lal H, Cunningham AL, et al. Efficacy of an adjuvant herpes zoster subunit vaccine in older adults. *N Engl J Med.* 2015;372:2087.

99. Advisory Committee on Immunization Practices. Updated recommendations for use of Tetanus Toxoid, Reduced Diphtheria Toxoid, and Acellular Pertussis (Tdap) vaccine in adults aged 65 years and older, ACIP 2012. *MMWR.* 2012;61:468. Available at http://www.cdc.gov/mmwr/preview/mmwrhtml/mm6125a4.htm. Accessed August 17, 2015.

100. American Geriatrics Society. Ten things physicians and patients should question—Choosing wisely, American Board of Internal Medicine, 2015. Available at http://www.choosingwisely.org/societies/american-geriatrics-society/. Accessed August 18, 2015.

101. Walter LC, Covinsky KE. Cancer screening in elderly patients—a framework for individualized decision making. *JAMA.* 2011;285:2750.

102. Wilt TJ, Harris RP, Qaseem A. Screening for cancer: advice for high value care from the American college of physicians. *Ann Intern Med.* 2015;162:718.

103. U.S. Preventive Services Task Force. Recommendations for primary care practice. Available at http://www.uspreventiveservicestaskforce.org/Page/Name/recommendations. Accessed August 18, 2015.

104. Park M, Unützer J. Geriatric depression in primary care. *Psych Clin North Am.* 2011;34:469.

105. U.S. Preventive Services Task Force. Draft recommendation statement. Depression in adults: screening. July, 2015. Available at http://www.uspreventiveservicestaskforce.org/Page/Document/draft-recommendation-statement115/depression-in-adults-screening1. Accessed August 19, 2015.

106. Taylor WD. Depression in the elderly. *N Engl J Med.* 2014;371:1228.

107. Maurer DM. Screening for depression. *Am Fam Physician.* 2012;85:139.

108. Arean PA, Niu G. Choosing treatment for depression in older adults and evaluating response. *Clin Geriatr Med.* 2014;30:535.

109. Lin JS, O'Connor, E, Rossom RC, et al. Screening for cognitive impairment in older adults: an evidence update for the U.S. Preventive Services Task Force. 2013 November. Evidence Syntheses No. 107. Available at http://www.ncbi.nlm.nih.gov/books/NBK174643/. Accessed August 18, 2015.

REFERENCES

110. Alzheimer's Association. 2015 Alzheimer's disease: facts and figures. Available at http://www.alz.org/facts/#prevalence. Accessed August 19, 2015.

111. Mayeux R. Early Alzheimer's disease. *N Engl J Med.* 2010;362:2194.

112. Blass DM, Rabins PV. In the clinic. Dementia. *Ann Intern Med.* 2014;161:ITC-2.

113. Marcantonio ER. In the clinic. Delirium. *Ann Intern Med.* 2011; 154:ITC6–1.

114. American Psychiatric Association. *Neurocognitive disorders, in Diagnostic and Statistical Manual of Mental Disorders.* 5th ed. Washington, DC: American Psychiatric Publishing; 2013:602.

115. Albert MS, DeKosky ST, Dickson D, et al. The diagnosis of mild cognitive impairment due to Alzheimer's disease: recommendations from the National Institute on Aging-Alzheimer's Association workgroups on diagnostic guidelines for Alzheimer's disease. *Alzheimers Dement.* 2011;7:270.

116. Markwick A, Zamboni G, Jager CA. Profiles of cognitive subtest impairment in the Montreal Cognitive Assessment (MoCA) in a research cohort with normal Mini-Mental State Examination (MMSE) scores. *J Clin Experimental Neuropsychology.* 2012;34:750.

117. Peters ME, Rosenberg PB, Steinberg M, et al. Neuropsychiatric symptoms as risk factors for progression from CIND to dementia: the Cache County Study. *Am J Geriatr Psychiatry.* 2013;21:1116.

118. McKhann GM, Knopman DS, Chertkow H, et al. The diagnosis of dementia due to Alzheimer's disease: recommendations from the National Institute on Aging–Alzheimer's Association workgroups on diagnostic guidelines for Alzheimer's disease. *Alzheimers Dement.* 2011;7:263.

119. Langa KM, Levine DA. The diagnosis and management of mild cognitive impairment: a clinical review. *JAMA.* 2014;312:2551.

120. Borson S, Scanlan JM, Chen P, et al. The Mini-Cog as a screen for dementia: validation in a population-based sample. *J Am Geriatr Soc.* 2003;51:1451.

121. Tsoi KK, Chan JY, Hirai HW, et al. Cognitive tests to detect dementia: a systematic review and meta-analysis. *JAMA Intern Med.* 2015;175(9):1450

122. Montreal Cognitive Assessment. 2015. Available at http://www.mocatest.org/. Accessed August 25, 2015.

123. Liew TM, Feng L, Gao Q, et al. Diagnostic utility of Montreal Cognitive Assessment in the Fifth Edition of Diagnostic and Statistical Manual of Mental Disorders: major and mild neurocognitive disorders. *J Am Med Dir Assoc.* 2015;16:144.

124. Roalf DR, Moberg PJ, Xie SX, et al. Comparative accuracies of two common screening instruments for classification of Alzheimer's disease, mild cognitive impairment, and healthy aging. *Alzheimers Demen.* 2013;9:529.

125. Rizzo M. Impaired driving from medical conditions: a 70-year-old man trying to decide if he should continue driving. *JAMA.* 2011; 305:1018.

126. Iverson DJ, Gronseth GS, Reger MA, et al. Practice Parameter update: evaluation and management of driving risk in dementia. Report of the Quality Standards Subcommittee of the American Academy of Neurology. *Neurology.* 2010;74:1316.

127. Martin AJ, Marottoli R, O'Neill D. Driving assessment for maintaining mobility and safety in drivers with dementia. *Cochrane Database Syst Rev.* 2013;8:CD006222.

128. Wang XM, Brisbin S, Loo T, et al. Elder abuse: an approach to identification, assessment and intervention. *CMAJ.* 2015;187:575.

129. Acierno R, Hernandez MA, Amstadter AB, et al. Prevalence and correlates of emotional, physical, sexual, and financial abuse and potential neglect in the United States: the National Elder Mistreatment Study. *Am J Public Health.* 2010;100:292.

130. National Center of Elder Abuse, Administration on Aging. Elder abuse: the size of the problem. Available at http://www.ncea.aoa.gov/Library/Data/index.aspx. Accessed August 21, 2015.

131. U.S. Preventive Services Task Force. Final recommendation statement. Intimate partner violence and abuse of elderly and vulnerable Adults: screening, January 2013. Available at http://www.uspreventiveservicestaskforce.org/Page/Document/UpdateSummaryFinal/intimate-partner-violence-and-abuse-of-elderly-and-vulnerable-adults-screening?ds = 1&s = elder abuse. Accessed August 21, 2015.

132. Moore AA, Siu AL. Screening for common problems in ambulatory elderly: clinical confirmation of a screening instrument. *Am J Med.* 1996;100:438.

133. Gorina Y, Schappert S, Bercovitz A, et al. Prevalence of incontinence among older Americans. National Center for Health Statistics. *Vital Health Stat.* 2014;3(36). Available at http://www.cdc.gov/nchs/data/series/sr_03/sr03_036.pdf. Accessed August 22, 2015.

134. Centers for Disease Control and Prevention. Older adult falls. Get the facts. Updated July 1, 2015. Available at http://www.cdc.gov/homeandrecreationalsafety/falls/adultfalls.html. Accessed August 23, 2015.

135. Panel on Prevention of Falls in Older Persons, American Geriatrics Society and British Geriatrics Society. Summary of the updated American Geriatrics Society/British Geriatrics Society clinical practice guideline for prevention of falls in older persons, 2010. *J Am Geriatr Soc.* 2011;59:148.

136. Stevens JA, Phelan EA. Development of STEADI: a fall prevention resource for health care providers. *Health Promot Pract.* 2013; 14:706.

137. Centers for Disease Control and Prevention. About CDC's STEADI (Stopping Elderly Accidents, Deaths, & Injuries) Tool Kit. Updated July 1, 2015. Available at http://www.cdc.gov/steadi/about.html. Accessed August 22, 2015.

138. Moyer VA; U.S. Preventive Services Task Force. Prevention of falls in community-dwelling older adults: U.S. Preventive Services Task Force recommendation statement. *Ann Intern Med.* 2012;157:197.

139. Tinetti ME, Kumar C. The patient who falls: "It's always a trade-off." *JAMA.* 2010;303:258.

140. Bjelakovic G, Gluud LL, Nikolova D, et al. Vitamin D supplementation for prevention of mortality in adults. *Cochrane Database Syst Rev.* 2014;1:CD007470.

141. Kalyani RR, Stein B, Valiyil R, et al. Vitamin D treatment for the prevention of falls in older adults: systematic review and meta-analysis. *J Am Geriatr Soc.* 2010;58:1299.

142. Gillespie LD, Robertson MC, Gillespie WJ, et al. Interventions for preventing falls in older people living in the community. *Cochrane Database Syst Rev.* 2012;9:CD007146.

143. James PA, Oparil S, Carter BL, et al. 2014 Evidence-based guidelines for the management of high blood pressure in adults: report from the panel members appointed to the eighth joint national committee (JNC8). *JAMA.* 2014;311:507.

144. Krakoff LR, Gillespie RL, Ferdinand KC, et al. 2014 hypertension recommendations from the eighth joint national committee panel members raise concerns for elderly black and female populations. *J Am Coll Cardiol.* 2014;64:394.

145. Benetos A, Rossignol P, Cherubini A, et al. Polypharmacy in the aging patient: management of hypertension in octogenarians. *JAMA.* 2015;314:170.

REFERENCES

146. Bangalore S, Gong Y, Cooper-DeHoff RM, et al. 2014 Eighth Joint National Committee panel recommendation for blood pressure targets revisited: results from the INVEST study. *J Am Coll Casrdiol.* 2014;64:784.

147. Weber MA, Bakris GL, Hester A, et al. Systolic blood pressure and cardiovascular outcomes during treatment of hypertension. *Am J Med.* 2013;126:501.

148. Kitzman DW, Taffet G. Kitzman DW, et al. Ch 74. Effects of aging on cardiovascular structure and function. In: Halter JB, Ouslander JG, Tinetti ME et al, eds. *Hazzard's Geriatric Medicine and Gerontology.* 6th ed. New York, NY: McGraw-Hill; 2009.

149. Freeman R, Wieling W, Axelrod FB, et al. Consensus statement on the definition of orthostatic hypotension, neutrally mediated syncope and the postural tachycardia syndrome. *Clin Auton Res.* 2011;21:69.

150. Vijayan J, Sharma VK. Neurogenic orthostatic hypotension - management update and role of droxidopa. *Ther Clin Risk Manag.* 2015;8:915.

151. Sathyapalan T, Aye MM, Atkin SL. Postural hypotension. *BMJ.* 2011: 342:d3128.

152. Perlmuter LC, Sarda G, Casavant V, et al. A review of the etiology, associated comorbidities, and treatment of orthostatic hypotension. *Am J Ther.* 2013;20:279.

153. Wilson JF. In the clinic. Herpes zoster. *Ann Intern Med.* 2011;154: ITC3–1.

154. Addis VM, DeVore HK, Summerfield ME. Acute visual changes in the elderly. *Clin Geriatr Med.* 2013;29:165.

155. Borooah S, Dhillon A, Dhillon B. Gradual loss of vision in adults. *BMJ.* 2015;350:h2093.

156. Liew G, Baker ML, Wong TY, et al. Differing associations of white matter lesions and lacunar infarction with retinal microvascular signs. *Int J Stroke.* 2014;9:921.

157. Wang JJ, Baker ML, Hand PJ, et al. Transient ischemic attack and acute ischemic stroke: associations with retinal microvascular signs. *Stroke.* 2011;42:404.

158. Vajaranant TS, Wu S, Torres M, et al. The changing face of primary open-angle glaucoma in the United States: demographic and geographic changes from 2011 to 2050. *Am J Ophthamol.* 2012;154:303.

159. Weinreb RN, Aung T, Medeiros FA. The pathophysiology and treatment of glaucoma: a review. *JAMA.* 2014;311:1901.

160. Ratnapriya R, Chew EY. Age-related macular degeneration-clinical review and genetics update. *Clin Genet.* 2013;84:160.

161. Friedman PK, Kaufman LB, Karpas SL. Oral health disparity in older adults: dental decay and tooth loss. *Dent Clin North Am.* 2014;58:757.

162. Yellowitz JA, Schneiderman MT. Elder's oral health crisis. *J Evid Based Dent Pract.* 2014;14(Suppl):191.

163. Gibson PG, McDonald VM, Marks GB. Asthma in older adults. *Lancet.* 2010;376:803.

164. Goldberg LR. In the clinic. Heart failure. *Ann Intern Med.* 2010; 152:ITC6–1.

165. Coffey S, Cox B, Williams MJ. The prevalence, incidence, progression, and risks of aortic valve sclerosis: a systematic review and meta-analysis. *J Am Coll Cardil.* 2014;63:2852.

166. Manning MJ. Asymptomatic aortic stenosis in the elderly: a clinical review. *JAMA.* 2013;310:1490.

167. Sandoval-Leon AC, Drews-Elger K, Gomez-Fernandez CR, et al. Paget's disease of the nipple. *Breast Cancer Res Treat.* 2013;141:1.

168. McDermott MM. Lower extremity manifestations of peripheral artery disease: the pathophysiologic and functional implications of leg ischemia. *Circ Res.* 2015;116;1540.

169. Miller KL, Baraldi CA. Geriatric gynecology: promoting health and avoiding harm. *Am J Obstet Bynecol.* 2012;207:355.

170. Zendell K, Edwards L. Lichen sclerosus with vaginal involvement: report of 2 cases and review of the literature. *JAMA Dermatol.* 2013;149:1199.

171. U.S. Preventive Services Task Force. Cervical cancer: screening (update in progress). March 2012. Available at http://www.uspreventiveservicestaskforce.org/Page/Document/UpdateSummaryFinal/cervical-cancer-screening. Accessed August 24, 2015.

172. Mahlknecht P, Kiechl S, Bloem BR, et al. Prevalence and burden of gait disorders in elderly men and women aged 60–97 years: a population-based study. *PLoS One.* 2013;8:e69627.

173. Lewis SJ. Neurological update: emerging issues in gait disorders. *J Neurol.* 2015;262:1590.

174. Jankovic J. Gait disorders. *Neurol Clin.* 2015;33:249.

175. Lam R. Office management of gait disorders in the elderly. *Can Fam Physician.* 2011;57:765.

176. Odenheimer G, Funkenstein HH, Beckett L, et al. Comparison of neurologic changes in "successful aging" persons vs. the total aging population. *Arch Neurol.* 1994;51:573.

177. Frank C, Pari G, Rossiter JP. Approach to diagnosis of Parkinson disease. *Can Fam Physician.* 2006;52:862.

178. Parkinson's Disease Foundation. Statistics on Parkinson's Available at http://www.pdf.org/en/parkinson_statistics. Accessed August 25, 2015.

179. Chahine LM, Stern MB. Diagnostic markers for Parkinson's disease. *Curr Opin Neurol.* 2011;24:309.

Index

Page numbers followed by f indicate figures; those followed by b indicate in-chapter boxed material; those followed by t indicate end-of-chapter tables. Items related to children, adolescents, and older adults can be found listed under those entries as well as the specific anatomic area.

A

ABCD method, for melanoma screening, 178, 178b–180b
Abdomen. *See also specific organs*
  anatomy of, 449–452
  examination techniques for, 470–487
    abdominal wall mass, 487
    in adolescents, 898
    aorta, 483, 483f
    appendicitis, 485–486, 486f
    ascites, 484–485, 484f, 485f
    auscultation, 472, 473f
    bladder, 483
    in children, 879–881
    cholecystitis, 486–487
    in infants, 838–840
    inspection, 471–472, 471f
    kidneys, 481–482
    liver, 475–478
    in older adults, 994
    palpation, 473–475, 474f
    percussion, 473
    during regnancy, 944–945
    spleen, 479–481
    ventral hernias, 487
  in health history, 453–464
    gastrointestinal tract and, 455–461
    urinary tract and, 461–464
  health promotion and counseling and, 464–470
  in physical examination, 22
  physiology of, 449–452
  protuberant, 500t
  pulses in, 512–513, 512f
  quadrants of, 450–451, 450b, 450f
  recording findings, 487, 487b
  sounds in, 501t
  tender, 502t–503t
  viscera, 450f
Abdominal aorta, anatomic considerations, 451
Abdominal aortic aneurysm (AAA), 483
  in older adults, 483
  risk factors for, 483
  screening for, 520–521
Abdominal bruits, 994
Abdominal fullness, 458
Abdominal masses
  assessment of, 487, 500t
  categories of, 474
Abdominal pain, 488t–489t
  gastrointestinal symptoms in, 457–458
  lower acute, 457
  lower chronic, 457
  rebound tenderness, 475b
  types of, 453–454
  upper acute, 455
  upper chronic, 455–456

Abdominal reflexes, 763, 763f
Abdominal striae, during pregnancy, 931b
Abdominal wall
  assessment of mass, 487, 500t
  localized bulges in, 499t
  tenderness of, 502t
Abducens nerve, 715, 715f, 716b
  examination of, 737
Abduction
  of fingers, 665, 665f
  of hip, 679b, 680, 681f
  of shoulder, 651b
  of thumb, 665–666, 666f
  of wrist, 662b
Abduction stress test, 689b
Abductor group, of hip muscles, 676, 676f
ABI. *See* Ankle–brachial index (ABI)
Abnormal blood pressure, 130, 130b
Abrasion of teeth with notching, 296t
Absence seizure, 781t
Absolute risk difference, 58
Abstract thinking, 166
Accessory muscle, 318
ACE. *See* Aid to Capacity Evaluation (ACE)
Acetabulum, 674, 674f
Achalasia, 490t
Achilles tendinitis, 688
Achilles tendon, 688, 691, 692
  ruptured, 688
Acholic stools, 461
ACL. *See* Anterior cruciate ligament (ACL)
Acne vulgaris, 204t
ACOG. *See* American College of Obstetricians and Gynecologists (ACOG)
Acoustic blink reflex, 826
Acoustic nerve, 715, 715f, 716b
  examination of, 739
Acral melanoma, 202t
Acral nevus, 202t
Acrocyanosis, in infants, 816, 818b, 918t
Acromegaly, facies in, 272t
Acromioclavicular arthritis, 701t
Acromioclavicular joint, 646f, 647, 649, 653b
  examination technique for, 653b
Acromion, 646–647, 646f, 648, 649
Actinic cheilitis, 290t
Actinic keratosis, 197t
Actinic purpura, 206t
Active listening, in interviewing, 68
Acute abdomen, 475
Acute bowel obstruction, 488t
Acute necrotizing ulcerative gingivitis, 295t
Acute pain, 134–137
Addiction, 96b
  of fingers, 665, 665f
  of thumb, 666, 666f

Adduction
  of hip, 679b, 681, 681f
  of shoulder, 651b
  stress test, 689b
  of wrist, 662b
Adductor group, of hip muscles, 676, 676f
Adductor tubercle, 682, 682f, 685
Adhesive capsulitis, 701t
Adie pupil, 277t
Adipose tissue, of breast, 420
Adnexa, 567
  masses, 592, 603t
  during pregnancy, 930, 947
Adolescent acne, 912t
Adolescents
  confidentiality issue in, 892
  contraception methods in, 581, 581b
  developmental tasks of, 890b–891b
  development of, 890
  examination techniques for, 894–906
    abdomen, 898
    breasts, 896–897
    ears, 895
    eyes, 895
    female genitalia, 900, 901b
    general survey, 894
    heart, 895–896
    male genitalia, 898–899
    musculoskeletal system, 901–905
    neck, 895
    nervous system, 906
    recording findings, 906, 906b–909b
    skin, 895
    throat, 895
    vital signs, 895
  health history in, 891–893
  health promotion and counseling and, 893, 894b
  health supervision visits, 894b
  sexual maturity assessment in, 569
Adult health history, components of, 8
Adult illness, in health history, 10
Adventitia, of artery, 509f, 510–511
Adventitious sounds, 325–326, 325b
Affect, in mental status examination, 155b, 159
Afferent fibers, 715, 717
African Americans
  breast cancer in women, 425
  cardiovascular disease in, 727b
Afterload, 353
Aid to Capacity Evaluation (ACE), 89
Air conduction (AC), 244, 739
Alcohol use
  CAGE questionnaire for, 151b, 465
  in health history, 10
  in older adults, 974, 974b
  screening for, 151b, 157, 464–466, 465b
  stroke and, 729b
Alertness, 769b